Textbook of Pleural Diseases

Textbook of Pleural Diseases

Second edition

Richard W Light MD FCCP
Professor of Medicine
Vanderbilt University
Nashville, Tennessee, USA

and

YC Gary Lee MBChB PhD FRACP FCCP
Consultant Chest Physician and Senior Lecturer
Oxford Centre for Respiratory Medicine and University of Oxford, Oxford, UK;
Research Team Leader
Centre for Respiratory Research, University College London, London, UK; and
Honorary Associate Professor
University of Western Australia, Perth, Australia

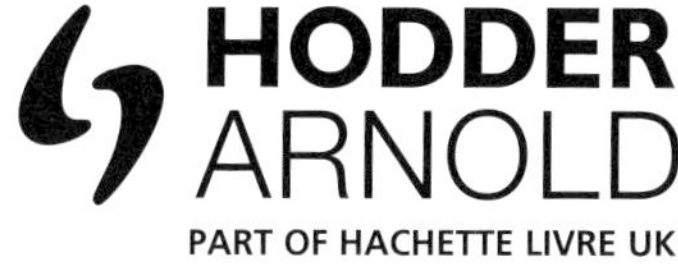

First published in Great Britain in 2003 by Arnold
This second edition published in 2008 by
Hodder Arnold, an imprint of Hodder Education and a member of the
Hachette Livre UK Group,
338 Euston Road, London NW1 3BH

www.hoddereducation.com

British Library Cataloguing in Publication Data
A catalogue record for this book is available from the British Library

Library of Congress Cataloging-in-Publication Data
A catalog record for this book is available from the Library of Congress

ISBN 978 0 340 94017 4

1 2 3 4 5 6 7 8 9 10

Commissioning Editor: Philip Shaw
Project Editor: Amy Mulick
Production Controller: Karen Tate
Cover Designer: Andrew Campling

Typeset in 10 on 12pt Minion by Phoenix Photosetting, Chatham, Kent
Printed and bound in Great Britain

Contents

PART TWO: CLINICAL SCIENCE

Contributors

Bekele Afessa
Division of Pulmonary and Critical Care Medicine, Mayo Clinic College of Medicine, Rochester, MN, USA

Steven M Albelda
Pulmonary, Allergy and Critical Care Division, Department of Medicine, University of Pennsylvania Medical Center, Philadelphia, PA, USA

Timothy C Allen
Department of Pathology, The University of Texas Health Center at Tyler, Tyler, TX, USA

Veena B Antony
Division of Pulmonary, Critical Care and Sleep Medicine, Department of Medicine, College of Medicine, University of Florida, Gainesville, FL, USA

Michael H Baumann
Division of Pulmonary and Critical Care Medicine, University of Mississippi Medical Center, Jackson, MS, USA

Brendan F Bellew
Division of Pulmonary, Critical Care and Sleep Medicine, Department of Medicine, College of Medicine, University of Florida, Gainesville, FL, USA

Chris T Bolliger
Division of Pulmonology, Department of Medicine, University of Stellenbosch, Cape Town, South Africa

Demosthenes Bouros
Department of Pneumonology, University Hospital of Alexandroupolis, Alexandropoulis, Greece

V Courtney Broaddus
Division of Pulmonary and Critical Care, San Francisco General Hospital, University of California, San Francisco, CA, USA

Philip T Cagle
Department of Pathology, Baylor College of Medicine, Houston, TX, USA

Blair Capitano
Department of Pharmacy and Therapeutics, Division of Infectious Diseases, University of Pittsburgh, Pittsburgh, PA, USA

Jose Castellote
Servicio Aparato Dipestivo, Hospital de Bellvitge, Barcelona, Spain

Henri Colt
Pulmonary and Critical Care Division, University of California, Orange, CA, USA

Helen E Davies
Oxford Centre for Respiratory Medicine, Oxford, UK

Robert JO Davies
Nuffield Department of Clinical Medicine, John Radcliffe Hospital, Headington, Oxford, UK

Nicholas H de Klerk
Centre for Child Health Research, University of Western Australia, Australia

Marc de Perrot
Division of Thoracic Surgery, Toronto General Hospital, University of Toronto, Toronto, ON, Canada

Andreas H Diacon
Division of Pulmonology, Department of Medicine, University of Stellenbosch, Cape Town, South Africa

Oner Dikensoy
Department of Pulmonary Diseases, Gaziantep University Hospital, Gaziantep, Turkey

Jeremy J Erasmus
University of Texas MD Anderson Cancer Center, Houston, TX, USA

Armin Ernst
Beth Israel Deaconess Medical Center, Boston, MA, USA

David Feller-Kopman
Interventional Pulmonology, Johns Hopkins Hospital, Baltimore, MD, USA

Jaume Ferrer
Respiratory Department, Hospital General Vall d'Hebron, Barcelona, Spain

Jocelyne Fleury-Feith
INSERM, Paris, France

Jose Garcia Valero
Departament de Biologia Cellular, Universitat de Barcelona, Barcelona, Spain

Fergus Gleeson
Nuffield Department of Surgery, John Radcliffe Hospital, Headington, Oxford, UK

John E Heffner
Providence Portland Medical Center, Oregon Health and Science University, Portland, OR, USA

Joost PJJ Hegmans
Department of Pulmonary Medicine, Erasmus Medical Center, Rotterdam, The Netherlands

Gunnar Hillerdal
Division of Respiratory Medicine, Karolinska University Hospital, Stockholm, Sweden

Steven Idell
Texas Lung Injury Institute, The University of Texas Health Center at Tyler, Tyler, TX, USA

Marie-Claude Jaurand
INSERM, Paris, France

Suresh C Jhanwar
Memorial Sloan-Kettering Cancer Center, New York, NY, USA

Joseph John
Department of Medicine, University of Texas Health Center at Tyler, Tyler, TX, USA

Kellie R Jones
Pulmonary Disease and Critical Care Medicine, Department of Medicine, Oklahoma Medical Research Foundation, Oklahoma City, OK, USA

Ioannis Kalomenidis
2nd Department of Pulmonary Medicine, Athens Medical School, "Atticon" Hospital, Haidari, Greece

Aryun Kim
Center for Antiinfective Research and Development, Hartford Hospital, Hartford, CT, USA

Gary T Kinasewitz
Pulmonary and Critical Care Medicine, Department of Medicin/UHSC, Oklahoma City, OK, USA

Coenraad FN Koegelenberg
Division of Pulmonology, Department of Medicine, University of Stellenbosch, Cape Town, South Africa

David Feller-Kopman
Johns Hopkins Hospital, Baltimore, MD, USA

Bart N Lambrecht
Department of Pulmonary Medicine, Erasmus Medical Center, Rotterdam, The Netherlands

YC Gary Lee
Oxford Centre for Respiratory Medicine and University of Oxford, Oxford, UK; Centre for Respiratory Research, University College London, London, UK; and University of Western Australia, Perth, Australia

Richard W Light
Vanderbilt University Medical School, Division of Allergy, Pulmonary and Critical Care Medicine, Nashville, TN, USA

Robert Loddenkemper
LungenKlinik Heckeshorn, HELIOS Klinikum Emil von Behring, Berlin, Germany

Gian Pietro Marchetti
Pulmonology Unit, Spedali Civili, Brescia, Italy

Edith M Marom
University of Texas MD Anderson Cancer Center, Houston, TX, USA

Antonio E Martin-Ucar
Department of Thoracic Surgery, Glenfield Hospital, Leicester, UK

Nick A Maskell
North Southmead Hospital, Westbury-on-Trym, Bristol, UK

Andew C Miller
Croydon Chest Clinic, London, UK

Juan F Montes
Departament de Biologia Cellular, Universitat de Barcelona, Barcelona, Spain

Paul E Moore
Pediatric Pulmonary Medicine, Vanderbilt University, Nashville, TN, USA

John Mullon
Division of Pulmonary and Critical Care Medicine, Mayo Clinic College of Medicine, Rochester, MN, USA

A William Musk
Department of Respiratory Medicine, Sir Charles Gairdner Hospital, Nedlands, Western Australia, Australia

Steven Mutsaers
PathWest and University of Western Australia, Crawley, WA, Australia

Delia Nelson
School of Biomedical Sciences, Curtin University, Bentley, WA, Australia

Charles H Nightingale
University of Connecticut School of Pharmacy, Storrs, CT, USA

Marc Noppen
University Hospital UZB, Brussels, Belgium

Edward F Patz Jr
Department of Radiology, Thoracic Imaging Division, Duke University Medical Center, Durham, NC, USA

Esteban Perez-Rodriguez
Respiratory Department, Ramón y Cajal Hospital and Alcalá de Henares University, Madrid, Spain

Elizabeth Perkett
Pediatric Pulmonary Medicine, Vanderbilt University, Nashville, TN, USA

José M Porcel
Department of Internal Medicine, Arnau de Vilanova University Hospital, Lleida, Spain

Xavier Xiol Quingles
Servicio de Aparato Digestivo, Hospital de Bellvitge, Barcelona, Spain

Najib M Rahman
Oxford Centre for Respiratory Medicine and University of Oxford, Headington, Oxford, UK

Francisco Rodriguez-Panadero
Unidad Médico-Quirúrgica de Enfermedades Respiratorias, Hospital Universitario Virgen del Rocio, Sevilla, Spain

Bruce WS Robinson
School of Medicine and Pharmacology, Sir Charles Gairdner Hospital Unit, Faculty of Medicine and Pharmacology, The University of Western Australia, Australia

Steven A Sahn
Division of Pulmonary, Critical Care, Allergy and Sleep Medicine, Medical University of South Carolina, Charleston, SC, USA

Sreerama Shetty
Texas Lung Injury Institute, The University of Texas Health Center at Tyler, Tyler, TX, USA

Georgios T Stathopoulous
Department of Critical Care and Pulmonary Services, General Hospital 'Evangelismos', School of Medicine, National and Kapodistrian University of Athens, Athens, Greece

Daniel Sterman
Pulmonary, Allergy and Critical Care Division, Department of Medicine, University of Pennsylvania Medical Center, Philadelphia, PA, USA

Charlie Strange
Medical University of South Carolina, Charleston, SC, USA

Gian Franco Tassi
Pulmonology Unit, Spedali Civili, Brescia, Italy

Lisete Ribeiro Teixeira
Pulmonary Division – Heart Institute, University of São Paulo Medical School, São Paulo, Brazil

Joseph R Testa
Fox Chase Cancer Center, Philadelphia, PA, USA

Francisco S Vargas
Pulmonary Division – Heart Institute, University of São Paulo Medical School, Brazil

Dimitris A Vassilakis
University of Crete, Crete, Greece

David A Waller
Department of Thoracic Surgery, Glenfield Hospital, Leicester, UK

Mark R Wick
Division of Surgical Pathology and Cytopathology, University of Virginia Medical Center, Charlottesville, VA, USA

Nicola A Wilson
Centre for Respiratory Research, University College London, UK

Preface

We have been most encouraged and delighted by the very positive responses received since the publication of the first edition of the *Textbook of Pleural Diseases* in 2003. It has been our aim to provide a comprehensive, yet easily readable, reference text that covers both basic and clinical science on pleural diseases. By doing so, we hope that this text will serve to stimulate much needed clinical and research interests in pleural diseases.

Knowledge concerning pleural diseases has grown in stature and complexity in the past few years. Seven new chapters have been added to this edition and the remaining chapters substantially updated to reflect the expansion in knowledge in the field. Ten of the fifty chapters in this edition are written by new expert authors providing fresh ideas and views. Recent years have seen the incorporation of new technologies in clinical management of pleural diseases, hence the new chapters on *Pleural ultrasound* and *Pleural manometry*. Likewise, new translational research techniques are likely to enhance our understanding of pathophysiology of pleural diseases (see *Proteomics in pleural disease*). Nonetheless, a definitive etiology remains elusive in many pleural effusions (see *Undiagnosed pleural effusions*), and serves as a reminder of the inadequacy of our current knowledge of pleural pathologies. Controversies have grown around how best to manage recurrent effusions and a separate chapter is introduced on *Pleurodesis*. A fascinating new chapter on *History of pleural diseases* provides us an opportunity to reflect on how far research on pleural diseases has progressed in the past centuries.

In this edition, we have kept the popular format of providing a bullet point summary in each chapter as well as highlighting seminal papers in the reference lists. We are confident that this edition will find a useful place in all hospitals and medical libraries.

Richard W Light
YC Gary Lee
March 2008

Preface to the first edition

Pleural disease affects over 3000 subjects per million population each year. While the pleural cavity is a confined space, pleural disease can originate from a broad spectrum of pathologies: from local diseases of the lung and pleura to systemic conditions such as collagen vascular diseases or drug reactions. Although the clinical presentations of pleural diseases are usually limited to pleuritic pain and dyspnea, the determination of the underlying cause(s) is frequently a clinical challenge despite the use of modern diagnostic modalities. Because the pleura is involved in such a wide range of conditions, contributions into pleural disease research have come from diverse backgrounds. Yet there are few comprehensive texts dedicated to pleural disease, and none that covers both the basic science and clinical aspects of the pleura.

This book provides a reference text for both clinicians and scientists whose clinical or research work involves the pleura. The 50 chapters are divided into the *Basic Science* and the *Clinical Science* sections. Experts on the respective topics from ten countries and four continents provide leading edge information in the context of their years of experience in the field. In each chapter, the author(s) has prepared a summary that underscores the 'take-home' messages. Interested readers can also pursue further readings from the highlighted references at the end of each chapter.

The *Basic Science* section covers the key aspects of preclinical topics involving the pleura. It contains state-of-the-art scientific knowledge but is written with sufficient clarity that it can easily be understood by clinicians with limited basic science background. The *Clinical Science* section begins with chapters general to pleural diseases, including the approach to patients, histology and radiology. The subsequent chapters discuss specific groups of pleural diseases in detail. Each of those chapters shares the same outline format, covering etiology, presentation, diagnosis, treatment and complications. Any published guidelines are also included. In the final chapter, we endeavor to make brave predictions of how we think the area of pleural disease may develop over the next decade or two.

It is our hope that this book will provide an easy reference for clinicians faced with specific management issues, yet allow interested readers to gather a comprehensive picture of the topic including the immuno-pathological validation behind the disease development. It is our hope that this book will stimulate interest in pleural disease, both in its research and clinical practice.

YC Gary Lee
Richard W Light
July 2002

Acknowledgements

We are grateful to the many readers who gave us extremely positive and constructive feedback on the first edition of this book. These encouragements have supported us through the many long hours spent in preparing this new edition.

We must thank all the authors for their energy and time in writing their superb chapters, without monetary reward but merely out of their passion on the subjects. The smooth production of this book would not have been possible without the help of the dedicated and experienced team at Hodder Arnold, in particular Amy Mulick and Philip Shaw, who worked tirelessly to ensure all aspects of the book met the highest standard we set.

Once again, our spouses (Audrey and Judi) have been most patient with us throughout the many months of production while we spent most evenings and weekends indulging in the pleasure of reading and thinking about pleural diseases.

YC Gary Lee
Richard W Light
March 2008

Glossary

α1AT	α1-antitrypsin
α-TOS	α-tocopheryl succinate
2D GE	two-dimensional gel electrophoresis
$AaPO_2$	alveolar-arterial oxygen gradient
AAV	*Adeno-associated virus*
ACCP	American College of Chest Physicians
Ad.HSVtk	adenovirus to deliver *Herpes simplex virus* thymidine kinase
ADA	adenosine deaminase
ADA2	adenosine deaminase isoenzyme 2
AFB	acid-fast bacilli
AIDS	acquired immmunodeficiency syndrome
ALT	alanine aminotransferase
ANA	antinuclear antibodies
AP	apurynic/apyrimidinic
APC	activated protein C
APD	all purpose drainage
Apo	apolipoprotein
ARDS	acute respiratory distress syndrome
ARNT	aryl hydrocarbon receptor nuclear translocator
AS	ankylosing spondylitis
ASGP	ascites sialoglycoprotein
ATRA	All-*trans*-retinoic acid
AUC	area under the curve
BAL	bronchoalveolar lavage
BAPE	benign asbestos pleural effusions
BCG	Bacille Calmette-Guérin
bFGF	basic fibroblast growth factor
BLP	bacteria lipoprotein
BNP	B-type natriuretic peptides
BSA	bovine serum albumin
BTS	British Thoracic Society
CABG	coronary artery bypass grafting
CALGB	Cancer and Leukemia Group B
CCPTC	clear cell papillary thyroid carcinoma
CCr5	C-C chemokine receptor-5
CEA	carcinoembryonic antigen
CEUS	contrast-enhanced ultrasound
CGH	comparative genomic hybridization
CHF	congestive heart failure
Cl	clearance
CLC	cardiotrophin-like cytokine
cM	centiMorgan
CMV	*Cytomegalovirus*
CNF	ciliary neurotrophic factor
COPD	chronic obstructive pulmonary disease
CPAP	continuous positive airway pressure
CPP	circumscribed pleural plaques
CPR	cardiopulmonary resuscitation
CRP	C-reactive protein
CSS	Churg–Strauss syndrome
CT	computed tomography
CT-1	cardiotrophin 1
CTA	computed tomographic angiography
CTD	connective tissue diseases
CTP	Child–Turcotte–Pugh
CTPA	computed tomography pulmonary angiogram
CXR	chest radiography
DC	dendritic cell
DCEMRI	dynamic contrast enhanced magnetic resonance imaging
DIGE	differential gel electrophoresis
DPT	diffuse pleural thickening
DSRCT	desmoplastic small round cell tumor
EBV	*Epstein–Barr virus*
ECG	electrocardiography
ECM	extracellular matrix
EGF	epidermal growth factor
EGFR	epidermal growth factor receptor
ELISA	enzyme-linked immunosorbent assay
EM	electron microscopy
EMA	epithelial membrane antigen
EMT	epithelial–mesenchymal transition
ENA-78	epithelial neutrophil-activating protein-78
EPIC	extrapancreatic inflammation on computed tomography score
EPP	extrapleural pneumonectomy
Eps	elastance of the pleural space
ERCP	endoscopic retrograde cholangiopancreatography
ERK	extracellular signal-regulated kinases
ERM	ezrin-radixin-moesin
ERP	estrogen receptor protein
ERS/ATS	European Respiratory Society/American Thoracic Society
ES	Ewing's sarcoma
ESI	electrospray ionization
ESR	erythrocyte sedimentation rate

FAK	focal adhesion kinase
FCS	fetal calf serum
FDA	Food and Drug Administration
FDG	fluorodeoxyglucose
FDP	fibrinogen degradation products
FEV_1	forced expiratory volume in one second
FGF	fibroblast growth factor
FRC	functional residual capacity
FT-ICR	Fourier transform ion cyclotron
FVC	forced vital capacity
GCDFP-15	gross cystic disease fluid protein-15
GCSF	granulocyte colony-stimulating factor
GCV	ganciclovir
GM-CSF	granulocyte macrophage-colony stimulating factor
GMS	Grocott's methenamine silver
GVHD	graft-versus-host disease
H&E	hematoxylin and eosin
HAART	highly active anti-retroviral therapy
HB-EGF	heparin-binding epidermal growth factor
HBSS	Hank's balanced salt solution
HCC	hepatocellular carcinoma
hCG	human chorionic gonadotropin
HGF	hepatocyte growth factor
HHV	*Human herpes virus*
HIF	hypoxia-inducible transcription factor
HIV	*Human immunodeficiency virus*
HPF	high power field
HPO	hypertrophic pulmonary osteoarthropathy
HRCT	high-resolution computed tomography
HSCT	hematopoietic stem cell transplantation
hsp65	heat shock protein 65
HSV	*Herpes simplex virus*
HSVtk	*Herpes simplex virus*-1 thymidine kinase
ICAM	intercellular adhesion molecules
ICAT	isotope-coded affinity tags
ICU	intensive care unit
IFN	interferon
Ig	immunoglobulin
IGF	insulin-like growth factor
IGFR	insulin-like growth factor receptor
IGSF CAM	immunoglobulin superfamily cell adhesion molecules
IL	interleukin
IMA	internal mammary artery
IMIG	International Mesothelioma Interest Group
IMRT	intensity modulated radiotherapy
INH	isoniazid
iNOS	inducible form of nitric oxide synthase
INR	international normalization ratio
IP	iatrogenic pneumothoraces
IPG	immobilized pH gradient
IR	insulin receptor
IR-A	insulin receptor isoform
ISPP	International Survey of Pleurodesis Practice
IT	ion trap
iTRAQ	tags for relative and absolute quantification
IVIG	intravenous immunoglobulin
JAK	janus kinase
KGF	keratinocyte growth factor
KS	Kaposi's sarcoma
LAK	lymphokine activated killer
LAM	lymphangioleiomyomatosis
LAM	lipoarabinomannan
LAP	latency associated peptide
LAT	limited axillary thoracotomy
LDH	lactate dehydrogenase
LE	Lupus erythematosus
LIF	leukemia inhibitory factor
LM	light microscopy
LMWH	low-molecular-weight heparin
LOH	loss of heterozygosity
LPS	lipopolysaccharide
LTA	lipoteichoic acid
LTBP	latent TGF-β binding protein
LVRS	lung volume reduction surgery
MALDI	matrix-assisted laser desorption-ionization
MALDI-TOF	matrix-assisted laser desorption-ionization-time of flight
MAP	mitogen-activated protein
MAPK	mitogen-activated protein kinases
MCP	monocyte chemoattractant protein
MDR	multidrug resistance
MEF	mouse embryonic fibroblasts
MELD	model of end-stage liver disease
MetAP2	methionine aminopeptidase-2
MHC	major histocompatibility complex
MHz	megahertz
MIC	minimum inhibitory concentration
MIP	macrophage inflammatory protein
MIST	Multi-center Intrapleural Streptokinase Trial
MM	malignant mesothelioma
MMP	matrix metalloproteinase
MMVF	man-made vitreous fibers
Mn-SOD	manganese-containing superoxide dismutase
MPE	malignant pleural effusions
MRI	magnetic resonance imaging
MRSA	methicillin-resistant *Staphylococcus aureus*
MS	mass spectrometry
MSCT	multislice computed tomography
MT1	membrane type 1
MTAP	methylthioadenosine phosphorylase gene
MT-MMP	membrane type matrix metalloproteinase
MTUOT	malignant tumors of uncertain origin and type
MudPIT	multidimensional protein identification technology
NAP	neutrophil activating protein
NB	neuroblastoma
N-cadherin	neural cadherin
NF	nuclear factor
NF2	neurofibromatosis type 2
NHL	non-Hodgkin's lymphoma
NK	natural killer
NO	nitric oxide

NPM	normal pleural mesothelial
NPN	neuropoietin
NSAID	non-steroidal anti-inflammatory drug
NSCLC	non-small cell lung cancer
NSE	neuron-specific enolase
OHSS	ovarian hyperstimulation syndrome
OHT	orthotopic heart transplant
OP-CABG	off-pump coronary artery bypass surgery
OSM	oncostatin M
OVA	ovalbumin
PA	plasminogen activators
PAI	plasminogen activator inhibitors
Pak	p21-activated kinase
PAMP	pathogen-associated molecular pattern
PAR	proteinase activated receptor
PARC	pulmonary and activation-regulated chemokine
PAS	periodic acid–Schiff
PBL	peripheral blood lymphocytes
PCIS	post-cardiac injury syndrome
PCP	*Pneumocystis jirovecii* pneumonia
PCR	polymerase chain reaction
PDGF	platelet-derived growth factor
PET	positron-emission tomography
PET-CT	positron emission tomography combined with computed tomography
PFE	pleural fluid eosinophilia
PG	proteoglycan
PGK	phosphoglycerate kinase
PGN	peptidoglycan
PI3K	phosphatidylinositol-3-kinase
PKC	protein kinase C
PLAP	placental alkaline phosphatase
PMF	peptide mass fingerprint
PNET	primitive neuroectodermal tumor
PPD	purified protein derivative
PPE	parapneumonic effusions
Ppl	intrapleural pressure
PRR	pattern recognition receptor
PSA	prostate-specific antigen
PSP	primary spontaneous pneumothorax
PT	prothrombin time
PTLD	post-transplant infection and lymphoproliferative disorder
PTT	partial thromboplastin time
Q	quadrupole
Q-TOF	quadrupole-time of flight
RA	rheumatoid arthritis
RA	rolled atelectasis
RalGDS	Ral guanine nucleotide dissociation stimulator
RANTES	regulated upon activation, normally T-cell expressed and secreted
Rb	retinoblastoma
RCF	refractory ceramic fibers
RECIST	response evaluation criteria in solid tumors
RH	refractory hydrothorax
RHAMM	receptor for hyaluronic acid mediated motility
rhDNase	recombinant human deoxyribonuclease
rhGH	recombinant human growth hormone
rhIL-11	recombinant human interleukin 11
RIETE	Registro Informatizado de la Enfermedad TromboEmbólica
RMS	rhabdomyosarcoma
RNI	reactive nitrogen intermediate
RNS	reactive nitrogen species
ROC	receiver operating characteristic
ROI	reactive oxygen intermediate
ROS	reactive oxygen species
ROSE	rapid on-site evaluation
RPE	re-expansion pulmonary edema
SAHA	superoylanilide and hydroxamic acid
SAPS II	simplified acute physiological score
SBEM	spontaneous bacterial empyema
SBP	spontaneous bacterial peritonitis
SCID	severe combined immunologically deficient
SCNC	small-cell neuroendocrine carcinoma
scuPA	(scuPA)
SDS-PAGE	sodium dodecyl sulfate–polyacrylamide gel electrophoresis
SELDI-TOF	surface-enhanced laser desorption/ionization-time of flight
SEM	scanning electron microscopy
SFT	solitary fibrous tumor
SFTP	solitary fibrous tumors of the pleura
sIL-2R	soluble interleukin 2 receptor
sIL-6R	soluble interleukin 6 receptor
SLE	systemic lupus erythematosus
SMC	sialomucin complex
SMRP	soluble mesothelin-related protein
SOCS	suppressor of cytokine signaling
SRCT	small round-cell tumors
SS	Sjögren's syndrome
SSAg	*Staphylococcal aureus* superantigen
SSc	systemic sclerosis
SSP	secondary spontaneous pneumothorax
SV	saphenous vein
SV40	*Simian virus 40*
SVC	superior vena cava
TACE	tumor necrosis factor α-converting enzyme
tag	t (transforming) antigen
Tag	large T antigen
TB	tuberculous
TCR	T-cell receptor
TEM	transmission electron microscopy
TF	tissue factor
TFPI	tissue factor pathway inhibitor
TGF	transforming growth factor
Th1	T-helper type 1
TIL	tumor infiltrating lymphocytes
TIM	tumor infiltrating macrophages
TIMP	tissue inhibitor of matrix metalloproteinases
TIPS	transjugular intrahepatic portosystemic shunt
TLR	toll-like receptor
TNF	tumor necross factor

TNM	tumor, node, metastasis
tPA	tissue plasminogen activator
TPB	transpulmonary bands
TPN	total parental nutrition
Treg	regulatory T-cells
TS	tumor suppressor
TSG	tumor suppressor gene
TTF1	thyroid transcription factor-1
TTFNA	transthoracic fine needle aspirations
TTNB	transthoracic needle biopsy
uPA	urokinase-type plasminogen activators
US	ultrasound
VATS	video-assisted thoracoscopic surgery
VCAM-1	vascular cell adhesion molecule-1
V_d	volume of distribution
VEGF	vascular endothelial growth factor
VLS	vascular leak syndrome
VPF	vascular permeability factor
VV	*Vaccinia virus*
WBC	white blood cell
WG	Wegener's granulomatosis
WHO	World Health Organization
WT-1	Wilm's tumor gene
XDR	extensive drug resistance

Reference annotation

The reference lists are annotated, where appropriate, to guide readers to key primary papers and major review articles as follows:

- Key primary papers are indicated by a ●
- Major review articles are indicated by a ◆
- Papers that represent the first formal publication of a management guideline are indicated by a *

We hope that this feature will render extensive lists of references more useful to the reader and help to encourage self-directed learning among both trainees and practicing physicians.

1

Pleural disease: historic perspective

GIAN FRANCO TASSI, GIAN PIETRO MARCHETTI

For centuries the pleura as an anatomical entity was either ignored or confused with the thoracic wall.[1] In ancient Greek, *pleuron* meant flank or side and was used generically in other fields such as mythology, zoology, geometry and botany. Pleuron was an important figure in Greek mythology (the brother of Calydon and son of Aetolus); in zoology, pleuron is the lateral part of the thorax of an insect; in Plato's *Timaeus* (c. 360BC) the side of a triangle is called a pleuron (Timaeus, 53c). There was also the city of Pleuron in Aetolia, cited by Homer in the *Iliad* (Book II, 639) and by Ovid in *Metamorphoses* (Book VII, 382), so-called perhaps because it was built on the side of a hill.

THE PLEURA AS AN ANATOMICAL ENTITY

There are no specific references to the pleura in the pre-Greek period, even though the ancient Egyptians could well have known of its existence, given their extensive knowledge of mummification and their practice of removing the organs from a body to be placed in their own funerary (canopic) jar. Having been extracted through the side of the diaphragm, the lungs were placed in a jar dedicated to the baboon-headed god Hapi.

The first to introduce the concept of a membrane was Aristotle (384–322BC). In his *History of Animals* he wrote '*In all sanguineous animals membranes are found. And membrane resembles a thin close-textured skin, but its qualities are different, as it admits neither of cleavage nor of extension. Membrane envelops each one of the bones and each one of the viscera, both in the larger and the smaller animals; though in the smaller animals the membranes are indiscernible from their extreme tenuity and minuteness.*'[2]

Another advance came from the School of Alexandria with Erasistratus (310–250BC), who distinguished between illnesses which affected only the lung and those which affected the *hymen hypezocota* (undergirding membrane) which covers the thorax.[3]

Pliny (23–79AD) said '*Nature, in its foresight, has enclosed all the principal viscera in membranes (membranae propriae) as if inside a special sheath.*'[4]

Soranus (98–138AD) and Galen (129–200AD) continued Erasistratus's approach, describing the '*membrana succingens*' (girding membrane): '*Nature created another structure of the same substance as the peritoneum and performing for the organs of the pneuma as does the peritoneum for the organs of assimilation. It is as fine as a spider's web; it is homogeneous and a true and real membrane.*' He attempted to define their function: '*These membranes are present on the inside of the entire thoracic cavity. They are located in order to provide protection for the lungs, preventing them from striking the bare bone during breathing.*'[5,6]

Aretaeus of Cappadocia (200AD) is more precise: '*Under the ribs, the spine, and the internal part of the thorax as far as the clavicles, there is stretched a thin strong membrane, adhering to the bones, which is named succingens*'.[7]

Avicenna (980–1037AD), a follower of the works of Aristotle, advanced the hypothesis in the book the *Canon of Medicine* that the pleura also covers the thoracic organs.[8]

However, it was only during the Renaissance when autopsies were carried out that a more accurate definition could be given. Mondino de Liuzzi (1275–1326), in his anatomical treatise *Anothomia* (1316), describes the parietal pleura. '*The membranes are three: the mediastinal pleura which divides the thoracic cavity medially in an anterior–posterior direction. Its function is that if for some reason an empyema, an accumulation of pus in the chest, forms, the pus does not drain to the other part. Then there is the costal-vertebral pleura, which is a strong membrane with a nervous structure; it is large and covers all the ribs and is thus in contact with all the organs of the thoracic cavity. Because of the sensitivity of the pleural membrane, an infection is followed by a sharp pain in the side of the body. The third membrane is the diaphragm.*'[9]

Thus the pleura begins to take on its own identity, being divided into its principal parts, each with its own characteristics, and with accurate anatomical references.

Three centuries later, Caspar Bauhin, in his *Theatrum Anatomicum* (1592), was still more precise when he accurately described visceral pleura. With him, the 'membrana costas succigens' definitely becomes 'pleura.'[10]

However, it was only in the monumental work of Francois Xavier Bichat (1771–1802) that the function of the pleura was considered, rather than being simply regarded as a covering. In his '*Traité des membranes en général et de diverses membranes en particulier*' (treatise on membranes in general and various membranes in particular), he wrote that '*The serous membranes are characterized by the lymphatic fluid which incessantly lubricates them and that every serous membrane represents a sack without an opening spread over the respective organs which it embraces. Their first function is doubtless to form about the essential organs a boundary which separates them from those of their vicinity. A second function is to facilitate the moving of the organs.*' Also, '*the surface of the pleura has a smooth and pale aspect because of a serous fluid of which the membrane is the source. This fluid is constantly produced and reabsorbed. It is so thin that the color of the underlying parts can be distinguished.*'[11]

PLEURAL DISEASES

It should be emphasized that the discussion of pleural infections in a historical context, and then making a systematic reconstruction, are extremely difficult owing to the imprecise nature of the terminology used. For example, the word 'empyema' was used not only to describe the disease but also for the operation performed to drain the empyema. The nature of the material removed in an intervention was not always specified, meaning that they could have been transudates, inflammatory exudates, or purulent effusions, since 'paracentesis thoracis' (thoracic paracentesis) was carried out in the presence of any accumulation of liquid, almost always with the broad definition of 'bad humor'. Also, an initially clear liquid often became purulent with the use of unsterile instruments.

The first recognized and described pleural disease was infectious pleurisy, both because the symptoms were often clear, such as fever and characteristic thoracic pain, and because of its frequent evolution into empyema.

The frequency, morbidity and mortality for this disease were extremely high until the twentieth century. An approximate attempt at quantification is that between 400BC and 1600AD, death was the result of 'pleural infection' in 80 percent of cases, in 70 percent between 1600 and 1800, in 50 percent until 1900, in 30 percent until 1950, with a gradual reduction to the present-day 3–5 percent. Each step of this improvement is the result of a significant therapeutic advance.

The first to illustrate pleurisy was Hippocrates of Kos (460–377BC), who frequently discussed it in his aphorisms and treatise on diseases. The symptoms described were: a constant fever, sweat, a cough and pain. He said '*When pleuritis arises, a person suffers the following: he has pain in his side, fever and shivering; he breathes rapidly and he has orthopnea …*'[12]

Many of his aphorisms – short sentences which were for many years the only source of information for practicing doctors – deal with pleurisy: '*Pleuritis that does not clear up in fourteen days results in empyema.*' '*Pneumonia coming on pleurisy is bad.*' '*Pains and fevers occur rather at the formation of pus than when it is already formed.*' Others refer to the prognosis: '*Persons who become affected with empyema after pleurisy, if they get clear of it in forty days from the breaking of it, escape the disease; but if not, it passes into phthisis.*' And therapy: '*When empyema is treated by the cautery or incision, if pure and white pus flow from the wound, the patients recover; but if mixed with blood, slimy and fetid, they die.*'[13]

Hippocrates recommended treating empyema by draining through the mouth, or with purgatives, or inducing vomiting, but also attempted a more 'modern' approach, advising an oblique cut in the lowest intercostals space, perforation or removal of a piece of rib, thereby creating the first open drainage system, and filling the incision with linen gauze. He suggested washing the cavity with oil and warm wine; an empyema can drain first from the lungs rather than from the thoracic wall; he describes (digital) clubbing in chronic suppuration. He also identified the most appropriate location for the incision in the thoracic wall with 'the sign of damp earth', which was achieved by covering the patient's thorax in mud and making the incision in the part which dried first. He was also responsible for 'hippocratic succussion', which involves shaking the patient by the shoulders in order to identify the sound of liquid inside the thorax. This maneuver only had positive results in the presence of a certain level of air and liquid, and was therefore only possible in the final stages of the disease.[14]

From the ancient Roman period there is not only documentary evidence regarding the history of pleural disease, but also archaeological discoveries from excavations at Pompei which have produced surgical instruments that were apparently used to drain purulent accumulations.

Aulus Cornelius Celsus (25BC to 50AD) identified the characteristics of inflammation (rubor, tumor, calor, dolor), applicable also to thoracic suppuration, and he describes pleurisy in his *De Medicina* (book IV): '*The stomach is girt about by the ribs, and in these also severe pains occur. And the commencement either is from a chill, or from a blow, or from excessive running, or from disease. But at times pain is all there is the matter, and this is recovered from be it slowly or quickly; at times it goes on until it is dangerous, and the acute disease arises which the Greeks call pleurisy. To the aforesaid pain in the side is added fever and cough; and by means of the cough, phlegm is expectorated when the disease is less serious, but blood when it is grave.*'[15] He suggests treatment by bleeding or cupping glass, advising walks and potions of hyssop with dried figs, rubbing the shoulder blades, light food, the application to the chest of a poultice of ground salt and abstinence from wine.

There is a curious but perhaps significant anecdote related by Pliny the Elder (23–79AD) in his *Naturalis Historia* in which he tells the story of the consul Publius Cornelius Rufus who, suffering from an empyema and convinced of his imminent end, launches himself boldly into battle and is struck by an enemy arrow in the thorax, causing the draining of the effusion and consequently his recovery.[4]

Soranus (98–138AD) offers some elementary epidemiological notions, confirming that pleurisy is more frequent in old age than in youth, in women than in men, and strikes mainly in winter months.

Galen (129–216AD) noted the importance of the pulse, which is faster in cases of inflammatory diseases of the thorax, and describes the occurrence of pleural effusion: '*A sense of heaviness can persist inside the ribs. This means a quantity of pus or other humor has gathered in the thoracic cavity causing dyspnea.*'[6]

There are numerous references to pleurisy in ancient Roman literature. For example Horace (65–8BC) called it '*laterum dolor*' (side pain) in his first book of the Satires. Vitruvius (c. 80–25BC) in his *De Architectura*, Book I, said that it is a disease common in areas exposed to winds. Aretaeus (c. 80AD), speaking of peripneumonia, writes: '*This is what we call Peripneumonia, being an inflammation of the lungs, with acute fever, when they are attended with heaviness of the chest, freedom from pain, provided the lungs alone are inflamed; for they are naturally insensible, being of loose texture, like wool. But branches of the aspera arteria are spread through them, of a cartilaginous nature, and these, also, are insensible; muscles there are nowhere, and the nerves are small, slender, and minister to motion. This is the cause of the insensibility to pain. But if any of the membranes, by which it is connected with the chest, be inflamed, pain also is present; respiration bad, and hot; they wish to get up into an erect posture, as being the easiest of all postures for the respiration.*'[7]

In subsequent centuries, references to pleurisy are less numerous, but in the *Regimen Sanitatis Salernitanum* (1000AD) is written: '*Pleuresia est vera cum spirandi gravitate, febreque continua, tussi, laterioque dolor*' (pleurisy is real if there is difficulty in breathing and constant fever, cough and lateral pain).[16] Avicenna (980–1037AD), in the third book of the Canon, described the clinical characteristics: '*The symptoms of simple pleurisy are clear: constant fever, violent pain under the ribs which sometimes only manifests itself when the patient breathes strongly… the third symptom is difficulty in breathing and frequency of breathing. The fourth symptom is a rapid and weak pulse. The fifth symptom is the cough.*'[8]

Until this time, descriptions of therapy tend to be brief and then in the twelfth and thirteenth centuries there appears to have been a proactive approach towards surgery by, among others, Henri de Mondeville (1260–1320).[17]

Ambrosie Paré (1510–1590) was a leading surgeon and specialist in battlefield surgery, and a pioneer in the medical field. (He was responsible for concocting an early 'antiseptic' for treating wounds, made from egg-yolk, oil of roses and turpentine.) He appears to have been particularly interested in empyema and had a series of instruments made for the drainage of effusions, and suggested the advantage of enlarging the breach in the thorax to facilitate the emptying of purulent substances and then washing the pleura with a disinfecting solution: '*the pus and matter must be evacuated little by little at several times, and the capacity of the chest cleansed by a detergent injection of barley water and honey of rose.*' He pointed out the serious effect of the entry of air into the thorax (so that the vital spirits do not escape). He also described subcutaneous emphysema resulting from a costal fracture (Figure 1.1).[18]

The work of Fabrizio d'Acquapendente (1537–1619) is also important. Having declared the empyema to be 'a collection of rotten material', he proposed '*manuariam operationem*' (manual operation) for removal, indicating that the effusion should be drained gradually, the thoracotomy breach left open, a perforated cannula introduced and the pleural cavity washed with wine and oil.[19]

In 1528 the first book entirely dedicated to pleurisy appeared, entitled *De incisione vene in pleuritide* by Andrea Turini. This was followed in 1536 by *Liber de pleuritide ad Galeni e Hippocratis scopum* by Benedetto Vittorio. Other books of note were *Tentamen medicum de pleuritide vera* by Leonardus Bardon di Montpellier (1777) and, in 1740, the systematic treatment of pleurisy in the volume *De pleuritide ejusque curatione* (Figure 1.2) written by Daniel Wilhelm Triller, a doctor and philosopher in Wittemberg. In 1664 the famous anatomist Frederik Ruysch graduated at Leiden with a thesis entitled *Disputatio medica inauguralis de pleuritide*.

In his *Armementarium Chirurgicum*, Johann Scultetus (1595–1645), student of Fabrizio d'Acquapendente, published some fine illustrations showing the operation of empyema, and underlined the active role the surgeon should have regarding drainage in thoracic diseases.[20]

In 1648, Riolano described thoracentesis of air '*flatus cum violentia displosus*' (violent expulsion of air). More incisive is the chapter on empyema in the excellent book of 1710 by Dionis, which has extensive and practical descriptions and is backed up by showing a set of surgical instruments made especially for the operation.[21]

In 1699, Giorgio Baglivi in *De praxi medica* followed Galen's line: '*If you would discover pleurisy, place your chief*

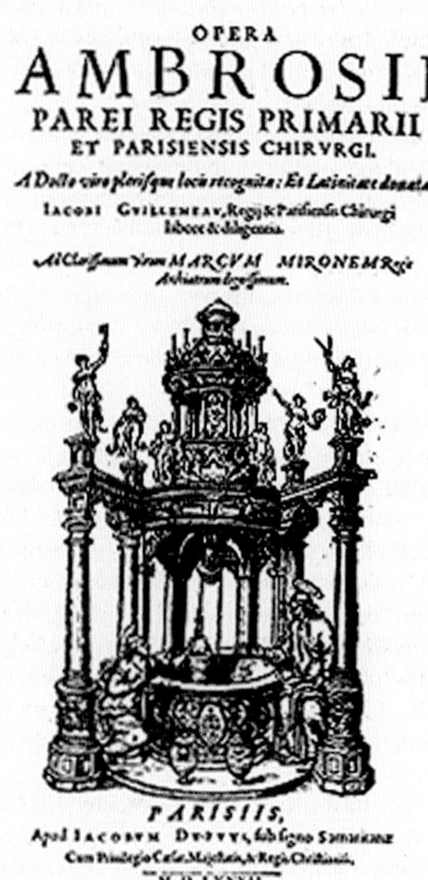

OPERA
AMBROSII
PAREI REGIS PRIMARII
ET PARISIENSIS CHIRVRGI.
A Docto viro plerisque locis recognita: Et Latinitate donata,
IACOBI GVILLEMEAV, Regij & Parisiensis Chirurgi [illegible]
Ad Clarissimum Virum MARCVM MIRONEM Regis
Archiatrum [illegible].
PARISIIS,
Apud IACOBVM DV PVYS, sub signo Samaritanae.
Cum Privilegio Caesar. Maiestatis, & Regis Christianiss.
M. D. LXXXII.

Figure 1.1 Ambroise Paré's 1582 book.

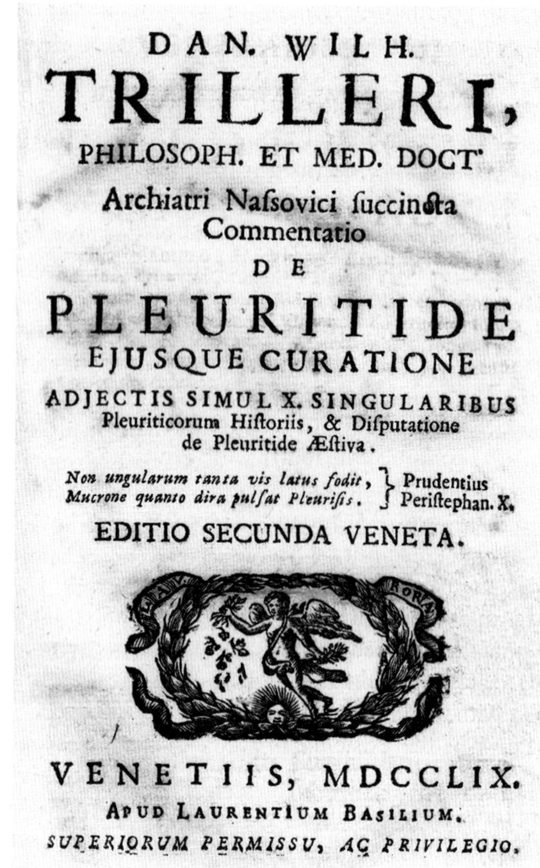

DAN. WILH.
TRILLERI,
PHILOSOPH. ET MED. DOCT.
Archiatri Nassovici succincta
Commentatio
DE
PLEURITIDE
EJUSQUE CURATIONE
ADJECTIS SIMUL X. SINGULARIBUS
Pleuriticorum Historiis, & Disputatione
de Pleuritide Æstiva.
Non ungularum tanta vis latus fodit, Mucrone quanto dira pulsat Pleurisis. } Prudentius Peristephan. X.
EDITIO SECUNDA VENETA.
VENETIIS, MDCCLIX.
APUD LAURENTIUM BASILIUM.
SUPERIORUM PERMISSU, AC PRIVILEGIO.

Figure 1.2 Triller's 1740 *De pleuritide ejusque curatione* (On pleurisy and its treatment).

care in observing the nature of the pulse. The hardness of the pulse is almost an infallible sign of all pleurisies'.[22]

In his *Observationes Medicae* (1676), Thomas Sydenham classified pleurisy as an epidemic disease. Willis (1621–1675) considered pleurisy and peripneumonia to be separate diseases. Boerhaave (1668–1738) described the variation in degrees of pain experienced by the patient caused by the act of breathing and pneumothorax following the rupture of the esophagus. In 1767, Hewson claimed that removal of air from the thorax was also possible.

Giambattista Morgagni, in 1761 in *De Sedibus et Causis Morborum* (Letters 20 and 21), discussed pleurisy at length and remarked on the frequency of adhesions. Their presence had already been noted in the sixteenth century, the period in which the practice of autopsy had become more widespread, and Isbrand di Diemerbroek, professor of Anatomy in Utrecht from 1651 to 1674, speculated that up to a third of the 'normal' population could be subject to this 'anomaly'. His contemporary, Nicolas Tulpius from Amsterdam, famous for being immortalized in a painting by Rembrandt, considered that a lung entirely free from adhesions was a rarity in adults. This opinion was shared by Morgagni, who, having observed their absence in fetuses, considered that they were not congenital, even though not necessarily the result of diseases such as pleurisy or pneumonia.

The origin of pleural adhesions gave rise to some fanciful theories, the most original of which was surely that of the French zoologist Duvernoy (1777–1855), who attributed them to laughter: '*le rire en effet n'appartient qu'aux seuls humains, et seulement après qu'ils sont nés*' (only humans laugh, and only after they are born).

In a series of 3000 autopsies in 1767, Joseph Lietaud described the presence of two pleural tumors, possibly mesothelioma: '*Reperitur in dextro thoracis latere tumor ingens pleuram occupans*' (On the right side of the thorax there was found a large tumor in the pleura).[23]

In the nineteenth century, more emphasis was placed on attempting early diagnosis. Until then interventions often took place when the symptoms of disease had become very obvious, i.e. at a very late stage.

Progress in this direction can be attributed to semeiotic respiration initiated by Leopold Auenbrugger and his '*Inventum Novum*' of 1761 (Figure 1.3) in which he presented chest percussion as a method of physical examination: '*The thorax of a healthy person sounds when struck. If a sonorous region of the chest appears, on percussion, entirely destitute of the natural sound, disease exists in that region*').

However, perhaps even more significant was *'De L'Auscultation Médiate'* by R.T.H. Laennec in 1819 in which he systematically described thoracic diseases.

Laennec distinguished between acute and chronic pleurisy, classified pleural disease, separates them from peripneumonia and described the hemorrhagic form and fibrothorax. With the introduction of the stethoscope, the presence of liquid in the thorax could be diagnosed at an earlier stage. He identified the major obstacle to the successful removal of liquid as being the pressure of the lung on the mediastinum and vertebral column and understood the danger of exposing the pleural cavity to the external environment, preferring repeated thoracentesis to trepanatation of the rib or an incision in the intercostal space. He considered the fourth–fifth intercostals space the ideal location for thoracentesis because of its centrality.[24]

In 1804 John Bell began to describe pneumothorax, even though it had not yet been called that. He considered the cause to be either thoracic traumas, putrefaction of the pleural cavity, or erosion of the lung.[25] The term 'pneumothorax' was coined by a student of Laennec, Jean Marc Gaspard Itard, who in 1803 described five cases of tuberculosis with air in the pleural cavity, even though he did not know of the existence of the spontaneous variant.[26] The latter form was described by his mentor: *'Aeriform fluid can be exhaled in the pleura without visible alterations in the membrane. I have twice seen an abundant simple pneumothorax accompanied by such dryness of the pleura that the membrane resembled parchment'*.[24]

LEOPOLDI AUENBRUGGER

MEDICINÆ DOCTORIS
IN CÆSAREO REGIO NOSOCOMIO NATIONUM
HISPANICO MEDICI ORDINARII.

INVENTUM NOVUM

EX

PERCUSSIONE THORACIS HUMANI

UT SIGNO

ABSTRUSOS INTERNI
PECTORIS MORBOS
DETEGENDI.

VINDOBONÆ,
TYPIS JOANNIS THOMÆ TRATTNER, CAS. REG.
MAJEST. AULÆ TYPOGRAPHI.

MDCCLXI.

Figure 1.3 *Inventum novum* (The new discovery) the first description of percussion by Leopold Auenbrugger.

After Laennec diagnosis became more accurate, and the identification of suspected pleurisy could be made earlier. In 1828 Piorry introduced indirect percussion and in 1843 Damoiseau, and later Ellis in 1874, identified the semi-elliptical curve, which is highest in the axilla, to define the limit of an effusion. In 1874 Garland described a paravertebral triangular area of relative resonance in the lower back between the spine and Damoiseau-line found in the same side as an effusion. In 1902 Grocco described a triangular area of dullness at the base of the chest near the spinal column on the side opposite a pleural effusion (Grocco's triangle) due to mediastinal shift caused by the effusion.

William Stokes (1804–1878), known for the eponymous 'periodic breathing' (Cheyne–Stokes respiration) and for atrioventricular block, described 20 cases of pleurisy treated successfully. He thought the results of thoracentesis were often not encouraging because it took place too late; he described contraindications in the presence of a fistula and considered that pleurisy was often caused by tuberculosis. Perhaps he was also the first to create a unidirectional valve. He proposed a higher position for the drain to facilitate spontaneous outflow of the liquid and prevent possible lesions to the diaphragm if entry was too low.[27]

Henry Bowditch (1808–1892) was an internist and physiologist from Boston who in 1852 published the results of paracentesis of the thorax in 65 cases. The treatment was used in the initial phases of exudate, based on clinical evidence of dyspnea and the presence of liquid, which was examined under a microscope, and in his opinion thoracentesis should not have been considered an extreme intervention, but a simple remedy.[28] This view was also held by his contemporary, Armand Trousseau (1801–1867), a French internist: *'I do not believe that I invented thoracentesis, in the same way that I did not invent the instruments to perform it, but I do think I am among the first to recommend its application in cases of excessive liquid in the thorax.'* He thought thoracentesis simple and that it could brilliantly resolve many clinical cases, even if often performed late, and that the introduction of air did not cause damage even if the pleura was inflamed.[29]

The physiology of pleura also became better understood. In 1863 Recklinghausen published an important study on the mesothelial stomata.[30] Carl Ludwig first made graphic recordings of intrapleural pressure in 1847 by use of a water-filled balloon placed in the pleural space and in 1900 Aron reported the first measurement of intrapleural pressure in a healthy human.[31] West proposed the hypothesis that the interface between the parietal wall and the lungs is separated by the pleurae.[31] Ernest Starling produced the equation which regulates hydrostatic and oncotic forces in 1895.[32] In 1870 Wagner gave the first anatomical–pathological description of a primary pleural tumor and in 1882 Ehrlich realized the possibility of identifying carcinoma cells in pleural liquid, describing the characteristic rosette-shaped aggregation.[33]

THORACOSCOPY

The first *in vivo* observation of the pleura was undoubtedly carried out by an Irish doctor, Samuel Gordon, who in the February edition of the 1866 Dublin Quarterly Journal refers to a clinical case: '*Most extensive pleuritic effusion rapidly becoming purulent; paracentesis; introduction of a drainage tube; examination of interior of pleura by the endoscope*' (Figure 1.4). With the aid of an expert endoscopist, Cruise, and a binocular instrument, he observed a '*granular surface*' and understood that: ' *This case is also very remarkable as being the first in which an examination of the interior of the chest has been made by the endoscope.*'[34]

His initiative remained isolated, as it would be more than 40 years before pleural endoscopy was mentioned again, when Hans Christian Jacobaeus (Figure 1.5), a Swedish internist, published '*On the possibility of using a cistoscope to examine the serous cavity*', dedicated to laparoscopy and thoracoscopy. He used a rigid cistoscope of Nitze n. 14 (14 Charrières = 4.6 mm), provided with a unidirectional automatic valve that prevented escapes of air both from the abdominal hollow and the thorax. The instrument had an overall diameter of 17 Chs. (5.6 mm including the trocar) with side vision to 90°, 22 cm long, and with a lamp at the end.

In the part dealing with the thorax, Jacobaeus says: '*In exudative pleurisy it is possible to reach the pleura without injuring the lung. Recently a treatment has been developed, in which the exudate is replaced by insufflated air. The quantity of air apparently small (half a liter) is certainly sufficient to perform a thoracoscopy. In two cases of exudative pleurisy I carried out an insufflation and afterwards I examined the pleura. The two cases demonstrate that the method has vast potential*'.[35]

The first real diagnostic applications were described in 1911 with 27 cases and a description of a normal pleural cavity and the pathological alterations in 15 cases of exudative pleurisy, three of empyema and nine of pneumothorax.

In 1913 Jacobaeus carried out the first attempt to free pleural adhesions, and in 1916 published a description of the technique which became known as 'Jacobaeus operation': thoracoscopic lysis of adhesions to obtain therapeutic pneumothorax (pleurolysis).[36]

The method achieved fruition with Felice Cova, 'the Paganini of the thoracoscope', who in 1928 published his '*Atlas Thoracoscopicon*' (Figure 1.6), with the principal endoscopic illustrations of pleural disease (Figure 1.7),

ART. VIII.—*Clinical Reports of Rare Cases, occurring in the Whitworth and Hardwicke Hospitals.* By SAMUEL GORDON, M.B., F.K. & Q.C.P.; Physician to the Hospitals, and Lecturer on the Practice of Medicine in the Carmichael School of Medicine.

(*Continued from Vol.* xxxiii., *page* 366.)

Most Extensive Pleuritic Effusion Rapidly Becoming Purulent; Paracentesis; Introduction of a Drainage Tube; Recovery; Examination of Interior of Pleura by the Endoscope.—I do not propose entering upon the history or details of the operation of *paracentesis thoracis* and the introduction of drainage tubes, but simply to record another case of recovery by this mode of treatment, and which has taken place under very adverse circumstances. I am induced to do so because I believe that this mode of treatment, originated by Dr. Goodfellow, of the Middlesex Hospital, has not met with sufficient favour on this side of the Channel.

Figure 1.4 Samuel Gordon article on 'Examination of interior of pleura by the endoscope'.

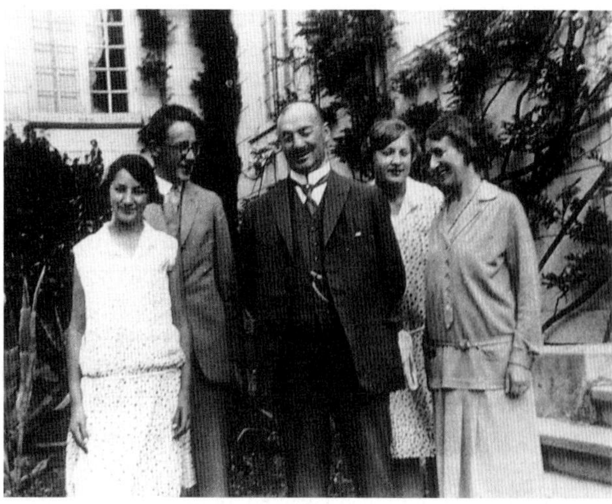

Figure 1.5 Hans Christian Jacobaeus with his family.

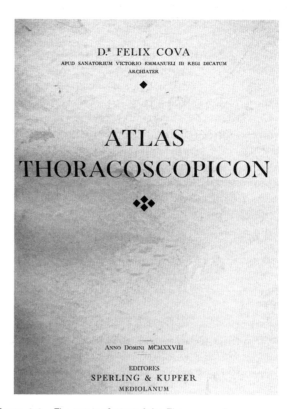

Figure 1.6 The cover of 1928 *Atlas Thoracoscopicon* (Thoracoscopy Atlas) of Felice Cova.

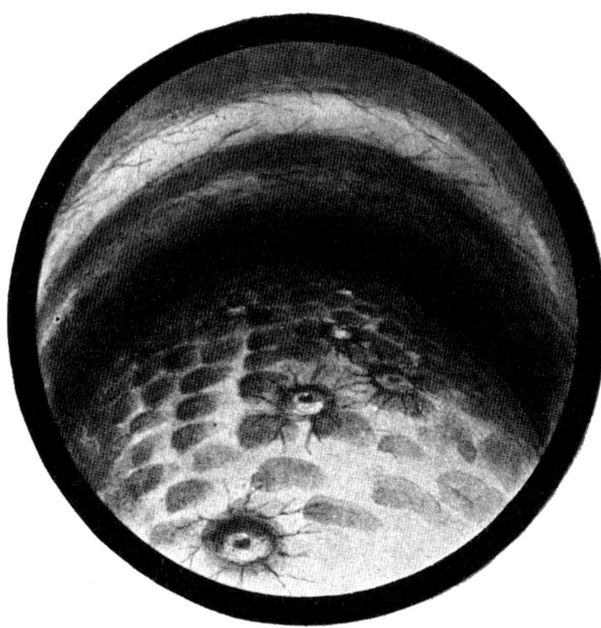

Figure 1.7 Illustration of neoplastic nodules on the lung surface taken from *Atlas Thoracoscopicon.* (See also Color Plate 1.)

written in Italian, German and English. This was the first systematic work on the subject, demonstrating its diffusion and reliability for habitual use.[37]

The 1940s saw the introduction of antibiotics and the first attempts to wash the pleural cavity with sulphonamides by Nicholson (1938) and Burford (1942), with penicillin by Keefer (1943), and with fibrinolythics by Tillet (1949).

In 1935 a Canadian thoracic surgeon by the name of Norman Bethune published an article (Figure 1.8) entitled '*Pleural poudrage – A new technique for the deliberate production of pleural adhesions as a preliminary lobectomy*'. '*Prepare iodized talc, using a fine commercial talc powder. Sterilize in autoclave. Under local anesthetic, insert the thoracoscopic cannula with an air-tight valve in the sixth or seventh space scapular line. Inspect the pleura. Take out the thoracoscope and insert through the same cannula the author's return-air powder blower. Give half a dozen puffs, then insert the thoracoscope again and inspect. Repeat as often as necessary to cover the surface of the lobe. When the lung is covered so as to resemble a cake sprinkled with confectioners' sugar, detach the blower and completely aspirate the air*'.[38]

PLEURAL POUDRAGE

A NEW TECHNIC FOR THE DELIBERATE PRODUCTION OF PLEURAL ADHESIONS AS A PRELIMINARY TO LOBECTOMY*

NORMAN BETHUNE,† M.D.(TOR.), F.R.C.S.(E)
MONTREAL, CANADA

Figure 1.8 Norman Bethune original article on 'Pleural poudrage'.

In 1937 Sattler studied pneumothorax endoscopically (Figure 1.9) and stated that the origin of the disease was connected with the spontaneous rupture of emphysematous bubbles.[39]

In 1939 Sergent and Kourilsky published '*Contribution a l' étude de l'endothéliome pleural, image radiologique e pleuroscopique*', which described the first case of mesothelioma to be investigated endoscopically in a patient with a history of repeated thoracentesis, parietal thoracic tumefaction and radiological confirmation of parietal pleural thickening.[40]

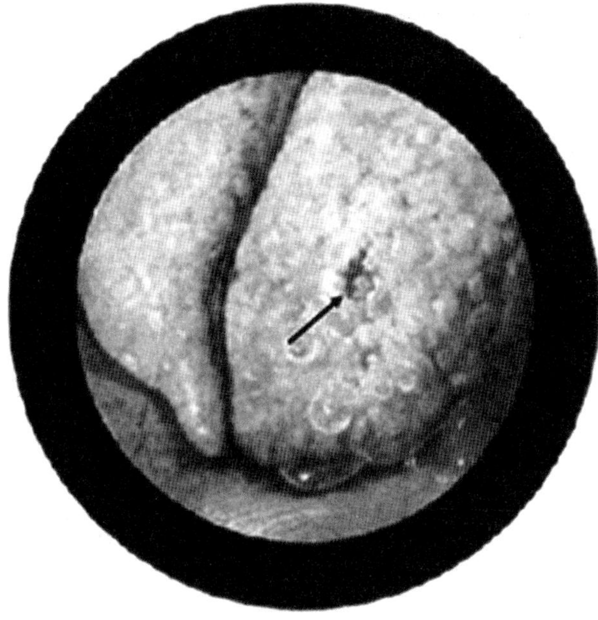

Figure 1.9 Sattler's illustration of the endoscopic aspect of the rupture of a lung emphysematous bulla (arrow). (See also Color Plate 2.)

OTHER DIAGNOSTIC AND THERAPEUTIC PROCEDURES

For hundreds of years empyema was treated using open drainage. In the middle of the nineteenth century, the first attempts were made to create a water-sealed drainage system. Trousseau was the first to develop one in 1850 and the distal end of the drain was submerged in the fluid drained. In 1867, Hiller applied underwater seal drainage for children. However, the pioneers responsible for the widespread use of underwater seal drainage systems were certainly Playfair who in 1872 introduced the water-seal, Hewett who in 1876 included the use of continuous chest drainage with a closed water-sealed system in the treatment of patients with empyemas, and Bülau, a German internist, who used the closed water-sealed drainage for empyema as early as 1875 and published his technique in 1891.[41]

The drainage system consisted of a cannula, introduced into the thorax via a trocar, the distal end of which was immersed in a bottle containing sodium and potassium permanganate (as an antiseptic). Pleural fluid could be drained slowly through the cannula and the force of aspiration could be increased by gradually lowering the bottle.

Gotthard Bülau, still today regarded as the leading pioneer of the water valve, described the application thus: '*I have always believed that the principal advantage of siphon-drainage is that it lowers the pressure within the pleural space, thereby bringing about re-expansion of the lung. The drain can function as a valve, allowing escape of pus and the air which has entered during the operation, while preventing entry of air. With each forcible expiration against a closed glottis, the air in the opposite (healthy) lung is forced into the partially collapsed one. With the next inspiration the valve closes, the lungs can expand, the expansion is maintained...* '.[41]

Another innovative concept was that introduced in 1877 by the Finn J.A. Estlander, who was the first to understand the beneficial effects on the lung of collapsing the thoracic wall in the treatment of chronic empyema. He designed the thoracoplasty which, with numerous variations, would be used until the 1950s for the treatment of suppurative lung diseases.[42] This procedure was further developed by the Swiss surgeon Edouard de Cérenville (1843–1915), who in 1885 widened its application to the tuberculous cavities, abscesses and suppurative infarcts, and proposed the total resection of one or more ribs.[43]

In 1893 the French surgeon Edmond Delorme performed the first decortication on a young French soldier suffering from tuberculous empyema and removed the visceral pleura to re-expand the lungs.[44]

In 1918 the world was ravaged by Spanish influenza, a terrible scourge which killed 20 million people worldwide. The disease was often complicated by development of a pleural empyema, which led to attempts to apply various techniques for therapeutic purposes. Within a short time the USA initiated a Commission for the study of empyema, and a brilliant young surgeon, Evarts Graham (1883–1957), was put in charge. He subsequently became famous for carrying out the first pneumonectomy for a pulmonary tumor on April 5, 1933. He noted that premature use of open drainage, in particular in the presence of streptococcus infection which produces 'liquid' pus, was detrimental because it might provoke a mediastinal shift that could be fatal. However, in empyemas in which the pus was more viscous and adhesions formed more rapidly, open drainage was less dangerous. He also noted that the first type of infection was more common in soldiers fighting in World War I, whilst the second was more common in civilians. Soldiers were therefore always treated with closed drainage and a water seal, and within a few months the mortality rate dropped from 30 to 4 percent.[45]

One further surgical approach to be considered is that of Leo Eloesser, who in 1935 developed 'skin flap open drainage', for the treatment of tuberculous empyema. A direct passage was made between the pleural cavity and the skin to allow open drainage of pus. The skin was folded back around the edges. This method is still used in a minority of cases which cannot be treated with less invasive methods.[46]

CONCLUSIONS

The famous French surgeon Guillaume Dupuytren (1777–1835) consulted five doctors when he felt ill with empyema. Having listened to their conflicting diagnoses, he said, 'I prefer to die by the hand of God than with the help of a surgeon.'

This chapter outlined the slow and difficult journey traveled in the development of better management strategies for patients with pleural diseases, especially in establishing interventions which were both simple and effective. Removing pathological material from an easily accessible (pleural) cavity would appear a simple task in theory. In reality, it has taken centuries of research to arrive at our current practices.[47]

KEY POINTS

- Parietal pleura was recognized as a separate anatomical entity and was subdivided into its principal parts (mediastinal, costal-vertebral and diaphragmatic pleura) in the treatise *Anothomia* (1316) by Mondino de Liuzzi.
- Visceral pleura was described in detail by Caspar Bauhin in his *Theatrum Anatomicum* (1592).
- The first to illustrate pleurisy was Hippocrates of Kos (460–377BC), who frequently discussed it in his aphorisms and treatise on diseases.
- A systematic treatment of pleurisy was demonstrated in the 1740 volume *De pleuritide ejusque curatione* (On pleurisy and its treatment) written by Daniel Wilhelm Triller, a doctor and philosopher in Wittemberg.
- Thoracoscopy was first started in 1910 by the Swedish internist Hans Christian Jacobaeus.
- Gotthard Bülau, a German internist, the leading pioneer of the water valve, introduced the closed water-seal drainage for empyema in 1875.
- Thoracoplasty in the treatment of chronic empyema was designed in 1877 by J.A. Estlander.
- The first decortication with removal of the visceral pleura to re-expand the lungs was performed in 1893 by the French surgeon E. Delorme on a young French soldier suffering from tuberculous empyema.

REFERENCES

● = Key primary paper
◆ = Major review article

◆1. Wilson A. On the history of disease concepts: the case of pleurisy. *History Sci* 2000; **38**: 271–319.
2. Aristotle. *On the parts of animals*. Translator Lennox JG. London: Oxford University Press, 2001.
3. Wilson LG. Erasistratus, Galen and the pneuma. *Bull Hist Med* 1959; **33**: 293–314.
4. Pliny. *The natural history*. Translators Bostock J and Riley HT. London: HG Bohn, 1855.
5. Ilberg J. *Vita Hippocratis secundum Soranum*. Leipzig, 1927.
6. Galen. *On anatomical procedures*. Translators Duckworth WLH , Lyons MC, B. Bowers. New York: Cambridge University Press, 1962.
7. Francis Adams LD (ed.). *The extant works of Aretaeus, The Cappadocian*. Boston: Milford House, 1972.
8. Avicenna. *Kitab al qanoun fi al toubb*. Romae: Typographia Medicea, 1593.
9. Mondino de Liuzzi. *Anothomia*. Bononia, 1316.
10. Bauhin C. *Theatrum anatomicum*. Frankfurt: typis Matthaei Beckeri, 1605.
◆11. Bichat X. *Traité des membranes en général et de diverses membranes en particulier*. Paris, 1799.
12. *The genuine works of Hippocrates*. Translator Charles Darwin Adams. New York: Dover, 1868.
13. Hippocrates. *The aphorisms*. Translator Coar T. London: Longman, 1822.
◆14. Littré E. *Oeuvres complètes* d' Hippocrate. Paris: chez Baillière, 1839.
15. Celsus Cornelius A. *On medicine*, vol. I. Books 1–4. Translator WG Spencer. Cambridge, MA: Harvard University Press, 1935.
16. Arnaldo di Villanuova (ed.). *Regimen sanitatis salernitanum*. Venetia, 1500.
17. Pagel JL. *Die chirurgie des Heinrich von Mondeville*. Berlin, 1892.
18. *Opera Ambrosii Parei regis primarii et parisiensis chirurgi*. Paris: apud Iacobum Dupuys, 1582.
19. D'Acquapendente F. *Opera omnia anatomica and physiologica*. Goezius, 1687.
20. Scultetus J. *Armamentarium chirurgicum*. Ulm, 1653.
21. Dionis P. *A course of chirurgical operations in the Royal Gardens*. London, 1710.
22. Baglivi G. *De praxi medica*. Roma, 1696.
23. Lietaud J. *Historia anatomico-medica*. Paris, 1767.
◆24. Laennec RTH. *De l'auscultation mediate*. Paris: chez Brosson JA et Chaudé JS, 1819.
25. Bell J. *Principles of surgery*. New York: Collins, 1812.
26. Itard JMG. *Dissertation sur le pneumothorax ou les collections gazeuses qui se forment dans la poitrine*. Thesis, Paris 1803.
27. Stokes W. *A treatise on the diagnosis and treatment of diseases of the chest*. Dublin, 1837.
●28. Bowditch H. On paracentesis thoracis. *Boston Surg J* 1857; **56**: 348–54.
29. Trousseau A. *De l'opération de l' empyème*. Presse Méd Belge 1850; **2**: 101–105.
30. Von Recklinghausen F. Zur fettresorption. *Arch f Path Anat and Physiol and f Klinische Med* 1862; **26**: 172–208.
31. Proctor FD (ed.). *A history of breathing physiology*. New York: Marcel Dekker, 1995.
32. Starling EH, Leathes JB. The absorption of salt solution from the pleural cavities. *J Physiol* 1895; **18**: 106–16.
33. Ehrlich P. Beitrage zur aetiologie und histologie pleuritischer exsudate. *Charité Ann* 1882; **7**: 199–230.
34. Gordon S. Clinical reports of rare cases. *Dublin Q J Med Sci* 1866; **41**: 83–99.
●35. Jacobaeus HC. Über die möglichkeit die Zystoskopie bei untersuchung seröser höhlungen anzuwenden. *Munch Med Woch* 1910; **57**: 2090–92.
36. Jacobaeus HC. Die thorakoskopie und ihre praktische bedeutung. *Ergebn ges Med* 1925; **7**: 112–66.
◆37. Cova F. *Atlas thoracoscopicon*. Milano: Sperling and Kupfer, 1928.
38. Bethune N. Pleural poudrage: a new technique for deliberate production of pleural adhesions as a preliminary to lobectomy. *J Thor Surg* 1935; **4**: 251–61.
39. Sattler A. Zur behandlung der spontapnumothorax mit besonderer berücksichtigung der thorakoskopie. *Beitr Klin Tuberk* 1937; **89**: 395–408.
40. Sergent E, Kourilsky R. Contribution a l' étude de l'endothéliome pleural. *La Presse Med* 1939; **14**: 257–9.
41. Bülau G. Für die heber-drainage bei behandlung des empyems. *Z Klin Med* 1891; **18**: 31–45.
42. Estlander JA. Sur la résection des côtes dans l'empyéme cronique. *R M Méd Chir* 1879; **3**: 885–8.
43. De Cérenville. De la résection des côtes dans le traitement des excavations des fistules consécutives a la pleurésie purulente. *Rev Méd* 1886; **6**: 7–8.
44. Delorme E. Nouveau traitement des empyèmes chroniques. *Gaz Hop Civ Milit* 1894; **67**: 94–6.
45. Empyema Commission. Case of empyema at Camp Lee,Virginia. *J Am Med Assoc* 1918; **71**: 366–73.
46. Eloesser L. An operation for tuberculous empyema. *Surg Gyn Obstet* 1935; **60**: 1096.
◆47. Yernault JC. The history of pleural disease. In: Bouros D. (ed.). *Pleural diseases*. New York: Marcel Dekker, 2004: 1–21.

PART 1

BASIC SCIENCE

2

Anatomy of the pleura

NAJIB M RAHMAN, NAI-SAN WANG†

INTRODUCTION

The precise structure and function of the pleural space is not fully understood. There is marked inter-species variation in the ultrastructure of the pleura; in humans the pleural cavities are separated by the mediastinum, whereas other mammals (e.g. mice, American buffalo) lack complete separation between the left and right pleurae, allowing free movement of air and fluid. The adult elephant is the only mammal that does not possess a pleural cavity – a normal pleural space is present *in utero*, but in late gestation the parietal pleural is replaced with a dense sheet of connective tissue.[1] The pleural space is then obliterated with loose connective tissue, permitting movement of the lung against the chest wall. Theories have been advanced as to why the elephant lacks a pleural space,[2] but the variations seen between mammals in the structure of the pleural cavity is as yet to be explained.

In humans, each hemithorax is constructed like a vertical, cone-shaped bellow with the diaphragm as the moving part at the caudal and widest end, and the trachea and nasal structures superiorly creating a narrow outlet/inlet and providing protection and functional adaptation for the lung. Within the thoracic cage, the lung must be able to both move and change volume with the respiratory cycle.

The lung expands during inhalation and deflates during exhalation, creating movement between the lung surface and the inner chest wall. In order to decrease friction generated between these two surfaces, the inner surface of the thoracic cage and the outer surface of the lung are covered by a serous, elastic membrane with a smooth lubricating surface – the pleura.

The pleural cavity describes the slit-like fluid filled space between these surfaces. It is thus an entirely sealed cavity inserted between the chest wall and lung, maintained at 10–20 μm across. This arrangement is crucial to the efficient function of the lung, in a manner analogous to the pericardium and pericardial space to the heart.

EMBRYOLOGY

All body cavities, including the pleural peritoneal and pericardial cavities, are derived from the coelom, the primitive body cavity. The coelom derives from the primitive mesoderm of the embryo and forms a cavity lined by serous membrane before all internal organs develop.

In the human embryo, the primitive mesoderm on both sides of the notochord divides first into the medial segmented and natural non-segmented plates. The left and right medial segmented plates later develop into the skull, vertebra, ribs and the thick muscles of the dorsal (rear) parts of the body wall.

In contrast, the lateral non-segmented plates split into the internal splanchnopleure (the precursor of the internal organs) and the lateral or external somatopleure (the precursor of the anterior and lateral body wall), between which structures a slit-like cavity is formed. The paired left and right splanchnopleure and somatopleure with their associated cavities extend along the length of the embryo in a cephalo-caudal direction, and out and over the surface of the yolk sacked ventrally or anteriorly. The fusion of the left and right somatopleure and two cavities ventrally (i.e. the fusion and closure of the ventral wall) creates a sealed primitive body cavity, an intra-embryonic coelom, in the seventh a week of gestation.[3] At this early stage the cavity is already completely covered by a layer of serous membrane with mesothelial cells on the surface.[4]

With the shrinkage of the yolk sack, the coelom expands. The internal organs move around within the embryo, changing in size and shape during development. Organs protrude as they develop into the body cavities and, as they protrude, are enveloped by a layer of serous membrane that covers the inner surface of the body cavities. Meanwhile, the coelom divides into the pleural and pericardial cavities by the fusion of the transverse septum arising from the ventral, as well as left and right, pleuroperitoneal folds from the dorsal walls. When the two pleuroperitoneal folds fuse, the two pleural cavities are completely separated from each other and from the pericardial cavity.[4] This arrangement allows flexibility for the organs to expand, retract, deform or displace each other as they develop and grow in the limited space of the four body cavities.

GROSS ANATOMY

To the naked eye, the normal pleural surfaces are smooth, wet and semi-transparent. In humans, the left and right pleural cavities are entirely separated from one another (by the mediastinum) and from the pericardial space. Although the visceral and parietal pleura originate from the same serous membrane of the coelom, they appear macroscopically different because of different underlying structures and topography (see section 'The regional difference').

The visceral pleura covers the entire surface of the lung, including the interlobular fissures. The parietal pleura covers the inner surface of the entire thoracic cage, including the mediastinal surfaces and diaphragm. The visceral and parietal pleura coalesce at the lung hilae, where the major airways and pulmonary vessels penetrate. The area of the entire pleural surface has been estimated to be 2000 cm^2 in an average adult male.

The visceral pleura adheres tightly to the lung surface throughout the thorax. The parietal pleura is further subdivided in to different anatomical regions as follows:

- the costal pleura, lining the inner surface of the ribs and intercostal muscles;
- the diaphragmatic pleura, covering the convex surface of the diaphragm;
- the cervical pleura, rising in to the neck and extending above the first rib;
- the mediastinal pleura, adherent to the mediastinal structures.

THE PLEURAL CAVITY

The pleural cavity is a sealed but expandable space that is formed between the visceral and parietal pleura.[5] The right and left pleural cavities in humans are completely separate from one another, and from the mediastinum and pericardial cavities. The dome, or cupola, of the pleural cavity extends above the first rib for 2–3 cm along the medial one-third of the clavicle behind the sternocleidomastoid muscles. The pleural space may therefore be entered in trauma to the lower neck, procedures such as central venous catheter insertion or surgical dissection of the lymph nodes, resulting in pneumothorax.

During development, several structures within the thoracic cavity acquire a double layer of parietal pleura. In the lower mediastinum, the dorsal and ventral mediastinal parietal pleura are pulled into the thoracic cavity as the lung develops, and form vertical structures from the hilum of the lung to the diaphragm, resulting in a pair of back-to-back layers of parietal pleura. These may persist into adulthood and are called the pulmonary ligaments. Pulmonary ligaments may divide the pleural space below the hilum into anterior and posterior compartments,[6] and may contain large lymphatic vessels. During surgery to the lung, incomplete ligation or damage to these lymphatic vessels may result in post-operative pleural effusion.[7] It has been suggested that their presence may prevent torsion of the lower lobes.

Inferiorly, the pleura reflect at the lower boundary of the thoracic cage, but often extend beyond the costal margin in the right infrasternal region and at the costovertebral angles bilaterally. A radiological study has demonstrated that the lung lies at or below the level of the 12th rib anteriorly in 80 percent of patients, and in 18 percent the lung reaches the level of the body of the L1 vertebra posteriorly.[8]

During deep inspiration, the lung fills the pleural cavity entirely. As the lung deflates during expiration, the most inferior and distal parts of the parietal pleura extend beyond the costal margins and may come into direct contact with one another to form the costophrenic recesses – any increase in the amount of fluid in the pleural cavity accumulates here first. Attempts to aspirate small amounts of pleural fluid within this recess, or approaching the upper abdominal structures (liver, adrenals or kidneys) posteriorly during medical or surgical procedures, may result in damage to the lung and pleura, and in iatrogenic pneumothorax or hemothorax.[8]

The visceral pleura extends into the interlobular space, and therefore each lobe of the lung may expand or collapse individually. Abnormal divisions of lobes and segments are common[5] and interlobar fissures may be incompletely or completely separated by septa. These altered fissures may appear radiologically as linear shadows, and occasionally cause 'vanishing tumours' when pleural fluid is trapped within them, due to conditions in which fluid may fluctuate such as heart failure.[9]

The major fissure of the lung extends obliquely downwards, posteriorly to anteriorly, paralleling the sixth rib. An intercostal tube placed through the fifth, sixth or seventh intercostal space may therefore enter the pleural cavity near the major fissure, and if the tube is directed centrally, may enter and become trapped within the fissure, resulting in ineffective drainage.[10]

MICROSCOPIC ANATOMY

Layers of the pleural membrane

The visceral and parietal pleura in humans are approximately 40 μm across. By light microscopy, the pleura is generally divided into five layers (see Figure 2.1), consisting of a single cellular layer and four subcellular layers. Proceeding from the pleural surface, the layers are as follows:

1 a single layer of mesothelial cells;
2 a thin subendothelial connective tissue layer, including a basal lamina;
3 a thin superficial and elastic layer (often merged with the second in layer);
4 a loose connective tissue layer (contains nerves, blood vessels, lymphatics);
5 a deep fibroelastic layer (often fused to underlying tissue).

The thickness of each layer is variable between species, and displays variation between regions in the pleural space in both animal and humans[5,11–15] (see section 'The regional difference').

The thickness and boundaries of the superficial connective and elastic fiber layers (i.e. the second and third layers) are usually imprecise. The loose fourth connective tissue layer contains adipose tissue, fibroblasts, mast cells and other mononuclear cells, blood vessels, nerves and lymphatics, and often serves as the cleavage plane at pleurectomy. The fifth deep fibroelastic layer often adheres tightly to, or is fused with, the underlying tissue (i.e. lung parenchyma, mediastinum, diaphragm, ribs or intercostal muscles). The fibroelastic layer is highly variable, according to its position within the pleural cavity. The overall amount, proportion and integration of the fibroelastic meshwork are directly proportional to the extent of pleural excursion during the respiratory cycle.[13]

MESOTHELIAL CELLS

A single layer of mesothelial cells covers the surface of both the parietal and visceral pleura. Although there are morphological differences in mesothelial cells found in different areas,[16] no significant differences have been identified

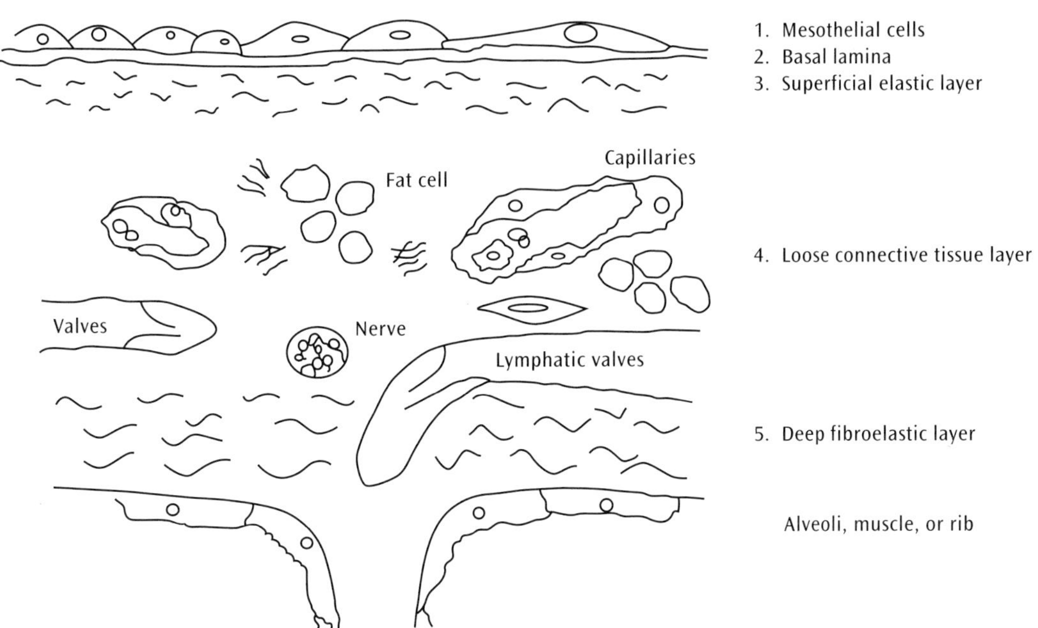

Figure 2.1 A schematic drawing of the pleura. On light microscopy, the pleura is divided into five layers. From the pleural surface, the layers are: first, a single layer of mesothelial cells; second, a thin submesothelial connective tissue lair, including a basal lamina; third, a thin superficial elastic layer; fourth, a loose connective tissue layer; and fifth, a deep fibroelastic layer. The thickness of each layer is markedly varied between species and between regions within the same individual.

between mesothelial cells found in the visceral or parietal pleura, or between cells found in the peritoneal pericardial and pleural cavities.

Human mesothelial cell ranges in size from 16.4 ± 6.8 to 41.9 ± 9.5 μm in diameter, and from less than 1 to greater than for 4 μm thick.[11,14] The mesothelial cell may therefore appear flattened, similar to endothelial cells, or more cuboidal, similar to epithelial cells.[16] The shape and size of the mesothelial cells often reflect the substructure of the pleura (see section 'The regional difference') or the functional status of the cells (see section 'The resting and reactive mesothelial cell').

Each mesothelial cell is covered with a bushy surface of microvilli, best visualized by transmission and scanning electron microscopy (Figures 2.2 and 2.3). The microvillus is approximately 0.1 μm in diameter and up to 3 μm or more in length. The microvilli often aggregate in clusters and appear wavy on transmission electron microscopy.[11,14,17–19]

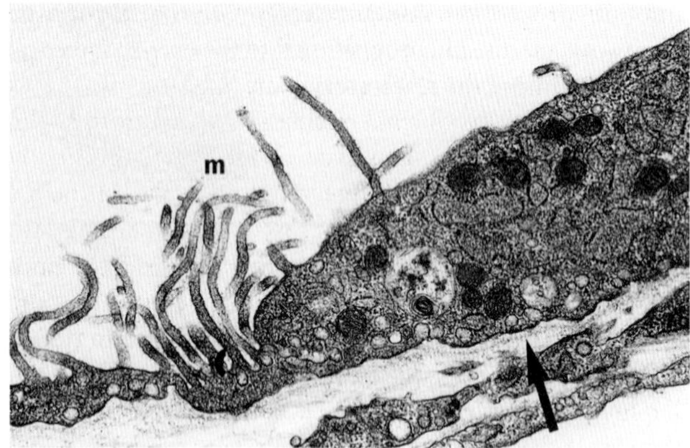

Figure 2.2 Surface microvilli on a mesothelial cell (rabbits visceral pleura, transmission electron microscopy, ×16 669). The microvillus is approximately 0.1 μm diameter and up to 3 μm or more in length. Many microvilli are often aggregated with each other and appear wavy (m). The cytoplasm of the mesothelial cell contains a moderate amount of organelles. A basal lamina is present beneath the cell (arrow). (With permission from Wang NS. Mesothelial cells *in situ.* In: Chretien J, Bignon J, Hirsch H (eds). *The pleura in health and disease.* New York: Marcel Dekker, 1985: 23–42.)

The microvilli are presumed to contribute to formation, absorption and organisation of the lubricating surface film of pleural fluid (see section 'The microvillus and lubricating membrane'). Under electron microscopy, numerous pinocytic vessels are identified within mesothelial cells, implying active secretion and absorption processes. Pinocytic vessels are often associated with microvilli on the cell membrane, especially at the pleural surface.[17,19]

The mesothelial cell nucleus is ovoid with a prominent nucleolus. The cytoplasm may be thin and scarce, or thick and abundant, but invariably contains a moderate to abundant amount of organelles including mitochondria, rough and smooth endoplasmic reticulum and dense

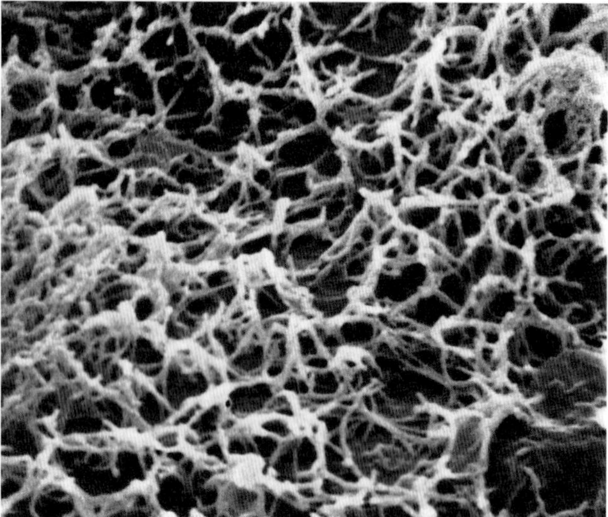

Figure 2.3 Microvilli are abundant, twisting and interwoven over the mesothelial cells in the lower thoracic wall. Rabbit parietal pleura, scanning electron microscopy, ×9375.

bodies (Figure 2.2). Evidence of metabolic activity is present, with polyribosomes, intermediate (pre-keratin) fibrils, golgi apparatus and glycogen granules identified[20] (see sections 'The resting and reactive mesothelial cell' and 'Subclinical alterations and repair of the pleura').

Mesothelial cells are always adherent to one another in their apical portion via tight junctions. Intermediate and desmosome junctions may be present but are not invariable.[20] At the basal cellular surface, cells are more loosely associated and are often overlapped, but are not attached to one another and are without intercellular junctions. During full inspiration, the overlap disappears,[20] suggesting that the mesothelial cells stretch and their cell bodies slide over each other during respiratory movements. The basal lamina is always present beneath the mesothelial cells and beneath the overlapped cytoplasmic processes.

The intra-membranous organization of the junctional complexes between parietal mesothelial cells is as loose as that of the venular endothelium.[20–22] This suggests that the parietal mesothelial layer is as fragile and leaky as the endothelial layer of a small vein. In contrast, the intra-membranous organization of the junctional complexes of the visceral mesothelial cell displays more complexity than that seen in the parietal mesothelial cell, at least in mice.[20,22] This finding suggests that the visceral mesothelial there is less likely to leak, or normally subjected to more tensile stretch and the parietal one.

THE MICROVILLUS AND LUBRICATING MEMBRANE

Microvilli are present diffusely over the entire pleural surface, on both parietal and visceral pleura. Each individual microvillus is oriented perpendicular to and projecting out from the cell surface, slightly twisting and interwoven with each other[13] (Figures 2.2 and 2.3).

The density of the carpet of microvilli varies according to position within the thoracic cavity, ranging from only a few to more than 600 per 100 μm^2, with an average of 300 per 100 μm^2.[11,14,18,19] A higher density of microvilli (in association with abundant hyaluronic acid) is found in the most actively moving parts of the lung, i.e. the lower thoracic cavity,[11,13,14] where the contraction and relation of the diaphragm and expansion and retraction of the lung and classic caged is highest. A higher density of microvilli is also found in the visceral rather than the parietal pleura at any given level.[11,13,14] The lowest density of microvilli is found on the inner surface of the ribs. Animal studies suggest that the microvilli carpet develops over the first few months of life, and subsequently changes and decays with increasing age.[23]

The function of microvilli is not completely clear. The cell surface area of the mesothelial cell layer is substantially increased by the presence of microvilli, and it is presumed that this also increases the cell membrane dependent functions, such as that of a variety of receptors ligands and enzyme productions such as metalloproteinases. As mentioned above, microvilli are associated with pinocytototic vessels, implying an important role in transcellular transport.[24] Given the apparent relationship between microvilli density and degree of movement of the lung, it seems likely that the microvilli's role in enmeshing glycoproteins rich in hyaluronic acid to lubricate the pleural surface and lesson friction between the lung and thorax is a key part of their function.[11,19]

Hyaluronic acid is secreted by the mesothelial cell, and by mesenchymal cells in the submesothelial interstitial tissue. Hyaluronic acid may be demonstrated by alcian blue or colloidal iron stains using light microscopy (LM) and electron microscopy (EM).[11]

THE BLOOD SUPPLY OF THE PLEURA

The blood supply of the parietal pleura

The parietal pleura is richly supplied with arterial blood, derived from multiple branches of adjacent systemic arteries according to region:[5,15,25]

- the costal pleura – supplied by the intercostal and internal mammary arteries;
- the mediastinal pleura – from the bronchial, upper diaphragmatic, internal mammary and mediastinal arteries;
- the cervical pleura – from the subclavian arteries and their collaterals;
- the diaphragmatic pleura – from the superior phrenic branches of internal mammary arteries, the posterior mediastinal arteries from the thoracic aorta and the inferior phrenic arteries of the abdominal aorta.

The venous drainage of the parietal pleura follows its arterial supply, with the majority eventually draining into the azygos vein and subsequently into the superior vena cava. Venous blood derived from the diaphragm drains either caudally into the inferior vena cava through the inferior phrenic veins or cranially into the superior vena cava through the superior phrenic veins, which run parallel with the internal mammary artery and thence into the brachiochepalic trunk.

The blood supply of the visceral pleura

The arterial blood supply of the visceral pleura in humans is still debated. Animals with thick pleura (such as horses, pigs or sheep), derive their arterial blood supply for the visceral pleura from the bronchial arteries. Animals with thin pleura (such as mice, rats and rabbits) tend to derive visceral pleural blood supply from the pulmonary circulation. Albertine *et al.*[14] have demonstrated that in young adult sheep the bronchial artery supplies the visceral pleura completely and exclusively.

Humans have thick visceral pleura, and therefore it is expected that the bronchial circulation should supply the human visceral pleura. However, this has not been clearly demonstrated.[26] There is agreement that the bronchial artery supplies most of the pleura facing the mediastinum, the pleura covering the interlobular surfaces, and a part of the diaphragmatic surface. The blood supply for the remaining visceral pleura (i.e. the entire convex costal lung surface including the apex and the greater part of the diaphragmatic surface) is less certain.[27] It has been suggested that these parts of the visceral pleura are supplied by pulmonary arteries which arise beneath the pleura from the pulmonary circulation.[5] Using techniques to delineate pulmonary and bronchial vessels, Milne and Pistolesi[28] concluded that the visceral pleural circulation is derived from and continuous with the pulmonary circulation. Disagreement continues about the blood supply of visceral pleura in humans (see section 'Shunting and pathological changes with age').

The greater part of the visceral pleura supplied by the bronchial artery is drained through the pulmonary veins, except for a small area around the hilum where the pleural veins drain into the bronchial veins.

Shunting and pathological changes with age

Shunts between the systemic and pulmonary arteries are known to exist in human lung, normally accounting for less than 5 percent of the circulation, but increasing with age and any chronic lung disease.[5] In aged human lungs, the bronchial arteries in the visceral pleura, especially those far from a hilum, are often sclerotic and obliterated (personal observation). It is therefore likely that the pulmonary circulation compensates for that part of the pleura which is deprived of the original bronchial blood supply. This phenomenon is most apparent in bullae of the lung.

Within the aged lung, and in association with many chronic lung and pleural diseases, the bronchial arteries proliferate around the airway and in the interlobular septum. Bronchial artery proliferation may be seen within the pleura in inflammation and fibrosis, and systemic arteries may invade into the visceral pleura from the parietal site, especially when adhesions between the lung and the chest wall develop.

INNERVATION

The costal parietal pleura and the peripheral part of the diaphragm are innervated by somatic intercostals nerves,[15,25] thus pain felt in these areas is referred to the adjacent chest wall. The central portion of the diaphragm is innervated by the phrenic nerve, resulting in referred pain to the ipsilateral shoulder tip during central diaphragm irritation.

The visceral pleura is extensively innervated by pulmonary branches of the vagus nerve and sympathetic trunk. However, the visceral pleural contains no pain fibers in contrast to the parietal pleura, and this is of clinical relevance. The presence of pleuritic chest pain therefore usually indicates involvement of the parietal pleural in the disease process.

CONTENTS OF THE PLEURAL SPACE

The volume and characteristics of liquid in the pleural space is determined by a combination of dynamic phenomenon, involving the pulmonary and systemic circulation, the lymphatic drainage, the mechanical movement of the thoracic cage and the movement of the heart.[6]

The volume of pleural fluid in health is small. Experiments in rabbits have demonstrated a total pleural fluid content of 0.2 mL, and previous data has suggested that the normal human pleural fluid volume is less than 1 mL.[29] In a subsequent study, the volume of pleural fluid collected from a single pleural cavity was 0.98 mL in the rabbit and 2.35 mL in the dog.[30] Noppen *et al.*,[31] using an interesting pleural lavage technique, estimated the mean pleural fluid volume in healthy human subjects undergoing medical thoracoscopy and found the mean pleural fluid volume in the right pleural cavity of healthy humans to be 8 mL. The amount of pleural fluid may be related to physical excursion of the chest, with Yamada[29] demonstrating an increase in the volume of pleural fluid in military recruits after exercise.

The small volume of pleural fluid forms a thin film between the visceral and parietal pleura, 10 μm thick at least.[32,33] This prevents contact between the visceral and parietal pleura throughout their surfaces. In support of this, experiments in sheep have demonstrated no direct contact between the visceral and parietal pleura,[34] suggesting that the pleural space is a real rather than a potential space.

Normal pleural fluid contains 1–2 g of protein per 100 mL, a figure similar to the concentration detected in the interstitial fluid of both animals and humans.[29,35] However, the concentration of large molecular weight proteins (e.g. lactate dehydrogenase, molecular weight 134 000) in pleural fluid is less than half that of serum, implying some regulation of molecular passage into the pleural cavity. There are 1400 to 4500 cells per microliter of pleural fluid in animals or humans,[29,30,35] largely made up of macrophages with a few leukocytes and red blood cells, again implying a restriction to cellular passage into the pleural cavity. (For further description of normal pleural fluid composition, see Chapter 4, Normal physiological fluid and cellular contents by M Noppen.)

TRANSPORT ACROSS THE MESOTHELIAL CELL AND PLEURA

Pleural fluid is produced by the parietal pleura, originating from the systemic circulation, and production occurs mostly in the less dependent region of the pleural cavity where blood vessels are closest to the mesothelial surface. Reabsorption of pleural fluid occurs mainly through lymphatic drainage in the most dependant part of the pleural cavity, and again occurs exclusively on the parietal pleural side. Drainage occurs from the parietal thoracic, mediastinal and diaphragmatic surfaces (see section 'The pleurolymphatic communication').[36,37]

Fluid filters out of parietal pleural capillaries and into the pleural space (or vice versa) according to the net hydrostatic–oncotic pressure gradient.[37] As fluid in the pleural space actively alters transpleural forces in respiration, optimal volume and thickness are closely maintained.[37,38]

Water and molecules less than 4 nm in size can freely pass between mesothelial cells. Intrapleural injections of hypotonic and hypertonic fluids have been demonstrated to induce an increase in the number and size of pinocytotic and cytoplasmic vesicles within mesothelial cells.[39] Intrapleural injection of larger particles, for example ferritin (11 nm), carbon (20–50 nm) and polystyrene (up to 1000 nm) result in the appearance of these substances within cytoplasmic vesicles of mesothelial cells.[40] Smaller particles are subsequently identified within the mesenchymal cells of the pleural wall.[20] Taken together, these findings suggest that transcytoplasmic transport is active within mesothelial cells.

Movement of fluid in between the pleural space and the alveolar or pulmonary interstitium is restricted by the presence of tight junctions between visceral mesothelial cells, as previously described (section 'Mesothelial cells'). However, during disease states, such as congestive cardiac failure or adult respiratory distress syndrome, both the endothelial and mesothelial barriers are damaged, permitting alveolar and pulmonary interstitial fluid movement into the pleural space. In this context, the pleural space is considered as one of the main important exits for lung edema fluid.[38]

Particles greater in size than 1000 nm are engulfed by mesothelial cells but are not transported across the basal lamina.[20] Effective removal of large particles or cells through the pleura is therefore unlikely, unless the basal lamina plus or minus deeper layers of the pleura have been damaged. However, the intrapleural injection of labeled red blood cells results in their appearance in the systemic circulation intact,[41,42] and large molecular weight proteins are absorbed rapidly through the pleural lymphatics.[42] Therefore, communication passages between the pleural cavity and the circulation system must exist, which are larger and faster than the cytoplasmic route (see section 'The pleuro-lymphatic communication').

LYMPHATICS

The lymphatics within the lung are divided into two systems: the superficial or pleural plexus, localized in the subpleural connective tissue layer of the visceral pleura, and the deep plexus located in the bronchovascular bundles. The deep plexus includes peribronchial, peripulmonary vascular and interlobular septum or connectivity tissue. Communications between the two plexuses exist only at the junction of the pleura and the interlobular septum.[5,15]

Lymphatic circulation of the visceral pleura

The superficial lymphatic plexus of the visceral pleura is composed of a network of lymphatic capillaries and collecting lymphatic vessels. Larger collecting lymphatic vessels are arranged mainly along the margin of the pleural bases of the respiratory lobules, forming a polyhedral and widely meshed network. There are smaller, blind-ending side-branches and capillaries unevenly distributed from this meshed network.[27] There are an increased number of lymphatic vessels in the dependant parts of the lung, associated with higher intravascular pressures.

Lymphatic flow may occur in any direction, governed by the pressure gradient. However, the larger visceral lymphatic vessels contain one-way valves, directing flow of lymph towards the hilar regions of the lung. All lymph draining from the visceral pleura therefore reaches the lung root, either through the lymphatic vessels of the lobular and lobar lung septae, all by flowing along visceral pleural surface to the lung hilum. The majority of large and small lymphatic vessels within the visceral pleura are located more closely to the alveolar than the pleural cavity side, and therefore most lymph drains into the vessels in the lobular septum.

Lymphatic circulation of the parietal pleura

The lymphatic drainage of the parietal pleura varies according to region. In the costal parietal pleura, lymphatic plexuses are confined to intercostal spaces and are absent or minimal over the inner surface of the ribs.[27] Lymph collected in the costal pleura drains ventrally towards nodes in the internal mammary nodes, or dorsally towards the intercostal lymph nodes near the heads of the ribs.

The lymphatic vessels of the mediastinal pleura are seen in areas with abundant fatty tissue, the lymph collected draining to the tracheobronchial and mediastinal nodes. In more caudal areas, the mediastinal lymphatics are often associated with Kampmeier's foci (see section 'Kampmeier's foci'). Lymphatic vessels from the diaphragmatic pleura drain into parasternal, middle phrenic and posteriorly mediastinal nodes.

The lymphatic system of the parietal pleura is more extensive, more complex and less restricted in direction and passage of flow than the visceral lymphatic system, mirroring the arterial and venous supply. The parietal lymphatics are therefore thought to play a key role in the formation and removal of pleural fluid. In normal and pathological states, the effective removal of fluid, cells and cellular debris relies upon the presence of the pleuro-lymphatic communications (see next section).

THE PLEURO-LYMPHATIC COMMUNICATION

Almost 150 years ago, von Recklinghausen[43] and Dybkowsky[44] inferred the presence of connections between serous cavities and the lymphatic channels. Demonstration of the absorption of red blood cells (8 μm in diameter) from the pleural space[41,42] argued for the existence of anatomical channels many years before morphological confirmation by ultrastructural studies in the 1970s.[45–47] There is direct evidence of transport of macromolecules through this system from studies in monkeys.[48] The pleuro-lymphatic channel consists of the components described below.

Stomata

Ovoid or round openings of 2–6 μm or greater in diameter, known as stomata, have been demonstrated on the parietal pleural surface of the anterior lower chest wall, mediastinum, and diaphragm in rabbits, mice and sheep (Figures 2.4–2.6).[13,20,45–47,49] The stomata connect the pleural cavity with the lacunae (see section 'Lacuna and lymphatic channels'), which are dilated lymphatic spaces in the parietal pleural wall that in turn drain into larger collecting lymphatic ducts.[20] Stomata appear to be unique to the parietal (and peritoneal) pleura.

The stoma may be single and isolated,[47] but is more often found in groups of between 10 and 20.[13] Shinohara[50] demonstrated a total of 1000 lymphatic stomata in a single thoracic hemisphere of a golden hamster, with around 85 percent in the dorso-caudal region, and the remaining 15 percent in the ventro-cranial region of the thoracic wall.[50] Lymphatic stomata were demonstrated along the costal margin in the ventro-cranial region and in the pre- and paravertebral fatty tissue in the dorsocaudal region. In this study, no lymphatic stomata were found on the pleural surface of the diaphragm.[50]

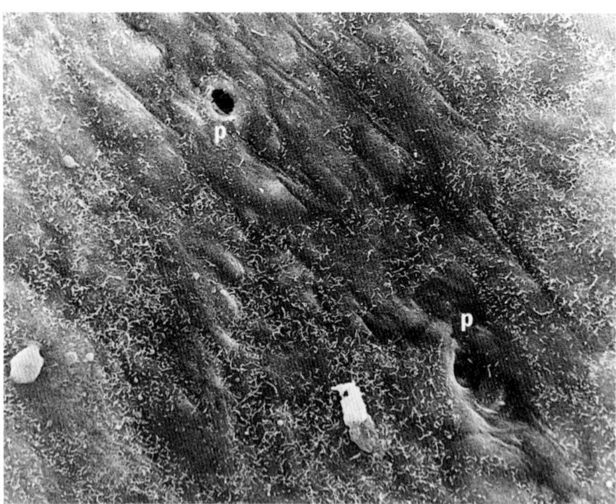

Figure 2.4 Two isolated round openings of the preformed stomata (p) are shown in the subcostal region of the parietal pleura. Mouse, scanning electron microscopy, ×1680. (With permission from Wang NS. Morphological data of pleura – normal conditions. In Chretien J, Hirsch H (eds). *Diseases of the pleura.* New York: Masson Publishing USA, Inc, 1983: 10–24.)

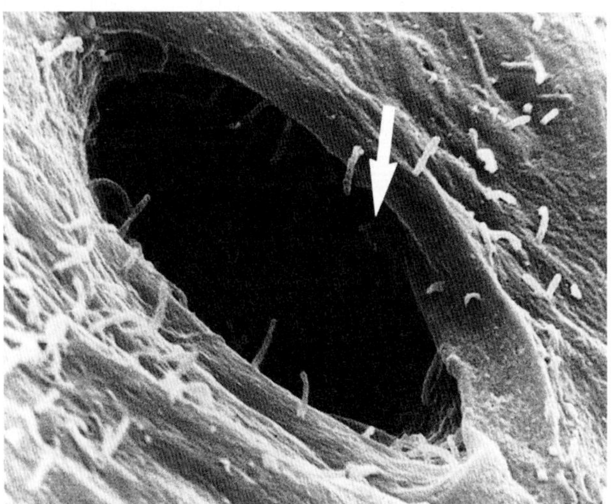

Figure 2.5 A high magnification view of a stoma. Mesothelial cells with surface microvilli extend into the stoma (arrow). Mouse parietal pleura, intercostal region of the lower thoracic wall, scanning electron microscopy, ×18060. (With permission from Wang NS. Morphological data of pleura – normal conditions. In Chretien J, Hirsch H (eds). *Diseases of the pleura.* New York: Masson Publishing USA, Inc, 1983: 10–24.)

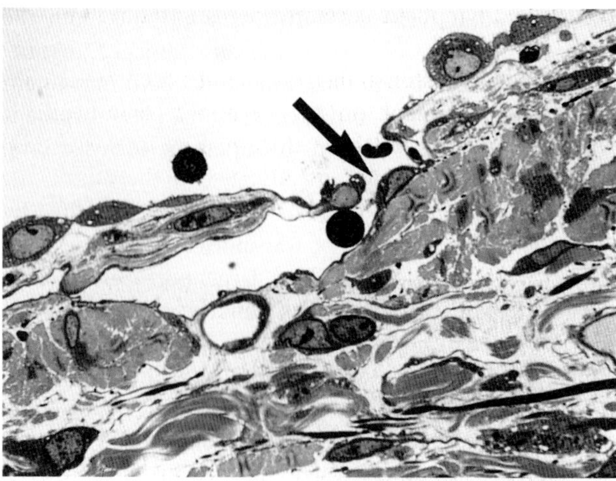

Figure 2.6 A red blood cell present at the stoma of a lacuna (arrow). The relatively bulky mesothelial cells on the pleural surface and the thin endothelial cell of the lymphatic appear to meet at the stoma. The diameters of the two large, dark-staining mononuclear cells are larger than the narrow opening of the stoma. Rabbit subcostal pleura, ×680. (With permission from Wang NS. The preformed stomas connecting the pleural cavity and the lymphatics in the parietal pleura. *Am Rev Respir Dis* 1975; **111**: 12–20.)

Other studies have demonstrated stomata in the parietal and diaphragmatic pleura, and stomata seem to be abundant in the diaphragmatic peritoneum of both humans and animals.[45–47,49] No study to date has demonstrated stomas in the visceral pleura.

The process of formation of the pleural stomata is as yet unknown. Studies in rats have suggested that parietal stoma appear in the first few days of life post delivery.[51] The diaphragmatic peritoneal stoma in rats are formed as a result of the breakdown of intercellular junctions in both the endothelial and mesothelial cell layers,[52] and it seems likely that the process in the parietal pleura is similar.

Membrana cribriformis (the cribriform lamina)

Beneath the stomal openings, the substructure of the parietal pleura is made of up a loosely knit layer of interweaving connective tissue bundles (Figures 2.7 and 2.8).[53,54] The membrana cribriformis forms the roof of a dilated lymphatic space – the lacuna (see section 'Lacuna and lymphatic channels'). The pleural surface of this connective tissue bundle network is covered with a layer of mesothelial cells, with the opposite surface covered with a layer of lymphatic endothelial cells (Figures 2.7 and 2.8).[47] The membrana cribriformis is therefore made up of lining cells bridging a connective tissue bundle mesh, and it is postulated that stomas are formed when the lining cells on both pleural and lymphatic surfaces are disrupted (Figures 2.7 and 2.8).

Similar to the stomal distribution, the membrana cribriformis is abundant on the peritoneal diaphragmatic surface,[55] and has not been documented in the visceral pleura of either humans or animals. In the rabbit, the membrane cribriformis has been measured at 7–60 μm in diameter.[56]

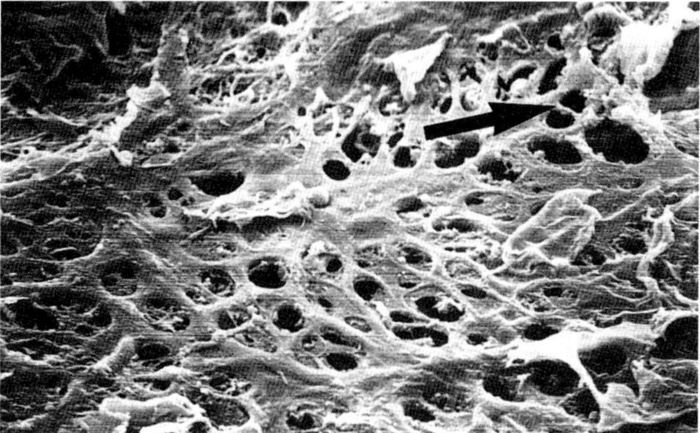

Figure 2.7 The covering mesothelial cells are mostly broken in the mediastinal pleura of this patient with massive pleural effusion, exposing the lamina cribriformis. The stomas between the collagen bundles are quite variable in size, as is the thickness of the collagen bundles. Rupture of the thin bundle (arrow) may change the adjacent stomas into much larger fenestrae. Scanning electron microscopy, ×8250. (With permission from Wang NS. Morphological data of pleura – normal conditions. In Chretien J, Hirsch H (eds). *Diseases of the pleura.* New York: Masson Publishing USA, Inc, 1983: 10–24.)

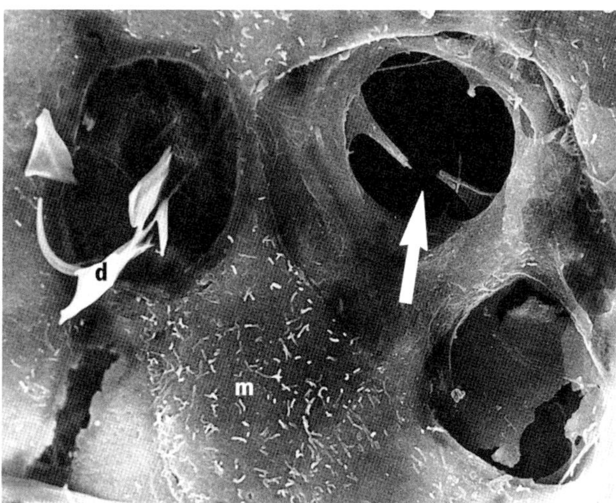

Figure 2.8 Mesothelial cells (m) with microvilli and lymphatic endothelial cells are in the process of disruption, or formation of stomas or fenestrae, on the lamina cribriformis. The stretched remnant of a lymphatic endothelial cell appears just broken (arrow). Debris of foreign particles (d) are present over a lymphatic endothelial cell, which is almost intact. Human parietal pleura, ×3105.

Lacuna and lymphatic channels

Beneath the stoma and membrana cribriformis is a lacuna, which is the terminal dilatation of a lymphatic channel. Each lacuna is connected at one end to the pleural cavity by a small number of stomas, and drains via a lymphatic channel with checking-valves at the other end (Figure 2.6).[20,47]

Movements of the lung and thoracic cage during respiration alter the rate of removal of particles, cells and fluid from the pleural cavity.[39,41,47] During inspiration, the chest wall expands and the intercostal spaces widen, resulting in the stomas and lacunae being pulled open. Fluid and particles enter the lacuna by a combination of the negative pressure generated within lacunae and the expanding lung pushing on the pleural contents. During expiration, the diameter of the stomas decrease as the chest wall contracts, resulting in compression of the lacunae and expulsion of fluid, particles and cells in to the draining lymphatic channels. Retrograde flow of material within the lymphatic channel is prevented during the next inspiratory movement by the presence of the lymphatic valves. Stomas and lacunae appear to function in a similar manner on the peritoneal diaphragmatic surface.[46,55]

Kampmeier's foci

In 1928, Kampmeier described small milky spots in the dorsal and caudal portion of the human mediastinum.[57] At light microscopy, these foci are made up of modified cuboidal mesothelial cells with stomas and are associated with an aggregate of lymphocytes, histiocytes, plasma cells and other mononuclear cells, located around a central lymphatic or vascular vessel. The mesothelial cells have increased cytoplasmic mass and granules, suggesting cellular activity (see section 'The resting and reactive mesothelial cell'). Under scanning electron microscopy, the foci appear as irregular, elevated mound-like structures.[20] Similar foci have been identified in the thoracic cavity of dogs and in the mesentery of many species.[58,59] It is postulated that these structures act as local host defence mechanisms, similar to the tonsils in the oropharynx or Peyer's patches in the gut. Infectious organisms and noxious particles may bypass these foci, and appear via the draining lymphatic channels in the parasternal lymph nodes.[60]

The crevices or fenestrae

Openings much larger than stomas, around 10–50 μm, have been documented in the mediastinal pleura of aged mice and are called crevices.[61] Similar structures have been observed in rabbits (personal observation). The precise mechanism of their formation is uncertain. However, crevices are only found in areas where stomas are normally present, and it is therefore postulated that they may be the result of fusion of adjacent stomas as a result of breakdown of the collagen bundle meshwork, perhaps owing to digestive enzyme release in pleuritis (Figure 2.8). This process is analogous to the development of pulmonary emphysema,[62,63] in which digestive enzyme-mediated breakdown of elastic fibers results in fusion of the interalveolar pores of Kohn.

The pleuro-lymphatic communication – does it exist?

Although several animal and human studies have demonstrated the presence of stomas connecting the pleural cavity with the lymphatics,[45–47,49,50] some studies have found no evidence of stomas in human pleura.[64] This may be due to their paucity, the limited availability of normal human tissue for study, or obscuration of the stomas by fibrin and cellular debris.[47,53,65]

Stomas are found readily in the peritoneal cavity,[46,66] with one study demonstrating around 250 stomas per mm^2 of diaphragmatic peritoneum.[66] In contrast, the pleural diaphragmatic density of stomas is as little as 1 per mm^2 in small mammals[47] and sheep.[65] The reason for this difference is unclear, but may reflect different demands on the pleural and abdominal cavities. The pleural space is sealed from the external environment in health, and relatively little fluid and cellular content requires removal. The peritoneal cavity is likely to require a greater capacity to remove fluid and cellular content, for example as the result of ovulation.

Stomas may therefore be relatively unimportant in health for the pleural cavity, but be recruited in disease states in which pleural fluid and cellular material clearance becomes important. Inflammation and chronic pleural effusion appears to easily disrupt the thin mesothelial and lymphatic lining cells covering the lamina cribriformis[47] (Figures 2.7 and 2.8), although no cause and effect relationship has been established. Stomas may increase in both size and number with age.[61]

THE PLEURO-PERITONEAL COMMUNICATION AND DIAPHRAGMATIC DEFECTS

The lymphatic plexuses of the diaphragmatic pleura and diaphragmatic peritoneum are separate, with communications between the two being poorly formed or infrequent. This is presumably an adaptation to prevent inflammatory or infected fluid from entering the pleural space and interfering with respiration.

Small diaphragmatic defects probably exist more often than is clinically suspected. Severe congenital diaphragmatic defects or anomalies may be fatal *in utero*, but are rare. Acquired defects are thought to arise from thinning and eventual separation of collagenous fibres within the tendinous part of the diaphragm.

Small diaphragmatic defects usually only become apparent clinically in the context of ascites associated with pleural effusion, for example hepatic hydrothorax,[67–69] continuous ambulatory peritoneal dialysis[70] or Meig's syndrome. Such defects may be demonstrated at thoracoscopy[69], by the injection of air[70] or labeled tracer into the peritoneal space with subsequent chest radiology, or at autopsy.[68]

In the absence of diaphragmatic defects, fluid may enter the pleural space from a peritoneal cavity distended with fluid (or rarely vice versa), through reversal of the normal pressure gradient within the lymphatics and valve insufficiency in the thoracic duct and its attributes. Peritonitis or subphrenic abscess is a recognized cause of pleural reaction, whereas lower lobe pneumonia resulting in intra-abdominal abscess is rare.

THE REGIONAL DIFFERENCE

There are substantial morphological differences in regions of the pleura. These differences include the mesothelial cell characteristics (e.g. size and shape, density of microvilli), the pleural substructure and the number of pleuro-lymphatic communications, including the Kapmeier's foci.[11,13,57]

Visceral pleura

In the apical portion of the hemithorax, the visceral pleura is relatively thin with flattened mesothelial cells and sparse microvilli, reflecting paucity of movement in the statically expanded upper lung. Beneath the mesothelial cell layer, the basal lamina and deeper three layers are often difficult to distinguish, especially in the apex where the systemic arterial supply is replaced by a pulmonary supply (see section 'The blood supply of the visceral pleura'). This thin pleura is the site of bleb formation seen in some patients with spontaneous pneumothorax and is often the site of bullae formation in chronic obstructive pulmonary disease. Rupture of these structures results in pneumothorax.

In more basal areas where the lung moves and stretches more, the visceral pleura is thicker with cuboidal mesothelial cells showing increased microvilli.[11,13,14] The amount of collagen and elastic fibers increases within the deeper layers toward the lower part of the lung.

Parietal pleura

Pleura overlying the inner rib surfaces is thin with flattened mesothelial cells, sparse microvilli and thin subcellular layers. The dense fifth layer of fibroelastic tissue fuses with the perichondrium or periosteum of the rib.

In areas of parietal pleura overlying loose substructures, for example the mediastinum, the costophrenic recesses and the subcostal margins, lining mesothelial cells are cuboidal and prominent. The second and third layers are well defined, whereas the fourth layer is often merged with a deeper and wider interstitial space, which contains a poorly formed or absent fifth layer. This loose fourth layer often serves as the cleavage plane in pleurectomy.

The pleura over the diaphragm and intercostal muscles is of moderate thickness, with characteristics somewhere between pleura overlying ribs and pleura overlying looser structures. The underlying tissue covered by the pleura therefore influences the cellular and non-cellular components of the pleural layers.

Albertine *et al.*[65] showed that unlike the varied thickness and appearance of the visceral pleura, the parietal pleura in sheep has a relatively uniform thickness over chest wall, diaphragm and mediastinum. There was a significant difference in the distance from capillary to pleural surface between parietal (10–12 μm) and visceral (18–56 μm, depending on region of the lung studied) pleura.[65] Transportation of fluid and large molecules is therefore anatomically easier through the parietal side.

THE RESTING AND REACTIVE MESOTHELIAL CELL

Resting mesothelial cells are cuboidal or flattened and their enzymes are predominantly those of the anaerobic pentose pathway.[71] In response to a variety of cytokines or thrombin, mesothelial cells become activated or reactive.[11,72] The cells become large and cuboidal or columnar in shape with increased microvilli, and use the enzymes of the oxidative pathway.[73] Surface membrane and mitochondrial enzyme activity, including 5′-nucleotidase, alkaline phosphatases, ATPase and cytochrome oxidase, is increased. Fibrinolytic activity increases and the synthesis of prostacylcins,[74] cytokines and hyaluronic acid-rich glycoproteins[75,76] are enhanced (see also Chapter 3, Mesothelial cells).

In inflammation of the pleura, mesothelial cell proliferation is increased as a response to a variety of growth and proliferation factors. Mesothelial cells from rats possess receptors for platelet derived growth factors (PDGFs), and human mesothelial cells have been shown *in vitro* to increase growth rate in response to PDGF and transforming growth factor-beta (TGF-β).[77] In chronic inflammation, cells in the deeper layers of pleura co-express cytokeratin and vimentin immunoreactivity. This suggests that in addition to proliferation, mesothelial cells migrate deep in to the pleura.[78]

The proliferative and invasive response of mesothelial cells is non-specific and occurs in response to many stimuli and in the subacute phase of lung injury. The responses may persist and progress to fibrosis in the presence of persistent pleural irritation, of which asbestos fiber is the clearest example.[78,79]

SUBCLINICAL ALTERATIONS AND REPAIR OF THE PLEURA

Pleural effusion or pleuritis may occur and regress spontaneously without the need for pleural intervention, for example in heart failure, pulmonary infarction and some cases of parapneumonic effusion. The course and mechanism of spontaneous resolution in pleural inflammation is not clear.[80] Experimental animal studies demonstrate that mesothelial cells become reactive, proliferate and migrate in response to injury. These changes appear to facilitate the removal of fibrin and inflammatory debris and to allow repair of the pleural surface, maintaining the integrity of the pleural cavity while preserving drainage.[75,81,82] Whether the pleura recovers completely or progresses to the development of fibrosis appears to be related to the degree of damage to the basal lamina.[83]

Human CT and MRI studies suggest that unsuspected pleural lesions are common, especially in smokers.[84] Pleural changes have been observed in patients with pneumonitis, lung cancer and myocardial ischaemia, without clinical or basic radiological evidence of pleural disease.[80] It is possible that minor damage and subsequent repair occur in the pleura frequently without any clinical manifestation and, in this case, the reactive and reparative properties of the mesothelial cell are important.

KEY POINTS

- The thoracic cage is constructed like a vertical cone-shaped bellow, with the diaphragm acting as a pump at the most caudal and widest end.
- The pleura is a sealed space inserted between the lung surface and thoracic cage/diaphragm, permitting easy movement of the lung during the respiratory cycle.
- Mesothelial cells enmesh hyaluronic acid-rich glycoproteins on surface microvilli, resulting in a lubricated pleural surface.
- Normally, a small amount of pleural fluid is present in the pleural space, regulated by hydrostatic–osmotic pressure and the pleurolymphatic drainage.
- Larger particles, cells and excess fluid are removed through a system of preformed stomata draining into the lymphatic system.
- Pleural injury appears to occur often, but a regulated repair process usually prevents clinically significant pleural fibrosis, or other complications. Mesothelial cells are active in constant damage repair and maintain the normal patent pleural space.

REFERENCES

● = Key primary paper
◆ = Major review article

1. West JB, Fu Z, Gaeth AP, Short RV. Fetal lung development in the elephant reflects the adaptations required for snorkeling in adult life. *Respir Physiol Neurobiol* 2003; **138**: 325–33.
2. West JB. Snorkel breathing in the elephant explains the unique anatomy of its pleura. *Respir Physiol* 2001; **126**: 1–8.
3. Patten BM, Carlson BW. *Foundations of embryology*, 3rd edn. New York: McGraw-Hill; 1974.
●4. Hesseldahl H, Larsen JF. Ultrastructure of human yolk sac: endoderm, mesenchyme, tubules and mesothelium. *Am J Anat* 1969; **126**: 315–35.
◆5. von Hayek H. *The parietal pleura and visceral pleura*. New York: Hafner; 1960.
6. Pistolesi M, Miniati M, Giuntini C. Pleural liquid and solute exchange. *Am Rev Respir Dis* 1989; **140**: 825–47.
7. Rabinowitz JG, Cohen BA, Mendleson DS. Symposium on nonpulmonary aspects in chest radiology. The pulmonary ligament. *Radiol Clin North Am* 1984; 22: 659–72.
8. Morrissey BM, Bisset RA. The right inferior lung margin: anatomy and clinical implication. *Br J Radiol* 1993; **66**: 503–5.
9. Satoh K, Sato A, Kobayashi T, *et al.* Septal structure of incomplete interlobar fissures of the lung. *Acad Radiol* 1996; **3**: 475–8.
10. Webb WR, LaBerge JM. Radiographic recognition of chest tube malposition in the major fissure. *Chest* 1984; **85**: 81–3.
●11. Wang NS. The regional difference of pleural mesothelial cells in rabbits. *Am Rev Respir Dis* 1974; **110**: 623–33.
12. Michailova KN. The serous membranes in the cat. Electron microscopic observations. *Ann Anat* 1996; **178**: 413–24.
13. Mariassy AT, Wheeldon EB. The pleura: a combined light microscopic, scanning, and transmission electron microscopic study in the sheep. I. Normal pleura. *Exp Lung Res* 1983; **4**: 293–314.
●14. Albertine KH, Wiener-Kronish JP, Roos PJ, Staub NC. Structure, blood supply, and lymphatic vessels of the sheep's visceral pleura. *Am J Anat* 1982; **165**: 277–94.
15. Nagaishi C. *Functional anatomy and histology of the lung*. Tokyo: Igaku Shoin; 1972.
16. Michailova K, Wassilev W, Wedel T. Scanning and transmission electron microscopic study of visceral and parietal peritoneal regions in the rat. *Ann Anat* 1999; **181**: 253–60.
17. Odor DL. Observations of the rat mesothelium with the electron and phase microscopes. *Am J Anat* 1954; **95**: 433–65.
●18. Legrand M, Pariente R, Andre J, Chretien J, Brouet G. [Ultrastructure of the human parietal pleura]. *Presse Med* 1971; **79**: 2515–20.
●19. Andrews PM, Porter KR. The ultrastructural morphology and possible functional significance of mesothelial microvilli. *Anat Rec* 1973; **177**: 409–26.
◆20. Wang NS. Mesothlelial cells *in situ*. In: Chretien J, Bignon J, Hirsch A (eds). *The pleura in health and disease*. New York: Marcel Dekker, 1985: 23–42.
21. Inoue T, Osatake H. Three-dimensional demonstration of the intracellular structures of mouse mesothelial cells by scanning electron microscopy. *J Submicrosc Cytol Pathol* 1989; **21**: 215–27.
●22. Simionescu M, Simionescu N. Organization of cell junctions in the peritoneal mesothelium. *J Cell Biol* 1977; **74**: 98–110.
23. Nomura K, Kida K, Kudoh S. [A morphological study to elucidate the differences in visceral pleura in young and old mice]. *Nippon Ika Daigaku Zasshi* 1998; **65**: 227–35.
24. Madison LD, Bergstrom-Porter B, Torres AR, Shelton E. Regulation of surface topography of mouse peritoneal cells. Formation of microvilli and vesiculated pits on omental mesothelial cells by serum and other proteins. *J Cell Biol* 1979; **82**: 783–97.
25. Clemente CD. *Anatomy of the human body*, 30th edn. Philadelphia: Lea & Febiger, 1985.
26. Davila RM, Crouch EC. Anatomic organisation and function of the human pleura. *Semin Respir Crit Care Med* 1979; **82**: 783–97.
27. Bernaudin JF, Fleury JY. Anatomy of the blood and lymphatic circulation of the pleural serosa. In: Chretien J, Bignon J, Hirsch A (eds). *The pleural in health and disease*. New York: Marcel Dekker; 1985: 101–24.
28. Milne ENC, Pistolesi M. *Reading the chest radiograph: a physiologic approach*. St Louis: Mosby; 1993.
●29. Yamada S. Uber die serose Flussigkeit in der Pleurahohle der gesunde Menschen. *Z Ges Exp Med* 1933; **90**: 342–8.
●30. Miserocchi G, Agostoni E. Contents of the pleural space. *J Appl Physiol* 1971; **30**: 208–13.
●31. Noppen M, De Waele M, Li R, *et al.* Volume and cellular content of normal pleural fluid in humans examined by pleural lavage. *Am J Respir Crit Care Med* 2000; **162**: 1023–6.
32. Butler JP, Huang J, Loring SH, *et al.* Model for a pump that drives circulation of pleural fluid. *J Appl Physiol* 1995; **78**: 23–9.
33. Agostoni E, Miserocchi G, Bonanni MV. Thickness and pressure of the pleural liquid in some mammals. *Respir Physiol* 1969; **6**: 245–56.
●34. Albertine KH, Wiener-Kronish JP, Bastacky J, Staub NC. No evidence for mesothelial cell contact across the costal pleural space of sheep. *J Appl Physiol* 1991; **70**: 123–34.
●35. Sahn SA, Willcox ML, Good JT Jr, Potts DE, Filley GF. Characteristics of normal rabbit pleural fluid: physiologic and biochemical implications. *Lung* 1979; **156**: 63–9.
36. Miserocchi G. Physiology and pathophysiology of pleural fluid turnover. *Eur Respir J* 1997; **10**: 219–25.
◆37. Staub NC. New concepts about the pathophysiology of pulmonary edema. *J Thorac Imaging* 1988; **3**: 8–14.
38. Miserocchi G, Venturoli D, Negrini D, Del Fabbro M. Model of pleural fluid turnover. *J Appl Physiol* 1993; **75**: 1798–806.
39. Shumko JZ, Feinberg RN, Shalvoy RM, DeFouw DO. Responses of rat pleural mesothelia to increased intrathoracic pressure. *Exp Lung Res* 1993; **19**: 283–97.
◆40. Wang NS. Morphological data of pleura – normal conditions. In: Chretien J, Hirsch A (eds). *The pleural in health and disease*. New York: Masson Publishing USA Inc; 1983: 10–24.
◆41. Courtice FC, Simmonds WJ. Physiological significance of lymph drainage of the serous cavities and lungs. *Physiol Rev* 1954; **34**: 419–48.
42. Wilson JL, Herrod CM, Scarle GL, *et al.* The absorption of blood from the pleural space. *Surgery* 1960; **48**: 766–74.
●43. von Recklinghausen FV. Zur Fettresorption. *Virchow Arch (Pathol Anat)* 1863; **26**: 172–278.
44. Dybkowsky. Ueber Aufsaugang und Absonderung der Pleurawand. *Ber d Kgl Sachs Gesellsch d Wissensch Math-physik Kl* 1866; **18**: 191–218.
45. Wheeldon EB, Mariassy AT, McSporran KD. The pleura: a combined light microscopic and scanning and transmission electron microscopic study in the sheep. II. Response to injury. *Exp Lung Res* 1983; **5**: 125–40.
46. Tsilibary EC, Wissig SL. Absorption from the peritoneal cavity: SEM study of the mesothelium covering the peritoneal surface of the muscular portion of the diaphragm. *Am J Anat* 1977; **149**: 127–33.
●47. Wang NS. The preformed stomas connecting the pleural cavity and the lymphatics in the parietal pleura. *Am Rev Respir Dis* 1975; **111**: 12–20.
48. Miura T, Shimada T, Tanaka K, Chujo M, Uchida Y. Lymphatic drainage of carbon particles injected into the pleural cavity of the monkey, as studied by video-assisted thoracoscopy and electron microscopy. *J Thorac Cardiovasc Surg* 2000; **120**: 437–47.
49. Li J. Ultrastructural study on the pleural stomata in human. *Funct Dev Morphol* 1993; **3**: 277–80.

50. Shinohara H. Distribution of lymphatic stomata on the pleural surface of the thoracic cavity and the surface topography of the pleural mesothelium in the golden hamster. *Anat Rec* 1997; **249**: 16–23.
51. Ohtani O, Ohtani Y, Li RX. Phylogeny and ontogeny of the lymphatic stomata connecting the pleural and peritoneal cavities with the lymphatic system – a review. *Ital J Anat Embryol* 2001; **106**: 251–9.
52. Nakatani T, Tanaka S, Mizukami S, *et al.* Peritoneal lymphatic stomata of the diaphragm in the mouse: process of their formation. *Anat Rec* 1997; **248**: 121–8.
53. Miura T, Shimada T, Tanaka K, Chujo M, Uchida Y. Lymphatic drainage of carbon particles injected into the pleural cavity of the monkey, as studied by video-assisted thoracoscopy and electron microscopy. *J Thorac Cardiovasc Surg* 2000; **120**: 437–47.
•54. Kihara T. Das extravasculare Saftbahn System. *Okazima Fol Anat Jpn* 1956; **28**: 601–21.
55. Oya M, Shimada T, Nakamura M, Uchida Y. Functional morphology of the lymphatic system in the monkey diaphragm. *Arch Histol Cytol* 1993; **56**: 37–47.
56. Li YY, Li JC. Ultrastructure and three-dimensional study of the lymphatic stomata in the costal pleura of the rabbit. *Microsc Res Tech* 2003; **62**: 240–6.
•57. Kampmeier OF. Concerning certain mesothelial thickenings and vascular plexus of the mediastinal pleura associated with histiocyte and fat cell production in the human newborn. *Anat Rec* 1928; **39**: 201–8.
58. Cooray GH. Defensive mechanisms in the mediastinum with special reference to the mechanics of pleural absorption. *J Pathol Bacteriol* 1949; 61: 551–67.
59. Lang J, Liebich HG. Uber eigenartige Kapillarkonvolute der Pleural parietalis. III. Elektronenmikroskopische Untersuchungen. *Z Mikrosk-Anat Forsch* 1976; **9**: 1092.
60. Burke HE, Wilson JA. A new method for establishing the diagnosis of pleural disease – parasternal lymph node biopsy. *Am Rev Respir Dis* 1966; **93**: 201–8.
♦61. Kanazawa K. Exchange through the pleura. Cells and particles. In: Chretien J, Bignon J, Hirsch A (eds). *The pleura in health and disease.* New York: Marcel Dekker; 1985: 195–231.
62. Wang NS. Scanning electron microscopy of the lung. In: Lenfant C, Schraunagel DE (eds). *Electron micsroscopy of the lung: lung biology in health and disease.* New York: Marcel Dekker; 1990: 517–55.
63. Boren HG. Alveolar fenestrae. Relationship to the pathology and pathogenesis of pulmonary emphysema. *Am Rev Respir Dis* 1962; **85**: 328–44.
64. Gaudio E, Rendina EA, Pannarale L, Ricci C, Marinozzi G. Surface morphology of the human pleura. A scanning electron microscopic study. *Chest* 1988; **93**: 149–53.
•65. Albertine KH, Wiener-Kronish JP, Staub NC. The structure of the parietal pleura and its relationship to pleural liquid dynamics in sheep. *Anat Rec* 1984; **208**: 401–9.
66. Negrini D, Del Fabbro M, Gonano C, Mukenge S, Miserocchi G. Distribution of diaphragmatic lymphatic lacunae. *J Appl Physiol* 1992; **72**: 1166–72.
67. Emerson PA, Davies JH. Hydrothorax complicating ascites. *Lancet* 1955; **268**: 487–8.
♦68. Alberts WM, Salem AJ, Solomon DA, Boyce G. Hepatic hydrothorax. Cause and management. *Arch Intern Med* 1991; **151**: 2383–8.
69. Nakamura A, Kojima Y, Ohmi H, Yamada J, Yamada Y. Peritoneal-pleural communications in hepatic hydrothorax demonstrated by thoracoscopy. *Chest* 1996; **109**: 579–81.
70. Nomoto Y, Suga T, Nakajima K, *et al.* Acute hydrothorax in continuous ambulatory peritoneal dialysis – a collaborative study of 161 centers. *Am J Nephrol* 1989; **9**: 363–7.
71. Whitaker D, Papadimitriou JM, Walters MN. The mesothelium: a histochemical study of resting mesothelial cells. *J Pathol* 1980; **132**: 273–84.
72. Hott JW, Sparks JA, Godbey SW, Antony VB. Mesothelial cell response to pleural injury: thrombin-induced proliferation and chemotaxis of rat pleural mesothelial cells. *Am J Respir Cell Mol Biol* 1992; **6**: 421–5.
73. Whitaker D, Papadimitriou JM, Walters MN. The mesothelium: a cytochemical study of 'activated' mesothelial cells. *J Pathol* 1982; **136**: 169–79.
74. Coene MC, Van Hove C, Claeys M, Herman AG. Arachidonic acid metabolism by cultured mesothelial cells. Different transformations of exogenously added and endogenously. *Biochim Biophys Acta* 1982; **710**: 437–45.
75. Whitaker D, Papadimitriou JM, Walters M. The mesothelium: its fibrinolytic properties. *J Pathol* 1982; **136**: 291–9.
♦76. Ryan GB, Grobety J, Majno G. Mesothelial injury and recovery. *Am J Pathol* 1973; **71**: 93–112.
77. Gabrielson EW, Gerwin BI, Harris CC, *et al.* Stimulation of DNA synthesis in cultured primary human mesothelial cells by specific growth factors. *FASEB J* 1988; **2**: 2717–21.
78. Adamson IY, Bakowska J, Bowden DH. Mesothelial cell proliferation: a nonspecific response to lung injury associated with fibrosis. *Am J Respir Cell Mol Biol* 1994; **10**: 253–8.
79. Adamson IY, Bakowska J, Bowden DH. Mesothelial cell proliferation after instillation of long or short asbestos fibers into mouse lung. *Am J Pathol* 1993; **142**: 1209–16.
80. Peng MJ, Wang NS, Vargas FS, Light RW. Subclinical surface alterations of human pleura. A scanning electron microscopic study. *Chest* 1994; **106**: 351–3.
81. Whitaker D, Papadimitriou J. Mesothelial healing: morphological and kinetic investigations. *J Pathol* 1985; **145**: 159–75.
82. Watters WB, Buck RC. Scanning electron microscopy of mesothelial regeneration in the rat. *Lab Invest* 1972; **26**: 604–9.
83. Davila RM, Crouch EC. Role of mesothelial and submesothelial stromal cells in matrix remodeling following pleural injury. *Am J Pathol* 1993; **142**: 547–55.
♦84. Kohda E, Suzuki K, Tanaka M, *et al.* [Radiological approach to the pleura and pleural cavity with CT and MRI]. *Nihon Kyobu Shikkan Gakkai Zasshi* 1994; **32**(Suppl): 148–54.

3

Mesothelial cells

MARIE-CLAUDE JAURAND, JOCELYNE FLEURY-FEITH

INTRODUCTION

Mesothelial cells form the monolayer mesothelium covering connective tissue over the basal lamina of the pleura. Morphological studies have shown that mesothelial cells may present different phenotypes, likely dependent on the various functions of the serosa that may differ between parietal, visceral and mediastinal pleura. Mesothelial cells also play a role in the maintenance of pleural homeostasis in response to stimuli (mechanical injury, inflammation). Mesothelial cells have secretary functions and can synthesize glycosaminoglycans and surfactant, providing lubrication between parietal and visceral pleura.[1] The main pleural pathologies are inflammatory processes (tuberculosis, other bacterial and viral infections) and cancers (e.g. mesothelioma). The aim of the chapter is to summarize our present knowledge on the morphology and biology of pleural mesothelial cells, focusing on functions and pathophysiological pathways involved in pleural diseases.

MESOTHELIAL CELL MORPHOLOGY

Mesothelial cells *in situ*

The pleural mesothelium consists of a single-layer epithelial sheet over a basal lamina, supported by the submesothelial connective tissue, covering the surfaces encompassing the pleural space (Figure 3.1a).[2] *In situ*, the apical surface of mesothelial cells is oriented in the pleural space, which is filled with a small volume of pleural fluid. According to Noppen *et al.*,[3] the volume of pleural fluid is 0.26 ± 0.1 mL/kg in human subjects and contains approximately 1.7×10^3 cells/mL, comprising approximately 75 percent macrophages, 23 percent lymphocytes, less than 3 percent polymorphonuclear cells and approximately 2 percent free mesothelial cells. (See also Chapter 4 for further discussions on normal physiological pleural fluid and its contents.)

Scanning electron microscopy (SEM) and transmission electron microscopy (TEM) studies have provided information on the structure and ultrastructure of mesothelial cells in different areas of the pleura. The apical surface shows heterogeneous morphology from long, randomly oriented microvilli to smoother surface with relatively few microvilli (Figure 3.1b). The diameter of the microvilli is approximately 0.1 μm and their lengths vary from 3 to 6 μm. According to Michailova and Usunoff,[1] microvilli in the rat are 0.05–0.08 μm in diameter and from 0.5 to 3.5–4.0 μm in length. The density of the microvilli is high (200–600 per 100 μm^2). Regional variations of the distribution of the microvilli have been reported: they are more numerous on the caudal than on the cranial portions of the pleura and are more numerous on the visceral than on the parietal pleura.[1,4] At the apical surface of mesothelial cells, a glycocalyx is interconnected with the microvilli.[5]

At least three functions are generally assigned to the microvilli: (i) they facilitate fluid absorption by increasing the exchange surface area in contact with the pleural fluid; (ii) together with the glycocalyx, they reduce the mechanical resistance to movement; (iii) by the adsorption of phospholipids at their apical part, they act to lubricate sites where liquid is absent or poor.[5,6] Singly, isolated cilia may be observed on both parietal and visceral mesothelial cells.

Mesothelial cell types can be divided into flat (squamous cells), cubic (cuboidal, high cells), as well as numerous intermediate cell forms. In adult Wistar rats, cubic cells cover the basal part of the lung; their mean apical surface is 13.0–37.6 μm^2, and that of flat cells is 43.2–182.7 μm^2.[1] Microvilli on cubic cells are more numerous

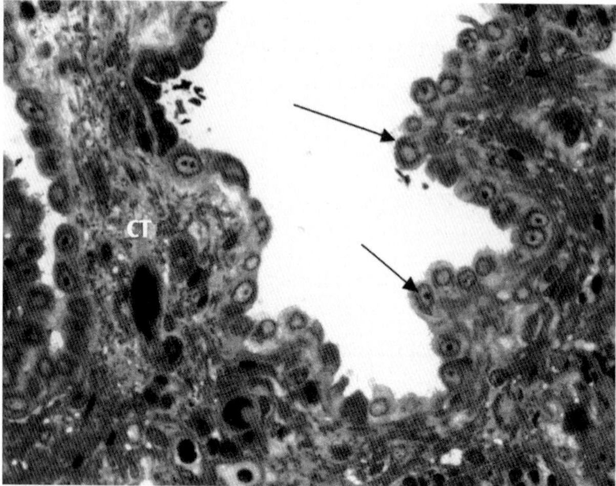

(a)

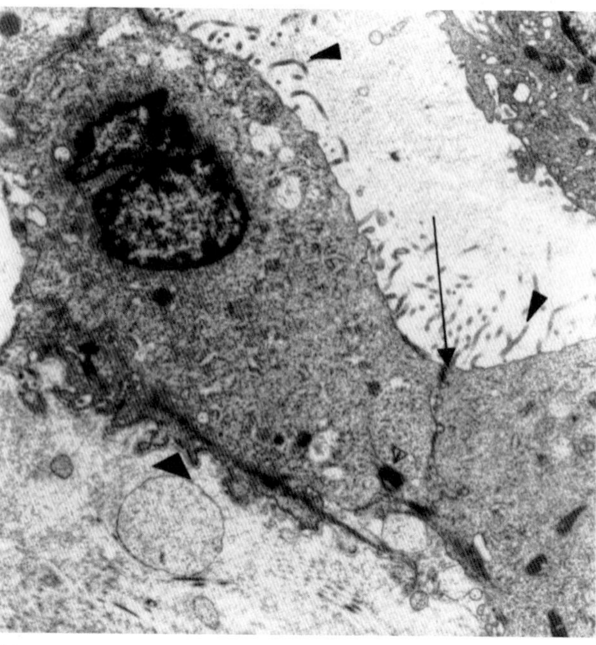

(b)

Figure 3.1 Mesothelial cells *in situ*. (a) Light micrograph of mesothelium: →, mesothelial cells (CT = submesothelial connective tissue, ×312). (b) Transmission electron microscopy: ►, microvilli; →, junctions; ▸, basal lamina (×3120).

and longer than those on the flat cells, which have few and short microvilli.[1] Cubic cells are located at the visceral mesothelial layer of the lung and the heart. Flat mesothelial cells are more numerous than cubic cells, and form the parietal sheet of the pleura and pericardium.

By TEM, cubic mesothelial cells have a large, rounded or ovoid nucleus with multiple and deep indentations, generally in the centre of the cell.[1] Organelles are well developed and form clusters or are perinuclearly and homogeneously distributed.[1] Cytoplasm of cubic mesothelial cells may be electron-dense or electron-lucent. Golgi apparatus is well developed. Flat mesothelial cells appear as elongated cells with a fusiform-like nucleus with single invagination, surrounded by a scant cytoplasm.[1]

The cytoplasm of mesothelial cells contains scattered microtubules, dispersed microfilaments and bundled intermediate filaments forming an extensive network consisting of actin, vimentin and mesothelial cytokeratins, particularly low molecular weight cytokeratins (CK5 and CK6). There are numerous plasmalemmal vesicles (60–70 nm diameter) throughout the cytoplasm; they are related to fluid-phase transport, permeability and absorption. Their presence suggests intense pinocytic and intracellular trafficking activity of mesothelial cells. Recently, in rat pleura, Von Ruhland *et al.*[7] demonstrated the presence of caveolae by immunostaining of caveolin-1, a protein located in some of this type of vesicles. These authors confirmed previous observations that the density of vesicular structures varies according to the mesothelial cell location. Visceral pleura contains higher numbers of caveolae than parietal pleura.[7,8] In rats, such vesicles are also abundant in the parietal pericardia and in the diaphragm.[7] Small membrane-bound vesicles, 20–25 mm in diameter, are mainly associated with the apical surface.[1]

Mesothelial cell interconnections consist of tight, adherens junctions (zonula adherens also called belt junctions, and desmosomes) and gap junctions (Figure 3.1b). The tight junctions, localized at the apical part of the mesothelial cells, separate the apical from the basolateral part of the cell.[9] Freeze-fracture studies in mice and intrapleural injection of peroxidase in the rat pleural space suggest that tight junctions are a constant feature in the visceral pleura but not in the parietal pleura.[2,10] Adherens junctions are less consistent and located at the basolateral part of the intercellular space; desmosomes are located at the more basal part of the cell.[9] Zonula adherens contain E-, P- and N-cadherins attached to actin microfilaments by catenins. These junctions play an important role to maintain cell-to-cell adhesion, cell form and permeability. Basal lamina is seen immediately below the mesothelial cells; its components are synthesized and secreted by the mesothelial cell and includes type IV collagen, fibronectin, laminin etc.[11]

In 1863, Recklinghausen demonstrated for the first time the existence of openings between the mesothelial cells and their connection with the lymphatic system.[1] Electron microscopy studies have confirmed the presence of pores between mesothelial cells, which communicate with the origin of lymphatics.[9] These stomas have been described specifically in the parietal and diaphragmatic pleura, but to date they have not been observed on the visceral pleura in any animals studied.

Malignant mesothelial cells

Malignant mesothelioma (MM) is the primary tumor arising from the neoplastic transformation of mesothelial cells. The major subtypes of MM are the epithelioid, sarcomatoid and biphasic forms,[12] which are also referred to as epithelial, sarcomatous, or mixed subtypes, respectively. These different features reflect the plasticity of mesothelial cells. In humans, epithelial subtype is predominant (approximately 55 percent) followed by sarcomatous (approximately 22 percent) and mixed (approximately 24 percent).[13] The typical light microscopy appearance of epithelioid mesothelioma is ill-defined tubular, papillary and loose solid nests of epithelial cells. The well-differentiated mesothelioma cells have similar phenotypes to normal cells, exhibiting cubic, polygonal, or flattened morphologies.[14,15]

The ultrastructural features of mesothelioma cells are characterized in the epithelia form by the presence of brush-like elongated, slender and branching microvilli (Figure 3.2).[16,17] The microvilli have a length to width ratio of approximately 12 within the range of that of normal cells.[18] Microvilli are found on the luminal surface, in the intercellular space, and also on the abluminal surface where, if abundant enough, they can disrupt the basal lamina.[19] Mesothelial characteristics of abundant cytoplasmic perinuclear intermediate filaments, multiple junctions including desmosomes, are found in epithelial malignant mesothelial cells. In the sarcomatous cells, these features are less typical or absent. Nevertheless, microvilli and desmosomes may be occasionally found by TEM analysis.

Immunohistochemical analysis of MM have demonstrated the presence of antigens usually present in normal mesothelial cells. Coexpression of cytokeratins and vimentin is characteristic of MM cells. Other membrane proteins – mesothelin, ME1 and HBME1 – are also present on these cells.

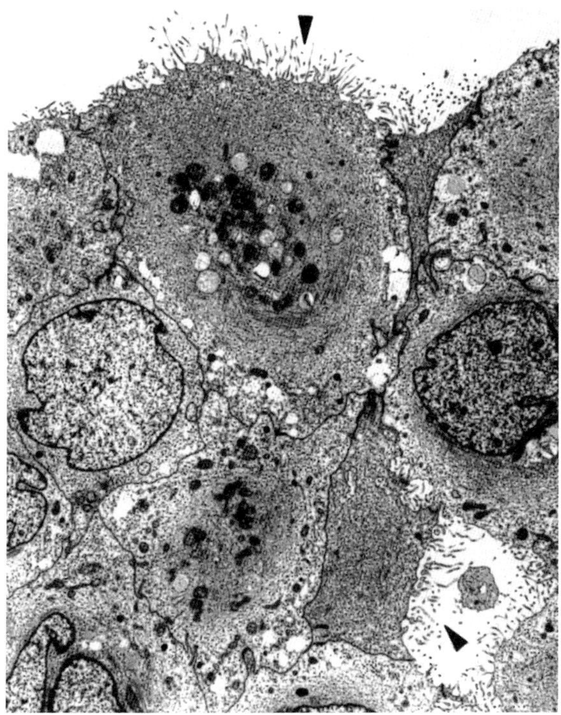

Figure 3.2 Transmission electron micrograph of human malignant mesothelial cells in culture. Mesothelial differentiation is demonstrated particularly by the occurrence of typical microvilli (▶) (×3276).

Mesothelial cells in culture

Pleural mesothelial cells have been successfully explanted and cultured. Early studies using imprint technique have permitted identification of some of the proteins expressed by mesothelial cells.[20] Rodent mesothelial cells can proliferate in culture and showed an ability to phagocytose asbestos fibres.[21] In culture, mesothelial cells form a monolayer with cobblestone morphology. *In vitro*, mesothelial cells maintain their morphological characteristics, i.e. presence of microvilli, perinuclear bundles of intermediate filaments and desmosomes.[22] Cell dedifferentiation occurs following a large number of population doublings. In rats, after approximately 40 passages (approximately 100 doublings), phenotypical changes appear in the culture layer, as foci of cells with looser contacts and loss of contact inhibition. However, these changes are not associated with the acquisition of tumorigenic potency, as assessed by inoculation in nude mice.[23]

More sophisticated culture medium, supplemented with transferrin, insulin and growth factors, has been made to grow human pleural mesothelial cells from noncancerous pleural fluids.[24] These systems of cultured mesothelial cells have helped researchers to explore the biological and physiological features of mesothelial cells, especially their participation in inflammatory processes and responses to asbestos fiber exposure. Long-term cultures for periods up to 5–6 months can be obtained by transfection of human normal pleural mesothelial cells with a plasmid containing the coding sequence of the simian virus (SV40) early region DNA.[25] These cells were not tumorigenic when injected subcutaneously in nude mice, even after a delay of 1 year.[25] One cell line (Met 5A) generated in this study is frequently used as a surrogate of normal pleural mesothelial cells.

Similarly, MM cells from tumors have been grown in culture. All mesothelioma cell lines showed strong immunoreactivity to anti-cytokeratin and -vimentin antibodies, and did not express carcinoembryonic antigen, factor VIII or Leu-M1 (Figure 3.3). Cultured cells of epithelial and sarcomatous morphological phenotypes both co-expressed cytokeratins and vimentin.[26] Ultrastructural features of mesothelioma cells in culture show a variety of differentiation status. While some cell lines exhibited well-differentiated microvilli, abundant perinuclear bundles of intermediate filaments and typical junctions, less differentiated cell lines were also found. These differences may be related to the original location of the mesothelial cells in the pleural space or to culture conditions. Interestingly, when injected subcutaneously in nude mice, some cell lines demonstrated higher differentiation

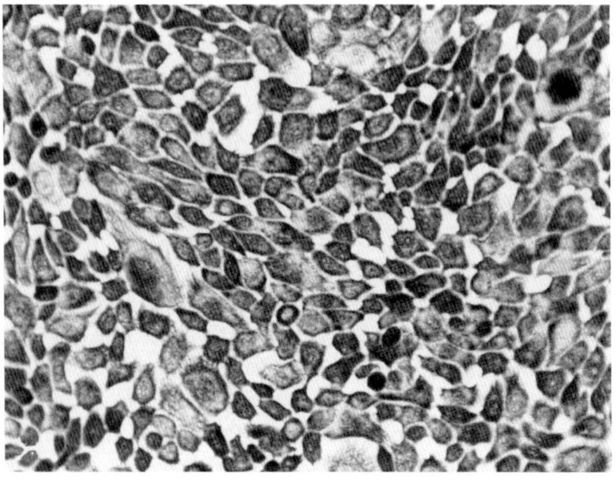

(a)

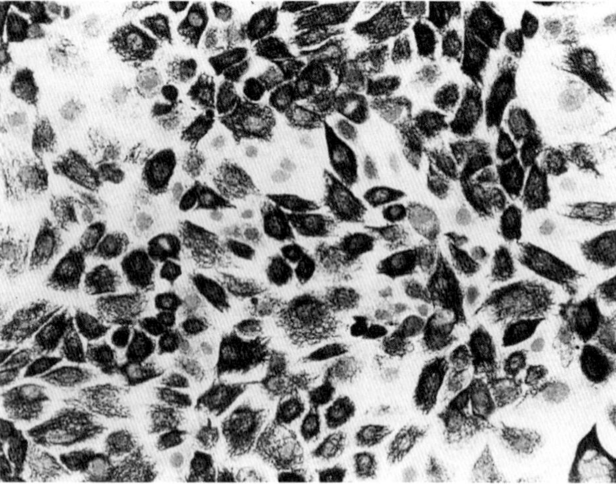

(b)

Figure 3.3 Immunocytochemistry of a human malignant mesothelioma cell line performed with cytokeratin (a) and vimentin (b) antibodies, showing positive cells with both antibodies (×268).

features than in tissue culture conditions, suggesting that the stromal or biochemical environment play a role in the modulation of morphological phenotype.[27]

REGULATION OF MESOTHELIAL CELL PROLIFERATION

Mesothelial cell turnover and mesothelium regeneration

The regeneration rate of normal mesothelial cells is slow. Mitotic figures of mesothelial cells are infrequent in the normal pleura. The percentage of cells undergoing mitosis at one time has been estimated to be 1 percent or less.[28,29] In rats, the estimated lifespan of mesothelial cells is 33 days.[30]

The cellular source involved in the regeneration of normal or damaged mesothelium is controversial. Mechanisms of mesothelium regeneration have been studied after chemical or mechanical abrasion of mesothelial surface, or after heat injury. It must be noted that mesothelium regeneration studies were mostly carried out on peritoneal serosa. While pleural and peritoneal serosa may have some differences, their overall pathological features are very similar. Several mechanisms have been proposed to explain mesothelium regeneration, including centripetal migration of mesothelial cells at the border of the damaged area, exfoliation of mature or proliferating mesothelial cells located at more or less distant sites, attachment of pre-existing free-floating serosal reserve cells, transformation of serosal macrophages, migration of submesothelial mesenchymal precursors, or implantation of bone marrow-derived circulating precursors.[31] From the different studies it was proposed that mesothelium regeneration requires the recruitment of inflammatory cells attracted by the release of inflammatory mediators at the damaged surface. Stimulation of mesothelial cell proliferation would permit both detachment and migration of mesothelial cells to reconstitute an intact mesothelial monolayer.[31] This mechanism differs from others suggested in that mesothelium regeneration originates from multipotent cells present in the submesothelial tissue.[32,33] This latter hypothesis was based on the presence of cytokeratin positive cells in the submesothelial compartment from injured serosa, contrasting with cytokeratin negative and vimentin positive cells in the normal serosa. This question of variability of mesothelial cell characteristics is complex, as mesothelial cells themselves can change their phenotype and undergo epithelial-mesenchymal transition. The process of epithelial–mesenchymal transition is demonstrated by both morphological changes and differential expression of cytokeratin and vimentin. A reversible morphological change from an epithelial to fusiform shape is expressed by mesothelial cells exposed to epidermal growth factor (EGF).[34,35] Moreover, cytokeratin content has been found to be regulated in culture, at least in peritoneal mesothelial cells. Connell and Rheinwald[36] reported changes in levels of cytokeratin and vimentin expression during *in vitro* growth of normal mesothelial cells obtained from an ovarian ascitis; cytokeratin expression was decreased during growth, and returned to high levels whenever growth slowed, while vimentin synthesis decreased in non-dividing cells.

The question of the existence of mesothelial progenitor cells is of great interest, and is presently debated. It has been suggested that mesothelial cells could be multipotent cells. This hypothesis is based on the mesothelial cells' ability to exhibit epithelial and mesenchymal phenotype, while retaining the properties of embryonic mesoderma.[37] The different studies on this subject have been recently summarized.[38] These authors report that epithelial mesothelial cells may convert into mesenchymal cells to repair serosal damage or during wound healing. So far, it is unknown which subtypes of mesothelial cells would be candidates, or whether mesothelial stem cells exist. Nevertheless, it remains that epithelial mesothelial cells have the capability to transdifferentiate from an epithelial to mesenchymal phenotype. This potential is illustrated in repair processes and in tumorigenesis, as it is not rare to observe not only sarcomatous differentiation, but also osseous and cartilaginous differentiation in human MM.[38] Murine models of MM also exhibit these differential features.[39]

Growth factors regulating cell growth

Proliferation of pleural mesothelial cells has been found to be modulated by several growth factors, including fibroblast growth factor (FGF), hepatocyte growth factor (HGF), keratinocyte growth factor (KGF), platelet-derived growth factor (PDGF) and vascular endothelial growth factor (VEGF). Productions of, and response to growth factors, have been investigated in the context of inflammatory processes following pleural injury, especially to explain the mechanism of pleural fibrosis. During the inflammatory process, macrophages release several factors such as hyaluronic acid, interleukin (IL)-1β, tumor necrosis factor (TNF)-α and interferon (IFN)-γ, which in turn may stimulate mesothelial cells to produce cytokines, chemokines and growth factors. EGF, basic FGF (bFGF) and PDGF have been shown to stimulate mesothelial cell proliferation *in vivo* and *in vitro*.[24,40–43] Cytokines such as TNF-α, transforming growth factor (TGF)-β and IL-1 stimulate mesothelial cells to produce growth factors.[31] TGF-β exerts inhibitory effect on normal pleural mesothelial (NPM) cell proliferation (Figure 3.4).[44]

Normal mesothelial cells from different individual donors have differential responses to growth factors, e.g. EGF.[24,42] Normal human mesothelial cells express low levels of mRNA of PDGF-A chain and the mRNA for PDGF-β was not detectable.[40] Messenger RNA transcripts for insulin-like growth factor (IGF)-I and its receptor, IGF-I receptor, were also expressed.[45] IGF-I appears to function as an autocrine growth stimulus in human mesothelial cells. IL-6 is another auto-regulatory factor in human mesothelial cell proliferation. A complete autocrine loop was demonstrated by the expression of IL-6 mRNA transcripts and IL-6 receptor subunits.[46] Platelet-derived growth factor-BB- or TGF-β1-stimulated normal human mesothelial cells express hyaluronan synthase and hyaluronan, an important constituent of the extracellular matrix.[47,48] Hyaluronan does not appear to be involved in proliferation of normal mesothelial cells since

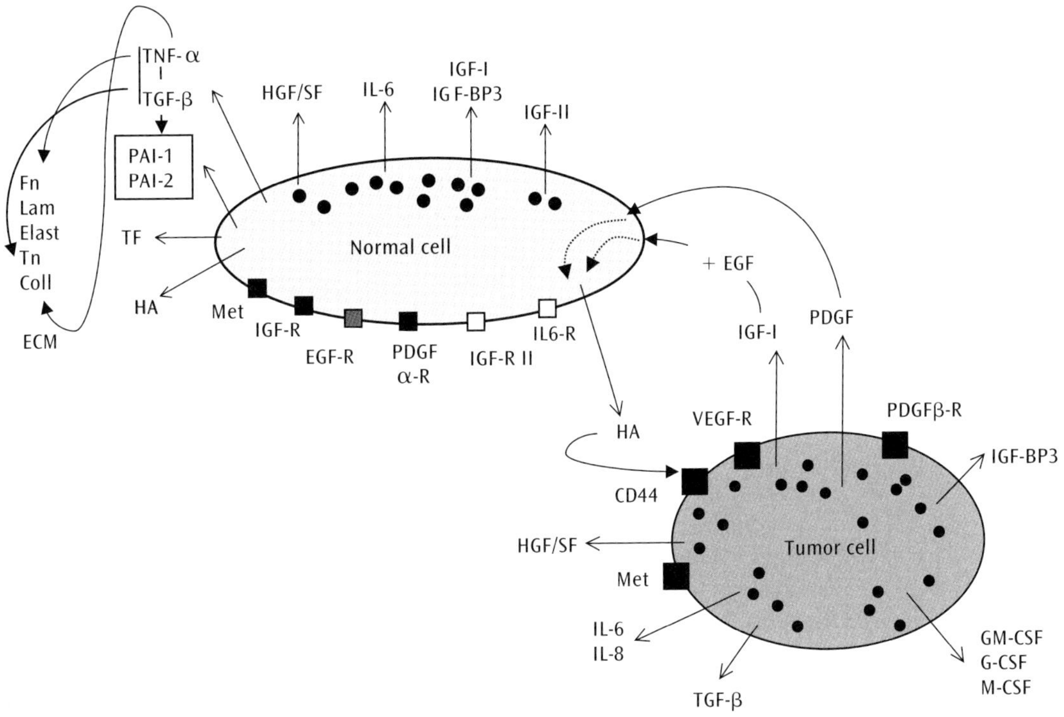

Figure 3.4 Schematic representation of the factors produce by mesothelial cells and receptors (human, ■; rat, □; both species, ▒) present in normal and malignant mesothelial cells. See text for details. Thin arrows indicate modulation of the expression of one factor (→) by another one (•). Coll, collagen; ECM, extracellular matrix; EGF, epidermal growth factor; EGF-R, epidermal growth factor receptor; Elast, elastin; Fn, fibronectin; G-, M- and GM-CSF, granulocyte-, macrophage- and granulocyte/macrophage colony stimulating factors, respectively; HA, hyaluronan; HGF/SF, hepatocyte growth factor/scattering factor; IGF-I, insulin-like growth factor receptor; IL-6, interleukin 6; IL-8, interleukin 8; Lam, laminine; PAI, plasminogen activator inhibitor; PDGF, platelet-derived growth factor; PDGF-R, platelet-derived growth factor receptor; TF, tissue factor; TGF-β, transforming growth factor β; Tn, tenascin; TNF-α, tumor necrosis factor α; VEGF-R, vascular endothelial growth factor receptor.

they do not express the hyaluronan receptor CD44.[49] Production of VEGF and its receptors is another feature of human mesothelial cells.[50,51] In contrast, no expression of scattering factor HGF/(SF) and the c-met receptor were detected in normal mesothelial cells.[52]

Normal mesothelial cells from the rat possess EGF receptors but the effect of EGF appears to depend on culture conditions, as proliferation is inhibited in serum free medium.[35] Like human cells, rat mesothelial cells produce IGF-I and IGF-II and autocrine growth stimulation by IGF-II has been suggested.[53] Other growth factors, PDGF, HGF and KGF, have also been demonstrated to stimulate the proliferation of rat mesothelial cells.[54,55]

Thus, normal pleural mesothelial cells have the capability to produce different growth factors which may in turn induce environment-dependent biological responses from the mesothelial cells. The mesothelial cells are also able to produce and respond to various inflammatory factors. These functions confirm that mesothelial cells play a crucial role in the maintenance of the pleural integrity.

To date, the mechanisms whereby mesothelial cells survive, or are committed to apoptosis, remain unknown. Recent data suggested a list of inhibitors of apoptosis expressed in a primary human mesothelial cell line.[56] Gene and protein analyses revealed inhibitors of apoptosis (IAPs), including IAP-1, IAP-2, XIAP, survivin and livin. Immunohistochemistry and Western blot analysis have demonstrated the production of IAP-1, IAP-2 and XIAP.[56]

Growth regulation in MM cells

Malignant mesothelioma cell growth may be linked to autocrine or paracrine stimulation. Platelet-derived growth factor has been suggested as a regulatory factor for proliferation of MM cells, either directly or indirectly via the hyaluronan/CD44 pathway.

Human MM cells express high level of PDGF-A and PDGF-B, as well as PDGF-β receptor.[40,57,58] Growth regulation in MM cells appears to be complex. Autocrine proliferation could occur via binding of homodimer of PDGF-B chains.[59] This process can occur in human MM cells.[44,57] PDGF-A-stimulated autocrine loop does not seem to play a positive role in mesothelioma proliferation *in vitro*. Nude mice injected with MM cells that over-express PDGF-A showed increased tumor incidence and reduced latency period to tumor formation.[60] These data suggest that PDGF-A could contribute to tumor formation via a paracrine mechanism to generate favorable environmental conditions, e.g. by stimulating angiogenesis, for tumor proliferation.[60] These processes would not seem to apply to rats, as neither PDFG-A nor PDGF-B chains were found to be expressed in asbestos-transformed rat peritoneal mesothelioma.[61] Alternatively, human MM cell growth could be the consequence of hyaluronan production and activation of hyaluronan synthase by PDGF, via interaction with the hyaluronan transmembrane receptor, CD44.[47,48]

Human MM cells produce mRNA transcripts for IGF-I, IGF-binding protein 3 and of IGF-I receptor; the expressions of IGF-I and IGF-binding protein 3 at a protein level have also been confirmed.[45] IGF-I appears to be an important regulator of MM cell growth (Figure 3.4).

The HGF/SF and c-Met pathway could be involved in an autocrine fashion in the control of MM cell proliferation. Several studies have demonstrated the expression of HGF/SF and c-Met in MM cell lines, and in paraffin sections.[52,62–67] Nevertheless, expression of HGF/SF could be limited to spindle-shaped cells.[63] In addition to the cell growth regulation, HGF/SF exerts stimulatory effect on the motility, spreading and proliferation of MM cells and stimulated the expression of matrix metalloproteinases.[52,63,65]

Vascular endothelial growth factor plays a role in the growth of mesothelioma. MM cells express both VEGF and VEGF receptors [fms-like tyrosine kinase (Flt-1) or fetal liver kinase (Flk-1)], and their expression appears to be enhanced in MM cells when compared with benign cells.[51] An autocrine role of VEGF has been suggested, using neutralizing antibodies against VEGF or the VEGF receptors Flt-1 and Flk-1.[50]

Malignant mesothelioma cells are resistant to apoptosis, but the mechanism remains to be elucidated. The anti-apoptotic factor, Bcl-x, seems to play a role in this resistance.[68–70] In MM cells, survival could be promoted by an activation of the AKT/PKB pathway.[71]

PHYSIOPATHOLOGY OF MESOTHELIAL CELLS

The mesothelium exerts physiological function as a barrier for exchange of ions and small molecules, and reacts to produce inflammatory molecules against several sorts of stimuli. Mesothelial cells secrete immunomodulatory, procoagulant and fibrinolytic molecules. Mesothelial cells have been shown to phagocytose foreign substances such as bacteria, mineral particles as asbestos fibers, and quartz or latex beads.[72] These multiple functions make the mesothelial cell crucial in maintaining pleural integrity.

The mesothelial cells in the inflammatory process

In response to pleural injury, or in the presence of foreign substances, mesothelial cells initiate pleural inflammation by the release of inflammatory factors. Production of chemokines induces the attraction of macrophages and leukocytes from the vascular compartment. Activated macrophages release mediators that stimulate mesothelial cells to release various cytokines and growth factors (see also Chapter 8, Immunology).

Migration of leukocytes from the systemic circulation to the pleura is facilitated by the expression of integrins and adhesion molecules such as intercellular adhesion molecule (ICAM)-1, vascular adhesion molecule

(VCAM)-1, E-cadherin and several types of selectins.[29,73] Release of growth factors TGF-β, b-FGF, PDGF and EGF stimulate cell proliferation and mesothelium regeneration. TGF-β is a multifunctional cytokine that may act as a chemotactic factor for lung fibroblasts that play a role in the synthesis of collagen and the development of fibrotic processes, and TGF-β2 and -β3 have been shown to upregulate mesothelial cell collagen expression.[74,75] TGF-β enhances pleural fluid formation in part by inducing the production of VEGF; it stimulates mesothelial cells to synthesize extracellular matrix components as well as to produce matrix metalloproteinases and inhibitors of metalloproteinases.[44,75] Pleural mesothelial cells may be activated to release inflammatory cytokines *in vitro* and to induce neutrophil recruitment *in vivo* by the stimulation of proteinase-activated receptor-2, a novel seven-transmembrane receptor with immunomodulatory roles.[76]

Transforming growth factor β also regulates the coagulation process, suppressing fibrinolysis by reduction of plasminogen activator production and stimulation of mesothelial cells to secrete plasminogen activator inhibitors. In addition, TGF-β can also induce angiogenesis via synthesis of VEGF by mesothelial cells.[51] VEGF is a key mediator in pleural effusion formation.[77]

Platelet-derived growth factor is a growth factor for fibroblasts and, as mentioned above, PDGF is mitogenic for mesothelial cells. Basic FGF has been shown to stimulate growth of both fibroblasts and mesothelial cells.

Mesothelial cells play an important role in the regulation of fibrin deposition in the pleura. Normal pleural mesothelial cells exhibit procoagulant activity due to their ability to release tissue factor, which initiates the coagulation cascade and the deposition of transitional fibrin. This process is facilitated by the production of plasminogen activator inhibitors (PAI), PAI-1 and PAI-2.[73,78] Mesothelial cells also secrete components of the fibrinolysis system. Fibrinolytic activity is mediated by tissue plasminogen activator (tPA) and urokinase PA (uPA) that activates plasminogen into plasmin, which degrades fibrin. Mesothelial cells are the main source of tPA in serosal cavities but also secretes lower levels of uPA.[29] (See also Chapter 9, Pleural fibrosis, for details on fibrinolytic pathways in the pleura.)

Phagocytosis

Mesothelial cells have been shown to phagocytose mineral particles such as asbestos fibers, talc and quartz, as well as glass microbeads.[72] It has been demonstrated that asbestos fibres can be translocated from the lung to the pleura; hence mesothelial cells can interact directly with fibers and respond to circulating mediators.[79–81] (See also Chapter 10, Pleural reaction to mineral dusts.) The response of mesothelial cells has been largely studied in the context of fibrogenic and carcinogenic potency of the fibers. Internalization of asbestos fibers by rat mesothelial cells results in a lysosomal degranulation in the phagocytic vacuole.[21] Human mesothelial cells also ingest asbestos fibers.[82,83] Fiber uptake is facilitated by the fiber coating with vitronectin, a serum component interacting with integrin receptors present in the mesothelial cell membrane.[84] Several forms of integrins, alpha2, alpha3, alpha 5, beta1, beta3 and alpha vbeta3, have been found to be highly expressed in cultures of primary pleural mesothelial cells.[85] In culture, the interaction between mesothelial cells and asbestos fibers results in the adaptation to oxidative stress, activation of signalling pathways and the release of cytokine and growth factor mediators already mentioned. Reactive oxygen species (ROS) and reactive nitrogen species (RNS) are generated in cells exposed to asbestos.[86] Activation of signaling pathways involved the activation of transcription factors, such as nuclear factor (NF)-κB and AP-1, that control expression of other genes, including those governing cell survival.[87] In serum-free conditions, EGF receptor appears to be activated by asbestos fibers, leading to signaling via the extracellular signal-regulated kinase (ERK) mitogen activated protein (MAP) kinase pathway.[87] In addition to production of ROS and RNS, cytokines and chemotactic factors are also expressed on mesothelial cells exposed to asbestos.[88–90]

Exposure of mesothelial cells to asbestos fibers results in cell injury that may be responsible for the carcinogenicity of the fibers. Fiber internalization can impair the progression of mitosis, as demonstrated by the formation of micronuclei, bi- and multi-nucleated mesothelial cells, induction of anaphase/telophase abnormalities and alteration of cytokinesis.[91,92] DNA damage, resulting from the production of ROS, has been demonstrated using methods allowing the detection of base oxidation and DNA breakage.[92,93] Indirectly, DNA damage has been demonstrated by the occurrence of DNA repair processes and activation of cell cycle control checkpoints.[92,94,95] Liu *et al.*[96] have reported that selective decrease in fiber uptake reduced the adverse effects of asbestos, including DNA strand breakage. These results indicate that the phagocytosis function of mesothelial cells is important and may contribute to the asbestos-induced fibrogenesis and cancer development in the pleura. (The molecular genetics of mesothelioma are also discussed in Chapter 11.)

Talc is a mineral used to induce pleurodesis in patients with malignant pleural effusions; its introduction in the pleural cavity produces pleural symphysis. Mesothelial cells stimulated with talc were found to release higher amount of b-FGF than untreated cells, in agreement with the fibrogenic process described above.[97] Use of talc pleurodesis remains controversial as it prevents further use of intrapleural therapy, a strategy that may be of interest for treatment of MM. (The clinical management of mesothelioma is detailed in Chapter 41, Malignant mesothelioma.)

Somatic genetic changes in malignant mesothelioma cells

Cytogenetic and loss of heterozygozity analysis of MM cells have shown the occurrence of multiple abnormalities and frequent deletions (see also Chapter 11, Genetics of malignant mesothelioma). Numerical and structural chromosome changes are shown in chromosomes 1, 3, 4, 6, 9, 13, 15 and 22.[98,99] These cytogenetic abnormalities could affect various initiation/progression steps of neoplastic progression. Candidate tumor suppressor genes in MM include *P16/CDKN2A*, *P14/ARF* and *P15/CDKN2B*, located at the *INK4* locus on chromosome 9, a frequently deleted region. In contrast, the *TP53* tumour suppressor gene is not frequently mutated.[100–102]

Malignant transformation of mesothelial cell is associated with abolishment of the G1 to S regulation of transition which may play a role in the genetic instability found in cancer cells. Nevertheless, MM cells appear to maintain the ability to control DNA damage, as the p53 protein remains wild type in most cases.

NF2 is another candidate tumor suppressor gene whose alterations have been found in approximately 50 percent of mesotheliomas.[103–105] This gene product helps link proteins from the cytoskeleton to membrane proteins. It plays a role in the stabilization of adherens junctions. So far, the role of the *NF2* protein in the physiology of mesothelial cells is unknown but it may hold specific pathophysiological functions.

The exact steps involved in the neoplastic transformation of mesothelial cells are unknown. However, inactivation of the tumor suppressor genes *P16/CDKN2A* and *P15/CDKN2B* has been proposed as an early event, followed by an inactivation of *NF2*, followed by other genes located on chromosomes 11, 6 and 3.[99] Accordingly, in a model of murine MM, we found that *NF2* does not appear to play a role in the initial steps of neoplastic progression.[106]

Hypotheses on the mechanism of mesothelial oncogenesis, especially in response to asbestos fibers, can be tested with experimental mesotheliomas in knockout mice. (Experimental models for mesothelioma are further discussed in Chapter 15.) Development of tumor models is a useful means to identify key genes related to specific oncogenic processes. MM models have been obtained by intraperitoneal inoculation of asbestos fibers or ceramic fibers in hemizygous $NF2^{+/-}$ mice.[39,106–108] Somatic genetic alterations were similar to those observed in human MM: frequent deletions of the orthologous genes at the *Ink4* locus, as well as a lower frequency of *Trp53* mutations, were detected. Further studies are needed to define the nature of other somatic genetic changes in murine fiber-induced MM, and provide data to better define the characteristics of this type of tumor.

CONCLUSIONS

A better knowledge of the biology of mesothelial cells is needed to improve our ability to treat pleural diseases. Further research should focus on the multipotent properties of mesothelial cells and better define the pathways regulating inflammatory responses, survival and apoptosis in normal mesothelial cells. Determination of the somatic genetic mutations in MM cells, and understanding the pathophysiology of alterations of cell regulation pathways, may explain how mesothelial cells acquire a neoplastic phenotype, and thereby allow better prevention and treatment of pleural diseases.

KEY POINTS

- The pleural mesothelium consists of a single-layer epithelial sheet over a basal lamina, supported by the submesothelial connective tissue. The apical surface of mesothelial cells shows heterogeneity from numerous randomly-oriented long microvilli to relatively few microvilli. The cytoplasm of mesothelial cells contains scattered microtubules, dispersed microfilaments and bundled intermediate filaments. Numerous plasmalemmal vesicles suggest intense pinocytic and intracellular trafficking activity of mesothelial cells.
- The mesothelium acts as a barrier for exchange of ions and small molecules. Mesothelial cells can secrete immunomodulatory molecules, procoagulants and fibrinolytic mediators. Mesothelial cells can phagocytose foreign particles. These multiple functions make the mesothelial cell crucial in maintaining pleural integrity.
- The cellular source involved in the regeneration of normal or damaged mesothelium is controversial. Mechanisms of mesothelium regeneration include centripetal migration of mesothelial cells at the border of the damaged area, and/or attachment of exfoliated mesothelial cells or precursor cells. It has been suggested that mesothelial cells could be multipotent cells.
- Multiple cytogenetic alterations, loss of heterozygozity and frequent deletions are common features in malignant mesothelioma cells. Exposure of mesothelial cells to asbestos fibers results in cell injury that may be responsible for the carcinogenicity of the fibers.
- Development of animal models of mesothelioma help identify key genes related to the underlying oncogenic processes. Somatic genetic alterations in malignant mesotheliomas obtained by intraperitoneal inoculation of asbestos or ceramic fibers in hemizygous $NF2^{+/-}$ mice were similar to those observed in human malignant mesothelioma.

REFERENCES

● = Key primary paper
◆ = Major review article

◆1. Michailova KN, Usunoff KG. Serosal membranes (pleura, pericardium, peritoneum). Normal structure, development and experimental pathology. *Adv Anat Embryol Cell Biol* 2006; **183**: 1-144.
◆2. Wang NS. Mesothelial cells *in situ*. In: Chrétien JB, Bignon J, Hirsch A (eds). *The pleura in health and disease*. New York: Marcell Dekker, 1985: 23-42.
●3. Noppen M, de Waele M, Li R, *et al*. Volume and cellular content of normal pleural fluid in humans examined by pleural lavage. *Am J Respir Crit Care Med* 2000; **162**: 1023-6.
●4. Wang NS. The preformed stomas connecting the pleural cavity and the lymphatics in the parietal pleura. *Am Rev Respir Dis* 1975; **111**: 12-20.
5. Andrews PM, Porter KR. The ultrastructural morphology and possible functional significance of mesothelial microvilli. *Anat Rec* 1973; **177**: 409-26.
◆6. Zocchi L. Physiology and pathophysiology of pleural fluid turnover. *Eur Respir J* 2002; **20**: 1545-58.
7. von Ruhland CJ, Campbell L, Gumbleton M, *et al*. Immunolocalization of caveolin-1 in rat and human mesothelium. *J Histochem Cytochem* 2004; **52**: 1415-25.
8. Wang NS. The regional difference of pleural mesothelial cells in rabbits. *Am Rev Respir Dis* 1974; **110**: 623-33.
9. Peng M, Wang NS. Embryology and gross structure. In: Light RW, Lee YCG (eds). *Textbook of pleural diseases*. London: Arnold; 2003: 3-16.
●10. Pinchon MC, Bernaudin JF, Bignon J. Pleural permeability in the rat. II. Ultrastructural basis. *Biol Cell* 1980; **37**: 269-72.
●11. Rennard SI, Jaurand MC, Bignon J, *et al*. Role of pleural mesothelial cells in the production of submesothelial connective tissue matrix of the lung. *Am Rev Respir Dis* 1984; **130**: 267-74.
12. Churg A, Roggli V, Galateau-Sallé F, *et al*. Mesothelioma. In: Travis WD, Brambilla E, Konrad Müller-Hermelink H, Harris CC (eds). *Pathology and genetics of the lung, pleura, thymus and heart*. Lyon: WHO Publications; 2004: 128-40.
13. Churg A, Cagle P, Roggli V. *Diffuse malignant tumors of the serosal membranes*. Washington, DC: American Registry of Pathology; 2006.
14. Chretien J, Danel CJ, Nebut M. Light microscopic examination of the pleura. Usual procedures and evaluation. In: Lenfant C (ed.). *Lung biology in health and disease*. New York: Marcel Dekker, 1985: 30: 697-711.
◆15. Wang NS. Pleural mesothelioma: An approach to diagnostic problems. *Respirology* 1996; **1**: 259-71.
16. Warhol MJ, Corson JM. An ultrastructural comparison of mesotheliomas with adenocarcinomas of the lung and breast. *Hum Pathol* 1985; **16**: 50-5.
17. Wick MR, Loy T, Mills SE, *et al*. Malignant epitheloid pleural mesothelioma versus peripheral pulmonary adenocarcinoma. A histo-chemical, ultrastructural and immunohistologic study of 103 cases. *Hum Pathol* 1990; **21**: 759-66.
18. Warhol MJ, Kickey WF, Corson JM. Malignant mesothelioma: ultrastructural distinction from adenocarcinoma. *Am J Surg Pathol* 1982; **6**: 307-14.
19. Dewar A, Valente M, Ring NP, Corrin B. Pleural mesothelioma of epithelial type and pulmonary adenocarcinoma: an ultrastructural and cytochemical comparison. *J Pathol* 1987; **152**: 309-16.
◆20. Whitaker D, Papadimitriou JM, Walters NI. The mesothelium: techniques for investigating the origin, nature and behaviour of mesothelial cells. *J Pathol* 1980; **132**: 263-71.
●21. Jaurand MC, Kaplan H, Thiollet J, *et al*. Phagocytosis of chrysotile fibers by pleural mesothelial cells in culture. *Am J Pathol* 1979; **94**: 529-38.
●22. Jaurand MC, Bernaudin JF, Renier A, *et al*. Rat pleural mesothelial cells in culture. *In vitro* 1981; **17**: 98-106.
23. Jaurand MC, Barrett JC. Neoplastic transformation of mesothelial cells. In: Jaurand MC, Bignon J (eds). *The mesothelial cell and mesothelioma*. New York, Basel: Marcel Dekker, Inc.; 1994: 207-21.
●24. Gabrielson EW, Gerwin BI, Harris CC, *et al*. Stimulation of DNA synthesis in cultured primary human mesothelial cells by specific growth factor. *Faseb J* 1988; **2**: 2717-21.
25. Ke Y, Reddel RR, Gerwin BI, *et al*. Establisment of human *in vitro* mesothelial cell model system for investigating mechanisms of asbestos-induced mesothelioma. *Am J Pathol* 1989; **134**: 979-91.
●26. Zeng L, Fleury-Feith J, Monnet I, *et al*. Immunocytochemical characterization of cell lines from human malignant mesothelioma – Characterization of human mesothelioma cell lines by immunocytochemistry with a panel of monoclonal antibodies. *Hum Pathol* 1994; **25**: 227-34.
27. Fleury-Feith J, Kheuang L, Zeng L, *et al*. Human malignant mesothelioma cells: Variability of ultrastructural features in established and nude mice transplanted cell lines. *J Pathol* 1995; **177**: 209-15.
28. Bryks S, Bertalanffy FD. Cytodynamic reactivity of the mesothelium. Pleural reaction to chrysotile asbestos. *Arch Env Health* 1971; **23**: 469-72.
29. Mutsaers SE. The mesothelial cell. *Int J Biochem Cell Biol* 2004; **36**: 9-16.
30. Masse R, Fritsch P, Chretien J. Renouvellement des cellules des bronches et du poumon. *Rev Fr Mal Respir* 1981; **9**: 85-112.
◆31. Mutsaers SE. Mesothelial cells: their structure, function and role in serosal repair. *Respirology* 2002; **7**: 171-91.
32. Bolen JW, Hammar SP, McNutt MA. Reactive and neoplastic serosal tissue. A light-microscopic, ultrastructural, and immunocytochemical study. *Am J Surg Pathol* 1986; **10**: 34-47.
33. Bolen JW, Hammar SP, McNutt MA. Serosal tissue: reactive tissue as a model for understanding mesotheliomas. *Ultrastruct Pathol* 1987; **11**: 251-62.
34. Kim KH, Stellmach V, Javors J, Fuchs E. Regulation of human mesothelial cell differentiation: opposing roles of retinoids and epidermal growth factor in the expression of intermediate filament proteins. *J Cell Biol* 1987; **105**: 3039-51.
35. Van der Meeren A, Levy F, Renier A, *et al*. Effect of epidermal growth factor on rat pleural mesothelial cell growth. *J Cell Physiol* 1990; **144**: 137-43.
●36. Connell ND, Rheinwald JG. Regulation of the cytoskeleton in mesothelial cells: Reversible loss of keratin and increase in vimentin during rapid growth in culture. *Cell* 1983; **34**: 245-53.
●37. Donna A, Betta PG. Differentiation towards cartilage and bone in a primary tumour of pleura. Further evidence in support of the concept of mesodermoma. *Histopathology* 1986; **10**: 101-8.
◆38. Herrick SE, Mutsaers SE. Mesothelial progenitor cells and their potential in tissue engineering. *Int J Biochem Cell Biol* 2004; **36**: 621-42.
39. Andujar P, Lecomte C, Renier A, *et al*. Clinico-pathological features and somatic gene alterations in refactory ceramic fibre-induced murine mesothelioma reveal mineral fibre-induced mesothelioma identities. *Carcinogenesis* 2007; **28**: 1599-605.
40. Gerwin BI, Lechner JF, Reddel RR, *et al*. Comparison of production of transforming growth factor-β and platelet-derived growth factor by normal human mesothelial cells and mesothelioma cell lines. *Cancer Res* 1987; **47**: 6180-4.
41. Laveck MA, Somers ANA, Moore LL, *et al*. Dissimilar peptide growth factors can induce normal human mesothelial cell multiplication. *In Vitro Cell Dev Biol* 1988; **24**: 1077-84.
42. Lechner JF, Laveck MA, Gerwin BI, Matis EA. Differential responses to growth factors by normal human mesothelial cultures from individual donors. *J Cell Physiol* 1989; **139**: 295-300.

43. Mutsaers SE, McAnulty RJ, Laurent GJ, *et al.* Cytokine regulation of mesothelial cell proliferation *in vitro* and *in vivo. Eur J Cell Biol* 1997; **72**: 24–9.
44. Zhong J, Gencay MM, Bubendorf L, *et al.* ERK1/2 and p38 MAP kinase control MMP-2, MT1-MMP, and TIMP action and affect cell migration: a comparison between mesothelioma and mesothelial cells. *J Cell Physiol* 2006; **207**: 540–52.
45. Lee TC, Zhang YH, Aston C, *et al.* Normal human mesothelial cells and mesothelioma cell lines express insulin-like growth factor-I and associated molecules. *Cancer Res* 1993; **53**: 2858–64.
46. Fujino S, Yokoyama A, Kohno N, Hiwada K. Interleukin 6 is an autocrine growth factor for normal human pleural mesothelial cells. *Am J Respir Cell Mol Biol* 1996; **14**: 508–15.
47. Heldin P, Asplund T, Ytterberg D, *et al.* Characterization of the molecular mechanisms involved in the activation of hyaluronan synthetase by platelet-derived growth factor in human mesothelial cells. *Biochem J* 1992; **283**: 165–70.
48. Jacobson A, Brinck J, Briskin MJ, *et al.* Expression of human hyaluronan synthases in response to external stimuli. *Biochem J* 2000; **348**: 29–35.
49. Asplund T, Heldin P. Hyaluronan receptors are expressed on human malignant mesothelioma cells but not on normal mesothelial cells. *Cancer Res* 1994; **54**: 4516–23.
50. Strizzi L, Catalano A, Vianale G, *et al.* Vascular endothelial growth factor is an autocrine growth factor in human malignant mesothelioma. *J Pathol* 2001; **193**: 468–75.
●51. Lee YCG, Melkerneker D, Thompson PJ, *et al.* Transforming growth factor β induces vascular endothelial growth factor elaboration from pleural mesothelial cells *in vivo* and *in vitro. Am J Respir Crit Care Med* 2002; **165**: 88–94.
52. Klominek J, Baskin B, Liu Z, Hauzenberger D. Hepatocyte growth factor/scatter factor stimulates chemotaxis and growth of malignant mesothelioma cells through c-met receptor. *Int J Cancer* 1998; **76**: 240–9.
53. Rutten AA, Bermudez E, Stewart W, *et al.* Expression of insulin-like growth factor II in spontaneously immortalized rat mesothelial and spontaneous mesothelioma cells : a potential autocrine role of insulin-like growth factor II. *Cancer Res* 1995; **55**: 3634–9.
54. Owens MW, Milligan SA. Growth factor modulation of rat pleural mesothelial cell mitogenesis and collagen synthesis – effects of epidermal growth factor and platelet-derived growth factor. *Inflammation* 1994; **18**: 77–87.
55. Adamson IYR, Bakowska J, Prieditis H. Proliferation of rat pleural mesothelial cells in response to hepatocyte and keratinocyte growth factors. *Am J Respir Cell Mol Biol* 2000; **23**: 345–9.
56. Gordon GJ, Mani M, Mukhopadhyay L, *et al.* Expression patterns of inhibitor of apoptosis proteins in malignant pleural mesothelioma. *J Pathol* 2007; **211**: 447–54.
57. Versnel MA, Claessonwelsh L, Hammacher A, *et al.* Human malignant mesothelioma cell lines express PDGF beta-receptors whereas cultured normal mesothelial cells express predominantly PDGF alpha-receptors. *Oncogene* 1991; **6**: 2005–11.
58. Ramael M, Buysse C, Vandenbossche J, *et al.* Immunoreactivity for the beta-chain of the platelet-derived growth factor receptor in malignant mesothelioma and non-neoplastic mesothelium. *J Pathol* 1992; **167**: 1–4.
♦59. Fredriksson L, Li H, Eriksson U. The PDGF family: four gene products form five dimeric isoforms. *Cytokine Growth Factor Rev* 2004; **15**: 197–204.
60. Metheny-Barlow LJ, Flynn B, van Gijssel HE, *et al.* Paradoxical effects of platelet-derived growth factor-A overexpression in malignant mesothelioma. Antiproliferative effects *in vitro* and tumorigenic stimulation *in vivo. Am J Respir Cell Mol Biol* 2001; **24**: 694–702.
61. Walker C, Bermudez E, Stewart W, *et al.* Characterization of patelet-derived growth factor and platelet-derived growth factor receptor expression in asbestos-induced rat mesothelioma. *Cancer Res* 1992; **52**: 301–6.
62. Harvey P, Warn A, Newman P, *et al.* Immunoreactivity for hepatocyte growth factor/scatter factor and its receptor, met, in human lung carcinomas and malignant meesotheliomas. *J Pathol* 1996; **180**: 389–94.
63. Harvey P, Warn A, Dobbin S, *et al.* Expression of HGF/SF in mesothelioma cell lines and its effects on cell motility, proliferation and morphology. *Br J Cancer* 1998; **77**: 1052–9.
64. Tolnay E, Kuhnen C, Wiethege T, *et al.* Hepatocyte growth factor/scatter factor and its receptor c-Met are overexpressed and associated with an increased microvessel density in malignant pleural mesothelioma. *J Cancer Res Clin Oncol* 1998; **124**: 291–6.
65. Harvey P, Clark IM, Jaurand MC, *et al.* Hepatocyte growth factor/scatter factor enhances the invasion of mesothelioma cell lines and the expression of matrix metalloproteinases. *Br J Cancer* 2000; **83**: 1147–53.
66. Thirkettle I, Harvey P, Hasleton PS, *et al.* Immunoreactivity for cadherins, HGF/SF, met, and erbB-2 in pleural malignant mesotheliomas. *Histopathol* 2000; **36**: 522–8.
67. Jagadeeswaran R, Ma PC, Seiwert TY, *et al.* Functional analysis of c-Met/hepatocyte growth factor pathway in malignant pleural mesothelioma. *Cancer Res* 2006; **66**: 352–61.
68. Cao XX, Mohuiddin I, Chada S, *et al.* Adenoviral transfer of mda-7 leads to BAX up-regulation and apoptosis in mesothelioma cells, and is abrogated by over-expression of BCL-XL. *Mol Med* 2002; **8**: 869–76.
69. Hopkins-Donaldson S, Cathomas R, Simoes-Wust AP, *et al.* Induction of apoptosis and chemosensitization of mesothelioma cells by Bcl-2 and Bcl-xL antisense treatment. *Int J Cancer* 2003; **106**: 160–6.
70. Ozvaran MK, Cao XX, Miller SD, *et al.* Antisense oligonucleotides directed at the bcl-xl gene product augment chemotherapy response in mesothelioma. *Mol Cancer Ther* 2004; **3**: 545–50.
71. Altomare DA, You H, Xiao GH, *et al.* Human and mouse mesotheliomas exhibit elevated AKT/PKB activity, which can be targeted pharmacologically to inhibit tumor cell growth. *Oncogene* 2005; **24**: 6080–9.
♦72. Jaurand MC, Pinchon MC, Bignon J. Mesothelial cells *in vitro*. In: Chrétien J, Bignon J, Hirsch A (eds). *The pleura in health and disease.* New York: Marcel Dekker Inc. 1985: 43–67.
♦73. Jantz MA, Antony VB. Pleural fibrosis. *Clin Chest Med* 2006; **27**: 181–91.
74. Kuwahara M, Kuwahara M, Bijwaard KE, *et al.* Mesothelial cells produce a chemoattractant for lung fibroblasts – role of fibronectin. *Am J Respir Cell Mol Biol* 1991; **5**: 256–64.
75. Lee YC, Lane KB, Zoia O, *et al.* Transforming growth factor-beta induces collagen synthesis without inducing IL-8 production in mesothelial cells. *Eur Respir J* 2003; **22**: 197–202.
76. Lee YC, Knight DA, Lane KB, *et al.* Activation of proteinase-activated receptor-2 in mesothelial cells induces pleural inflammation. *Am J Physiol Lung Cell Mol Physiol* 2005; **288**: L734–40.
♦77. Grove CS, Lee YC. Vascular endothelial growth factor: the key mediator in pleural effusion formation. *Curr Opin Pulm Med* 2002; **8**: 294–301.
78. Idell S, Zwieb C, Kumar A, *et al.* Pathways of fibrin turnover of human pleural mesothelial cells *in vitro. Am J Respir Cell Mol Biol* 1992; **7**: 414–26.
●79. Boutin C, Dumortier P, Rey F, *et al.* Black spots concentrate oncogenic asbestos fibers in the parietal pleura: thoracoscopic and mineralogic study. *Am J Respir Crit Care Med* 1996; **153**: 444–9.
80. Gelzleichter TR, Bermudez E, Mangum JB, *et al.* Pulmonary and pleural responses in Fischer 344 rats following short-term inhalation of a synthetic vitreous fiber. II. Pathobiologic responses. *Fundam Appl Toxicol* 1996; **30**: 39–46.
81. Mitchev K, Dumortier P, De Vuyst P. 'Black Spots' and hyaline pleural plaques on the parietal pleura of 150 urban necropsy cases. *Am J Surg Pathol* 2002; **26**: 1198–206.

●82. Lechner JF, Tokiwa T, LaVeck M, *et al.* Asbestos-associated chromosomal changes in human mesothelial cells. *Proc Natl Acad Sci, USA* 1985; **82**: 3884–8.
83. Pelin K, Kivipensas P, Linnainmaa K. Effects of asbestos and man-made vitreous fibers on cell division in cultured human mesothelial cells in comparison to rodent cells. *Environ Mol Mutagen* 1995; **25**: 118–25.
84. Wu J, Liu W, Koenig K, *et al.* Vitronectin adsorption to chrysotile asbestos increases fiber phagocytosis and toxicity for mesothelial cells. *Am J Physiol Lung Cell Mol Physiol* 2000; **279**: L916–23.
85. Liaw YS, Yu CJ, Shun CT, *et al.* Expression of integrins in human cultured mesothelial cells: the roles in cell-to-extracellular matrix adhesion and inhibition by RGD-containing peptide. *Respir Med* 2001; **95**: 2216.
◆86. Kamp DW, Graceffa P, Pryor WA, Weitzman SA. The role of free radicals in asbestos-induced diseases. *Free Rad Biol Med* 1992; **12**: 293–315.
87. Ramos-Nino ME, Haegens A, Shukla A, Mossman BT. Role of mitogen-activated protein kinases (MAPK) in cell injury and proliferation by environmental particulates. *Mol Cell Biochem* 2002; **234–235**: 111–8.
◆88. Antony VB, Owen CL, Hadley KJ. Pleural mesothelial cells stimulated by asbestos release chemotactic activity for neutrophils in vitro. *Am Rev Respir Dis* 1989; **139**: 199–206.
89. Boylan AM, Ruegg C, Kim KJ, *et al.* Evidence of a role for mesothelial cell-derived interleukin-8 in the pathogenesis of asbestos-induced pleurisy in rabbits. *J Clin Invest* 1992; **89**: 1257–67.
90. Kuwahara M, Kuwahara M, Verma K, *et al.* Asbestos exposure stimulates pleural mesothelial cells to secrete the fibroblast chemoattactant, fibronectin. *Am J Respir Cell Mol Biol* 1994; **10**: 167–76.
●91. Yegles M, Saint-Etienne L, Renier A, *et al.* Induction of metaphase and anaphase/telophase abnormalities by asbestos fibers in rat pleural mesothelial cells *in vitro. Am J Respir Cell Mol Biol* 1993; **9**: 186–91.
92. Jaurand MC. Use of *in-vitro* genotoxicity and cell transformation assays to evaluate potential carcinogenicity of fibres. In: Kane AB, Boffetta P, Sarracci R, Wilbourn JD (eds). *Mechanisms in fiber carcinogenesis.* Lyon: IARC, 1996: 55–72.
●93. Jaurand MC, Broaddus C. Asbestos fibers and their interaction with mesothelial cells *in vitro* and *in vivo.* In: Robinson BWS, Chahinian A (eds). *Mesothelioma.* London: Martin Dunitz, 2002: 273–94.
94. Levresse V, Renier A, Fleury-Feith J, *et al.* Analysis of cell cycle disruptions in cultures of rat pleural mesothelial cells exposed to asbestos fibres. *Am J Respir Cell Mol Biol* 1997; **17**: 660–71.
95. Levresse V, Moritz S, Renier A, *et al.* Effect of simian virus large T antigen expression on cell cycle control and apoptosis in rat pleural mesothelial cells exposed to DNA damaging agents. *Oncogene* 1998; **16**: 1041–53.
96. Liu W, Ernst JD, Broaddus VC. Phagocytosis of crocidolite asbestos induces oxidative stress, DNA damage, and apoptosis in mesothelial cells. *Am J Respir Cell Mol Biol* 2000; **23**: 371–8.
97. Antony VB, Nasreen N, Mohammed KA, *et al.* Talc pleurodesis: basic fibroblast growth factor mediates pleural fibrosis. *Chest* 2004; **126**: 1522–8.
98. Murthy SS, Testa JR. Asbestos, chromosomal deletions, and tumor suppressor gene alterations in human malignant mesothelioma. *J Cell Physiol* 1999; **180**: 150–7.
◆99. Sandberg AA, Bridge JA. Updates on the cytogenetics and molecular genetics of bone and soft tissue tumors. Mesothelioma. *Cancer Genet Cytogenet* 2001; **127**: 93–110.
100. Metcalf RA, Welsh JA, Bennett WP, *et al.* p53 and Kirsten-ras mutations in human mesothelioma cell lines. *Cancer Res* 1992; **52**: 2610–5.
101. Mor O, Yaron P, Huszar M, *et al.* Absence of p53 mutations in malignant mesothelioma. *Am J Respir Cell Mol Biol* 1997; **16**: 9–13.
102. Vivo C, Lecomte C, Levy F, *et al.* Cell cycle checkpoint status in human malignant mesothelioma cell lines: response to gamma radiation. *Br J Cancer* 2003; **88**: 388–95.
103. Arakawa H, Hayashi N, Nagase H, *et al.* Alternative splicing of the NF2 gene and its mutation analysis of breast and colorectal cancers. *Hum Mol Genet* 1994; **3**: 565–8.
●104. Bianchi AB, Mitsunaga S, Cheng J, *et al.* High frequency of inactivating mutations in the neurofibromatosis type 2 gene (NF2) in primary malignant mesothelioma. *Proc Natl Acad Sci USA* 1995; **92**: 10854–8.
105. Yaegashi S, Sachse R, Ohuchi N, *et al.* Low incidence of a nucleotide sequence alteration of the neurofibromatosis 2 gene in human breast cancers. *Jpn J Cancer Res* 1995; **86**: 929–33.
●106. Fleury-Feith J, Lecomte C, Renier A, *et al.* Hemizygosity of Nf2 is associated with increased susceptibility to asbestos-induced peritoneal tumours. *Oncogene* 2003; **22**: 3799–805.
107. Altomare DA, Vaslet CA, Skele KL, *et al.* A mouse model recapitulating molecular features of human mesothelioma. *Cancer Res* 2005; **65**: 8090–5.
108. Lecomte C, Andujar P, Renier A, *et al.* Similar tumor suppressor gene alteration profiles in asbestos-induced murine and human mesothelioma. *Cell Cycle* 2005; **4**: 1862–9.

4

Normal physiological fluid and cellular contents

MARC NOPPEN

In normal conditions, the pleural space contains a small amount of pleural fluid.[1] This small volume of pleural fluid is maintained in the pleural space by a complex interplay of hydrostatic pressures and lymphatic drainage, which allows for steady liquid and protein turnover.[1,2] Pathological processes may lead to the development of pleural effusions by causing disequilibrium between the rates of pleural fluid formation, pleural permeability and pleural fluid absorption. The focus here is on the normal pleural fluid volume, cellular and solute content in normal, physiological circumstances. Normal pleural fluid is a microvascular filtrate; its volume and composition are tightly controlled. Liquid enters the pleural space through the parietal pleura down a net filtering pressure gradient, and is removed by an absorptive pressure gradient through the visceral pleura, by lymphatic drainage through parietal pleura stomas and by cellular mechanisms (active transport of solutes by mesothelial cells).[3,4] The main function of the normal pleural fluid is thought to be lubrication of the pleural surfaces, enabling transmission of the forces of breathing between the lung and the chest wall. Together with the presence of subatmospheric pressures within the pleural space, this lubrication function enables respiratory movements by a mechanical coupling between lung and chest wall. This lubrication function is supported by the presence of surfactant lipids in normal pleural fluid, which are efficient in terms of boundary lubrication and adherence to biological surfaces, and of hyaluran.[3,5] Most of what is known about the volume, composition and dynamics of normal pleural fluid has been obtained from animal studies. Retrieval of the few milliliters of normal pleural fluid in humans is indeed difficult without traumatically disturbing the pleural space: therefore, only a few human studies are available.

ANIMAL STUDIES

Data derived from animal studies are summarized in Table 4.1. Although there is a certain degree of concordance as to the total volume and total white blood cell count of normal rabbit and dog pleural fluid, there is a large disparity between the various differential cell counts between the various animal models. The reasons for this disparity include differences in identification of and distinction between macrophages, monocytes and mesothelial cells, and methodological differences in fixation, staining and fluid retrieval techniques (aspiration or lavage), and possible genuine interspecies differences.[6]

Miserocchi and Agostoni[7] collected pleural fluid from the costodiaphragmatic sinuses of rabbits and dogs. In rabbits, 0.46 mL of free fluid could be retrieved from both pleural spaces (0.2 mL/kg). In dogs, 0.55 mL or 0.15 mL/kg could be collected. When the volume of fluid adherent to the lung surfaces was assessed and included, volumes of pleural fluid rose to 0.4 mL/kg and 0.26 mL/kg, respectively. Total and differential white blood cell counts were performed using a cell counting chamber and May–Grünwald–Giemsa stained cell smears. In rabbits, 2442 ± 595 cells/μL were present, including 31.8 percent mesothelial cells, 60.8 percent monocytes and 7.4 percent lymphocytes. In dogs, 2208 ± 734 cells/μL were present, including 69.6 percent mesothelial cells, 28.2 percent monocytes and 2.2 percent lymphocytes. Stauffer *et al.*[8] compared different cytopreparations and different methods of fluid collection in rabbits: aspiration of the free fluid versus irrigation with 10 mL Hanks solution. The total volume of aspirated pleural fluid volume for both pleural spaces was 0.45 ± 0.12 mL (0.13 mL/kg). Total white blood cell count for the original aspirated fluid was 1503 ± 281 cells/μL.

Table 4.1 Data derived from animal studies

Study (ref)	Species	Mean volume (right and left pleural space) (mL/kg)	Total white blood cell count (cells/μL)	Macrophages (%)	Monocytes (%)	Mesothelial cells (%)	Lymphocytes (%)
7	Rabbits	0.2[a]	2442 ± 595	NR	60.8	31.8	7.4
7	Dogs	0.15[a]	2208 ± 734	NR	28.2	69.8	8.2
8	Rabbits	0.13	1503 ± 281	7.6–16	38.6–70.1	3.7–25.4	10–10.6
9	Rabbits	0.13	1503 ± 414	7.5 ± 1.5	70.1 ± 3.6	8.9 ± 1.6	10.6 ± 1.8
10	Rabbits[b]	NR	NR	9.25	66.5	8	9.75
10	Rabbits[c]	NR	NR	5	60.17	10	11
11	Rabbits	0.1	1216 ± 800	NR	NR	NR	NR
12	Rabbits	0.09	NR	NR	NR	NR	NR
13	Rabbits	0.22	NR	NR	NR	NR	NR
14	Dogs	0.1	NR	NR	NR	NR	NR
15	Sheep	0.12	NR	NR	NR	NR	NR
16	Sheep	0.04	NR	NR	NR	NR	NR
17	Rats	0.6	NR	NR	NR	NR	NR
17	Puppies	1.33	NR	NR	NR	NR	NR
17	Cats	0.28	NR	NR	NR	NR	NR
17	Pigs	0.22	NR	NR	NR	NR	NR

[a]Not including fluid adherent to lung surfaces; [b]fluid retrieved by aspiration; [c]fluid retrieved by lavage; NR = not reported.

Differential cell counts varied with the different methods of fixation (95 percent alcohol and Papinacolaou stain versus 50 percent alcohol, 1 percent polyethylene glycol and Papinicolaou stain) between 38.6 and 70.1 percent monocytes, 10 and 10.6 percent lymphocytes and 5.5 and 16.6 percent macrophages. Sahn *et al.*[9] aspirated costodiaphragmatic fluid in rabbits. Total volume of the free pleural fluid in both pleural spaces was 0.45 ± 0.90 mL (0.13 mL/kg). Total white blood cell count was 1503 ± 414 cells/μL, with 70.1 ± 3.6 percent monocytes, 10.6 ± 1.8 percent lymphocytes, 8.9 ± 1.6 percent mesothelial cells and 7.5 ± 1.5 percent macrophages. Novakov and Peshev[10] performed aspiration and lavage in rabbits. Volumes and total white blood cell counts were not reported; differential cell counts included 9.25 percent macrophages, 66.5 percent monocytes, 8 percent mesothelial cells and 9.75 percent lymphocytes after aspiration, and 5 percent macrophages, 60.17 percent monocytes, 10 percent mesothelial cells and 11.08 percent lymphocytes after lavage. Other measurements of pleural fluid volume have been made by Broaddus and Araya,[11],Wang and Lai-Fook[12] and Agostoni and Zocchi[13] in rabbits, Mellins *et al.*[14] in dogs, Wiener-Kronish *et al.*[15] and Broaddus *et al.*[16] in sheep and Miserocchi *et al.*[17] in various animal models (cats, dogs and pigs), as part of studies for purposes other than actual volume measurements. All measurements (except those in puppies) yielded total volumes between 0.04 and 0.28 mL/kg.

The solute composition of normal pleural fluid is similar to that of interstitial fluid of other organs and contains 1–2 g/100 mL, mainly consisting of albumin (50 percent), globulins (35 percent) and fibrinogen.[3,9] Levels of large molecular weight proteins, such as lactate dehydrogenase, in the pleural fluid are less than half of that found in serum.

HUMAN STUDIES

Reliable data on the volume and cellular content of pleural fluid in normal humans are scarce because of the obvious difficulties in retrieving this small amount of fluid without 'disturbing' the pleural environment. The first study addressing this issue was that of Yamada,[18] published in 1933, who punctured the ninth or tenth intercostals space on the dorsal axillary line in a group of healthy Japanese soldiers. In approximately 30 percent of cases, some fluid was aspirated after a period of rest, whereas in approximately 70 percent of cases some fluid was retrieved after exercise. Usually only a few drops of foam was aspirated but, in a few cases, up to 20 mL could be retrieved. Total white blood cell count was 4500 cells/μL (range 1700–6200). Differential cell count showed 53.7 percent cells similar to monocytes, 10.2 percent lymphocytes, 3 percent mesothelial cells, 3.6 percent granulocytes and 29.5 percent 'deteriorated cells of difficult classification'. More recently, a pleural lavage technique was used to retrieve the few milliliters of pleural fluid present in the pleural space of otherwise healthy participants undergoing thoracoscopic sympathectomy for the treatment of essential hyperhidrosis.[19] In analogy with bronchoalveolar lavage (a technique enabling retrieval of small volumes of epithelial lining fluid from the lung), 150 mL of prewarmed saline was injected in, and immediately aspirated from, the right pleural space, after induction of a pneumothorax in the setting of a thoracoscopic sympathectomy performed for the treatment of essential hyperhidrosis.[20] With urea used as an endogenous marker of dilution, measured mean right-sided pleural fluid volume was 8.4 ± 4.3 mL. In a subgroup of subjects, right- and left sided pleural fluid volumes were shown to be similar. Expressed per kg of body mass, total pleural fluid volume in non-smoking, healthy subjects is 0.26 mL/kg, which corresponds well with values obtained in animal studies. Total white blood cell count in the pleural fluid of normal non-smoking subjects was 1716 cells/μL. Differential cell count yielded a predominance of macrophages (median 75 percent, interquartile range 16 percent) and lymphocytes (median 23 percent, interquartile range 18 percent). Mesothelial cells, neutrophils and eosinophils were only marginally present. A typical image of a cell smear is shown in Figure 4.1. In a second study using a similar lavage technique, lymphocyte subtyping showed a lower proportion of CD4+ T cells (30 percent versus 45.8 percent) and a higher proportion of CD8+ T cells (11.78 versus 9.6 percent) and regulatory (CD4+CD25+) T cells in pleural fluid in normal subjects compared with blood, which may suggest that previously described abnormalities in lymphocyte subsets in pleural effusions may not only be a result of the pleural disease but may also be a characteristic of the pleural compartment itself.[21] Interestingly, a small but statistically significant increase in pleural fluid neutrophils was observed in smoking subjects. In addition to revealing the volume and cellular composition of normal pleural fluid (which may be helpful in understanding cellular events occurring in disorders characterized by pleural effusions), this pleural lavage technique allows the study of the pathophysiological events in pleural disorders that typically are not associated with pleural effusions, such as pneumothorax[22] and asbestos-related pleurisy.[23]

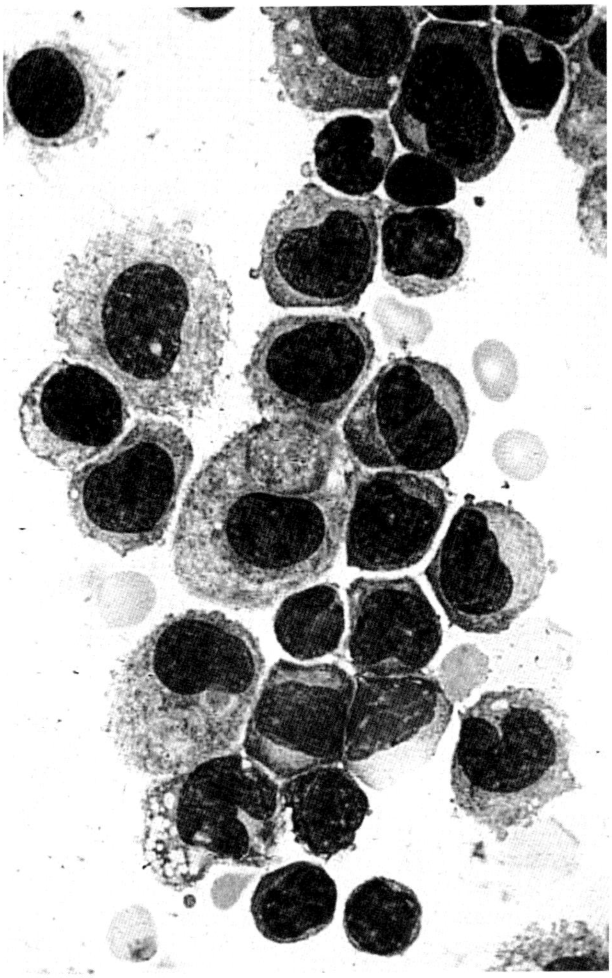

Figure 4.1 Typical cell smear of a pleural lavage sample from a normal, non-smoking subject; showing predominance of macrophages and lymphocytes (hematoxylin-eosin stain, ×320). (See also Color Plate 3.)

KEY POINTS

- In normal animals and humans, the pleural space contains a small volume of pleural fluid. In different adult animal species this volume varies between 0.04 and 0.60 mL/kg. In normal humans, the pleural fluid volume is 0.26 mL/kg.
- This fluid has the solute characteristics of all interstitial fluids, and contains a total of 1000 to 2500 white blood cells per μL. Macrophages/monocytes and lymphocytes are the predominant cell types.
- Pleural lavage is a safe and simple technique allowing the study of normal pleural fluid, and of pleural disease which is not characterized by pleural effusions

REFERENCES

● = Key primary paper
◆ = Major review article

◆1. Miserocchi G. Physiology and pathophysiology of pleural fluid turnover. *Eur Respir J* 1997; **10**: 219–25.
2. Miserocchi G, Venturoli D, Negrini D, Del-Fabbro M. Model of pleural fluid turnover. *J Appl Physiol* 1993; **75**: 1798–806.
◆3. Lai-Fook S. Pleural mechanics and fluid exchange. *Physiol Rev* 2004; **84**: 385–410.
◆4. Zocchi L. Physiology and pathophysiology of pleural fluid turnover. *Eur Respir J* 2002; **20**: 1545–58.

5. Mills PC, Chen Y, Hills YC, Hills BA. Comparison of surfactant lipids between pleural and pulmonary lining fluids. *Pulm Pharmacol Ther* 2006; **19**: 292–6.
6. Noppen M. Normal volume and cellular contents of pleural fluid. *Curr Opin Pulm Med* 2001; **7**: 180–82.
●7. Miserocchi G, Agostoni E. Contents of pleural space. *J Appl Physiol* 1971; **30**: 208–13.
8. Stauffer JL, Potts DE, Sahn SA. Cellular contents of the normal rabbit pleural space. *Acta Cytol* 1978; **22**: 570–74.
9. Sahn SA, Willcox ML, Good JT , Potts DE, Filley DF. Characteristics of normal rabbit pleural fluid: physiologic and biochemical implications. *Lung* 1979; **156**: 63–9.
10. Novakov IP, Peshev ZP. Cell types in the normal pleural fluid from rabbits. *Trakia J Sci* 2005; **3**: 22–5.
11. Broaddus VC, Araya M. Liquid and protein dynamics using a new minimally invasive pleural catheter in rabbits. *J Appl Physiol* 1992; **72**: 851–7.
12. Wang PM, Lai-Fook SJ. Pleural tissue hyaluran produced by post-mortem ventilation in rabbits. *Lung* 2000; **178**: 1–12.
13. Agostoni E, Zocchi L. Starling forces and lymphatic drainage in pleural liquid and protein exchanges. *Respir Physiol* 1991; **86**: 271–81.
14. Mellins RB, Levine OR, Fishman AP. Effects of systemic and pulmonary venous hypertension on pleural and pericardial fluid accumulation. *J Appl Physiol* 1970; **29**: 546–9.
15. Wiener-Kronish JP, Albertine KH, Licko V, Staub NC. Protein egress and entry rates in pleural fluid and plasma in sheep. *J Appl Physiol* 1984; **56**: 459–63.
16. Broaddus VC, Araya M, Carlton DP, Bland RD. Developmental changes in pleural liquid protein concentration in sheep. *Am Rev Respir Dis* 1991; **143**: 38–41.
17. Miserocchi G, Negrini D, Mortola J. Comparative features of Starling-lymphatic interaction at the pleural level in mammals. *J Appl Physiol* 1984; **56**: 1151–6.
●18. Yamada S. Uber die seröse Flüssigkeit in der Pleurahöhle der gesunden Menschen. *Z Ges Exp Med* 1933; **90**: 342–8.
●19. Noppen M, De Waele M, Li R, *et al.* Volume and cellular content of normal pleural fluid in humans examined by pleural lavage. *Am J Respir Crit Care Med* 2001; **7**: 180–82.
20. Noppen M, Herregodts P, D'haese J, Vincken W, Dhaens J. A simplified thoracoscopic sympathicolysis technique for essential hyperhidrosis: results in 100 consecutive patients. *J Laparoendosc Surg* 1996; **6**: 151–9.
21. Scherpereel A, Madsen P, Chahine B, *et al.* T cell subsets in pleural fluid of healthy subjects. *Am J Respir Crit Care Med* 2007; **175**: A452.
22. De Smedt A, Vanderlinden E, Demanet C, *et al.* Characterisation of pleural inflammation occurring after primary spontaneous pneumothorax. *Eur Respir J* 2004; **23**: 896–900.
23. Noppen M, Vanderlinden E, Demanet C, De Waele M. Pleural lavage in non-exudative benign asbestos-related pleural disease. *Am J Respir Crit Care Med* 2002; **165**: A33.

5

Physiology: fluid and solute exchange in normal physiological states

V COURTNEY BROADDUS

INTRODUCTION

The major function of the pleura and the pleural space may be to permit the lungs to expand and deflate easily within the chest. The pleural coverings allow the lungs to move with minimal friction and adjust their shape during changes in size. Because the space is under subatmospheric pressure with no internal barriers to liquid movement, the pleural space can also accommodate large volumes of liquid. These collections, pleural effusions, are a common clinical issue. In this chapter, we will discuss what is known about normal movement of liquid and solutes into and out of the pleural space.

The division of the pleura into visceral and parietal membranes is based primarily upon the structures each envelops, though structural histological differences between the two exist. The visceral pleura encloses the lungs and interlobar fissures before turning back on itself to form the parietal pleura covering the inner wall of the chest, the diaphragm and the mediastinum. In the normal state, a subatmospheric intrapleural pressure keeps the visceral pleura, which is firmly attached to the lung parenchyma, mechanically coupled to the parietal pleura, which is attached to the chest wall. Indeed, it is the subatmospheric pressure that allows the pleural space to act as a sump for the collection of excess liquid produced elsewhere in the body. The balance of pleural pressures keeps the mediastinum midline and, if the mediastinum is not fixed in position, a rise in intrapleural pressure due to the presence of intrapleural liquid or air will cause a shift of the mediastinum to the contralateral side.

Under normal conditions, the pleural space is home to a small amount of fluid, recently quantified in humans by pleural lavage to be 0.26 mL/kg of body weight, which translates roughly to less than 12 mL per hemithorax.[1] This small amount of liquid is distributed along the pleural space with an average thickness of approximately 20 μm, with the thickest portion in the dependent regions.[2] The liquid has been shown to separate the pleural membranes over the entire surface of the lungs, because, in studies of frozen pleura, no area of contact has been identified.[2] The pleural space is thus a real, not a potential, space but one that has been particularly difficult to study by virtue of its extremely thin (20 μm) and wide (1–2 m^2) extent.

Owing to the difficulty of study, there has been controversy regarding the normal source and movement of pleural fluid. For example, at one time, normal pleural liquid was proposed to arise from secretion by mesothelial cells or from filtration from the systemic (high pressure) circulation with absorption into the pulmonary (low pressure) circulation. A consensus has now arisen that the pleural liquid flows by filtration from systemic vessels and is absorbed into lymphatics, in a manner analogous to other interstitial spaces of the body.[3,4]

This view is supported by many lines of evidence, often obtained via studies using non-invasive or minimally invasive experimental approaches in animals, such as sheep, that have pleural anatomy similar to that of humans.[5–8]

PLEURAL FLUID PRODUCTION

Based on studies in animals, normal human pleural liquid probably contains between 1 and 2 g/dL of protein.[9] It is notable that the collection of a pleural effusion, even with transudative liquid with a protein concentration between 2–3 g/dL, represents a definite increase in the protein concentration above the normal level. The low protein concentration of normal liquid indicates a high degree of sieving of the protein molecules during fluid filtration from the microvasculature. The concentration, which represents a protein ratio of 0.15–0.2, is in keeping with systemic interstitial liquids of the body and is very different from the higher protein ratio of pulmonary filtrate (0.6–0.7).[10,11] Thus, the low protein concentration is strong evidence that normal pleural liquid arises from systemic vessels.

Additional evidence for the systemic origin of pleural liquid derives from studies in animals in which systemic pressure is found to vary. In animals with an increased systemic arterial (and microvascular) pressure, filtration at the microvessels and the sieving of protein would be expected to be higher and, if systemic vessels were the source of pleural liquid, the pleural protein concentration ratio (pleural/plasma) would be expected to be lower than in animals with a lower systemic pressure. In the first study, spontaneously hypertensive rats were found to have lower total protein and albumin concentration ratios and a higher pleural space thickness than in the control, normotensive rats.[12] In the second study, sheep were studied at different stages of development. As mammals grow from fetal to newborn to adult life, systemic arterial pressure increases while pulmonary arterial pressure decreases. Thus, if pleural liquid arose from the systemic circulation, pleural liquid protein concentrations would be expected to decrease; if pleural liquid arose from the pulmonary circulation, the opposite would be expected. In pleural liquid collected from sheep at different ages, pleural liquid protein concentration ratios decreased progressively; in fetuses, the ratio was 0.50, in newborns 0.27 and in adults 0.15, supporting a systemic origin of the liquid.[13]

The likely systemic sources of liquid lie in the adjacent pleural membranes themselves (Figures 5.1 and 5.2). In effect, the pleural space is sandwiched between two systemic circulations: the intercostal arterial circulation of the parietal pleura (Figure 5.1, see B) and the bronchial arterial

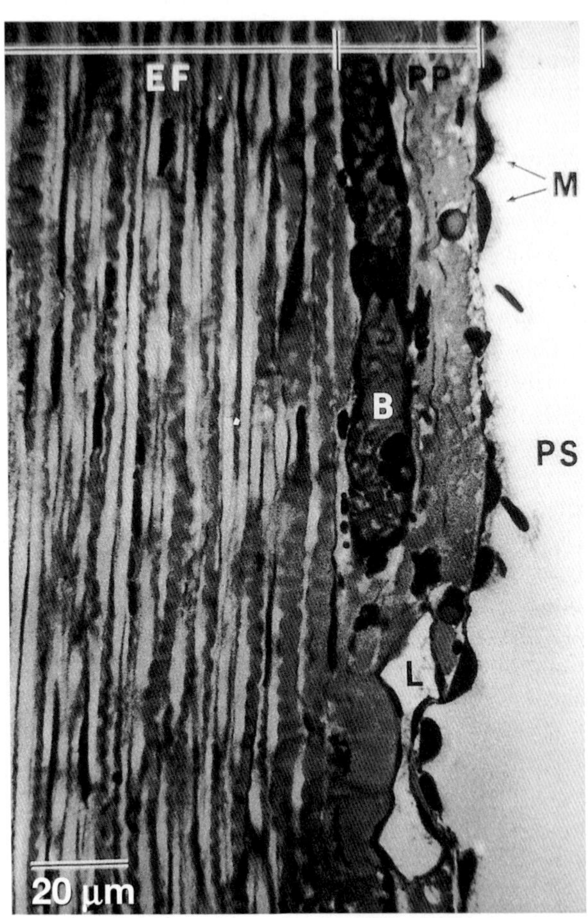

Figure 5.1 Parietal pleura. The parietal pleura is lined by mesothelial cells (M) adjacent to the pleural space (PS). The blood supply is via the intercostal arteries (B). The parietal pleura, but not the visceral pleura, contains the lymphatics (L) that drain pleural liquid via stomata that open into the pleural space.

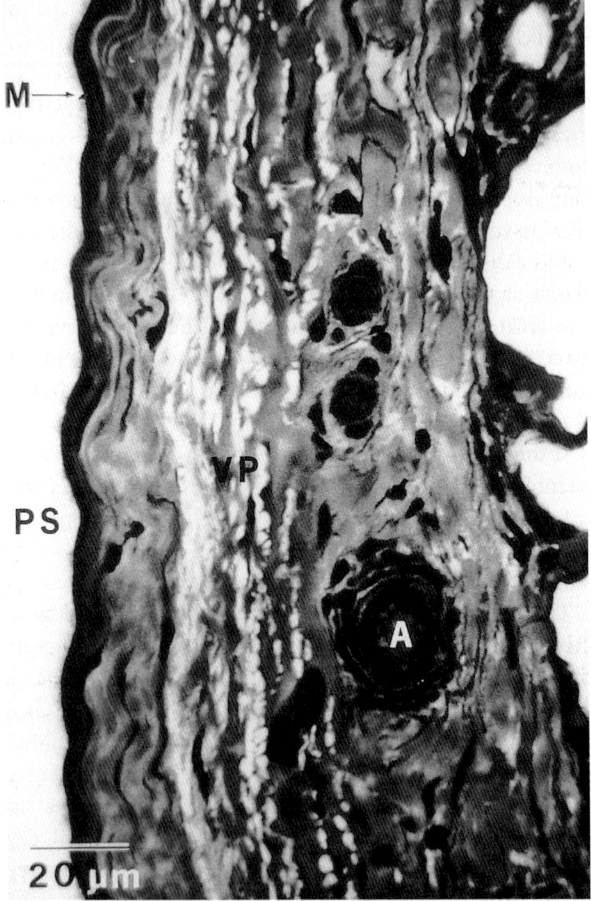

Figure 5.2 Visceral pleura. The visceral pleura (VP) lies between the pleural space (PS) and the alveoli of the lung parenchyma, and is lined by mesothelial cells (M). The blood supply to the visceral pleura is via the bronchial arteries (A). (Reproduced from Reference 3 by courtesy of Marcel Dekker, Inc.)

circulation of the visceral pleura (Figure 5.2, see A). It is interesting that the parietal pleural circulation is constant among species with a morphology almost interchangeable from small mammals to humans.[7] By contrast, the visceral pleural circulation changes drastically depending on whether the visceral pleura is 'thick' as in humans, sheep and most large animals, or is 'thin' as in smaller mammals like dogs, rabbits and mice.[6] Thick visceral pleura has a systemic bronchial blood supply while the thin visceral pleura has no systemic circulation itself but is nourished by the underlying pulmonary circulation. For several reasons, the systemic blood supply of the parietal pleura is thought to be the major source of normal pleural liquid. First, despite the great differences in visceral pleural anatomy and blood supply, measured rates of pleural liquid production are similar among different species, suggesting the constant parietal pleura as the source.[9,14] Second, the parietal pleural microvessels are closer to the pleural space (10–15 μm) than are those of the visceral pleura (20–50 μm).[6,7] Finally, the parietal pleural vessels are likely to have a higher microvascular pressure due to their drainage into systemic venules while the visceral bronchial vessels drain into lower resistance pulmonary venules.[3]

Once the liquid filters across the systemic vessels, it can then flow along a pressure gradient across the mesothelial layer into the pleural space (Figure 5.3). The pressure gradient exists from the high pressure pleural systemic microvessels into its surrounding interstitial tissue and from the interstitial tissues into the subatmospheric pleural space.[15] The mesothelial layer separating the interstitial tissue from the pleural space is leaky, especially relative to other barriers such as the epithelial barriers of the alveoli or the kidney. Mesothelium has been shown, both in *in vitro* and *in situ* studies, to offer little resistance to the movement of liquid and protein.[8,16] Thus, the liquid and protein filtered from the pleural microvessels (as well as liquid arising anywhere in the body) can flow across the mesothelium along a pressure gradient into the pleural space. By virtue of its large size and surface area, its subatmospheric pressure and its relative leaky borders, the pleural space is clearly vulnerable to the accumulation of liquids.

The mesothelium has been proposed to be capable of active transport. This possibility is particularly intriguing when examining the distribution of ions in pleural liquid and serum because pleural concentrations of some ionic solutes such as bicarbonate have been noted to be slightly different from those in serum.[17,18] Although a higher pleural concentration has raised the possibility of an active transport mechanism for bicarbonate into the pleural space, the distribution of ions may also be explained by a passive process, the Donnan equilibrium. In such an equilibrium, differences in protein concentrations may passively alter ionic balances between two electrolytic solutions separated by a semipermeable membrane. Such a mechanism has been proposed to explain similar differences in ion concentrations between body fluids and serum in patients.[19] Thus, passive forces alone may be sufficient to explain the small difference in ionic concentrations between pleural liquid and serum and are more consistent with the leaky nature of the mesothelium.[8,20]

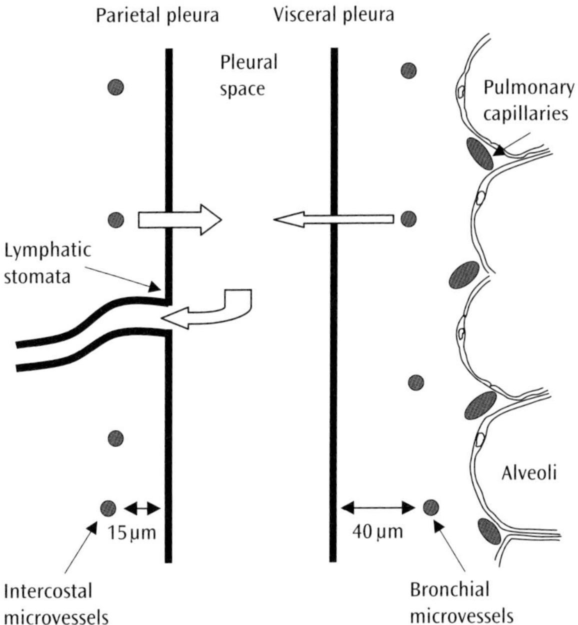

Figure 5.3 Schema of pleural liquid entry and exit in the normal state. The microvascular filtrate of the arterial blood supply flows across the leaky mesothelial layer into the lower pressure pleural space. From the pleural space pleural liquid exits via the lymphatic stomata into the parietal pleural lymphatics.

Once it enters the pleural space, pleural liquid very slowly flows toward the dependent regions of the pleural space.[21] Such flow has been proposed based on findings of pleural pressure gradients. Pleural pressure has been exceedingly difficult to measure: even by placing a small catheter into the pleural space, the space is greatly widened and pressures are measured consistent with a static column of liquid. However, when pleural pressures are measured with micropipettes that do not distort the space, pleural pressure gradients are consistent with a gradual flow of liquid from the top to bottom.[22,23]

Based on noninvasive studies in different species, the production of pleural liquid is normally slow. In earlier studies, measured flows were probably overestimated due to inflammation and distortion caused by invasive techniques used to measure the fluid turnover. Based upon radiolabel studies or minimally invasive techniques that leave the pleural space intact, pleural liquid production has been measured at approximately 0.01 mL/(kg × h) in awake sheep[9] and 0.02 in rabbits.[14] The half-time of pleural liquid turnover in sheep and rabbits is 6–8 hours.[14] At these rates, there would be an entry (and exit) of 15 mL per day in a 60 kg human.

PLEURAL FLUID ABSORPTION

Studies and clinical experience suggest that the majority of pleural fluid exits the pleural space by bulk flow, and not by diffusion or other routes. If liquid were absorbed by diffusion or via solute channels, proteins would be expected to diffuse via different pathways at a slower rate and the protein concentration of the remaining liquid would progressively increase. Clinically, however, the protein concentration of pleural effusions does not change as a hydrothorax is absorbed. With bulk flow, liquid and protein are removed at the same rates and the protein concentration of the liquid remaining in the pleural space does not change. This constancy is fortuitous, as it has allowed the protein concentration to be a useful clinical guide to the mechanism of formation of an effusion by indicating whether the vasculature of origin was normal, in which case there would be low protein as in a transudate, or whether the vasculature was injured or leaky, resulting in an exudate with high protein.

Sodium channels and other ion transport have been implicated in fluid absorption from the pleural space,[24] although this cannot explain the clearance of particulates. In addition, the agents used to accelerate (e.g. terbutaline) or inhibit (e.g. amiloride) the activity of such pumps may also affect lymphatic contractility and flow. In particular, amiloride, used as an inhibitor of sodium channels, has also been shown to decrease lymph flow.[25] To date, the contribution of active transcellular processes to overall clearance has not been established although it may account for a small movement of fluid. Similarly, transcytosis of albumin across the mesothelial cell layer may account for a small amount of clearance of protein.[26] Nonetheless, as in other interstitial spaces of the body, lymphatic clearance would best explain the bulk clearance of fluid, protein and particulates from the pleural space.

The lymphatics have direct connections to the pleural space via stomata, which have now been described in many species by ultrastructural studies. They were first reported in mice and rabbits as being 2–6 μm in diameter in the resting state,* and it was assumed that they would stretch to a larger diameter with inspiration and expansion of the chest wall.[27] Injected red blood cells were seen at the orifice and inside the lymphatic lacunae. No lymphatic stomata were found on the visceral pleura. On the parietal pleura in sheep, lymphatic stomata were described as 1–3 μm in diameter, again in the resting state.[7] Injected chicken red blood cells, identified by their nuclei, and carbon black entered the lymphatic lacunae. In golden hamsters, lymphatic stomata have been noted on the costal pleura, at approximately 1000 lymphatic stomata per thoracic hemisphere. Approximately 15 percent of them are distributed in the ventro-cranial regions of the thoracic wall, with approximately 85 percent in the dorso-caudal region.[28] In rabbits, stomata have been found on the costal pleura at a density of 120 per mm^2.[29] In the rat, colloidal particulates were found to clear via lymphatics primarily via the parietal pleura[30] where stomata have been described.[31] In humans, there has been some confusion concerning the presence and location of lymphatic stomata. In some reports, the human pleura appeared to have micropores or clefts[32] while in other studies stomata with a diameter of approximately 6 μm have been described on the diaphragmatic pleura.[33] A careful study of lymphatic clearance of carbon particles in monkeys by direct observation using videothoracoscopy has shown that carbon particles enter lymphatics in the costal, mediastinal and diaphragmatic pleura in 10–15 minutes and are drained to collecting lymphatics within 30 minutes.[34] Study of the pleura by electron microscopy (EM) showed a network of sievelike submesothelial lymphatic structures suggesting a rich lymphatic drainage of the pleural space.[34]

Stomata have not been described on the visceral pleura, although many studies do not mention whether the lung surface was examined for them. In studies in which the lung was examined after injection of intrapleural carbon ink, carbon particulates were described to enter the parietal, but not the visceral, pleura.[7]

There has also been confusion about the route of lymphatics in the diaphragm, where some have speculated that connections exist between the peritoneal and pleural spaces. Recent studies have described two separate networks of lymphatic systems in the diaphragm that do not connect to each other[35,36] supporting the general concept that the fluid dynamics of the peritoneal and pleural spaces in the physiological state are separate.

The physiological function of pleural stomata is demonstrated by the clearance of artificial hydrothoraces containing labeled erythrocytes. Indeed, the erythrocytes are absorbed intact, almost in the same proportion as the liquid and protein,[5] indicating that the major route of exit is through openings large enough to accommodate sheep erythrocytes (6–8 μm diameter). The similar rate of absorption of these particulates, along with the fluid and protein, argues that the major route of clearance for all components is the same, by bulk flow via lymphatics.

Notably, the pleural lymphatics have a large capacity for absorption. When artificial effusions were instilled into the pleural space of awake sheep, the exit rate [0.28 mL/(kg × h)] was nearly 30 times the baseline exit rate [0.01 mL/(kg × h)].[5] In a rare study of pleural liquid turnover in patients, Leckie and Tothill[37] demonstrated, using labeled tracers, that mean lymphatic flow was 0.22 mL/(kg × h) in patients with congestive heart failure, though there was great variation among subjects. In the balance between maximal clearance and production, this large reserve capacity serves to resist effusion formation. Nonetheless, there is a maximal absorptive capacity that limits absorp-

*Owing to a typesetting error, the measurements in this original paper were incorrectly listed as nanometers (nm) instead of the correct unit of measurement, micrometers (μm), leading to some confusion over the years (Nai-San Wang, personal communication).

tion beyond that point. Although over time this maximal rate could increase, for example by increases in stomata number or size or increases in lymphatic contractility, lymphatic capacity would set a definite limit in the ability of the pleural space to handle liquid.

Water channels have been investigated as a possible means of clearance of pleural fluid.[38,39] Aquaporins (AQP) present in mesothelial cells, particularly AQP1, have been shown to participate in the rapid osmotic shifts that mediate movement of pure water. However, pleural clearance of isoosmotic fluids, such as saline, is not affected by the presence or absence of aquaporins. Therefore the main route of clearance of fluid and protein is still most likely via the lymphatics.

KEY POINTS

- Intrapleural pressure is lower than the interstitial pressure of either of the pleural tissues. This pressure difference constitutes a gradient for liquid movement into, but not out of, the pleural space.
- The pleural membranes are leaky to liquid and protein providing little resistance to protein movement.
- The entry of pleural liquid is normally slow and is compatible with known interstitial flow rates, approximately 0.5 mL hourly in a grown man.
- Most liquid exits the pleural space by bulk flow, not by diffusion. This is evident because the protein concentration of pleural effusions does not change as the effusion is absorbed.
- The major exit of liquid and protein is via the parietal pleural stomata (2–6 μm diameter) and the pleural lymphatics. These lymphatics have a large capacity for absorption, increasing up to 30 times the baseline exit rate, effusion and thereby resisting formation.

REFERENCES

● = Key primary paper
◆ = Major review article

1. Noppen M, De Waele M, Li R, *et al.* Volume and cellular content of normal pleural fluid in humans examined by pleural lavage. *Am J Respir Crit Care Med* 2000; **162**: 1023–6.
2. Albertine KH, Wiener-Kronish JP, Bastacky J, Staub NC. No evidence for mesothelial cell contact across the costal pleural space of sheep. *J Appl Physiol* 1991; **70**: 123–4.
◆3. Staub NC, Wiener-Kronish JP, Albertine KH. Transport through the pleura: physiology of normal liquid and solute exchange in the pleural space. In: Chretien J, Bignon J, Hirsch A (eds). *The pleura in health and disease.* New York: Marcel Dekker, Inc., 1985: 174–5.
◆4. Broaddus VC, Light RW. Pleural effusion. In: Mason RJ, Murray JF, Broaddus VC, Nadel JA (eds). *Murray Nadel's Textbook of Respiratory Medicine*, 4th ed. Philadelphia: Saunders, 2000: 1913–60.
●5. Broaddus VC, Wiener-Kronish JP, Berthiaume Y, Staub NC. Removal of pleural liquid and protein by lymphatics in awake sheep. *J Appl Physiol* 1988; **64**: 384–90.
6. Albertine KH, Wiener-Kronish JP, Roos PJ, Staub NC. Structure, blood supply, and lymphatic vessels of the sheep's visceral pleura. *Am J Anat* 1982; **165**: 277–94.
7. Albertine KH, Wiener-Kronish JP, Staub NC. The structure of the parietal pleura and its relationship to pleural liquid dynamics in sheep. *Anat Rec* 1984; **208**: 401–9.
8. Kim KJ, Critz AM, Crandall ED. Transport of water and solutes across sheep visceral pleura. *Am Rev Resp Dis* 1979; **120**: 883–92.
●9. Wiener-Kronish JP, Albertine KH, Licko V, Staub NC. Protein egress and entry rates in pleural fluid and plasma in sheep. *J Appl Physiol* 1984; **56**: 459–63.
10. Erdmann AJ, Vaughan TR, Brigham KL, Woolverton WC, Staub NC. Effect of increased vascular pressure on lung fluid balance in unanesthetized sheep. *Circ Res* 1975; **37**: 271–84.
◆11. Wiener-Kronish JP, Broaddus VC. Interrelationship of pleural and pulmonary interstitial liquid. *Annu Rev Physiol* 1993; **55**: 209–26.
12. Lai-Fook SJ, Kaplowitz MR. Pleural protein concentration and liquid volume in spontaneously hypertensive rats. *Microv Res* 1988; **35**: 101–8.
13. Broaddus VC, Araya M, Carlton DP, Bland RD. Developmental changes of pleural liquid protein concentration in sheep. *Am Rev Resp Dis* 1991; **143**: 38–41.
14. Broaddus VC, Araya M. Liquid and protein dynamics using a new, minimally invasive pleural catheter in rabbits. *J Appl Physiol* 1992; **72**: 851–7.
15. Bhattacharya J, Gropper MA, Staub NC. Interstitial fluid pressure gradient measured by micropuncture in excised dog lung. *J Appl Physiol* 1984; **56**: 271–7.
16. Parameswaran S, Brown LV, Ibbott GS, Lai-Fook SJ. Hydraulic conductivity, albumin reflection and diffusion coefficients of pig mediastinal pleura. *Microvasc Res* 1999; **58**: 114–27.
17. D'Angelo E, Heisler N, Agostoni E. Acid-base balance of pleural liquid in dogs. *Respir Physiol* 1979; **37**: 137–49.
18. Rolf LL, Travis DM. Pleural fluid-plasma bicarbonate gradients in oxygen-toxic and normal rats. *Am J Physiol* 1973; **224**: 857–61.
19. Gilligan DR, Volk MC, Blumgart HL. Observations on the chemical and physical relation between blood serum and body fluids. *J Clin Invest* 1934; **13**: 365–81.
20. Payne DK, Kinasewitz GT, Gonzalez E. Comparative permeability of canine visceral and parietal pleura. *J Appl Physiol* 1988; **65**: 2558–64.
21. Lai-Fook S. Pleural mechanics and fluid exchange. *Physiol Rev* 2004; **84**: 385–410.
22. Lai-Fook SJ, Rodarte JR. Pleural pressure distribution and its relationship to lung volume and interstitial pressure. *J Appl Physiol* 1991; **70**: 967–78.
23. Lai-Fook S, Price D, Staub N. Liquid thickness vs vertical pressure gradient in a model of the pleural space. *J Appl Physiol* 1987; **62**: 1747–54.
24. Agostoni E, Zocchi L. Active Na+ transport and coupled liquid outflow from hydrothoraces of various size. *Respir Physiol* 1993; **92**: 101–13.
25. Negrini D, Ballard ST, Benoit JN. Contribution of lymphatic myogenic activity and respiratory movements to pleural lymph flow. *J Appl Physiol* 1994; **76**: 2267–76.
26. Agostoni E, Bodega F, Zocchi L. Albumin transcytosis from the pleural space. *J Appl Physiol* 2002; **93**: 1806–12.
●27. Wang N-S. The preformed stomas connecting the pleural cavity and the lymphatics in the parietal pleura. *Am Rev Respir Dis* 1975; **111**: 12–20.
28. Shinohara H. Distribution of lymphatic stomata on the pleural surface of the thoracic cavity and the surface topography of the

pleural mesothelium in the golden hamster. *Anat Rec* 1997; **249**: 16–23.

29. Li Y-Y, Li J-C. Ultrastructure and three-dimensional study of the lymphatic stomata in the costal pleura of the rabbit. *Micros Res Techn* 2003; **62**: 240–46.
30. Liu J, Wong HL, Moselhy J, *et al.* Targeting colloidal particulates to thoracic lymph nodes. *Lung Cancer* 2006; **51**: 377–86.
31. Wang Q, Ohtani O, Saitoh M, Ohtani Y. Distribution and ultrastructure of the stomata connecting the pleural cavity with lymphatics in the rat costal pleura. *Acta Anat (Basel)* 1997; **158**: 255–65.
32. Gaudio E, Rendina EA, Pannarale L, Ricci C, Marinozzi G. Surface morphology of the human pleura. A scanning electron microscopic study. *Chest* 1988; **93**: 149–53.
33. Li J. Ultrastructural study on the pleural stomata in human. *Funct Develop Morphol* 1993; **3**: 277–80.
●34. Miura T, Shimada T, Tanaka K, Chujo M, Uchida Y. Lymphatic drainage of carbon particles injected into the pleural cavity of the monkey, as studied by video-assisted thoracoscopy and electron microscopy. *J Thorac Cardiovasc Surg* 2000; **120**: 437–47.
35. Shinohara H, Kominami R, Taniguchi Y, Yasutaka S. The distribution and morphology of lymphatic vessels on the peritoneal surface of the adult human diaphragm, as revealed by an ink-absorption method. *Okajimas Folia Anat Jpn* 2003; **79**: 175–83.
36. Grimaldi A, Moriondo A, Sciacca L, *et al.* Functional arrangement of rat diaphragmatic initial lymphatic network. *Am J Physiol Heart Circ Physiol* 2006; **291**: H876–85.
37. Leckie WJH, Tothill P. Albumin turnover in pleural effusions. *Clin Sci* 1965; **29**: 339–52.
●38. Song Y, Yang B, Matthay MA, Ma T, Verkman AS. Role of aquaporin water channels in pleural fluid dynamics. *Am J Physiol Cell Physiol* 2000; **279**: C1744–50.
39. Jiang J, Hu J, Bai CX. Role of aquaporin and sodium channel in pleural water movement. *Respir Physiol Neurobiol* 2003; **139**: 83–8.

6

Physiology: changes with pleural effusion and pneumothorax

RICHARD W LIGHT

In this chapter the effects of pleural fluid or pleural air on pleural pressures, the lung, the diaphragm, the heart, pulmonary gas exchange and exercise tolerance will be discussed.

EFFECTS OF EFFUSION ON THE PLEURAL PRESSURE

When pleural fluid is present, its volume must be compensated for by an increase in the size of the thoracic cavity, a decrease in the size of the lung or the heart, or a combination of these changes. The thoracic cavity, the lungs and the heart are all distensible objects, which means that the volume of each is dependent upon the pressure inside minus the pressure outside. The presence of pleural fluid increases the pleural pressure. Since the distending pressure of the thoracic wall is the atmospheric pressure minus the pleural pressure, an increase in the pleural pressure will lead to an increase in the distending pressure of the thoracic cavity and an increase in the volume of the thoracic cavity. In contrast, the distending pressure of the lungs is the alveolar pressure minus the pleural pressure. Therefore, an increase in the pleural pressure will lead to a decreased lung volume. The distending pressure of the heart is the intracardiac pressure minus the pleural pressure, so an increase in the pleural pressure will lead to a decrease in the size of the heart.

The pleural pressure is normally negative. However, when more than minimal pleural fluid accumulates, the pleural pressure becomes positive. When there is sufficient pleural fluid such that the lung is separated from the chest wall, there is a vertical gradient of 1 cm H_2O per cm vertical height because of the weight of the fluid.[1] If there is a hydrostatic column 40 cm high in a hemithorax, then the pressure at the bottom of the column would be expected to be approximately 40 cm H_2O.

In one older study we measured the pleural pressure in 52 patients with significant pleural effusions (median amount of fluid greater than 1000 mL). Overall, the mean pleural pressure was approximately 0, but there was a wide range in the pleural pressures with a range of −21 cmH_2O to +8 cmH_2O (Figure 6.1).[2] Pleural pressures of −5 cmH_2O and lower were only seen with a trapped lung or with malignancy. Villena *et al.*[3] measured the pleural pressure in 61 patients with pleural effusions of varying etiology. These workers found that the initial pleural pressure ranged from −12 to +25 cmH_2O and the mean pressure in their patients was approximately +5 cmH_2O. The reason that the pleural pressures were not more positive in the above two studies is probably due to the insertion of the thoracentesis needle closer to the superior than the inferior end of the hydrostatic column. The pleural pressure at times can be quite positive with a pleural effusion. Neff and Buchanan[4] reported that the initial pleural pressure was 76 cmH_2O in a patient with a pleural effusion secondary to pneumothorax therapy for tuberculosis many years previously.

When pleural fluid is removed with thoracentesis, the fluid volume removed is compensated for by an increase in

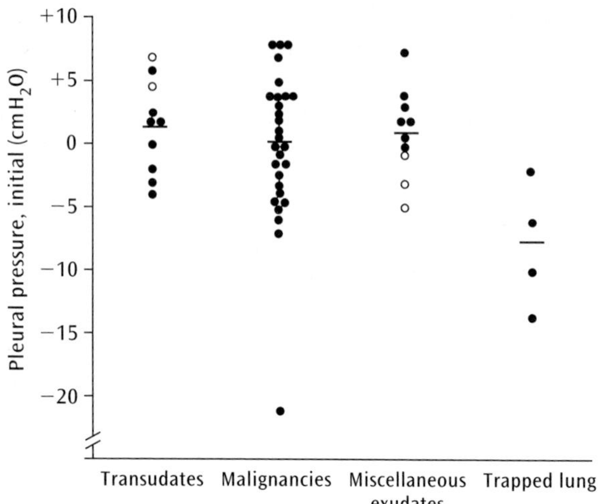

Figure 6.1 Initial pleural pressures for 52 patients at the time of thoracentesis. Each patient is represented by a single point. The open circles in the category of transudates represent the patients with hepatic hydrothorax. The closed circles in the category of miscellaneous exudates represent patients with pleural infection. Reprinted with permission from Reference 2.

the volume of the lung and/or a decrease in the volume of the hemithorax. When the volume of either of these structures changes in these directions, there must be a decrease in the pleural pressure. When the pleural pressure is monitored during pleural fluid removal, there is tremendous variability from patient to patient.[2,3] The pleural space elastance has been defined as the change in pleural pressure (cmH_2O) divided by the amount of fluid removed (liters).[2] The larger this number, the greater the pressure change. In our original series, the pleural space elastance varied from 2 to >150 cmH_2O/L with a mean elastance of approximately 15 cmH_2O.[2] Patients with trapped lungs due to malignancy or benign disease had pleural space elastances that exceeded 25 cmH_2O. Villena *et al.*[3] reported similar values for pleural space elastances. If one looks at the plot of the pleural pressures versus the volume of fluid removed (Figure 6.2), the elastance (the negative slope of the line) tends to be higher during the latter part of the thoracentesis.[2,3]

Measurement of the pleural pressure can be useful clinically. The demonstration of a pleural elastance greater than 25 cmH_2O can be used to establish the diagnosis of trapped lung.[2,3] It has also been suggested that thoracentesis can continue safely as long as the pleural pressure is greater than −20 cmH_2O.[2,3] Indeed, on several occasions I have removed more than 5000 mL pleural fluid from patients when the pleural pressure remained above −20 cmH_2O and the patients suffered no ill consequences. Feller-Kopman *et al.*[5] have shown that there is no relationship between the amount of pleural fluid withdrawn during a thoracentesis and the development of symptoms. However, patients who develop chest discomfort during thoracentesis have a significantly lower pleural pressure than do patients who were asymptomatic or who developed cough.

Measurements of the pleural space elastance appear to be useful in predicting whether or not a pleurodesis will be successful.[6] The theory is that if the pleural pressure falls rapidly when fluid is removed from the pleural space, then the creation of a pleurodesis is unlikely because it will be difficult to keep the two pleural surfaces together (which is necessary to create a pleurodesis). Lan *et al.*[6] measured the change in pleural pressure after 500 mL of pleural fluid had been withdrawn in 65 patients with a pleural malignancy. They then inserted a chest tube and continued to drain the effusion until: (a) the drainage was less than 150 mL per day; (b) the drainage was less than 250 mL per day for four consecutive days; or (c) the drainage had continued for 10 days. After one of the above three criteria was met, they attempted pleurodesis if the lung had expanded.

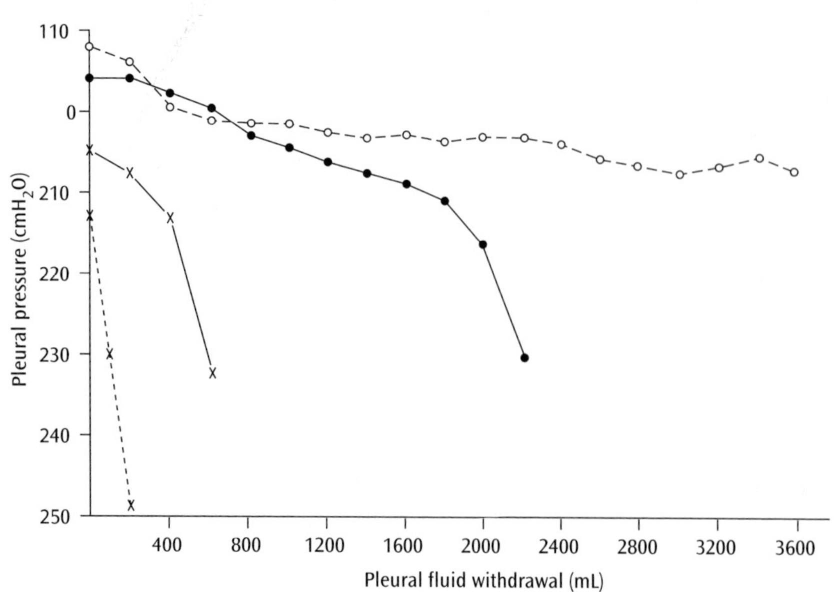

Figure 6.2 The relationship between the pleural pressure and the amount of pleural fluid withdrawn in two patients with malignancy (circles) and two patients with trapped lung (Xs). Reprinted with permission from Reference 2.

They reported that the lung did not re-expand (trapped lung) in 11 of the 14 patients that had a pleural elastance greater than 19 cmH_2O. Pleurodesis was attempted in the other three patients with a high pleural elastance and it failed in all three. In contrast, only three of 51 patients with pleural elastance less than 19 cmH_2O had a trapped lung, and pleurodesis was successful in 42 of 43 patients (98 percent) who returned for evaluation.[6]

EFFECTS OF EFFUSION ON PULMONARY FUNCTION

The effects of a pleural effusion on pulmonary function are difficult to determine. Many diseases that cause pleural effusions, such as congestive heart failure, malignancy, pneumonia and pulmonary embolism, also affect the pulmonary parenchyma. Therefore, it is difficult to determine what part of the pulmonary dysfunction is caused by the pleural effusion and what part is caused by disease in the underlying lung.

There have been limited studies of the effects of a pleural effusion on the pulmonary function of animals. Krell and Rodarte[7] studied the volume changes in the lung and hemithorax after 200 to 1200 mL pleural fluid was added to the right hemithorax of dogs. They found that the decrease in lung volume at functional residual capacity (FRC) was approximately one-third of the added saline volume, while the decrease in the lung volume at total lung capacity (TLC) was one-fifth of the added saline volume. Consequently, the chest wall volume increased by two-thirds the added saline volume at FRC and by four-fifths of the added saline volume at TLC.[7] At a given esophageal pressure (which is taken as a measure of pleural pressure), the chest wall volume was higher and the lung volume was lower when saline had been added to the hemithorax. There was a larger decrease in the lower lobe volume than in upper lobe volume.[7]

There have been several studies evaluating the pulmonary function of patients with pleural effusions. We performed pulmonary function tests before and 24 hours after thoracentesis in 26 patients from whom a mean of 1740 mL pleural fluid was withdrawn (Table 6.1).[8] We found that the mean forced vital capacity (FVC) and the forced expiratory volume in one second (FEV_1) each increased approximately 400 mL. In other words, for every 1000 mL pleural fluid removed, the FVC and FEV_1 improve approximately 200 mL. In this study the TLC increased almost twice as much as did the FVC or FEV_1. This is in contrast to the dog study outlined above where the TLC was affected less than the FRC. One possible explanation for the varying results in humans and in dogs is that in humans the lower lobe is frequently completely atelectatic when a large pleural effusion is present. When fluid is then removed, the lower lobe re-expands and the residual volume in the reexpanded lobe increases the TLC more than just the increase in the vital capacity of that lobe.

Although there is approximately a 20 mL increase in the FVC for every 100 mL of pleural fluid withdrawn, there is much inter-individual variability (Figure 6.3). Changes in the FVC are related to pressure measurements during thoracentesis.[8] Patients with higher initial pleural pressures and patients with smaller changes in the pleural pressure as fluid is removed are more likely to have larger increases in their vital capacity. Nevertheless, even by taking into consideration the amount of fluid removed, the initial pleural pressure and the pleural elastance, the multiple regression coefficient with the FVC as the dependent variable never exceeded 0.60. This indicates that less than 40 percent of the variance in the change in the FVC was related to the amount of fluid removed and the measures of pleural pressure. Possible explanations for the poor correlation are: (a) the pulmonary function testing was not performed until 24 hours after the thoracentesis and the fluid might have reaccumulated to a variable degree during this time period; (b) the pleural pressure changes recorded reflected the elastance of the pleural space during the thoracentesis and if the lung had been atelectatic for a prolonged period, it may take several hours or days for the lung to re-expand; and (c) in some patients with large effusions, there is mediastinal shift to the opposite side, but this does not always occur with malignancy because of fixation of the mediastinum by the malignant process.[8]

Estenne and colleagues[9] measured the changes in respiratory mechanics in nine patients 2 hours after the removal of a mean 1818 mL pleural fluid. They reported a mean increase of 300 mL in the vital capacity, which was

Table 6.1 Mean pulmonary functions baseline and 24 hours after therapeutic thoracentesis

Test	Before	After	Change ± SEM
FVC (mL), $n = 26$	2060	2470	410 ± 76[a]
FEV_1 (mL), $n = 26$	1360	1640	380 ± 55[a]
TLC (mL), $n = 12$	4580	5280	700 ± 196[a]
Sgaw, $n = 12$	0.18	0.14	−0.04 ± 0.02
DLCO, $n = 9$	13.4	14.1	0.7 ± 0.70

FVC, forced vital capacity; FEV_1, forced expiratory volume in 1 second; TLC, total lung capacity; Sgaw, specific airway conductance; DLCO, diffusion capacity of the lung.
[a]$p < 0.001$.

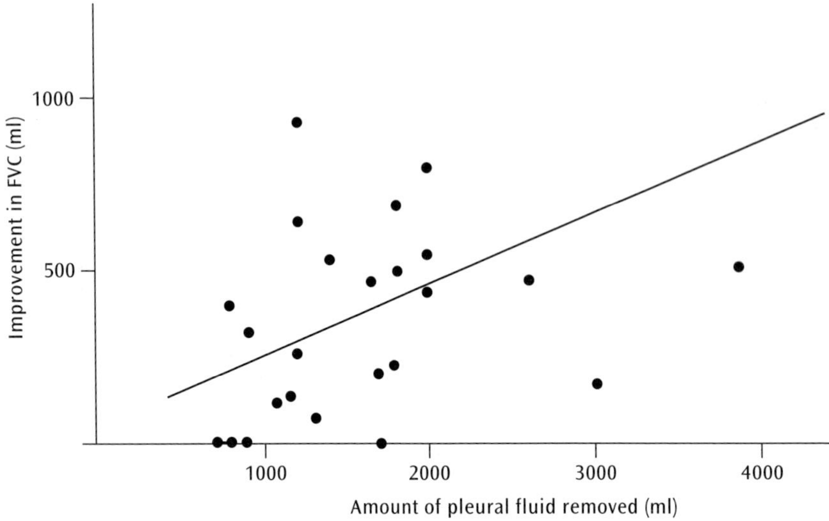

Figure 6.3 Relationship between the amount of pleural fluid removed during thoracentesis and the improvement in the forced vital capacity (FVC) 24 hours after thoracentesis. Reprinted with permission from Reference 8.

similar to what we reported. They also found that the TLC increased approximately twice as much as did the FVC.[9] In addition, they studied the maximal pressures generated by the inspiratory muscles and found that the pressures were much greater post thoracentesis at a given lung volume. The greater inspiratory pressures were attributed to a decrease in the thoracic cage volume.[9] For example, the maximal inspiratory pressure (MIP) at TLC was $-16\ cmH_2O$ before thoracentesis and increased to $-25\ cmH_2O$ after thoracentesis, while the highest MIP went from $-41\ cmH_2O$ before thoracentesis to $-52\ cmH_2O$ post thoracentesis.[9] I believe that relief of the downward displacement of the diaphragm by the pleural fluid is probably the primary explanation for the improvement in the ability of the patient to generate more negative inspiratory pressures after thoracentesis.[10]

Some support for the last statement has been provided by Wang and Tseng.[11] These researchers selected 21 patients who had a pleural effusion and an inverted diaphragm and measured pulmonary function before and 24 hours after the removal of a mean of 1610 mL pleural fluid. They found that the mean FVC increased by 317 mL while the mean FEV_1 increased by 234 mL, which were changes similar to those observed by Estenne *et al.*[9] and our group.[8] Interestingly, the patients in this study were very dyspneic prior to thoracentesis and their dyspnea improved markedly following the thoracentesis. They attributed the decreased dyspnea to the fact that the diaphragm was no longer inverted.

A therapeutic thoracentesis has essentially no effect on the diffusion capacity of the lung (DLCO)[8] or the specific airway conductance.[8,9]

EFFECTS OF EFFUSION ON BLOOD GASES

Although patients with pleural effusions frequently have abnormal arterial blood gas results, the performance of a therapeutic thoracentesis has relatively little effect on the arterial blood gas results.

When experimental bilateral pleural effusions were induced in pigs, there was a mild decrease in the partial pressure of arterial O_2 (PaO_2) while the partial pressure of arterial CO_2 ($PaCO_2$) remained stable as the total amount of pleural fluid was increased to 30 mL/kg (Figure 6.4).[12] However, after the amount of pleural fluid exceeded 30 mL/kg, the PaO_2 dropped precipitously and the $PaCO_2$ started to increase. When the amount of pleural fluid reached 80 mL/kg, the PaO_2 (on 100 percent oxygen) was less than 80 mmHg while the $PaCO_2$ had increased from 34 to 51 mmHg. When the pleural fluid was removed in these normal pigs, the PaO_2 and $PaCO_2$ rapidly returned to normal (Fig. 6.4).[13]

Things seem more complicated in humans. In an early study of 16 patients with pleural effusions, Brandstetter and Cohen[13] obtained blood gases before, and then 20 minutes, two hours and 24 hours after a thoracentesis in which 150 to 1600 mL pleural fluid was removed. They reported that the mean PaO_2 at baseline was 70.4 mmHg, and this decreased significantly to 61.2 mmHg 20 minutes following thoracentesis. In every patient there was a decrease in the PaO_2 over this 20-minute period. The PaO_2 remained significantly reduced at 2 hours (64.4 mmHg) but had returned to baseline 24 hours later. In this study there were no significant changes in the pH or the $PaCO_2$.[13]

The effects of a therapeutic thoracentesis on the blood gases of patients on mechanical ventilation is not clear. In one study[14] a chest tube was placed in 19 patients with acute respiratory distress syndrome (ARDS) who had pleural effusions and refractory hypoxemia.[14] After placement of the chest tube, the compliance of their lungs improved immediately, and 24 hours after insertion of the chest tube, the PaO_2/fraction of inspired air that is O_2 (FIO_2) had improved to 245 ± 29 from 151 ± 13.[14] However, in a second study, nine patients on mechanical

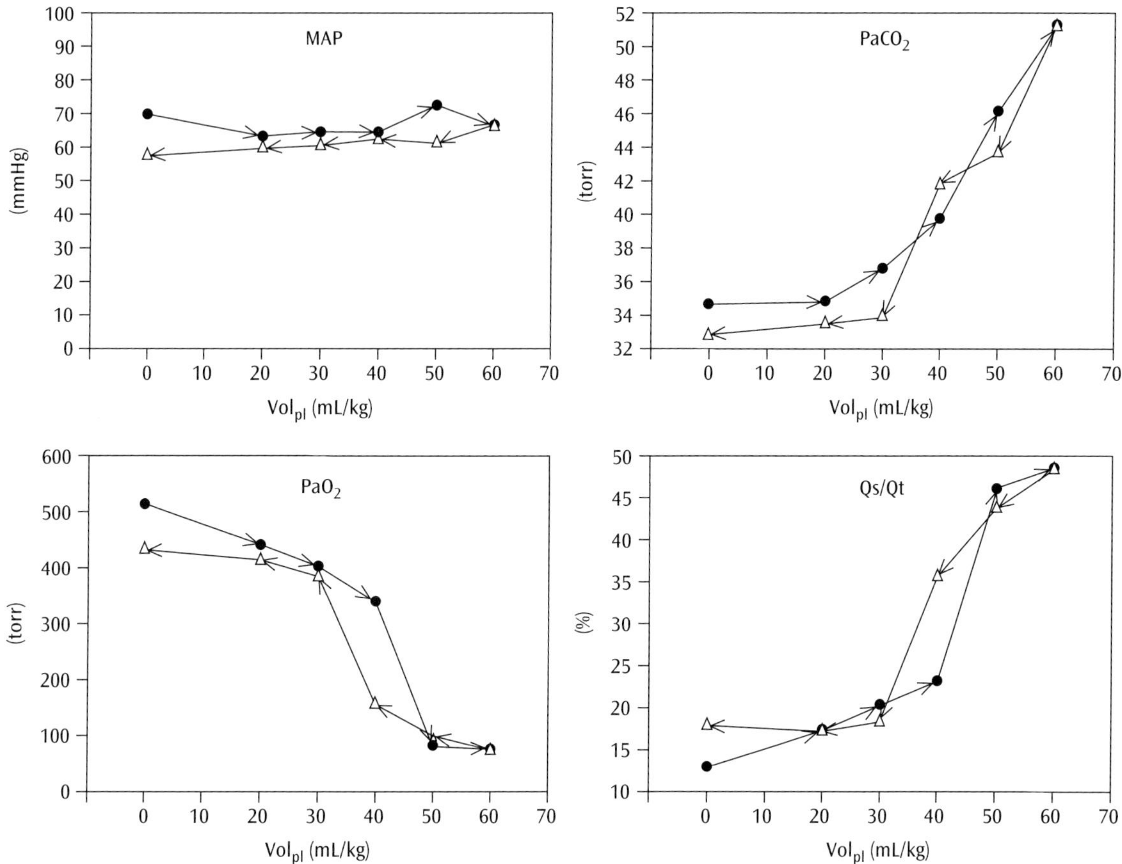

Figure 6.4 Mean arterial pressure (MAP), arterial partial pressure of O_2 and CO_2 (PaO_2, $PaCO_2$) and intrapulmonary shunt (Qs/Qt) in pigs. Solid circles indicate increasing intrapleural volume (Vol$_{pl}$) and open triangles indicate decreasing Vol$_{pl}$. Reprinted with permission from Reference 12.

ventilation were subjected to a therapeutic thoracentesis (mean 1495 mL pleural fluid) and immediately after thoracentesis there was no significant change in the lung compliance or the alveolar–arterial oxygen gradient ($AaPO_2$).[15] The dissimilar results in the two studies may be due to the time the measurements were obtained or the poorer oxygenation status of the patients in the first study.

Agusti *et al.*[16] attempted to determine the mechanisms for the hypoxemia associated with pleural effusions and the effects of thoracentesis on the hypoxemia by studying the oxygenation status of nine patients before and immediately after thoracentesis (mean 693 ± 424 mL) with the multiple inert gas technique. They reported that the mean difference in the $AaPO_2$ was 29 mmHg before thoracentesis and remained at 29 mmHg post thoracentesis. These investigators also showed that the main mechanism underlying arterial hypoxemia in patients with pleural effusion is an intrapulmonary shunt, which does not change significantly after thoracentesis.

There have been four separate studies that examined the effects of position on the oxygenation status of patients with pleural effusions.[17–20] In each of the four studies the oxygenation status was slightly better when the patients were positioned with the side of the effusion superior (Table 6.2). The improvement was thought to be due to gravity distributing more blood to the lung that was not partially compressed by the pleural effusion. However, the differences in the mean levels of the oxygenation were not statistically significant in any of the studies and are probably not clinically significant either.

Table 6.2 Effects of position on oxygenation status of patients with pleural effusion

Study	*n*	Effusion side down	Effusion side up
Sonnenblick *et al.*[17]	8	66.7 ± 8.7 mmHg (PO_2)	71.9 ± 9.3 mmHg (PO_2)
Chang *et al.*[19]	21	66.0 ± 66.0 mmHg (PO_2)	69.6 ± 14.6 mmHg (PO_2)
Romero *et al.*[20]	33	78.0 ± 12.5 mmHg (PO_2)	81.4 ± 8.5 mmHg (PO_2)
Neagley *et al.*[18]	10	93.4 ± 2.1% (SaO_2)	94.7 ± 2.1% (SaO_2)

PO_2, partial pressure of O_2; SaO_2, arterial O_2 saturation.

EFFECTS OF EFFUSION ON EXERCISE TOLERANCE

There has been limited research on the effects of a pleural effusion on the exercise tolerance of patients. We obtained maximum exercise tests on 15 patients before and after they underwent a therapeutic thoracentesis. The symptom-limited exercise tests were conducted on a bicycle ergometer with 15 watt increments every minute.[21,22] The mean age of the patients was 64.7 and most of them had malignant pleural effusions. Pre-thoracentesis, the mean FEV_1 and FVC were only 43 ± 17 percent and 49 ± 17 percent of predicted, respectively. Seven of the 15 had obstructive lung disease, as reflected by an FEV_1/FVC ratio of less than 0.70.

The exercise tolerance of these elderly patients was significantly reduced prior to the thoracentesis. The mean maximum workload prior to thoracentesis was only 79 watts (43 percent of predicted) while the mean maximum oxygen consumption per minute ($\dot{V}O_2$) was only 907 mL/minute (37 percent of predicted) (Table 6.3). When the individual exercise tests were examined, the explanation for the reduced exercise tolerance was not obvious. Eight of the patients appeared to be ventilatory limited (minute ventilation at maximum exercise [$\dot{V}_E$ max] greater than 80 percent of predicted maximum at exhaustion), and four of these also appeared to be cardiac limited (maximum heart rate greater than 80 percent of predicted at exhaustion). There were two additional patients who appeared to be only cardiac limited. At the maximum tolerated workload (Emax) the remaining five patients appeared to be neither ventilatory nor cardiac limited. In general, the patients' ventilation was inefficient, as shown by their high ventilatory equivalents for oxygen ($\dot{V}_E/\dot{V}O_2$) and carbon dioxide ($\dot{V}_E/\dot{V}CO_2$) (Table 6.3). In addition, the patients' cardiac function appeared to be impaired, as indicated by the high resting pulse (Table 6.3) and the reduced oxygen pulse (O_2 pulse), which is a reflection of the stroke volume.

The performance of a therapeutic thoracentesis (mean 1612 mL) had relatively little influence on the exercise tolerance of the 15 patients (Table 6.3). Although the mean FEV_1 and FVC both improved significantly (Table 6.3), there was no significant change in the maximum workload or the mean maximum oxygen consumption per minute ($\dot{V}O_2$max). Overall, after thoracentesis, five patients had an improvement in their workload, five patients had a decrease in the workload and five patients had no change in the workload. The change in exercise capacity was not significantly correlated with the amount of fluid removed or with the changes in pleural pressure. However, there was a significant correlation between changes in the $\dot{V}O_2$max and changes in the FEV_1 ($r = 0.576$, $p < 0.05$), changes in the FVC ($r = 0.610$, $p < 0.05$) and changes in the maximum O_2 pulse ($r = 0.78$, $p < 0.05$).

In summary, based on this series, elderly patients with moderate to large pleural effusions have a marked reduction in their exercise capacity. The lung function, as reflected by the FEV_1 and the FVC, and the cardiac function, as reflected by the O_2 pulse, are both reduced and contribute to the exercise limitation. However, the performance of a therapeutic thoracentesis does not result in a significant improvement in exercise tolerance of many patients.

EFFECTS OF EFFUSION ON THE DIAPHRAGM

When pleural fluid is present, the diaphragm on the side of the effusion is profoundly affected by the weight of the fluid on the diaphragm. The changes in the diaphragm have been classified into three categories by Mulvey[23]

Table 6.3 Results of maximal exercise tests before and after a therapeutic thoracentesis in 15 patients from whom a mean of 1612 mL pleural fluid was removed

	Pre	Post	Change	*p*
FEV_1, L (%pred)	1.56 ± 0.63 (43%)	1.74 ± 0.69 (47%)	0.18 ± 0.23	0.007
FVC, L (%pred)	2.32 ± 0.76 (49%)	2.63 ± 0.81 (56%)	0.31 ± 0.43	0.013
Max Work, watts (%pred)	77.7 ± 44.5 (43%)	79.0 ± 40.7 (44%)	1.3 ± 19.4	0.794
$\dot{V}O_2$ max, mL/min (%pred)	992 ± 431 (41%)	1038 ± 395 (43%)	46 ± 226	0.449
$\dot{V}_E$ max, L/min (%pred)	45.1 ± 20.2 (79%)	48.2 ± 18.8 (77%)	3.1 ± 11.8	0.321
$\dot{V}_E/\dot{V}O_2$ max (%pred)	46.1 ± 9.9 (158%)	47.3 ± 12.0 (162%)	1.2 ± 5.2	0.394
$\dot{V}_E/\dot{V}CO_2$ max (%pred)	45.6 ± 7.4 (172%)	44.7 ± 8.1 (1.68%)	−0.9 ± 4.7	0.454
HR rest, bpm	93.4 ± 16.6	93.6 ± 17.2	0.2 ± 12.9	0.953
HR max, bpm (%pred)	120.7 ± 15.6 (78%)	114.6 ± 17.3 (74%)	−6.1 ± 10.6	0.049
O_2 pulse rest, mL/beat	3.28 ± 0.72	3.38 ± 0.53	0.11 ± 0.67	0.547
O_2 pulse SW, mL/beat	8.02 ± 2.94	8.59 ± 2.68	0.58 ± 1.14	0.083
O_2 pulse max, mL/beat (%pred)	8.21 ± 2.99 (61%)	9.04 ± 3.00 (67%)	0.83 ± 1.57	0.070

FEV_1, forced expiratory volume in 1 second; FVC, forced vital capacity; $\dot{V}O_2$, oxygen consumption per minute; $\dot{V}_E$ max, minute ventilation at maximum exercise; $\dot{V}CO_2$, CO_2 respired per minute.

based on the findings on the plain film and fluoroscopy. In the first, or least severe category, the hemidiaphragm is domed and functions normally. Patients in this category are usually asymptomatic even though the effusion may be large. In the second category, the diaphragm is flattened and does not move with respiration. Patients in this category frequently complain of dyspnea, which is likely to be relieved with a therapeutic thoracentesis. In the third category, the diaphragm is inverted and there may be paradoxical movements on respiration. Patients in this category usually have severe dyspnea that is markedly relieved with a therapeutic thoracentesis.

The percentage of patients in each of the three categories has not been studied carefully. It is likely that inversion of the diaphragm may be more common than is generally realized. Wang and Tseng[11] were able to document diaphragmatic inversion in 21 patients over a 3-year period. Interestingly, when these patients underwent therapeutic thoracentesis they experienced marked relief of their dyspnea.

EFFECTS OF EFFUSION ON THE HEART

The presence of pleural fluid may also adversely influence cardiac function because the increase in the pleural pressure can decrease the distending pressures of the heart chambers. Vaska *et al.*[24] studied seven spontaneously breathing dogs with a two-dimensional echocardiograph during infusions of saline into both pleural spaces. They reported that right ventricular diastolic collapse began when the mean pleural pressure increased by 5 mmHg. When the méan pleural pressure had increased by 15 mmHg, the stroke volume had fallen by nearly 50 percent and the cardiac output had fallen by 33 percent.[24] In contrast, Nishida *et al.*[12] reported that the infusion of 20 mL/kg saline into each pleural space had no effect on the cardiac output in anesthetized pigs. It should be noted that Vaska *et al.*[24] infused more than 50 mL/kg into the pleural spaces of their dogs.

It appears that the presence of a large effusion frequently adversely affects cardiac function. In a study of 27 patients who had more than a hemithorax occupied by pleural fluid, Traylor *et al.*[25] reported that eight subjects had elevated jugular venous pressure, eight had pulsus paradoxus, six had right ventricular diastolic collapse and 23 had flow velocity paradoxus. Post thoracentesis or chest tube placement, all these abnormalities resolved in all patients but one in whom only 900 mL pleural fluid was withdrawn.[25] Sadaniantz *et al.*[26] reviewed the echocardiograms of 116 patients with pleural effusion and observed cardiac chamber collapse in 21 (18 percent). All had right atrial collapse while one had concomitant right ventricular collapse, four had left atrial collapse and none had left ventricular collapse.[26] Of the 21 patients with chamber collapse, 13 had large, three had moderate, two had small and three had unknown amounts of left pleural effusion (no chest X-ray).[26] It was unusual to have chamber collapse with isolated right pleural effusion. Hemodynamics were studied in 22 mechanically ventilated patients with moderate to large pleural effusions before and after they underwent drainage of the effusions with a pigtail catheter by Ahmed *et al.*[27] They reported that the mean cardiac output increased from 7.7 to 8.4 L/minute, but that this change was not statistically significant. However, the pulmonary capillary wedge pressure and the central venous pressure both decreased significantly after the pleural fluid was drained.

There have been three reports of patients with compromised cardiac output attributed to large pleural effusions.[28–30] Negus *et al.*[28] reported a 60-year-old woman who presented with a large left sided pleural effusion with marked mediastinal shift to the right. Shortly after presentation, her blood pressure became unobtainable and her carotid and femoral pulses were very weak. When a chest tube was placed and 1125 mL of pleural fluid was withdrawn, the blood pressure rose to 140/86 and the pulses became bounding.[28]. Kisanuki *et al.*[29] reported a 68-year-old man who presented with a blood pressure of 90/60 and a large left encapsulated pleural effusion. A two-dimensional echocardiogram revealed that the pleural effusion compressed the lateral wall of the left ventricle. With M-mode echocardiogram, the left ventricular collapse was observed throughout diastole. After drainage of 500 mL of pleural fluid, the blood pressure rose from 90/60 to 120/80 and the left ventricular collapse during diastole resolved.[29] Kopterides *et al.*[30] reported two patients who had hemodynamic compromise with large left-sided effusions in whom left ventricular diastolic collapse was demonstrated by transthoracic echocardiograph. It is interesting that all four of the patients in the above three reports had left sided effusions. It is probable that the increased pleural pressure resulting from the pleural fluid is responsible for the decreased cardiac output.

EFFECTS OF PNEUMOTHORAX ON PLEURAL PRESSURE

When a pneumothorax is present, the pleural pressure increases as it does with the presence of a pleural effusion. However, with a pneumothorax, the pressure is the same throughout the entire pleural space. In contrast, with a pleural effusion there is a gradient in the pleural pressure due to the hydrostatic column of fluid so that the pleural pressure in the dependent part of the hemithorax is much greater than it is in the superior part of the hemithorax. Another way to look at this is that with a pneumothorax the lung sinks to the bottom of the hemithorax because it is heavier than air, while with a pleural effusion, the lung rises to the top of the hemithorax because it is lighter than fluid and is floating in the fluid. The net result is that with a pneumothorax, the upper lobe is affected more than the lower lobe while with a pleural effusion the lower lobe is affected more than the upper lobes.

EFFECTS OF PNEUMOTHORAX ON PULMONARY FUNCTION

When there is a communication between the alveoli and the pleural space or between the ambient air and the pleural space, air will enter the pleural space because the pleural pressure is normally negative.[10] As air enters the pleural space, the pleural pressure gradually increases. Air will continue to enter the pleural space until the pleural pressure becomes zero or the communication is closed. Since both the hemithorax and the lung are distensible objects whose volume depends upon their distending pressure, the hemithorax will enlarge while the lung will become smaller as the pleural pressure increases due to air entering the pleural space.

Since patients with significant pneumothoraces are usually symptomatic, there is a dearth of information available concerning their pulmonary function. In general, when a pneumothorax is present, the increase in the volume of the hemithorax is less than the decrease in the volume of the lung. For example, if a volume of air equal to 33 percent of the vital capacity is introduced into the pleural space, the volume of the lung will decrease by 25 percent of the vital capacity while the volume of the hemithorax will increase by 8 percent of the vital capacity (Figure 6.5).[10]

EFFECTS OF PNEUMOTHORAX ON BLOOD GASES

The presence of a pneumothorax adversely affects the oxygenation status in experimental animals. When Rutherford *et al.*[31] induced pneumothoraces in 10 awake, standing dogs with the intrapleural administration of 50 mL/kg N_2, the mean PaO_2 fell from 86 ± 6 mmHg to 51 ± 5 mmHg. When a tension pneumothorax is produced in animals breathing room air spontaneously, there is a profound deterioration in the oxygenation status. In one study in goats the mean PaO_2 fell from 85 to 28 mmHg, while in monkeys the PaO_2 fell from 90 to 22 mmHg before the animals became apneic.[32] There was a linear reduction in the PaO_2 as the volume of pleural air was increased.[32] The reduction in the PaO_2 appeared to be caused by the continued perfusion of the side with the pneumothorax despite decreased ventilation.[31] The cardiac output was relatively well preserved in the animals with a tension pneumothorax.[32] Anthonisen[33] reported that the lung underlying a pneumothorax in humans demonstrated uniform airway closure at low lung volumes, and suggested that airway closure is the chief cause of ventilation maldistribution in spontaneous pneumothorax. When the air is evacuated from the pleural space in experimental animals, the oxygenation status returns to normal almost immediately.[31]

The presence of a pneumothorax in humans also adversely affects the blood gases. In one study of 12 patients,[34] the PaO_2 was below 80 mmHg in nine (75 percent) and was below 55 mmHg in two patients. In this same series, 10 of the 12 patients had an increased $AaPO_2$. Not unexpectedly, patients with secondary spontaneous pneumothorax and patients with a larger pneumothorax tend to have a lower PaO_2.[34] In the VA cooperative pneumothorax study, blood gases were obtained in 118 patients with spontaneous pneumothorax. In these patients the mean PaO_2 was below 55 mmHg in 20 (17 percent) and below 45 in five (4 percent), while the mean $PaCO_2$ exceeded 50 mmHg in 19 (16 percent) exceeded 60 mmHg

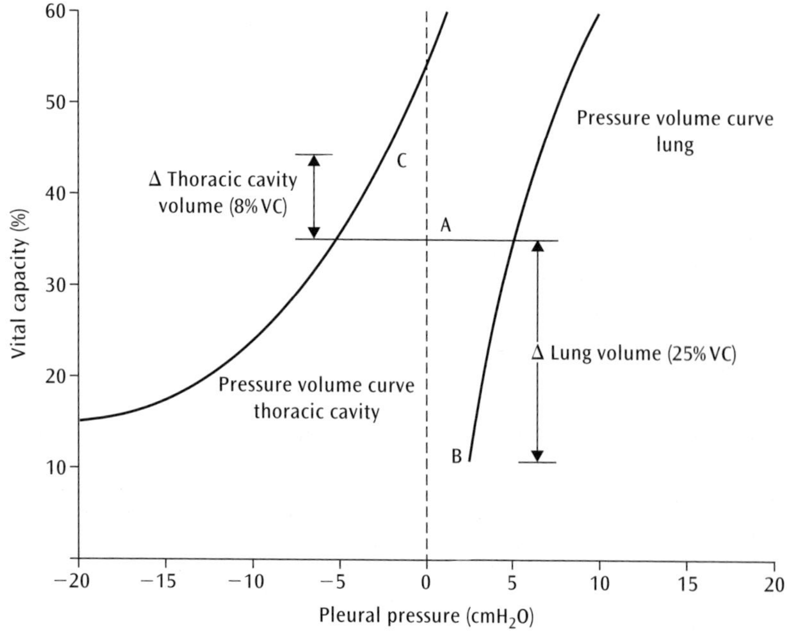

Figure 6.5 Influence of a pneumothorax on the volumes of the lung and hemithorax. In this example, enough air entered the pleural space to increase the pleural pressure from −5.0 to −2.5 cmH_2O. The end-expiratory volume of the lung moved from point A to point B, which represents a volume change equal to 25 percent of the vital capacity. The end-expiratory volume of the hemithorax moved from point A to point C, which represents a volume change equal to 8 percent of the vital capacity. VC, vital capacity. Reprinted with permission from Reference 10.

in five (4 percent).[35] Of course, the abnormalities in the blood gases may have been due at least in part to the underlying lung disease in this study.[35]

When the air is evacuated from patients with a pneumothorax, the oxygenation levels return to normal more slowly than they do in the experimental animals. Norris *et al.*[34] reported that in patients with an initial anatomic shunt above 20 percent, there was a reduction of at least 10 percent in their shunt 30–90 minutes after tube thoracostomy was performed. Nevertheless, all patients had a shunt above 5 percent at 90 minutes. Moreover, three additional patients with anatomic shunts between 10 and 20 percent had no change in their shunt when the air was removed.[34]

EFFECTS OF PNEUMOTHORAX ON DIAPHRAGMATIC FUNCTION

To my knowledge, there have been no studies evaluating the effects of a pneumothorax on diaphragmatic function. I would anticipate that the presence of a pneumothorax would have less effect on the diaphragmatic function than would a pleural effusion of comparable volume, since the pleural pressure would increase much more with the pleural fluid. The diaphragmatic inversion, which is seen relatively frequently with a pleural effusion, is not seen with pneumothorax. With a tension pneumothorax, the diaphragm may be displaced inferiorly due to the increased pleural pressure but the functional significance of this displacement is not known.

EFFECTS OF PNEUMOTHORAX ON EXERCISE TOLERANCE

There have been no studies on the effects of a pneumothorax on the exercise tolerance of either animals or man. However, it would be anticipated that the exercise tolerance would be markedly impaired since many patients are dyspneic at rest.

EFFECTS OF PNEUMOTHORAX ON CARDIAC FUNCTION

The presence of a small to moderate pneumothorax has very little influence on cardiac function. When Moran *et al.*[32] introduced 50 mL/kg N_2 into the pleural spaces of dogs, the cardiac output was not significantly affected. However, when tension pneumothoraces are induced in mechanically ventilated animals, there is a marked reduction in cardiac output. Carvalho *et al.*[36] produced right-sided tension pneumothoraces with mean pleural pressures of +10 and +25 cmH_2O in 10 mechanically ventilated adult sheep. In these animals the mean cardiac output fell from 3.5 L/minute to approximately 1.2 L/minute and the mean blood pressure fell from 80 mmHg to less than 40 mmHg. The development of a tension pneumothorax in man is also associated with impaired hemodynamics. Beards and Lipman[37] recorded the hemodynamics of three patients who developed a tension pneumothorax while on mechanical ventilation. The mean cardiac outputs, which were 7.3, 4.8 and 3.6 L/minute/m^2 at baseline, fell to 3.0, 3.1 and 1.4 L/minute/m^2 with the development of the tension pneumothorax. In a similar manner, the mean arterial pressures that were 97, 96 and 68 mmHg fell to 33, 68 and 57 mmHg, respectively. The probable mechanism for the decreased cardiac output is decreased venous return due to the increased pleural pressures.

KEY POINTS

- When fluid or air is present in the pleural space, the lung must get smaller or the hemithorax must get larger, or a combination of the two must occur.
- When the patient is upright, the presence of fluid in the pleural space affects mostly the lower lobes while the presence of air in the pleural space affects the upper lobes more than the lower lobes.
- When a thoracentesis is performed, the vital capacity increases by an average of 20 mL for each 100 mL fluid removed, but there is marked inter-individual variation.
- A thoracentesis has variable effects on blood gases.
- The exercise tolerance of many patients with pleural effusion does not improve after a therapeutic thoracentesis.
- The presence of a pleural effusion can lead to diaphragmatic inversion which is associated with marked dyspnea.
- The presence of a pleural effusion can compress the heart and lead to a compromised cardiac output.

REFERENCES

● = Key primary paper
◆ = Major review article

1. Agostoni E, D'Angelo E. Thickness and pressure of the pleural liquid at various heights and with various hydrothoraces. *Respir Physiol* 1969; **6**: 330–42.
●2. Light RW, Jenkinson SG, Minh VD, George RB. Observations on pleural fluid pressures as fluid is withdrawn during thoracentesis. *Am Rev Respir Dis* 1980; **121**: 799–804.
3. Villena V, Lopez-Encuentra A, Pozo F, De-Pablo A, Martin-Escribano P. Measurement of pleural pressure during therapeutic thoracentesis. *Am J Respir Crit Care Med* 2000; **162**: 1534–8.

4. Neff TA, Buchanana BD. Tension pleural effusion: a delayed complication of pneumothorax therapy in tuberculosis. *Am Rev Respir Dis* 1973; **111**: 543–8.
5. Feller-Kopman D, Walkey A, Berkowitz D, *et al.* The relationship of pleural pressure to symptom development during therapeutic thoracentesis. *Chest* 2006; **129**: 1556–60.
●6. Lan RS, Lo SK, Chuang ML, *et al.* Elastance of the pleural space: a predictor for the outcome of pleurodesis in patients with malignant pleural effusion. *Ann Intern Med* 1997; **126**: 768–74.
●7. Krell WS, Rodarte JR. Effects of acute pleural effusion on respiratory system mechanics in dogs. *J Appl Physiol* 1985; **59**: 1458–63.
8. Light RW, Stansbury DW, Brown SE. The relationship between pleural pressures and changes in pulmonary function following therapeutic thoracentesis. *Am Rev Respir Dis* 1986; **133**: 658–61.
9. Estenne M, Yernault J-C, De Troyer A. Mechanism of relief of dyspnea after thoracocentesis in patients with large pleural effusions. *Am J Med* 1983; **74**: 813–9.
◆10. Light RW. *Pleural diseases*, 5th edn. Baltimore: Lippincott, Williams and Wilkins, 2007.
●11. Wang JS, Tseng CH. Changes in pulmonary mechanics and gas exchange after thoracentesis on patients with inversion of a hemidiaphragm secondary to large pleural effusion. *Chest* 1995; **107**: 1610–14.
●12. Nishida O, Arellano R, Cheng DC, DeMajo W, Kavanagh BP. Gas exchange and hemodynamics in experimental pleural effusion. *Crit Care Med* 1999; **27**: 583–7.
●13. Brandstetter RD, Cohen RP. Hypoxemia after thoracentesis: a predictable and treatable condition. *J Am Med Assoc* 1979; **242**: 1060–61.
14. Talmor M, Hydo L, Gershenwald JG, Barie PS. Beneficial effects of chest tube drainage of pleural effusion in acute respiratory failure refractory to positive end-expiratory pressure ventilation. *Surgery* 1998; **123**: 137–43.
15. Doelken P, Abreu R, Sahn SA, *et al.* Effect of thoracentesis on respiratory mechanics and gas exchange in the patient receiving mechanical ventilation. *Chest* 2006; **130**: 1354–61.
16. Agusti AG, Cardus J, Roca J, *et al.* Ventilation-perfusion mismatch in patients with pleural effusion: effects of thoracentesis. *Am J Respir Crit Care Med* 1997; **156**: 1205–9.
17. Sonnenblick M, Melzer E, Rosin AJ. Body positional effect on gas exchange in unilateral pleural effusion. *Chest* 1983; **83**: 784–6.
18. Neagley SR, Zwillich CW. The effect of positional changes on oxygenation in patients with pleural effusions. *Chest* 1985; **88**: 714–17.
19. Chang SC, Shiao GM, Perng RP. Postural effect on gas exchange in patients with unilateral pleural effusions. *Chest* 1989; **96**: 60–3.
20. Romero S, Martin C, Hernandez L, *et al.* Effect of body position on gas exchange in patients with unilateral pleural effusion: influence of effusion volume. *Respir Med* 1995; **89**: 297–301.
21. Shinto RA, Stansbury DW, Brown SE, Light RW. Does therapeutic thoracentesis improve the exercise capacity of patients with pleural effusion? *Am Rev Respir Dis* 1987; **135**: A244.
22. Shinto RA, Stansbury DW, Fischer CE, Light RW. The effect of thoracentesis on central respiratory drive in patients with large pleural effusions. *Am Rev Respir Dis* 1988; **137**: A112.
●23. Mulvey RB. The effect of pleural fluid on the diaphragm. *Radiology* 1965; **84**: 1080–86.
●24. Vaska K, Wann LS, Sagar K, Klopfenstein HS. Pleural effusion as a cause of right ventricular diastolic collapse. *Circulation* 1992; **86**: 609–17.
25. Traylor JJ, Chan K, Wong I, *et al.* Large pleural effusions producing signs of cardiac tamponade resolved by thoracentesis. *Am J Cardiol* 2002; **89**: 106–8.
26. Sadaniantz A, Anastacio R, Verma V, *et al.* The incidence of diastolic right atrial collapse in patients with pleural effusion in the absence of pericardial effusion. *Echocardiography* 2003; **20**: 211–15.
27. Ahmed SH, Ouzounian SP, Dirusso S, *et al.* Hemodynamic and pulmonary changes after drainage of significant pleural effusions in critically ill, mechanically ventilated surgical patients. *J Trauma* 2004; **57**: 1184–8.
28. Negus RA, Chachkes JS, Wrenn K. Tension hydrothorax and shock in a patient with a malignant pleural effusion. *Am J Emerg Med* 1990; **8**: 205–7.
29. Kisanuki A, Shono H, Kiyonaga K, *et al.* Two-dimensional echocardiographic demonstration of left ventricular diastolic collapse due to compression by pleural effusion. *Am Heart J* 1991; **122**: 1173–5.
30. Kopterides P, Lignos M, Papanikolaou S, *et al.* Pleural effusion causing cardiac tamponade. Report of two cases and review of the literature. *Heart Lung* 2006; **35**: 66–7.
●31. Rutherford RB, Hurt HH, Brickman RD, Tubb JM. The pathophysiology of progressive, tension pneumothorax. *J Trauma* 1968; **8**: 212–27.
32. Moran JF, Jones RH, Wolfe WG. Regional pulmonary function during experimental unilateral pneumothorax in the awake state. *J Thorac Surg* 1977; **74**: 396–402.
33. Anthonisen NR. Regional function in spontaneous pneumothorax. *Am Rev Respir Dis* 1977; **115**: 873–6.
34. Norris RM, Jones JG, Bishop JM. Respiratory gas exchange in patients with spontaneous pneumothorax. *Thorax* 1968; **23**: 427–33.
35. Light RW, O'Hara VS, Moritz TE, *et al.* Intrapleural tetracycline for the prevention of recurrent spontaneous pneumothorax. *J Am Med Assoc* 1990; **264**: 2224–30.
36. Carvalho P, Hilderbrandt J, Charan NB. Changes in bronchial and pulmonary arterial blood flow with progressive tension pneumothorax. *J Appl Physiol* 1996; **81**: 1664–9.
37. Beards SC, Lipman J. Decreased cardiac index as an indicator of tension pneumothorax in the ventilated patient. *Anaesthesia* 1994; **49**: 137–41.

7

Pleural inflammation and infection

VEENA B ANTONY, BRENDAN F BELLEW

INTRODUCTION

The pleural mesothelium is a monolayer of cells that may vary in shape from flattened ovoid to columnar or cuboidal. The mesothelium adheres to a basement membrane that comprises a matrix of connective tissue.[1] The basement membrane of the pleura is a complex structure that plays an important role in inflammation of the pleural space.[2] The visceral pleura is nourished by a large network of capillaries that originate from the bronchial arteries. The parietal and diaphragmatic surfaces of the pleura are supplied by the blood vessels local to those areas. Together, the visceral, parietal and diaphragmatic surfaces of the pleura form a closed boundary around the pleural space. Under normal conditions the volume of fluid in the pleural space is very small, in the range of 0.2–0.5 mL. The pleural space may expand to accommodate much larger volumes under certain conditions, such as pleural effusion. Although the pleural space is drained by lymphatic vessels, they are not present in large numbers. Indeed, the lymphatic vessels draining the pleural space may grow in size and number according to need.[3] Among the lymph nodes that drain pleural structures are the mediastinal, intercostal and sternal lymph nodes. Normally, pleural fluid is characterized by low protein concentration and low cellularity with an absence of inflammatory cells.[4]

The development of pleural infections depends on the balance between immune pleural responses and the virulence of the organism. Pleural infections were recognized over 300 years ago and pleural empyema was described in great detail in 1685 by Thomas Willis.[5] Sources of pleural infection may be several. A classic mechanism whereby organisms enter the pleural space is pneumonia, where the invasion of the alveolar air space by organisms is followed by a breach of the pleural barrier with the development of parapneumonic effusions. Other mechanisms where the pleura may be contaminated by infecting organisms are the rupture of subpleural tuberculous foci or granuloma, or dissemination of infectious particles and toxins via the bloodstream. Intra-abdominal infections may enter the pleural space through the diaphragm and penetrating injury to the chest wall may also result in introduction of organisms into the pleura. A devastating and dangerous form of pleural infection is seen in Boerhaave's syndrome where there is rupture of the esophagus and contamination of the pleural space with mouth and stomach flora.

Upon infection, the microorganism is recognized by the pleural mesothelial cell which remains the first line of defense. Pleural responses to infection include those of innate immunity as well as adaptive or acquired immunity. Innate immunity was formerly thought to be a nonspecific immune response characterized by engulfment and digestion of microorganisms by mucosal cells, mesothelial cells, macrophages and other leukocytes. It is now recognized that innate immunity possesses specificity. Also, mesothelial cells and other phagocytic cells are capable of discriminating between pathogens and self. Importantly, innate immune responses and acquired immune responses are closely linked and innate immune responses can be a prerequisite for the presence of adaptive immunity.[6] In this review, we consider both innate immune responses and acquired immune responses against invading organisms in the pleural space as well as the virulence factors that contribute to the establishment of an infection.

MICROBIAL VIRULENCE FACTORS

The capacity of an organism to cause pleural inflammation and disease is often determined by its ability to produce a variety of virulence factors.[7] The first step in this process is the adherence of the microorganism to the pleural mesothelial surface.[8] However, if highly virulent and able to produce toxins, the microorganism does not necessarily have to be in contact with the pleural mesothelium to initiate the changes of inflammation.[9] Classically, the attachment process of an organism to the mesothelial monolayer allows it to establish a beachhead from which cell penetration of surface anatomic barriers can occur.[10] Not only do organisms produce toxins that allow them to kill and damage host cells, but organisms such as staphylococci produce factors such as the staphylococcal protein-A which facilitate intracellular survival as well as disarm host defense mechanisms.[11] Among some of the toxins produced by bacteria are the ADP-ribosylating toxins which include exotoxin A produced by *Pseudomonas aeruginosa*, which has the biological effect of inhibiting protein synthesis and causing early cell death of the infected membrane. Other organisms can cause inhibition of signal transduction mediated by G-protein targets.[12] Gram-negative organisms produce toxins which may or may not be released in soluble form, but are sometimes delivered to the target cell while contained in a vesicle of the outer membrane.[13] Other toxins, such as the hemolytic phospholipases, are bacterial exoenzymes that appear to interact with the external surface of host cell membranes by catalyzing their specific reactions and can achieve their toxic effect without entering the cell.[14] *Staphylococcus aureus* and group-A streptococci produce toxins that elicit significant systemic reactions.[15] Streptococcal M-protein and streptococcal enterotoxins share the ability to stimulate T-cells and are thereby designated superantigens. This interaction of superantigens on immune and mesothelial cells cause the production of cytokines such as interleukin-1 (IL-1) and tumor necrosis factor (TNF) and may, in part, be responsible for the subsequent inflammatory changes.[16]

The process of pleural infection is a complex one and involves a concerted effort by microbes to attach to the appropriate surface. This allows them to acquire nutrients, proliferate and survive. Virulence factors may be directed at overcoming the anatomic barrier of the pleura.[17] This allows invasion of the mesothelial cell membrane and paracellular movement of the organism from the alveolar airspace compartment into the pleural space.[18] Virulence factors may be directed at disrupting or avoiding humoral factors, for example by degradation of antibodies, inhibition of lysozymes and assimilation of mesothelial proteins on the microbial surface, or molecular mimicry of the host's own molecular stryctures.[19] A secondary line of pleural mesothelial defense against microbial infection is provided by the humoral factors released by mesothelial cells such as antibodies, complement-induced mediators and other host proteins such as clotting factors, β-lysin and transferrin.[20] Bacterial enzymes can degrade antibodies or modify their own external surface to avoid interaction with these antibodies.[21] Some organisms can elaborate factors that degrade fibrin or other clotting factors and this may be associated with increased virulence.[22]

Once the microbe attaches to the pleural surface, it may induce apoptosis of the pleural mesothelial cell. When this occurs, there may be desquamation of the mesothelium.[23] On the pleural surface, as well as on other mucosal surfaces, desquamation imposes an additional selective pressure for bacterial attachment.[24] The colonizing bacteria may become dislodged and be transiently present in the pleural fluid, but then reattach to new mesothelial surface resulting in further desquamation. Certain bacteria may exhibit tropism for the pleural surface. Although not clearly defined, this may, in part, explain why pleural effusions are more common with certain organisms than with others.

Bacteria possess proteinaceous ligands called adhesins on their surface that allow them to bind to complementary molecules called receptors on the surface of the pleural mesothelium.[25] Adhesin–receptor interactions involve complementary molecules and can be viewed as a lock-and-key mechanism at the molecular level.[26] These are similar to antibody–antigen or enzyme–substrate interactions.[27] An example of an adhesin is lipoteichoic acid (LTA), which is involved in the attachment of *S. aureus* to epithelial cells, including mesothelial cells.[28] The pleural tissue receptors that interact with organisms are just being elucidated. These include toll-like receptors, manosyl containing receptors and glycoproteins on the surface of the pleural mesothelial cell.[29] Another mechanism for evasion of local defenses is the production of proteases by a variety of bacteria, parasites and fungi, which degrade components of the immune system. A non-selective proteolysis may be induced by *P. aeruginosa*, which degrades antibodies, cell-surface receptors and complement molecules.[30] Another example is group-A streptococci which produce a protease that inactivates C5a. Other mechanisms for microbial evasion include membrane components that are present on organisms, such as certain types of mycobacteria and *Legionella*, which direct the organism to enter macrophages via receptors for the third component of complement.[31] These receptors are not linked to production of a respiratory burst and oxidant generation.[32] Thus, the organisms can, like a Trojan horse, enter the phagocytic cell without provoking a defensive respiratory burst. Other organisms, such as *Mycobacterium tuberculosis*, inhibit phagosome–lysosome fusion, thus preventing formation of a phagolysosome and thereby inhibiting intracellular killing.[33]

DEFENSE MECHANISMS OF THE PLEURA

Consequences of microbial invasion of the pleural space

A massive attack by microbial factors in the pleural space has several deleterious consequences if not aggressively countered. Microbial invasion of the pleural space results in increased volume of pleural fluid with increased protein concentration and cellularity. Pleural infection also results in structural and functional changes of the mesothelium and its basement membrane. Clearly, pleural infection is a continuum from the early development of a small sterile parapneumonic effusion to the actual invasion of the pleural space by microorganisms. Under favourable conditions, infection of the pleural space resolves with sterilization of the pleural fluid and a return to normal homeostasis with normal pleural fluid and normal pleural structure. Under unfavorable circumstances, infection of the pleural space resolves with residual pockets of infected proteinaceous fluid contained by thickened fibrotic pleura and adhesions between opposing pleural surfaces.

Drainage of the pleural space prior to the development of significant adhesions is a critical method of removing large numbers of bacteria from the pleural space, as well as proteolytic material that may cause further damage to the mesothelium. The use of fibrinolytics is also based on the same principles, namely lysis of fibrin pockets which allows for removal of pus and proteases from the infected pleural space. Appropriate antibiotic therapy, initiated early in the process of development of pleural infection, however, remains the major mechanism of achieving microbial killing and mitigating their effect on the pleura. (For management of empyema, see also Chapter 26, Effusions from infections: parapneumonic effusions and empyema.)

The pleural mesothelium as a physical barrier

The pleural mesothelium is an important host defense. As a physical barrier the pleura may be seen to comprise multiple elements: the basement membrane, the mesothelial cell monolayer, the extracellular domain of the mesothelium and the pleural fluid bathing the pleural surface. The physical properties of each element are critically important to preventing the entry of organisms into the pleural space.

The pleural basement membrane comprises proteins, laminin, fibronectin, elastin and collagen types I, III and IV,[2] and the hyaluronan (a glycosaminoglycan).

The pleural mesothelium is an intact monolayer of cells that adhere to each other and the basement membrane. The integrity of the pleural mesothelium is dependent on the organization of the intermesothelial adherens junctions. Human mesothelial cells express a large number of integrins which play a critical role in the adherence of mesothelial cells to the extracellular matrix and to other cell types.[34] Mesothelial cells express α2, α3, α5, β1, β3, and αvβ 3 integrins in high quantities. Expression of α1 is noted in intermediate quantities, while expression of α6 is low and seen in less than 30 percent of mesothelial cells.[35] The ability of mesothelial cells to adhere to its extracellular matrix is a function of some of these integrins.

Importantly, mesothelial cells also express membrane type matrix metalloproteinase (MT-MMP)-1, 2, 3 and 9, and tissue inhibitor of metalloproteinase (TIMP)-I, -II and -III. In mesothelial cells, the differential expression of MMPs and TIMPs is influenced by the pro-inflammatory cytokine IL-1β and the anti-inflammatory cytokine TGF-β1.[36,37] A balance of these factors is important in inhibiting adherence of other cells as well as in maintaining the integrity of the pleural monolayer.

Multiple membrane-bound mucin-like molecules have been demonstrated on the pleural surface. Pleural mesothelial cells produce a significant amount of sialomucins and proteoglycans that coat the surface of the mesothelium.[38] The membrane-bound mucins have a hydrophobic membrane-spanning domain and an extracellular domain containing numerous serine and threonine residues. The extracellular domain of the mucins is abundantly glycosylated by oligosaccharides *O*-linked to the serine and threonine residues.[39–43] Thus, mucins are very large molecules that contain 60–80 percent carbohydrate by weight.[44] Mucins serve as lubricants and protect the underlying mesothelial cells. The extracellular domain of the mucins is anionic, thus the free surface of the mesothelium has a negative charge. Mutual repulsion of the negatively charged surfaces maintains the pleural cavity. The negative charge also repels bacteria.[45] Mesothelial cells also produce fibronectin. Fibronectin is a large glycoprotein that resists adherence of microbes, such as *P. aeruginosa* and others.

Sialomucin complex (SMC) is a family of heterodimeric glycoproteins expressed by mesothelial cells on their surface. These sialomucins contain abundant sialic acid, accordingly they are strongly anionic and they resist the adherence of bacteria and inflammatory cells. Members of the SMC family include CD34, ascites sialoglycoprotein (ASGP)-1 and podocalyxin.[46] CD34 is important for its ability to act as a ligand of L-selectin.

The pleural membrane is also bathed in secretions containing microbicidal proteins, such as lysozyme. Lysozyme is an enzyme that degrades the peptidoglycan in the cell wall of Gram-positive bacteria by hydrolyzing the β-(1,4)-glycosidic linkage from *N*-acetyl muramic acid to *N*-acetyl glucosamine.[47] Normal pleural fluid also contains immunoglobulins, principally IgG and IgA. Pleural fluid contains complement which is a group of proteins that interact with each other in a cascade when activated.[48] Complement activation can lead to microbial lysis and may also play a role in amplifying inflammation with cytokine production and increased phagocytosis of cells.[49] Although the formation of pleural fluid has been thought to represent a detrimental effect of pleural infection, it might be considered as an appropriate response to infection inasmuch as there is an exuberant flow of proteins and cells into the pleural space that may kill or inactivate the infectious organism.

Immune responses of mesothelial cells

The inflammatory stimuli to the mesothelium include microbes or microbial products, allergens, autoantigens, alloantigens, tumor cells, etc. Interaction between the inflammatory stimuli and the mesothelial cell are mediated by membrane-spanning proteins expressed on the mesothelial cell surface. In the presence of inflammatory stimuli, the mesothelial cell itself may act as an effector cell or it may signal other cell types to participate in a coordinated reaction. Immune responses of the mesothelial cell orchestrate a combined response comprising both innate and acquired immunity.

The various classes of pathogens (Gram-negative bacteria, Gram-positive bacteria, mycobacteria, fungi, parasites, viruses, etc.) have characteristic molecular structures upon their surfaces, such as lipopolysaccharide (LPS), bacteria lipoprotein (BLP), flagellin, peptidoglycan (PGN), LTA, lipoarabinomannan (LAM), viral glycoproteins, etc. Collectively, these microbial molecular structures are called pathogen-associated molecular patterns (PAMPs). Pleural mesothelial cells express pattern recognition receptors (PRRs).[50] These allow the mesothelial cell to respond to the various classes of pathogen with specificity.[51] Among the PRRs on pleural mesothelial cells are β2 integrins (CD11, CD18) complement receptors, C-type lectins and toll-like receptors (TLRs).[52] Interaction of PAMPs with PRRs triggers a defensive reaction mobilizing the both innate and adaptive immune responses, which could include the release of reactive oxygen intermediates (ROIs) or reactive nitrogen intermediates (RNIs), or secretion of antimicrobial peptides, inflammatory cytokines and chemokines.[53]

One of the innate immune responses of the pleural mesothelial cell is the release of ROIs and RNIs. The nitric oxide radical (•NO) is a diatomic molecule containing an unpaired electron that permits it to react with other molecules.[54,55] The reaction of •NO with superoxide anion leads to formation of the peroxynitrite anion ($ONOO^-$) and peroxynitrous acid. The inducible form of NO synthase (iNOS) is capable of producing micromolar quantities of •NO over a prolonged period. Pleural mesothelial cells produce large quantities of •NO in response to stimulation with cytokines, LPS and particulates.[56] Thus the inducible isoform of NO synthase contributes to the control of a variety of infections in the pleural space.

Pleural mesothelial cells are actively phagocytic cells.[57] This phenomenon of phagocytosis by mesothelial cells is not very well recognized, but is a critical response to the presence of microbes. As a consequence of phagocytosis, a number of responses are initiated by the mesothelial cell. An important and immediate response is the release of toxic oxygen metabolites such as hydrogen peroxide, superoxide and nitric oxide.[58] The release of oxygen radicals is also associated with the release of other antibacterial molecules such as cathepsin-G and defensins, which kill microbes and some viruses by permeabilizing their membranes.[59] Phagocytosis of the microbe may be made more efficient by the coating of particles with antibody. All three classes of IgG Fc receptors can mediate phagocytosis.[60] When a microbe is coated with antibody as well as complement, even encapsulated bacteria will be phagocytosed by mesothelial cells and phagocytic cells.[61] Antibodies produced by mesothelial cells also inhibit the ability of extracellular viruses to infect either the recruited phagocyte or the mesothelial cell. Antibody responses, however, are less effective against viruses such as the human immunodeficiency virus (HIV), which can enter the mesothelial cell through multiple receptors, including C-C chemokine receptor-5 (CCR5).

Pleural mesothelial cells also recruit inflammatory cells to the pleural space by secreting chemokines and regulate their activity by secreting cytokines. Pleural mesothelial cells can secrete several critically important chemokines of both the C-X-C, C-C and C-X3-C families. Human pleural mesothelial cells activated by LPS secrete monocyte chemotactic protein-1 (MCP-1) and interleukin-8 (IL-8).[62] MCP-1 is a member of the C-C chemokine family and is chemotactic for monocytes. IL-8 is a member of the C-X-C family and is chemotactic for neutrophils. Mesothelial cells also express fractalkine, the only known member of the C-X3-C chemokine family. In its soluble form, fractalkine is chemotactic for T-cells, natural killer (NK) cells and monocytes; in its membrane bound form it promotes adhesion by those cell types.[63] Mesothelial cells also coordinate with the acquired immune response by presentation of antigen.[64]

Apoptosis, or programmed cell death, is thought to contribute to the homeostasis of the functional leukocyte pool in the pleural space. Interestingly, pleural fluid of patients with complicated parapneumonic effusions contain significantly high levels of granulocyte/macrophage colony stimulating factor (GM-CSF), and neutrophils in empyema pleural fluids demonstrate a decrease in apoptosis when compared with neutrophils in uncomplicated parapneumonic effusions.[65] Neutrophils exposed to mesothelial cells express the *Bcl-x_L* gene, which is an anti-apoptotic gene.[66] This anti-apoptotic gene is the counterpart of *Bak* gene expression.[67] Thus, mesothelial cells can control the initiation of the inflammatory response to infection in the pleural space, and may also control the resolution of the inflammatory response by regulating the changes in the level of the *Bak* gene expression.

Invasion by phagocytic cells

Over 100 years ago Elie Metchnikoff described the acute inflammatory response as a reaction of phagocytes against a harmful agent.[68] This theory is classically demonstrated in the pleural space, since there is a rapid and site-directed movement of leukocytes into the pleura following inflammation. This transfer of leukocytes from the vascular compartment into the pleural space involves a multistep paradigm of leukocyte recruitment involving margination, capture of the free-flowing leukocytes in the vascular compartment via leukocyte rolling, activation and movement to the surface of the pleura. When the leukocyte encounters the pleura, it initiates a similar process, but with the pleural mesothelial cell instead of the endothelial cell, and initiates movement under the direction of chemokines, from the basilar surface of the mesothelium out onto the apical surface of the mesothelium and into the pleural space. Malignant cells that invade the pleural space activate similar responses.[69] Mesothelial cell expression of adhesion molecules, including the immunoglobulin superfamily cell adhesion molecules (IGSF CAMs), such as the intercellular adhesion molecules (ICAMs), selectins, such as L-, P- and E-selectin, and other adhesion molecules, such as CD44, come into play during the movement of cells into the pleural space. L-selectin is constitutively expressed on almost all leukocytes as well as mesothelial cells. Selectins are monomeric molecules that span the plasma membrane and contain complement-controlled protein-like repeats.[70] The calcium-dependent lectin domain at the NH_2-terminus defines their ability to bind to specific ligands. Integrin expression by leukocytes allows for firm adhesion between the invading phagocytic and the mesothelial cell. In particular, β2 integrin (CD11/CD18) on the surface of neutrophils binds to the ICAMs that are expressed by mesothelial cells. These ICAMs, namely ICAM-1 (CD54), ICAM-2 (CD102), ICAM-3 (CD50) and VCAM-1 (CD106), are upregulated on mesothelial cells during transfer of neutrophils, mononuclear cells and lymphocytes into the pleural space.[71]

Acquired immune responses in the pleural space

Acquired immunity is characterized by specificity and memory and is mediated via clonally distributed T and B lymphocytes as well as mesothelial cells. It is important to recognize that certain proteins may link innate and acquired immunity. Although innate immunity was initially considered to control infections caused by intracellular microbes, it is now clear that these cells and products play a pivotal role in regulating multiple levels of the immune response in an orchestrated manner. The γδ T cells and NK cells and macrophages are important subsets of all aspects of immunity. Evidence of the connections linking innate and acquired immunity are multiple. The TLRs, which function as pattern recognition receptors on mesothelial cells, play an essential role in recognition of microbial components. These TLRs allow the cells to present antigen to naive T cells, which in turn regulate the development of Th1/Th2 cell development. The TLRs induce the production of cytokines such as IL-12 and IL-18 in antigen-presenting cells. These cytokines are instructive cytokines and drive the naive T cell to differentiate into Th1 cells. The TLRs also recognize the presence of LPS, PGN and glycolipids. Activation of TLRs is involved in the recognition of *M. tuberculosis* as well as in the killing of these organisms.[72] Th1 T cells can produce interferon-gamma (IFN-γ) in the presence of effector cytokines, while Th2 cells will produce IL-4, IL-5, IL-10 and IL-13. T cells can be functionally divided into cells that provide help for other immune cell types such as B cells and cells that mediate cytotoxicity.[73] Helper T cells express the glycoprotein CD4 while cytotoxic T cells express CD8. CD4+ and CD8+ T cells can be selectively called into the pleural space in response to infections, such as tuberculosis. When mature T cells are exposed to an antigen, such as a mycobacterial antigen, e.g. the 65 kilodalton mycobacterial heat shock protein or lipoarabinomannan (LAM), their function and phenotype changes and remains persistently changed thenceforth. Enhanced responses by these T cells can be observed for decades after the initial exposure to the antigen. These CD4+ αβ T cells are contained predominantly within a subset that comprises approximately 40 percent of these cells in the adult circulation.

Monocytes and macrophages are important sources of a specific group of cytokines. A classic example of this is IFN-γ, which, in tuberculous effusions, is found in very high quantities in the pleural space, as are CD4+ T cells.[74] IFN-γ not only improves phagocytosis and killing of mycobacteria, it may also mediate the level of expression of chemokine receptors on the recruited mononuclear phagocyte. Thus, while in the vascular compartment, the mononuclear cell has a high level of CCR2 expression when it enters the pleural space, the presence of IFN-γ downregulates the expression of CCR2, in effect capturing it and localizing it to the pleural space. T lymphocytes are important sources of other cytokines, such as IL-2 and IL-9, and lymphotoxins.

PLEURAL INFLAMMATORY CELLS

Neutrophils

Under normal conditions, it is rare to find neutrophils in the pleural space. During inflammation and infection there is an abundant movement of neutrophils into the pleural space. The granulocytic cells are the most numerous leukocytes found in pleural fluid in the process of acute inflammation. They are derived from pluripotent stem cells in the bone marrow. Several low molecular weight proteins such as colony-stimulating factor are responsible for the production, maturation and proliferation of these cells.[75] Neutrophils are armed with an azurophil or primary granules as well as specific or secondary granules. These granules contain peroxidases, phosphatases and gelatinases that, when in contact with the microorganism, allow for microbial killing and digestion.[76] Secondary granules are true lysosomes and contain acid hydrolases as well as proteases and cationic proteins.[77]

Neutrophils enter the pleural space via diapedesis across the pleural monolayer. The pattern of migration is not unique since it closely follows the migratory patterns and pathways in inflammation where recruited neutrophils traffic.

Specific granules contain the CD11b/CD18 receptor. CD11b/CD18 receptor mediates neutrophil chemotactic activity. Although only approximately 5 percent of the granulocyte pool is in the intravascular compartment, the granulocytes can move from the vascular compartment into the pleural space in as little as 2 hours. The classical description of the phagocytic cell moving out of the vasculature involves rolling adhesion, firm adhesion and transmigration. Similar processes occur at the level of the pleural mesothelium, however, as phagocytes move from the basilar surface of the pleura towards the apical surface along paracellular channels and out into the pleural space. Mesothelial cells express intercellular adhesion molecules (ICAM-1) integrins and interdigitate with the CD11/CD18 integrin on the surface of the neutrophil.[78]

Although the intravascular half-life of neutrophils is 6–8 hours, they may persist far longer in the pleural space. The lifespan of a neutrophil is short compared with other leukocytes and neutrophils are constitutively committed to apoptosis. Interestingly, the mesothelial cell regulates the process of neutrophil apoptosis by the release of factors, such as GM-CSF, granulocyte colony-stimulating factor (G-CSF) or IL-8.[79] In particular, GM-CSF inhibits neutrophil apoptosis during pleural responses to infections.[80] GM-CSF inhibits neutrophil apoptosis via modulation of Bcl-x_L.

Mononuclear cells

Mesothelial cells recruit significant numbers of mononuclear cells to the pleural space during a variety of infections. This influx may be strong and persistent in response to infections such as tuberculosis.[81] Mesothelial cells release several C-C chemokines, which recruit mononuclear cells to the pleural space. Among the C-C chemokines are regulated upon activation, normally T-cell expressed and secreted (RANTES) and MCP-1, -2 and -3. The expression of C-C receptors, specifically CCR2 on mononuclear cells, is regulated in part by factors produced at local sites of inflammation such as the pleural space. Thus, CCR2 expression is high while the mononuclear cells are in the peripheral blood circulation, but is significantly reduced when the mononuclear cells reach the pleural space. This mechanism serves to localize and immobilize the monocytes once they reach the pleural cavity.[82] Also, the C-X3-C chemokine fractalkine in its soluble form is chemotactic for monocytes and in its membrane-bound form promotes strong adhesion by monocytes.[83]

Eosinophils

Eosinophils are identified as playing an important role in the pathogenesis of idiopathic or allergic responses to pleural injury, parasitic diseases, the presence of air or blood in the pleural space and in hypersensitivity responses to certain drugs.[84] The mechanisms and control of the accumulation of these cells in the pleural space is unclear.

Lymphocytes

The pleural space has a small population of lymphocytes, both B-lymphocytes and T-lymphocytes.[85] The T-lymphocytes include $\gamma\delta$-T cells and CD4-/CD8-$\alpha\beta$-T cells. During granulomatous inflammation, the number of lymphocytes can increase dramatically reflecting either a Th-1, CD4 T-cell predominant response in diseases such as tuberculosis, or a CD8+ response in some diseases as in certain lymphomas, etc. The production of antibodies by B cells and associated lymphoid tissue is important for resistance to infectious processes; however, little is known about this immune processing pathway in the pleural space.

INITIATION OF INFLAMMATION

The mesothelial cell plays a critical role in the initiation of inflammatory responses in the pleural space because it is the first cell to recognize the invasion of the pleural space. Pleural inflammation is not only associated with an influx of a large number of inflammatory cells, but also with a transfer of proteins and a change in the permeability of the pleura. Pleural mesothelial cells release chemokines in a polar fashion, with a higher concentration being released on the apical surface, which leads to directed migration of phagocytic cells into the pleural space. However, the mechanisms whereby pleural integrity to proteins and fluid is breached with the development of an exudative high-protein-containing effusion are beginning to be elucidated. An infectious agent can initiate a cascade of events which include release of nitric oxide and production of vascular permeability factor (VPF)/vascular endothelial growth factor (VEGF) through the accumulation of HIF-1α. VEGF downregulates both cadherins and catenins, which leads to increased pleural permeability and movement of cells, proteins and fluid across the intermesothelial gaps, leading to pleural effusion formation.

Pleural mesothelial cell release of RNIs has been demonstrated to lead to the accumulation of transcription factors such as hypoxia-inducible transcription factor (HIF)-1α as well as nuclear factor (NF)-κB. HIF-1 is a heterodimer. Both subunits are basic helix-loop-helix proteins containing a PAS domain containing proteins. The first subunit is HIF-1α; the second subunit is aryl hydrocarbon receptor nuclear translocator (ARNT), also known as HIF-1β.[86–90] HIF-1α accumulates under multiple pathophysiological conditions, including hypoxia, hence its name. It has been documented, however, to accumulate in pleural mesothelial cells that have been stimulated via release of •NO and other inflammatory mediators. The availability of HIF-1β is mainly determined by HIF-1α. HIF-1α dimerizes with HIF-1β, translocates to the nucleus, and binds to the target DNA sequence in the promoter region of various genes. HIF-1α response correlates with •NO formation, and administration of the iNOS inhibitor carboxy-2-phenyl-4,4,5,5-tetramethylimidazide-1-oxyl-3-oxide (carboxy PTIO) to scavenge •NO suppresses HIF-1α accumulation. Among the various factors that cause an increase in accumulation of HIF-1α are thrombin, platelet-derived growth factor and angiotensin-2.

A critically important regulatory cytokine in the pleural space is VPF/VEGF.[91] This is upregulated in mesothelial cells through an HIF-1 dependent pathway. VPF/VEGF is a 35–43 kDa dimeric polypeptide expressed in several isoforms that result from alternative mRNA splicing of a single gene.[92] It was initially discovered because of its ability to increase vascular permeability. The molecule was first called vascular permeability factor. It is now recognized as a pivotal angiogenic factor mediating neovascularization under many conditions, but remains an extremely potent inducer of permeability.[93] Recent reports demonstrate that VPF/VEGF plays a central role in the formation of ascites and pleural effusions in animal models.[94] In patients with inflammatory pleural effusions such as empyema and tuberculosis, a significant amount of VEGF is found in the pleural fluids. Interestingly, recent investigations suggest that VEGF is essential for sufficient formation of pleural fluid in animal models of lung cancer-induced pleural effusions.[95]

Bacteria such as *S. aureus* have been shown to cause gap formation between mesothelial cells.[96] The major ubiquitous type of mesothelial cell–cell junction are adherens junctions. In the mesothelium the adherens junctions are predominantly neural cadherin (*n*-cadherin) and β-catenins.[97] Dysregulation of these proteins causes intercellular gap formation and increases permeability to cells, fluids and proteins. The mesothelium is a continuous monolayer of cells linked by adhesive structures which are involved in the control of pleural permeability to plasma proteins, phagocytic cells, and allow for cell polarity.[98] It is the most common connecting cell–cell link between mesothelial cells. This cadherin family of proteins is a major class of homophilic cell adhesion molecules that mediate calcium-dependent cell–cell interactions.[99] These transmembrane cadherin proteins function as a zipper between cells allowing for a change in permeability to occur via signaling mechanisms that lead to contraction of the intracellular actin cytoskeletal filaments and to gap formation between mesothelial cells.[100] When adherens junctions are stabilized under normal conditions, the majority of *n*-cadherin loses tyrosine phosphorylation and combines with plakoglobin and actin; however, when cells have weak junctions, *n*-cadherin is heavily phosphorylated in tyrosine and there is also decreased expression of β-catenin.[101] Thus, *n*-cadherin and β-catenin are critical determinants of mesothelial paracellular permeability. This interaction is a dynamic one, since permeability is reversible. Monoclonal antibodies directed against *n*-cadherin modulate pleural permeability.

PERPETUATION OF INFLAMMATION

Following initiation of the inflammatory process, several mediators – cells and extracellular matrix components – play a critical role in perpetuating the process of inflammation. An example of an extracellular matrix component that plays a role in perpetuation of inflammation is hyaluronan. Hyaluronan is a high molecular weight nonsulfated glycosaminoglycan produced by mesothelial cells, under both normal and inflammatory conditions. Hyaluronan is present in the pericellular and extracellular matrix of mesothelial cells. Hyaluronan is a linear polysaccharide composed of repeating alternation of *N*-acetyl glucosamine and glucuronide with each *N*-acetyl glucosamine joined to gluconuride by a β-1,4 glycosidic linkage and each glucuronide joined to the next *N*-acetyl glucosamine by a β-1,3 glycosidic linkage.[102] Each molecule of hyaluronan may contain 10 000 or more disaccharide repeats and have a molecular mass of several million Daltons. This high molecular weight hyaluron is a relatively inactive component but when it undergoes hydrolysis it produces fragments of low molecular weight, which may mediate multiple processes. Low molecular weight fragments of hyaluronan induce mesothelial cells to express the chemokines MCP-1 and IL-8.[103] Hyaluronan interacts with specific malignant cell receptors, such as CD44 and the receptor for hyaluronic acid mediated motility (RHAMM).[104] We have demonstrated that the standard isoform, CD44s, which does not contain variant exon product and is highly expressed in malignant breast cancer cells, is a specific mechanism whereby breast cancer cells adhere to pleural mesothelial cells.[105] Addition of CD44s antibody to the media blocks adherence of malignant breast cancer MCF7 cells to mesothelial monolayers.[106] Regulation of the degree of adherence can be regulated by the presence or absence of the variant exon products. The

CD44–hyaluron complex is internalized by the malignant cells, whereupon acid hydrolases in lysosomal compartments break it down via hydrolysis to several small, activated low molecular weight fragments that then can participate in the migration process of a malignant cell through the pleural surface. Hyaluronan is acted upon by lysosomal hyaluronidase allowing for the cleavage of *N*-acetyl hexosaminidic linkages[107] with a series of saccharides being formed. The oligosaccharides are chemoattractant for tumor cells. They are also growth factors for malignant cells and can mediate permeability of the monolayer. These fragments of hyaluronan, because of their ability to perpetuate the process of inflammation by attracting malignant cells and mononuclear cells, change the cell population in the pleural space during the process of development of metastatic pleural effusions.[108]

RESOLUTION AND REPAIR

The process of resolution of pleural inflammation is just beginning to be elucidated. It is recognized that the lifespan of the inflammatory responses in the pleural space is in part regulated by the mesothelial cell through secretion of antiinflammatory cytokines and regulation of apoptosis of neutrophils, monocytes and lymphocytes.

It is important to note that pleural space inflammation may eventually result in either a normal pleural mesothelial monolayer without the presence of remodeling and fibrosis or in the development of multiple adhesions, fibrosis and loss of integrity of the pleural membranes. The factors that direct the process of remodeling of the pleura remain unclear. Resolution of pleural inflammation and pleural remodeling and fibrosis may be mediated in part by transforming growth factor beta (TGF-β). TGF-β is an anti-inflammatory cytokine. TGF-β_2 induces mesothelial cells to synthesize collagen.[109]

Importantly, under certain circumstances, pleural sclerosis is a defined therapeutic goal. In patients with malignant effusions or in patients with pneumothorax, inflammation is produced via the introduction of talc or other agents into the pleural space. An exuberant fibrotic response develops on both the surfaces of the pleura, connecting the two and obliterating differentiating margins. The study of this process has allowed some insight into the mechanisms of pleural fibrosis. Patients that had pleurodesis attempted via talc insufflation had a rapid and marked increase in the amount of basic fibroblast growth factor in the pleural fluid.[110] Pleural mesothelial cells stimulated by talc also release basic fibroblast growth factor (b-FGF) *in vitro*. This process is inhibited *in vitro* through the use of cycloheximide, which prevents protein synthesis, or by the use of colchicine, which prevents phagocytosis and adherence of talc. Thus, it appears that when studied *in vitro*, mesothelial cells were required to phagocytose or adhere to talc particles prior to the release of b-FGF; b-FGF was also actively synthesized by mesothelial cells. An interesting and important finding was that in patients there was a significant inverse correlation between the release of b-FGF into the pleural fluids and the tumor size, as evaluated by an objective grading scale during thoracoscopy. This implies that pleurodesis requires the presence of normal mesothelial cells to release growth factors for fibroblasts. Recent evidence suggests that talc also causes pleural mesothelial cells to secrete endostatin, which inhibits angiogenesis, thus changing the milieu of the pleural space from angiogenic to angiostatic.[111]

Importantly, mesothelial cells also express MT-MMP-1, 2, 3 and 9, and TIMP-I, -II and -III. In mesothelial cells, the differential expression of MMPs and TIMPs is influenced by the pro-inflammatory cytokine IL-1β and the anti-inflammatory cytokine TGF-β1.[36,37] Under normal conditions, the balance of these factors is important in maintaining the integrity of the pleural monolayer; in the context of recovery from infection the balance of these factors determines the outcome of remodeling and repair.

INHIBITION OF PLEURAL INFLAMMATORY RESPONSES

Under certain circumstances, such as malignancy and acquired immune deficiency syndrome (AIDS), there is an inhibition of normal pleural inflammatory responses leading to deleterious end results for the host. The interaction of malignant and mesothelial cells, as well as their extracellular matrix, is an example of one of the multiple pathways that allow malignant cells to elude control by the host and local regulatory cells, such as the mesothelial cell. Tumor cells, for example, may themselves produce large amounts of VEGF and growth factors that allow autocrine regulation of their ability to grow. Mesothelioma cells may themselves produce IL-8 which contains the Glu-Leu-Arg (ELR) motif making it an autocrine growth factor and an angiogenic factor.[112] During angiogenesis, new vessels emerge from existing endothelial vessels. This invasive process allows feeder blood vessels to be generated near and within the tumor tissue. Although mesothelial cells have recently been recognized as producing significant anti-angiogenic factors, such as endostatin, their role in defense mechanisms against invasion by malignant cells is still unclear. In diseases such as AIDS, multiple systemic responses are weakened which make the patient susceptible to opportunistic infections. Patients with AIDS have a higher incidence of development of parapneumonic effusions, both uncomplicated and complicated, as well as a higher incidence of effusions secondary to diseases such as tuberculosis,[96] where delayed hypersensitivity responses are key. Kaposi's sarcoma is also known to metastasize from the lung into the pleural space with great ease. It appears that the mesothelial cell loses its regulatory capabilities when the host is immunocompromised. In patients with tuberculous pleural effusions, the mechanisms of development of pleural effusions are now being described. It appears that not only is there loss of Th-1 cells and cytokines, but other local immune responses regulated by the mesothelial cell are abnormal.

KEY POINTS

- During pleural inflammation, mesothelial cells play an active role secreting cytokines and chemokines that attract and activate multiple inflammatory cell types.
- During pleural inflammation there is a flow of inflammatory cells and protein into the pleural space.
- Pleural inflammation may resolve with restoration of normal pleural structure and return to normal function; alternatively, resolution of pleural inflammation may lead to pleural fibrosis and gross distortion of pleural architecture.
- Microbial virulence factors are aimed at overcoming specific host-defense mechanisms.
- The outcome of pleural infection depends upon the virulence of the invading microbe and the pleural defense mechanisms.
- Passive pleural defenses against pleural infection include the microbicidal proteins within the pleural fluid, the biophysical properties of the extracellular domain at the mesothelium surface, the structural integrity of the mesothelial cell monolayer itself and the pleural basement membrane.
- Microbial invasion of the pleural space provokes both innate and adaptive immune responses; the pleural mesothelial cell participates in and coordinates both the innate and the adaptive immune responses.
- The consequences of pleural infection may include pleural effusion, empyema and pleural fibrosis.

REFERENCES

● = Key primary paper
◆ = Major review article

1. Wang NS. Mesothelial cells *in situ*. In: Chrétien J, Bignon J, Hirsch A (eds). *The pleura in health and disease*, Vol. 30. New York: Marcel Dekker, 1985: 23–42.
2. Rennard S, Jaurand M-C, Bignon J, Ferrans V, Crystal R. Connective tissue matrix of the pleura. In: Chrétien J, Bignon J, Hirsch A (eds). *The pleura in health and disease*, Vol. 30. New York: Marcel Dekker, 1985: 69–85.
3. Wang NS. The preformed stomas connecting the pleural cavity and the lymphatics in the parietal pleura. *Am Rev Respir Dis* 1975; **111**: 12–20.
◆4. Sahn SA. State of the art. The pleura. *Am Rev Respir Dis* 1988; **138**: 184–234.
5. Willis T. The London practice of physics. In: *Classics of medicine*. New York: Library Division of Gryphon, 1992: 113–20.
6. Anderson KV. Toll signaling pathways in the innate immune response. *Curr Opin Immunol* 2000; **12**: 13–19.
7. Hewlett EL. Toxins and other virulence factors. In: Mandell G, Douglas R, Bennett J (eds). *Principles and practice of infectious diseases*, Vol. 1. New York, Edinburgh: Churchill Livingstone, 1995: 2–11.
8. Christensen GD, Simpson WA, Beachey EH. Adhesion of bacteria to animal tissues: complex mechanisms. In: Savage DCFM (ed). *Bacterial adhesion*. New York: Plenum Press, 1985: 279–306.
9. Ofek I. General concepts and principles of bacterial adherence in animals and man. In: Beachey EH. (ed.) *Bacterial adherence*. London: Chapman and Hall, 1980: 1–29.
10. Arp L. Bacterial infection of mucosal surfaces: an overview of cellular and molecular mechanisms. In: Roth J (ed). *Virulence mechanisms of bacterial pathogens*. Washington DC: American Society of Microbiology, 1988: 3–27.
11. Schlievert PM. Role of superantigens in human disease. *J Infect Dis* 1993; **167**: 997–1002.
12. Birnbaumer LM, Yatani, A. Recent advances in the understanding of multiple roles of G proteins in coupling of receptors to ionic channels and other effectors. In: Moss J, Vaughan M (eds). *ADP-ribosylating toxins and G proteins: insights into signal transduction*. Washington, DC: American Society for Microbiology, 1990: 225–66.
13. Middeldorp JM, Witholt B. K88-mediated binding of *Escherichia coli* outer membrane fragments to porcine intestinal epithelial cell brush borders. *Infect Immun* 1981; **31**: 42–51.
14. Mollby R. Bacterial phospholipases. In: Jeljaszewicz JWT (ed). *Bacterial toxins and cell membranes*. New York: Academic Press, 1978: 367–424.
15. Lee PK, Vercellotti GM, Deringer JR, Schlievert PM. Effects of staphylococcal toxic shock syndrome toxin 1 on aortic endothelial cells. *J Infect Dis* 1991; **164**: 711–19.
16. Marrack P, Kappler J. The staphylococcal enterotoxins and their relatives. *Science* 1990; **248**: 705–11.
17. Smith H, Huggins M. Further observations on the association of the colicine V plasmic of *Escherichia coli* with pathogenicity and with survival in the alimentary tract. *J Gen Microbiol* 1976; **92**: 335–50.
18. Mohammed KA, Nasreen N, Ward MJ, Antony VB. Induction of acute pleural inflammation by *Staphylococcus aureus*. I. CD4+ T cells play a critical role in experimental empyema. *J Infect Dis* 2000; **181**: 1693–9.
19. Brubaker RR. Mechanisms of bacterial virulence. *Annu Rev Microbiol* 1985; **39**: 21–50.
20. Meyer TF. Pathogenic *Neisseriae* – model of bacterial virulence and genetic flexibility. *Immun Infekt* 1989; **17**: 113–23.
21. McCutchan JA, Katzenstein D, Norquist D, *et al.* Role of blocking antibody in disseminated gonococcal infection. *J Immunol* 1978; **121**: 1884–8.
22. Hirakata Y, Kaku M, Mizukane R, *et al.* Potential effects of erythromycin on host defense systems and virulence of *Pseudomonas aeruginosa*. *Antimicrob Agents Chemother* 1992; **36**: 1922–7.
23. Nasreen N, Mohammed KA, Dowling PA, *et al.* Talc induces apoptosis in human malignant mesothelioma cells *in vitro*. *Am J Respir Crit Care Med* 2000; **161**: 595–600.
24. Eidels L, Proia RL, Hart DA. Membrane receptors for bacterial toxins. *Microbiol Rev* 1983; **47**: 596–620.
25. Falkow S, Small P, Isberg R, Hayes SF, Corwin D. A molecular strategy for the study of bacterial invasion. *Rev Infect Dis* 1987; **9** (Suppl 5): S450–5.

26. Finlay BB, Falkow S. Common themes in microbial pathogenicity. *Microbiol Rev* 1989; **53**: 210–30.
27. Jones GW, Isaacson RE. Proteinaceous bacterial adhesins and their receptors. *Crit Rev Microbiol* 1983; **10**: 229–60.
28. Beachey EH, Ofek I. Epithelial cell binding of group A streptococci by lipoteichoic acid on fimbriae denuded of M protein. *J Exp Med* 1976; **143**: 759–71.
29. Ohtsuka A, Yamana S, Murakami T. Localization of membrane-associated sialomucin on the free surface of mesothelial cells of the pleura, pericardium, and peritoneum. *Histochem Cell Biol* 1997; **107**: 441–7.
30. Heinzel F. Antibodies. In: Mandell G, Douglas R, Bennett J (eds). *Principles and practice of infectious diseases*, Vol. 1. New York, Edinburgh: Churchill Livingston, 1995: 36–57.
31. Payne NR, Horwitz MA. Phagocytosis of *Legionella pneumophila* is mediated by human monocyte complement receptors. *J Exp Med* 1987; **166**: 1377–89.
32. Dowling JN, Saha AK, Glew RH. Virulence factors of the family Legionellaceae. *Microbiol Rev* 1992; **56**: 32–60.
33. Hacker J, Ott M, Ludwig B, Rdest U. Intracellular survival and expression of virulence determinants of *Legionella pneumophila*. *Infection* 1991; **19** (Suppl 4): 198–201.
34. Spurzem J, Rennard S, Romberger D. Interactions between pulmonary epithelial cells and extracellular matrix. In: Ward P, Fantone J (eds). *Adhesion molecules and the lung*, Vol. 89. New York: Marcel Dekker, 1996: 127–46.
35. Liaw YS, Yu CJ, Shun CT, *et al.* Expression of integrins in human cultured mesothelial cells: the roles in cell-to-extracellular matric adhesion and inhibition by RGD-containing peptide. *Respir Med* 2001; **95**: 221–6.
36. Ma C, Tarnuzzer RW, Chegini N. Expression of matrix metalloproteinases and tissue inhibitor of matrix mettaloproteinases in mesothelial cells and their regulation by transforming growth factor-beta 1. *Wound Repair Regen* 1999; 7:477–85.
37. Martin J, Yung S, Robson RL, Steadman R, Davies M. Production and regulation of matrix metalloprotienases and their inhibitors by human peritoneal mesothelial cells. *Perit Dial Int* 2000; **20**: 5.
38. Price-Schiavi SA, Zhu X, Aquinin R, Carraway KL. Sialomucin complex (rat Muc4) is regulated by transforming growth factor beta in mammary gland by a novel post-translational mechanism. *J Biol Chem* 2000; **275**: 17800–7.
39. Zannettino AC, Buhring HJ, Niutta S, *et al.* The sialomucin CD164 (MGC-24v) is an adhesive glycoprotein expressed by human hematopoietic progenitors and bone marrow stromal cells that serves as a potent negative regulator of hematopoiesis. *Blood* 1998; **92**: 2613–28.
40. Ohtsuka A, Yamana S, Murakami T. Localization of membrane-associated sialomucin on the free surface of mesothelial cells of the pleura, pericardium, and peritoneum. *Histochem Cell Biol* 1997; **107**: 441–7.
41. Sassetti C, van Zante A, Rosen SD. Identification of endoglycan, a member of the CD34/podocalyxin family of sialomucins. *J Biol Chem* 2000; **275**: 9001–10.
42. Doyonnas R, Kershaw DB, Duhme C, *et al.* Anuria, omphalocele, and perinatal lethality in mice lacking the CD34-related protein podocalyxin. *J Exp Med* 2001; **194**: 13–27.
43. Hilkens J, Ligtenberg MJ, Vos HL, Litvinov SV. Cell membrane-associated mucins and their adhesion-modulating property. *Trends Biochem Sci* 1992; **17**: 359–63.
44. Hjelle JT, Golinska BT, Waters DC, *et al.* Lectin staining of peritoneal mesothelial cells *in vitro*. *Perit Dial Int* 1991; **11**: 307–16.
45. Leak LV. Distribution of cell surface charges on mesothelium and lymphatic endothelium. *Microvasc Res* 1986; **31**: 18–30.
46. Andrews PM, Porter KR. The ultrastructural morphology and possible functional significance of mesothelial microvilli. *Anat Rec* 1973; **177**: 409–26.
47. Frank MM, Joiner K, Hammer C. The function of antibody and complement in the lysis of bacteria. *Rev Infect Dis* 1987; **9** (Suppl 5): S537–45.
48. Fearon D, Austen K. The alternative pathway of complement: a system for host resistance to microbial infection. *N Engl J Med* 1980; **303**: 259–63.
49. Joiner KA. Complement evasion by bacteria and parasites. *Annu Rev Microbiol* 1988; **42**: 201–30.
50. Medzhitov R, Janeway CA Jr. Innate immunity: impact on the adaptive immune response. *Curr Opin Immunol* 1997; **9**: 4–9.
51. Gorbach S, Bartlett J, Blacklow N. Infectious diseases. In: Blacklow N (ed). *Host factors*. Philadelphia: Saunders, 1992: 37.
52. Zhang G, Ghosh S. Toll-like receptor-mediated NF-kappaB activation: a phylogenetically conserved paradigm in innate immunity. *J Clin Invest* 2001; **107**: 13–19.
53. Toews GB. Pulmonary clearance of infectious agents. In: Fishman AP, Elias JA (eds). *Pulmonary diseases and disorders*. New York: McGraw-Hill 1997: 1891–904.
54. Arriero MM, Rodriguez-Feo JA, Celdran A, *et al.* Expression of endothelial nitric oxide synthase in human peritoneal tissue: regulation by *Escherichia coli* lipopolysaccharide. *J Am Soc Nephrol* 2000; **11**: 1848–56.
55. Chen JY, Chiu JH, Chen HL, *et al.* Human peritoneal mesothelial cells produce nitric oxide: induction by cytokines. *Perit Dial Int* 2000; **20**: 772–7.
56. Owens MW, Grisham MB. Nitric oxide synthesis by rat pleural mesothelial cells: induction by cytokines and lipopolysaccharide. *Am J Physiol* 1993; **265**: L110–16.
57. Antony VB. Pathogenesis of malignant pleural effusions and talc pleurodesis. *Pneumologie* 1999; **53**: 493–8.
58. Owens MW, Milligan SA, Grisham MB. Nitric oxide synthesis by rat pleural mesothelial cells: induction by growth factors and lipopolysaccharide. *Exp Lung Res* 1995; **21**: 731–42.
59. Lehrer RI, Barton A, Daher KA, *et al.* Interaction of human defensins with *Escherichia coli*. Mechanism of bactericidal activity. *J Clin Invest* 1989; **84**: 553–61.
60. Burton DR, Woof JM. Human antibody effector function. *Adv Immunol* 1992; **51**: 1–84.
61. Spitznagel J. Non-oxidative antimicrobial reactions of leukocytes. *Contemp Top Immunobiol* 1984; **14**: 283.
62. Antony VB, Hott JW, Kunkel SL, *et al.* Pleural mesothelial cell expression of C-C (monocyte chemotactic peptide) and C-X-C (interleukin 8) chemokines. *Am J Respir Cell Mol Biol* 1995; **12**: 581-8.
63. Bazan JF, Bacon KB, Hardiman G, *et al.* A new class of membrane chemokine with a CX3C motif. *Nature* 1997; **385**: 640–4.
64. Hausmann MJ, Rogachev B, Weiler M, Chaimovitz C, Douvdevani A. Accessory role of human peritoneal mesothelial cells in antigen presentation and T-cell growth. *Kidney Int* 2000; **57**: 476-86.
•65. Nasreen N, Mohammed KA, Sanders KL, *et al.* Differential expression of C-phos, C-June, and apoptosis in pleural mesothelial cells exposed to *Staph. aureus*. *Am J Respir Crit Care Med* 2001; **163**: A772.
66. Payne CM, Glasser L, Tischler ME, *et al.* Programmed cell death of the normal human neutrophil: an *in vitro* model of senescence. *Microsc Res Technol* 1994; **28**: 327–44.
67. Weinmann P, Gaehtgens P, Walzog B. Bcl-Xl- and Bax-alpha-mediated regulation of apoptosis of human neutrophils via caspase-3. *Blood* 1999; **93**: 3106–15.
68. Metchnikoff M. *Lectures on the comparative pathology of inflammation*. London: Kegan Paul, Trench, Trubner & Co., 1893: 1845–916.
69. Antony VB. Pathogenesis of malignant pleural effusions and talc pleurodesis. *Pneumologie* 1999; **53**: 493–8.
70. Barclay A, Brown M, Law S, *et al.* *The leukocyte antigen facts book*. San Diego: Academic Press, 1997.

71. Jonjic N, Peri G, Bernasconi S, *et al.* Expression of adhesion molecules and chemotactic cytokines in cultured human mesothelial cells. *J Exp Med* 1992; **176**: 1165–74.
72. Krieger M, Stern DM. Series introduction: multiligand receptors and human disease. *J Clin Invest* 2001; **108**: 645–7.
73. Locksley R, Wilson C. Cell-mediated immunity and its role in host defense. In: Mandell G, Douglas R, Bennett J (eds). *Principles and practice of infectious diseases*, Vol. 1. New York: Churchill Livingstone, 1995: 102–49.
74. Ellner JJ, Barnes PF, Wallis RS, Modlin RL. The immunology of tuberculous pleurisy. *Semin Respir Infect* 1988; **3**: 335–42.
◆75. Malech H. Phagocytic cells: egress from marrow and diapedesis. In: Gallin J, Goldstein I, Snyderman R (eds). *Inflammation: basic principles and clinical correlates*. New York: Raven Press, 1988; 297–308.
76. Weiss J, Elsbach P, Olsson I, Odeberg H. Purification and characterization of a potent bactericidal and membrane active protein from the granules of human polymorphonuclear leukocytes. *J Biol Chem* 1978; **253**: 2664–72.
77. Ganz T, Selsted ME, Szklarek D, *et al.* Defensins. Natural peptide antibiotics of human neutrophils. *J Clin Invest* 1985; **76**: 1427–35.
78. Nasreen N, Hartman D, Mohammed K, Antony V. Talc induces pleural mesothelial cell expression of proinflammatory cytokines and intracellular adhesion molecule-1 (ICAM-1). *Am J Respir Crit Care Med* 1998; **158**: 971–8.
79. Cox G, Gauldie J, Jordana M. Bronchial epithelial cell-derived cytokines (G-CSF and GM-CSF) promote the survival of peripheral blood neutrophils *in vitro*. *Am J Respir Cell Mol Biol* 1992; **7**: 507–13.
80. Coxon A, Tang T, Mayadas TN. Cytokine-activated endothelial cells delay neutrophil apoptosis *in vitro* and *in vivo*. A role for granulocyte/macrophage colony-stimulating factor. *J Exp Med* 1999; **190**: 923–34.
81. Antony VB, Sahn SA, Antony AC, Repine JE. Bacillus Calmette–Guerin-stimulated neutrophils release chemotaxis for monocytes in rabbit pleural spaces and *in vitro*. *J Clin Invest* 1985; **76**: 1514–21.
82. Mantovani A, Garlanda C. Novel pathways for negative regulation of inflammatory cytokines centered on receptor expression. *Dev Biol Stand* 1999; **97**: 97–104.
83. Imai T, Heishima K, Haskell C, *et al.* Identification and molecular characterization of fractaline receptor CX3CR1, which mediates both leukocyte migration and adhesion. *Cell* 1997; **91**: 1-20
84. Klein A, Talvani A, Silva PM, *et al.* Stem cell factor-induced leukotriene B4 production cooperates with eotaxin to mediate the recruitment of eosinophils during allergic pleurisy in mice. *J Immunol* 2001; **167**: 524–31.
85. Light RW. Parapneumonic effusions and infections of the pleural space. In: Light RW (ed). *Pleural diseases*. Philadelphia: Lea and Febiger, 1990.
86. Wang GL, Jiang BH, Rue EA, Semenza GL. Hypoxia-inducible factor 1 is a basic-loop-helix-loop-PAS hetero dimmer regulated by cellular O2 tension. *Proc Natl Acad Sci USA* 1995; **92**: 5510–4.
87. Marti HJ, Bernaudin M, Bellail A, *et al.* Hypoxia-induced vascular endothelial growth factor expression precedes neovascularization after cerebral ischemia. *Am J Pathol* 2000; **156**: 965–76.
88. Richard DE, Berra E, Pouyssegur J. Nonhypoxic pathway mediates the induction of hypoxia-inducible factor 1alpha in vascular smooth muscle cells. *J Biol Chem* 2000; **275**: 26765–71.
89. Sandau KB, Fandrey J, Brune B. Accumulation of HIF-1alpha under the influence of nitric oxide. *Blood* 2001; **97**: 1009–15.
90. Semenza GL. HIF-1 and human disease: one highly involved factor. *Gene Dev* 2000; **14**(16): 1983–91.
●91. Yano S, Shinohara H, Herbst RS, *et al.* Production of experimental malignant pleural effusions is dependent on invasion of the pleura and expression of vascular endothelial growth factor/vascular permeability factor by human lung cancer cells. *Am J Pathol* 2000; **157**: 1893–903.
92. Mazure NM, Chen EY, Laderoute KR, Giaccia AJ. Induction of vascular endothelial growth factor by hypoxia is modulated by a phosphatidylinositol 3-kinase/Akt signaling pathway in *Ha-ras*-transformed cells through a hypoxia inducible factor-1 transcriptional element. *Blood* 1997; **90**: 3322–31.
93. Becker PM, Alcasabas A, Yu AY, Semenza GL, Bunton TE. Oxygen-independent upregulation of vascular endothelial growth factor and vascular barrier dysfunction during ventilated pulmonary ischemia in isolated ferret lungs. *Am J Respir Cell Mol Biol* 2000; **22**: 272–9.
94. Thickett DR, Armstrong L, Millar AB. Vascular endothelial growth factor (VEGF) in inflammatory and malignant pleural effusions. *Thorax* 1999; **54**: 707–10.
95. D'Arcangelo D, Facchiano F, Barlucchi LM, *et al.* Acidosis inhibits endothelial cell apoptosis and function and induces basic fibroblast growth factor and vascular endothelial growth factor expression. *Circ Res* 2000; **86**: 312–18.
96. Mohammed KA, Nasreen N, Ward MJ, Antony VB. Induction of acute pleural inflammation by *Staphylococcus aureus*. I. CD4+ T cells play a critical role in experimental empyema. *J Infect Dis* 2000; **181**: 1693–9.
97. Zhang XY, Pettengell R, Nasiri N, *et al.* Characteristics and growth patterns of human peritoneal mesothelial cells: comparison between advanced epithelial ovarian cancer and non-ovarian cancer sources. *J Soc Gynecol Invest* 1999; **6**: 333–40.
98. Nasreen N, Mohammed KA, Hardwick J, *et al.* Polar production of interleukin-8 by mesothelial cells promotes the transmesothelial migration of neutrophils: role of intercellular adhesion molecule-1. *J Infect Dis* 2001; **183**: 1638–45.
99. Corada M, Liao F, Lindgren M, *et al.* Monoclonal antibodies directed to different regions of vascular endothelial cadherin extracellular domain affect adhesion and clustering of the protein and modulate endothelial permeability. *Blood* 2001; **97**: 1679–84.
100. Blankesteijn WM, van Gijn ME, Essers-Janssen YP, Daemen MJ, Smits JF. Beta-catenin, an inducer of uncontrolled cell proliferation and migration in malignancies, is localized in the cytoplasm of vascular endothelium during neovascularization after myocardial infarction. *Am J Pathol* 2000; **157**: 877–83.
101. Dejana E. Endothelial adherens junctions: implications in the control of vascular permeability and angiogenesis. *J Clin Invest* 1996; **98**: 1949–53.
102. Bourguignon LY, Lokeshwar VB, Chen X, Kerrick WG. Hyaluronic acid-induced lymphocyte signal transduction and HA receptor (GP85/CD44)-cytoskeleton interaction. *J Immunol* 1993; **151**: 6634–44.
103. Haslinger B, Mandl-Weber S, Sellmayer A, Sitter T. Hyaluronan fragments induce the synthesis of MCP-1 and IL-8 in cultured human peritoneal mesothelial cells *Cell Tissue Res* 2001; **305**:79–86.
104. Ponta H. The CD44 protein family. *Int J Biochem Cell Biol* 1998; **30**: 299–305.
105. Hott J, Godbey S, Antony V. The role of the mesothelial cell in pleural metastasis: inhibition of breast carcinoma cell adherence to pleural cells by hyaluronidase. *FASEB J* 1992; **6**: 1919.
106. Hott J, Godbey S, Antony VB. The role of the mesothelial cell in pleural metastasis: breast carcinoma cell adherence to pleural mesothelial cells by a mechanism involving hyaluronate and CD44. *Am Rev Respir Dis* 1993; **147**: A794.
107. Johnson JP. Cell adhesion molecules of the immunoglobulin supergene family and their role in malignant transformation and progression to metastatic disease. *Cancer Metastasis Rev* 1991; **10**: 11–22.
108. Underhill C. CD44: the hyaluronan receptor. *J Cell Sci* 1992; **103** (Pt 2): 293–8.
109. Lee YCG, Lane, KB, Zoia O, *et al.* Transforming growth factor-β induces collagen synthesis without inducing IL-8 production in mesothelial cells. *Eur Respir J* 2003; **22**:197–202.

110. Antony VB, Nasreen N, Mohammed KA, *et al.* Talc pleurodesis: basic fibroblast growth factor mediates pleural fibrosis. *Chest* 2004; **126**:1522-8
111. Nasreen N, Mohammed, KA, Brown S, *et al.* Talc mediates angiostasis in malignant pleural effusions via endostatin induction. *Eur Respir J* 2007; **29**: 761–9.
112. Galffy G, Mohammed K, Ward M, Dowling PA, Antony V. Interleukin-8: an autocrine growth factor for malignant mesothelioma. *Am Cancer Res* 1999; **59**: 367–71.

8

Immunology

NICOLA A WILSON, STEVEN E MUTSAERS, YC GARY LEE

INTRODUCTION

The term 'cytokine' was first used in 1974 to describe the group of low molecular weight molecules that are secreted by one cell to mediate cell–cell interaction and regulate the behavior of the same or other nearby cells. The last decade has seen an explosion of literature on cytokine research. The majority of cytokines are multifunctional, share overlapping functions, and their actions are often cell- and environment-specific. Disruption of the balances of the cytokine network underlies the pathogenesis of disease states. Therapeutic manipulation of cytokine profiles are increasingly used in clinical trials.

The presence of many cytokines has been demonstrated in pleural fluids or in the pleura. Resident mesothelial cells, as well as infiltrating inflammatory and cancer cells, are known to produce a vast variety of cytokines. Cytokines can also reach the pleural space from the systemic circulation. Actual evidence of cytokine actions in the pleura is limited and their functions in the pleura are often extrapolated from results in other systems. Several cytokines of interest are described below and are arbitrarily divided into groups according to their reported functions in the pleura.

CYTOKINE GROWTH FACTORS IN PLEURAL FIBROSIS

A host of cytokine growth factors have been demonstrated in the pleura, and are likely to be of biological significance.

Transforming growth factor beta

Transforming growth factor beta (TGF-β) is currently considered the most potent pro-fibrotic cytokine and its effects on the pleura have attracted attention. TGF-β is produced by and can act on mesothelial cells, as well as most cells which infiltrate the pleura (e.g. inflammatory and malignant cells). TGF-β is also present in pleural effusions of infective and malignant etiologies, indicating that it may have a role in the inflammatory and pro-fibrotic pathogenesis of many pleural diseases.[1] It is also present in high levels in asbestos-induced pleural fibrosis[2] and in parapneumonic effusions, suggesting a pathogenic role. Early evidence shows that TGF-β has a role in the granulomatous inflammation process and in the pleural fibrosis in tuberculosis (TB) pleuritis.[3]

PLEURAL EFFUSION

Pleural effusions of various etiologies contain all three TGF-β isoforms: β_1, β_2 and β_3. Significantly higher TGF-β levels are found in exudative and loculated effusions (of malignant, empyema and tuberculous origins), compared with transudative and free-flowing effusions, but TGF-β levels cannot distinguish exudative effusions of different etiologies.[4] Pleural concentrations of TGF-β are usually significantly higher than corresponding serum levels, implying a localized release of the cytokine to stimuli during pleural diseases.

PLEURAL FIBROSIS

Overproduction of TGF-β is the principal abnormality in most fibrotic diseases, and its direct administration potently induces fibrosis.[5] After tissue injury, a repair process is initiated with increased expression of TGF-β by parenchymal cells, infiltrating macrophages and lymphocytes.[6] Latent TGF-β can be activated within 1 hour, followed by a second wave of activation several days later.[7] TGF-β induces fibrosis by increasing the expression of most extracellular matrix proteins, as well as by inhibiting their degradation[8] (Figure 8.1).

Excessive formation of adhesions and resultant pleural fibrosis are commonly seen in pleural diseases (e.g. empyema, fibrothorax following tuberculosis). Increased levels of TGF-β have been observed in the pleural fluid during these pathologies. During the progression of empyema, pleural fluid TGF-β1 increases. This correlates with the pleural fibrosis that takes place, measured by microscopic thickness and fibroblast score.[9] TGF-β is a potent chemoattractant for fibroblasts, which are important in the synthesis and deposition of collagen, leading to the progression of pleural fibrosis. However, the mesothelium itself also participates in the matrix turnover and deposition. Upon stimulation by TGF-β, mesothelial cells can synthesize matrix proteins and collagen,[10] matrix metalloproteinase (MMP)-1, MMP-9 and tissue inhibitor of matrix metalloproteinases (TIMP)-2.[11,12] TGF-β can contribute to the profibrotic environment by also suppressing fibrinolysis via reduction of tissue plasminogen activators and via increasing the mesothelial cell production of plasminogen activator inhibitor (PAI)-1 and -2.[13,14] Collagen, PAI-1 and fibronectin production by stimulated mesothelial cells can be downregulated by TGF-β1 short hairpin RNA.[15]

Strategies to antagonize TGF-β activity therefore hold promise to prevent pleural fibrosis. Significant reductions in bleomycin-induced pulmonary fibrosis,[16] glomerulosclerosis,[17] wound scarring[18] and intra-abdominal adhesions[19] have been achieved in animal models by neutralizing TGF-β functions, or by increasing the levels of inhibitory Smad proteins.[20]

The use of pan-specific neutralizing anti-TGF-β antibodies have been shown to decrease the volume of pus and the adhesions formed during *Pasteurella multocida*-induced empyema in rabbits.[21] Importantly, the microscopic pleural thickness and fibroblast scores were also decreased. Similarly, the volume of pleural effusion and recruitment of inflammatory cells to the pleural cavity were decreased by neutralizing pan anti-TGF-β antibodies during *Mycobacterium tuberculosis* antigen-specific pleural effusion formation.[22]

PLEURODESIS

Although the potent pro-fibrotic properties of TGF-β are implicated in the pathogenesis of excessive pleural fibrosis, these properties can be utilized for therapeutic pleurodesis (i.e. iatrogenic induction of pleural fibrosis to obliterate the pleural space). Pleurodesis is generally performed by intrapleural administration of a chemical agent or by mechanical abrasion during surgery. These processes aim to provoke acute pleural inflammation,[1] which, if intense enough, will result in pleural fibrosis (Figure 8.2).

Direct intrapleural administration of TGF-β2 and -β3 induce excellent pleurodesis in different animal models[23–27] (Figure 8.3). Histologically, intrapleural deliv-

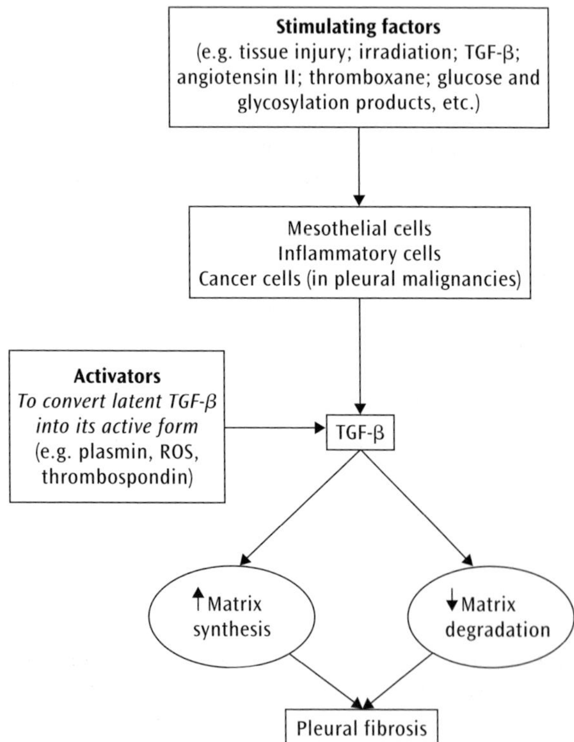

Figure 8.1 A simplified diagram of the role of transforming growth factor (TGF)-β in pleural fibrosis. ROS, reactive oxygen species.

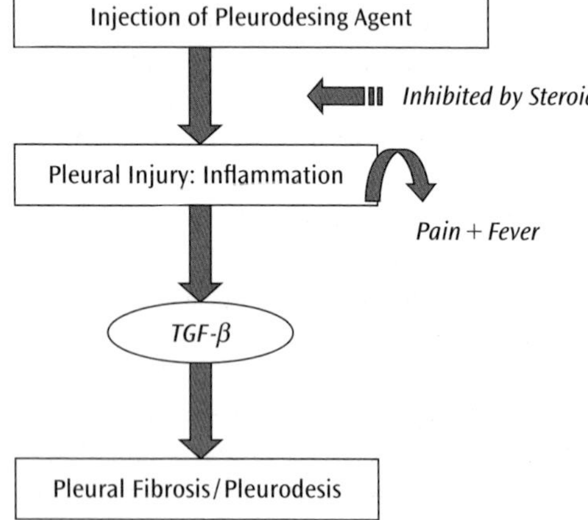

Figure 8.2 The intrapleural administration of conventional pleurodesing agents induces an acute pleural injury and inflammation. This process is inhibited by corticosteroids. Pain and fever associated with pleurodesis are presumed to be a result of the acute pleural inflammation. The inflammation may heal with restoration of normal pleura (failed pleurodesis). However, if the inflammation is sufficiently intense, it will progress to chronic inflammation and pleural fibrosis (successful pleurodesis). Transforming growth factor (TGF)-β is most likely the mediator of the fibrotic process.[21] Reprinted from Lee YCG, Lane KB. *Curr Opin Pulm Med* 2001; **7**: 173–9, with permission from the publisher, Lippincott, Williams & Wilkins.

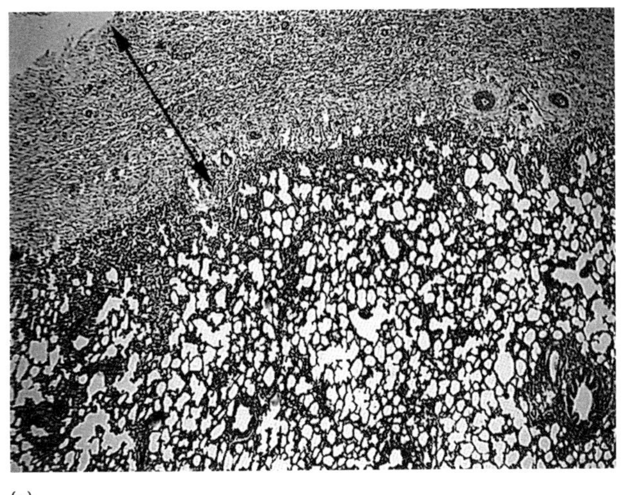

(a)

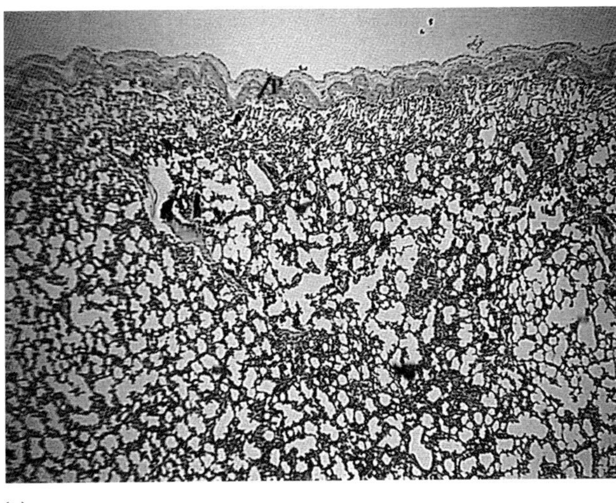

(b)

Figure 8.3 The pleura (indicated by the arrows) following treatment with transforming growth factor (TGF)-β2 injection (a) is significantly thickened with a large amount of collagen and fibrous tissue deposition compared with pleura from the control side (b). Reprinted from Lee YCG, Lane KB, Parker RE, *et al. Thorax* 2000; **55**: 1058–62 with permission from the publisher, the BMJ Publishing Group.

ery of TGF-β2 stimulates marked collagen deposition,[24] resulting in dramatic pleural fibrosis and adhesions,[26] more rapidly than talc (Figure 8.3). Injection of fibronectin, a downstream matrix protein induced by TGF-β, fails to reproduce the fibrotic effects of TGF-β in the pleura.[28] TGF-β upregulation of mesothelial cell collagen synthesis is at least as potent as talc and doxycycline.[24] Interestingly, intrapleural introduction of TGF-β2 and -β3 in rabbit models induces an increase in pleural fluid volume before pleurodesis ensues.[27,29]

Intrapleural administration of TGF-β in low doses appears safe. No acute cardiopulmonary abnormalities or histological extrapulmonary abnormalities at 14 days are found in sheep after TGF-β pleurodesis.[30] The systemic levels of TGF-β1 and -β2 in sheep that received TGF-β2 pleurodesis are no different from those given talc or bleomycin.[30] In humans, regular intravenous therapy with TGF-β2 was shown to be safe in a phase I clinical trial in multiple sclerosis patients.[31]

The concept of administration of TGF-β to initiate fibrosis has the advantage of bypassing the pleural inflammatory process (Figure 8.2). Additionally, TGF-β has potent anti-inflammatory properties. The pleural fluid induced after the intrapleural injection of TGF-β has significantly lower inflammatory indices[23,24] and IL-8 levels[32] when compared with those after talc or doxycycline administration. After intrapleural talc introduction, TGF-β1 steadily increases over time.[33] In cultured mesothelial cells, talc and doxycycline, but not TGF-β, stimulates significant IL-8 release.[32] Systemic corticosteroids reduce the pleural inflammation and hence the efficacy of talc and doxycycline pleurodesis in animal models.[34,35] However, TGF-β-induced pleurodesis remains effective in the presence of corticosteroids,[25] supporting the notion that TGF-β can induce pleurodesis without necessitating significant pleural inflammation. TGF-β therefore carries a theoretical advantage of producing pleurodesis with less pain or fever than conventional agents (Figure 8.2).

Although TGF-β appears promising as a pleurodesing agent, its long-term effects and effectiveness in abnormal (e.g. malignant) pleural surfaces requires evaluation in humans.[1] Importantly, results to date challenge the traditional concept that creation of pleurodesis must be accompanied with pleural injury and inflammation.[1]

IMMUNE MODULATION

Transforming growth factor-β plays a critical role in the immune regulation. Most commonly, it behaves as a potent anti-inflammatory cytokine[36] and suppresses the production of tumor necrosis factor alpha (TNF-α), interleukin (IL)-1[37–39] and IL-8,[40] thus deactivating neutrophil and macrophage functions. TGF-β1 knockout mice succumb to overwhelming systemic inflammation mediated by lymphocytes[41] with significantly elevated levels of TNFα and IL-1. TGF-β inhibits the production of and the response to cytokines associated with both Th1 and Th2 lymphocytes.[42] In addition, TGF-β inhibits natural killer cell functions and the generation of lymphokine-activated killer cells.[36,43] TGF-β also blocks leukocyte adhesion and recruitment to inflammation sites.[44]. While IL-1 can stimulate TGF-β in cultured mesothelial cell,.[45,46] TGF-β in turn suppresses the mesothelial production of IL-8[32] and nitric oxide,[47] in keeping with its anti-inflammatory role. The therapeutic potential of the anti-inflammatory properties of TGF-β in inflammatory pleural conditions warrant investigation.

CARCINOGENESIS

Transforming growth factor-β bears a biphasic 'love-hate' relationship with cancer. It is a potent inhibitor of cell proliferation. TGF-β acts as a tumor suppressor by also promoting cellular differentiation or apoptosis[48] in normal human cells, including mesothelial cells,[49] and during the early stage of carcinogenesis. However, advanced tumors are often resistant to such TGF-β-mediated growth arrest, probably as a result of reduced TGF-β signaling secondary to mutations in genes encoding TGF-β signaling mediators.[48] Once resistance develops, the more aggressive forms of cancer cells can make use of TGF-β to enhance their growth and metastasis in several ways. TGF-β signaling in the tumor microenvironment significantly affects carcinoma initiation, progression and metastasis via epithelial cell autonomous and interdependent stromal–epithelial interactions (see review[50]). TGF-β can promote angiogenesis essential for tumor growth, and increases extracellular matrix synthesis by cancer cells, allowing their binding to cell-adhesion molecules, thereby facilitating distant metastasis. The immunosuppressive functions of TGF-β may enable cancer cells to escape immune surveillance.[48]

The effect of TGF-β on pleural malignancies is largely unknown. In mesothelioma cells, TGF-β increases the synthesis of matrix protein[10] and urokinase-type plasminogen activator. Antagonizing TGF-β activity can inhibit mesothelioma cell proliferation and tumor growth *in vivo*.[51] Small molecule inhibitor of ALK5 kinase (TBR-I) can prevent tumor recurrence in a malignant mesothelioma model which overexpresses TGF-β.[52]

Given the complex relationship between TGF-β and cancer, the potential application of TGF-β or its antagonists as cancer therapy require careful clinical assessments.[1]

TGF-β ACTIVATION

Transforming growth factor-β is secreted in trimeric or dimeric latent form, according to cell type and environment. The dimer consists of the TGF-β itself, and the latency associated peptide (LAP), which confers inactivity on the molecule. In the trimeric form, this dimer, also known as the small latent complex, is bound to extracellular matrix by the latent TGF-β binding protein (LTBP). The most crucial step of TGF-β bioavailability is post-translational activation, taking the form of the separation of the TGF-β from the LAP, allowing it to become active. Proteolytic cleavage and conformational change can bring this about, and there is a diverse range of activators including matrix metalloproteinases (MMPs), integrins αvβ6 and αvβ8, thrombospondin (TSP)-1, and physiological extremes such as low pH or mechanical stress. The post-translational regulation of TGF-β activity in the pleura has not been explored, but may represent a target point for therapeutic intervention.

GENETICS

The TGF-β1 gene is located on human chromosome 19q13. There are at least five polymorphisms in the TGF-β1 gene and several others in its promoter region[53] and can be associated with variation in circulating TGF-β levels.[54] Homozygosity for arginine at codon 25 of the leader sequence of TGF-β1 correlates with higher TGF-β production *in vitro*, and is associated with fibrotic lung pathology before lung transplantation and with the development of fibrosis in the graft.[55] The effect of these polymorphisms on pleural fibrosis awaits investigation.

Hepatocyte growth factor

Hepatocyte growth factor (HGF), also known as scatter factor and tumor cytotoxic factor, is a multifunctional polypeptide involved in embryonic development, tissue repair and cancer growth. HGF forms part of a family of plasminogen-related growth factors along with HGF-like/macrophage stimulating protein, plasminogen and apolipoprotein – all of which are thought to have evolved from the same ancestral gene.[56]

STRUCTURE

The gene encoding HGF maps on chromosome 7q21.1 in humans and is composed of 18 exons interrupted by 17 introns spanning approximately 70 kb. The protein is derived from a biologically inactive single chain propeptide (pro-HGF) of 728 amino acids, with a similar amino acid sequence as plasminogen.[56,57] The propeptide is cleaved extracellularly by serine proteases, such as plasminogen activator, to give an active heterodimeric glycoprotein consisting of an α and β chain held together by a disulfide bond.[58]

Hepatocyte growth factor is produced not only by hepatocytes but also by a wide variety of cell types including mesothelial cells, platelets, monocytes, fibroblasts and certain tumor cells including malignant mesothelioma.[59] Inflammatory cytokines and mediators produced by tumor cells including IL-1β, IL-6, IL-8, TNF-α, prostaglandin E_2, basic fibroblast growth factor (b-FGF), epidermal growth factor (EGF) and platelet-derived growth factor (PDGF) can stimulate HGF production,[60] whereas TGF-β has been shown to downregulate HGF expression.[61]

The HGF receptor is the met protein, a product of the c-met proto-oncogene (p190 met) found principally on epithelial and endothelial cells, mesothelial cells and a variety of tumors, including mesothelioma.[62] c-met consists of a transmembrane 145-kDa β-chain and an extracellular 50-kDa α-chain to form a dimeric 190 kDa protein with structural features of a tyrosine kinase receptor. HGF also binds to cell surface heparan sulfate proteoglycans that serve as low affinity HGF receptors and modulate the interaction between HGF and c-met receptor. c-met signals largely via the Ras signaling pathway. Data has shown that activation of the Ras pathway leads to cell proliferation whereas the PI3 kinase pathway is needed to induce mitogenesis. Both pathways are essential for invasive growth. Dysregulation of c-met signaling is observed in carcinogenesis. Point mutations in c-met detected in the catalytic domain of the receptor have been associated with carcinomas and overexpression of the c-met gene in transgenic mice leads to carcinomas of the thyroid gland, breast, liver, pancreas and ovary. Increased expression of c-met is associated with a poor prognosis.[56,63]

BIOLOGICAL FUNCTIONS

Hepatocyte growth factor acts as an endocrine, paracrine and autocrine factor and regulates a wide range of cellular processes such as cell survival, proliferation, migration and differentiation.[63] Mice genetically deficient in HGF are embryonic lethal with severe placental insufficiency, reduction of sensory nerves and developmental defects in the liver and muscle.[64–67] During organogenesis, HGF plays a key role in epithelial–mesenchymal transition (EMT), and helps regulate lung morphogenesis.[68,69] Administration of HGF to the airways of mice also reduces airway inflammation, hyper-responsiveness and remodeling in injury models.[70] In addition, HGF suppresses dendritic cell functions, thus down-regulating antigen-induced Th1- and Th2-type immune responses.[71] Transgenic mice that overexpress HGF develop diverse tumors, polycystic kidney disease and inflammatory bowel disease.

TISSUE REPAIR

Hepatocyte growth factor is a potent growth factor and protects from fibrosis in many tissues but its role in the pleura and other serosal tissues is unclear. Mesothelial cells both secrete HGF and express c-met on their surface, suggesting an autocrine loop of self-stimulation.[59] HGF induces proliferation, migration and EMT-like responses in normal mesothelial cells and stimulates production of types I and III collagen *in vitro*.[72] After intratracheal instillation of asbestos in rats, increased mesothelial cell proliferation is associated with increased levels of HGF and keratinocyte growth factor in the pleural fluid.[73] Although HGF may be associated with various pathologies linked with asbestos exposure such as mesothelioma, its role in normal tissues is more likely to be associated with repair.

Administration of HGF to various animal models of tissue injury, including the lung, enhanced repair and retarded the progression of tissue fibrosis,[74–81] whereas application of neutralizing antibodies to HGF increased fibrosis.[82,83] HGF ameliorates fibrosis by stimulating tissue repair mechanisms. In addition, HGF inhibits apoptosis, protects epithelial cells against DNA damaging agents, promotes angiogenesis and antagonizes the profibrotic actions of TGF-β1, possibly through enhancing extracellular matrix catabolism via both MMP and the plasminogen activator/plasmin proteolytic pathways.[84] The possible protective role of HGF against pleural/peritoneal fibrosis is being examined.

MESOTHELIOMA

High levels of activated HGF and c-met have been observed in mesothelioma and other cancers, and in some tumor types these levels correlate with disease relapse and poor prognosis.[85–88] Tumors positive for HGF also have a higher microvessel density and hence may have a role in mesothelioma angiogenesis.[88] Transgenic mice that overexpress HGF develop diverse tumors, suggesting that HGF may promote tumor development and progression.[89]

Recent studies suggest that *Simian virus 40* (SV40) may be a cause or be a cofactor in mesothelioma development. SV40 positive mesothelioma cells show evidence of c-met activation associated with cell cycle progression into S-phase, acquisition of a fibroblastoid morphology and the assembly of viral particles.[90] In infected cells, c-met activation and subsequent biological effects appear to be mediated by an autocrine HGF circuit which can be blocked using HGF neutralizing antibodies.[90] Mesothelioma frequently express elevated AKT activity associated with HGF activation. Early studies inhibiting the downstream phosphatidylinositol 3-kinase (PI3K)/AKT signaling pathway blocked cell growth and induced apoptosis and this effect was enhanced when combined with standard chemotherapeutic agents.[91]

Hepatocyte growth factor has also been implicated in dissemination of mesothelioma and other tumors by disrupting cell–cell adhesion and inducing mesothelial cells to round up and detach from the serosal surface. The exposed underlying matrix is an ideal substrate for attachment and invasion of the tumor cell.[92–94] HGF may be secreted by the tumors themselves or by surrounding stromal cells in response to the tumor or inflammatory mediators released following surgical resection.[93,94] HGF also stimulates mesothelioma cells *in vitro* to secrete MMP-1, -9 and membrane type 1 (MT1)-MMP which may induce extracellular matrix degradation and subsequent tumor invasion and spread.[92] Adenoviral transfection of peritoneal mesothelial cells with the HGF antagonist NK4 has been used therapeutically in mice to demonstrate the potential for targeting HGF activity in inhibiting dissemination of pancreatic and gallbladder cancer cell lines.[95,96]

Epidermal growth factor

The epidermal growth factor family consists of six structurally related polypeptides; EGF, TGF-α, amphiregulin, heparin-binding EGF (HB-EGF), betacellulin and epiregulin. These factors all contain a conserved three-loop compact structure, known as the EGF-like domain, and their soluble forms are proteolytically derived from their membrane precursors. Neuregulins are a subfamily of proteins also related to the EGF family of growth factors.[97]

The EGF receptor (EGFR) is a transmembrane glycoprotein which belongs to the erbB family of tyrosine kinase receptors. Activation of EGFR leads to receptor dimerization and internalization followed by auto- or trans-phosphorylation of the receptor tyrosine kinase domains, which initiates multiple intracellular signaling pathways, including the Ras-Raf-mitogen-activated protein kinase (MAPK) pathway and the phosphatidylinositol 3-kinase-Akt pathway.[98] Activation of ErbB receptors is important in regulating cell proliferation, differentiation, migration and survival in different tissues, with migration also requiring the activation of integrins for some cells.[99]

Epidermal growth factor is a potent mitogen for human, rat and mouse mesothelial cells *in vitro*[100–104] but has no mitogenic effect on confluent monolayers of mouse mesothelial cells *in vivo*.[105] The mitogenic effect on injured mesothelial cells has not been determined *in vivo*. EGF, together with TGF-β, can also induce EMT of cultured mesothelial cells from a cobblestone into a fibroblastoid spindle-shaped morphology and stimulate collagen production (Lee, unpublished results). HB-EGF mRNA is upregulated in mesothelial cells treated with the inflammatory cytokines IL-1β and TNF-α[106] and HB-EGF induces mesothelial cells to adhere to collagen type I, express β1 integrins and migrate.[107] Taken together, these findings suggest a role for EGF family proteins in repair of the pleura and other serosal surfaces.

PLEURAL INFLAMMATION

Epidermal growth factor participates in eliciting inflammatory responses in the pleura. Pretreatment of mesothelial cells with EGF greatly enhanced mononuclear leukocyte adhesion.[108] Prolonged co-culture for 3 weeks stimulated proliferation and differentiation of monocytes/macrophages on the mesothelial surface. Adhesion was not related to EGF-induced upregulation of ICAM-1 or CD44 expression on mesothelial cells.[108] Proliferation of the mononuclear leukocytes was most likely due to EGF-stimulated mesothelial cell production of macrophage colony-stimulating activity, shown to be due predominantly to macrophage colony-stimulating factor.[108]

Epidermal growth factor alone does not induce nitric oxide (NO) production by mesothelial cells but does augment NO synthesis induced by endotoxin.[109] In addition, EGFR ligands can act as chemoattractants on normal mesothelial cells.[99]

Epidermal growth factor also promotes adhesion of malignant cells to the mesothelium *in vitro* and may therefore be important in tumor deposition in the pleura/peritoneum *in vivo*.[104] It may also have a role in effusion formation. Peritoneal infusion of EGF via osmotic minipumps resulted in dose-dependent formation of bloody ascites. The EGF-induced ascites were significantly inhibited using indomethacin or dexamethasone.[110] EGF also activates the NA^+–H^+ exchanger in human pleural mesothelial cells, a mechanism requiring protein kinase C (PKC) activation.[111]

MESOTHELIOMA

The EGF receptor has been associated with the pathogenesis of asbestos-related pleural disease. Crocidolite and erionite fibers stimulate increases in EGFR synthesis[112,113] and elevated serum levels of secreted EGFR are found in retired asbestos workers when compared with non-exposed individuals.[114] Intense patterns of EGFR protein expression are linked to mesothelial cells phagocytosing long fibers[112] and previous studies have shown a correlation between asbestos fiber length and carcinogenicity.[115] The asbestos fibers induce autophosphorylation of EGFR in pleural mesothelial cells which activates the MAPK signaling pathway and induction of the AP-1 family members c-fos and c-jun,[112,116–118] leading to cell proliferation and carcinogenesis.

Overexpression of EGFR plays an important role in the pathogenesis and progression of a variety of malignancies. EGFR are expressed on normal mesothelial cells[99] and is overexpressed in many malignant mesotheliomas, with reports varying from 44 to 97.6 percent.[119–123] EGFR positivity has been associated with improved survival[121,122] but this was not supported by other studies.[119,120,123] The discrepancies in the findings may be partly explained by the greater expression of EGFR in the epithelioid mesothelioma, which has a better prognosis than the sarcomatoid tumors.[121,122] EGF also upregulates MMP-3 and -9 production by mesothelioma cells which may participate in the local invasion and spread of the tumor.[124]

The therapeutic potential of EGFR inhibitors in the treatment of mesothelioma is unclear. Several *in vitro* studies using small molecule tyrosine kinase inhibitors (e.g. PD153035 and gefitinib) have shown significant inhibition of EGFR-dependent cell signaling, including Akt phosphorylation and extracellular signal-regulated kinases 1 and 2 in mesothelioma cell lines examined. This has led to the suppression of mesothelioma cell motility, invasion and proliferation.[125,126] Gefitinib also increased tumor responsiveness to radiation therapy in an animal model of mesothelioma.[127] Another tyrosine kinase inhibitor, tyrphostin AG-1478, significantly ameliorated asbestos-induced increases in the mRNA of the protooncogene c-fos. Pretreatment of mesothelial cells with AG-1478 also reduced apoptosis in cells exposed to asbestos.[113]

However, a recent phase II study by the Cancer and Leukemia Group B (CALGB) using gefitinib failed to provide benefits in 43 patients with previously untreated mesothelioma.[122] This may be explained by the absence of common EGFR tyrosine kinase domain mutations in mesotheliomas which recently has been shown to confer sensitivity to gefitinib in lung cancers.[128] A similar study by the Southwest Oncology Group examined the effect of the tyrosine kinase inhibitor erlotinib in 63 previously untreated mesothelioma patients, with the same outcome as the CALGB study.[129] Activation of the extracellular signal-regulated kinase (ERK) and phosphatidylinositol 3-kinase/Akt downstream pathways were suggested as possible resistance mechanisms to EGFR tyrosine kinase inhibitors.[129]

The effect of farnesyltransferase inhibitors on mesothelioma cell growth has also been examined *in vitro*. Farnesylation of Ras (downstream molecule in EGFR signaling) is the obligatory first step in the switch from an inactive to an active Ras-GTP bound form. Preventing Ras farnesylation was proposed to inhibit Ras functions and hence block downstream effects resulting from EGFR activation. Growth of mesothelioma cell lines were not effected by a number of farnesyltransferase inhibitors, highlighting the concept that the same signaling pathway can be regulated in different ways and these regulations can differ between different cells of different origin.[130] EGFR status in malignant cells recovered from pleural effusions may have prognostic implications. In one study, breast cancer patients with negative EGFR status in the malignant cells in pleural fluids had the longest survival time, whereas patients with positive EGFR but negative estrogen and progesterone receptor status had the worst prognosis.[131]

Basic fibroblast growth factor

Basic fibroblast growth factor is present in pleural effusions of various etiologies.[132,133] Mesothelial cells synthesize and release considerable amounts of b-FGF.[106,134] The majority (80 percent) of b-FGF is localized intracellularly, and the remainder is associated with extracellular matrix components on the mesothelial cell surface.[134] b-FGF is known to stimulate mesothelial cell proliferation *in vitro* and *in vivo*.[105] Early evidence to date suggests a role of b-FGF in pleural fibrosis and malignant pleural diseases.

PLEURAL FIBROSIS

In vitro talc-stimulated mesothelial cells increased their b-FGF transcription and secretion.[135] Pleural fibroblasts proliferate when incubated with conditioned medium from talc stimulated mesothelial cells – this response is diminished by neutralizing antibodies against b-FGF.[135] A higher pleural level of b-FGF was seen in patients who had a successful talc-induced pleurodesis, compared with those in whom talc pleurodesis failed.[135]

MALIGNANT PLEURAL DISEASES

Basic fibroblast growth factor is a potent angiogenic factor, and is implicated in cancer growth and metastasis. Protein expression of b-FGF in solid tumors is correlated with heparanase expression, their co-expression is thought to allow heparanase mediated release of b-FGF from the extracellular matrix.[136] Mesothelioma proliferation *in vitro* can be inhibited using α-tocopheryl succinate (α-TOS) which downregulates FGF-2 transcription, thereby interrupting the FGF autocrine growth loop.[137] One study reported that the mean b-FGF level is significantly lower in malignant effusions (including mesotheliomas) compared with nonmalignant ones. Significantly, an inverse correlation is observed between b-FGF levels found in mesothelioma effusions and patient survival. High serum b-FGF levels are also associated with reduced survival.[133] However, another study reported a negative correlation between b-FGF and tumor size observed during thoracoscopy.[135]

Interleukin-1 induced mesothelial cell production of b-FGF in one study[134] but not in another.[106] In both studies, TNFα did not stimulate b-FGF release. IL-2, however, can produce a marked suppression of b-FGF expression.[106] In mesothelioma cells, b-FGF increases glycosaminoglycans production but has no significant effect on heparan sulfate synthesis.[138]

Platelet-derived growth factor

The platelet-derived growth factor family of cytokines consists of dimers of two related polypeptide chains designated A, B, C and D that can exist as heterodimers (PDGF-AB) or homodimers (PDGF-AA, PDGF-BB, PDGF-CC and PDGF-DD).[139–141] These factors exert their cellular effects through structurally similar PDGF protein tyrosine kinase receptors (PDGFR-α and -β). The PDGFR-α binds to A-, B- and C- chains with high affinity, whereas PDGFR-β only binds the B- and D- chains. PDGF-C and PDGF-D require proteolytic activation before binding to and activating PDGFR. A heterodimeric PDGF-α/β complex has also been identified which can be activated by PDGF-AB, PDGF-BB and PDGF-CC.[139–142]

Platelet-derived growth factor ligand binding induces dimerization of both receptors and subsequently autophosphorylation of the tyrosine kinase domain. This in turn phosphorylates numerous signaling molecules that initiate intracellular signaling cascades, including the ras/MAPK and PI3K/Akt pathways, ultimately promoting cell migration, proliferation, differentiation and survival, and tumor resistance to radiotherapy and chemotherapy.[142]

This factor is produced by a variety of cells including mesothelial cells, macrophages, smooth muscle cells, endothelial cells, fibroblasts and many types of tumors, and large stores of PDGF-AB are found in α granules of platelets. PDGF exerts its potent mitogenic and chemotactic effects in a variety of mesenchymal cells such as fibroblasts, vascular smooth muscle cells, glomerular mesangial cells and brain glial cells.[142]

In the pleura, PDGF is thought to have active roles in normal and pathologic conditions. Mesothelial cells produce PDGF which has potent mitogenic effects on fibroblasts and mesothelial cells.[102,105] PDGF is a potent mediator of asbestos-induced pleural fibroblast proliferation.[143] Fibroblast proliferation was blocked using neutralizing antibodies against PDGF.[143] PDGF is also a chemoattractant for neutrophils and monocytes and stimulates the activation of macrophages.[144,145] It upregulates fibronectin gene expression,[146] hyaluronan synthesis,[147] procollagen synthesis[102,148] and increases collagenase activity,[149] processes essential for connective tissue remodeling and fibrosis. The combination of EGF and PDGF produce a synergistic effect in stimulating collagen production by mesothelial cells.[102] PDGF also induces the expression of TGF-β further potentiating the fibrotic response.[150]

MESOTHELIOMA

Elevated levels of PDGF-AB are also seen in patients with pleural mesothelioma compared with high risk and normal controls, and positive PDGF-AB levels were associated with lower survival.[151] Mesotheliomas produce significant amounts of PDGF. The PDGF-A chain, and less frequently the PDGF-B chain, is highly overexpressed in mesothelioma compared with normal mesothelial cells, suggesting a role for PDGF in the pathogenesis of mesothelioma.[152,153] This is supported by studies showing that the SV40 T antigen-immortalized human mesothelial cells were only tumorigenic after ectopic PDGF-A overexpression.[154]

Normal mesothelial cells predominantly express one PDGF receptor, PDGFR-α, but have weak to undetectable expression of another receptor, PDGFR-β.[155,156] Stimulation with TGF-β1 decreases PDGFR-α mRNA expression in normal mesothelial cells.[157]

On the other hand, most mesothelioma cells express PDGFR-β with little PDGFR-α.[155,158,159] It has been suggested that mesothelioma cells in effusions may express the receptor and therefore possess an autocrine stimulatory loop.[160] However, such an autocrine loop is likely to only exist for PDGF-B. PDGF-B, acting in conjunction with integrin α3β1, is a chemoattractant for mesothelioma cells.[161] Overexpression studies also showed that PDGF-A is tumorigenic *in vivo* through paracrine, but not autocrine, mechanisms of cell proliferation.[155]

Platelet-derived growth factor has also been recovered in higher levels in pleural effusions from adenocarcinomas of the lung than those from small cell lung cancers or benign effusions.[162]

THERAPEUTIC APPROACHES TO INHIBIT PDGF

Studies applying dipyridamole on mesothelial cells demonstrated inhibition of PDGF-induced proliferation through attenuated ERK activity, preservation of p27(Kip1) and decreased pRB phosphorylation,[163] This may represent a potential therapeutic strategy against pleural fibrosis.

Imatinib mesylate selectively blocks tyrosine kinases, including PDGFR-β. Imatinib induces cytotoxicity and apoptosis selectively on PDGFR-β positive mesothelioma cells, via blockade of receptor phosphorylation and interference with the Akt pathway.[164] However, phase II clinical trials using imatinib mesylate alone against mesothelioma showed no obvious benefits.[165] Imatinib synergises with gemcitabine and pemetrexed[164] and combinational chemotherapy for mesothelioma using imatinib mesylate awaits evaluation. Several other tyrosine kinase inhibitors are now available which will block PDGFR but their use in pleural disease has not been reported.[166]

Insulin-like growth factor

The insulin-like growth factors (IGF-I and IGF-II) are single-chain polypeptides with structural homology to proinsulin. They are produced by most cells in the body and are abundant in the circulation, usually bound to high affinity binding proteins (IGFBP), of which six have been identified.[167] These binding proteins protect IGF from proteolysis and modulate its interaction with the IGF receptor (IGFR). The liver is the major source of circulating IGFs, which are synthesized in response to growth hormone, and controls the growth and differentiation of most tissues of the body.[168]

The IGFs bind with high affinity to two cell surface receptors, IGF-RI (or type I receptor) and IGF-RII (or type II receptor). The IGF-RI receptor has a high degree of homology to the insulin receptor and binds IGF-I with higher affinity than either IGF-II or insulin.[167,169] It exists at the cell surface as a heterotetramer consisting of two α and two β subunits joined by disulfide bonds. When the ligand binds to the extracellular α subunit there is a conformational change that induces autophosphorylation of tyrosine residues within the intracellular segment of the β subunit. This leads to receptor tyrosine kinase activity and the induction of various intracellular signaling cascades, including MAP kinase and phosphoinositide 3′-kinase pathways, which leads to growth and metabolic responses.[169]

The IGF-RII is identical to the cation-independent mannose 6-phosphate receptor. It exhibits higher affinity for IGF-II than IGF-I and does not bind insulin.[168] The IGF-RII has no intrinsic tyrosine kinase activity, hence the intracellular mechanisms by which the receptor can mediate its biological effects, including lysosomal enzyme trafficking, clearance and/or activation of a variety of growth factors and endocytosis-mediated degradation of IGF-II, is unclear.[169]

MESOTHELIOMA

Normal human mesothelial cells, as well as mesothelioma cell lines, express IGF-I, IGF-II, some of the IGF binding proteins (IGFBP), IGF-RI and IGF-RII,[124,170,171] and IGF-1 is mitogenic for mesothelial cells *in vitro*.[170] SV40-induced transformation of mesothelial cells requires the presence of a functional IGFR, suggesting an important role for IGF in the development of mesothelioma.[172] This is supported by studies showing decreased growth and tumorigenicity of SV40-induced hamster mesotheliomas following treatment with antisense IGFR transcripts.[173] More recently, a novel IGF-R1 inhibitor, NVP-AEW541, has shown concentration-dependent inhibitory effects on cultured mesothelioma cells.[174] Further evaluation of NVP-AEW541 is required for its possible therapeutic potential *in vivo*. The IGFR adaptor proteins, insulin receptor substrate (IRS)-1 and -2, also appear to play roles in the phenotype of mesothelioma. Mesotheliomas that signal through IRS-1 have increased cellular growth whereas those that signal through IRS-2 have increased motility.[170] This may affect tumor pathology as preferential signaling through IRS-1 may lead to increased local spread of the tumor whereas utilization of IRS-2 may promote metastases.[175]

Mesotheliomas express IGFBP 2, 4 and 5 but not 1, 3 or 6. The absence of the beneficial IGFBP-3 together with the presence of the deleterious IGFBP-4 would allow for a more aggressive phenotype.[176] However, in another study, IGFBP1-4 were overexpressed whereas IGFBP-5 was underexpressed.[177] In this case, IGFBP-5 may be an inhibitor of IGF-1 activation and its decrease could lead to over stimulation of the receptor and autocrine stimulation or growth.[170] More studies need to confirm these observations.

SOLITARY FIBROUS TUMOR OF THE PLEURA

Solitary fibrous tumor (SFT) is a mesenchymal tumor which arises at a variety of sites including the pleura (see Chapter 38). Approximately 10–15 percent of tumors behave in a malignant fashion.[178]

Many SFTs secrete IGF-II which is believed to be the cause of intermittent hypoglycemia present in 4–5 percent of patients. In several case studies, high levels of IGF-II were reported in the patient's serum prior to surgery.[179–181] Larger amounts of high molecular weight IGF-II were also found in the tumor cystic fluid than in the serum.[182] The high molecular weight IGF-II ('big' IGF-II) is most likely an incompletely processed IGF-II precursor (pro-IGF-II). In all cases, the hypoglycemia resolved upon removal of the tumor[183] and IGF-II levels in the serum returned to normal.[182] Others have suggested that altered IGF-1 activity may also play a role in hypoglycemia associated with these tumors, although varying results have been reported for IGF-1.[184] Chang and colleagues[184] found that serum IGF-I levels were normal in patients with SFT and IGF-1R was highly expressed on tumor cells. However, Li and coworkers[185] failed to find IGF-IR expression on these tumors.

The downstream oncogenic pathways of IGF-II are not clear but a recent study showed that insulin receptor (IR) signaling pathways are constitutively activated in SFTs.[185] IGF-II has been thought to mediate many of its biological effects through IGF-IR, however this study did not find expression of IGF-IR in these tumors. IGF-II is known to bind to an IR isoform (IR-A), with an affinity similar to that of insulin. It was shown that the IGF-II binding IR-A was the predominant isoform in SFTs suggesting that IGF-II/IR signaling plays an oncogenic role in SFTs.[185]

The hypersecretion of pro-IGF-II is associated with suppression of growth hormone secretion. Application of recombinant human growth hormone (rhGH), and in some studies with glucocorticoid treatment, reverses the suppression and has been successfully used as an alternative to surgery in a small number of patients to alleviate hypoglycemia.[186,187] The mechanism by which the rhGH controls hypoglycemia in non-islet cell tumors, including SFT, is unclear, but it is likely to involve multiple pathways, one of which is through reduction of the bioavailability of IGF-II.[187]

The possible use of IGF-1 and IGFBP-2 as potential markers of malignant effusions has also been suggested.[188] In 25 patients with malignant, infective or congestive heart failure effusions, IGF-1 and IGFBP-2 levels in effusions of malignant solid tumors were significantly higher than in lymphoma, followed by infection and transudative effusion of congestive heart failure. In effusion of solid tumors, IGFBP-2 levels were higher than those in corresponding sera, which suggests local production of this binding protein.[188]

CYTOKINES IN PLEURAL FLUID FORMATION

Vascular endothelial growth factor

Vascular hyperpermeability and plasma leakage is fundamental to the development of most exudative pleural effusions. Compelling experimental evidence demonstrates that vascular endothelial growth factor (VEGF) is a crucial mediator in pleural fluid formation, and clinical trials are underway using VEGF antagonists in the management of malignant pleural effusions (see review[189]).

This factor, initially known as vascular permeability factor, is a potent inducer of vascular permeability and the permeability of the mesothelial monolayer.[190] VEGF promotes microvascular permeability by enhancing the activity of vesicular vacuolar organelles, through which macromolecules extravazate. It can also increase active trans-endothelial transport via pinocytotic vesicles. VEGF increases the capillary and venular leakage by opening the endothelial intercellular junctions and by inducing fenestrae development in endothelia. *In vivo* it is also a vasodilator. Exogenous VEGF administration induces a reversible increase in vascular permeability within minutes. VEGF also has diverse effects on vascular endothelial cells and is capable of inducing morphological changes, stimulating cell proliferation and migration, altering their gene expression and inhibiting apoptosis.

VEGF LEVELS IN PLEURAL EFFUSIONS

Vascular endothelial growth factor is present in significant quantities in pleural and peritoneal effusions of varying etiologies, and its level is consistently higher in exudative than in transudative pleural effusions.[190–193] Although

VEGF levels are higher in malignant than in benign effusions,[194] the VEGF level is of limited use as a diagnostic tool[191,192] for malignant effusions, or to predict cancer staging[193] and histological cancer cell types.[193]

Different isoforms of VEGF have been shown to be involved in the evolution of malignant pleural effusions with different characteristics by the implantation of lung cancer cells transfected with these isoforms.[195] VEGF-A promotes tumor cells dissemination, capillary neogenesis and bloody effusions, while VEGF-D promotes both pleural and lymph node tumor dissemination.[195]

The majority of VEGF in the effusions is believed to originate from local pleural or peritoneal production.[196,197] Quiescent mesothelial cells produce large amounts of VEGF, which can be increased at mRNA and protein level by FGF-2.[198] Mesothelial cells are likely to represent the principal source of pleural fluid VEGF,[29,190] but infiltrating inflammatory cells and malignant cells (in malignant pleuritis) also contribute to VEGF production.[189]

Most malignant cell types overexpress VEGF.[199,200] This includes lung[201] and breast[202] carcinomas and mesothelioma.[203] Immunohistochemistry has confirmed the presence of VEGF in malignant cells in human pleural tissue,[194] suggesting that they may be a source of the consistently high VEGF in malignant pleural effusions. VEGF is likely to be an autocrine growth factor in mesothelioma.[197] Functional coexpression of VEGF-C (a protein closely related to VEGF), as well as its receptor VEGFR-3, has been demonstrated in malignant mesothelioma.[204]

Empyema fluids contain high levels of VEGF,[191,205] significantly above those in uncomplicated parapneumonic effusions.[190] *Staphylococcus aureus*, a common causative organism in empyema, can stimulate a dose- and time-dependent VEGF release from mesothelial cells.[190] Acidosis[206] and hypoglycemia,[207] common biochemical characteristics of empyema fluids, are also known to induce VEGF. VEGF is also elevated and correlated with other cytokines such as IL-1β and TNFα in tuberculous pleural effusions.[208]

In post-coronary artery bypass grafting (CABG) pleural effusions, VEGF levels correlate with inflammatory cells and lactate dehydrogenase (LDH) levels, as well as with protein levels which reflect the degree of vascular hyperpermeability.[209] VEGF is likely to contribute to the generalized hyperpermeability and the resultant formation of large effusions in ovarian hyperstimulation syndrome[210] and in Meigs' syndrome.[211]

Hypoxia and ischemia are amongst the most established stimulators of VEGF[212–215] and may contribute to the pathogenesis of pleural effusion from pulmonary emboli.[191]

TARGETING VEGF TO CONTROL PLEURAL OR PERITONEAL EFFUSIONS

Vascular endothelial growth factor is essential in malignant effusion formation.[216] When cancer cells are injected into mice, lung lesions from adenocarcinoma (high VEGF output) express more VEGF and the tumors are more vascular than the squamous cell cancer (which produce lower VEGF) lesions. VEGF expression correlates directly with the volume of effusion formed. Importantly, transfection of adenocarcinoma cells with antisense VEGF[165] gene, significantly reduces the vascular permeability and pleural effusions. Conversely, transfecting the squamous cancer cells with sense VEGF gene increases their VEGF production, and results in significantly more fluid accumulation. Similar results apply to malignant ascites development.[217]

Promising results are rapidly accumulating on the use of VEGF inhibition in preventing pleural and peritoneal fluid accumulation.[189] VEGF activity can be antagonized with various techniques, including antibodies that block VEGF binding to its receptors, inhibitors of the tyrosine kinase functions of the VEGF receptors, and antisense nucleic acids to disrupt cellular VEGF production.[218,219] Many of these methods have been successfully used to inhibit tumor growth in animals and are now in phase II/III clinical trials.[219] Antisense oligonucleotide (ODN), inhibiting VEGF and VEGF-C expression, is capable of specifically inhibiting mesothelioma cell growth. VEGF-R2 and VEGF-R3 blocking antibodies act synergistically to inhibit mesothelioma cell growth.[204]

Several VEGF receptors have been described, amongst which two signaling tyrosine kinase receptors, Flt-1 (VEGFR-1) and KDR/Flk-1 (VEGFR-2), are most studied.[213,220] VEGF-R3 is the receptor for VEGF-C, a molecule closely related to VEGF.[204] VEGF receptors are expressed primarily on endothelial cells, but are also found in many diverse normal and malignant cell types.[213] Pleural tissues, in both healthy and diseased states, express significant levels of VEGF receptors.[205] Upon ligand binding to the receptors, the intracellular signaling for various VEGF functions are mediated via the MAPK, PKC and PI/Akt pathways,[221] which are potential target points for inhibition of VEGF activities.[222]

Phosphorylation blockade of the VEGF receptor (with an oral inhibitor of tyrosine kinase phosphorylation of KDR/Flk-1 and Flt-1 receptors) inhibits the formation of malignant effusion in mice with lung adenocarcinomas by reducing vascular permeability.[223] A neutralizing antibody (A4.6.1) that blocks VEGF access to *both* its receptors completely inhibits ascites formation, tumor growth and prolongs the survival in mice inoculated intraperitoneally with human ovarian cancer cells.[224] Antibodies against the KDR/Flk-1 receptors (DC101) and exogenous soluble human Flt-1 receptors (as an inhibitor of VEGF binding) also effectively inhibit malignant ascites accumulation in mice.[225,226]

A VEGF tyrosine kinase inhibitor (SU5416) is under clinical trial against recurrent pleural effusion and ascites formation.[227] ZD6474, an antagonist of VEGFR-2 tyrosine kinase, can inhibit formation of malignant pleural effusions resulting from adenocarcinoma cells inoculated into nude mice.[228] Further clinical studies are anticipated to evaluate other VEGF antagonists in controlling pleural/peritoneal effusions. While most investigations focus on VEGF inhibition in the setting of malignant effusion, the results are likely to be also applicable for most other exudative effusions. At present, the oral and systemic administration of VEGF inhibitors has been tried. The intrapleural route of delivery of VEGF antagonists is another method worth exploring.

Gene transfer of soluble Flt-1 (VEGFR-1) attenuated peritoneal fibrosis formation in mice treated with adenovirus encoding active TGF-β.[229] Gene therapy to halt VEGF production in the setting of malignant pleural effusion warrants investigation.

Interferon suppresses VEGF production *in vitro* but a pilot study using intrapleural interferon for the management of malignant effusions showed disappointing results.[193]

Targeting upstream cytokine stimulators of VEGF is another approach worth pursuing.[189] VEGF production can be stimulated by various cytokines, amongst which TGF-β appears to be the most potent and consistent.[230] TGF-β induces a dose-dependent increase in VEGF release from pleural mesothelial cells and *in vivo*.[29] In human pleural effusions, the levels of TGF-β1 and -β2 both correlate with those of VEGF,[29] in keeping with the animal experiment data that TGF-β contributes to intrapleural VEGF accumulation.

Other inflammatory mediators, including IL-1, IL-6, TNF-α, PDGF, FGF-2, keratinocyte growth factor (KGF), EGF, IGF-1, platelet-activating factor (PAF) and nitric oxide can also stimulate VEGF synthesis *in vitro*.[212,213,231–238] Angiotensin II[239] and inhibitors of the mitochondrial electron transport chain also promote VEGF expression.[207] Conversely, angiotensin-converting enzyme (ACE) inhibitors can inhibit IL-1- and TNF-α-induced VEGF expression by mesothelial cells.[240] The role of these molecules in pleural VEGF accumulation is unknown.

Many other compounds (e.g. octreotide,[241] corticosteroids[236,242] and cyclooxygenase [COX]-2 inhibitors[243]) are capable of reducing VEGF activities but their role in pleural diseases has not been assessed. Genetic polymorphisms of the VEGF gene have been associated with changes in plasma VEGF levels,[244] and may potentially predispose patients to the development of pleural effusions in disease conditions.

Whether the inhibition of malignant effusion formation by anti-VEGF treatment is entirely a result of reduced vascular permeability or represents an indirect consequence of reducing tumor load (secondary to the anti-angiogenic effects of VEGF inhibition) requires further elaboration. However, research on VEGF biology represents an exciting and rapidly expanding area, and is likely to provide further insight into the pathophysiology of pleural fluid formation. An increasing number of case series have successfully demonstrated that bevacizumab, an anti-VEGF antibody, can inhibit effusions of non-malignant etiologies, e.g. from amyloidosis.[245,246]

IMMUNOMODULATORY CYTOKINES

Many cytokines participate in the inflammatory process, and the majority is likely to have a role in pleural inflammation. A comprehensive review of all these cytokines is outside the scope of this chapter. The key inflammatory cytokines and their effects in the setting of pleural pathology have been included in Chapter 7, Pleural inflammation and infection. Several important pro-inflammatory cytokines and their pertinent actions in the pleura are highlighted below.

TNF-α and IL-1

Tumor necross factor- and IL-1 play predominant roles in inflammatory responses.[247] TNF-α increases neutrophil margination and activates neutrophils, monocytes, macrophages and eosinophils. TNF-α often elicits acute-phase reactions characterized by fever and anorexia.[247] IL-1 is a strong immune adjuvant and contributes to stimulating non-specific host responses and promotes wound healing. It enhances blood flow and induction of chemoattractants, which bring the key inflammatory cells (e.g. neutrophils and macrophages) to the injury sites. In animal models, administration of high doses of these cytokines produce clinical pictures of systemic inflammation, mimicking septic shock.[247]

Recombinant human TNF-α and IL-1α can both induce chemotactic activity for polymorphonuclear cells in a dose-dependent manner in the mesothelium[248]. Similarly, IL-1β can induce leukocyte adhesion and migration across cultured human peritoneal mesothelial monolayers,[249] while TNFα can increase mesothelial expression of ICAM-1 to which migrating cells attach.[250] In human mesothelial cells, interferon (IFN)-γ inhibits basal and TNF-α- or IL-1β-induced IL-8 release, and therefore reduces IL-1β mediated migration of polymorphonuclear cells *in vivo*.[251]

In vitro exposure of mesothelial cells to TNFα and IL-1 stimulates the production of a wide variety of cytokines, including IL-6,[252] IL-8,[252] monocyte chemoattractant protein-1, regulated upon activation, normally T-cell expressed and secreted (RANTES),[251] TGF-β[253] and a dose-dependent release of VEGF.[238] IL-1 and TNF-α both induce MMP-1 and MMP-3 production by mesothelial cells.[254] Diltiazem, a calcium channel antagonist, can suppress IL-1β induced mesothelial TGF-β production.[253]

In turn, mesothelial cells produce TNF-α and IL-1 in response to a variety of stimuli. Activation of proteinase activated receptor (PAR)-2 by coagulation proteinase Xa, trypsin or tryptase potently initiates dose-dependent release of inflammatory cytokines including TNF-α *in vitro* and in mice.[255]

In addition to their inflammatory roles, TNF-α and IL-1 can alter mesothelial cell cycle progression and proliferation.[256] IL-1 induces mesothelial cell progression into S-phase and, with IFN-γ, induces proliferation. In contrast, TNF-α causes mesothelial cell cycle arrest in the G0/G1 phase.[256]

HUMAN PLEURAL EFFUSIONS

Both TNF-α and IL-1β are present in pleural effusions of various causes. Their levels are significantly higher in exudates than transudates, and in loculated than in free-flowing pleural effusions.[256] In tuberculous and empyema effusions their levels correlate with each other.[257] Their levels in pleural fluids likely reflect the degree of local inflammation. Very high IL-1 levels have been reported in empyema fluids.[257] However, the pleural fluid levels of TNF-α and IL-1 are not diagnostically useful as considerable overlap exists among effusions of various etiologies.

Mesothelial cells are likely the major source of pleural fluid TNF-α and IL-1β. Pleural fluid TNF-α is significantly higher than serum TNF-α in the malignant and in parapneumonic effusions.[258,259] Conflicting results exist for IL-1: its concentrations were higher in serum than in pleural fluids in one study,[259] but the reverse was reported in another.[257]

PLEURAL FIBROSIS

Amongst its pleiotropic nature, TNF-α is known to stimulate fibroblast proliferation and regulate collagen production.[260] TNF-α induce epithelial–mesenchymal transformation of mesothelial cells, altering expression of cytokeratins 8 and 18, MMP-9 and collagen, but not that of vimentin.[261] It is likely that TNF-α has a role in the fibrotic processes in the pleura. *In vitro*, TNF-α has been shown to stimulate and reduce mesothelial cell production of plasminogen activator inhibitor (PAI)-1 and tissue-type plasminogen activator (tPA).[262] Experimentally, anti-TNF-α antibodies inhibit talc pleurodesis.[263] In clinical studies, pleural fibrosis from tuberculous pleuritis occurs more commonly in patients with higher pleural fluid TNF-α and IL-1 levels.[257]

Polymorphisms of TNF-α have recently been associated with silicosis[264] and asbestosis[265] and genetic predisposition may have a role in pleural fibrosis.

PLEURAL MALIGNANCY

The role of TNF-α in the biology of mesothelioma is complicated. Recent evidence suggests a critical role of TNF-α in asbestos-induced malignant transformation of mesothelial cells. Although asbestos is usually cytotoxic to mesothelial cells, treatment with TNF-α significantly reduced asbestos cytotoxicity via activation of nuclear factor (NF)-κB. This protective mechanism allows more asbestos-damaged mesothelial cells to survive and undergo malignant transformation.[266] TNF-α and IL-1β are involved in malignant transformation of human benign mesothelial cells induced by erionite.[267]

Tumor necrosis factor-α has also been shown to enhance SN38-mediated apoptosis in malignant mesothelioma cells *in vitro*.[268] TNF-α and IL-1β both enhance attachment of colon and pancreatic carcinoma cell adhesion to mesothelial monolayers *in vitro*.[269,270] TNF-α has also been shown to promote peritoneal metastasis *in vivo*.[271] Recently, the role of TNF-α in malignant effusion formation has been confirmed in a murine model of malignant pleural effusion using lung cancer cell lines, raising the possibility of TNF-α as a novel therapeutic target in the management of pleural malignancies.[272]

THERAPEUTIC INHIBITION OF TNF-α

Anti-TNF-α agents are now available and their anti-inflammatory effect in the pleura has been confirmed in animal models. TNF-α-converting enzyme (TACE) cleaves the precursor form of TNF, allowing the mature form to be secreted into the extracellular space. In the pleural space, a TACE inhibitor significantly reduces the pleural fluid TNF-α accumulation in zymosan-induced pleural inflammation.[273] Similarly, GW3333, a dual inhibitor of TACE and MMPs, effectively inhibits the increase in TNF-α and the associated influx of inflammatory cells in zymosan-induced pleuritis.[274]

Steroids can also inhibit TNF-α and IL-1 production in the pleura. FR167653, a cytokine synthesis inhibitor, also suppresses TNF-α and IL-1β accumulation in the pleura in rat carrageenin-induced pleurisy. As a result, it inhibits plasma exudation and leukocyte infiltration and significantly lowered the prostanoid levels in the exudates.[275] These agents thus may have a role in treating pleural inflammation and may also prevent the development of subsequent fibrothorax. Anti-IL-1 strategies are available but little is known about their clinical effectiveness in the pleural setting.

IL-2

Interleukin 2 is a pleiotropic cytokine with a variety of effects on the immune system. Its effects are often environment-specific; hence conflicting accounts have been reported.

The interaction of IL-2 with the IL-2 receptor induces proliferation and differentiation of various T lymphocyte subsets, and stimulates a cytokine cascade that includes various interleukins, interferons and TNF-α. IL-2 induces mesothelial cell expression of CCR2 and cell proliferation. Intrapleural IL-2 administration induces nitric oxide accumulation in the pleural fluid.[276] Haptotactic migration is upregulated when mesothelial cells are cultured with IL-2 (see Chapter 7, Pleural inflammation and infection).

IL-2 LEVELS IN PLEURAL EFFUSIONS

Levels of IL-2 as well as of soluble IL-2 receptor (sIL-2R) are higher in tuberculous effusions than in malignant ones, though the large degree of overlap precludes their use as a diagnostic tool.[277–279] sIL-2R is a marker of T-lymphocyte activity: high levels of sIL-2R are present in other inflammatory effusions, especially rheumatoid pleuritis.[280] It has been suggested that effusion levels of sIL-2R and IFN-γ are useful post-treatment markers of pleural thickening.[278]

THERAPEUTIC APPLICATION OF IL-2 IN PLEURAL MALIGNANCIES

Recombinant IL-2s (e.g. aldesleukin, teceleukin) are non-glycosylated, modified forms of the endogenous compound. High-dose IL-2 results in objective regression of metastatic melanoma and renal cell carcinoma in approximately 15 percent of patients,[281] though response rates are lower in other malignancies.[282] The growth inhibitory effect of IL-2 on cancer cells varies with the proliferative status of these cells. In highly proliferating mesothelioma cells, a reduction of malignant cells in the S-phase, with an accumulation in G0/G1 of the cell cycle followed by apoptosis, is observed. In cells proliferating at a lower rate, IL-2 produces late cytotoxic effects with resultant apoptosis, without obvious influence on the cell cycle.[276]

Interleukin-2 has anti-proliferative effects on human malignant mesothelioma cells and thus has been used for the management of malignant pleural effusions[283] and mesothelioma. IL-2 also augmented the *in vitro* cytolytic activity of mesothelial cells and cytolytic T-cells, isolated from malignant pleural effusions, against autologous tumors. Lymphocytes recovered from malignant pleural effusions show depressed proliferation, IFN-γ production and cytolytic activity, as compared with lymphocytes from tuberculous effusions. Both IL-7 and IL-12, as well as TCR-CD3 (T-cell receptor-CD3), in the presence of IL-2, can restore the immunosuppressed cytolytic activity of the lymphocytes of malignant effusions against autologous tumors.[284,285]

In a murine model of mesothelioma, intratumoral injection of IL-2 induced tumor regression in part via CD8+ T-cells. Complete regression was seen with small tumors, but less so with bulky lesions.[286,287]

In humans, IL-2 as a palliative therapy for malignant effusions has been reported in case series. Intracavitary administration of low-dose IL-2, as an initial treatment, resulted in an objective clinical response in 72 percent for a median duration of 5 months in 100 patients with malignant (68 percent pleural) effusions. The response is better in pleural than in peritoneal effusion control.[288] Similar results were achieved in another study of 21 patients with malignant pleural effusions from non-small cell lung carcinomas. Complete response was achieved in 33 percent, and partial response in 29 percent, with a median duration of 8 months (range 4–10 months).[289] Treatment was well tolerated in both studies. The effectiveness of IL-2 has yet to be compared with conventional therapies for malignant pleural effusions.

Interleukin-2 has been used in the treatment of mesothelioma via different routes of delivery, though the results were generally disappointing. Thirty-one patients were given repeated intrapleural instillation of IL-2 for 4 weeks, followed by regular subcutaneous IL-2 injections for up to 6 months. Only one patient had a complete, and six a partial, tumor response. Interestingly, 90 percent of patients had no further or minimal (asymptomatic) pleural fluid collection. Side effects included fever (19 percent) and cardiac failure (3 percent) and occurred mainly after intrapleural instillations.[290] In another study using intrapleural IL-2 for 5 days in 22 mesothelioma patients, 11 partial responses and one complete response were detected after 36 days.[291]

Intravenous IL-2 therapy, followed by regular subcutaneous injections, was well tolerated by 29 previously untreated mesothelioma patients, but only two patients achieved a partial response.[292] Combining IL-2 with epirubicin results in significant toxicity, without improving the response rate (5 percent).[293] IL-2 has also been applied to malignant pleural mesothelioma during a phase II study of a four-modality treatments that included preoperative IL-2, pleurectomy/decortication, intrapleural IL-2, adjuvant radiotherapy, systemic chemotherapy and long-term subcutaneous IL-2. The median survival was 26 months for patients with stage II/III mesothelioma.[294]

VASCULAR LEAK SYNDROME

When high dose intravenous IL-2 is used to treat metastatic diseases, vascular leak syndrome (VLS) can occur which often limits the dosage that can be administered. VLS is characterized by an increase in vascular permeability accompanied by significant extravazation of fluids and proteins resulting in interstitial edema, anasarca and, at times, cardiovascular or respiratory failure. Pleural, pericardial and peritoneal effusions occur as part of the generalized vascular hyperpermeability.[295] VLS is generally believed to involve endothelial cell damage and is mediated by nitric oxide. CD4+/CD25+ T-regulatory cells have an important regulatory role, as their depletion in murine models demonstrates a significant increase in IL-2 induced VLS.[296] Natural killer (NK) and polymorphonuclear cells are important in late events, including edema, of VLS.[297] The potential role of IL-2 in vascular leakage and pleural fluid formation in other conditions has not been explored.

IL-6

Interleukin-6 is a member of a family of closely related pleiotropic cytokines which also include IL-11, IL-27, IL-31, leukemia inhibitory factor (LIF), oncostatin M (OSM), ciliary neurotrophic factor (CNF) and cardiotrophin 1 (CT-1), cardiotrophin-like cytokine (CLC) and neuropoietin (NPN).[298] Individual family members play important roles in the immune, nervous, cardiovascular and hemopoietic systems, as well as bone metabolism, inflammation, wound repair, the acute phase response and development of the embryo.[299] Their actions are mediated through specific cell surface receptors, consisting of a unique α or β chain and the shared signal transducing subunit, glycoprotein β-subunit (gp)130 as part of a multimeric (α, β) receptor complex.[300,301] By itself, gp130 does not provide high-affinity binding to any of the IL6-family cytokines, but rather converts low-affinity binding to 'specific' α-subunit receptors into a high-affinity receptor complex.[302]

Soluble forms of the α-subunits lacking the transmembrane and cytoplasmic domains have been identified for IL-6, IL-11 and LIF, as well as gp130.[302] The soluble IL-6 receptor (sIL-6R) is generated either by limited proteolysis of the IL-6R[303] or translation from alternatively spliced mRNA.[304] sIL-6R can only bind its ligand, IL-6, however the complex of IL-6 and sIL-6R can bind to and activate gp130 on cells which do not express the membrane-bound IL-6R, thereby initiating signaling.[305]

Gp130 has no intrinsic tyrosine kinase activity and thus requires recruitment and activation of specific kinases and docking proteins. Following binding of the cytokine to its α or β subunit and subsequent dimerization with gp130, cytoplasmic janus kinases (JAKs) are recruited and phosphorylate gp130.[306] The subsequent activation of intracellular signaling is dependent on specific phosphotyrosine residues on gp130, which act as docking sites for SH2 domain-containing intermediate signaling molecules. For example, the Src homology protein tyrosine phosphatase 2 (SHP2) binds to membrane proximal tyrosine residues (Y759 in humans, Y757 in mice) and is necessary and sufficient for activation of the MAPK/ERK pathway. In contrast, members of the STAT transcription factors dock to several membrane distal phosphotyrosine residues. Once phosphorylated, STAT proteins form a homodimer, translocate to the nucleus and activate target genes.[307] This system is negatively regulated by a number of inhibitory molecules, most notably the family of suppressor of cytokine signaling (SOCS) proteins.

ROLE OF IL-6 IN INFLAMMATION

Interleukin-6 plays important pro-inflammatory roles. In the acute inflammation phase, IL-6 stimulates hepatocytes to produce acute phase proteins, e.g. C-reactive protein, fibrinogen, α_1-antitrypsin and serum amyloid A, and simultaneously suppresses albumin production. It also induces the secretion of the iron regulatory protein hepcidin, hence excessive production of IL-6 leads to hypoferremia of inflammation.[299,308] Overexpression of IL-6 also causes leukocytosis and fever and promotes the production of VEGF.[308] When exposed to carrageenan-induced pleuritis, knockout mice exhibit reduced pleural exudation and polymorphonuclear cell migration. Downstream inflammatory changes, including lung myeloperoxidase activity, lipid peroxidation and the expression of inducible nitric oxide synthase and cylco-oxygenase-2, are significantly reduced in IL-6 knockout mice compared with wild-type controls.[309] Pretreatment of the wild-type mice with IL-6 neutralizing antibodies before carrageenan treatment results in the same responses as for the knockout animals.[309]

Interleukin-6 dictates the transition from acute to chronic inflammation by changing the nature of the leukocyte infiltrate (from polymorphonuclear neutrophils to monocytes/macrophages).[310–312] IL-6 is also involved in the development of specific cellular and humoral immune responses, including B cell proliferation and differentiation, immunoglobulin secretion and T-cell activation, thus favoring chronic inflammatory responses.[313]

IL-6 LEVELS IN PLEURAL EFFUSIONS

Interleukin-6 is produced by various cell types including T cells, B cells, monocytes, fibroblasts, keratinocytes, endothelial cells, mesangial cells and some tumor cells.[308] In serosal tissues, IL-6 is also secreted by mesothelial and malignant mesothelioma cells.[252,314–318] Elevated IL-6 levels have been demonstrated in the pleura and other serosal cavities following injury or disease. High levels of pleural fluid IL-6 is associated with pleural tuberculosis (TB). Initial IL-6 levels prior to treatment correlates with the number of febrile days and the percentage change of cytokines after 2 weeks of treatment helps to predict residual pleural scarring.[319] Elevated IL-6 levels together with increases in other known inflammatory cytokines was measured in the pleural lavage of patients suffering from primary spontaneous pneumothorax showing that this condition is associated with a substantial pleural inflammatory reaction.[320] Elevated pleural IL-6 has also been shown in experimental animal models using zymosan and carrageenan to induce pleuritis.[321,322] Intrapleural instillation of TNF-α in rats caused a sharp rise in plasma IL-6 which stimulated an increase in T-kininigen. Similarly, in a clinical trial involving mesothelioma patients, intrapleural administration of TNF-α induced a rise in IL-6 levels both in pleural fluid and serum.[322] IL-6 levels were also markedly increased in the pleural fluid following intrapleural tetracycline injection in patients with malignant pleural effusion.[323] Surgery can also stimulate production of IL-6 in serosal cavities. In the peritoneum 1 hour after laparotomy, the levels of IL-6 were significantly greater than immediately after the procedure.[324] Mesothelioma patients who underwent pleurectomy or extrapleural pneumonectomy followed by intraoperative photodynamic therapy also showed significant increases in serum IL-6 levels.[325]

In disease states, IL-6 levels are consistently higher in the pleural fluid than in the corresponding sera or plasma, with no direct correlation between pleural effusions and peripheral blood.[326–328] In one study, the IL-6 concentration in the pleural fluid of patients with adenocarcinoma was 60 to 1400 times higher than in the serum.[327] These data suggest that IL-6 is locally produced, probably by mesothelial and inflammatory cells, rather than from diffusion from the systemic circulation.

Pleural fluid IL-6 is higher in exudative versus transudative effusions, malignant versus benign effusions and TB pleuritis versus malignant or other parapneumonic effusions.[259,326,328,329] The concentration of IL-6 is also higher in effusions from mesotheliomas than those from adenocarcinomas.[330] However, the sensitivity and specificity of IL-6 in any of these conditions is inadequate for it to be used diagnostically.

Pleural effusion levels of IL-6 clearly reflect disease states but changes in the concentration of serum IL-6 is not so obvious. Serum IL-6 is not significantly different in patients with exudates compared with those with transudates[329] and is only slightly raised in patients with tuberculous pleurisy compared with controls.[331] However, patients with malignant pleurisy more frequently had elevated serum IL-6, fibrinogen, fibrinogen degradation products (FDP) and C-reactive protein levels compared with lung cancer patients without malignant pleurisy.[332] This suggests that the pleural IL-6 is absorbed systemically, which induces increases in plasma fibrinogen and subsequently FDP. In contrast to IL-6, sIL-6R concentrations are much higher in serum than in corresponding pleural fluids in patients with malignant or infective pleural effusions.[327,333] sIL-6R levels are also low in pleural effusions when the levels of IL-6 are high, which may reflect a downregulation of sIL-6R expression in the presence of excessive amounts of IL-6.[333]

A role for IL-6 in pleural fluid formation has also been suggested in several gynecological conditions. Increased amounts of pleural fluid and elevated IL-6 levels have been observed in Meigs' syndrome[132] and in severe ovarian hyperstimulation syndrome.[334]

MESOTHELIOMA

Normal mesothelial cells produce IL-6 in response to stimuli and express gp130.[314] Therefore, it has been predicted that IL-6 acts as an autocrine factor for mesothelial cells.[314] However, mesothelial cells do not express the IL-6R, therefore activation of mesothelial cells by IL-6 must occur when complexed to the sIL-6R, possibly shed by neutrophils following initiation of inflammation.[310]

Mesothelioma cells produce and secrete high levels of IL-6[317,335,336] but express only low levels of IL-6R mRNA.[337] It was recently shown that IL-6 together with sIL-6R stimulated mesothelioma cell growth and induced expression of vascular endothelial growth factor *in vitro*, via STAT3 signaling.[337] This suggests an autocrine role for IL-6 in the development of mesothelioma. A high incidence of thrombocytosis (48 percent) and a significant correlation between platelet count and serum IL-6 levels have been reported in mesothelioma patients.[330] This is consistent with the observation that in patients with tuberculous pleurisy, high levels of IL-6 in the pleural fluid are also associated with thrombocytosis.[330] It has been hypothesized that large amounts of IL-6 from the pleural fluid of patients with mesothelioma leak into the systemic circulation and induce the systemic inflammatory reactions related to mesothelioma,[330] including thrombocytosis, fever and cachexia.[338]

Production of IL-6 by mesotheliomas has also been measured as a way to predict tumor response to chemotherapy. Gemcitabine, and to a lesser extant irinotecan, but not most other agents, inhibit IL-6 secretion at low doses but stimulate a surge in IL-6 at higher doses.[315] These results suggest a palliative role for low doses of these chemotherapeutic agents in non-responders by decreasing the secretion of IL-6.

OTHER PLEURAL DISEASES

There is growing evidence for a role of the IL-6 family of cytokines in fibrosis of various tissues, in particular IL-6, IL-11 and OSM.[339] To date, there have been no published studies examining the effect of these molecules on pleural fibrosis but it is likely that they will play a significant role in the fibrotic pathway in pleural and other serosal cavities.

OTHER IL-6 FAMILY PROTEINS IN PLEURAL DISEASE

Very few studies have examined any of the IL-6 family cytokines, other than IL-6, in pleural or serosal biology. LIF is present in higher levels in infective and malignant pleural effusions than in transudates. Pleural fluid levels of LIF correlated with IL-8 levels in malignant effusions and with IL-4 in infective effusions.[340] Mesothelioma cells have been shown to secrete LIF as well as IL-6[341] and mesothelial cells express the OSM receptor.[327,331] However, it is likely that other IL-6 family proteins play important roles in maintaining pleural and serosal hemostasis and tissue repair, as well as in the pathogenesis of pleural disease.

IL-8

Interleukin-8 is one of the most studied chemokines, and its role in pleural inflammation is well established. Mesothelial cells express IL-8 basally.[342,343] Inflammatory stimuli,[344] asbestos fibers[345] and infective agents,[346,347] among others, are known to stimulate significant increases in mesothelial cell production of IL-8.

Interleukin-8 is a downstream cytokine from TNF-α and IL-1. In humans, significant elevation of pleural levels of IL-8 is seen after intrapleural administration of TNF-α in mesothelioma patients.[348] *In vitro*, exposure of mesothelial cells to TNF-α or IL-1β stimulates IL-8 release in a time- and dose-dependent fashion,[248,252,342,343,345,349–352] which is diminished by IFN-γ.[353] The stimulatory effects of TNF-α and IL-1 can be synergistic.[342] IL-8 secretion from pleural fibroblast is also induced by IL-1, TNF-α and

LPS.[354] Conversely, antibodies to TNF-α or IL-1 inhibit IL-8 release in mesothelial cells.[352] The neutrophil chemotactic activity of supernatants from mesothelial cells stimulated with either TNF-α or IL-1 is completely neutralized with IL-8 antiserum.[248] IL-1 receptor antagonist also inhibits asbestos-induced IL-8 production from mesothelial cells.[351] Similarly, in animal models of LPS-induced pleuritis, IL-8 release is inhibited by anti-TNF-α antibodies, but the production of TNF-α is not affected by anti-IL-8 treatment.[355]

CHEMOTAXIS

Interleukin-8 plays a crucial role in neutrophil influx and also participates in the recruitment of monocytes and lymphocytes from the vascular compartment to the pleural space.[356,357] *In vitro*, mesothelial cells produce IL-8 in a polar fashion[358] by releasing more IL-8 toward the apical surface, providing a gradient to attract neutrophils from the basal side of the mesothelium towards the pleural cavity.[358] Similarly, IL-8 derived from peritoneal mesothelial cells contributes to the intraperitoneal recruitment of leukocytes during peritoneal inflammation. Neutrophil migration was significantly reduced in the presence of IL-8 antibody.[344]

Pleural fluid levels of IL-8 are consistently higher than its serum levels, supporting local production as the predominant source of IL-8 in the pleura.[259,331,359] Consistent with its role as a neutrophil chemotaxin, IL-8 concentrations in empyema are higher than in effusions of other causes,[356,359–361] and the pleural fluid neutrophil count correlates with pleural fluid IL-8 levels in most studies.[356,359,361] *In vitro*, conditioned media from *Mycobacterium tuberculosis* infected pleural macrophages induce IL-8 secretion from mesothelial cells, which may explain the high IL-8 concentrations detected in tuberculous pleural effusions.[362]

Antagonizing IL-8 activity can effectively reduce inflammatory cell influx and pleural inflammation. Anti-IL-8 antibodies decrease chemotactic activity in empyema liquids,[356,361] significantly inhibit neutrophil recruitment in endotoxin-induced pleurisy[346] and diminish the neutrophil chemotaxis into the pleural space following local instillation of crocidolite asbestos.[345]

ANGIOGENESIS AND TUMOR GROWTH

Interleukin-8 has angiogenic properties and has been shown to play a critical role in endotoxin-induced vascular permeability.[355] IL-8 induced angiogenesis is likely to be important in tumor-related neovascularization.

Interleukin-8 also possesses a direct growth-potentiating effect on certain tumors. In mesothelioma cell lines, IL-8 causes a dose-dependent increase in proliferating activity, and can also function as an autocrine growth factor in tumors. Concurrently, neutralization of IL-8 significantly abrogates mesothelioma proliferation.[363,364] Similarly, an autocrine growth inhibitory circuit, involving α-melanocyte stimulating hormone, has been shown in mesothelioma cells. Interruption of this circuit enhanced IL-8 expression on mesothelioma cells.[365]

PLEURODESIS

As discussed in previous sections (see under TGF-β), the conventional method of pleurodesis involves inducing acute pleural inflammation, which then progresses to chronic inflammation and pleural fibrosis. As such, most pleurodesing agents stimulate an acute pleural injury, and hence production of IL-8, which holds an important role in successful pleurodesis.

Intrapleural instillations of talc,[366,367] tetracycline[323,368] and OK-432[369,370] have all been shown to stimulate a rapid rise in mesothelial cell production of IL-8, or pleural IL-8 accumulation in humans, which is then followed by pleural neutrophilia. A good correlation between IL-8 levels and neutrophil chemotactic response has been observed.[367,369] Specific neutralization or removal of IL-8 by antibody column significantly inhibited the neutrophil chemotaxis[366,369] and is likely to inhibit pleural fibrosis/pleurodesis. However, the intrapleural administration of IL-8 itself was ineffective in producing pleurodesis or facilitating the pleurodesis with talc (Vargas and Light, personal communications).

IL-10

Interleukin-10 is an antiinflammatory cytokine with potent immunosuppressive properties. In humans, the main sources of IL-10 are lymphocytes and monocytes, but macrophages, mast cells and eosinophils also synthesize IL-10.[371,372] Circulating levels of IL-10 are elevated in patients with sepsis and have been associated with an adverse clinical outcome. Experimental studies show that exogenous IL-10, as an anti-inflammatory agent, can improve outcome in sepsis[372] and inhibit airway inflammation in asthma.[371] IL-10 also carries strong immunosuppressive actions mediated through the downregulation of pro-inflammatory cytokines, the major histocompatibility complex (MHC) class II molecules and T-cell mediated inflammatory responses, including delayed hypersensitivity and Th2-driven allergic responses.[372]

It is likely IL-10 plays a role during the early phases of pleural inflammation, in mediating cell trafficking to the pleura and vascular leak.[373,374] Intrapleural IL-10 inhibits the early phase of carrageenan-induced pleural inflammation in a murine model.[373] IL-10 null mice had enhanced rates of pleural exudation and polymorphonuclear cell trafficking; while mice injected with anti-IL-10 neutralizing antibodies had increased leukocyte influx and vascular leakage in the early phase of carrageenan-induced pleural inflammation.[373]

Interleukin-10 is present in tuberculous and malignant pleural effusions. Its pleural fluid concentrations are significantly higher than the corresponding serum levels, suggesting that local production is its principal source.[375] Resident pleural macrophages may be a source of pleural IL-10, as macrophage ablation in a murine model of carrageenan pleurisy has demonstrated a reduced level of IL-10 as well as other inflammatory cytokines.[376] Alveolar macrophages isolated from older rats produce less IL-10 than those isolated from young rats.[377] These rats also exhibit significantly reduced pleural fluid IL-10 levels during carrageenan-induced pleurisy than younger rats. However, the effusion IL-10 level does not correlate with lymphocyte subpopulations in the pleural fluids or in blood[378] and does not predict survival in malignant effusions.[375]

Tumor cells can produce IL-10, which is known to suppress the production of anti-tumor cytokines (such as TNF-α and IL-1β) by pleural macrophages.[379] IL-10 is reported to promote the growth of activated or neoplastic B lymphocytes[380] and its expression has been shown in high levels in cell lines of primary effusion lymphoma[381] and in pyothorax-associated lymphoma.[382]

In tuberculous effusions, IL-10 levels decrease over the course of the disease.[383] IL-10 may be induced in the early stages of chronic disease by Th1 type cytokine profiles, but its host-protective downregulatory effects on immune response may allow the mycobacterium to persist.[383] An inverse correlation also exists between IL-10 and mononuclear cell proliferation in tuberculous pleuritis[384] and high IL-10 levels have been associated with pleural necrosis.

In murine models of *Staphylococcus aureus* empyema, IFN-γ levels rise in the controls, whereas the interleukin-10 level increases significantly in the CD4 knockout mice.

Therapeutic use of IL-10, especially in sepsis, has been explored in phase I and II trials.[385] Further investigations on its potential use in pleural diseases would be worthwhile.

IL-12

Interleukin-12 is a heterodimeric cytokine that enhances cell-mediated and cytotoxic immune responses to intracellular pathogens and tumors.[210] IL-12 is produced primarily by antigen presenting cells. It is considered crucial in promoting Th1 responses and subsequent cell mediated immunity. These functions are facilitated by the ability of IL-12 to stimulate T lymphocyte and NK cell proliferation, their cytotoxicity and IFN-γ production. IL-12 receptors comprise of two subunits IL-12R-β1 and -β2, which are expressed mainly on activated T and NK cells.[386,387]

TUBERCULOUS PLEURITIS

The role of IL-12 in TB pleuritis has been studied. IL-12 contributes to the anti-mycobacterial immune response by enhancing production of IFN-γ, facilitating the development of Th1 cells and augmenting cytotoxicity of antigen-specific T cells and NK cells. Knockout mice with disrupted IL-12 or IL-12Rβ1 genes have defective cell mediated immunity, fail to develop granulomatous reactions and are prone to develop TB.[387] In TB patients, the percentage of T cells expressing IL-12 receptors is significantly decreased, and IFN-γ production by peripheral monocytes is also reduced.[388] In TB pleuritis, the mean IL-12 concentrations are tenfold higher in pleural fluid than in serum.[389] *In vitro*, pleural fluid cells have been shown to proliferate and produce bioactive IL-12 when stimulated with *M. tuberculosis*.[389] IL-12 in turn induces mononuclear cells in pleural effusions to increase their killing activity dose-dependently and enhances their production of IFN-γ.[390]

Pleural malignancy

Interleukin-12 is considered to have potent anti-tumor effects. Systemic administration of recombinant IL-12 induces a significant and persistent anti-tumor immune response, mediated by CD4 and CD8 T lymphocytes, and results in growth inhibition or even regression in a murine model of mesothelioma.[391] IL-12 may also be useful as a candidate for gene therapy in malignant pleural diseases. Paracrine secretion of IL-12, generated by gene transfer, can induce immunity against mesothelioma locally and at a distant site, without causing significant systemic complications.[392]

A Th2 to Th1 shift is observed when lymphocytes from malignant effusions are treated with IL-12. The use of lymphocytes treated in this fashion as a novel adoptive immunotherapy for cancer has been suggested.[393] Other studies have reported that, upon IL-12/IL-2 co-stimulation, monocytes isolated from malignant pleural effusions are able to produce cytokines of both the Th1 and Th2 types.[394]

Interleukin-12 also serves to augment the anti-cancer effects of other cytokines. *In vitro*, IL-12, in the presence of IL-2, can restore the cytolytic activity of the lymphocytes in malignant pleural effusion against autologous tumor.[284] *In vivo*, co-administration of IL-15 with IL-12 activates the CD8+ T lymphocytes and NK cells, providing strong anti-tumor activity against malignant pleuritis in mice. The therapeutic effect is probably mainly due to enhanced IFN-γ production as the administration of anti-IFN-γ antibodies inhibits the beneficial effect of IL-15 and IL-12.[395] IL-12 has also been shown to promote pleural and blood monocyte cytotoxic activity against a small cell lung cancer cell line.[394]

Interleukin-12 has now been used in small clinical trials against a variety of malignancies. Whether it has a therapeutic value against pleural mesothelioma awaits investigation.

Interferons

There are two types of interferon: type I and type II. The type I IFNs consist of seven classes, of which the

IFN-α and IFN-β are the most studied. There is only one human IFN-β but there are multiple IFN-α species. Type II interferon consists of IFN-γ only. In addition, four IFN-like cytokines have been reported.[396] Type I IFNs are secreted by virus infected cells while the type II IFN is secreted mainly by T cells, NK cells and macrophages.[396] Toll-like receptors play an important role in the expression of IFNs[397] as well as monocyte-derived pro-inflammatory cytokines such as IL-12, IL-15 and IL-18, especially in combination.[394,398,399]

The interferons and IFN-like molecules signal through the Jak-Stat pathway. The type I interferons all share the same receptor complex, whereas type II IFN-γ binds to a distinct receptor. The type I IFNs predominantly signal through Stat1 and Stat2 but IFN-α and IFN-β pathways can involve Stat3, Stat4, Stat5 and IFN regulatory factors in various cells under different conditions. IFN-γ activates Jak1, Jak2 and Stat1 that in turn induce genes containing the γ-activation sequence in the promoter. IFN-γ can also activate Stat3 and Stat5. The IFNs can also activate other pathways including PI3K, Akt, NF-κB, MAPK and others.[396]

The type I interferons exhibit a wide array of biological activities including antiviral, antiproliferative and cytotoxicity, on a wide variety of immune cells to increase the expression of tumor-associated antigens and other surface molecules such as MHC class I antigens, activation of pro-apoptotic proteins, modulation of differentiation and antiangiogenic activity.[396]

TUBERCULOUS PLEURITIS

Tuberculosis pleural effusion is common (see Chapter 27) and the pleural fluid is exudative with a mononuclear cell predominance. High levels of IFN-γ are present in the pleural fluid which is thought to be important in the pathogenesis of TB.[400]

Interferon-γ stimulates mesothelial cells to secrete MIP-1α and MCP-1 which mediates recruitment of mononuclear cells to the pleural space.[401] A positive correlation has also been seen between IFN-γ and the proliferative response of mononuclear cells induced by *M. tuberculosis*.[384] IFN-γ-mediated pathways are extremely important in cell-mediated protective immunity against *M. tuberculosis* antigen. The cell-mediated immune response in TB originates predominantly from IFN-γ-releasing CD4 and CD8 effector T cells. This Th1 response helps to limit mycobacterial replication and spread, however, it can also lead to significant immunopathology. IFN-γ also inhibits the proliferation of Th2 cells and thereby modulates Th2 mediated responses (see review[402]). NK cells extravazate to the site of TB infection. The $CD56^{dim}CD16^{+}$ subset has an increased susceptibility to undergo apoptosis induced by heat-stable/labile mediators present in tuberculous effusions, leading to an enrichment of $CD56^{bright}$ cells. These NK cells cannot lyse *M. tuberculosis*-infected target cells, but are larger producers of IFN-γ upon *M. tuberculosis* contact, contributing to regulation of the immune response toward the Th1 profile. Because $CD56^{bright}$ cells retain homing receptors for lymph nodes, they maintain their capacity to migrate to them. Therefore, these findings may explain why tuberculous pleurisy results in the clearance of *M. tuberculosis* and resolves without treatment.[403]

Polymorphisms within the IFN-γ/IFN-γ receptor (IFN-γR) complex have been identified which, depending on the polymorphism or combination of polymorphisms, can confer susceptibility or protection from disease.[404–408] Recent studies on genetics and TB have also examined gene variants involved in iron acquisition. In one study examining the iron regulatory genes haptoglobin and NRAMP1, common polymorphic variants showed functionally distinct biochemical phenotypes that would be predicted to influence the course of TB infection in humans.[409,410]

Pleural fluid INF-γ is important not only in the pathogenesis but also in the diagnosis of TB (see Chapter 27 on TB pleural effusions).

PLEURAL INFLAMMATION

Interferon-γ has anti-inflammatory properties and can inhibit basal and IL-1β- and TNF-α-induced production of IL-8. In addition, it can antagonize the polymorphonuclear cell influx induced by IL-1β.[251] IFN-γ also controls polymorphonuclear cell infiltration and modulates IL-6 signaling through sIL-6R to promote their apoptosis and clearance.[411] Therefore, IFN-γ plays a role in controlling the phenotype of infiltrating leukocytes during inflammation through regulation of resident cell cytokine and chemokine synthesis.

MESOTHELIOMA

There is growing evidence that immunotherapy may be useful in the treatment of mesothelioma. Several studies have shown that IFN-α and IFN-γ inhibits the growth of human mesothelioma cell lines which is further enhanced by the combination with other cytokines or chemotherapeutic agents.[412–416] A combination of IFN-α and IFN-γ augments the response of mesothelioma cells to methotrexate by as much as 75 percent.[413] Interestingly however, the sensitivity to IFN-γ alone was shown to be cell line dependent.[413] The antiproliferative effect of IFN-γ on mesothelioma cell lines appears to be mediated through the JAK–STAT pathway.[417] Failure of cells to respond to IFN-γ was related to the limited transcriptional activity of STAT1, or a defect in JAK2 expression.[417] Studies of the gene expression profiles of human mesothelioma cell lines in response to IFN-γ treatment revealed many differences between IFN-γ-resistant and -sensitive pathways, including features other than just the antiproliferative response.[418]

Gene transfer of IFN-γ or IFN-β into established murine mesotheliomas has demonstrated significant tumor regression and long-term survival. This may be due to peripheral tumor infiltration by CD4+ and CD8+ lymphocytes. The combination of IFN-β with cyclooxygenase-2 inhibition or surgical debulking further reduced tumor growth and recurrence.[419,420]

Despite the promise that IFN therapy had in treating patients with malignant mesothelioma, the clinical trial results have been disappointing. IFN, given singly or in combination with chemotherapeutic agents, has shown no significant clinical response or survival benefits.[421–430] Toxicity, in particular myelosuppression and fatigue, is significant which further limits its application.

To minimize systemic toxicity, intrapleural administration has been tried. In a multicenter study, recombinant human IFN-γ was instilled into the pleural cavity of 89 patients with Butchart disease stages I and II, epithelial or mixed mesotheliomas. The overall response rate was relatively low at 20 percent with most responders having early stage disease.[431] Drug tolerance was acceptable via the intrapleural route, though systemic side effects of hyperthermia, liver toxicity and neutropenia were still seen.

The mechanisms of action of IFN-γ in the pleura are poorly understood but in six patients with mesothelioma, IFN-γ treatment induced a marked decrease in intrapleural IL-6 levels and produced *in situ* activation of macrophages and cytotoxic T-lymphocytes.[338] However, IFN-γ showed no effect on reducing IL-6 production by mesothelial cells *in vitro* suggesting that the systemic manifestations of mesothelioma may be related to the production of IL-6 by malignant cells.[338]

Intracavitary administration of IFN-α and IFN-β has also been tried as palliative therapy for malignant effusions, with efficacy on reducing pleural fluid reaccumulation, though they are not as effective as IL-2.[432] These results have not been compared with conventional pleurodesing agents prospectively.

KEY POINTS

- Cytokines play a crucial role in both normal and pathological states of the pleura.
- Transforming growth factor-β holds a significant role in pleural fibrosis. Therapeutic intrapleural administration of TGF-β can induce excellent pleurodesis in animal models.
- Vascular endothelial growth factor is a potent stimulator of vascular hyperpermeability, and its overexpression is key to increased pleural fluid formation. Various strategies aiming to antagonize VEGF activity have shown success in inhibiting malignant effusion formation in experimental models. Clinical trials are underway.
- Tumor necrosis factor-α, IL-1 and IL-8 have well-established roles in pleural inflammation.
- Intrapleural administration of cytokines with anti-tumor activities has been used in the management of pleural malignancies and in the control of malignant effusions with mixed results.
- Cytokine research is a rapidly expanding area, and is likely to enhance our understanding of the pathophysiology and may provide novel treatment for various pleural diseases.

SUMMARY

A comprehensive understanding of the cytokine network is crucial to the understanding of the pathophysiology of pleural diseases. However, the complex range of overlapping functions of the ever-expanding number of cytokines and their diverse inter-relations make the study of cytokine behavior in pleural disease an extremely challenging task. It is anticipated that in the rapid expansion of our knowledge in cytokines and their intracellular pathways, breakthroughs in the diagnosis and management of pleural diseases will be made.

REFERENCES

● = Key primary paper
◆ = Major review article

◆1. Lee YCG, Lane KB. The many faces of transforming growth factor beta in pleural diseases. *Curr Opin Pulm Med* 2001; **7**: 173–9.
2. Jagirdar J, Lee TC, Reibman J, *et al.* Immunohistochemical localization of transforming growth factor beta isoforms in asbestos-related diseases. *Environ Health Perspect* 1997; **105** (Suppl 5): 1197–203.
3. Maeda J, Ueki N, Ohkawa T, *et al.* Local production and localization of transforming growth factor-beta in tuberculous pleurisy. *Clin Exp Immunol* 1993; **92**: 32–8.
4. Cheng D-S, Lee YC, Roger JT, *et al.* Vascular endothelial growth factor level correlates with transforming growth factor-beta isoform levels in pleural effusions. *Chest* 2000; **118**: 1747–53.
5. Martin M, Lefaix J, Delaniau S. TGF-beta 1 and radiation fibrosis: a master switch and a specific therapeutic target? *Int J Radiat Oncol Biol Phys* 2000; **47**: 277–90.
6. Branton MH, Kopp JB. TGF-β and fibrosis. *Microbes Infect* 1999; **1**: 1349–65.
7. Yang L, Qiu CX, Ludlow A, Ferguson MW, Brunner G. Active transforming growth factor-beta in wound repair: determination using a new assay. *Am J Pathol* 1999; **154**: 105–11.
◆8. Sheppard D. Transforming growth factor beta. A central modulator of pulmonary and airway inflammation and fibrosis. *Proc Am Thorac Soc* 2006; **3**: 413–7.
9. Sasse SA, Jadus MR, Kukes GD. Pleural fluid transforming growth factor β-1 correlates with pleural fibrosis in experimental empyema. *Am J Respir Crit Care Med* 2003; **168**: 700–5.
10. Kinnula V, Linnala A, Viitala E, Linniainmaa K, Virtanen I. Tenascin and fibronectin expression in human mesothelial cells and pleural

mesothelioma cell-line cells. *Am J Respir Cell Mol Biol* 1998; **19**: 445–52.
11. Rougier JP, Moullier P, Piedaguel R, Ronco PM. Hyperosmolality suppresses but TGF beta 1 increases MMP9 in human peritoneal mesothelial cells. *Kidney Int* 1997; **51**: 337–47.
12. Ma C, Tarnuzzer RW, Chegini N. Expression of matrix metalloproteinases and tissue inhibitors of matrix metalloproteinases in mesothelial cells and their regulation by transforming growth factor-beta 1. *Wound Repair Regen* 1999; **7**: 477–85.
13. Idell S, Zweib C, Kumar A, Koenig KB, Johnson AR. Pathways of fibrin turnover of human pleural mesothelial cells *in vitro*. *Am J Respir Cell Mol Biol* 1992; **7**: 414–26.
14. Falk P, Ma C, Chegini N, Holmdahl L. Differential regulation of mesothelial cells fibrinolysis by transforming growth factor beta 1. *Scan J Clin Lab Invest* 2000; **60**: 439–47.
15. Liu F, Liu H, Peng Y, *et al.* Inhibition of transforming growth factor beta (TGFbeta1) expression and extracellular matrix secretion in human peritoneal mesothelial cells by pcDU6 vector-mediated TGFbeta1 shRNA and by pcDNA3.1(-)-mediated antisense TGFbeta1 RNA. *Adv Petit Dial* 2005; **21**: 41–52.
16. Wang Q, Wang Y, Hyde DM, *et al.* Reduction of bleomycin induced lung fibrosis by transforming growth factor soluble receptor in hamsters. *Thorax* 1999; **54**: 805–12.
17. Border WA, Okuda S, Languino LR, Sporn MB, Ruoslahti E. Suppression of experimental glomerulonephritis by antiserum against transforming growth factor β1. *Nature* 1990; **346**: 371–4.
18. Shah M, Foreman DM, Ferguson MW. Control of scarring in adult wounds by neutralising antibody to transforming growth factor β. *Lancet* 1992; **339**: 213–4.
19. Lucas PA, Warejcka DJ, Young HE, Lee BY. Formation of abdominal adhesions is inhibited by antibodies to transforming growth factor-beta 1. *J Surg Res* 1996; **65**: 135–8.
20. Nakao A, Fujii M, Matsumura R, *et al.* Transient gene transfer and expression of Smad 7 prevents bleomycin-induced lung fibrosis in mice. *J Clin Invest* 1999; **104**: 5–11.
●21. Kunz CR, Jadus MR, Kukes GD, *et al.* Intrapleural injection of transforming growth factor-β antibody inhibits pleural fibrosis in empyema. *Chest* 2004; **126**: 1636–44.
●22. Allen SS, Cassone L, Lasco TM, McMurray DN. Effect of neutralizing transforming growth factor beta 1 on the immune response against mycobacterium tuberculosis in guinea pigs. *Infect Immun* 2004; **72**: 1358–63.
●23. Light RW, Cheng DS, Lee YCG, *et al.* A single intrapleural injection of transforming growth factor beta-2 produces an excellent pleurodesis in rabbits. *Am J Respir Crit Care Med* 2000; **162**: 98–104.
24. Lee YCG, Teixeira LR, Devin CJ, *et al.* Transforming growth factor-β2 induces pleurodesis significantly faster than talc. *Am J Respir Crit Care Med* 2001; **163**: 640–4.
25. Lee YCG, Devin CJ, Teixiera LR, *et al.* Transforming growth factor beta-2 induced pleurodesis is not inhibited by corticosteroids. *Thorax* 2001; **56**: 643–8.
26. Lee YCG, Lane KB, Parker RE, *et al.* Transforming growth factor beta-2 (TGFβ2) produces effective pleurodesis in sheep with no systemic complications. *Thorax* 2000; **55**: 1058–62.
27. Kalomenidis I, Guo Y, Lane KB, Hawthorne M, Light RW. Transforming growth factor-beta3 induces pleurodesis in rabbits and collagen production of human mesothelial cells. *Chest* 2005; **127**: 1335–40.
28. Lee YCG, Malkerneker D, Devin CJ, *et al.* Comparing transforming growth factor beta-2 and fibronectin as pleurodesing agents. *Respirology* 2001; **6**: 281–6.
29. Lee YCG, Malkerneker D, Thompson PJ, Light RW, Lane KB. Transforming growth factor-β induces vascular endothelial growth factor elaboration from pleural mesothelial cells *in vivo* and *in vitro*. *Am J Respir Crit Care Med* 2002; **165**: 88–94.
30. Lee YCG, Yasay JR, Johnson JE, *et al.* Comparing transforming growth factor (TGF)-b2, talc and bleomycin as pleurodesing agents in sheep. *Respirology* 2002; **7**: 209–16.
31. Calabresi PA, Fields NS, Maloni HW, *et al.* Phase I trial of transforming growth factor beta 2 in chronic progressive MS. *Neurology* 1998; **51**: 289–92.
32. Lee YCG, Lane KB, Zoia O, *et al.* Transforming growth factor-beta induces collagen synthesis without inducing IL-8 production in mesothelial cells. *Eur Respir J* 2003; **22**: 197–202.
33. Marchi E, Vargas FS, Acencio MM, *et al.* Evidence that mesothelial cells regulate the acute inflammatory response in talc pleurodesis. *Eur Respir J* 2006; **28**: 929–32.
34. Teixeira LR, Wu W, Cheng DS, Light RW. The effect of corticosteroids on pleurodesis induced by doxycycline in rabbits. *Chest* 2002; **121**: 216–9.
35. Teixeira LR, Vargas FS, Acencio MM, *et al.* Influence of antiinflammatory drugs (methylprednisolone and diclofenac sodium) on experimental pleurodesis induced by silver nitrate or talc. *Chest* 2005; **128**: 4041–5.
36. Kelley J. Transforming growth factor-beta. In: Kelley J (ed.). *Cytokines of the lung*. New York: Marcel Dekker, 1993: 101–37.
37. Link J, He B, Navikas V, *et al.* Transforming growth factor-beta 1 suppresses autoantigen-induced expression of pro-inflammatory cytokines but not of interleukin-10 in multiple sclerosis and myasthenia gravis. *J Neuroimmunol* 1995; **58**: 21–35.
38. Zissel G, Schlaak J, Schlaak M, Muller-Quernheim J. Regulation of cytokine release by alveolar macrophages treated with interleukin-4, interleukin-10, or transforming growth factor beta. *Eur Cytokine Netw* 1996; **7**: 59–66.
39. Karres I, Kremer JP, Steckholzer U, Kenney JS, Ertel W. Transforming growth factor-beta 1 inhibits synthesis of cytokines in endotoxin-stimulated human whole blood. *Arch Surg* 1996; **131**: 1310–6.
40. Smith WB, Noack L, Khew-Goddall Y, *et al.* Transforming growth factor-beta 1 inhibits the production of IL-8 and the transmigration of neutrophils through activated endothelium. *J Immunol* 1996; **157**: 360–8.
41. Diebold RJ, Eis MJ, Yin M, *et al.* Early-onset multifocal inflammation in the transforming growth factor beta 1-null mouse is lymphocyte mediated. *Proc Natl Acad Sci U S A* 1995; **92**: 12215–9.
42. Letterio JJ, Roberts AB. Regulation of immune responses by TGF-β. *Annu Rev Immunol* 1998; **16**: 137–61.
43. Chen W, Wahl SM. Manipulation of TGF-b to control autoimmune and chronic inflammatory diseases. *Microbes Infect* 1999; **1**: 1367–80.
44. Gamble JR, Khew-Goodall Y, Vadas MA. Transforming growth factor-β inhibits E-selectin expression on human endothelial cells. *J Immunol* 1993; **150**: 4494–503.
45. Denk PO, Roth-Eichhorn S, Gressner AM, Knorr M. Effect of cytokines on regulation of the production of transforming growth factor beta-1 in cultured human Tenon's capsule fibroblasts. *Eur J Ophthalmol* 2000; **10**: 110–5.
46. Offner FA, Feichtinger H, Stadlmann S, *et al.* Transforming growth factor-beta synthesis by human peritoneal mesothelial cells. Induction by interleukin-1. *Am J Pathol* 1996; **148**: 1679–88.
47. Owens MW, Milligan SA, Grisham MB. Inhibition of rat pleural mesothelial cell nitric oxide synthesis by transforming growth factor-beta 1. *Inflammation* 1996; **20**: 637–46.
48. Blobe GC, Schiemann WP, Lodish HF. Role of transforming growth factor (beta) in human disease. *N Engl J Med* 2000; **342**: 1350–8.
49. Ikubo A, Morisaki T, Katano M, *et al.* A possible role of TGF-beta in the formation of malignant effusions. *Clin Immunol Immunopathol* 1995; **77**: 27–32.
◆50. Stover DG, Bierie B, Moses HL. A delicate balance: TGF-beta and the tumor microenvironment. *J Cell Biochem* 2007; **101**: 851–61.
51. Marzo AL, Fitzpatrick DR, Robinson BW, Scott B. Antisense oligonucleotides specific for transforming growth factor beta2 inhibit the growth of malignant mesothelioma both *in vitro* and *in vivo*. *Cancer Res* 1997; **57**: 3200–7.

●52. Suzuki E, Kim S, Cheung HK, *et al.* A novel small-molecule inhibitor of transforming growth factor beta type 1 receptor kinase (SM16) inhibits murine mesothelioma tumor growth *in vivo* and prevents tumor recurrence after surgical resection. *Cancer Res* 2007; **67**: 2351–9.
53. Cambien F, Ricard S, Troesch A, *et al.* Polymorphisms of the transforming growth factor-beta 1 gene in relation to myocardial infarction and blood pressure. The Etude Cas-Temon de l'Infarctus du Myocarde (ECTIM) study. *Hypertension* 1996; **28**: 881–7.
54. Awad MR, El-Gamel A, Hasleton P, *et al.* Genotype variation in the transforming growth factor-beta 1 gene. *Transplantation* 1998; **66**: 1014–20.
55. El-Gamel A, Awad MR, Hasleton PS, *et al.* Transforming growth factor-beta (TGF-beta1) genotype and lung allograft fibrosis. *J Heart Lung Transplant* 1999; **18**: 517–23.
56. Stella MC, Comoglio PM. HGF: a multifunctional growth factor controlling cell scattering. *Int J Biochem Cell Biol* 1999; **31**: 1357–62.
57. Weidner KM, Arakaki N, Hartmann G, *et al.* Evidence for the identity of human scatter factor and human hepatocyte growth factor. *Proc Natl Acad Sci U S A* 1991; **88**: 7001–5.
58. Naldini L, Tamagnone L, Vigna E, *et al.* Extracellular proteolytic cleavage by urokinase is required for activation of hepatocyte growth factor/scatter factor. *Embo J* 1992; **11**: 4825–33.
59. Warn R, Harvey P, Warn A, *et al.* HGF/SF induces mesothelial cell migration and proliferation by autocrine and paracrine pathways. *Exp Cell Res* 2001; **267**: 258–66.
60. Jiang W, Hiscox S, Matsumoto K, Nakamura T. Hepatocyte growth factor/scatter factor, its molecular, cellular and clinical implications in cancer. *Crit Rev Oncol Hematol* 1999; **29**: 209–48.
61. Matsumoto K, Tajima H, Okazaki H, Nakamura T. Negative regulation of hepatocyte growth factor gene expression in human lung fibroblasts and leukemic cells by transforming growth factor-beta 1 and glucocorticoids. *J Biol Chem* 1992; **267**: 24917–20.
●62. Bottaro DP, Rubin JS, Faletto DL, *et al.* Identification of the hepatocyte growth factor receptor as the c-met proto-oncogene product. *Science* 1991; **251**: 802–4.
63. Funakoshi H, Nakamura T. Hepatocyte growth factor: from diagnosis to clinical applications. *Clin Chim Acta* 2003; **327**: 1–23.
64. Bladt F, Riethmacher D, Isenmann S, Aguzzi A, Birchmeier C. Essential role for the c-met receptor in the migration of myogenic precursor cells into the limb bud. *Nature* 1995; **376**: 768–71.
65. Maina F, Hilton MC, Andres R, *et al.* Multiple roles for hepatocyte growth factor in sympathetic neuron development. *Neuron* 1998; **20**: 835–46.
66. Schmidt C, Bladt F, Goedecke S, *et al.* Scatter factor/hepatocyte growth factor is essential for liver development. *Nature* 1995; **373**: 699–702.
67. Uehara Y, Minowa O, Mori C, *et al.* Placental defect and embryonic lethality in mice lacking hepatocyte growth factor/scatter factor. *Nature* 1995; **373**: 702–5.
68. Ohmichi H, Koshimizu U, Matsumoto K, Nakamura T. Hepatocyte growth factor (HGF) acts as a mesenchyme-derived morphogenic factor during fetal lung development. *Development* 1998; **125**: 1315–24.
69. Padela S, Cabacungan J, Shek S, *et al.* Hepatocyte growth factor is required for alveologenesis in the neonatal rat. *Am J Respir Crit Care Med* 2005; **172**: 907–14.
70. Ito W, Kanehiro A, Matsumoto K, *et al.* Hepatocyte growth factor attenuates airway hyperresponsiveness, inflammation, and remodeling. *Am J Respir Cell Mol Biol* 2005; **32**: 268–80.
71. Okunishi K, Dohi M, Nakagome K, *et al.* A novel role of hepatocyte growth factor as an immune regulator through suppressing dendritic cell function. *J Immunol* 2005; **175**: 4745–53.
72. Rampino T, Cancarini G, Gregorini M, *et al.* Hepatocyte growth factor/scatter factor released during peritonitis is active on mesothelial cells. *Am J Pathol* 2001; **159**: 1275–85.
73. Adamson IY, Bakowska J. KGF and HGF are growth factors for mesothelial cells in pleural lavage fluid after intratracheal asbestos. *Exp Lung Res* 2001; **27**: 605–16.
74. Dworkin LD, Gong R, Tolbert E, *et al.* Hepatocyte growth factor ameliorates progression of interstitial fibrosis in rats with established renal injury. *Kidney Int* 2004; **65**: 409–19.
75. Hattori N, Mizuno S, Yoshida Y, *et al.* The plasminogen activation system reduces fibrosis in the lung by a hepatocyte growth factor-dependent mechanism. *Am J Pathol* 2004; **164**: 1091–8.
76. Matsuda Y, Matsumoto K, Yamada A, *et al.* Preventive and therapeutic effects in rats of hepatocyte growth factor infusion on liver fibrosis/cirrhosis. *Hepatology* 1997; **26**: 81–9.
77. Matsuo K, Maeda Y, Naiki Y, *et al.* Possible effects of hepatocyte growth factor for the prevention of peritoneal fibrosis. *Nephron Exp Nephrol* 2005; **99**: e87–94.
78. Mizuno S, Kurosawa T, Matsumoto K, *et al.* Hepatocyte growth factor prevents renal fibrosis and dysfunction in a mouse model of chronic renal disease. *J Clin Invest* 1998; **101**: 1827–34.
79. Mizuno S, Matsumoto K, Li MY, Nakamura T. HGF reduces advancing lung fibrosis in mice: a potential role for MMP-dependent myofibroblast apoptosis. *FASEB J* 2005; **19**: 580–2.
80. Watanabe M, Ebina M, Orson FM, *et al.* Hepatocyte growth factor gene transfer to alveolar septa for effective suppression of lung fibrosis. *Mol Ther* 2005; **12**: 58–67.
81. Yaekashiwa M, Nakayama S, Ohnuma K, *et al.* Simultaneous or delayed administration of hepatocyte growth factor equally represses the fibrotic changes in murine lung injury induced by bleomycin. A morphologic study. *Am J Respir Crit Care Med* 1997; **156**: 1937–44.
82. Gong R, Rifai A, Tolbert EM, *et al.* Hepatocyte growth factor ameliorates renal interstitial inflammation in rat remnant kidney by modulating tubular expression of macrophage chemoattractant protein-1 and RANTES. *J Am Soc Nephrol* 2004; **15**: 2868–81.
83. Liu Y, Rajur K, Tolbert E, Dworkin LD. Endogenous hepatocyte growth factor ameliorates chronic renal injury by activating matrix degradation pathways. *Kidney Int* 2000; **58**: 2028–43.
84. Gong R, Rifai A, Tolbert EM, Centracchio JN, Dworkin LD. Hepatocyte growth factor modulates matrix metalloproteinases and plasminogen activator/plasmin proteolytic pathways in progressive renal interstitial fibrosis. *J Am Soc Nephrol* 2003; **14**: 3047–60.
85. Harvey P, Warn A, Dobbin S, *et al.* Expression of HGF/SF in mesothelioma cell lines and its effects on cell motility, proliferation and morphology. *Br J Cancer* 1998; **77**: 1052–9.
86. Harvey P, Warn A, Newman P, *et al.* Immunoreactivity for hepatocyte growth factor/scatter factor and its receptor, met, in human lung carcinomas and malignant mesotheliomas. *J Pathol* 1996; **180**: 389–94.
87. Lengyel E, Prechtel D, Resau JH, *et al.* C-Met overexpression in node-positive breast cancer identifies patients with poor clinical outcome independent of Her2/neu. *Int J Cancer* 2005; **113**: 678–82.
88. Tolnay E, Kuhnen C, Wiethege T, *et al.* Hepatocyte growth factor/scatter factor and its receptor c-Met are overexpressed and associated with an increased microvessel density in malignant pleural mesothelioma. *J Cancer Res Clin Oncol* 1998; **124**: 291–6.
89. Takayama H, LaRochelle WJ, Sharp R, *et al.* Diverse tumorigenesis associated with aberrant development in mice overexpressing hepatocyte growth factor/scatter factor. *Proc Natl Acad Sci U S A* 1997; **94**: 701–6.
90. Cacciotti P, Libener R, Betta P, *et al.* SV40 replication in human mesothelial cells induces HGF/Met receptor activation: a model for viral-related carcinogenesis of human malignant mesothelioma. *Proc Natl Acad Sci U S A* 2001; **98**: 12032–7.
91. Altomare DA, You H, Xiao GH, *et al.* Human and mouse mesotheliomas exhibit elevated AKT/PKB activity, which can be targeted pharmacologically to inhibit tumor cell growth. *Oncogene* 2005; **24**: 6080–9.

92. Harvey P, Clark IM, Jaurand MC, Warn RM, Edwards DR. Hepatocyte growth factor/scatter factor enhances the invasion of mesothelioma cell lines and the expression of matrix metalloproteinases. *Br J Cancer* 2000; **83**: 1147–53.
93. Uchiyama A, Morisaki T, Beppu K, *et al.* Hepatocyte growth factor and invasion-stimulatory activity are induced in pleural fluid by surgery in lung cancer patients. *Br J Cancer* 1999; **81**: 721–6.
94. Yashiro M, Chung YS, Inoue T, *et al.* Hepatocyte growth factor (HGF) produced by peritoneal fibroblasts may affect mesothelial cell morphology and promote peritoneal dissemination. *Int J Cancer* 1996; **67**: 289–93.
95. Saimura M, Nagai E, Mizumoto K, *et al.* Intraperitoneal injection of adenovirus-mediated NK4 gene suppresses peritoneal dissemination of pancreatic cancer cell line AsPC-1 in nude mice. *Cancer Gene Ther* 2002; **9**: 799–806.
96. Tanaka T, Shimura H, Sasaki T, *et al.* Gallbladder cancer treatment using adenovirus expressing the HGF/NK4 gene in a peritoneal implantation model. *Cancer Gene Ther* 2004; **11**: 431–40.
97. Xian CJ. Roles of epidermal growth factor family in the regulation of postnatal somatic growth. *Endocr Rev* 2007; **28**: 284–96.
98. Carpenter G. The EGF receptor: a nexus for trafficking and signaling. *Bioessays* 2000; **22**: 697–707.
99. Palmer U, Liu Z, Broome U, Klominek J. Epidermal growth factor receptor ligands are chemoattractants for normal human mesothelial cells. *Eur Respir J* 1999; **14**: 405–11.
100. Gabrielson EW, Gerwin BI, Harris CC, *et al.* Stimulation of DNA synthesis in cultured primary human mesothelial cells by specific growth factors. *FASEB J* 1988; **2**: 2717–21.
101. Goodglick LA, Vaslet CA, Messier NJ, Kane AB. Growth factor responses and protooncogene expression of murine mesothelial cell lines derived from asbestos-induced mesotheliomas. *Toxicol Pathol* 1997; **25**: 565–73.
102. Owens MW, Milligan SA. Growth factor modulation of rat pleural mesothelial cell mitogenesis and collagen synthesis. Effects of epidermal growth factor and platelet-derived factor. *Inflammation* 1994; **18**: 77–87.
103. Pache JC, Janssen YM, Walsh ES, *et al.* Increased epidermal growth factor-receptor protein in a human mesothelial cell line in response to long asbestos fibers. *Am J Pathol* 1998; **152**: 333–40.
104. van Rossen ME, Hofland LJ, van den Tol MP, *et al.* Effect of inflammatory cytokines and growth factors on tumour cell adhesion to the peritoneum. *J Pathol* 2001; **193**: 530–7.
105. Mutsaers SE, McAnulty RJ, Laurent GJ, *et al.* Cytokine regulation of mesothelial cell proliferation *in vitro* and *in vivo*. *Eur J Cell Biol* 1997; **72**: 24–9.
106. Jayne DG, Perry SL, Morrison E, Farmery SM, Guillou PJ. Activated mesothelial cells produce heparin-binding growth factors: implications for tumour metastases. *Br J Cancer* 2000; **82**: 1233–8.
107. Faull RJ, Stanley JM, Fraser S, Power DA, Leavesley DI. HB-EGF is produced in the peritoneal cavity and enhances mesothelial cell adhesion and migration. *Kidney Int* 2001; **59**: 614–24.
108. Muller J, Yoshida T. Interaction of murine peritoneal leukocytes and mesothelial cells: in vitro model system to survey cellular events on serosal membranes during inflammation. *Clin Immunol Immunopathol* 1995; **75**: 231–8.
109. Owens MW, Milligan SA, Grisham MB. Nitric oxide synthesis by rat pleural mesothelial cells: Induction by growth factors and lipopolysaccharide. *Exp Lung Res* 1995; **21**: 731–42.
110. Ohmura E, Tsushima T, Kamiya Y, *et al.* Epidermal growth factor and transforming growth factor alpha induce ascitic fluid in mice. *Cancer Res* 1990; **15**: 4915–7.
111. Liaw YS, Yang PC, Yu CJ, *et al.* PKC activation is required by EGF-stimulated Na(+)-H+ exchanger in human pleural mesothelial cells. *Am J Physiol* 1998; **274**(5 Pt 1): L665–L72.
112. Faux SP, Houghton CE, Hubbard A, Patrick G. Increased expression of epidermal growth factor receptor in rat pleural mesothelial cells correlates with carcinogenicity of mineral fibres. *Carcinogenesis* 2000; **21**: 2275–80.
113. Zanella CL, Timblin CR, Cummins A, *et al.* Asbestos-induced phosphorylation of epidermal growth factor receptor is linked to c-fos and apoptosis. *Am J Physiol* 1999; **277**(4 Pt 1): L684–L93.
114. Lahat N, Froom P, Kristal-Boneh E, *et al.* Increased serum concentrations of growth factor receptors and Neu in workers previously exposed to asbestos. *Occup Environ Med* 1999; **56**: 114–7.
115. Stanton MF, Layard M, Tegeris A, *et al.* Relation of particle dimension to carcinogenicity in amphibole asbestoses and other fibrous minerals. *J Natl Cancer Inst* 1981; **67**: 965–75.
116. Heintz NH, Janssen YM, Mossman BT. Persistent induction of c-fos and c-jun expression by asbestos. *Proc Natl Acad Sci U S A* 1993; **90**: 3299–303.
117. Janssen YM, Heintz NH, Mossman BT. Induction of c-fos and c-jun proto-oncogene expression by asbestos is ameliorated by *N*-acetyl-L-cysteine in mesothelial cells. *Cancer Res* 1995; **55**: 2085–9.
118. Zanella CL, Posada J, Tritton TR, Mossman BT. Asbestos causes stimulation of the extracellular signal-related kinase 1 mitogen-activated protein kinase cascade after phosphorylation of the epidermal growth factor receptor. *Cancer Res* 1996; **56**: 5334–8.
119. Dazzi H, Hasleton PS, Thatcher N, *et al.* Malignant pleural mesothelioma and epidermal growth factor receptor (EGF-R). Relationship of EGF-R with histology and survival using fixed paraffin embedded tissue and the F4, monoclonal antibody. *Br J Cancer* 1990; **61**: 924–6.
120. Destro A, Ceresoli GL, Falleni M, *et al.* EGFR overexpression in malignant pleural mesothelioma. An immunohistochemical and molecular study with clinico-pathological correlations. *Lung Cancer* 2006; **51**: 207–15.
121. Edwards JG, Swinson DE, Jones JL, Waller DA, O'Byrne KJ. EGFR expression: associations with outcome and clinicopathological variables in malignant pleural mesothelioma. *Lung Cancer* 2006; **54**: 399–407.
122. Govindan R, Kratzke RA, Herndon JE, 2nd, *et al.* Gefitinib in patients with malignant mesothelioma: a phase II study by the Cancer and Leukemia Group B. *Clin Cancer Res* 2005; **11**: 2300–4.
123. Ramael M, Segers K, Buysse C, Van den Bossche J, Van Marck E. Immunohistochemical distribution patterns of epidermal growth factor receptor in malignant mesothelioma and non-neoplastic mesothelium. *Virchows Arch A Pathol Anat Histopathol* 1991; **419**: 171–5.
124. Liu Z, Klominek J. Regulation of matrix metalloprotease activity in malignant mesothelioma cell lines by growth factors. *Thorax* 2003; **58**: 198–203.
125. Cole GW Jr, Alleva AM, Reddy RM, *et al.* The selective epidermal growth factor receptor tyrosine kinase inhibitor PD153035 suppresses expression of prometastasis phenotypes in malignant pleural mesothelioma cells *in vitro*. *J Thorac Cardiovasc Surg* 2005; **129**: 1010–7.
126. Janne PA, Taffaro ML, Salgia R, Johnson BE. Inhibition of epidermal growth factor receptor signaling in malignant pleural mesothelioma. *Cancer Res* 2002; **62**: 5242–7.
127. She Y, Lee F, Chen J, *et al.* The epidermal growth factor receptor tyrosine kinase inhibitor ZD1839 selectively potentiates radiation response of human tumors in nude mice, with a marked improvement in therapeutic index. *Clin Cancer Res* 2003; **9**(10 Pt 1): 3773–8.
128. Cortese JF, Gowda AL, Wali A, *et al.* Common EGFR mutations conferring sensitivity to gefitinib in lung adenocarcinoma are not prevalent in human malignant mesothelioma. *Int J Cancer* 2006; **118**: 521–2.
129. Garland LL, Rankin C, Gandara DR, *et al.* Phase II study of erlotinib in patients with malignant pleural mesothelioma: a Southwest Oncology Group Study. *J Clin Oncol* 2007; **25**: 2406–13.
130. Cesario A, Catassi A, Festi L, *et al.* Farnesyltransferase inhibitors and human malignant pleural mesothelioma: a first-step

comparative translational study. *Clin Cancer Res* 2005; **11**: 2026–37.

131. Athanassiadou P, Athanassiades P, Kyrkou K, *et al.* Expression of vimentin and epidermal growth factor receptor in effusions from patients with breast cancer; correlation with oestrogen and progesterone receptor status. *Cytopathology* 1993; **4**: 91–8.
132. Abramov Y, Anteby SO, Fasouliotis SJ, Barak V. Markedly elevated levels of vascular endothelial growth factor, fibroblast growth factor, and interleukin 6 in Meigs syndrome. *Am J Obstet Gynecol* 2001; **184**: 354–5.
133. Strizzi L, Vianale G, Catalano A, *et al.* Basic fibroblast growth factor in mesothelioma pleural effusions: correlation with patient survival and angiogenesis. *Int J Oncol* 2001; **18**: 1093–8.
134. Cronauer MV, Stadlmann S, Klocker H, *et al.* Basic fibroblast growth factor synthesis by human peritoneal mesothelial cells: induction by interleukin-1. *Am J Pathol* 1999; **155**: 1977–84.
135. Antony VB, Nasreen N, Mohammed KA, *et al.* Talc pleurodesis: basic fibroblast growth factor mediates pleural fibrosis. *Chest* 2004; **126**: 1522–8.
136. Davidson B, Vintman L, Zcharia E, *et al.* Heparanase and basic fibroblast growth factor are co-expressed in malignant mesothelioma. *Clin Exp Metastasis* 2004; **21**: 469–76.
137. Stapelberg M, Gellert N, Swettenham E, *et al.* Alpha-tocopheryl succinate inhibits malignant mesothelioma by disrupting the fibroblast growth factor autocrine loop: mechanism and the role of oxidative stress. *J Biol Chem* 2005; **280**: 25369–76.
138. Tzanakakis GN, Hjerpe A, Karamanos NK. Proteoglycan synthesis induced by transforming and basic fibroblast growth factors in human malignant mesothelioma is mediated through specific receptors and the tyrosine kinase intracellular pathway. *Biochimie* 1997; **79**: 323–32.
139. Bergsten E, Uutela M, Li X, *et al.* PDGF-D is a specific, protease-activated ligand for the PDGF beta-receptor. *Nat Cell Biol* 2001; **3**: 512–6.
140. Fredriksson L, Li H, Eriksson U. The PDGF family: four gene products form five dimeric isoforms. *Cytokine Growth Factor Rev* 2004; **15**: 197–204.
141. Li X, Ponten A, Aase K, *et al.* PDGF-C is a new protease-activated ligand for the PDGF alpha-receptor. *Nat Cell Biol* 2000; **2**: 302–9.
142. Li M, Jendrossek V, Belka C. The role of PDGF in radiation oncology. *Radiat Oncol* 2007; **2**: 5.
143. Adamson IYR, Prieditis H, Young L. Lung mesothelial cell and fibroblast responses to pleural and alveolar macrophage supernatants and to lavage fluids from crocidolite-exposed rats. *Am J Respir Cell Mol Biol* 1997; **16**: 650–6.
144. Deuel TF, Senior RM, Huang JS, Griffin GL. Chemotaxis of monocytes and neutrophils to platelet-derived growth factor. *J Clin Invest* 1982; **69**: 1046–9.
145. Tzeng DY, Deuel TF, Huang JS, Baehner RL. Platelet-derived growth factor promotes human peripheral monocyte activation. *Blood* 1985; **66**: 179–83.
146. Blatti SP, Foster DN, Ranganathan G, Moses HL, Getz MJ. Induction of fibronectin gene transcription and mRNA is a primary response to growth-factor stimulation of AKR-2B cells. *Proc Natl Acad Sci U S A* 1988; **85**: 1119–23.
147. Heldin P, Asplund T, Ytterberg D, Thelin S, Laurent TC. Characterization of the molecular mechanism involved in the activation of hyaluronan synthetase by platelet-derived growth factor in human mesothelial cells. *Biochem J* 1992; **283**: 165–70.
148. Butt RP, Laurent GJ, Bishop JE. Collagen production and replication by cardiac fibroblasts is enhanced in response to diverse classes of growth factors. *Eur J Cell Biol* 1995; **68**: 330–5.
149. Bauer EA, Cooper TW, Huang JS, Altman J, Deuel TF. Stimulation of in vitro human skin collagenase expression by platelet-derived growth factor. *Proc Natl Acad Sci U S A* 1985; **82**: 4132–6.
150. Pierce GF, Mustoe TA, Lingelbach J, *et al.* Platelet-derived growth factor and transforming growth factor-beta enhance tissue repair activities by unique mechanisms. *J Cell Biol* 1989; **109**: 429–40.
151. Filiberti R, Marroni P, Neri M, *et al.* Serum PDGF-AB in pleural mesothelioma. *Tumour Biol* 2005; **26**: 221–6.
152. Gerwin BI, Lechner JF, Reddel RR, *et al.* Comparison of production of transforming growth factor-beta and platelet-derived growth factor by normal human mesothelial cells and mesothelioma cell lines. *Cancer Res* 1987; **47**: 6180–4.
153. Versnel MA, Hagemeijer A, Bouts MJ, van der Kwast TH, Hoogsteden HC. Expression of c-sis (PDGF B-chain) and PDGF A-chain genes in ten human malignant mesothelioma cell lines derived from primary and metastatic tumors. *Oncogene* 1988; **2**: 601–5.
154. Van der Meeren A, Seddon MB, Betsholtz CA, Lechner JF, Gerwin BI. Tumorigenic conversion of human mesothelial cells as a consequence of platelet-derived growth factor-A chain overexpression. *Am J Respir Cell Mol Biol* 1993; **8**: 214–21.
155. Metheny-Barlow LJ, Flynn B, van Gijssel HE, Marrogi A, Gerwin BI. Paradoxical effects of platelet-derived growth factor-A overexpression in malignant mesothelioma. Antiproliferative effects *in vitro* and tumorigenic stimulation *in vivo*. *Am J Respir Cell Mol Biol* 2001; **24**: 694–702.
156. Ramael M, Buysse C, van den Bossche J, Segers K, van Marck E. Immunoreactivity for the beta chain of the platelet-derived growth factor receptor in malignant mesothelioma and non-neoplastic mesothelium. *J Pathol* 1992; **167**: 1–4.
157. Langerak AW, De Laat PA, Van Der Linden-Van Beurden CA, *et al.* Expression of platelet-derived growth factor (PDGF) and PDGF receptors in human malignant mesothelioma *in vitro* and *in vivo*. *J Pathol* 1996; **178**: 151–60.
158. Langerak AW, van der Linden-van Beurden CA, Versnel MA. Regulation of differential expression of platelet-derived growth factor alpha- and beta-receptor mRNA in normal and malignant human mesothelial cell lines. *Biochim Biophys Acta* 1996; **1305**: 63–70.
159. Versnel MA, Claesson-Welsh L, Hammacher A, *et al.* Human malignant mesothelioma cell lines express PDGF beta-receptors whereas cultured normal mesothelial cells express predominantly PDGF alpha-receptors. *Oncogene* 1991; **6**: 2005–11.
160. Ascoli V, Scalzo CC, Facciolo F, Nardi F. Platelet-derived growth factor receptor immunoreactivity in mesothelioma and nonneoplastic mesothelial cells in serous effusions. *Acta Cytol* 1995; **39**: 613–22.
161. Klominek J, Baskin B, Hauzenberger D. Platelet-derived growth factor (PDGF) BB acts as a chemoattractant for human malignant mesothelioma cells via PDGF receptor beta-integrin alpha3beta1 interaction. *Clin Exp Metastasis* 1998; **16**: 529–39.
162. Safi A, Sadmi M, Martinet N, *et al.* Presence of elevated levels of platelet-derived growth factor (PDGF) in lung adenocarcinoma pleural effusions. *Chest* 1992; **102**: 204–7.
163. Hung KY, Chen CT, Yen CJ, *et al.* Dipyridamole inhibits PDGF-stimulated human peritoneal mesothelial cell proliferation. *Kidney Int* 2001; **60**: 872–81.
164. Bertino P, Porta C, Barbone D, *et al.* Preliminary data suggestive of a novel translational approach to mesothelioma therapy: Imatinib mesylate with gemcitabine or pemetrexed. *Thorax* 2007; **62**: 690–5..
165. Mathy A, Baas P, Dalesio O, van Zandwijk N. Limited efficacy of imatinib mesylate in malignant mesothelioma: a phase II trial. *Lung Cancer* 2005; **50**: 83–6.
166. Board R, Jayson GC. Platelet-derived growth factor receptor (PDGFR): a target for anticancer therapeutics. *Drug Resist Updat* 2005; **8**:75–83.
167. Duan C. Specifying the cellular responses to IGF signals: roles of IGF-binding proteins. *J Endocrinol* 2002; **175**: 41–54.
168. Laviola L, Natalicchio A, Giorgino F. The IGF-I signaling pathway. *Curr Pharm Des* 2007; **13**: 663–9.
169. Hawkes C, Kar S. The insulin-like growth factor-II/mannose-6-phosphate receptor: structure, distribution and function in the central nervous system. *Brain Res Brain Res Rev* 2004; **44**: 117–40.

170. Hoang CD, Zhang X, Scott PD, *et al.* Selective activation of insulin receptor substrate-1 and -2 in pleural mesothelioma cells: association with distinct malignant phenotypes. *Cancer Res* 2004; **64**: 7479–85.
171. Lee TC, Zhang Y, Aston C, *et al.* Normal human mesothelial cells and mesothelioma cell lines express insulin-like growth factor I and associated molecules. *Cancer Res* 1993; **53**: 2858–64.
172. Porcu P, Ferber A, Pietrzkowski Z, *et al.* The growth-stimulatory effect of simian virus 40 T antigen requires the interaction of insulinlike growth factor 1 with its receptor. *Mol Cell Biol* 1992; **12**: 5069–77.
173. Pass HI, Mew DJ, Carbone M, *et al.* The effect of an antisense expression plasmid to the IGF-1 receptor on hamster mesothelioma proliferation. *Dev Biol Stand* 1998; **94**: 321–8.
174. Whitson BA, Jacobson BA, Frizelle S, *et al.* Effects of insulin-like growth factor-1 receptor inhibition in mesothelioma. *Ann Thorac Surg* 2006; **82**: 996–1001.
175. Whitson BA, Kratzke RA. Molecular pathways in malignant pleural mesothelioma. *Cancer Lett* 2006; **239**: 183–9.
176. Hodzic D, Delacroix L, Willemsen P, *et al.* Characterization of the IGF system and analysis of the possible molecular mechanisms leading to IGF-II overexpression in a mesothelioma. *Horm Metab Res* 1997; **29**: 549–55.
177. Hoang CD, D'Cunha J, Kratzke MG, *et al.* Gene expression profiling identifies matriptase overexpression in malignant mesothelioma. *Chest* 2004; **125**: 1843–52.
178. Briselli M, Mark EJ, Dickersin GR. Solitary fibrous tumours of the pleura: eight new cases and review of 360 cases in the literature. *Cancer* 1981; **47**: 2678–89.
179. Cole FH Jr, Ellis RA, Goodman RC, Weber BC, Courington DP. Benign fibrous pleural tumor with elevation of insulin-like growth factor and hypoglycemia. *South Med J* 1990; **83**: 690–4.
180. Fukasawa Y, Takada A, Tateno M, *et al.* Solitary fibrous tumor of the pleura causing recurrent hypoglycemia by secretion of insulin-like growth factor II. *Pathol Int* 1998; **48**: 47–52.
181. Masson EA, MacFarlane IA, Graham D, Foy P. Spontaneous hypoglycaemia due to a pleural fibroma: role of insulin like growth factors. *Thorax* 1991; **46**: 930–1.
182. Kishi K, Homma S, Tanimura S, Matsushita H, Nakata K. Hypoglycemia induced by secretion of high molecular weight insulin-like growth factor-II from a malignant solitary fibrous tumor of the pleura. *Intern Med* 2001; **40**: 341–4.
183. Rena O, Filosso PL, Papalia E, *et al.* Solitary fibrous tumour of the pleura: surgical treatment. *Eur J Cardiothorac Surg* 2001; **19**: 185–9.
184. Chang ED, Lee EH, Won YS, *et al.* Malignant solitary fibrous tumor of the pleura causing recurrent hypoglycemia; immunohistochemical stain of insulin-like growth factor i receptor in three cases. *J Korean Med Sci* 2001; **16**: 220–4.
185. Li Y, Chang Q, Rubin BP, *et al.* Insulin receptor activation in solitary fibrous tumours. *J Pathol* 2007; **211**: 550–4.
186. Bourcigaux N, Arnault-Ouary G, Christol R, *et al.* Treatment of hypoglycemia using combined glucocorticoid and recombinant human growth hormone in a patient with a metastatic non-islet cell tumor hypoglycemia. *Clin Ther* 2005; **27**: 246–51.
187. Drake WM, Miraki F, Siddiqi A, *et al.* Dose-related effects of growth hormone on IGF-I and IGF-binding protein-3 levels in non-islet cell tumour hypoglycaemia. *Eur J Endocrinol* 1998; **139**: 532–6.
188. Olchovsky D, Shimon I, Goldberg I, *et al.* Elevated insulin-like growth factor-1 and insulin-like growth factor binding protein-2 in malignant pleural effusion. *Acta Oncol* 2002; **41**: 182–7.
189. Grove CS, Lee YCG. Vascular endothelial growth factor: the key mediator in pleural effusion formation. *Curr Opin Pulm Med* 2002; **8**: 294–301.
190. Mohammed KA, Nasreen N, Hardwick J, *et al.* Bacterial induction of pleural mesothelial monolayer barrier dysfunction. *Am J Physiol Lung Cell Mol Physiol* 2001; **281**: L119–L25.
191. Cheng D, Rodriguez RM, Perkett EA, *et al.* Vascular endothelial growth factor in pleural fluid. *Chest* 1999; **116**: 760–5.
192. Cheng DS, Lee YC, Rogers JT, *et al.* Vascular endothelial growth factor level correlates with transforming growth factor beta isoform levels in pleural effusions. *Chest* 2000; **118**: 1747–53.
193. Yanagawa H, Takeuchi E, Suzuki Y, *et al.* Vascular endothelial growth factor in malignant pleural effusion associated with lung cancer. *Cancer Immunol Immunother* 1999; **48**: 396–400.
194. Ishimoto O, Saijo Y, Narumi K, *et al.* High level of vascular endothelial growth factor in hemorrhagic pleural effusion of cancer. *Oncology* 2002; **63**: 70–5.
195. Ishii H, Yazawa T, Sato H, *et al.* Enhancement of pleural dissemination and lymph node metastasis of intrathoracic lung cancer cells by vascular endothelial growth factors (VEGFs). *Lung Cancer* 2004; **45**: 325–37.
196. Kraft A, Weindel K, Ochs A, *et al.* Vascular endothelial growth factor in the sera and effusions of patients with malignant and nonmalignant disease. *Cancer* 1999; **85**: 178–87.
197. Strizzi L, Catalano A, Vianale G, *et al.* Vascular endothelial growth factor is an autocrine growth factor in human malignant mesothelioma. *J Pathol* 2001; **193**: 468–75.
198. Sako A, Kitayama J, Yamaguchi H, *et al.* Vascular endothelial growth factor synthesis by human omental mesothelial cells is augmented by fibroblast growth factor-2: possible role of mesothelial cell on the development of peritoneal metastasis. *J Surg Res* 2003; **115**: 113–20.
199. Brown LF, Detmar M, Claffey K, Nagy JA. Vascular permeability factor/vascular endothelial growth factors: A multifunctional angiogenic cytokine. *EXS* 1997; **79**: 233–69.
200. Ferrara N, Keyt B. Vascular endothelial growth factor: Basic biology and clinical implications. *EXS* 1997; **79**: 209–32.
201. Takahama M, Tsutsumi M, Tsujiuchi T, *et al.* Enhanced expression of Tie2, its ligand angiopoietin-1, vascular endothelial growth factor, and CD31 in human non-small cell lung carcinomas. *Clin Cancer Res* 1999; **5**: 2506–10.
202. Yoshiji H, Gomez DE, Shibuya M, Thorgeirsson UP. Expression of vascular endothelial growth factor, its receptor, and other angiogenic factors in human breast cancer. *Cancer Res* 1996; **56**: 2013–6.
203. Cacciotti P, Strizzi L, Vianale G, *et al.* The presence of simian-virus 40 sequences in mesothelioma and mesothelial cells is associated with high levels of vascular endothelial growth factor. *Am J Respir Cell Mol Biol* 2002; **26**: 189–93.
204. Masood R, Kundra A, Zhu S, *et al.* Malignant mesothelioma growth inhibition by agents that target the VEGF and VEGF-C autocrine loops. *Int J Cancer* 2003; **104**: 603–10.
205. Thickett DR, Armstrong L, Millar AB. Vascular endothelial growth factor (VEGF) in inflammatory and malignant pleural effusions. *Thorax* 1999; **54**: 707–10.
206. D'Arcangelo D, Facchiano F, Barlucchi LM, *et al.* Acidosis inhibits endothelial cell apoptosis and function and induces basic fibroblast growth factor and vascular endothelial growth factor expression. *Circ Res* 2000; **86**: 312–8.
207. Clauss M, Schaper W. Vascular endothelial growth factor: a jack of all trades or a nonspecific stress gene? *Circ Res* 2000; **86**: 251–2.
208. Momi H, Matsuyama W, Inoue K, *et al.* Vascular endothelial growth factor and proinflammatory cytokines in pleural effusions. *Respir Med* 2002; **96**: 817–22.
209. Kalomenidis I, Stathopoulos GT, Barnette R, *et al.* Vascular endothelial growth factor levels in post-CABG pleural effusions are associated with pleural inflammation and permeability. *Respir Med* 2007; **101**: 223–9.
210. Light RW. *Pleural diseases*, 4th edn. Baltimore: Lippincott, Williams & Wilkins, 2001.
211. Ishiko O, Yoshida H, Sumi T, Hirai K, Ogita S. Vascular endothelial growth factor levels in pleural and peritoneal fluid in Meigs' syndrome. *Eur J Obstet Gynecol Reprod Biol* 2001; **98**: 129–30.
212. Ferrara N. Molecular and biological properties of vascular endothelial growth factor. *J Mol Med* 1999; **77**: 527–43.

213. Neufeld G, Cohen T, Gengrinovitch S, Poltorak Z. Vascular endothelial growth factor and its receptors. *FASEB J* 1999; **13**: 9–22.
214. Kranz A, Rau C, Kochs M, Waltenberger J. Elevation of vascular endothelial growth factor-A serum levels following acute myocardial infarction. Evidence for its origin and functional significance. *J Mol Cell Cardiol* 2000; **32**: 65–72.
215. Lee SH, Wolf PL, Escudero R, *et al.* Early expression of angiogenesis factors in acute myocardial ischemia and infarction. *N Engl J Med* 2000; **342**: 626–33.
216. Yano S, Shinohara H, Herbst RS, *et al.* Production of experimental malignant pleural effusions is dependent on invasion of the pleura and expression of vascular endothelial growth factor/vascular permeability factor by human lung cancer cells. *Am J Pathol* 2000; **157**: 1893–903.
217. Yeo K-T, Wang HH, Nagy JA, *et al.* Vascular permeability factor (vascular endothelial growth factor) in guinea pig and human tumor and inflammatory effusions. *Cancer Res* 1993; **53**: 2912–8.
218. Margolin K. Inhibition of vascular endothelial growth factor in the treatment of solid tumors. *Curr Oncol Rep* 2002; **4**: 20–8.
219. Schlaeppi JM, Wood JM. Targeting vascular endothelial growth factor (VEGF) for anti-tumor therapy, by anti-VEGF neutralizing monoclonal antibodies or by VEGF receptor tyrosine-kinase inhibitors. *Cancer Metastasis Rev* 1999; **18**: 473–81.
220. Robinson CJ, Stringer SE. The splice variants of vascular endothelial growth factor (VEGF) and their receptors. *J Cell Sci* 2001; **114**: 853–65.
221. Zachary I, Gliki G. Signaling transduction mechanisms mediating biological actions of the vascular endothelial growth factor family. *Cardiovasc Res* 2001; **49**: 568–81.
222. Giles FJ. The vascular endothelial growth factor (VEGF) signaling pathway: A therapeutic target in patients with hematologic malignancies. *Oncologists* 2001; **6** (Suppl 5): 32–9.
●223. Yano S, Herbst RS, Shinohara H, *et al.* Treatment for malignant pleural effusion of human lung adenocarcinoma by inhibition of vascular endothelial growth factor receptor tyrosine kinase phosphorylation. *Clin Cancer Res* 2000; **6**: 957–65.
224. Mesiano S, Ferrara N, Jaffe RB. Role of vascular endothelial growth factor in ovarian cancer: inhibition of ascites formation by immunoneutralization. *Am J Pathol* 1998; **153**: 1249–56.
225. Yoshiji H, Kuriyama S, Hicklin DJ, *et al.* The vascular endothelial growth factor receptor KDR/Flk-1 is a major regulator of malignant ascites formation in the mouse hepatocellular carcinoma model. *Hepatology* 2001; **33**: 841–7.
226. Stoelcker B, Echtenacher B, Weich HA, *et al.* VEGF/Flk-1 interaction, a requirement for malignant ascites recurrence. *J Interferon Cytokine Res* 2000; **20**: 511–7.
227. Verheul HMW, Hoekman K, Jorna AS, Smit EF, Pinedo HM. Targeting vascular endothelial growth factor blockade: ascites and pleural effusion formation. *Oncologist* 2000; **5**: 45–50.
228. Matsumori Y, Yano S, Goto H, *et al.* ZD6474, an inhibitor of vascular endothelial growth factor receptor tyrosine kinase, inhibits growth of experimental lung metastasis and production of malignant pleural effusions in a non-small cell lung cancer model. *Oncol Res* 2006; **16**: 15–26.
●229. Motomura Y, Kanbayashi H, Khan WI, *et al.* The gene transfer of soluble VEGF type I receptor (Flt-1) attenuates peritoneal fibrosis formation in mice but not soluble TGF-beta type II receptor gene transfer. *AJP – Gastrointestinal Liver Physiol* 2005; **288**: G143–G50.
230. Boussat S, Eddahibi S, Coste A, *et al.* Expression and regulation of vascular endothelial growth factor in human pulmonary epithelial cells. *Am J Physiol Lung Cell Mol Physiol* 2000; **279**: L371–8.
231. Cohen T, Nahari D, Cerem LW, Neufeld G, Levi BZ. Interleukin 6 induces the expression of vascular endothelial growth factor. *J Biol Chem* 1996; **271**: 736–41.
232. Ravindranath N, Wion D, Brachet P, Djakiew D. Epidermal growth factor modulates the expression of vascular endothelial growth factor in the human prostate. *J Androl* 2001; **22**: 432–43.
233. Punglia RS, Lu M, Hsu J, *et al.* Regulation of vascular endothelial growth factor expression by insulin-like growth factor I. *Diabetes* 1997; **46**: 1619–26.
234. Schams D, Kosmann M, Berisha B, Amselgruber WM, Miyamoto A. Stimulatory and synergistic effects of luteinising hormone and insulin like growth factor 1 on the secretion of vascular endothelial growth factor and progesterone of cultured bovine granulosa cells. *Exp Clin Endocrinol Diabetes* 2001; **109**: 155–62.
235. Ryuto M, Ono M, Izumi H, *et al.* Induction of vascular endothelial growth factor by tumor necrosis factor alpha in human glioma cells. Possible roles of SP-1. *J Biol Chem* 1996; **271**: 28220–8.
236. Nauck M, Roth M, Tamm M, *et al.* Induction of vascular endothelial growth factor by platelet-activating factor and platelet-derived growth factor is downregulated by corticosteroids. *Am J Respir Cell Mol Biol* 1997; **16**: 398–406.
237. Saadeh PB, Mehrara BJ, Steinbrech DS, *et al.* Mechanisms of fibroblast growth factor-2 modulation of vascular endothelial growth factor expression by osteoblastic cells. *Endocrinology* 2000; **141**: 2075–83.
238. Mandl-Weber S, Cohen CD, Haslinger B, Kretzler M, Sitter T. Vascular endothelial growth factor production and regulation in human peritoneal mesothelial cells. *Kidney Int* 2002; **61**: 570–8.
239. Gruden G, Thomas S, Burt D, *et al.* Interaction of angiotensin II and mechanical stretch on vascular endothelial growth factor production by human mesangial cells. *J Am Soc Nephrol* 1999; **10**: 730–7.
240. Sauter M, Cohen CD, Wörnle M, *et al.* ACE inhibitor and AT1-receptor blocker attenuate the production of VEGF in mesothelial cells. *Perit Dial Int* 2007; **27**: 162–72.
241. Cascinu S, Del Ferro E, Ligi M, *et al.* Inhibition of vascular endothelial growth factor by octreotide in colorectal cancer patients. *Cancer Invest* 2001; **19**: 8–12.
242. Fischer S, Renz D, Schaper W, Karliczek GF. *In vitro* effects of dexamethasone on hypoxia-induced hyperpermeability and expression of vascular endothelial growth factor. *Eur J Pharmacol* 2001; **411**: 231–43.
243. Kirschenbaum A, Liu X-H, Yao S, Levine AC. The role of cyclooxygenase-2 in prostate cancer. *Urology* 2001; **58** (Suppl. 2A): 127–31.
244. Renner W, Kotschan S, Hoffmann C, Obermayer-Pietsch B, Pilger E. A common 936 C/T mutation in the gene for vascular endothelial growth factor is associated with vascular endothelial growth factor plasma levels. *J Vasc Res* 2000; **37**: 443–8.
245. Hoyer RJ, Leung N, Witzig TE, Lacy MQ. Treatment of diuretic refractory pleural effusions with bevacizumab in four patients with primary systemic amyloidosis. *Am J Hematol* 2007; **82**: 409–13.
246. Pichelmayer O, Zielinski C, Raderer M. Response of a nonmalignant pleural effusion to bevacizumab. *N Engl J Med* 2005 **353**: 740–1.
247. Moldawer LL. Biology of proinflammatory cytokines and their antagonists. *Crit Care Med* 1994; **22**: S3–S7.
248. Goodman RB, Wood RG, Martin TR, Hanson-Painton O, Knasewitz GT. Cytokine-stimulated human mesothelial cells produce chemotactic activity for neutrophils including NAP-1/IL-8. *J Immunol* 1992; **148**: 457–65.
249. Zeillemaker AM, Mul FP, Hoynck van Papendrecht AA, *et al.* Neutrophil adherence to and migration across monolayers of human peritoneal mesothelial cells. The role of mesothelium in the influx of neutrophils during peritonitis. *J Lab Clin Med* 1996; **127**: 279–86.
250. Alkhamesi NA, Ziprin P, Pfistermuller K, Peck DH, Darzi AW. ICAM-1 mediated peritoneal carcinomatosis, a target for therapeutic intervention. *Clin Exp Metastasis* 2005; **22**: 449–59.
251. Robson RL, McLoughlin RM, Witowski J, *et al.* Differential regulation of chemokine production in human peritoneal mesothelial cells: IFN-gamma controls neutrophil migration across the mesothelium *in vitro* and *in vivo*. *J Immunol* 2001; **167**: 1028–38.

252. Zhang XY, Guckian M, Nasiri N, *et al.* Normal and SV40 transfected human peritoneal mesothelial cells produce IL-6 and IL-8: implication for gynaecological disease. *Clin Exp Immunol* 2002; **129**: 288–96.
253. Fang CC, Yen CJ, Chen YM, *et al.* Diltiazem suppresses collagen synthesis and IL-1beta-induced TGF-beta1 production on human peritoneal mesothelial cells. *Nephrol Dial Transplant* 2006; **21**: 1340–7.
254. Braundmeier AG, Nowak RA. Cytokines regulate matrix metalloproteinases in human uterine endometrial fibroblast cells through a mechanism that does not involve increases in extracellular matrix metalloproteinase inducer. *Am J Reprod Immunol* 2006; **56**: 201–14.
255. Lee YCG, Knight DA, Lane KB, *et al.* Activation of Proteinase Activated Receptor-2 in mesothelial cells induces pleural inflammation. *Am J Physiol Lung Cell Mol Physiol* 2005; **288**: L734–L40.
256. Stadlmann S, Pollheimer J, Renner K, *et al.* Response of human peritoneal mesothelial cells to inflammatory injury is regulated by interleukin-1beta and tumor necrosis factor-alpha. *Wound Repair Regen* 2006; **14**: 187–94.
257. Hua CC, Chang LC, Chen YC, Chang SC. Proinflammatory cytokines and fibrinolytic enzymes in tuberculous and malignant pleural effusions. *Chest* 1999; **116**: 1292–6.
258. Odeh M, Sabo E, Srugo I, Oliven A. Tumour necrosis factor alpha in the diagnostic assessment of pleural effusion. *QJM* 2000; **93**: 819–24.
259. Alexandrakis MG, Coulocheri SA, Bouros D, *et al.* Evaluation of inflammatory cytokines in malignant and benign pleural effusions. *Oncol Rep* 2000; **7**: 1327–32.
260. Rochester CL, Elias JA. Cytokines and cytokine networking in the pathogenesis of interstitial and fibrotic lung disorders. *Semin Respir Med* 1993; **14**: 389–416.
261. Zhu Z, Yao J, Wang F, Xu Q. TNF-alpha and the phenotypic transformation of human peritoneal meosthelioma cell. *Chin Med J (Engl)* 2002; **115**: 513–7.
262. Haslinger B, Kleemann R, Toet KH, Kooistra T. Simvastatin suppresses tissue factor expression and increases fibrinolytic activity in tumor necrosis factor-alpha-activated human peritoneal mesothelial cells. *Kidney Int* 2003; **63**: 2065–74.
263. Cheng DS, Rogers JT, Wheeler A, *et al.* The effects of intrapleural polyclonal anti-tumor necrosis factor alpha (TNF alpha) Fab fragments on pleurodesis in rabbits. *Lung* 2000; **178**: 19–29.
264. Corbett EL, Mozzato-Chamay N, Butterworth AE, *et al.* Polymorphisms in the tumor necrosis factor-alpha gene promoter may predispose to severe silicosis in black South African miners. *Am J Respir Crit Care Med* 2002; **165**: 690–3.
265. Musk AW, Wong KCC, De Klerk NH, Cookson WO, Moffatt MF. Candidate gene polymorphism and pulmonary fibrosis in subjects with asbestos exposure. *Am J Respir Crit Care Med* 2001; **163**: A44.
•266. Yang H, Bocchetta M, Kroczynska B, *et al.* TNF-alpha inhibits asbestos-induced cytotoxicity via a NF-kappaB-dependent pathway, a possible mechanism for asbestos-induced oncogenesis. *Proc Natl Acad Sci* 2006; **103**: 10397–402.
267. Wang Y, Faux SP, Hallden G, *et al.* Interleukin-1beta and tumour necrosis factor-alpha promote the transformation of human immortalised mesothelial cells by erionite. *Int J Oncol* 2004; **25**: 173–8.
268. Russo P, Catassi A, Malacarne D, *et al.* Tumor necrosis factor enhances SN38-mediated apoptosis in mesothelioma cells. *Cancer* 2005; **103**: 1503–18.
269. van Grevenstein WM, Hofland L, Jeekel J, van Eijck CH. The expression of adhesion molecules and the influence of inflammatory cytokines on the adhesion of human pancreatic carcinoma cells to mesothelial monolayers. *Pancreas* 2006; **32**: 396–402.
270. van Grevenstein W, Hofland L, van Rossen M, *et al.* Inflammatory cytokines stimulate the adhesion of colon carcinoma cells to mesothelial monolayers. *Dig Dis Sci* 2007; **52**: 2775–83.
271. Mochizuki Y, Nakanishi H, Kodera Y, *et al.* TNF-α promotes progression of peritoneal metastasis as demonstrated using a green fluorescence protein (GFP)-tagged human gastric cancer cell line. *Clin Exp Metastasis* 2004; **21**: 39–47.
•272. Stathopoulos GT, Kollintza A, Moschos C, *et al.* Tumor necrosis factor-alpha promotes malignant pleural effusion. *Cancer Res* 2007; **67**: 9825–34.
273. Rabinowitz MH, Andrews RC, Becherer JD, *et al.* Design of selective and soluble inhibitors of tumor necrosis factor-alpha converting enzyme (TACE). *J Med Chem* 2001; **44**: 4252–67.
274. Conway JG, Andrews RC, Beaudet B, *et al.* Inhibition of tumor necrosis factor-alpha (TNF-alpha) production and arthritis in the rat by GW3333, a dual inhibitor of TNF-alpha-converting enzyme and matrix metalloproteinases. *J Pharmacol Exp Ther* 2001; **298**: 900–8.
275. Hatanaka K, Kawamura M, Murai N, *et al.* FR167653, a cytokine synthesis inhibitor, exhibits anti-inflammatory effects early in rat carrageenin-induced pleurisy but no effect later. *J Pharmacol Exp Ther* 2001; **299**: 519–27.
276. Porta C, Danova M, Orengo AM, *et al.* Interleukin-2 induces cell cycle perturbations leading to cell growth inhibition and death in malignant mesothelioma cells *in vitro*. *J Cell Physiol* 2000; **185**: 126–34.
277. Chang SC, Hsu YT, Chen YC, *et al.* Usefulness of soluble interleukin 2 receptor in differentiating tuberculous and carcinomatous pleural effusions. *Arch Intern Med* 1994; **154**: 1097–101).
278. Kim YK, Lee SY, Kwon SS, *et al.* Gamma-interferon and soluble interleukin 2 receptor in tuberculous pleural effusion. *Lung* 2001; **179**: 175–84.
279. Porcel JM, Gazquez I, Vives M, *et al.* Diagnosis of tuberculous pleuritis by the measurement of soluble interleukin 2 receptor in pleural fluid. *Int J Tuberc Lung Dis* 2000; **4**: 975–9.
280. Pettersson T, Soderblom T, Nyberg P, *et al.* Pleural fluid soluble interleukin 2 receptor in rheumatoid arthritis and systemic lupus erythematous. *J Rheumatol* 1994; **21**: 1820–4.
281. Schwartzentruber DJ. Guidelines for the safe administration of high-dose interleukin-2. *J Immunother* 2001; **24**: 287–93.
282. Whittington R, Faulds D. Interleukin-2. A review of its pharmacological properties and therapeutic use in patients with cancer. *Drugs* 1993; **46**: 446–514.
283. Yanagawa H, Sone S, Munekata M, *et al.* IL-6 in malignant pleural effusions and its augmentation by intrapleural instillation of IL-2. *Clin Exp Immunol* 1992; **88**: 207–12.
284. Chen YM, Tsai CM, Whang-Peng J, Perng RP. Interleukin-7 and interleukin-12 have different effects in rescue of depressed cellular immunity: comparison of malignant and tuberculous pleural effusions. *J Interferon Cytokine Res* 2001; **21**: 249–56.
285. Chen YM, Ting CC, Peng JW, *et al.* Restoration of cytotoxic T lymphocyte function in malignant pleural effusion: interleukin-15 vs. interleukin-2. *J Interferon Cytokine Res* 2000; **20**: 31–9.
286. van Bruggen I, Nelson DJ, Currie AJ, Jackaman C, Robinson BW. Intratumoral poly-*N*-acetyl glucosamine-based polymer matrix provokes a prolonged local inflammatory response that, when combined with IL-2, induces regression of malignant mesothelioma in a murine model. *J Immunother* 2005; **28**: 359–67.
287. Jackaman C, Bundell CS, Kinnear BF, *et al.* IL-2 Intratumoral immunotherapy enhances CD8+ T cells that mediate destruction of tumor cells and tumor-associated vasculature: A novel mechanism for IL-2. *J Immunol* 2003; **171**: 5051–63.
288. Lissoni P, Mandala M, Curigliano G, *et al.* Progress report on the palliative therapy of 100 patients with neoplastic effusions by intracavitary low-dose interleukin-2. *Oncology* 2001; **60**: 308–12.
289. Masotti A, Fumagalli L, Morandini GC. Intrapleural administration of recombinant interleukin-2 in non-small cell lung cancer with neoplastic pleural effusion. *Monaldi Arch Chest Dis* 1997; **52**: 225–8.
290. Castagneto B, Zai S, Mutti L, *et al.* Palliative and therapeutic activity of IL-2 immunotherapy in unresectable malignant pleural

mesothelioma with pleural effusion: Results of a phase II study on 31 consecutive patients. *Lung Cancer* 2001; **31**: 303–10.

291. Astoul P, Picat-Joossen D, Viallat JR, Boutin C. Intrapleural administration of interleukin-2 for the treatment of patients with malignant pleural mesothelioma: a Phase II study. *Cancer* 1998; **83**: 2099–104.
292. Mulatero C, Surentheran T, Breuer J, Rudd RM. Simian virus 40 and human pleural mesothelioma. *Thorax* 1999; **54**: 60–1.
293. Bretti S, Berruti A, Dogliotti L, *et al.* Combined epirubicin and interleukin-2 regimen in the treatment of malignant mesothelioma: a multicenter phase II study of the Italian Group on Rare Tumors. *Tumori* 1998; **84**: 558–61.
294. Lucchi M, Chella A, Melfi F, *et al.* A phase II study of intrapleural immuno-chemotherapy, pleurectomy/decortication, radiotherapy, systemic chemotherapy and long-term sub-cutaneous IL-2 in stage II-III malignant pleural mesothelioma. *Eur J Cardiothorac Surg* 2007; **31**: 529–33.
295. Baluna R, Vitetta ES. Vascular leak syndrome: a side effect of immunotherapy. *Immunopharmacology* 1997; **37**: 117–32.
296. Melencio L, McKallip RJ, Guan H, *et al.* Role of CD4+CD25+ T regulatory cells in IL-2-induced vascular leak. *Int Immunol* 2006; **18**: 1461–71.
297. Assier E, Jullien V, Lefort J, *et al.* NK cells and polymorphonuclear neutrophils are both critical for IL-2-induced pulmonary vascular leak syndrome. *J Immunol* 2004; **172**: 7661–8.
298. Rose-John S, Scheller J, Elson G, Jones SA. Interleukin-6 biology is coordinated by membrane-bound and soluble receptors: role in inflammation and cancer. *J Leukoc Biol* 2006; **80**: 227–36.
299. Kishimoto T. The biology of interleukin-6. *Blood* 1989; **74**: 1–10.
300. Kishimoto T, Akira S, Narazaki M, Taga T. Interleukin-6 family of cytokines and gp130. *Blood* 1995; **86**: 1243–54.
301. Scheller J, Rose-John S. Interleukin-6 and its receptor: from bench to bedside. *Med Microbiol Immunol* 2006; **195**: 173–83.
302. Heinrich PC, Behrmann I, Haan S, *et al.* Principles of interleukin (IL)-6-type cytokine signalling and its regulation. *Biochem J* 2003; **374** (Pt 1): 1–20.
303. Mullberg J, Schooltink H, Stoyan T, Heinrich PC, Rose-John S. Protein kinase C activity is rate limiting for shedding of the interleukin-6 receptor. *Biochem Biophys Res Commun* 1992; **189**: 794–800.
304. Horiuchi S, Koyanagi Y, Zhou Y, *et al.* Soluble interleukin-6 receptors released from T cell or granulocyte/macrophage cell lines and human peripheral blood mononuclear cells are generated through an alternative splicing mechanism. *Eur J Immunol* 1994; **24**: 1945–8.
305. Mackiewicz A, Schooltink H, Heinrich PC, Rose-John S. Complex of soluble human IL-6-receptor/IL-6 up-regulates expression of acute-phase proteins. *J Immunol* 1992; **149**: 2021–7.
306. Rodig SJ, Meraz MA, White JM, *et al.* Disruption of the Jak1 gene demonstrates obligatory and nonredundant roles of the Jaks in cytokine-induced biologic responses. *Cell* 1998; **93**: 373–83.
307. Zhong Z, Wen Z, Darnell JE Jr. Stat3: a STAT family member activated by tyrosine phosphorylation in response to epidermal growth factor and interleukin-6. *Science* 1994; **264**: 95–8.
◆308. Nishimoto N, Kishimoto T. Interleukin 6: from bench to bedside. *Nat Clin Pract Rheumatol* 2006; **2**: 619–26.
309. Cuzzocrea S, Sautebin L, De Sarro G, *et al.* Role of IL-6 in the pleurisy and lung injury caused by carrageenan. *J Immunol* 1999; **163**: 5094–104.
310. Hurst SM, Wilkinson TS, McLoughlin RM, *et al.* IL-6 and its soluble receptor orchestrate a temporal switch in the pattern of leukocyte recruitment seen during acute inflammation. *Immunity* 2001; **14**: 705–14.
311. McLoughlin RM, Hurst SM, Nowell MA, *et al.* Differential regulation of neutrophil-activating chemokines by IL-6 and its soluble receptor isoforms. *J Immunol* 2004; **172**: 5676–83.
312. McLoughlin RM, Jenkins BJ, Grail D, *et al.* IL-6 trans-signaling via STAT3 directs T cell infiltration in acute inflammation. *Proc Natl Acad Sci USA* 2005; **102**: 9589–94.
313. Gabay C. Interleukin-6 and chronic inflammation. *Arthritis Res Ther* 2006; **8** (Suppl 2): S3.
314. Fujino S, Yokoyama A, Kohno N, Hiwada K. Interleukin 6 is an autocrine growth factor for normal human pleural mesothelial cells. *Am J Respir Cell Mol Biol* 1996; **14**: 508–15.
315. McLaren BR, Robinson BW, Lake RA. New chemotherapeutics in malignant mesothelioma: effects on cell growth and IL-6 production. *Cancer Chemother Pharmacol* 2000; **45**: 502–8.
316. Menet E, Corbi P, Ancey C, *et al.* Interleukine-6 (IL-6) synthesis and gp130 expression by human pericardium. *Eur Cytokine Netw* 2001; **12**: 639–46.
317. Schmitter D, Lauber B, Fagg B, Stahel RA. Hematopoietic growth factors secreted by seven human pleural mesothelioma cell lines: interleukin-6 production as a common feature. *Int J Cancer* 1992; **51**: 296–301.
318. Yao V, Platell C, Hall JC. Peritoneal mesothelial cells produce inflammatory related cytokines. *ANZ J Surg* 2004; **74**: 997–1002.
319. Wong CF, Yew WW, Leung SK, *et al.* Assay of pleural fluid interleukin-6, tumour necrosis factor-alpha and interferon-gamma in the diagnosis and outcome correlation of tuberculous effusion. *Respir Med* 2003; **97**: 1289–95.
320. De Smedt A, Vanderlinden E, Demanet C, *et al.* Characterisation of pleural inflammation occurring after primary spontaneous pneumothorax. *Eur Respir J* 2004; **23**: 896–900.
321. Torres SR, Frode TS, Nardi GM, *et al.* Anti-inflammatory effects of peripheral benzodiazepine receptor ligands in two mouse models of inflammation. *Eur J Pharmacol* 2000; **408**: 199–211.
322. Utsunomiya I, Ito M, Oh-ishi S. Generation of inflammatory cytokines in zymosan-induced pleurisy in rats: TNF induces IL-6 and cytokine-induced neutrophil chemoattractant (CINC) *in vivo*. *Cytokine* 1998; **10**: 956–63.
323. Lin CC, Liu CC, Lin CY. Changes in cell population and tumor necrosis factor, interleukin-6, and interleukin-8 in malignant pleural effusions after treatment with intrapleural tetracycline. *Am Rev Respir Dis* 1993; **147**: 1503–6.
324. Yahara N, Abe T, Morita K, Tangoku A, Oka M. Comparison of interleukin-6, interleukin-8, and granulocyte colony-stimulating factor production by the peritoneum in laparoscopic and open surgery. *Surg Endosc* 2002; **16**: 1615–9.
325. Yom SS, Busch TM, Friedberg JS, *et al.* Elevated serum cytokine levels in mesothelioma patients who have undergone pleurectomy or extrapleural pneumonectomy and adjuvant intraoperative photodynamic therapy. *Photochem Photobiol* 2003; **78**: 75–81.
326. Alexandrakis MG, Kyriakou DS, Bouros D, *et al.* Interleukin-6 and its relationships to acute phase proteins in serous effusion differentiation. *Oncol Rep* 2001; **8**: 415–20.
327. Marie C, Losser MR, Fitting C, *et al.* Cytokines and soluble cytokine receptors in pleural effusions from septic and nonseptic patients. *Am J Respir Crit Care Med* 1997; **156**: 1515–22.
328. Xirouchaki N, Tzanakis N, Bouros D, *et al.* Diagnostic value of interleukin-1alpha, interleukin-6, and tumor necrosis factor in pleural effusions. *Chest* 2002; **121**: 815–20.
329. Alexandrakis MG, Coulocheri SA, Bouros D, Eliopoulos GD. Evaluation of ferritin, interleukin-6, interleukin-8 and tumor necrosis factor alpha in the differentiation of exudates and transudates in pleural effusions. *Anticancer Res* 1999; **19**: 3607–12.
330. Nakano T, Chahinian AP, Shinjo M, *et al.* Interleukin 6 and its relationship to clinical parameters in patients with malignant pleural mesothelioma. *Br J Cancer* 1998; **77**: 907–12.
331. Hoheisel G, Izbicki G, Roth M, *et al.* Compartmentalization of pro-inflammatory cytokines in tuberculous pleurisy. *Respir Med* 1998; **92**: 14–7.
332. Yamaguchi T, Kimura H, Yokota S, *et al.* Effect of IL-6 elevation in malignant pleural effusion on hyperfibrinogenemia in lung cancer patients. *Jpn J Clin Oncol* 2000; **30**: 53–8.

333. Hoheisel G, Izbicki G, Roth M, *et al.* Proinflammatory cytokine levels in patients with lung cancer and carcinomatous pleurisy. *Respiration* 1998; **65**: 183–6.
334. Loret de Mola JR, Arredondo-Soberon F, Randle CP, Tureck RT, Friedlander MA. Markedly elevated cytokines in pleural effusion during the ovarian hyperstimulation syndrome: transudate or ascites? *Fertil Steril* 1997; **67**: 780–2.
335. Higashihara M, Sunaga S, Tange T, Oohashi H, Kurokawa K. Increased secretion of interleukin-6 in malignant mesothelioma cells from a patient with marked thrombocytosis. *Cancer* 1992; **70**: 2105–8.
336. Kimura N, Ogasawara T, Asonuma S, *et al.* Granulocyte-colony stimulating factor- and interleukin 6-producing diffuse deciduoid peritoneal mesothelioma. *Mod Pathol* 2005; **18**: 446–50.
337. Adachi Y, Aoki C, Yoshio-Hoshino N, *et al.* Interleukin-6 induces both cell growth and VEGF production in malignant mesotheliomas. *Int J Cancer* 2006; **119**: 1303–11.
338. Monti G, Jaurand MC, Monnet I, *et al.* Intrapleural production of interleukin 6 during mesothelioma and its modulation by gamma-interferon treatment. *Cancer Res* 1994; **54**: 4419–23.
339. Knight DA, Ernst M, Anderson GP, Moodley YP, Mutsaers SE. The role of gp130/IL-6 cytokines in the development of pulmonary fibrosis: critical determinants of disease susceptibility and progression? *Pharmacol Ther* 2003; **99**: 327–38.
340. Heymann D, L'Her E, Nguyen JM, *et al.* Leukaemia inhibitory factor (LIF) production in pleural effusions: comparison with production of IL-4, IL-8, IL-10 and macrophage-colony stimulating factor (M-CSF). *Cytokine* 1996; **8**: 410–6.
341. Meysman M, Schoors DF, Noppen M, Vincken W, Dewilde P. Tuberculous pleural effusion following coronary artery bypass graft. *Acta Clin Belg* 1995; **50**: 305–9.
342. Topley N, Brown Z, Jorres A, *et al.* Human peritoneal mesothelial cells synthesize interleukin-8. Synergistic induction by interleukin-1 beta and tumor necrosis factor-alpha. *Am J Pathol* 1993; **142**: 1876–86.
343. Arici A, Tazuke SI, Attar E, Kliman HJ, Olive DL. Interleukin-8 concentration in peritoneal fluid of patients with endometriosis and modulation of interleukin-8 expression in human mesothelial cells. *Mol Hum Reprod* 1996; **2**: 40–5.
344. Li FK, Davenport A, Robson RL, *et al.* Leukocyte migration across human peritoneal mesothelial cells is dependent on directed chemokine secretion and ICAM-1 expression. *Kidney Int* 1998; **54**: 2170–83.
345. Boylan AM, Ruegg C, Kim KJ, *et al.* Evidence of a role for mesothelial cell-derived interleukin-8 in the pathogenesis of asbestos-induced pleurisy in rabbits. *J Clin Invest* 1992; **89**: 1257–67.
346. Broaddus VC, Boylan AM, Hoeffel JM, *et al.* Neutralization of IL-8 inhibits neutrophil influx in a rabbit model of endotoxin-induced pleurisy. *J Immunol* 1994; **152**: 2960–7.
347. Visser CE, Steenbergen JJ, Betjes MG, *et al.* Interleukin-8 production by human mesothelial cells after direct stimulation with staphylococci. *Infect Immun* 1995; **63**: 4206–9.
348. Stam TC, Swaak AJ, Kruit WH, Stoter G, Eggermont AM. Intrapleural administration of tumour necrosis factor-alpha (TNFalpha) in patients with mesothelioma: cytokine patterns and acute-phase protein response. *Eur J Clin Invest* 2000; **30**: 336–43.
349. Witowski J, Thiel A, Dechend R, *et al.* Synthesis of C-X-C and C-C chemokines by human peritoneal fibroblasts: induction by macrophage-derived cytokines. *Am J Pathol* 2001; **158**: 1441–50.
350. Antony VB, Hott JW, Kunkel SL, *et al.* Pleural mesothelial cell expression of C-C (monocyte chemotactic peptide) and C-X-C (interleukin 8) chemokines. *Am J Respir Cell Mol Biol* 1995; **12**: 581–8.
351. Griffith DE, Miller EJ, Gray LD, Idell S, Johnson AR. Interleukin-1-mediated release of interleukin-8 by asbestos-stimulated human pleural mesothelial cells. *Am J Respir Cell Mol Biol* 1994; **10**: 245–52.
352. Betjes MG, Tuk CW, Struijk DG, *et al.* Interleukin-8 production by human peritoneal mesothelial cells in response to tumor necrosis factor-alpha, interleukin-1, and medium conditioned by macrophages cocultured with *Staphylococcus epidermidis*. *J Infect Dis* 1993; **168**: 1202–10.
353. Man L, Lewis E, Einbinder T, *et al.* Major involvement of CD40 in the regulation of chemokine secretion from human peritoneal mesothelial cells. *Kidney Int* 2003; **64**: 2064–71.
354. Loghmani F, Mohammed K, Nasreen N, *et al.* Inflammatory cytokines mediate C-C (monocyte chemotactic protein 1) and C-X-C (interleukin 8) chemokine expression in human pleural fibroblasts. *Inflammation* 2002; **26**: 73–82.
355. Fukumoto T, Matsukawa A, Yoshimura T, *et al.* IL-8 is an essential mediator of the increased delayed-phase vascular permeability in LPS-induced rabbit pleurisy. *J Leukoc Biol* 1998; **63**: 584–90.
356. Antony VB, Godbey SW, Kunkel SL, *et al.* Recruitment of inflammatory cells to the pleural space. Chemotactic cytokines, IL-8, and monocyte chemotactic peptide-1 in human pleural fluids. *J Immunol* 1993; **151**: 7216–23.
357. Pace E, Gjomarkaj M, Melis M, *et al.* Interleukin-8 induces lymphocyte chemotaxis into the pleural space. Role of pleural macrophages. *Am J Respir Crit Care Med* 1999; **159**: 1592–9.
358. Nasreen N, Mohammed KA, Hardwick J, *et al.* Polar production of interleukin-8 by mesothelial cells promotes the transmesothelial migration of neutrophils: role of intercellular adhesion molecule-1. *J Infect Dis* 2001; **183**: 1638–45.
359. Ceyhan BB, Ozgun S, Celikel T, Yalcin M, Koc M. IL-8 in pleural effusion. *Respir Med* 1996; **90**: 215–21.
360. Segura RM, Alegre J, Varela E, *et al.* Interleukin-8 and markers of neutrophil degranulation in pleural effusions. *Am J Respir Crit Care Med* 1998; **157**: 1565–72.
361. Broaddus VC, Hebert CA, Vitangcol RV, *et al.* Interleukin-8 is a major neutrophil chemotactic factor in pleural liquid of patients with empyema. *Am Rev Respir Dis* 1992; **146**: 825–30.
362. Park JS, Kim YS, Jee YK, Myong NH, Lee KY. Interleukin-8 production in tuberculous pleurisy: Role of mesothelial cells stimulated by cytokine network involving tumour necrosis factor-α; and interleukin-1β. *Scand J Immunol* 2003; **57**: 463–9.
363. Galffy G, Mohammed KA, Nasreen N, Ward MJ, Antony VB. Inhibition of interleukin-8 reduces human malignant pleural mesothelioma propagation in nude mouse model. *Oncol Res* 1999; **11**: 187–94.
364. Galffy G, Mohammed KA, Dowling PA, *et al.* Interleukin 8: an autocrine growth factor for malignant mesothelioma. *Cancer Res* 1999; **59**: 367–71.
365. Catania A, Colombo G, Carlin A, *et al.* Autocrine inhibitory influences of α-melanocyte-stimulating hormone in malignant pleural mesothelioma. *J Leukoc Biol* 2004; **75**: 253–9.
366. Nasreen N, Hartman DL, Mohammed KA, Antony VB. Talc-induced expression of C-C and C-X-C chemokines and intercellular adhesion molecule-1 in mesothelial cells. *Am J Respir Crit Care Med* 1998; **158**: 971–8.
367. van den Heuvel MM, Smit HJ, Barbierato SB, *et al.* Talc-induced inflammation in the pleural cavity. *Eur Respir J* 1998; **12**: 1419–23.
368. Miller EJ, Kajikawa O, Pueblitz S, *et al.* Chemokine involvement in tetracycline-induced pleuritis. *Eur Respir J* 1999; **14**: 1387–93.
369. Tsuchiya I, Kasahara T, Yamashita K, *et al.* Induction of inflammatory cytokines in the pleural effusion of cancer patients after the administration of an immunomodulator, OK-432: role of IL-8 for neutrophil infiltration. *Cytokine* 1993; **5**: 595–603.
370. Kataoka M, Morishita R, Hiramatsu J, *et al.* OK-432 induces production of neutrophil chemotactic factors in malignant pleural effusion. *Intern Med* 1995; **34**: 352–6.
371. Bellinghausen I, Knop J, Saloga J. The role of interleukin 10 in the regulation of allergic immune responses. *Int Arch Allergy Immunol* 2001; **126**: 97–101.
372. Oberholzer A, Oberholzer C, Moldawer LL. Interleukin-10: a complex role in the pathogenesis of sepsis syndromes and its

potential as an anti-inflammatory drug. *Crit Care Med* 2002; **30** (1 Suppl): S58–63.

373. Frode TS, Souza GE, Calixto JB. The effects of IL-6 and IL-10 and their specific antibodies in the acute inflammatory responses induced by carrageenan in the mouse model of pleurisy. *Cytokine* 2002; **17**: 149–56.

374. Fine JS, Rojas-Triana A, Jackson JV, *et al.* Impairment of leukocyte trafficking in a murine pleuritis model by IL-4 and IL-10. *Inflammation* 2003; **27**: 161–74.

375. Chen YM, Yang WK, Whang-Peng J, Tsai CM, Perng RP. An analysis of cytokine status in the serum and effusions of patients with tuberculous and lung cancer. *Lung Cancer* 2001; **31**: 25–30.

●376. Cailhier JF, Sawatzky DA, Kipari T, *et al.* Resident pleural macrophages are key orchestrators of neutrophil recruitment in pleural inflammation. *Am J Respir Crit Care Med* 2006; **173**: 540–7.

377. Corsini E, Di Paola R, Viviani B, *et al.* Increased carrageenan-induced acute lung inflammation in old rats. *Immunology* 2005; **115**: 253–61.

378. Chen YM, Yang WK, Whang-Peng J, Kuo BI, Perng RP. Elevation of interleukin-10 levels in malignant pleural effusion. *Chest* 1996; **110**: 433–6.

379. Yanagawa H, Takeuchi E, Suzuki Y, *et al.* Presence and potent immunosuppressive role of interleukin-10 in malignant pleural effusion due to lung cancer. *Cancer Lett* 1999; **136**: 27–32.

380. Kanno H, Naka N, Yasunaga Y, *et al.* Production of the immunosuppressive cytokine interleukin-10 by Epstein–Barr-virus-expressing pyothorax-associated lymphoma: possible role in the development of overt lymphoma in immunocompetent hosts. *Am J Pathol* 1997; **150**: 349–57.

381. Drexler HG, Uphoff CC, Gaidano G, Carbone A. Lymphoma cell lines: in vitro models for the study of HHV-8+ primary effusion lymphomas (body cavity-based lymphomas). *Leukemia* 1998; **12**: 1507–17.

382. Kanno H, Naka N, Yasunaga Y, Aozasa K. Role of an immunosuppressive cytokine, interleukin-10, in the development of pyothorax-associated lymphoma. *Leukemia* 1997; **11** (Suppl 3): 525–6.

383. Barbosa T, Arruda S, Chalhoub M, *et al.* Correlation between interleukin-10 and in situ necrosis and fibrosis suggests a role for interleukin-10 in the resolution of the granulomatous response of tuberculous pleurisy patients. *Microbes Infect* 2006; **8**: 889–97.

384. Arruda S, Chalhoub M, Cardoso S, Barral-Netto M. Cell-mediated immune responses and cytotoxicity to mycobacterial antigens in patients with tuberculous pleurisy in Brazil. *Acta Trop* 1998; **71**: 1–15.

385. Huber TS, Gaines GC, Welborn MBR, *et al.* Anticytokine therapies for acute inflammation and the systemic inflammatory response syndrome: IL-10 and ischemia/reperfusion injury as a new paradigm. *Shock* 2000; **13**: 425–34.

386. Park AY, Scott P. IL-12: Keeping cell-mediated immunity alive. *Scand J Immunol* 2001; **53**: 529–32.

387. Dorman SE, Holland SM. Interferon-γ and interleukin-12 pathway defects and human disease. *Cytokine Growth Factor Rev* 2000; **11**: 321–33.

388. Zhang M, Gong J, Presky DH, Xue W, Barnes PF. Expression of the IL-12 receptor beta 1 and beta 2 subunits in human tuberculosis. *J Immunol* 1999; **162**: 2441–7.

389. Zhang M, Gately MK, Wang E, *et al.* Interleukin 12 at the site of disease in tuberculosis. *J Clin Invest* 1994; **93**: 1733–9.

390. Hiramatsu K, Yanagawa H, Haku T, Sone S. Generation of killer activity by interleukin-12 of mononuclear cells in malignant pleural effusions due to lung cancer. *Cancer Immunol Immunother* 1998; **46**: 1–6.

391. Caminschi E, Venetsanakos E, Leong CC, *et al.* Interleukin-12 induces an effective antitumor response in malignant mesothelioma. *Am J Respir Cell Mol Biol* 1998; **19**: 738–46.

392. Caminschi I, Venetsanakos E, Leong CC, *et al.* Cytokine gene therapy of mesothelioma. Immune and antitumor effects of transfected interleukin-12. *Am J Respir Cell Mol Biol* 1999; **21**: 347–56.

393. Chen YM, Yang WK, Ting CC, *et al.* Cross regulation by IL-10 and IL-2/IL-12 of the helper T cells and the cytolytic activity of lymphocytes from malignant effusions of lung cancer patients. *Chest* 1997; **112**: 960–6.

394. Takeuchi E, Yanagawa H, Suzuki Y, *et al.* IL-12-induced production of IL-10 and interferon-gamma by mononuclear cells in lung cancer-associated malignant pleural effusions. *Lung Cancer* 2002; **35**: 171–7.

395. Kimura K, Nishimura H, Matsuzaki T, *et al.* Synergistic effect of interleukin-15 and interleukin-12 on antitumor activity in a murine malignant pleurisy model. *Cancer Immunol Immunother* 2000; **49**: 71–7.

◆396. Pestka S, Krause CD, Walter MR. Interferons, interferon-like cytokines, and their receptors. *Immunol Rev* 2004; **202**: 8–32.

397. Ozato K, Tsujimura H, Tamura T. Toll-like receptor signaling and regulation of cytokine gene expression in the immune system. *Biotechniques* 2002; **Suppl**: 66–8, 70, 2 passim.

398. Baccala R, Kono DH, Theofilopoulos AN. Interferons as pathogenic effectors in autoimmunity. *Immunol Rev* 2005; **204**: 9–26.

399. Okamoto M, Kawabe T, Iwasaki Y, *et al.* Evaluation of interferon-gamma, interferon-gamma-inducing cytokines, and interferon-gamma-inducible chemokines in tuberculous pleural effusions. *J Lab Clin Med* 2005; **145**: 88–93.

400. Gopi A, Madhavan SM, Sharma SK, Sahn SA. Diagnosis and treatment of tuberculous pleural effusion in 2006. *Chest* 2007; **131**: 880–9.

401. Mohammed KA, Nasreen N, Ward MJ, *et al.* Mycobacterium-mediated chemokine expression in pleural mesothelial cells: role of C-C chemokines in tuberculous pleurisy. *J Infect Dis* 1998; **178**: 1450–6.

◆402. Yew WW, Leung CC. Update in tuberculosis 2006. *Am J Respir Crit Care Med* 2007; **175**: 541–6.

403. Schierloh P, Yokobori N, Aleman M, *et al.* Increased susceptibility to apoptosis of CD56dimCD16+ NK cells induces the enrichment of IFN-gamma-producing CD56bright cells in tuberculous pleurisy. *J Immunol* 2005; **175**: 6852–60.

404. Bulat-Kardum L, Etokebe GE, Knezevic J, *et al.* Interferon-gamma receptor-1 gene promoter polymorphisms (G-611A; T-56C) and susceptibility to tuberculosis. *Scand J Immunol* 2006; **63**: 142–50.

405. Cooke GS, Campbell SJ, Sillah J, *et al.* Polymorphism within the interferon-gamma/receptor complex is associated with pulmonary tuberculosis. *Am J Respir Crit Care Med* 2006; **174**: 339–43.

406. Etokebe GE, Bulat-Kardum L, Johansen MS, *et al.* Interferon-gamma gene (T874A and G2109A) polymorphisms are associated with microscopy-positive tuberculosis. *Scand J Immunol* 2006; **63**: 136–41.

407. Ferrara G, Losi M, D'Amico R, *et al.* Use in routine clinical practice of two commercial blood tests for diagnosis of infection with *Mycobacterium tuberculosis*: a prospective study. *Lancet* 2006; **367**: 1328–34.

408. Henao MI, Montes C, Paris SC, Garcia LF. Cytokine gene polymorphisms in Colombian patients with different clinical presentations of tuberculosis. *Tuberculosis (Edinb)* 2006; **86**: 11–9.

409. Krithika R, Marathe U, Saxena P, *et al.* A genetic locus required for iron acquisition in *Mycobacterium tuberculosis*. *Proc Natl Acad Sci U S A* 2006; **103**: 2069–74.

410. McDermid JM, Prentice AM. Iron and infection: effects of host iron status and the iron-regulatory genes haptoglobin and NRAMP1 (SLC11A1) on host-pathogen interactions in tuberculosis and HIV. *Clin Sci (Lond)* 2006; **110**: 503–24.

411. McLoughlin RM, Witowski J, Robson RL, *et al.* Interplay between IFN-gamma and IL-6 signaling governs neutrophil trafficking and apoptosis during acute inflammation. *J Clin Invest* 2003; **112**: 598-607.

412. Gattacceca F, Pilatte Y, Billard C, *et al.* Ad-IFN gamma induces antiproliferative and antitumoral responses in malignant mesothelioma. *Clin Cancer Res* 2002; **8**: 3298–304.

413. Hand A, Pelin K, Mattson K, Linnainmaa K. Interferon (IFN)-alpha and IFN-gamma in combination with methotrexate: *in vitro* sensitivity studies in four human mesothelioma cell lines. *Anticancer Drugs* 1995; **6**: 77–82.

414. Hand AM, Husgafvel-Pursiainen K, Pelin K, *et al.* Interferon-alpha and -gamma in combination with chemotherapeutic drugs: *in vitro* sensitivity studies in four human mesothelioma cell lines. *Anticancer Drugs* 1992; **3**: 687–94.

415. Hand AM, Husgafvel-Pursiainen K, Tammilehto L, Mattson K, Linnainmaa K. Malignant mesothelioma: the antiproliferative effect of cytokine combinations on three human mesothelioma cell lines. *Cancer Lett* 1991; **58**: 205–10.

416. Phan-Bich L, Buard A, Petit JF, *et al.* Differential responsiveness of human and rat mesothelioma cell lines to recombinant interferon-gamma. *Am J Respir Cell Mol Biol* 1997; **16**: 178–86.

417. Buard A, Vivo C, Monnet I, *et al.* Human malignant mesothelioma cell growth: activation of janus kinase 2 and signal transducer and activator of transcription 1alpha for inhibition by interferon-gamma. *Cancer Res* 1998; **58**: 840–7.

418. Kettunen E, Vivo C, Gattacceca F, Knuutila S, Jaurand MC. Gene expression profiles in human mesothelioma cell lines in response to interferon-gamma treatment. *Cancer Genet Cytogenet* 2004; **152**: 42–51.

419. DeLong P, Tanaka T, Kruklitis R, *et al.* Use of cyclooxygenase-2 inhibition to enhance the efficacy of immunotherapy. *Cancer Res* 2003; **63**: 7845–52.

420. Kruklitis RJ, Singhal S, Delong P, *et al.* Immuno-gene therapy with interferon-beta before surgical debulking delays recurrence and improves survival in a murine model of malignant mesothelioma. *J Thorac Cardiovasc Surg* 2004; **127**: 123–30.

421. Altinbas M, Er O, Ozkan M, *et al.* Ifosfamide, mesna, and interferon-alpha2A combination chemoimmunotherapy in malignant mesothelioma: results of a single center in central anatolia. *Med Oncol* 2004; **21**: 359–66.

422. Ardizzoni A, Pennucci MC, Castagneto B, *et al.* Recombinant interferon alpha-2b in the treatment of diffuse malignant pleural mesothelioma. *Am J Clin Oncol* 1994; **17**: 80–2.

423. Bard M, Ruffie P. Malignant mesothelioma. Medical oncology: standards, new trends, trials – the French experience. *Lung Cancer* 2004; **45** (Suppl 1): S129–31.

424. Metintas M, Ozdemir N, Ucgun I, *et al.* Cisplatin, mitomycin, and interferon-alpha2a combination chemoimmunotherapy in the treatment of diffuse malignant pleural mesothelioma. *Chest* 1999; **116**: 391–8.

425. Monnet I, Breau JL, Moro D, *et al.* Intrapleural infusion of activated macrophages and gamma-interferon in malignant pleural mesothelioma: a phase II study. *Chest* 2002; **121**: 1921–7.

426. Parra HS, Tixi L, Latteri F, *et al.* Combined regimen of cisplatin, doxorubicin, and alpha-2b interferon in the treatment of advanced malignant pleural mesothelioma: a Phase II multicenter trial of the Italian Group on Rare Tumors (GITR) and the Italian Lung Cancer Task Force (FONICAP). *Cancer* 2001; **92**: 650–6.

427. Pass HI, Temeck BK, Kranda K, *et al.* Phase III randomized trial of surgery with or without intraoperative photodynamic therapy and postoperative immunochemotherapy for malignant pleural mesothelioma. *Ann Surg Oncol* 1997; **4**: 628–33.

428. Soulie P, Ruffie P, Trandafir L, *et al.* Combined systemic chemoimmunotherapy in advanced diffuse malignant mesothelioma. Report of a phase I-II study of weekly cisplatin/interferon alfa-2a. *J Clin Oncol* 1996; **14**: 878–85.

429. Tansan S, Emri S, Selcuk T, *et al.* Treatment of malignant pleural mesothelioma with cisplatin, mitomycin C and alpha interferon. *Oncology* 1994; **51**: 348–51.

430. Upham JW, Musk AW, van Hazel G, Byrne M, Robinson BW. Interferon alpha and doxorubicin in malignant mesothelioma: a phase II study. *Aust N Z J Med* 1993; **23**: 683–7.

431. Boutin C, Nussbaum E, Monnet I, *et al.* Intrapleural treatment with recombinant gamma-interferon in early stage malignant pleural mesothelioma. *Cancer* 1994; **74**: 2460–7.

432. Lissoni P, Barni S, Tancini G, *et al.* Intracavitary therapy of neoplastic effusions with cytokines: comparison among interferon alpha, beta and interleukin-2. *Support Care Cancer* 1995; **3**: 78–80.

9

Pleural fibrosis

SREERAMA SHETTY, JOSEPH JOHN, STEVEN IDELL

OVERVIEW: THE PATHOGENESIS OF PLEURAL FIBROSIS AND DISORDERED FIBRIN TURNOVER

The pathogenesis of pleural fibrosis resembles that of fibrosis in other organ systems. The basic derangements recapitulate those associated with the development of fibrotic repair during wound healing.[1] In all these situations, the inflammatory response is potentiated by activation of multiple proinflammatory pathways including cellular, humoral, immunological, cytokine and other mediator networks. Complex interactions between components of these proinflammatory pathways contribute to the remodeling process and scarring. The role of selected pathways implicated in pleural inflammation and repair are considered in other chapters of this volume (see Chapter 7, Pleural inflammation and infection and Chapter 8, Immunology).

A large body of clinical, preclinical and basic investigation lends strong support to the hypothesis that disordered fibrin turnover and specific pathways of coagulation and fibrinolysis are integral to pleural remodeling and fibrosis.[2] It has long been postulated that fibrin strands within organizing pleural exudates are responsible for loculation, and that clearance of intrapleural fibrin by intrapleural administration of fibrinolysins is of therapeutic value. For example, in the 1940s, Tillett and Sherry[3] used preparations of streptokinase or streptodornase to break up pleural loculations attributable to parapneumonic effusions or hemothoraces. Their approach was in part predicated on surgical observations that intrapleural adhesions appeared to be fibrinous and might therefore be cleared by fibrinolytic agents. The early success of this approach was pursued over the next several decades using a variety of fibrinolysins. Recently, a consensus statement endorsed intrapleural intervention with fibrinolytic agents as an appropriate interventional option for patients with loculated parapneumonic effusions at risk for poor outcome.[4] More recent clinical investigation has challenged this approach and the use of fibrinolytic therapy is undergoing reassessment, as described later in this chapter.

It is clear that many proinflammatory pathways are activated during the continuum of evolving pleural injury and fibrosis. Nonetheless, morphological findings strongly suggest that disordered fibrin turnover plays a central role in the pathogenesis of pleural fibrosis.[5] While intrapleural fibrin is not observed in the absence of pleural disease, extravascular fibrin deposition that occurs at the visceral and parietal pleural surfaces is a hallmark of early pleural injury.[2,6] Adhesions between the visceral and parietal pleural surfaces that form within 1 day after pleural injury are fibrinous, as confirmed by immunohistochemical analyses.[6] Collagen within the fibrils is detectable within 3 days of pleural injury induced by intrapleural administration of tetracycline in rabbits.[7] These observations confirm that fibrin deposition characterizes pleural injury, suggesting that intrapleural fibrin formation and/or clearance could contribute to the development of pleural fibrosis.

Interestingly, the prominence of extravascular fibrin deposition in pleural injury and repair parallels the situation in fibrosing lung injury.[2] In acute respiratory distress syndrome (ARDS), fibrin deposition is likewise characteristic in the alveolar compartment.[2,8,9] Alveolar fibrin deposition commonly accompanies diffuse alveolar damage, which is the histologic constellation that commonly occurs in ARDS.[10,11] Prominent fibrin deposition is similarly observed in a variety of acute lung injuries, indicating that formation of a fibrinous neomatrix is a consistent feature of acute alveolitis.[12–15] Alveolar fibrin deposition also characterizes interstitial lung diseases, including idiopathic pulmonary fibrosis with active alveolitis,[16,17] further supporting a link between extravascular fibrin deposition and subsequent fibrosis.

LINKAGE BETWEEN DISORDERED FIBRIN TURNOVER AND FIBROSIS

Fibrosis after tissue injury evolves through remodeling and organization of transitional fibrin.[2] This paradigm is not unique to injury in the pleural compartment. It is now well established that a wide range of inflammatory and neoplastic diseases is associated with disordered fibrin turnover and fibrin deposition.[18] Formation and subsequent remodeling of the transitional fibrin neomatrix follows a common progression in virtually all forms of tissue injury. Acute inflammation initially promotes increased microvascular permeability, facilitating the passage of plasma coagulation substrates into the injured tissue or inflamed body compartment. Next, coagulation at sites of tissue injury is initiated, primarily by tissue factor (TF) associated with activated coagulation factor VII (Figure 9.1). The TF-VIIa, or extrinsic pathway complex, is primarily responsible for amplification of downstream coagulation following tissue injury and initiates formation of a fibrin neomatrix.[1] Remodeling of the transitional fibrin next occurs via the elaboration and release of proteases from inflammatory cells, including macrophages, and fibroblasts that invade the neomatrix. While persistent fibrin deposition occurs in ongoing pleural and parenchymal lung injury, continued formation and resorption of extravascular fibrin is facilitated by cytokines and other mediators in the inflammatory microenvironment. These mediators can increase local expression of tissue factor and induce expression of the plasminogen activator inhibitors (PAI) as well as plasminogen activators (PA), including both tissue-type PA (tPA) and urokinase-type PA (uPA).[2]

The major PA implicated in clearance of extravascular fibrin in the lung is uPA (Figure 9.1).[8] The relative expression of uPA versus that of PAIs and antiplasmins is a key determinant of local fibrinolytic capacity. With ongoing remodeling of transitional fibrin, collagen deposition eventually leads to progressive scarring and fibrotic repair. The desmoplastic response associated with solid neoplasms is predicated on a similar sequence of events,[1,19] as is accelerated pulmonary fibrosis following ARDS[2,8,20] and in various interstitial lung diseases.[18,21,22]

There is good evidence to support the hypothesis that extravascular fibrin in pleural (or other) diseases is pathophysiologic rather than incidental.[1,2,8,23–26] Perturbations of either coagulation or fibrinolytic pathways can influence inflammation and tissue repair in several different ways. For example, components of coagulation and fibrinolytic pathways are interactive with other proinflammatory pathways, and interactions with the complement and kinin systems can amplify the local inflammatory response.[2] The expression of tissue factor can also be stimulated by a variety of cytokines now known to be elaborated in pleural diseases.[6,27] Thrombin can influence cytokine expression and increase vascular permeability via cellular signaling.[28,29] In addition, fibrin and its derivatives can independently influence the inflammatory response. For example, fibrin and its products can disrupt endothelial cell organization,[30] suppress lymphocyte proliferation,[31] and promote directed migration of macrophages and fibroblasts.[32] In addition, proteolytic fragments of fibrin(ogen) can effect increased vascular permeability.[30,33,34] Plasmin, which is generated from plasminogen through the action of PAs, including uPA, can also activate transforming growth factor (TGF)-β and thereby promote fibrotic repair.[26] The induction of PAI-1 by TGF-β is likely to be involved in this process. These observations strongly support the concept that disordered fibrin turnover is central to the pathogenesis of pleural inflammation and repair.

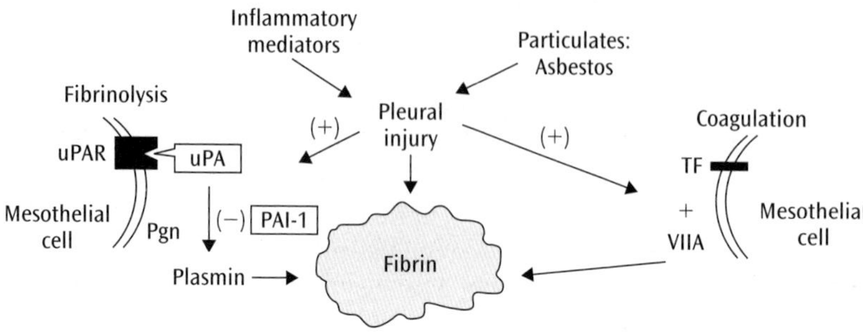

Figure 9.1 Procoagulant and uPA-dependent fibrinolytic pathways are illustrated. + indicates facilitation; – indicates inhibition; Pgn, plasminogen; VIIA, activated factor VII.

COAGULATION AND PLEURAL INJURY

The major procoagulant activity present in pleural effusions that form after injury is tissue factor (Figure 9.1), which likely originates from resident cell types in the pleural compartment.[2,6,35] Several cell types residing in the pleural compartment express tissue factor, including macrophages,[36–38] pleural mesothelial cells,[39] and fibroblasts.[40] Pleural effusions also contain appreciable levels of coagulation proteins,[41] including fibrinogen, so that coagulation initiated by tissue factor associated with factor VIIa can be amplified in the pleural compartment.[6] When intrapleural coagulation is activated by chemical or inflammatory stimuli, fibrinogen is converted to fibrin, forming the transitional intrapleural neomatrix.[1,19]

Apart from creating transitional fibrin, the conversion of fibrinogen to fibrin can also influence mesothelial cell function. Fibrinopeptide A, which is liberated via the cleavage of fibrinogen by α-thrombin, or α-thrombin itself, stimulates the proliferation of pleural mesothelial cells.[42] Pleural mesothelial cells can in turn augment intrapleural tissue factor expression via the elaboration of a number of cytokines.[43–49] These cells and fibroblasts also express adhesion molecules which facilitate interactions with fibrin or fibrinogen.[34,50] Fibrinogen has been shown to facilitate the adhesion of U937 myeloid cells to pleural mesothelial cells and the mechanism involves a bridging interaction between mesothelial cell intercellular adhesion molecule (ICAM)-1, fibrinogen and CD11b/CD18 of U937 monocytic cells.[50] This scenario occurs *in vivo* in rabbits with fibrosing pleuritis.[50]

Tissue factor pathway inhibitor (TFPI) has been identified in pleural effusions from patients and in pleural effusions from rabbits with tetracycline-induced pleural fibrosis.[6,35] Pleural mesothelial cells, as well as lung fibroblasts, elaborate both tissue factor as well as TFPI *in vitro* and *in vivo*.[51] It appears that intrapleural elaboration of tissue factor exceeds that of TFPI under these circumstances, given the strong activation of coagulation and intrapleural fibrin deposition that occurs concurrently in pleural injury. The relative imbalance by which tissue factor related procoagulant activity exceeds that of anticoagulant activity because TFPI recapitulates that occurring in bronchoalveolar lavage fluids of patients with ARDS.[52]

Intrapleural coagulation is upregulated in patients with exudative pleural effusions versus patients with transudative effusions caused by congestive heart failure. These observations confirm that the balance of intrapleural fibrin turnover is changed to favor initiation of fibrin formation in the setting of pleural injury. The upregulation of tissue factor-mediated coagulation in pleural injury parallels the findings observed in bronchoalveolar lavage fluids of patients with ARDS, pneumonia, or the interstitial lung diseases.[22,53–57] Selective reversal of this procoagulant-procoagulant inhibitor balance has recently been used to attenuate acute lung injury in baboons with ARDS induced by septic challenge.[58] Whether this approach can successfully be extended to block pleural inflammation and fibrosis remains unclear.

FIBRINOLYSIS AND PLEURAL INJURY

The uPA-PAI-1-urokinase receptor (uPAR) system has also been implicated in the pathogenesis of pleural injury and fibrosis (Figure 9.1).[2] The form of uPA released from cells is a relatively inactive single polypeptide chain proenzyme, prouPA, also called single-chain uPA (scuPA). scuPA is then converted by limited proteolysis into active two chain uPA; tcuPA, otherwise known as uPA. Both scuPA and uPA bind to uPAR with high affinity and either bound form retains PA activity.[59–61] Binding of scuPA to uPAR enables it to resist irreversible inactivation by PA inhibitors, while unbound uPA remains susceptible. scuPA can be converted to the more active tcuPA by plasmin while it is receptor-bound and receptor-bound tcuPA efficiently activates plasminogen.[59,60,62]

The components of the uPA–uPAR-mediated fibrinolytic system are likely present within the pleural compartment in health and disease. Plasminogen is present in pleural fluids in a form that can be activated by either uPA or tPA. Both uPA and tPA are also detectable in pleural effusions, both in free form and complexed to their inhibitors PAI-1 or PAI-2.[35] In addition, both uPA and tPA are elaborated by cultured human pleural mesothelial cells.[39] tPA is mainly responsible for effecting intravascular thrombolysis, while uPA is mainly involved in extravascular proteolysis and tissue remodeling.[26] Localized generation of plasmin by uPA, either in free form in pleural fluids or interacting with its specific cell surface receptor, uPAR, permits mesothelial and other cells to degrade extracellular matrix (ECM).[26,63] uPAR is expressed at the surface of pleural mesothelial cells,[64,65] macrophages,[21,66] and lung fibroblasts.[67] Interestingly, uPAR expression is differentially increased in lung fibroblasts harvested from fibrotic versus histologically normal human lungs.[68] uPAR is similarly overexpressed in several malignant lung carcinoma and mesothelioma cell lines.[69] uPA is also a chemotaxin and is mitogenic for mesothelial cells and lung fibroblasts.[64,65,68] In addition, the regulation of several cytokines is likewise effected, either directly or indirectly, via expression of uPA and uPAR.[26] uPA and uPAR are involved in the regulation of cell traffic and cytokine-mediated cell-to-cell signaling.[24,70,71] Thus, the uPA–uPAR system is integrally involved in inflammatory responses germane to matrix remodeling and cellular proteolysis.

The plasminogen activator inhibitors, PAI-1 and PAI-2, are the major inhibitors of uPA.[72] In pleural fluids, the expression of uPA-related fibrinolytic activity is inhibited in series by PAIs, in particular PAI-1, and by antiplasmins.[35] The fibrinolytic defect in these conditions is implicated in the development of accelerated pleural organization and fibrosis, by inhibiting intrapleural fibrin clearance. It also appears that the expression of uPAR is a major determinant of proteolysis and inflammatory cell traffic, as occurs in the injured pleural space.[2,8] Cytokines expressed in the course of pleural injury (see also Chapter 8, Immunology), including tumor necrosis factor (TNF)-α and TGF-β can upregulate uPAR at the surface of cell types expressed in pleural injury.[2] Exposure of mesothelial cells to particulates can also influence uPAR expression. Along these lines, chrysotile or crocidolite asbestos induce uPAR expression at the surface of rabbit pleural mesothelial or MeT5A mesothelial cells.[73] These observations indicate that pleural disease caused by asbestos exposure involves alterations of the mesothelial uPA–uPAR system. It has also been shown that expression of uPA and uPAR by endothelial or epithelial cells is increased by asbestos exposure.[74–76] In all, these studies demonstrate that the uPA–uPAR system plays a role in the pathogenesis of a range of pleural disorders.

Recent studies suggest that PAI-1, in particular, plays an important role in the pathogenesis of pulmonary fibrosis.[77,78] Overexpression of PAI-1 promotes alveolar and small airway fibrosis in lung injury induced by bleomycin.[79] Evidence developed by our laboratory and other investigators likewise strongly implicates PAI-1 as being central to the pathogenesis of pleural injury and repair.[2] Fibrinolytic activity is virtually undetectable in pleural effusions of patients with exudative pleuritis and in tetracycline-induced pleural injury where much of the uPA expressed in pleural fluids is bound to PAI-1.[35] Interaction between uPA and PA-inhibitors irreversibly blocks expression of uPA activity. In addition, in pleural fluids in patients with exudative pleuritis and in tetracycline-induced pleural injury, PAI-1 is also disproportionately (up to 1000-fold) increased compared with plasma levels, strongly suggesting that it is a major inhibitor of fibrinolytic activity in exudative pleural fluids.[35] Both PAI-1 and PAI-2 are products of mesothelial cells, lung fibroblasts and several other cell types,[39,40,80] so that these inhibitors can be locally elaborated in the setting of pleural injury. PAI-1, but not PAI-2, is usually present in plasma, so that increased microvascular permeability may also influence levels of this inhibitor in pleural fluids. PAI-1 is also relatively overexpressed in asbestos-mediated pleural injury.[75,81,82] Levels of PAI-1 in pleural fluids of patients with congestive heart failure approximate those found in plasma, whereas the PAI-1 concentrations in exudative fluids are, as noted above, markedly increased.

NEWLY DEFINED POST-TRANSCRIPTIONAL PATHWAYS BY WHICH uPA, uPAR AND PAI-1 ARE REGULATED

Since expression of PAI-1, uPA and uPAR are all linked to disordered fibrin clearance, the mechanisms by which these proteins are regulated in the pleural compartment are germane to pleural repair. Using cultured pleural mesothelial and mesothelioma cells, novel mechanisms involving 'switch-off' rather than gene activation have been shown to be involved. These mechanisms operate at the post-transcriptional level of mRNA stability. At this level, the stability of the respective mRNAs are contingent on the interactions between mRNA sequences that contain regulatory information and newly recognized mRNA binding proteins that bind one or more of the coding or untranslated mRNA regions (Figure 9.2).

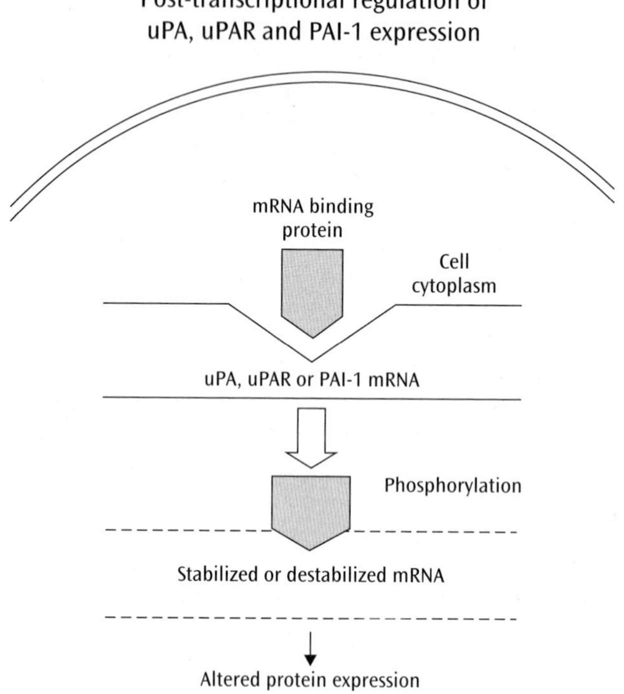

Figure 9.2 Post-transcriptional regulation of uPA, uPAR and PAI-1 expression.

Post-transcriptional regulation of PAI-1

Regulation of PAI-1 expression has been shown to occur at multiple levels. In HepG2 cells, for example, expression of the PAI-1 gene is regulated at both the transcriptional and post-transcriptional levels.[83] In HepG2 cells, PAI-1 mRNA exists in two forms; a labile 3.2 kb (half-life 0.85 hours) and a relatively more stable 2.2 kb (half-life 2.5 hours) species. Post-transcriptional control is involved in the regulation of both species. Steady-state levels of PAI-1 mRNA increase in these cells in response to treatment with insulin and insulin-like growth factor-I (IGF-1).[84] IGF-I stabilizes both PAI-1 mRNA species while insulin stabilizes the 3.2 kb PAI-1 mRNA form. mRNA-binding multiprotein complexes with molecular masses ranging from 38 to 76 kDa interact with cAMP responsive sequences to regulate PAI-1 mRNA.[85] These observations indicate that a post-transcriptional component contributes to expression of PAI-1 in selected cell types and that PAI-1 mRNA-binding protein interactions can influence PAI-1 mRNA stability.

We previously found that human tracheal epithelial cells express PAI-1[80] and recently determined that selected lung carcinoma cells express more PAI-1 antigen compared with normal lung epithelial cells. Post-transcriptional regulation accounts for, at least in part, the increased PAI-1 expression in lung cancer cells, attested to by increased PAI-1 mRNA stability after transcriptional blockade. Cytokines, including TNF-α and TGF-β, increase the stability of PAI-1 mRNA, an effect that is also regulated at the post-transcriptional level.[86] uPA also induces PAI-1 expression via post-transcriptional stabilization of PAI-1 mRNA.[87] Apart from its role in lung and pleural inflammation, the regulation of PAI-1 appears to be of clinical importance in neoplasia, as previous reports suggest that increased PAI-1 expression relates to poor outcome in lung cancer patients.[88,89]

While the regulatory mechanism is incompletely understood at the present time, the interaction between a sequence within the untranslated region of PAI-1 mRNA and a 60 kDa PAI-1 mRNA binding protein appears to regulate the stability of PAI-1 mRNA. In small airway epithelial cells this interaction is readily detectable and correlates with a relatively short PAI-1 mRNA half-life. In cytokine-treated cells or malignant lung carcinoma derived cells the binding interaction is attenuated or undetectable. This inverse relationship between PAI-1 mRNA stability and the PAI-1 mRNA binding protein-PAI-1 mRNA interaction suggests that the interaction is destabilizing. The precise binding sequence within PAI-1 mRNA that interacts with the protein remains to be elucidated and the regulatory consequences of the binding interaction are yet to be confirmed.

We determined that post-transcriptional regulation of PAI-1 similarly occurs in MeT5A human pleural mesothelial cells and in primary cultures of rabbit pleural mesothelial cells (Shetty and Idell, unpublished results). In these cells, PAI-1 mRNA stability is increased by cytokine stimulation. In MeT5A cells, the 60 kDa PAI-1 mRNA binding protein-PAI-1 mRNA interaction appears to be involved in the regulation of PAI-1 gene expression. These observations indicate that regulation of PAI-1 expression by pleural mesothelial cells involves a post-transcriptional component. PAI-1 mRNA is also regulated at the post-transcriptional level by 8-bromo-cAMP and cAMP-mediated destabilization of PAI-1 mRNA and involves association of the 3′-most 134 nt PAI-1 mRNA sequence with a 50 kDa PAI-1-mRNA binding protein.[90] Whether this regulatory pathway contributes to regulation of PAI-1 in pleural mesothelial cells remains to be determined.

Post-transcriptional regulation of uPAR

It is now well-established that uPAR expression is regulated at the transcriptional level.[91–93] Alternative, novel post-transcriptional mechanisms have recently been shown to regulate uPAR expression in pleural mesothelial and mesothelioma cells. uPAR mRNA stability is increased in these cells by treatment with cytokines and translational inhibitors.[94] The ability of translational inhibitors to augment the stability of uPAR mRNA in mesothelial cells suggests that a protein is involved in the regulatory process. In fact, a 50-kDa moiety; phosphoglycerate kinase (PGK) selectively interacts with a coding region sequence of the uPAR mRNA.[95] The binding sequence for PGK on uPAR mRNA has been mapped and encompasses a 51 nucleotide sequence within the coding region.[94] It also appears that a 40 kDa protein, hnRNPC,[96] and the 30 kDa protein HuR[97] likewise regulate uPAR mRNA stability. The PGK–uPAR mRNA coding region interaction destabilizes uPAR mRNA whereas the hnRNPC–3′UTR interaction decreases uPAR mRNA degradation. However, the role of Hur on uPAR mRNA turnover is not well established but most likely involves stabilization of uPAR mRNA.[97] Based on chimeric gene analyses, it appears that both the PGK binding uPAR coding region and the hnRNPC-binding 3′UTR determinants contain information for uPAR mRNA degradation. The relative contribution of these determinants to the regulation of uPAR mRNA stability was further confirmed by creation of deletion mutant mRNAs lacking either coding or 3′UTR or both determinants. It was found that both the coding and 3′UTR determinants contain information for uPAR mRNA destabilization and deletion of both the determinants additively stabilizes uPAR mRNA (Shetty, unpublished results). Interaction of PGK with the 51 nt coding region determinant enhances the degradation of uPAR mRNA and proinflammatory agents inhibit PGK binding to uPAR mRNA by tyrosine phosphorylation of PGK.[98] Alternatively, the binding of hnRNPC to the 110 nt 3′UTR binding sequence promotes uPAR mRNA stability.[96]

Unstimulated MeT5A or primary human pleural mesothelial or mesothelioma cells demonstrate interaction between the 5′ coding region and PGK.[94] TGF-β and TNF-α, cytokines known to participate in the pathogenesis of pleural injury, block or attenuate the binding interaction and concurrently increase stability of uPAR mRNA. These same changes in the binding interaction occur in rabbit pleural mesothelial cells,[67] malignant mesothelioma cells and lung carcinoma cells.[69] uPA similarly induces uPAR expression through post-transcriptional stabilization of uPAR mRNA in lung epithelial cells,[99] but this pathway has yet to be demonstrated in pleural mesothelial cells.

Post-transcriptional regulation of uPA

Pleural mesothelial cells express uPA as well as uPAR, and the expression of uPA by these cells is increased by cytokines including TNF-α.[39] Expression of uPA by human malignant mesothelioma cells also facilitates matrix remodeling by these cells. The mechanisms by which uPA is regulated by these cells remain to be elucidated but recent evidence in other cell types raises the possibility that this molecule may, like uPAR or PAI-1, be subject to post-transcriptional control. In normal renal epithelial cells, uPA mRNA has been shown to be regulated at this level in a number of studies.[100–103] It appears that the 3′ untranslated region of uPA mRNA contains multiple instability determinants that regulate the half-life of uPA mRNA.[104] A 40 kDa AU-binding protein has been identified in breast cancer cells that may be involved in the regulatory mechanism.[105] Epithelial cells from the lung also regulate uPA gene expression at the post-transcriptional level.[106] Interaction of a 30 kDa uPA mRNA-binding protein with a 66 nucleotide sequence of the 3′ untranslated region of uPA mRNA appears to regulate uPA mRNA expression in Beas2B cells. By chimeric gene analyses, in which this binding sequence is inserted in β-globin mRNA, the binding interaction is destabilizing and shortens the decay of uPA mRNA. Interestingly, the binding protein is found in the cytoplasm of Beas2B cells but not in lung carcinoma cells. In carcinoma-derived cells, which exhibit a longer uPA mRNA half-life and express more uPA, the binding protein is found in the nucleus. These observations suggest that the nuclear–cytoplasmic distribution of the protein is a key determinant of the post-transcriptional regulatory mechanism. Proinflammatory cytokines including TNF-α enhance uPA expression at the post-transcriptional level by altering the interaction of uPA mRNA with a 30 kDa uPA mRNA-binding protein that is yet to be characterized.[107] The role of this pathway in fibrin clearance in the pleural compartment remains to be determined.

INTERVENTIONAL FIBRINOLYSINS AND ANTICOAGULANTS TO PREVENT PLEURAL INJURY

The introduction of fibrinolysins to treat pleural loculation occurred over 50 years ago.[3] These agents continue to be used in clinical practice today. Intrapleural fibrinolysins upregulate local fibrinolytic activity and thereby reverse the fibrinolytic defect found in exudative pleuritis.[2,35,61] Interestingly, increased pleural fluid fibrinolytic activity is associated with failure of pleurodesis, further suggesting that pathways of fibrin clearance are related to the outcome of pleural fibrosis.[108] From a pathophysiology perspective, the ability of fibrinolysins to clear pleural loculation underscores the importance of intrapleural fibrin in the pathogenesis of pleural organization and scarring.[109,110]

Streptokinase and urokinase have frequently been used as the interventional agents in recently reported literature.[111–115] Several reports indicate the efficacy of this approach in a variety of circumstances, including pleural empyemas, complicated parapneumonic effusions with loculation, malignant effusions with loculation and hemothorax with pleural organization.[111–121] The clinical endpoints of efficacy in these studies included improvement in radiographic evidence of pleural injury, pleural drainage and the need for further surgical procedures. The intrapleural administration of fibrinolysins appears to be well tolerated, generally does not cause clinically important systemic fibrinolysins and reduces the need for surgery.[110–114,122,123] Other reports have shown that the increased volume of pleural drainage associated with use of thrombolytic therapy does not uniformly alter the morbidity or mortality of underlying empyema.[115] In 2000, an evidence-based guideline on the management of parapneumonic effusions from the American College of Chest Physicians (ACCP) supported the optional use of fibrinolytic interventions if the effusion was large, loculated or was associated with thickened pleura, positive culture, pus, or pH was < 7.2. Fibrinolytic therapy was associated with lower mortality and a decreased need for second intervention in patients with empyema and extensive disease and at risk for poor outcome.[4] A Cochrane review assessed the evidence for efficacy of fibrinolytic therapy from available randomized controlled trials in 2004. The review concluded that intrapleural fibrinolytic interventions is an adjunctive therapy for patients with empyema or complicated parapneumonic effusions as it confers significant benefits in terms of hospital stay, duration of fever, radiographic improvement and the need for surgical treatment. However, the routine use of fibrinolysins was not recommended because the numbers of patients in these randomized trials were small and study designs heterogeneous.[124,125]

More recently, a randomized controlled trial in 53 subjects showed improved outcomes and decreased need for surgery when fibrinolysins with streptokinase was used in adjunction to drainage.[126] However, a large randomized controlled clinical trial (MIST1) including 454 subjects with pleural infection treated with intrapleural streptokinase or placebo[127] recently challenged the prevailing favorable view of the efficacy of intrapleural fibrinolytic therapy. In this trial, streptokinase did not alter mortality, the need for surgery at 3 and 12 months, radiological appearance, or length of stay. A meta-analysis of all trials using fibrinolysins for pleural infection arrived at results similar to MIST1, in large part because the MIST1 trial contributed 75 percent of the subjects in the analysis.[128] These new results have sparked discussions to explain the differences between these results and those of multiple trials supporting the use of intrapleural fibrinolysins.[129–133] While the basis for the disparity is unclear, differences in outcomes may relate to enrolment of subjects with early effusions versus those with relatively protracted illness and well-established pleural reaction where fibrinolysins may be less likely to be efficacious. The advanced age of subjects and commitment to intrapleural fibrinolysis because of limited availability of surgery may have contributed to masking of potential benefits of fibrinolysins in patients with pleural loculations (see also Chapter 24, Effusions from cardiac diseases).

A recent report comparing video-assisted thoracoscopy with intrapleural streptokinase in post-traumatic retained hemothorax showed thoracoscopy to be associated with shorter hospitalization and a decreased need for decortication.[134] A randomized controlled trial comparing the two strategies for empyema also showed higher efficacy, shorter hospitalization and lower costs for thoracoscopy compared with catheter directed fibrinolytic therapy.[135] These data support the use of early thoracoscopy in complicated parapneumonic effusions, reserving fibrinolytics for poor surgical candidates or circumstances where thoracoscopy is not available. Further studies are needed to clarify if there are specific clinical circumstances in which fibrinolytic therapy with currently available or new agents can yield superior outcomes versus tube thoracostomy or thoracoscopy.

The results of studies in adults may not be applicable to the pediatric population with pleural infection. In children with complicated parapneumonic effusion, fibrinolysis has been achieved with streptokinase, urokinase, or alteplase. Several reports show fibrinolytic therapy to be efficacious, safe and a less invasive option in children.[136–140] Few randomized controlled trials of intrapleural fibrinolytic agents have been carried out in children. In one randomized controlled trial in children, urokinase reduced hospital stay.[141] Another randomized controlled trial showed benefit in terms of decreased pleural thickening at 1 month that was attributable to fibrinolytic treatment in the subset of children with multiloculated empyema.[142] A prospective randomized trial comparing primary video-assisted thoracoscopic surgery (VATS) with tube thoracostomy for treatment of parapneumonic effusions showed decreased length of hospital stay, number of chest tube days, narcotic use, number of radiographic procedures and interventional procedures when children underwent VATS. No patient in the VATS surgery group required fibrinolytic therapy.[143] Conversely, a recent randomized trial including 60 patients demonstrated comparable length of hospital stay, failure rate, or radiologic outcome after 6 months of follow-up in children with empyema who were treated with either video-assisted thoracoscopy or intrapleural urokinase. Treatment costs were lower in the urokinase treatment group.[144] The authors concluded that urokinase represents the preferred option given its advantage of economy and equivalent efficacy. Larger randomized controlled studies may better delineate the role of fibrinolytic therapy versus surgical treatment for pleural infections in children.

Ongoing studies are being carried out to evaluate the ability of new fibrinolysins to clear intrapleural fibrinous loculations. At this stage, these agents are being tested in preclinical models. In many forms of pleural injury, increased pleural fluid procoagulant activity is accompanied by a profound decrement in fibrinolytic activity that occurs despite local elaboration of uPA as well as that of tPA.[2] A comparable paucity of pleural fluid fibrinolytic activity is also seen in experimental pleural injury induced by tetracycline in rabbits.[27] Interestingly, intrapleural administration of either the anticoagulant heparin or the low molecular weight uPA, the form of uPA that was until recently most commonly used for clinical applications, attenuated pleurodesis in rabbits with tetracycline-induced pleural fibrosis.[27] Presumably, the effects relate to the blockade of intrapleural fibrin, although it is possible that the attenuation of tissue injury could be attributable to altered cytokine networking or cross-talk, or cellular signaling. These studies suggest that the balance of plasminogen activators versus their inhibitors in organizing pleuritis can therefore be altered to prevent fibrotic sequelae of pleural injury.

Due to increased PAI-1 appearing to play a major role in the downregulation of pleural fluid fibrinolytic activity, a fibrinolytic agent that resists inhibition by PAI-1 would be desirable for intrapleural administration. Single-chain uPA exhibits this property when bound to uPAR. scuPA is the form of urokinase secreted by cells and it can be cleaved by proteases such as plasmin to the more active tcuPA. Both forms of urokinase bind uPAR with high affinity.[59,60] tcuPA is susceptible to inhibition by PAI-1 but scuPA activity is increased when bound to uPAR and it is relatively resistant to inhibition by either PAI-1 or PAI-2.[60,62,145] Thus, binding of scuPA to uPAR protects it from conversion to tcuPA, potentiates its enzymatic activity and retards its inhibition by PAI-1. Interestingly, this agent has been used as an intervention for stroke, where plasma fibrinogen concentrations were preserved and bleeding complications were reduced compared with other fibrinolysins including tPA.[146] scuPA also binds rabbit pleural mesothelial cells and lung fibroblasts with kinetics comparable to that exhibited with binding to human cells (Mazar and Idell, unpublished data). In tetracycline-induced pleurodesis in the rabbit, intrapleural administration of scuPA was found to be as effective as scuPA bound to its recombinant receptor in terms of prevention of intrapleural adhesion formation.[147] More recently, single dose scuPA was found to provide excellent protection against pleural adhesion formation in the same model, whether given before, during, or after adhesion formation.[148]

It is possible that interventions for malignant mesothelioma may similarly be predicated on changing the local fibrinolytic milieu. While the role of fibrinolysins and their inhibitors in the pathogenesis of malignant mesothelioma remains to be clarified, there is good reason to speculate that they may play a role in the remodeling of the stroma of this neoplasm. Fibrous and epithelioid subtypes of this malignancy express uPA, uPAR and PAI-1.[149] Extravascular fibrin is commonly found at the leading edge of tumor stroma invading the normal pleura, suggesting that locally disordered fibrin turnover is central to the spread of this neoplasm.[149] Whether these observations can be exploited for therapeutic gain remains to be determined, but uPA and uPAR expression have been linked to the growth or invasiveness of tumors, including malignant mesothelioma.[64,150–152] Blockade of their expression has been used to reduce the invasiveness of solid neoplasms, including malignant mesothelioma cells *in vitro*.[59,153–155] Whether an antifibrinolytic strategy can be of clinical value for the treatment of patients with malignant mesothelioma remains to be determined.

Anticoagulants have been used in preclinical pleural injury to prevent pleural loculation. The use of these agents is based upon the inference that preventing increased expression of intrapleural procoagulant activity could block pleural scarring. Intrapleural coagulation is initiated by tissue factor.[27] Local elaboration of TFPI in pleural injury occurs but appears to be inadequate to block intrapleural fibrin deposition.[6,35] Along these lines, the administration of intrapleural heparin attenuates pleural loculation in tetracycline-induced pleural injury in rabbits.[27] Whether other intrapleural anticoagulants could be of clinical value in organizing pleuritis is currently unclear.

The derangements in systemic sepsis involve an increase in tissue factor related procoagulant activity and a decrement in systemic fibrinolysis.[156,157] These derangements thereby recapitulate the local changes that are observed in organizing pleural injury.[2] Recent reports that activated protein C (APC) and tissue factor pathway inhibitor can attenuate end-organ dysfunction, and mortality in sepsis suggests the possibility that these agents might attenuate or prevent pleural injury. APC is an anticoagulant that inhibits factors VIIIa and Va and exerts other proinflammatory properties that might be useful in preventing pleural loculation.[158] APC also inhibits PAI-1 and thereby promotes fibrinolysis and exerts anti-inflammatory properties, including decreased production of TNF-α, interleukin (IL)-1 and IL-6.[156,159,160] The ability of APC to protect against pleural injury remains to be evaluated in preclinical models.

KEY POINTS

- Pleural injury and repair is characterized by disordered fibrin turnover, which contributes to the pathogenesis of pleural fibrosis.
- Intrapleural coagulation is initiated by increased local expression of tissue factor and fibrinolysis is concurrently downregulated, owing mainly to increased expression of PAI-1 and downstream anti-plasmins.
- Formation of adhesions between the visceral and parietal pleural surfaces occurs in association with intrapleural coagulation and downregulation of fibrinolysis.
- As the process of pleural loculation evolves, the fibrinous adhesions progressively exhibit more collagen, following the traditional progression of events associated with wound healing.
- Fibrinolysins have been used to exploit the derangements of intrapleural fibrin turnover and are capable of clearing pleural loculations.
- While the broad use of fibrinolysins has recently been challenged, they provide a therapeutic option that can be of value for selected patients who are poor surgical candidates and who have extensive pleural loculations that place them at risk for poor outcome.
- New fibrinolytic strategies are now being evaluated for potential application to clinical practice.

REFERENCES

● = Key primary paper
◆ = Major review article
* = Paper that represents the first formal publication of a management guideline

◆1. Dvorak HF. Tumors: wounds that do not heal. Similarities between tumor stroma generation and wound healing. *N Engl J Med* 1986; **315**:1650–9.
2. Idell S. Coagulation, fibrinolysis and fibrin deposition in lung injury and repair. Pulmonary fibrosis. In: Lenfant C (ed.). *Lung biology in health and disease.* New York: Marcel Dekker, 1995: 743–76.
●3. Tillett WS, Sherry S. The effect in patients of streptococcal fibrinolysin (streptokinase) and streptococcal desoxyribonuclease on fibrinous, purulent, and sanguinous pleural exudations. *J Clin Invest* 1949; **28**: 173–90.
*4. Colice GL, Curtis A, Deslauriers J, *et al.* Medical and surgical treatment of parapneumonic effusions: an evidence-based guideline. *Chest* 2000; **118**: 1158–71.
5. Bignon J, Gee JB. Pleural fibrogenesis. The pleura in health and disease. In Lenfant C (ed.). *Lung biology in health and disease.* New York: Marcel Dekker, 2001: 417–43.
6. Idell S, Pendurthi U, Pueblitz S, *et al.* Tissue factor pathway inhibitor in tetracycline-induced pleuritis in rabbits. *Thromb Haemost* 1998; **79**: 649–55.
7. Miller EJ, Kajikawa O, Pueblitz S, *et al.* Chemokine involvement in tetracycline-induced pleuritis. *Eur Respir J* 1999; **14**: 1387–93.
◆8. Idell S. Extravascular coagulation and fibrin deposition in acute lung injury. *New Horiz* 1994; **2**: 566–74.
9. Bachofen M, Weibel ER. Structural alterations of lung parenchyma in the adult respiratory distress syndrome. *Clin Chest Med* 1982; **3**: 35–56.
10. Idell S, James KK, Coalson JJ. Fibrinolytic activity in bronchoalveolar lavage of baboons with diffuse alveolar damage: trends in two forms of lung injury. *Crit Care Med* 1992; **20**: 1431–40.
11. Idell S, Peters J, James KK, *et al.* Local abnormalities of coagulation and fibrinolytic pathways that promote alveolar fibrin deposition in the lungs of baboons with diffuse alveolar damage. *J Clin Invest* 1989; **84**: 181–93.
12. Idell S, Kumar A, Koenig KB, Coalson JJ. Pathways of fibrin turnover in lavage of premature baboons with hyperoxic lung injury. *Am J Respir Crit Care Med* 1994; **149**: 767–75.

13. Idell S, James KK, Gillies C, *et al.* Abnormalities of pathways of fibrin turnover in lung lavage of rats with oleic acid and bleomycin-induced lung injury support alveolar fibrin deposition. *Am J Pathol* 1989; **135**: 387–99.
14. Idell S, Peterson BT, Gonzalez KK, *et al.* Local abnormalities of coagulation and fibrinolysis and alveolar fibrin deposition in sheep with oleic acid-induced lung injury. *Am Rev Respir Dis* 1988; **138**: 1282–94.
15. Idell S, Gonzalez KK, MacArthur CK, *et al.* Bronchoalveolar lavage procoagulant activity in bleomycin-induced lung injury in marmosets. Characterization and relationship to fibrin deposition and fibrosis. *Am Rev Respir Dis* 1987; **136**: 124–33.
16. Jackson LK. Idiopathic pulmonary fibrosis. *Clin Chest Med* 1982; **3**: 579–92.
17. Kuhn C III, Boldt J, King TE Jr, *et al.* An immunohistochemical study of architectural remodeling and connective tissue synthesis in pulmonary fibrosis. *Am Rev Respir Dis* 1989; **140**: 1693–703.
18. Brown LF, Dvorak AM, Dvorak HF. Leaky vessels, fibrin deposition, and fibrosis: a sequence of events common to solid tumors and many other types of disease. *Am Rev Respir Dis* 1989; **140**: 1104–7.
◆19. Dvorak HF, Senger DR, Dvorak AM. Fibrin as a component of the tumor stroma: origins and biological significance. *Cancer Metastasis Rev* 1983; **2**: 41–73.
20. Marshall R, Bellingan G, Laurent G. The acute respiratory distress syndrome: fibrosis in the fast lane. *Thorax* 1998; **53**: 815–17.
21. Chapman HA Jr, Bertozzi P, Reilly JJ Jr. Role of enzymes mediating thrombosis and thrombolysis in lung disease. *Chest* 1988; **93**: 1256–63.
◆22. Dabbagh K, Chambers RC, Laurent GJ. From clot to collagen: coagulation peptides in interstitial lung disease. *Eur Respir J* 1998; **11**: 1002–5
◆23. Dano K, Andreasen PA, Grondahl-Hansen J, *et al.* Plasminogen activators, tissue degradation, and cancer. *Adv Cancer Res* 1985; **44**: 139–266.
◆24. Chapman HA. Plasminogen activators, integrins, and the coordinated regulation of cell adhesion and migration. *Curr Opin Cell Biol* 1997; **9**: 714–24.
25. Abraham E. Coagulation abnormalities in acute lung injury and sepsis. *Am J Respir Cell Mol Biol* 2000; **22**: 401–4.
◆26. Vassalli JD, Sappino AP, Belin D. The plasminogen activator/plasmin system. *J Clin Invest* 1991; **88**: 1067–72.
27. Strange C, Baumann MH, Sahn SA, Idell S. Effects of intrapleural heparin or urokinase on the extent of tetracycline-induced pleural disease. *Am J Respir Crit Care Med* 1995; **151**: 508–15.
28. Stevens T, Garcia JG, Shasby DM, *et al.* Mechanisms regulating endothelial cell barrier function. *Am J Physiol Lung Cell Mol Physiol* 2000; **279**: L419–22.
◆29. Narayanan S. Multifunctional roles of thrombin. *Ann Clin Lab Sci* 1999; **29**: 275–80.
30. Dang CV, Bell WR, Kaiser D, Wong A. Disorganization of cultured vascular endothelial cell monolayers by fibrinogen fragment D. *Science* 1985; **227**: 1487–90.
31. Edgington TS, Curtiss LK, Plow EF. A linkage between the hemostatic and immune systems embodied in the fibrinolytic release of lymphocyte suppressive peptides. *J Immunol* 1985; **134**: 471–7.
32. Ciano PS, Colvin RB, Dvorak AM, *et al.* Macrophage migration in fibrin gel matrices. *Lab Invest* 1986; **54**: 62–70.
33. Rowland FN, Donovan MJ, Picciano PT, *et al.* Fibrin-mediated vascular injury. Identification of fibrin peptides that mediate endothelial cell retraction. *Am J Pathol* 1984; **117**: 418–28.
34. Colvin RB, Gardner PI, Roblin RO, *et al.* Cell surface fibrinogen-fibrin receptors on cultured human fibroblasts. Association with fibronectin (cold insoluble globulin, LETS protein) and loss in SV40 transformed cells. *Lab Invest* 1979; **41**: 464–73.
35. Idell S, Girard W, Koenig KB, *et al.* Abnormalities of pathways of fibrin turnover in the human pleural space. *Am Rev Respir Dis* 1991; **144**: 187–94.
36. Chapman HA, Stahl M, Allen CL, *et al.* Regulation of the procoagulant activity within the bronchoalveolar compartment of normal human lung. *Am Rev Respir Dis* 1988; **137**: 1417–25.
37. Drake TA, Morrissey JH, Edgington TS. Selective cellular expression of tissue factor in human tissues. Implication for disorders of hemostasis and thrombosis. *Am J Pathol* 1989; **134**: 1087–97.
38. McGee MP, Rothberger H. Tissue factor in bronchalveolar lavage fluids. Evidence for an alveolar macrophage source. *Am Rev Respir Dis* 1985; **131**: 331–6.
39. Idell S, Zwieb C, Kumar A, *et al.* Pathways of fibrin turnover of human pleural mesothelial cells in vitro. *Am J Respir Cell Mol Biol* 1992; **7**: 414–26.
40. Idell S, Zwieb C, Boggaram J, *et al.* Mechanisms of fibrin formation and lysis by human lung fibroblasts: influence of TGF-beta and TNF-alpha. *Am J Physiol* 1992; **263**: L487–94.
41. Wyshock EG, Idell S, Colman RW. The contribution of factor V to the coagulant property of pleural fluid. *J Lab Clin Med* 1992; **120**: 726–34.
42. Griffith DE, Johnson AR, Kumar A, *et al.* Growth factors for human pleural mesothelial cells in soluble products from formed clots. *Thromb Res* 1994; **74**: 207–18.
43. Jonjic N, Peri G, Bernasconi S, *et al.* Expression of adhesion molecules and chemotactic cytokines in cultured human mesothelial cells. *J Exp Med* 1992; **176**: 1165–74.
44. Griffith DE, Miller EJ, Gray LD, *et al.* Interleukin-1-mediated release of interleukin-8 by asbestos-stimulated human pleural mesothelial cells. *Am J Respir Cell Mol Biol* 1994; **10**: 245–52.
45. Gerwin BI, Lechner JF, Reddel RR, *et al.* Comparison of production of transforming growth factor-beta and platelet-derived growth factor by normal human mesothelial cells and mesothelioma cell lines. *Cancer Res* 1987; **47**: 6180–4.
46. Gerwin BI. Cytokine signaling in mesothelial cells: Receptor expression closes the autocrine loop. *Am J Respir Cell Mol Biol* 1996; **14**: 505–7.
47. Fujino S, Yokoyama A, Kohno N, Hiwada K. Interleukin 6 is an autocrine growth factor for normal human pleural mesothelial cells. *Am J Respir Cell Mol Biol* 1996; **14**: 508–515.
48. Fitzpatrick DR, Peroni DJ, Bielefeldt-Ohmann H. The role of growth factors and cytokines in the tumorigenesis and immunobiology of malignant mesothelioma. *Am J Respir Cell Mol Biol* 1995; **12**: 455–60.
49. Antony VB, Hott JW, Kunkel SL, *et al.* Pleural mesothelial cell expression of C-C (monocyte chemotactic peptide) and C-X-C (Interleukin 8) chemokines. *Am J Respir Cell Mol Biol* 1995; **12**: 581–8.
50. Shetty S, Kumar A, Pueblitz S, *et al.* Fibrinogen promotes adhesion of monocytic to human mesothelioma cells. *Thromb Haemost* 1996; **75**: 782–90.
51. Bajaj MS, Pendurthi U, Koenig K, *et al.* Tissue factor pathway inhibitor expression by human pleural mesothelial and mesothelioma cells. *Eur Respir J* 2000; **15**: 1069–78.
52. Sabharwal AK, Bajaj SP, Ameri A, *et al.* Tissue factor pathway inhibitor and von Willebrand factor antigen levels in adult respiratory distress syndrome and in a primate model of sepsis. *Am J Respir Crit Care Med* 1995; **151**: 758–67.
53. Bertozzi P, Astedt B, Zenzius L, *et al.* Depressed bronchoalveolar urokinase activity in patients with adult respiratory distress syndrome. *N Engl J Med* 1990; **322**: 890–7.
54. Idell S, James KK, Levin EG, *et al.* Local abnormalities in coagulation and fibrinolytic pathways predispose to alveolar fibrin deposition in the adult respiratory distress syndrome. *J Clin Invest* 1989; **84**: 695–705.
55. Idell S, Koenig KB, Fair DS, *et al.* Serial abnormalities of fibrin turnover in evolving adult respiratory distress syndrome. *Am J Physiol* 1991; **261**: L240–8.
56. Nakstad B, Lyberg T, Skjonsberg OH, Boye NP. Local activation of

the coagulation and fibrinolysis systems in lung disease. *Thromb Res* 1990; **57**: 827–38.

57. Saldeen T. The microembolism syndrome, a review. In: *The microembolism syndrome*. Stockholm: Almqvist and Wiskell, 1979: 7–44.
58. Welty-Wolf KE, Carraway MS, Miller DL, *et al.* Coagulation blockade prevents sepsis-induced respiratory and renal failure in baboons. *Am J Resp Crit Care Med* 2001; **164**: 1988–96.
59. Mazar AP, Henkin J, Goldfarb RH. The urokinase plasminogen activator system in cancer: implications for tumor angiogenesis and metastasis. *Angiogenesis* 1999; **3**: 15–32.
60. Higazi AA, Bdeir K, Hiss E, *et al.* Lysis of plasma clots by urokinase-soluble urokinase receptor complexes. *Blood* 1998; **92**: 2075–83.
61. Agrenius V, Chmielewska J, Widstrom O, Blomback M. Pleural fibrinolytic activity is decreased in inflammation as demonstrated in quinacrine pleurodesis treatment of malignant pleural effusion. *Am Rev Respir Dis* 1989; **140**: 1381–5.
62. Ellis V, Behrendt N, Dano K. Plasminogen activation by receptor-bound urokinase: A kinetic study with both cell-associated and isolated receptor. *J Biol Chem* 1991; **266**: 12752–8.
63. Alfano D, Iaccarino I, Stoppelli MP. Urokinase signaling through its receptor protects against anoikis by increasing BCL-xL expression levels. *J Biol Chem* 2006; **281**: 17758–67.
64. Shetty S, Kumar A, Johnson A, *et al.* Urokinase receptor in human malignant mesothelioma cells: role in tumor cell mitogenesis and proteolysis. *Am J Physiol* 1995; **268**: L972–82.
65. Shetty S, Kumar A, Johnson AR, Idell S. Regulation of mesothelial cell mitogenesis by antisense oligonucleotides for the urokinase receptor. *Antisense Res Dev* 1995; **5**: 307–14.
66. Sitrin RG, Todd RF III, Albrecht E, Gyetko MR. The urokinase receptor (CD87) facilitates CD11b/CD18-mediated adhesion of human monocytes. *J Clin Invest* 1996; **97**: 1942–51.
67. Shetty S, Idell S. A urokinase receptor mRNA binding protein from rabbit lung fibroblasts and mesothelial cells. *Am J Physiol* 1998; **274**: L871–82.
68. Shetty S, Kumar A, Johnson AR, *et al.* Differential expression of the urokinase receptor in fibroblasts from normal and fibrotic human lungs. *Am J Respir Cell Mol Biol* 1996; **15**: 78–87.
69. Shetty S, Idell S. Post-transcriptional regulation of urokinase receptor gene expression in human lung carcinoma and mesothelioma cells *in vitro*. *Mol Cell Biochem* 1999; **199**: 189–200.
70. Gyetko MR, Sitrin RG, Fuller JA, *et al.* Function of the urokinase receptor (CD87) in neutrophil chemotaxis. *J Leukoc Biol* 1995; **58**: 533–8.
71. Gyetko MR, Chen GH, McDonald RA, *et al.* Urokinase is required for the pulmonary inflammatory response to *Cryptococcus neoformans*. A murine transgenic model. *J Clin Invest* 1996; **97**: 1818–26.
72. Sprengers ED, Kluft C. Plasminogen activator inhibitors. *Blood* 1987; **69**: 381–7.
73. Perkins RC, Broaddus VC, Shetty S, *et al.* Asbestos upregulates expression of the urokinase-type plasminogen activator receptor on mesothelial cells. *Am J Respir Cell Mol Biol* 1999; **21**: 637–46.
74. Barchowsky A, Roussel RR, Krieser RJ, *et al.* Expression and activity of urokinase and its receptor in endothelial and pulmonary epithelial cells exposed to asbestos. *Toxicol Appl Pharmacol* 1998; **152**: 388–96.
75. Lenz SP, Green FH, Murphy PG, *et al.* Expression of plasminogen activator and plasminogen activator inhibitor by rat mesothelioma induced by asbestos. *Cancer Lett* 1993; **68**: 119–27.
76. Bajaj MS, Pendurthi U, Koenig K, *et al.* Tissue factor pathway inhibitor expression by human pleural mesothelial and mesothelioma cells. *Eur Respir J* 2000; **15**: 1069–78.
77. Barazzone C, Belin D, Piguet PF, *et al.* Plasminogen activator inhibitor-1 in acute hyperoxic mouse lung injury. *J Clin Invest* 1996; **98**: 2666–73.
78. Olman MA, Mackman N, Gladson CL, *et al.* Changes in procoagulant and fibrinolytic gene expression during bleomycin-induced lung injury in the mouse. *J Clin Invest* 1995; **96**: 1621–30.
79. Eitzman DT, McCoy RD, Zheng X, *et al.* Bleomycin-induced pulmonary fibrosis in transgenic mice that either lack or overexpress the murine plasminogen activator inhibitor-1 gene. *J Clin Invest* 1996; **97**: 232–7.
80. Idell S, Kumar A, Zwieb C, *et al.* Effects of TGF-beta and TNF-alpha on procoagulant and fibrinolytic pathways of human tracheal epithelial cells. *Am J Physiol* 1994; **267**: L693–703.
81. Li XY, Brown GM, Lamb D, Donaldson K. Increased production of plasminogen activator inhibitor *in vitro* by pleural leukocytes from rats intratracheally instilled with crocidolite asbestos. *Environ Res* 1991; **55**: 135–44.
82. Donaldson K, Brown GM, Bolton RE, Davis JM. Fibrinolysis by rat mesothelial cells *in vitro*: the effect of mineral dusts at non-toxic doses. *Br J Exp Pathol* 1988; **69**: 487–94.
83. Bosma PJ, Kooistra T. Different induction of two plasminogen activator inhibitor 1 mRNA species by phorbol ester in human hepatoma cells. *J Biol Chem* 1991; **266**: 17845–9.
84. Fattal PG, Schneider DJ, Sobel BE, Billadello JJ. Post-transcriptional regulation of expression of plasminogen activator inhibitor type 1 mRNA by insulin and insulin-like growth factor 1. *J Biol Chem* 1992; **267**: 12412–15.
85. Tillmann-Bogush M, Heaton JH, Gelehrter TD. Cyclic nucleotide regulation of PAI-1 mRNAStability. Identification of cytosolic proteins that interact with an a-rich sequence. *J Biol Chem* 1999; **274**: 1172–9.
86. Shetty S, Idell S. Post-transcriptional regulation of plasminogen activator inhibitor-1 in human lung carcinoma cells *in vitro*. *Am J Physiol Lung Cell Mol Physiol* 2000; **278**: L148–56.
87. Shetty S, Bdeir K, Cines DB, Idell S. Induction of plasminogen activator inhibitor-1 by urokinase in lung epithelial cells. *J Biol Chem* 2003; **278**: 18124–31.
88. Pedersen H, Brunner N, Francis D, *et al.* Prognostic impact of urokinase, urokinase receptor, and type 1 plasminogen activator inhibitor in squamous and large cell lung cancer tissue. *Cancer Res* 1994; **54**: 4671–5.
89. Pedersen H, Grondahl-Hansen J, Francis D, *et al.* Urokinase and plasminogen activator inhibitor type 1 in pulmonary adenocarcinoma. *Cancer Res* 1994; **54**: 120–3.
90. Heaton JH, Dlakic WM, Dlakic M, Gelehrter TD. Identification and cDNA cloning of a novel RNA-binding protein that interacts with the cyclic nucleotide-responsive sequence in the Type-1 plasminogen activator inhibitor mRNA. *J Biol Chem* 2001; **276**: 3341–7.
91. ◆ Saksela O, Rifkin DB. Cell-associated plasminogen activation: regulation and physiological functions. *Annu Rev Cell Biol* 1988; **4**: 93–126.
92. Duggan C, Maguire T, McDermott E, *et al.* Urokinase plasminogen activator and urokinase plasminogen activator receptor in breast cancer. *Int J Cancer* 1995; **61**: 597–600.
93. Blasi F, Vassalli JD, Dano K. Urokinase-type plasminogen activator: proenzyme, receptor, and inhibitors. *J Cell Biol* 1987; **104**: 801–4.
94. Shetty S, Kumar A, Idell S. Post-transcriptional regulation of urokinase receptor mRNA: identification of a novel urokinase receptor mRNA binding protein in human mesothelioma cells. *Mol Cell Biol* 1997; **17**: 1075–83.
95. Shetty S, Muniyappa H, Halady PK, Idell S. Regulation of urokinase receptor expression by phosphoglycerate kinase. *Am J Respir Cell Mol Biol* 2004; **31**: 100–6.
96. Shetty S. Regulation of urokinase receptor mRNA stability by hnRNP C in lung epithelial cells. *Mol Cell Biochem* 2005; **272**: 107–18.
97. Tran H, Maurer F, Nagamine Y. Stabilization of urokinase and urokinase receptor mRNAs by HuR is linked to its cytoplasmic accumulation induced by activated mitogen-activated protein kinase-activated protein kinase 2. *Mol Cell Biol* 2003; **23**: 7177–88.

98. Shetty S, Idell S. Urokinase receptor mRNA stability involves tyrosine phosphorylation in lung epithelial cells. *Am J Respir Cell Mol Biol* 2004; **30**: 69–75.
99. Shetty S, Idell S. Urokinase induces expression of its own receptor in Beas2B lung epithelial cells. *J Biol Chem* 2001; **276**: 24549–56.
100. Altus MS, Pearson D, Horiuchi A, Nagamine Y. Inhibition of protein synthesis in LLC-PK1 cells increases calcitonin-induced plasminogen-activator gene transcription and mRNA stability. *Biochem J* 1987; **242**: 387–2.
101. Altus MS, Nagamine Y. Protein synthesis inhibition stabilizes urokinase-type plasminogen activator mRNA. Studies *in vivo* and in cell-free decay reactions. *J Biol Chem* 1991; **266**: 21190–6.
102. Ziegler A, Knesel J, Fabbro D, Nagamine Y. Protein kinase C down-regulation enhances cAMP-mediated induction of urokinase-type plasminogen activator mRNA in LLC-PK1 cells. *J Biol Chem* 1991; **266**: 21067–74.
103. Ziegler A, Hagmann J, Kiefer B, Nagamine Y. Ca^{2+} potentiates cAMP-dependent expression of urokinase-type plasminogen activator gene through a calmodulin- and protein kinase C-independent mechanism. *J Biol Chem* 1990; **265**: 21194–201.
104. Nanbu R, Menoud PA, Nagamine Y. Multiple instability-regulating sites in the 3' untranslated region of the urokinase-type plasminogen activator mRNA. *Mol Cell Biol* 1994; **14**: 4920–8.
105. Nanbu R, Montero L, D'Orazio D, Nagamine Y. Enhanced stability of urokinase-type plasminogen activator mRNA in metastatic breast cancer MDA-MB-231 cells and LLC-PK $_1$ cells down-regulated for protein kinase C-correlation with cytoplasmic heterogeneous nuclear ribonucleoprotein C. Eur *J Biochem* 1997; **247**: 169–74.
106. Shetty S, Idell S. Post-transcriptional regulation of urokinase mRNA. Identification of a novel urokinase mRNA-binding protein in human lung epithelial cells *in vitro*. *J Biol Chem* 2000; **275**: 13771–9.
107. Shetty S. Cytoplasmic-nuclear shuttling of the urokinase mRNA binding protein regulates message stability. *Mol Cell Biochem* 2002; **237**: 55–67.
108. Rodriguez-Panadero F, Segado A, Martin Juan J, *et al.* Failure of talc pleurodesis is associated with increased pleural fibrinolysis. *Am J Respir Crit Care Med* 1995; **151**: 785–90.
109. Bouros D, Schiza S, Siafakas N. Utility of fibrinolytic agents for draining intrapleural infections. *Semin Respir Infect* 1999; **14**: 39–47.
110. Sahn SA. Use of fibrinolytic agents in the management of complicated parapneumonic effusions and empyemas. *Thorax* 1998; **53** (Suppl 2): S65–S72.
111. Bouros D, Schiza S, Patsourakis G, *et al.* Intrapleural streptokinase versus urokinase in the treatment of complicated parapneumonic effusions: a prospective, double-blind study. *Am J Respir Crit Care Med* 1997; **155**: 291–5.
112. Davies RJ, Traill ZC, Gleeson FV. Randomised controlled trial of intrapleural streptokinase in community acquired pleural infection. *Thorax* 1997; **52**: 416–21.
113. Tuncozgur B, Ustunsoy H, Sivrikoz MC, *et al.* Intrapleural urokinase in the management of parapneumonic empyema: a randomised controlled trial. *Int J Clin Pract* 2001; **55**: 658–60.
114. Bouros D, Schiza S, Tzanakis N, *et al.* Intrapleural urokinase versus normal saline in the treatment of complicated parapneumonic effusions and empyema. A randomized, double-blind study. *Am J Respir Crit Care Med* 1999; **159**: 37–42.
115. Chin NK, Lim TK. Controlled trial of intrapleural streptokinase in the treatment of pleural empyema and complicated parapneumonic effusions. *Chest* 1997; **111**: 275–9.
116. Basile A, Boullosa-Seoane E, Dominguez Viguera L, *et al.* Intrapleural fibrinolysis in the management of empyemas and haemothoraces. Our experience. *Radiol Med (Torino)* 2003; **105**: 12–16.
117. Laisaar T, Puttsepp E, Laisaar V. Early administration of intrapleural streptokinase in the treatment of multiloculated pleural effusions and pleural empyemas. *Thorac Cardiovasc Surg* 1996; **44**: 252–6.
118. Davies CW, Traill ZC, Gleeson FV, Davies RJ. Intrapleural streptokinase in the management of malignant multiloculated pleural effusions. *Chest* 1999; **115**: 729–33.
119. Kemper P, Kohler D. Current value of intrapleural fibrinolysis in the treatment of exudative fibrinous pleural effusions in pleural empyema and hemothorax. *Pneumologie* 1999; **53**: 373–84.
120. Jerjes-Sanchez C, Ramirez-Rivera A, Elizalde JJ, *et al.* Intrapleural fibrinolysis with streptokinase as an adjunctive treatment in hemothorax and empyema: a multicenter trial. *Chest* 1996; **109**: 1514–19.
121. de Gregorio MA, Ruiz C, Alfonso ER, *et al.* Drainage of loculated and/or multiloculated pleural effusions using a small caliber catheter and urokinase (pleuro-fibrinolysis). *Arch Bronconeumol* 1996; **32**: 510–5.
122. Davies CW, Lok S, Davies RJ. The systemic fibrinolytic activity of intrapleural streptokinase. *Am J Respir Crit Care Med* 1998; **157**: 328–330.
123. Berglin E, Ekroth R, Teger-Nilsson AC, William-Olsson G. Intrapleural instillation of streptokinase. Effects on systemic fibrinolysis. *Thorac Cardiovasc Surg* 1981; **29**: 124–6.
◆124. Cameron R, Davies HR. Intra-pleural fibrinolytic therapy versus conservative management in the treatment of parapneumonic effusions and empyema. *Cochrane Database Syst Rev* 2004; **2**: CD002312.
◆125. Cameron R. Intrapleural fibrinolytic therapy vs. conservative management in the treatment of parapneumonic effusions and empyema. Cochrane Database Syst Rev 2000; **3**: CD002312.
126. Diacon AH, Theron J, Schuurmans MM, *et al.* Intrapleural streptokinase for empyema and complicated parapneumonic effusions. *Am J Respir Crit Care Med* 2004; **170**: 49–53.
●127. Maskell NA, Davies CW, Nunn AJ, *et al.* UK Controlled trial of intrapleural streptokinase for pleural infection. *N Engl J Med* 2005; **352**: 865–74.
128. Tokuda Y, Matsushima D, Stein GH, Miyagi S. Intrapleural fibrinolytic agents for empyema and complicated parapneumonic effusions: a meta-analysis. *Chest* 2006; **129**: 783–90.
129. Idell S. Update on the use of fibrinolysins in pleural disease. *Clin Pulm Med* 2005; **12**: 184–90.
130. Lee YC. Ongoing search for effective intrapleural therapy for empyema: is streptokinase the answer? *Am J Respir Crit Care Med* 2004; **170**:1–2.
131. Antoniou KM, Pataka A, Bourous D, Siafakas NM. Pathogenetic pathways and novel pharmacotherapeutic targets in idiopathic pulmonary fibrosis. *Pulm Pharmacol Ther* 2007; **20:** 453–61.
132. Heffner JE. Multicenter trials of treatment for empyema – after all these years. *N Engl J Med* 2005; **352**: 926–8.
133. Bouros D, Antoniou KM, Light RW. Intrapleural streptokinase for pleural infection. *BMJ* 2006; **332**: 133–4.
134. Oguzkaya F, Akcali Y, Bilgin M. Videothoracoscopy versus intrapleural streptokinase for management of post traumatic retained haemothorax: a retrospective study of 65 cases. *Injury* 2005; **36**: 526–9.
135. Wait MA, Sharma S, Hohn J, Dal Nogare A. A randomized trial of empyema therapy. *Chest* 1997; **111**: 1548–51.
136. Cochran JB, Tecklenburg FW, Turner RB. Intrapleural instillation of fibrinolytic agents for treatment of pleural empyema. *Pediatr Crit Care Med* 2003; **4**: 39–43.
137. Wells RG, Havens PL. Intrapleural fibrinolysis for parapneumonic effusion and empyema in children. *Radiology* 2003; **228**: 370–8.
138. Yao CT, Wu JM, Liu CC, *et al.* Treatment of complicated parapneumonic pleural effusion with intrapleural streptokinase in children. *Chest* 2004; **125**: 566–71.
139. Barnes NP, Hull J, Thomson AH. Medical management of parapneumonic pleural disease. *Pediatr Pulmonol* 2005; **39**: 127–34.

140. Chen JP, Lue KH, Liu SC, *et al.* Intrapleural urokinase treatment in children with complicated parapneumonic effusion. *Acta Paediatr Taiwan* 2006; **47**: 61–6.
141. Thomson AH, Hull J, Kumar MR, *et al.* Randomised trial of intrapleural urokinase in the treatment of childhood empyema. *Thorax* 2002; **57**: 343–7.
142. Singh M, Mathew JL, Chandra S, *et al.* Randomized controlled trial of intrapleural streptokinase in empyema thoracis in children. *Acta Paediatr* 2004; **93**: 1443–5.
●143. Kurt BA, Winterhalter KM, Connors RH, *et al.* Therapy of parapneumonic effusions in children: video-assisted thoracoscopic surgery versus conventional thoracostomy drainage. *Pediatrics* 2006; **118**: e547–53.
●144. Sonnappa S, Cohen G, Owens CM, *et al.* Comparison of urokinase and video-assisted thoracoscopic surgery for treatment of childhood empyema. *Am J Respir Crit Care Med* 2006; **174**: 221–7.
145. Higazi AA, Mazar A, Wang J, *et al.* Single-chain urokinase-type plasminogen activator bound to its receptor is relatively resistant to plasminogen activator inhibitor type 1. *Blood* 1996; **87**: 3545–9.
146. Vermeer F, Bosl I, Meyer J, *et al.* Saruplase Is a safe and effective thrombolytic agent; observations in 1,698 patients: results of the PASS Study. *J Thromb Thrombolysis* 1999; **8**: 143–50.
147. Idell S, Mazar A, Cines D, *et al.* Single-chain urokinase alone or complexed to its receptor in tetracycline-induced pleuritis in rabbits. *Am J Respir Crit Care Med* 2002; **166**: 920–6.
148. Idell S, Allen T, Chen S, *et al.* Intrapleural activation, processing, efficacy and duration of protection of single-chain urokinase in evolving tetracycline-induced pleural injury in rabbits. *Am J Physiol Lung Cell Mol Physiol* 2007; **292**: L25–32.
149. Strange C, Baumann MH, Sahn SA, Idell S. Effects of intrapleural heparin or urokinase on the extent of tetracycline-induced pleural disease. *Am J Respir Crit Care Med* 1995; **151**: 508–15.
150. Bruckner A, Filderman AE, Kirchheimer JC, *et al.* Endogenous receptor-bound urokinase mediates tissue invasion of the human lung carcinoma cell lines A549 and Calu-1. *Cancer Res* 1992; **52**: 3043–7.
151. Bianchi E, Cohen RL, Thor AT, *et al.* The urokinase receptor is expressed in invasive breast cancer but not in normal breast tissue. *Cancer Res* 1994; **54**: 861–6.
152. Achbarou A, Kaiser S, Tremblay G, *et al.* Urokinase overproduction results in increased skeletal metastasis by prostate cancer cells in vivo. *Cancer Res* 1994; **54**: 2372–7.
153. Crowley CW, Cohen RL, Lucas BK, *et al.* Prevention of metastasis by inhibition of the urokinase receptor. *Proc Natl Acad Sci U S A* 1993; **90**: 5021–5.
154. Min HY, Doyle LV, Vitt CR, *et al.* Urokinase receptor antagonists inhibit angiogenesis and primary tumor growth in syngeneic mice. *Cancer Res* 1996; **56**: 2428–33.
155. Shetty S, Idell S. A urokinase receptor mRNA binding protein-mRNA interaction regulates receptor expression and function in human pleural mesothelioma cells. *Arch Biochem Biophys* 1998; **356**: 265–79.
156. Vervloet MG, Thijs LG, Hack CE. Derangements of coagulation and fibrinolysis in critically ill patients with sepsis and septic shock. *Semin Thromb Hemost* 1998; **24**: 33–44.
◆157. ten Cate H. Pathophysiology of disseminated intravascular coagulation in sepsis. *Crit Care Med* 2000; **28**: S9–11.
158. Esmon CT. Introduction: Are natural anticoagulants candidates for modulating the inflammatory response to endotoxin? *Blood* 2000; **95**: 1113–16.
159. de Fouw NJ, de Jong YF, Haverkate F, Bertina RM. Activated protein C increases fibrin clot lysis by neutralization of plasminogen activator inhibitor – no evidence for a cofactor role of protein S. *Thromb Haemost* 1988; **60**: 328–33.
160. Bajzar L, Nesheim ME, Tracy PB. The profibrinolytic effect of activated protein C in clots formed from plasma is TAFI-dependent. *Blood* 1996; **88**: 2093–100.

10

Pleural reaction to mineral dusts

JAUME FERRER, JOSÉ GARCÍA-VALERO, JUAN F MONTES

INTRODUCTION

Inhalation of mineral dusts can cause pleural disease. Pleural abnormalities can occur in patients with pneumoconioses, and on occasions the pleura may be affected without lung involvement. Inorganic pleural disease includes several pathological disorders, ranging from pleural fibrosis and calcification to malignant transformation.

Mesothelial cell damage has been studied *in vitro* and *in vivo*, particularly after exposure to asbestos and man-made mineral fibers. However, despite considerable research efforts, the mechanisms by which the pleura are affected by mineral dusts remain poorly understood. In addition to secondary involvement as a result of mineral dust inhalation, the pleura can also be directly exposed from therapeutic intrapleural administration of talc. Talc is currently the most commonly used agent for human pleurodesis (see also Chapter 25, Effusions from malignance and Chapter 46, Pleurodesis). Consequently, the effects of talc on mesothelial cells will also be discussed.

In this chapter we focus on current knowledge of pleural involvement by inhaled and intrapleurally introduced mineral dusts.

PLEURAL INVOLVEMENT BY SILICA AND NON-FIBROUS SILICATES

Inhalation of dust with high silica content can produce silicosis. Occupations at risk are mainly mining, granite, sandstone and slate quarrying, tunneling, stone-working, abrasives and foundry work, among others.[1] Silica-induced pleural changes consist of macroscopically visible nodular lesions in visceral pleura, known as candlewax lesions, with or without pulmonary involvement. By light microscopy, these lesions correspond to silicotic nodules containing silica and silicates.[2] Radiologically, diffuse pleural fibrosis and pleural thickening with occasional calcification are frequent findings.[1] It has been proposed that silica exposure can cause pleural effusion,[3] but this possibility remains to be proved.

In coal workers' pneumoconiosis, pathological black-stained pleural surface is often observed. Subpleural nodules can also occur, but radiological pleural thickening is only detected in cases of progressive massive fibrosis.[4] In a study of 765 anthracite workers, 43 (6 percent) showed detectable pleural changes on chest X-rays such as pleural thickening and costophrenic sinus obliteration. Moreover, costophrenic obliteration was associated with exposure to coal dust with a high silica content.[5]

Evidence of pleural involvement for the other minerals mentioned is scarce. Kaolin workers have occasional thickening, nodules and adhesions of the pleura, but no radiological alterations have been described.[6,7] Mixed dust fibrosis caused by inhalation of dust containing silica and less fibrogenic minerals can produce pleural thickening and subpleural nodules.[8] In talc workers, parietal and visceral pleural thickening, pleural plaques affecting thoracic and diaphragmatic parietal pleura (which are often calcified) and obliteration of costophrenic angles, have been described;[9] however, in some reports, talc was contaminated by asbestos.[10–12] In a study of 121 workers of talc contaminated with antophylite and tremolite, pleural thickening affected 31 percent of individuals exposed for more than 15 years, while the overall prevalence of pleural calcification was 3.4 percent.[10] Pleural calcification and pleural plaques are also seen in workers exposed to mica;[11–13] in a survey of 302 cases, five (1.6 percent) showed pleural calcification.[11] Inhalation of non-fibrous minerals has not been shown to cause pleural malignancies.

Fibrous silicates are more harmful for the pleura. Sepiolite exposure was associated with calcified pleural plaque in Bulgaria,[14] but there was no pleural involvement in 218 sepiolite workers studied in Spain.[15] Erionite, of the zeolite family, was related to fibrosis, plaques and mesothelioma in Turkey[16] and wollastonite produced bilateral pleural thickening in 13 out of 46 (28 percent) workers exposed for a mean of 22 years.[17] The highest potential for injury to the pleura corresponds to asbestos. Up to 82 percent of 2907 asbestos insulators with an exposure time equal or greater than 40 years had pleural fibrosis[18] (see also Chapter 40, Asbestos-related pleural diseases).

DYNAMICS OF FIBERS AND PARTICLES IN LUNG AND PLEURA

Inhaled mineral dust progresses through the airways depending on the physical characteristics of the particles and the characteristics of the inhaled dust. Only particles with a mean diameter of less than 5 μm reach the alveoli, while larger particles are lodged at bronchial bifurcations. Particles and fibers deposited in the respiratory tract are cleared by host defense mechanisms. The mucociliary 'escalator', comprising of ciliated epithelial cells and their covering of mucous fluid, helps remove the particles from the airways, where they are expectorated or swallowed. Uncleared particles are phagocytosed by alveolar macrophages and epithelial cells and eliminated by ciliary movement or via the lymphatic system, if the loaded macrophages penetrate the lung interstitium. Accumulation of mineral deposits in the lung parenchyma appears to occur when the amount of inhaled dust exceeds the capacity of the clearance system.[19]

Part of the inhaled dust is deposited in the subpleural lung.[20] Increased silicon deposition has been described in the visceral pleura of individuals with silicosis and in non-silicotic individuals exposed to silica dust compared with the reference population.[21] In asbestos-exposed workers chrysotile is always found in the pleura; in contrast, amphiboles, the most pathogenic fibers, are rarely detected,[22] see below.

The mechanism by which inhaled inorganic particles or fibers reach the pleura is not well understood. It has been proposed that asbestos fibers migrate towards the peripheral lung and visceral pleura, and the parietal pleura is subsequently eroded during respiratory movements.[23] This theory is not supported by the fact that crocidolite fibers, which are larger and more pathogenic than chrysotile fibers, and thus more able to irritate the parietal pleura, are rarely found in pleural samples of exposed individuals.[22] Particles or fibers could also reach the parietal pleura from the lung retrogadely by the lymphatic system. Once hiliar and mediastinal lymph nodes are overloaded by mineral material, dust would be carried towards the bronchomediastinal lymphatic trunk, and backwards to the intercostal vessels, leading to lymphangitis and reactive fibrosis. The finding of coal dust in intercostal vessels in cases of coal pneumoconiosis supports this theory.[24]

MECHANISMS OF MESOTHELIAL DAMAGE

Asbestos

Asbestos consists of fibrous hydrated silicates which include serpentines and amphiboles (see Chapter 40, Asbestos-related pleural diseases). The most common serpentine is chrysotile, while amphiboles include crocidolite, amosite, anthophilite, actinolite and tremolite. Chemically, the various asbestos fibers differ. Crocidolite contains a considerable amount of iron, while chrysotile contains mostly magnesium. Although both amphiboles and chrysotile are harmful *in vitro* for the mesothelial cell, crocidolite is the one mostly found in pleural samples of patients with mesothelioma.[25] This is thought to be due to the superior biopersistence of crocidolite in the lung compared with chrysotile (biopersistence being the physical durability and chemical stability of fibers in tissue over a particular period of time). This is because chrysotile is soluble in organic fluids, more fragmentable and therefore eliminated more quickly. It is accepted that fibers measuring less than 0.25 μm in diameter and more than 8 μm long are more carcinogenic.[26]

Asbestos appears to damage the pleura by direct and indirect mechanisms. Inhalation or intratracheal administration of asbestos in rats induces epithelial cell proliferation[27] and phagocytosis of asbestos fibers in the first 24 hours.[28] Mesothelial cells start to proliferate from 24 hours up to 14 days,[27] while fibroblast proliferation persists for 6 weeks.[29] In addition, inflammatory cells increase in pleural lavage fluid at 1 week.[29] Supernatants of alveolar and pleural macrophages taken at 1 week stimulate proliferation of mesothelial cells and fibroblasts, but by 6 weeks only fibroblasts are stimulated. Fibroblast growth was reduced by antibodies against platelet-derived growth factor (PDGF), whereas mesothelial proliferation was blocked by an antibody to keratinocyte growth factor (KGF)[29] (see also Chapter 8, Immunology). No correlation was found between cell proliferation and the number of fibers in the pleura,[27] and asbestos fibers were not found in pleural macrophages.[29] Taken together, these data suggest that mediators from asbestos-phagocytozing cells induce pleural accumulation of inflammatory cells and thereby mesothelial cell proliferation. However, the studies mentioned do not support the idea that asbestos directly stimulates the mesothelium.

Since a percentage of asbestos fibers reach the pleura after being inhaled, fiber–mesothelium interaction merits special mention. *In vitro* studies have shown that mesothelial cells can phagocytose asbestos fibers, which are then incorporated into phagosomes.[30] Vitronectin, and perhaps other serum adhesive proteins, covers asbestos fibers and permit their binding to vitronectin receptors of the mesothelial cell: integrins $\alpha_v\beta_3$ and $\alpha_v\beta_5$. The covering by vitronectin increases asbestos fiber phagocytosis, and could therefore increase the tissue damage via an oxidative effect.[31] *In vivo*, phagocytosis of asbestos fibers probably occurs at the apical domain of mesothelial cells, which is the region of the cell membrane facing the pleural space.

In addition to internalizing fibers, mesothelial cells exposed to asbestos would recruit inflammatory cells by secreting interleukin (IL)-8 and monocyte chemoattractant protein-1 (MCP-1).[32–34] This process is potentiated in the presence of IL-1 and MCP-1. It has been shown that asbestos exposure increases the adhesion of pleural leukocytes to rat pleural mesothelial cells, and upregulates the expression of vascular cell adhesion molecule-1 (VCAM-1) on rat pleural mesothelial cells.[35] This effect, which is dose-dependent and potentiated by IL-1, supports the idea that asbestos induces an early pleural cellular response leading to additional oxidative and inflammatory damages. Finally, mesothelial cells can also recruit fibroblasts by secreting fibronectin and promote collagen synthesis.[36] The pathogenesis of benign asbestos pleural diseases is probably the result of a pleural inflammation involving the direct and indirect mechanisms mentioned. Pleural inflammation can provoke collagen deposition, as occurs in plaques, fibrosis and rounded atelectasis of the pleura. Alternatively, asbestos-induced pleural inflammation can lead to an increase in the capillary permeability in the pleura, resulting in the development of an effusion. The reason(s) why any patient develops certain type(s) of asbestos-induced pleural disease but not the others is unknown.

Other *in vitro* effects of asbestos on mesothelial cells include cell proliferation,[37] cytotoxicity,[38] genetic changes such as aneuploidy and diverse chromosomal alterations,[39] mitotic damage consisting of anaphase and telophase abnormalities,[40] and DNA breakage (see also Chapter 11, Genetics of malignant mesothelioma).[41,42] However, asbestos-related genetic effects are not necessarily irreversible or transmitted to daughter cells. Data from other studies reflect a regulatory reaction of mesothelial cells after previous asbestos genetic damage. The finding that asbestos-exposed rat pleural mesothelial cells are arrested in G0/G1, G1/S and G2/M stages[43,44] suggests that the cell cycle of damaged cells is interrupted to permit repairs. Conversely, expression of the DNA-repairing enzyme apurynic/apyrimidinic (AP) endonuclease in mesothelial cells by crocidolite[44] further supports the idea that the asbestos-damaged DNA may be repaired.[45]

Apoptosis, or programmed cell death, is thought to be a physiological mechanism for eliminating damaged cells, and is therefore an important cell-regulating phenomenon. Asbestos-damaged mesothelial cells undergo apoptosis,[46,47] and this effect is mediated by reactive oxygen species (ROS) and by internalization of fibers by mesothelial cells.[47] Moreover, increased DNA synthesis and apoptosis are in dynamic balance in asbestos-exposed mesothelial cells.[37] Apoptosis is the key mechanism for eliminating mesothelial cells damaged by asbestos, ensuring the removal of cells carrying genetic abnormalities with potential harmful biological effects.

Attention has recently been paid to the role of ROS in cell toxicity caused by asbestos. Iron present in the surface of asbestos fibers and other silicates drive local generation of ROS via redox reactions.[48] Oxidation also occurs after the respiratory burst of phagocytosis of large asbestos fibers.[44] The participation of ROS in asbestos mesothelial damage has been suggested by recent *in vitro* studies. Culture medium from asbestos-exposed mesothelial cells contains dose-dependent increases of oxidant-induced base modifications such as 8-oxo-2′-deoxyguanosine and 8-hydroxydeoxyguanosine, thereby indicating DNA damage.[49,50] However, overexpression of the antioxidant enzymes heme oxygenase and manganese-containing superoxide dismutase (Mn-SOD) in asbestos-exposed human mesothelial cells suggests a reaction against oxidative damage.[51]

Recent *in vitro* data have contributed to the elucidation of the signal transduction cascade, through which asbestos fibers regulate gene expression in mesothelial cells. Phosphorylation of the epidermal growth factor receptor (EGF-R) on mesothelial cells by asbestos, especially the longest fibers,[52] appears to be the initial step, since it is known to induce cell proliferation.[53] Phosphorylation of the mitogen-activated protein (MAP) kinases and extracellular signal-regulated kinases (ERK) 1 and 2 would then occur, and these activated kinases would translocate to the nucleus to induce c-fos transactivation.[54] In a recent study, crocidolite was shown to be able to induce activation of the p38 arm of the MAP pathway in rat mesothelial cells.[55]

After activation by MAPK signaling cascades, the proliferative effect of asbestos on mesothelial cells can be mediated by upregulation of the early response proto-oncogenes *c-fos* and *c-jun*.[56] The c-fos and c-jun proteins form the AP-1 transcription factor, which binds to AP-1 DNA sites and regulates transition of the G1 to S phase of the cell cycle.[57]

It is probable that biopersistence of asbestos, mainly amphiboles, in lung and pleura cause a low-grade but sustained inflammation and cell proliferation via c-fos and c-jun and protein kinase C (PKC) pathways. Regulatory mechanisms such as DNA repair and apoptosis would be bypassed, favoring uncontrolled cell growth in certain cases and after a long latency period.

Alternative mechanisms of DNA modification have been proposed. Mechanical interference of asbestos fibers with chromosomes, including severing, piercing or disruption of the mitotic spindle, are known to occur.[30,40] Another possibility is transfection of exogenous DNA into mesothelial cells. Transfection of plasmid DNA into mesothelial cells by asbestos fibers has been carried out *in vitro*,[58] but the role of this mechanism in asbestos pleural disease remains unknown.

Man-made vitreous fibers

Man-made or synthetic mineral fibers include slag, rock or glass wools, continuous filament glass and refractory ceramic fibers. These fibers are mainly used for thermal and acoustic insulation. *In vitro* studies show that exposure to man-made vitreous fibers (MMVF) induces cytotoxicity,[38] cell division,[59] cell proliferation[60] and oxidative DNA damage[61] in mesothelial cells. *In vivo*, intrapleural introduction of MMVF with a high length–diameter ratio causes malignant mesothelioma, but these studies cannot predict human carcinogenicity, owing to differences in dose, fiber length and their pleural deposition.[62] In animal studies (using the inhalatory route), only refractory ceramic fibers are able to induce mesothelioma.[63]

The occurrence of pleural plaques in workers exposed to refractory ceramic fibers, with greater risk associated with latency time, duration, and intensity of exposure, has recently been described either in cross-sectional[64] and longitudinal studies.[65] However, the industrial use of refractory ceramic fibers is relatively recent and further studies with longer latency period are required to ascertain the potential to cause benign pleural disease of these fibers. Regarding mesothelioma in humans, there are no data supporting the hypothesis that it can occur as a consequence of the exposure to MMVF.[66] In conclusion, we believe that the International Association for Research on Cancer's statement that MMVF are a possible human carcinogen, with classification in group 2B,[67] remains valid. This category is used to classify agents with limited or inadequate evidence of carcinogenicity in humans, and sufficient or insufficient evidence of carcinogenicity in animals. The lower pathogenicity of MMVF compared with asbestos could be due to their lower lung biopersistence.[68]

Silica and non-asbestos silicates

The most important clinical effect of inhaled silica and non-asbestos silicates in the pleura is pleural fibrosis. However, information on the effects of silica and non-asbestos silicates on the mesothelium is scarce. Intratracheal silica instillation induces mesothelial proliferation.[69] In cultured mesothelial cells, silica exposure reduces protein and collagen synthesis[70] and fibrinolytic activity,[71] and supernatant of silica-treated mesothelial cells increase collagen synthesis in mesothelial cells and fibroblasts.[70]

It is likely, therefore, that mesothelial cells can drive pleural inflammation in individuals exposed to silica and non-asbestos silicates. As mentioned previously for asbestos, the mesothelial reaction can be caused by direct contact with particles translocated to the pleura[21] or indirectly through pulmonary mediators and influx of inflammatory cells. Oxidant mechanisms are probably involved in direct mesothelial damage by silica and non-fibrous silicates.[72]

To our knowledge, non-fibrous particles are not toxic to mesothelial cells[73] and do not produce genetic changes. Mesothelioma has not been associated with silica or non-asbestos silicate human inhalation, and this tumor has not developed in animals after intrapleural administration of quartz.[74]

LOCAL AND SYSTEMIC REACTIONS ASSOCIATED WITH TALC PLEURODESIS

Background

Talc is currently the most common agent used for pleurodesis. Talc pleurodesis can be performed either by insufflating talc powder by thoracoscopy or by introducing a slurry through a chest tube. Despite its high efficacy, concerns are now focused on the possible development of acute respiratory distress syndrome (ARDS) after intrapleural talc administration.

Although talc is used worldwide for pleurodesis, the cellular and molecular basis of talc-induced pleural symphysis has not been fully established. Local and systemic inflammatory reactions, extrapleural talc dissemination, and their relationship with talc particle characteristics and the dose used, are of special interest (see also Chapter 46, Pleurodesis).

Talc particle characteristics

Talc is a pulverized, natural, sheet-like, hydrated magnesium silicate with the approximate chemical formula of $Mg_3(Si_2O_5)_2(OH)_2$, although calcium, manganese, aluminum and iron are always present in variable amounts depending on the geographical origin of the talc. Non-talc minerals associated with commercial talc vary from deposit to deposit and may include calcite, magnesite, dolomite, chlorite, serpentine, quartz and others.[75]

During the treatment process, talc ore is first crushed and ground to a fineness which liberates it from other associated non-talc minerals. After washing, the talc is passed through mesh to eliminate the larger-sized talc particles. The final talc may be 200-, 325- or 400-mesh. With a 400-mesh, 90–95 percent of the particles are smaller than 37 μm, while with a 200-mesh 95–99 percent of the particles are under 74 μm. In a study by Ferrer *et al.*,[75] particle size of talcs used for pleurodesis from different countries was measured. The mean diameter ranged between 10.8 and 33.6 μm, and USA talcs had the lowest diameters (between 10.8 and 20.1 μm). The pattern of contaminant minerals among the different talc preparations also showed a marked variation.[75]

Talc as an inflammatory agent

TALC PARTICLE–MESOTHELIUM INTERACTION

In humans, the intrapleural administration of talc provokes an inflammatory response characterized by an increase in the production of IL-8 (up to 68.9 ng/mL at 24 hours) and MCP-1 (up to 29.0 ng/mL at 6 hours) in pleural fluids.[76] It has been suggested that IL-8 and MCP-1 are involved in the chemotaxis of neutrophils and monocytes in the pleural cavity of humans undergoing talc pleurodesis.[76,77]

Results from animal models concur with data from human pleurodesis. It has been shown that, following talc pleurodesis, high concentrations of IL-8[78–82] and MCP-1[78] accumulated in the pleural fluids in rabbits.

Pioneering work carried out by Nasreen *et al.*[83] showed that primary cultures of human pleural mesothelial cells exposed to several talc concentrations increased the release of IL-8 and MCP-1 in a time- and dose-dependent manner. Further, the observed effects were specific for talc particles, since parallel cultured cells exposed to glass microbeads of a similar size did not stimulate mesothelial chemokine production as much as did talc. These authors also showed that talc exposure induced IL-8 and MCP-1 mRNA expression and the protein products possessed biological activity.

Likewise, *in vitro* studies have shown that talc also induces significant increase in IL-8 production in primary cultures of rabbit pleural mesothelial cells.[79]

Interleukin-8, expressed by mesothelial cells, macrophages, fibroblasts, endothelial cells and a number of tumor cell lines, is chemotactic for neutrophil granulocytes. Monocyte chemoattractant protein-1 is expressed by mesothelial cells, monocytes, vascular endothelial cells, smooth muscle cells and human pulmonary type 2-like epithelial cells in culture. It is chemotactic for monocytes but not for neutrophils.

In addition to mesothelial cells, pleural macrophages can contribute to driving the pleurodesis process. *In vitro* experiments reveal that interaction of macrophages with polyethylene particles is followed by an increase in the secretion of signaling molecules, particularly cytokines. Green *et al.*[84] observed the induced secretion of tumor necrosis factor (TNF)-α, IL-1β and IL-6 after phagocytosis of polyethylene particles, especially when the particles had a diameter less than 10 μm.

It is therefore likely that pleural or interstitial macrophages could also secrete *in vivo*, after interaction with talc particles, proinflammatory cytokines such as TNF-α, or IL-β, which are active on the mesothelium, thereby promoting, in an indirect manner, its activation.[85,86]

PLEURAL INFLAMMATION

To our knowledge, only one study has focused on the pleural histopathological effects of the application of talc to achieve therapeutic pleurodesis in humans.[87] Histomorphological findings after talc pleurodesis show the development of talc-containing granulation tissue with giant-cell foreign-body reaction, evolving to connective tissue formation and obliteration of the pleural cavity.

Although several animal models have been used to characterize the pleural inflammatory effects of talc application, the widespread animal model used for this target has been the rabbit.[88–95] Rabbits that underwent experimental pleurodesis showed inflammatory effects in both pleural surfaces. Talc caused mesothelial denudement and an exudative neutrophilic pleural effusion, which resolved after 48 hours. These effects were accompanied by a mononuclear cell infiltration into the subpleural tissue matrix.[88] Later, reactive cuboidal mesothelial cells covered a thickened loose connective tissue matrix that extended above and below the discontinuous fibroelastic lamina. Finally, flattened mesothelial cells proliferated to cover the thickened connective tissue layer, which often contained talc particles and associated multinucleated giant cells.[88,93,95] (For animal models for pleurodesis, see also Chapter 14.)

Talc-treated animals showed an active process of vascularization in this fibrotic pleural thickening.[91,93,96] Thus, at 1 week, capillary sprouting and small neovessels were detected in the newly-developed submesothelial tissue. These blood vessels were located close to both the pleural and parenchymal sides of the elastic layer. By 1 month, a rich vascular network, originating in the subjacent parenchymal vascularization, had developed in the fibrotic pleural thickening[96] (Figure 10.1). The pivotal role of angiogenesis in the production of pleurodesis has been clearly demonstrated by Guo *et al.*[97] who, by inhibiting angiogenesis with anti-vascular endothelial growth factor (VEGF) antibody, reported a significant reduction in the pleurodesis score in a rabbit model.

When the effects of different doses and talc particle size used to perform pleurodesis in rabbits were compared, the histopathological effects were quite similar to the findings described above. However, thickening of pleural fibrotic tissue was dose- and particle diameter-dependent. Greater thickening was obtained with the highest doses[95] and smallest talc particle size.[93]

PLEURAL SYMPHYSIS: A MODEL OF FIBRINOUS INFLAMMATION

Talc particles can activate the mesothelium, the pleural macrophages and the endothelium of both the visceral and parietal pleurae, resulting in the production of a fibrinous exudate bridging both surfaces. This exudate evolves to form a fibrin network, a process modulated by the activators and inhibitors affecting both the coagulation and the

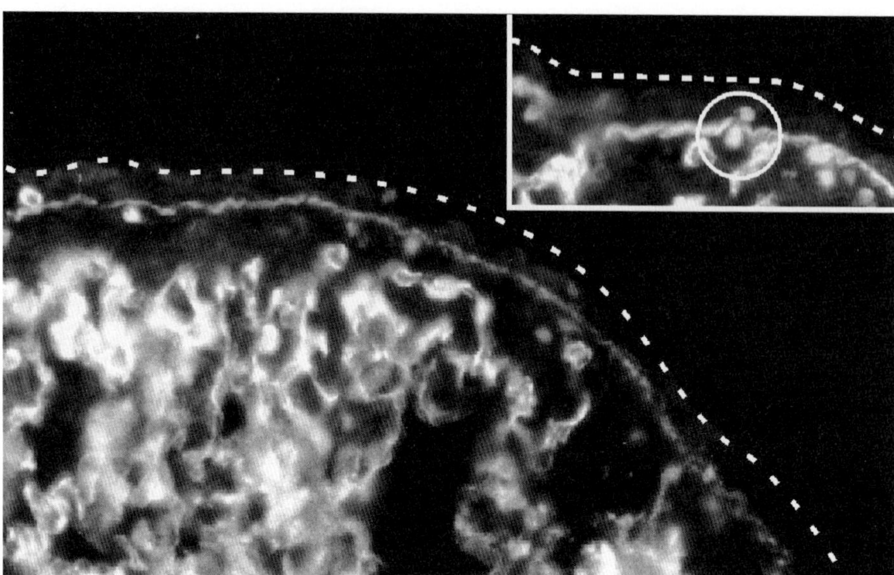

Figure 10.1 Immunolocalization of platelet/endothelial cell adhesion molecule (PECAM)-1 allows one to observe the marginal vascularization of pulmonary parenchyma (×138). Inset shows a newly formed vessel (circled) crossing the elastic layer to supply the fibrotic tissue of the pleura. Dotted line marks the external limit of the tissue under repair.

fibrinolytic cascades, such as thrombin-antithrombin III complex and plasminogen activator inhibitor-1.[98] Stabilization of this fibrin network[99] and increased levels of basic fibroblast growth factor (bFGF) result in the recruitment and proliferation of fibroblasts.[100,101] Fibroblast proliferation is negatively regulated by transforming growth factor (TGF)-β1, although, in contrast, this growth factor promotes the synthesis of numerous matrix molecules such as collagen, proteoglycans, fibronectin, thrombospondin and osteonectin, and can simultaneously inhibit the expression of matrix metalloproteases. TGF-β can be expressed by several cell effectors involved in the pleurodesis, including the mesothelial cells, macrophages, endothelial cells and lymphocytes. The importance of this growth factor resides in its role in the regulation of the fibrotic process. Light *et al.*[102] and Lee *et al.*[103] showed that intrapleural injections of TGF-β2 induced excellent pleurodesis in rabbits and in sheep, without producing an inflammatory pleural effusion. Further, *in vitro* studies revealed that TGF-β2 stimulated collagen synthesis in primary cultures of rabbit pleural mesothelial cells.[79] The maturation of fibrotic tissue of the newly formed adhesion is associated with mesothelial re-epithelialization of their surface.[96] (See Chapter 8, Immunology, for a detailed discussion of cytokines in pleural diseases.)

Although adhesions are considered to play a critical role in the establishment of pleural symphysis, little is known about their histopathogenesis. In a recent morphological and ultrastructural study following talc pleurodesis, all rabbit pleural adhesions examined were mesothelial-covered fibrovascular bands containing well-developed blood and lymphatic vessels establishing a structural continuity between both pleural layers, more resembling newly formed pleural tissue than a simple scar.[96] Strikingly, nerves were present in adhesions from 20 percent of the rabbits. They consisted of a single fascicle containing 5 to 20 thin myelinated axons of various diameters (1–6 μm) uniformly distributed throughout the nerve section. Nerves were always observed in association with blood vessels, mainly arterioles, and followed a sinuous course along the longitudinal axis of the adhesion. It has been suggested that this association is a consequence of the control role played by the angiogenic process in nerve growth during adhesion formation.[104] Nerve fibers appeared to originate from the parietal pleura, which is mainly innervated by the internal intercostal nerves (costal pleura and peripheral part of the diaphragmatic pleura) and the phrenic nerves (central portion of the diaphragmatic pleura and mediastinal pleura). Nerve fibers have also been found in murine[105] and human[104,106–108] peritoneal adhesions. Although the effect of innervation on adhesion function is unknown, an interesting clinical question is whether talc-induced pleural adhesions are potentially capable of conducting pain sensation.

SYSTEMIC REACTIONS

There is currently little information on the systemic effects of talc pleurodesis. Available data indicate that a systemic inflammatory response can develop early after talc pleurodesis. In humans, the intrapleural administration of talc has been associated with increases in both the percentage of leukocytes,[109–111] the erythrocyte sedimentation rate[110] and the levels of C-reactive protein (CRP)[110–112] in peripheral blood. Further, leukocytosis (34×10^9/L) has been reported in a patient suffering an acute respiratory failure following talc pleurodesis.[109] It is interesting to note that a recent trial involving 48 patients has shown that pleurodesis with mixed talc (50 percent of the particles <15 μm) produces more systemic inflammation and more hypoxemia than pleurodesis with graded talc (50 percent of the particles >25 μm).[112] Nine of 22 (41 percent) patients receiving mixed talc developed fever, whereas fever was almost absent (1 of 24, 4 percent) in those receiving graded talc. In addition, the rise in plasma CRP was significantly greater after mixed-talc pleurodesis than it was after graded-talc pleurodesis.

Data from animal models concur with these findings. The intrapleural administration of talc in the rabbit model has been associated with a transient increase in the count of leukocytes,[80,81] the percentage[80,81] and count[95] of neutrophils, the count of monocytes,[95] the count of platelets,[95] the levels of IL-8,[80,81] the levels of VEGF[80,81] and the activity of angiotensin-converting enzyme[91] in peripheral blood. Further, hyperplasia of the white periarteriolar substance of the spleen was observed 24 h following 200-mg/kg talc dose administration in rabbits.[93] It has been reported that this systemic inflammatory response is a dose-related phenomenon.[95]

Extrapleural talc deposition

Acute respiratory distress syndrome is a potentially lethal respiratory failure that can develop very soon after talc administration either as a slurry[113–118] or by insufflation[115,118–124] in up to 9 percent of patients.[115] In a recent international survey of 859 pulmonologists, 58 percent reported cases of respiratory failure after talc pleurodesis.[125] Although the pathogenesis of talc-induced ARDS is uncertain, it has been suggested that extrapleural talc dissemination results in cytokine release and increased permeability-type pulmonary edema.[126,127] It has been postulated that talc particles of small sizes are more likely to be absorbed via the parietal lymphatics into the systemic circulation following intrapleural administration of talc.

The detection of talc particles in a sample can be carried out without destroying the sample or by removing the organic fraction by incineration or enzymatic degradation. Methods to observe talc particles include light and electron microscopy, polarized light microscopy and X-ray diffraction, among others, but a description of each method is beyond the scope of this chapter. It has to be taken into account that detection of the total number of talc particles in a sample requires the use of electron microscopy, because particles smaller than 1 μm can be missed by light microscopy. Particle analysis, in order to detect the characteristic elemental composition of talc, is achieved by energy-dispersive X-ray analysis.

After therapeutic pleurodesis with talc, some patients showed dissemination of particles in lung parenchyma[87,123] or in air spaces after bronchoalveolar lavage (BAL).[121,123,124] In one patient who died of ARDS after talc pleurodesis, necropsy revealed talc crystals in almost every organ examined including lung, brain, liver, kidney, heart and skeletal muscle.[123] However, no talc particles have been found either in BAL samples[128,129] or lung tissues[130] from patients with no respiratory complications after talc administration.

Several attempts to assess safety following intrapleural talc administration have been made in animal models. Werebe *et al.*[131] detected talc particles by light microscopy in every organ studied (chest wall, lungs, heart, brain, spleen and kidney) in 100 percent of rats undergoing pleurodesis with two doses of talc (33 or 67 mg/kg). However, Fraticelli *et al.*[132] only found few talc particles in the liver (6 percent of total animals), spleen (3 percent) and brain (3 percent) after intrapleural administration of a 40-mg/kg talc dose containing large particles in rats. No talc particles were found in the blood, kidneys and contralateral lung.

With respect to the rabbit model, only some rabbits undergoing experimental pleurodesis with a dose of 70 mg/kg showed talc dissemination to mediastinal lymph nodes (17 percent of total animals), kidney (17 percent) and spleen (40 percent), although no particles were detected in lung parenchyma.[88] In addition, it has been shown that in rabbits the probability of dissemination of talc particles to thoracic (lung, mediastinum and pericardium) and extrathoracic organs (liver, spleen and kidney) was related to dose[95] and particle diameter[93] (Figure 10.2). Greater extrapleural talc dissemination was

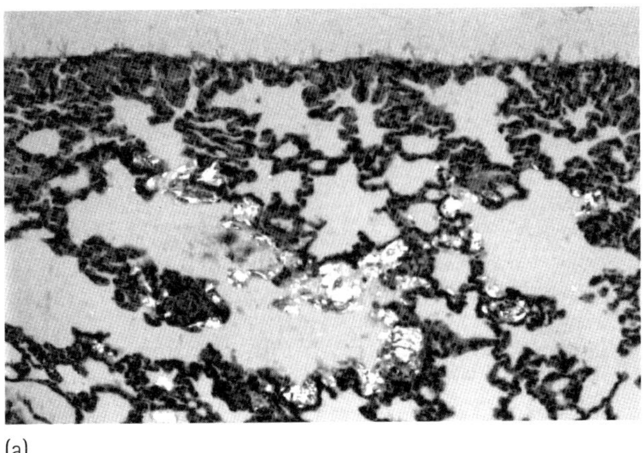
(a)

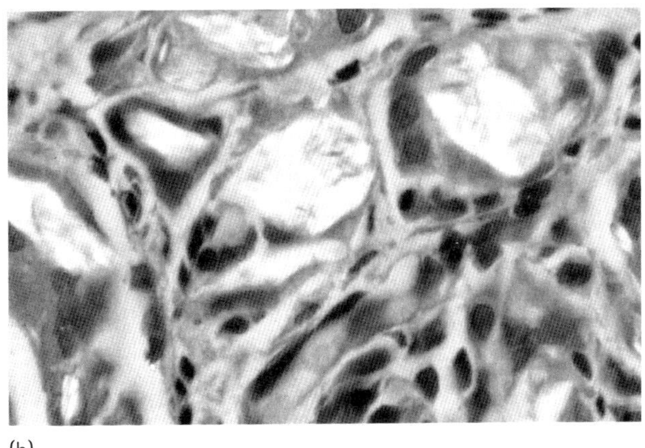
(b)

Figure 10.2 Extrapleural dissemination of talc to pulmonary parenchyma (a, ×40) and mediastinum (b, ×200). Talc particles are seen as bright structures when observed by means of 45° polarized light microscopy.

observed with the highest doses and smallest talc particle size.

Taking into account this evidence, it remains possible that lung dissemination of talc particles leads to ARDS. However, the precise underlying causes and mechanisms of post-talc ARDS are still unknown.

KEY POINTS

- Inhaled inorganic dusts can cause pleural disease. Asbestos and other fibrous silicates such as erionite and wollastonite may induce benign and malignant pleural diseases. Patients exposed to non-fibrous minerals, such as silica, talc and mica, may develop pleural thickening and calcification.
- Among various types of asbestos fibers, amphiboles are more dangerous than chrysotile, because of their greater biopersistence in pulmonary tissue.
- Upon ingestion of asbestos, phagocytes in the respiratory tract release mediators that induce mesothelial cell proliferation. Asbestos fibers are also endocytosed by mesothelial cells, triggering the release of proinflammatory factors such as IL-8 and MCP-1.
- Direct or indirect asbestos-related mesothelial inflammation is probably involved in benign asbestos pleural diseases. Asbestos can also induce genetic changes. Sustained inflammation and cell proliferation via c-fos, c-jun and protein kinase C pathways would explain the carcinogenic effect of asbestos.
- Talc is currently the most common agent used for pleurodesis. Talc particle size and contaminants vary markedly among talc preparations used in different countries.
- In the animal model, talc-induced pleural inflammation is driven by mesothelial cells and macrophages, which release chemotactic factors for neutrophils and monocytes, e.g. IL-8 and MCP-1. Pleural inflammation results in the production of a fibrinous exudate bridging both pleural surfaces. This is followed by fibroblast infiltration and collagen deposition, which results in adhesion formation and pleural symphysis.
- After talc pleurodesis, talc particles can disseminate to extrapleural organs including the lung. It is possible that acute respiratory distress syndrome induced after talc pleurodesis is caused by talc deposition in the lung.

REFERENCES

● = Key primary paper
◆ = Major review article

1. Weill H, Jones RN, Parkes WR. Silicosis and related diseases. In: Parkes WR (ed.). *Occupational lung diseases.* London: Butterworth-Heinemann, 1994: 285–339.
◆2. Craighead JE and the Silicosis and Silicate Disease Committee. Diseases associated with exposure to silica and nonfibrous silicate minerals. *Arch Pathol Lab Med* 1988; **112**: 673–720.
3. Zeren EA, Colby TV, Roggli VL. Silica-induced pleural disease. An unusual case mimicking malignant mesothelioma. *Chest* 1997; **112**: 1436–8.
4. Green FHY, Vallyathan V. Coal worker's pneumoconiosis and pneumoconiosis due to other carbonaceous dusts. In: Churg A, Green FHY (eds). *Pathology of occupational lung disease.* Baltimore: Williams & Wilkins, 1998:129–207.
5. Orriols R, Muñoz X, Sunyer J, *et al.* Radiologically recognized pleural changes in nonpneumoconiotic silica-exposed coal miners. *Scand J Work Environ Health* 2005; **31**: 115–21.
6. Hale LW, Gough J, King EJ, Nagelschmidt G. Pneumoconiosis of kaolin workers. *Br J Ind Med* 1956; **13**: 251–9.
7. Lapenas D, Gale P, Kennedy T, Rawlings W. Dietrich P. Kaolin pneumoconiosis. Radiologic, pathologic, and mineralogic findings. *Am Rev Respir Dis* 1984; **130**: 282–8.
8. Gibbs AR, Wagner JC. Diseases due to silica. In: Churg A, Green FHY (eds). *Pathology of occupational lung disease.* Baltimore: Williams & Wilkins, 1998: 209–33.
9. Vallyathan NV, Craighead JE. Pulmonary pathology in workers exposed to nonasbestiform talc. *Hum Pathol* 1981; **12**: 28–35.
10. Gamble JF, Fellner W, Dimeo MJ. An epidemiologic study of a group of talc workers. *Am Rev Respir Dis* 1979; **119**: 741–53.
11. Ross Smith A. Pleural calcification resulting from exposure to certain dusts. *Am J Roentgnol* 1952; **67**: 375–82.
12. Kleinfeld M. Pleural calcification as a sign of silicatosis. *Am J Med* 1966; **251**. 215–24.
13. Skulberg KR, Gylseth B, Skaug V, Hanoa R. Mica pneumoconiosis. A literature review. *Scand J Work Environ Health* 1985; **11**: 65–74.
14. Burilkov T, Michailova L. Sepiolite content of the soil in regions with endemic pleural calcifications. *Int Arch Arbeitsmed* 1972; **29**: 95–101.
15. McConnochie K, Bevan C, Newcombe RG, *et al.* A study of spanish sepiolite workers. *Thorax* 1993; **48**: 370–374.
16. Baris YI, Simonato L, Saracci R, Skidmore JW, Artvinli M. Malignant mesothelioma and radiological chest abnormalities in two villages in central Turkey. *Lancet* 1981; i: 984–7.
17. Huuskonen MS, Tossavainen A, Koskinen H, *et al.* Wollastonite exposure and lung fibrosis. *Environ Res* 1983; **30**: 291–304.
18. Lilis R, Miller A, Godbold J, Chan E, Selikoff IJ. Radiographic abnormalities in asbestos insulators: effects of duration from onset of exposure and smoking. Relationships of dyspnea with parenchymal and pleural fibrosis. *Am J Ind Med* 1991; **20**: 1–15.
19. Rom WN, Crystal RG. Consequences of chronic inorganic dust exposure. In: Crystal RG, West JB (eds). *The lung.* New York: Raven Press, 1991: 1885–97.
20. Dodson RF, Ford JO. Early response to the visceral pleura following asbestos exposure. *J Toxicol Environ Health* 1985; **15**: 673–86.
21. Ferrer J, Orriols R, Tura JM, *et al.* Energy-dispersive X-ray analysis and scanning electron microscopy of pleura. Study of reference, non-pneumoconiotic and silicosis populations. *Am J Respir Crit Care Med* 1994; **149**: 888–92.
22. Sebastien P, Janson X, Gaudichet A. Asbestos retention in human respiratory tissues. Comparative measurements in lung parenchyma and in parietal pleura. In: Wagner JC. (ed.). *Biological effects of mineral fibers,* vol 1. Lyon: IARC Scientific publications No 30, 1980: 237–46.

23. Heard BE, Williams R. The pathology of asbestosis with reference to lung function. *Thorax* 1961; **16**: 264–81.

•24. Taskinen E, Ahlman K, Wiikeri M. A current hypothesis of the lymphatic transport of inspired dust to the parietal pleura. *Chest* 1973; **64**: 193–6.

25. Browne K. Asbestos-related disorders. In: Parkes WR (ed.). *Occupational lung diseases*. London: Butterworth-Heineman, 1994: 411–504.

•26. Stanton MF, Layard M, Tegeris A, *et al*. Relation of particle dimension to carcinogenicity in amphibole asbestoses and other fibrous minerals. *J Natl Cancer Inst*. 1981; **67**: 965–75.

27. Sekhon H, Wright J, Churg A. Effects of cigarette smoke and asbestos on airway, vascular and mesothelial cell proliferation. *Int J Exp Pathol* 1995; **76**: 411–8.

28. Brodi AR, Hill LH, Adkins B, O'Connor RW. Chrysotile asbestos inhalation in rats: deposition pattern and reaction of alveolar epithelium and pulmonary macrophages. *Am Rev Respir Dis* 1981; **123**: 670–9.

29. Adamson IY. Early mesothelial cell proliferation after asbestos exposure: *in vivo* and *in vitro* studies. *Environ Health Perspect* 1997; **105** (Suppl 5): 1205–8.

30. Wang NS, Jaurand MC, Magne L, *et al*. The interactions between asbestos fibers and metaphase chromosomes of rat pleural mesothelial cells in culture. A scanning electron microscopy study. *Am J Pathol* 1987; **126**: 343–9.

31. Boylan AM, Sanan DA, Sheppard D, Broaddus VC. Vitronectin enhaces internalization of crocidolite asbestos by rabbit pleural mesothelial cells via the integrin alpha v beta 5. *J Clin Invest* 1995; **96**: 1987–2001.

32. Tanaka S, Choe N, Iwagaki A, Hemenway DR, Kagan E. Asbestos exposure induces MCP-1 secretion by pleural mesothelial cells. *Exp Lung Res* 2000; **26**: 241–55.

33. Antony VB, Owen CL, Hadley KJ. Pleural mesothelial cells stimulated by asbestos release chemotactic activity for neutrophils in vitro. *Am Rev Respir Dis* 1898; **139**: 199–206.

34. Griffith DE, Miller EJ, Gray LD, Idell S, Johnson AR. Interleukin-1 mediated release of interleukin-8 by asbestos-stimulated human pleural mesothelial cells. *Am J Respir Cell Mol Biol* 1994; **10**: 245–52.

35. Choe N, Zhang J, Iwagaki A, *et al*. Asbestos exposure upregulates the adhesion of pleural leukocytes to pleural mesothelial cells via VCAM-1. *Am J Physiol* 1999; **277**: 292–300.

36. Kuwahara M, Kuwahara M, Bijwaard KE, *et al*. Mesothelial cells produce a chemoattractant for lung fibroblasts: role of fibronectine. *Am J Respir Cell Mol Biol* 1991; **5**: 256–64.

37. Goldberg JL, Zanella CL, Janssen YM, *et al*. Novel cell imaging techniques show induction of apoptosis and proliferation in mesothelial cells by asbestos. *Am J Respir Cell Mol Biol*. 1997; **17**:265–71.

38. Wang QE, Han CH, Wu WD, *et al*. Biological effects of man-made fibers (I) – Reactive oxygen species production and calcium homeostasis in alveolar macrophages. *Ind Health* 1999; **37**: 62–7.

•39. Lechner JF, Tokiwa T, LaVeck M, *et al*. Asbestos-associated chromosomal changes in human mesothelial cells. *Proc Natl Acad Sci U S A*. 1985; **82**:3884–8.

40. Yegles M, Saint-Etienne L, Renier A, Janson X, Jaurand MC. Induction of metaphase/telophase abnormalities by asbestos fibers in rat pleural mesothelial cells *in vitro*. *Am J Respir Cell Mol Biol* 1993; **9**: 186–91.

41. Levresse V, Renier A, Levy F, Broaddus VC, Jaurand M. DNA breakage in asbestos-treated normal and transformed (TSV40) rat pleural mesothelial cells. *Mutagenesis* 2000; **15**: 239–44.

42. Ollikainen T, Linnainmaa K, Kinnula VL. DNA single strand breaks induced by asbestos fibers in human pleural mesothelial cells *in vitro*. *Environ Mol Mutagen* 1999; **33**: 153–60.

43. Levresse V, Renier A, Fleury-Feith J, *et al*. Analysis of cell cycle disruptions in cultures of rat pleural mesothelial cells exposed to asbestos fibers. *Am J Respir Cell Mol Biol*. 1997; **17**: 660–71.

44. Liu W, Ernst JD, Broaddus VC. Phagocytosis of crocidolite asbestos induces oxidative stress, DNA damage, and apoptosis in mesothelial cells. *Am J Respir Cell Mol Biol* 2000; **23**: 371–8.

45. Fung H, Kow YW, Van Houten B, *et al*. Asbestos increases mammalian AP-endonuclease gene expression, protein levels, and enzyme activity in mesothelial cells. *Cancer Res* 1998; **58**: 189–94.

•46. Broaddus VC, Yang L, Scavo LM, Ernst JD, Boylan AM. Asbestos induces apoptosis of human and rabbit pleural mesothelial cells via reactive oxygen species. *J Clin Invest* 1996; **98**: 2050–9.

47. BeruBe KA, Quinlan TR, Fung H, *et al*. Apoptosis is observed in mesothelial cells after exposure to crocidolite asbestos. *Am J Respir Cell Mol Biol*. 1996;**15**:141–7.

48. Weitzman SA, Graceffa P. Asbestos catalyzes hydroxyl and superoxide radical generation from hydrogen peroxide. *Arch Biochem Biophys* 1984; **228**: 373–6.

49. Chen Q, Marsh J, Ames B, Mossman BT. Detection of 8-oxo-2′-deoxyguanosine, a marker of oxidative DNA damage, in culture medium from human mesothelial cells exposed to crocidolite asbestos. *Carcinogenesis* 1996; **17**: 2525–7.

50. Fung H, Kow YW, Van Houten B, Mossman BT. Patterns of 8-hydroxydeoxyguanosine formation in DNA and indications of oxidative stress in rat and human pleural mesothelial cells after exposure to crocidolite asbestos. *Carcinogenesis* 1997; **18**: 825–32.

51. Janssen YM, Marsh JP, Absher MP, *et al*. Oxidant stress responses in human pleural mesothelial cells exposed to asbestos. *Am J Respir Crit Care Med*. 1994; **149**: 795–802.

52. Pache JC, Janssen YM, Walsh ES, *et al*. Increased epidermal growth factor-receptor protein in a human mesothelial cell line in response to long asbestos fibers. *Am J Pathol* 1998;**152**: 333–40.

53. Faux SP, Houghton CE, Hubbard A, Patrick G. Increased expression of epidermal growth factor receptor in rat pleural mesothelial cells correlates with carcinogenicity of mineral fibers. *Carcinogenesis* 2000; **21**: 2275–80.

54. Zanella CL, Posada J, Tritton TR, Mossman BT. Asbestos causes stimulation of the extracellular signal-regulated kinase Y mitogen-activated protein kinase after phosphorylation of the epidermal growth factor receptor. *Cancer Res 1996*; **65**: 5334–8.

55. Swain WA, O'Byrne J, Faux SP. Activation of p38 MAP Kinase by asbestos in rat mesothelial cells is mediated by oxidative stress. *Am J Physiol* 2004; **286**: 859–65.

•56. Heintz NH., Janssen YM., Mossman BT. Persistent induction of c-fos and c-jun expression by asbestos. *Proc Natl Acad Sci U S A* 1993; **90**: 3299–303.

57. Angel P, Karin M. The role of Jun, Fos and the AP-1 complex in cell-proliferation and transformation. *Biochem Biophys Acta* 1991; **1072**:129–57

58. Gan L, Savransky EF, Fasy TM, Johnson EM. Transfection of human mesothelial cells mediated by different asbestos fiber types. *Environ Res* 1993; **62**: 28–42.

59. Pelin K, Kivipensas P, Linnainmaa K. Effects of asbestos and man-made vitrous fibers on cell division in cultured human mesothelial cells in comparison to rodent cells. *Environ Mol Mutagen* 1995; **25**: 118–25.

60. Rutten AA, Bermudez E, Mangum JB, *et al*. Mesothelial cell proliferation induced by intrapleural instillation of man-made fibers in rats and hamsters. *Fundam Appl Toxicol* 1994; **23**: 107–16.

61. Cavallo D, Campopiano A, Cardinally G, *et al*. Cytotoxic and oxidative effects induced by man-made vitreius fibers (MMVFs) in human mesothelial cell line. *Toxicology* 2004; **201**: 219–29.

62. Gibbs AR, Wagner JC, Churg A. Diseases due to synthetic fibers. In: Churg A, Green FHY (eds). *Pathology of occupational lung disease*. Baltimore: Williams & Wilkins, 1998: 393–402.

63. Mast RW, Hesterberg TW, Glass LR, *et al*. Chronic inhalation and biopersistence of refractory ceramic fiber in rats and hamsters. *Environ Health Perspect*. 1994; **102**(Suppl 5): 207–9.

64. Lockey J, Lemasters G, Rice C, *et al.* Refractory ceramic fiber exposure and pleural plaques. *Am J Respir Crit Care Med* 1996; **154**:1405–10.
65. Lockey JE, Lemasters GK, Levin L, *et al.* A longitudinal study of chest radiographic changes of workers in the refractory ceramic fiber industry. *Chest* 2002; **121**: 2044–51.
◆66. De Vuyst P, Dumortier P, Swaen GMH, Pairon JC, Brochard P. Respiratory health effects man-made vitreous fibres. *Eur Respir J* 1995; **8**: 2149–73.
◆67. IARC. Man-made mineral fibers and radon. In: *IARC monographs in the evaluation of the carcinogenic risk of chemicals to humans*, vol. 43. Lyon: International Agency for Reasearch on Cancer, 1988.
68. Hesterberg TW, Miiler WC, Musselman RP, *et al.* Biopersistence of man-made vitreous fibers and crocidolite asbestos in the rat lung following inhalation. *Fundam Appl Toxicol* 1996; **29**: 267–79.
69. Adamson IYR, Bakowska J, Bowden DH. Mesothelial cell proliferation: a non-specific response to lung injury associated with fibrosis. *Am J Respir Cell Mol Biol* 1994; **10**: 253–8.
70. Aalto M, Kulonen E, Penttinen R, Renvall S. Collagen synthesis in cultured mesothelial cells. Response to silica. *Acta Chir Scand* 1981; **147**: 1–6.
71. Donaldson K, Brown GM, Bolton RE, Davis JM. Fibrinolysis by rat mesothelial cells *in vitro*: the effect of mineral dusts at non-toxic doses. *Br J Exp Pathol* 1988; **69**: 487–94.
72. Ghio AJ, Kennedy TP, Schapira RM, Crumbliss AL, Hoidal JR. Hypothesis: is lung disease after silicate inhalation caused by oxidant generation? *Lancet* 1990; **336**: 967–9.
73. Jaurand MC, Bastie-Sigeac Y, Renier A, Bignon J. Comparative toxicities of different forms of asbestos on rat pleural mesothelial cells. *Environ Health Perspect* 1983; **51**: 153–8.
74. Jaurand MC, Fleury J, Monchaux G, Nebut M, Bignon J. Pleural carcinogenic potency of mineral fibers (asbestos, attapulgite) and their cytotoxicity on culture cells. *J Natl Cancer Inst* 1987; **79**: 797–804.
75. Ferrer J, Villarino MA, Tura JM, Traveria A, Light RW. Talc preparations used for pleurodesis vary markedly from one preparation to another. *Chest* 2001; **119**: 1901–5.
76. van den Heuvel MM, Smit HJM, Barbierato SB, *et al.* Talc-induced inflammation in the pleural cavity. *Eur Respir J* 1998; **12**: 1419–23.
●77. Antony VB, Godbey SW, Kunkel SL, *et al.* Recruitment of inflammatory cells to the pleural space. Chemotactic cytokines, IL-8, and monocyte chemotactic peptide-1 in human pleural fluids. *J Immunol* 1993; **151**: 7216–23.
78. Miller EJ, Kajikawa O, Pueblitz S, *et al.* Chemokine involvement in tetracycline-induced pleuritis. *Eur Respir J* 1999; **14**: 1387–93.
79. Lee YCG, Lane KB, Zoia O, *et al.* Transforming growth factor-β induces collagen synthesis without inducing IL-8 production in mesothelial cells. *Eur Respir J* 2003; **22**: 197–202.
80. Marchi E, Vargas FS, Acencio MMP, *et al.* Talc and silver nitrate induce systemic inflammatory effects during the acute phase of experimental pleurodesis in rabbits. *Chest* 2004; **125**: 2268–77.
●81. Marchi E, Vargas FS, Teixeira LR, *et al.* Intrapleural low-dose silver nitrate elicits more pleural inflammation and less systemic inflammation than low-dose talc. *Chest* 2005; **128**: 1798–804.
82. Marchi E, Vargas FS, Acencio MM, *et al.* Evidence that mesothelial cells regulate the acute inflammatory response in talc pleurodesis. *Eur Respir J* 2006; **28**: 929–32.
●83. Nasreen N, Hartman DL, Mohammed KA, Antony VB. Talc-induced expression of C-C and C-X-C chemokines and intercellular adhesion molecule-1 in mesothelial cells. *Am J Respir Crit Care Med* 1998; **158**: 971–8.
84. Green TR, Fisher J, Stone M, Wroblewski BM, Ingham E. Polyethylene particles of a 'critical size' are necessary for the induction of cytokines by macrophages *in vitro. Biomaterials* 1998; **19**: 2297–302.
85. Antony VB, Hott JW, Kunkel SL, *et al.* Pleural mesothelial cell expression of C-C (monocyte chemotactic peptide) and C-X-C (interleukin 8) chemokines. *Am J Respir Cell Mol Biol* 1995; **12**: 581–8.
86. Mohammed KA, Nasreen N, Ward MJ, Antony VB. Macrophage inflammatory protein-1 C-C chemokine in parapneumonic pleural effusions. *J Lab Clin Med* 1998; **132**: 202–9.
87. Krismann M, Pieper K, Müller K-M. Pleurale reaktionsmuster nach talcum-pleurodese. *Pathologe* 1998; **19**: 214–20.
88. Kennedy L, Harley RA, Sahn SA, Strange C. Talc slurry pleurodesis. Pleural fluid and histologic analysis. *Chest* 1995; **107**: 1707–12.
89. Light RW, Wang NS, Sassoon CSH, Gruer SE, Vargas FS. Talc slurry is an effective pleural sclerosant in rabbits. *Chest* 1995; **107**: 1702–6.
90. Xie C, Teixeira LR, McGovern JP, Light RW. Systemic corticosteroids decrease the effectiveness of talc pleurodesis. *Am J Respir Crit Care Med* 1998; **157**: 1441–4.
91. Mitchem RE, Herndon BL, Fiorella RM, *et al.* Pleurodesis by autologous blood, doxycycline, and talc in a rabbit model. *Ann Thorac Surg* 1999; **67**: 917–21.
92. Lee YC, Teixeira LR, Devin CJ, *et al.* Transforming growth factor-beta$_2$ induces pleurodesis significantly faster than talc. *Am J Respir Crit Care Med* 2001; **163**: 640–4.
93. Ferrer J, Montes JF, Villarino MA, Light RW, García-Valero J. Influence of particle size on extrapleural talc dissemination after talc slurry pleurodesis. *Chest* 2002; **122**: 1018–27.
94. Vargas FS, Teixeira LR, Antonangelo L, *et al.* Experimental pleurodesis in rabbits induced by silver nitrate or talc. 1-year follow-up. *Chest* 2001; **119**: 1516–20.
95. Montes JF, Ferrer J, Villarino MA, *et al.* Influence of talc dose on extrapleural talc dissemination after talc pleurodesis. *Am J Respir Crit Care Med* 2003; **168**: 348–55.
96. Montes JF, García-Valero J, Ferrer J. Evidence of innervation in talc-induced pleural adhesions. *Chest* 2006; **130**: 702–9.
97. Guo YB, Kalomenidis I, Hawthorne M, *et al.* Pleurodesis is inhibited by anti-vascular endothelial growth factor antibody. *Chest* 2005; **128**: 1790–7.
98. Rodríguez-Panadero F, Segado A, Martín Juan J, *et al.* Failure of talc pleurodesis is associated with increased pleural fibrinolysis. *Am J Respir Crit Care Med* 1995; **151**: 785–90.
◆99. Kroegel C, Antony VB. Immunobiology of pleural inflammation: potential implications for pathogenesis, diagnosis and therapy. *Eur Respir J* 1997; **10**: 2411–8.
100. Antony VB, Kamal MA, Godbey S, Loddenkemper RW. Talc induced pleurodesis: role of basic fibroblast growth factor (bFGF). *Eur Respir J* 1997; **10**: 403S.
101. Antony VB, Nasreen N, Mohammed KA, *et al.* Talc pleurodesis. Basic fibroblast growth factor mediates pleural fibrosis. *Chest* 2004; **126**: 1522–8.
102. Light RW, Cheng D-S, Lee YC, *et al.* A single intrapleural injection of transforming growth factor-beta$_2$ produces an excellent pleurodesis in rabbits. *Am J Respir Crit Care Med* 2000; **162**: 98–104.
103. Lee YC, Lane KB, Parker RE, *et al.* Transforming growth factor beta$_2$ (TGF-β_2) produces effective pleurodesis in sheep with no systemic complications. *Thorax* 2000; **55**: 1058–62.
104. Sulaiman H, Gabella G, Davis C, *et al.* Presence and distribution of sensory nerve fibers in human peritoneal adhesions. *Ann Surg* 2001; **234**: 256–61.
105. Sulaiman H, Gabella G, Davis C, *et al.* Growth of nerve fibres into murine peritoneal adhesions. *J Pathol* 2000; **192**: 396–403.
106. Kligman I, Drachenberg C, Papadimitriou J, Katz E. Immunohistochemical demonstration of nerve fibers in pelvic adhesions. *Obstet Gynecol* 1993; **82**: 566–8.
107. Tulandi T, Chen MF, Al-Took S, Watkin K. A study of nerve fibers and histopathology of postsurgical, postinfectious, and endometriosis-related adhesions. *Obstet Gynecol* 1998; **92**: 766–8.
108. Herrick SE, Mutsaers SE, Ozua P, *et al.* Human peritoneal adhesions are highly cellular, innervated, and vascularized. *J Pathol* 2000; **192**: 67–72.

109. Lineau C, Le Coz A, Quinquenel ML, *et al.* Insuffisance respiratoire aiguë après talcage pleural d'un pneumothorax. *Rev Pneumol Clin* 1993; **49**: 153–55.

110. Ukale V, Agrenius V, Widström O, Hassan A, Hillerdal G. Inflammatory parameters after pleurodesis in recurrent malignant pleural effusions and their predictive value. *Respir Med* 2004; **98**: 1166–72.

111. Froudarakis ME, Klimathianaki M, Pougounias M. Systemic inflammatory reaction after thoracoscopic talc poudrage. *Chest* 2006; **129**: 356–61.

●112. Maskell NA, Lee YCG, Gleeson FV, *et al.* Randomized trials describing lung inflammation after pleurodesis with talc of varying particle size. *Am J Respir Crit Care Med* 2004; **170**: 377–82.

113. Rinaldo JE, Owens GR, Rogers RM. Adult respiratory distress syndrome following intrapleural instillation of talc. *J Thorac Cardiovasc Surg* 1983; **85**: 523–6.

114. Kennedy L, Rusch VW, Strange C, Ginsberg RJ, Sahn SA. Pleurodesis using talc slurry. *Chest* 1994; **106**: 342–6.

115. Rehse DH, Aye RW, Florence MG. Respiratory failure following talc pleurodesis. *Am J Surg* 1999; **177**: 437–40.

116. Brant A, Eaton T. Serious complications with talc slurry pleurodesis. *Respirology* 2001; **6**: 181–5.

117. Bondoc AYP, Bach P, Vander Els N. Talc pneumonitis: incidence, clinical features and outcome. *Chest* 1999; **116**: 358S–9S.

118. Dresler CM, Olak J, Herndon JE, *et al.* Phase III intergroup study of talc poudrage vs talc slurry sclerosis for malignant pleural effusion. *Chest* 2005; **127**: 909–15.

119. Nandy P. Recurrent spontaneous pneumothorax; an effective method of talc poudrage. *Chest* 1980; **77**: 493–5.

120. Todd TR, Delarue NC, Ilves R, Pearson FG, Cooper JD. Talc poudrage for malignant pleural effusion. *Chest* 1980; **78**: 542–3.

121. Bouchama A, Chastre J, Gaudichet A, Soler P, Gibert C. Acute pneumonitis with bilateral pleural effusion after talc pleurodesis. *Chest* 1984; **86**: 795–7.

122. Petrou M, Kaplan D, Goldstraw P. Management of recurrent malignant pleural effusions. The complementary role of talc pleurodesis and pleuroperitoneal shunting. *Cancer* 1995; **75**: 801–5.

123. Milanez JR, Werebe EC, Vargas FS, Jatene FB, Light RW. Respiratory failure due to insufflated talc. *Lancet* 1997; **349**: 251–2.

124. Milanez JR, Vargas FS, Werebe EC, *et al.* Thoracoscopy talc poudrage. A 15-year experience. *Chest* 2001; **119**: 801–6.

●125. Lee YCG, Baumann MH, Maskell NA, *et al.* Pleurodesis practice for malignant pleural effusions in five English-speaking countries. Survey of pulmonologists. *Chest* 2003; **124**: 2229–38.

126. Light RW, Vargas FS. Pleural sclerosis for the treatment of pneumothorax and pleural effusion. *Lung* 1997; **175**: 213–23.

◆127. Light RW. Diseases of the pleura: the use of talc for pleurodesis. *Curr Opin Pulm Med* 2000; **6**: 255–8.

128. Boutin C, Mathlouthi A, Espinasse P, *et al.* Perméabilité alvéolaire au cours des épanchements et aprés symphyse pleurale au talc. *Rev Fr Mal Respir* 1988; **5**: R125.

129. Viallat JR, Rey F, Astoul P, Boutin C. Thoracoscopic talc poudrage pleurodesis for malignant effusions: a review of 360 cases. *Chest* 1996; **110**: 1387–93.

130. Rodríguez-Panadero F. Current trends in pleurodesis. *Curr Opin Pulm Med* 1997; **3**: 319–25.

131. Werebe EC, Pazetti R, Milanez JR, *et al.* Systemic distribution of talc after intrapleural administration in rats. *Chest* 1999; **115**: 190–3.

132. Fraticelli A, Robaglia-Schlupp A, Riera H, *et al.* Distribution of calibrated talc after intrapleural administration. An experimental study in rats. *Chest* 2002; **122**: 1737–41.

11

Genetic alterations in mesothelioma pathogenesis

JOSEPH R TESTA, SURESH C JHANWAR

Malignant mesothelioma (MM) is a tumor of adult life that mostly affects individuals older than 50 years of age and occurs more commonly in men than in women.[1] Approximately 3000 patients are diagnosed with MM in the USA each year. MMs arise from serosal surfaces and are approximately four times more common in the pleural than in the peritoneal cavity. MM manifests as a diffuse or localized growth, with the former accounting for approximately 75 percent of all cases.[1] The increasing frequency of this disease over the last 40 years is a reflection of exposure to asbestos fibers in industrialized countries, particularly in connection with the mining and shipyard industries.[2] A history of asbestos exposure is associated with approximately 80 percent of the cases, and a lag phase of 20–40 years between exposure and tumor development is usual. In pleural MM, the first symptoms are typically dyspnea and chest pain, and radiological examination often reveals a pleural effusion. Cytological discrimination between MM, benign inflammatory or reactive effusions, and metastatic carcinoma is not always clear.[1] On the other hand, recurrent cytogenetic and molecular genetic abnormalities have been identified in MM, which can aid in discriminating neoplastic disease from benign mesothelioma. Besides asbestos, some evidence has implicated *Simian virus 40* (SV40) in the etiology of some MMs.[3,4] (See also Chapter 41, Malignant mesothelioma.)

In this chapter, we provide an overview of both cytogenetic and molecular genetic alterations in MM, mechanisms by which asbestos and other carcinogenic mineral fibers contribute to MM pathogenesis, and briefly discuss potential signaling pathways by which alterations of certain tumor suppressor genes (TSGs) play a role in the multistep tumorigenic process. We also discuss potential therapeutic approaches that target molecular alterations found in this disease.

MECHANISMS OF ASBESTOS CARCINOGENICITY

Whether asbestos fibers act directly on mesothelial cells or indirectly via induction of reactive oxygen species (ROS) and growth factors[5,6] is not fully understood. *In vitro* studies have demonstrated that asbestos can physically interact with the mitotic spindle apparatus, which could result in aneuploidy and other forms of chromosome damage.[7] *In vivo*, however, iron-rich crocidolite asbestos fibers may lead to the release of ROS when hydrogen peroxide and superoxide react to form hydroxyl radicals. Asbestos fibers induce expression and enzymatic activation of the mammalian DNA repair enzyme, apurinic/apyrimidinic endonuclease, suggesting that ROS generated by asbestos may produce DNA damage such as G to T transversions.[8] Recent evidence indicates that G to T transversions, often induced by the premutagenic DNA adduct 8-hydroxydeoxyguanosine, are among the most prevalent mutations detected following crocidolite treatment of omenta from lacI transgenic rats.[9] Moreover, the inflammatory response to asbestos leads to the generation of various cytokines responsible for the local and systemic immunosuppressive activity of asbestos.[10] In addition, asbestos can induce autophosphorylation of the epidermal growth factor (EGF) receptor, which results in increased expression of c-*fos* and c-*jun*, which encode transcription factors that activate genes critical in the initiation of DNA synthesis.[5] Induction of these transcription activators may enhance cellular proliferation and, thus, render cells more susceptible to subsequent mutations in TSGs. The enhanced expression of proto-oncogenes and inactivation of TSGs may cooperate in a multistep process leading to mesothelial cell oncogenesis.

In vivo, macrophages are known to phagocytose asbestos and, in response, release tumor necrosis factor alpha (TNF-α) and other cytokines that play a role in carcinogenesis through poorly understood mechanisms. *In vitro*, asbestos does not induce transformation of primary human mesothelial cells, but instead causes extensive cell death. Yang *et al.*[11] recently reported that asbestos induces the secretion of TNF-α and the expression of TNF-α receptor in primary human mesothelial cells.[11] TNF-α was found to activate nuclear factor (NF)-κB and that NF-κB activation led to resistance to the cytotoxic effects of asbestos. TNF-α/NF-κB signaling increased cell survival following asbestos exposure, permitting increased susceptibility of mesothelial cells to malignant transformation. Cytogenetics supported this hypothesis, showing only rare, aberrant metaphases in mesothelial cells exposed to asbestos and an increased mitotic rate with fewer irregular metaphases in mesothelial cells exposed to both TNF-α and asbestos. These data provide a mechanistic rationale for the paradoxical inability of asbestos to transform mesothelial cells *in vitro* and suggest that TNF-α plays a significant role in asbestos pathogenesis in humans.

RECURRENT CYTOGENETIC ABNORMALITIES

Conventional cytogenetic analysis of MMs, using chromosome banding techniques, has revealed that most MMs have complex karyotypes (reviewed in refs. 12 and 13). All of the 39 MMs we karyotyped (reviewed in ref. 14; A. Elahi and S.C. Jhanwar, unpublished data) displayed extensive aneuploidy and structural rearrangements of various chromosomes, particularly the short (p) arms of chromosomes 1, 3 and 9 and the long (q) arm of chromosome 6. Loss of a copy of chromosome 22 is the single most consistent numerical change seen in MMs. In some series, losses or rearrangements of chromosomes 4, 14 and 17 and gain of chromosome 7 have also been commonly observed. In the series by Taguchi *et al.*[14] and an additional 19 cases analyzed by A. Elahi and S.C. Jhanwar (unpublished data), deletions and unbalanced rearrangements accounted for overlapping losses from the chromosome region 1p21–22 in 32 of 39 (82 percent) cases. MMs also had interstitial deletions or other rearrangements that resulted in losses from 3p21. Twenty cases (51 percent) showed losses from 6q, with the shortest region of overlap (SRO) being 6q15–21. Losses involving 9p were observed in 31 (79 percent) cases, with the SRO being 9p21–22. Loss or relative deficiency of chromosome 17 was detected in 11 of 39 (28 percent) cases. Loss of a copy of chromosome 22 was documented in 26 cases (67 percent). These recurrent losses of 1p, 3p, 6q, 9p, 17 and 22 frequently occurred in combination in a given tumor. The complexity of the cytogenetic alterations observed suggest the emergence of tumor progression-associated changes. However, because cytogenetic data are lacking for early mesothelial lesions, it is not possible to distinguish between alterations associated with tumor initiation and those associated with progression of the disease. In any case, the accumulated loss of DNA sequences from chromosomes 1p, 3p, 6q, 9p, 17 and 22 appears to play a fundamental role in the pathogenesis of MM.

We also employed comparative genomic hybridization (CGH) analysis to detect recurrent genomic imbalances in MM. CGH is a DNA-based molecular cytogenetic technique that permits the identification of chromosome gains and losses in the entire tumor genome in a single experiment. We performed metaphase-based CGH analyses on 24 MM cell lines derived from American patients;[15] each of these cell lines exhibited multiple (6–25) genomic imbalances. Losses involving 22q were the most consistent change, being detected in 14 of 24 (58 percent) cell lines. The analyses also confirmed earlier conventional cytogenetic findings, with losses of 1p, 3p, 6q and 9p each being detected in approximately 30–40 percent of cell lines. Moreover, the CGH analysis uncovered other recurrent chromosome losses not detected by conventional cytogenetic studies. Especially noteworthy, 13 of 24 MMs (54 percent) showed losses of part or all of 15q, with the SRO being 15q11.1–21. Additionally, losses of 14q24.2-qter and 13q12–14 were each observed in 42 percent of the cell lines. The most common overrepresented chromosomal arm was 5p (54 percent of cases), suggesting the involvement of a putative oncogene(s) in this region.

Similar recurrent genomic imbalances were identified in MM specimens from Finland.[16] However, three prominent imbalances reported in the series from the USA, i.e. losses of 15q11.1–21.1, 8p21-pter and 3p21, were each observed in only one of 42 Finnish cases. Discrepancies between the data from Finland and the USA may reflect dissimilarities in the type of asbestos exposure or genetic differences in the study populations.

DELETION MAPPING OF RECURRENT CHROMOSOMAL LOSSES

The pattern of recurrent genomic losses observed in MMs is consistent with the possibility of a recessive mechanism of oncogenesis. The common sites of chromosomal loss are thought to represent the locations of putative TSGs that contribute to the development and/or progression of MM. As an initial approach to isolate these putative TSGs, the commonly deleted regions defined by cytogenetic studies of MM were mapped at the molecular genetic level by loss of heterozygosity (LOH) analysis using numerous polymorphic DNA markers. Results of these investigations have been reviewed in detail elsewhere[12,13] and are briefly summarized below.

Chromosome 1p22

In order to map the critically deleted segment of 1p, LOH analyses were performed on 50 MMs using a large panel of DNA markers distributed along the short arm of chromosome 1.[17] Allelic losses at 1p21–22 were observed in 36 cases (72 percent), and we were able to localize the SRO of deletions to a 4-centiMorgan (cM) region in 1p22. We ruled out the involvement of *BCL10*,[18,19] a gene located at 1p22 that encodes a protein containing an *N*-terminus caspase recruitment domain homologous to the motif found in several regulatory and effector apoptotic molecules. DNA analysis of other candidate TSGs in 1p22 have not revealed any mutations, although expression of several genes in this region are often downregulated in MM cells compared with that observed in normal mesothelial cells (JR Testa, unpublished data).

Chromosome 3p21

Two independent research groups demonstrated that 3p is a common site of allelic loss in MM.[20,21] For example, we detected LOH from 3p in 15 of 24 (63 percent) MMs, with the highest frequency of allelic loss being at 3p21.3. Losses from this region have also been reported in other forms of cancer, particularly lung tumors, suggesting that perturbation of a TSG(s) located at this site may play a role in the development of multiple tumor types. The nature of the TSG(s) located in this region is not known, although a homozygous deletion of the beta-catenin gene (*CTNNB1*), located at 3p21.3, has been reported in one MM cell line.[22] None of the remaining nine MM cell lines and tumor specimens examined showed deletions or aberrant expression of *CTNNB1*.

Chromosome 6q14–25

A LOH analysis of 6q in MMs has revealed a complex pattern of allelic loss.[23] LOH at 6q occurs in *c.* 60 percent of MMs, and deletions fall into several discrete regions including 6q14–21, 6q16.3–21, 6q21–23.2 and 6q25. Multiple non-overlapping regions of 6q loss have also been described in other types of cancer, such as non-Hodgkin's lymphoma.

Chromosome 9p21

We performed gene dosage studies on a series of MM cell lines, 83 percent of which showed homozygous or hemizygous deletions involving an approximately 1-megabase segment located between the interferon gene cluster and the marker D9S171 in 9p21.[24] The *CDKN2A/ARF* locus, which encodes the alternative TSG products $p16^{INK4a}$ and $p14^{ARF}$, is located within this region. The cellular function of $p16^{INK4a}$ and $p14^{ARF}$ and their potential role in MM pathogenesis are discussed below.

Chromosome 13q13.3–14.2

Some cytogenetic investigations of MM have revealed frequent losses in chromosomes 13 and 14. To define the SRO of deletions from these chromosomes, we performed LOH analyses on 30 MMs using 25 microsatellite markers in 13q and 21 markers in 14q.[25] Twenty of the 30 MMs (67 percent) showed allelic loss of at least one marker in 13q. The SRO of deletions was delineated as an approximately 7-cM region located at 13q13.3–14.2. Thirteen of the 30 MMs (43 percent) displayed allelic losses from 14q, with at least three distinct regions of LOH located at segments q11.2–13.2, q22.3–24.3 and q32.12. These data highlight a single region of chromosomal loss in 13q in many MMs, implicating the involvement of a TSG that is critical to the pathogenesis of this malignancy. In contrast, the lower incidence and diffuse pattern of allelic losses in 14q suggest that several TSGs in this chromosome arm may contribute to tumorigenic progression in some MMs.

Chromosome 15q15

Our CGH analyses demonstrated losses from 15q in 13 of 24 (54 percent) MM cell lines examined, and LOH analyses showed allelic losses from one or more 15q loci in 10 of these 13.[15] The SRO was located at 15q11.1–15. Losses overlapping this region have also been observed in other types of cancer, such as metastatic tumors of the breast, lung and colon, suggesting that this region harbors a TSG that may contribute to the progression of a variety of epithelial cancer types. In subsequent studies, we performed a high density LOH analysis of 15q in 46 MMs. These studies have defined a minimally deleted region of approximately 3cM, which was confirmed to reside at 15q15 by fluorescence *in situ* hybridization analysis with DNA probes known to map to this region.[25]

Chromosome regions 17p13 and 17q21.3–25

Preliminary studies have revealed abnormalities of 17p in 11 of 20 (55 percent) MM cell lines examined either by cytogenetics alone or in combination with RFLP analysis (S.C. Jhanwar, unpublished data). The abnormalities included either relative deficiency or rearrangements of 17p, as determined by cytogenetic analysis, or allelic loss. In addition, 14 of 20 (70 percent) cell lines also showed loss of alleles from 17q, eight (40 percent) of which sustained allelic losses from both arms, indicating that concurrent loss from both arms of chromosome 17 may be common in MM. The relative deficiencies of either 17p or whole chromosome 17 were not detected by CGH analysis; the reason for this appears to be that abnormalities of chromosome 17 arise by either uniparental disomy or trisomy, as determined by cytogenetic and restriction fragment length polymorphism (RFLP) analyses performed on the same specimens (SC Jhanwar and A Elahi, unpublished data).

Recurrent cytogenetic and molecular genetic abnormalities observed in MM are summarized in Table 11.1. A depiction of frequently deleted chromosomal regions and the location of TSGs known or potentially involved in MM is presented in Figure 11.1.

INVOLVEMENT OF TUMOR SUPPRESSOR GENES

p16^{INK4a}

One product of the *CDKN2A/ARF* locus, p16^{INK4a}, is capable of binding to and inhibiting the cyclin-dependent kinase CDK4. Shortly after being cloned, the *p16*^{INK4a} gene was identified as the 9p21 TSG, and homozygous deletions of *p16*^{INK4a} were detected at high frequencies in cell lines derived from various types of cancer.[26] To assess the possible involvement of *p16*^{INK4a} in MM, we performed deletion mapping studies of 40 MM cell lines;[27] 34 (85 percent) of the lines had homozygous deletions of one or more

Table 11.1 Summary of allelic losses and tumor suppressor genes associated with multistep tumorigenesis in human malignant mesothelioma

Chromosome region	Incidence of allelic loss[a] (%)	Tumor suppressor genes
1p22	72	–
3p21.3	63	–
6q14-25	60	–
9p21	83[b]	*p16*^{INK4a}, *p14*^{ARF}, *p15*^{INK4b}
13q13.2–14.2	67	–
15q15	48	–
17p13	40	*TP53*
17q21–25	70	–
22q12	72	*NF2*

[a]Percentages shown reflect incidence of allelic loss observed in mesothelioma cell lines examined by the authors. Note: each of these common sites of allelic loss was confirmed in a subset of cases for which corresponding tumor tissue was available.

[b]At the *p16*^{INK4a}/*p14*^{ARF} locus, 85 percent of cell lines exhibited homozygous losses, nearly all of which affected both *p16*^{INK4a} and *p14*^{ARF}; 78 percent of these cell lines also showed homozygous loss of *p15*^{INK4b}.

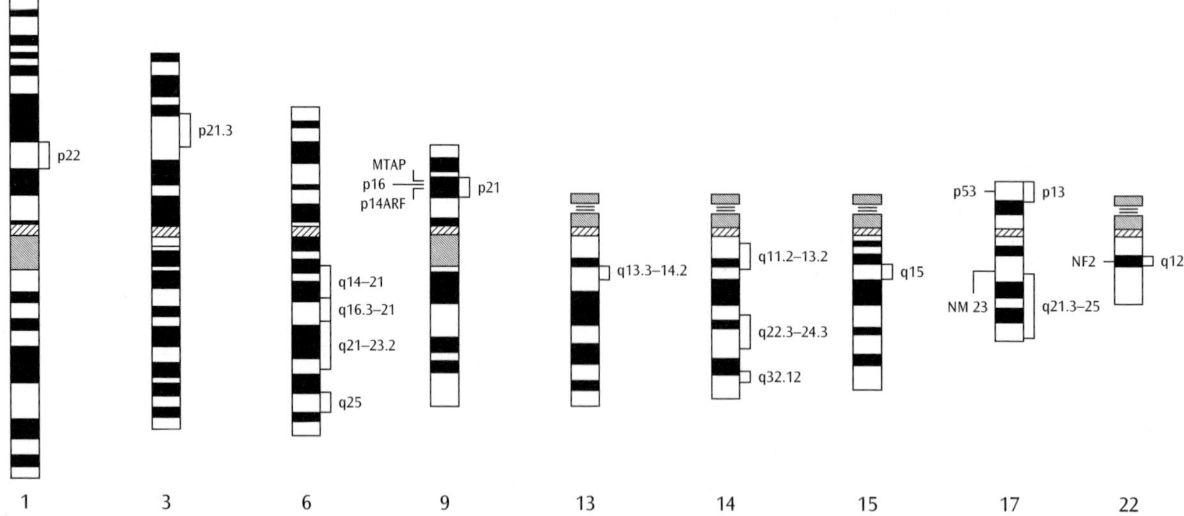

Figure 11.1 Idiograms of chromosomes frequently altered in malignant mesothelioma (MM), indicative of multistep tumorigenesis in this disease. Brackets demarcate minimally deleted regions (SROs) in each chromosome. Locations of TSGs (*p14*^{ARF}, *p16*^{INK4a}, *TP53* and *NF2*) known to be either mutated or homozygously deleted in MM are shown; other candidate genes (*MTAP*, *NM23*) are also indicated. (See also Color Plate 4.)

p16^{INK4a} exons and another had a point mutation in *p16^{INK4a}*. Downregulation of *p16^{INK4a}* was observed in four of the remaining cell lines. Homozygous deletions of *p16^{INK4a}* were identified in 5 of 23 (22 percent) MM tumor specimens. The higher frequency of *p16^{INK4a}* alterations in MM cell lines than in tumor samples may be associated with a selective growth advantage provided by *p16^{INK4a}* loss during cell culturing. On the other hand, MM samples often contain a significant amount of contaminating normal stroma, which can mask the existence of a homozygous deletion in the malignant cell population. Downregulation of *p16^{INK4a}* in MM cells may result from 5′CpG island hypermethylation, as has been observed in other kinds of cancer.[28] At the protein level, abnormal expression of *p16^{INK4a}* has been reported in 12 of 12 MM specimens and 15 of 15 MM-derived cell lines examined by immunohistochemistry.[29]

p14^{ARF}

In most cases, homozygous deletion of the *CDKN2A/ARF* locus also leads to inactivation of another putative TSG, *p14^{ARF}*, because *p16^{INK4a}* and *p14^{ARF}* share exons two and three, although their reading frames differ. p14^{ARF} is essential for the activation of p53 in response to the action of certain oncogene products such as Ras or Myc.[30] The *p16^{INK4a}* product, on the other hand, induces cell cycle arrest at the G1 phase by inhibiting the phosphorylation of the retinoblastoma protein, pRb. Therefore, homozygous loss of *p14^{ARF}* and *p16^{INK4a}* would collectively affect both p53- and pRb-dependent growth regulatory pathways, respectively. *CDKN2B* (*p15^{INK4b}*), another gene located near the *CDKN2A/ARF* locus, is also frequently deleted in human MMs,[31] although to date a critical role for *p15^{INK4b}* in MM has not been clearly defined.

The methylthioadenosine phosphorylase gene (*MTAP*) is also frequently co-deleted with the *CDKN2A/ARF* locus in MM. For example, in one study of 95 MM cases, 70 tumors showed homozygous deletions of *p16^{INK4a}*, 64 (91 percent) of which exhibited co-deletion of *MTAP*.[32] Whether loss of MTAP expression plays a fundamental role in MM pathogenesis is unknown at this time, but this enzyme may represent an interesting therapeutic target (see below).

TP53

While loss of p14^{ARF} is frequently observed in MM, mutations of the p53 gene (*TP53*) are less commonly reported in this malignancy.[33–35] *TP53* is located at chromosome 17p13, and loss or relative deficiency of the short arm of chromosome 17 is a recurrent change in MM. Immunohistochemical staining of p53 protein in MM cell lines was performed by one of us (SCJ). Mutant p53 protein was detected in a significant percentage (>50 percent) of cells by immunohistochemistry in 8 of 20 (40 percent) cell lines examined.

While the *TP53* gene is associated with 17p loss, the putative TSG involved in 17q losses in MM is not known. The human nm23 gene (*NME1*), located at 17q21.3, represents one candidate gene in this region. Reduced expression of nm23 is associated with a high potential for metastasis in some tumor types. In MM, we have detected LOH at the *NME1* locus in 8 of 20 (40 percent) cell lines, four of which also showed downregulated expression compared with control mesothelial cells (SC Jhanwar, unpublished data).

NF2

As noted earlier, numerical loss of a copy of chromosome 22 is a frequent occurrence in MM. Although germline mutations of the neurofibromatosis type 2 TSG, *NF2*, predispose affected individuals to tumors of neuroectodermal origin, somatic mutations of *NF2* have occasionally been identified in seemingly unrelated malignancies.[36] Therefore, two groups independently embarked on mutational studies of *NF2* in MM. We identified nucleotide mutations in 8 of 15 (53 percent) MM cell lines.[37] The mutations, which included deletions and insertions and one nonsense mutation, predicted truncated forms of the NF2 protein, known as merlin or schwannomin. Similarly, Sekido and colleagues[38] detected somatic mutations in one MM specimen and in 7 of 17 (41 percent) MM cell lines. In our study, the mutations observed in cDNAs from MM cell lines were confirmed in genomic DNA from six matched primary tumor specimens.[37] The two cDNA alterations that could not be confirmed by genomic analysis were both splicing related: i.e., deletion of exon 10 in one cell line, and a 43-bp insertion between exons 13 and 14 in the other.

In a follow-up investigation, mutations in the *NF2* coding region were detected in 12 of 23 (52 percent) additional MM cell lines.[39] Western blot analyses revealed loss of merlin expression in each of the 12 cell lines having alterations of the *NF2* gene. In addition, two cell lines with *NF2* mutations reported in an earlier study were also examined, both of which lacked NF2 expression. LOH analyses were performed on the entire 25 MM cell lines using two polymorphic DNA markers residing at or near the *NF2* locus in chromosome 22q12. Eighteen of the 25 cell lines showed losses at one or both of these loci. All cases exhibiting mutation and aberrant expression of NF2 displayed LOH, consistent with bi-allelic inactivation of NF2 in MM.

Merlin exhibits significant homology to the ezrin–radixin–moesin (ERM) family of proteins known to play a role in cell surface dynamics by linking the cytoskeleton to components of the cell membrane. However, the mechanisms by which merlin exerts its tumor suppressor activity are incompletely understood. One mechanism involves the inhibition of cellular proliferation by repressing cyclin D1 expression.[40] Thus, we found that adenovirus-mediated expression of merlin in *NF2*-deficient MM cells led to cell cycle arrest at G1 phase, concomitant with decreased expression of cyclin D1, inhibition of CDK4 activity, and dephosphorylation of pRB. The effect of merlin on cell cycle progression was partially overridden by ectopic expression of cyclin D1. RNA interference experiments with *NF2*-positive cells showed that silencing of the endogenous *NF2* gene results in up-regulation of cyclin D1 and S-phase entry.

Because Rho GTPase-mediated signaling phosphorylates ERM proteins, we and others tested whether merlin is also regulated by members of the Rho family of GTPases. These investigations showed that merlin is phosphorylated in response to expression of activated Rac and activated Cdc42.[41,42] Furthermore, we demonstrated that merlin phosphorylation is mediated by p21-activated kinase (Pak), a common downstream target of both Rac and Cdc42.[42] Various kinase assays demonstrated that Pak can directly phosphorylate merlin at serine 518, a site that affects merlin activity and localization. In other experiments, we found that Pak1-stimulated cyclin D1 promoter activity was repressed by co-transfection of *NF2*, and Pak activity was inhibited by expression of merlin.[40] Interestingly, a S518A mutant form of merlin, which is refractory to phosphorylation by Pak, was more efficient than the wild-type protein in inhibiting cell cycle progression and in repressing cyclin D1 promoter activity. Collectively, our data indicate that merlin exerts its antiproliferative effect, at least in part, via repression of Pak-induced cyclin D1 expression.

Other data indicate that merlin and Pak participate in a feedback loop, because merlin has been shown to inhibit activation of Pak1.[43,44] Thus, loss of merlin expression results in the inappropriate activation of Pak1, whereas overexpression of merlin in cells with high basal activity of Pak1 inhibited Pak1 activation. Merlin's inhibitory function is mediated by impeding Pak1 recruitment to focal adhesions.[43]

Importantly, Pak has been shown to regulate motility in mammalian cells,[45] which raised the intriguing possibility that merlin loss of function may contribute to invasiveness and/or metastasis in MM. We recently showed that re-expression of merlin in *NF2*-null MM cells inhibits invasiveness and negatively regulates focal adhesion kinase (FAK).[46] Re-expression of merlin markedly inhibited cell motility, spreading and invasiveness, properties connected with the malignant phenotype of MM cells. To test directly whether merlin inactivation promotes invasion in a non-malignant system, we used small interfering RNA to silence *Nf2* in mouse embryonic fibroblasts (MEFs) and found that downregulation of merlin resulted in enhanced cell spreading and invasion. To delineate signaling events connected with this phenotype, we investigated the effect of merlin expression on FAK, a key component of cellular pathways affecting migration and invasion. Expression of merlin attenuated FAK phosphorylation at the critical phosphorylation site Tyr397 and disrupted the interaction of FAK with its binding partners Src and p85, the regulatory subunit of phosphatidylinositol-3-kinase (PI3K). In addition, *NF2*-null MM cells stably overexpressing FAK showed increased invasiveness, which decreased significantly when merlin expression was restored. Altogether, these findings suggest that merlin inactivation is a critical step in MM pathogenesis and is related, at least in part, with upregulation of FAK activity.

Recently, merlin has also been shown to suppress cellular proliferation by inhibiting the activation of the small G-protein Ras.[47] Merlin was found to counteract the ERM-dependent activation of Ras, which correlated with the formation of a complex comprising ERM proteins, Grb2, SOS, Ras and filamentous actin. Thus, part of the tumor suppressor function of merlin appears to be its interference with Ras- and Rac-dependent oncogenic signaling.

Merlin has also been shown to interact with Ral guanine nucleotide dissociation stimulator (RalGDS), a downstream molecule of Ras, and to inhibit its activity.[48] Functional studies revealed that merlin inhibits RalGDS-induced RalA activation, colony formation and cell migration in mammalian cells.

AN *NF2* MOUSE MODEL RECAPITULATING MOLECULAR FEATURES OF HUMAN MALIGNANT MESOTHELIOMA

To better understand the significance of *NF2* inactivation in MM and identify tumor suppressor gene alterations that cooperate with NF2 loss of function in MM pathogenesis, we treated *Nf2*(+/−) knockout mice with asbestos to induce MMs.[31] Asbestos-exposed *Nf2*(+/−) mice exhibited markedly accelerated MM tumor formation compared with asbestos-treated wild-type littermates. Loss of the wild-type *Nf2* allele, leading to bi-allelic inactivation, was observed in all nine asbestos-induced MMs from *Nf2*(+/−) mice and in 50 percent of MMs from asbestos-exposed wild-type mice. For a detailed comparison with the murine model, DNA analyses were also carried out on a series of human MM samples. Remarkably, similar to human MM, tumors from *Nf2*(+/−) mice showed frequent homologous deletions of the *Cdkn2a/Arf* locus and adjacent *Cdkn2b* tumor suppressor gene, as well as reciprocal inactivation of the p53 gene, *Tp53*, in a subset of tumors that retained the *Arf* locus. As in the human disease counterpart, MMs from *Nf2*(+/−) mice also showed frequent activation of Akt kinase, which plays a central role in tumorigenesis and therapeutic resistance. Thus, this murine model of environmental carcinogenesis faithfully recapitulated many of the molecular features of human MM and has significant implications for the further characterization of MM pathogenesis and preclinical testing of novel therapeutic drugs.

AKT/Akt KINASE ACTIVATION IN MALIGNANT MESOTHELIOMA

The PI3K/AKT pathway has been implicated in tumor aggressiveness, in part by mediating cell survival and reducing sensitivity to chemotherapy. Using antibodies recognizing the phosphorylated (active) form of AKT, we observed elevated phospho-AKT staining in 17 of 26 (65 percent) human MM specimens.[49] In addition, AKT phosphorylation was repeatedly observed in MMs arising in asbestos-treated mice and in xenografts of human MM cells. Consistent with reports implicating hepatocyte growth factor (HGF)/Met receptor signaling in MM, all 14 human and murine MM cell lines had HGF-inducible AKT activity. One of nine human MM cell lines had elevated AKT activity under serum-starvation conditions, which was connected with a homozygous deletion of *PTEN*. Treatment of this cell line with the mTOR inhibitor rapamycin resulted in growth arrest in G1 phase. Treatment of MM cells with the PI3K inhibitor LY294002 in combination with cisplatin had greater efficacy in inhibiting cell proliferation and inducing apoptosis than either agent alone. Taken together, these findings indicate that both human and murine MMs frequently express elevated AKT activity, which may be targeted pharmacologically to enhance chemotherapeutic efficacy.

ERIONITE AND POSSIBLE GENETIC PREDISPOSITION TO MALIGNANT MESOTHELIOMA

In the small villages of Karain, Tuzkoy and 'Old' Sarihidir in Cappadocia, a region in Central Anatolya, Turkey, characterized by volcanic tuffs and natural caves, nearly 50 percent of deaths are caused by MM. This extremely high incidence of MM is associated with exposure to erionite, a form of zeolite that causes MM in rodents.[50,51] However, houses in the nearby village of Karlik were built with the same type of stones, yet no MMs were observed. Moreover, in Karain and Tuzkoy, cancer occurred mostly in certain houses where entire families had succumbed to MM. The amount of erionite in stone samples from these houses was found to be comparable to that of other houses in MM or non-MM villages, suggesting the possible involvement of a genetic susceptibility factor.[51,52] Pedigree analysis suggested that MM was genetically transmitted, possibly as an autosomal dominant disease.[52] Approximately 50 percent of the descendents of affected parents developed MM, whereas MM was absent in other families. When members of unaffected families married into affected families, MM appeared in their descendents.[52] The X-ray diffraction pattern and crystal structure of erionite did not appear to differ in households with high or no incidence of MM.[53] Thus, it appears that in Karain, Tuzkoy and 'Old' Sarihidir, MM is genetically transmitted and that erionite is a cofactor. The isolation of the putative MM susceptibility gene could lead to the development of therapeutic approaches for members of these families. Moreover, it is possible that the same gene may be a target in sporadic MMs associated with exposure to asbestos and, thus, the eventual isolation of this gene might enhance our understanding of molecular mechanisms involved in the pathogenesis of MM generally.

POTENTIAL THERAPEUTIC TARGETS IN MALIGNANT MESOTHELIOMA

During the last three decades, much has been learned about the genetic alterations associated with various cancers. This has led to the realization that the same genetic changes involved in the development of a particular cancer may also serve as markers of disease susceptibility, initiation and progression. In addition, some of these alterations have also provided a genetic basis for targeted therapy. It is only in recent years that scientists have begun to utilize this information with reasonable success to develop clinical trials to treat some of the cancers refractory to standard therapies (see also Chapter 41, Malignant mesothelioma).

Considering the fact that the initial clinical presentation of MM is localized only to the pleural or peritoneal cavity[1] and that there is a lack of any effective treatment for this lethal disease,[54] in theory, gene replacement therapy in MM is an attractive option. In order to achieve success, however, it will be necessary to overcome various impediments to gene therapy.[55] If obstacles such as toxicity and delivery can be effectively addressed, molecularly-based therapies could become practical.

As an initial approach to developing and testing such therapy, investigators have utilized MM cell lines that have sustained complete loss of a TSG to determine if the transfer of a normal copy of that gene inhibits growth and restores other biological features of normal mesothelial cells. For example, it has been shown that adenovirus-mediated gene transfer of $p16^{INK4a}$ in MM cells results in cell-cycle arrest and cell death, as well as tumor suppression and regression.[54] Similarly, adenovirus-mediated replacement of $p14^{ARF}$ in MM cell lines restored p53 function, inducing cell cycle arrest in G1 phase and cell death.[56] We have utilized retroviral vectors and adenovirus to re-express the *NF2* gene in MM cell lines, and various experiments outlined above have shown that restoring expression of merlin results in an altered cell phenotype and tumor suppression.[41]

The chemotherapeutic drug L-alanosine, a strong inhibitor of *de novo* AMP synthesis, has been used in various clinical trials to treat patients with leukemia and various solid tumors. It has been suggested that this drug is particularly effective in selectively killing tumor cells deficient in methythioadenosine phosphorylase (MTAP), an important enzyme for the salvage of adenine and methionine.[57] Furthermore, it has been demonstrated that

MTAP-deficient cells are highly sensitive to L-alanosine treatment (reviewed in reference 57). It is, therefore, not unreasonable to propose that MMs with homozygous deletion of 9p21 encompassing *MTAP* may be candidates for such a therapeutic choice along with conventional therapies employed to treat MMs.

As discussed earlier, NF2 has been shown to directly inhibit Pak1, which is thought to be essential for Ras transformation. Furthermore, certain Pak1 inhibitors are known to selectively inhibit the growth of *NF2*-null cancer cells, but not *NF2*-positive cells.[44] These results suggest that Pak1-specific blocking drugs could potentially be useful for the treatment of *NF2*-deficient MM. Moreover, the frequent activation of AKT signaling observed in human MMs suggests that this pathway could represent an attractive therapeutic target for the treatment of this highly aggressive form of cancer. Importantly, numerous groups are attempting to identify specific chemical inhibitors of proteins implicated in MM tumorigenesis, such as Pak and AKT, by high throughput screening of unbiased chemical libraries. The identification of such lead compounds is likely to provide biologically meaningful approaches for novel targeted therapeutic strategies. Moreover, the fact that TNF-α inhibits asbestos-induced cytotoxicity via a NF-κB-dependent survival pathway (see also Chapter 8, Immunology) suggests that TNF-α/NF-κB may also serve as targets for chemoprevention in high-risk groups, such as asbestos workers or Cappadocian villagers exposed to erionite.

CONCLUSIONS

Multiple genetic changes are involved in the development of most cancers. Asbestos is known to cause genetic damage. In a normal cell, mitosis is controlled through a delicate balance of phosphorylation and dephosphorylation events. Autophosphorylation of the EGF receptor results in phosphorylation of MEK1 kinase, which in turn phosphorylates ERK (MAP kinases). The activation of these kinases causes activation of other intermediaries, and this in turn stimulates c-fos and c-jun and other members of the AP-1 family and induces cell division.[5] Downregulation of AP-1 activity is achieved through the phosphatase PP2A, which dephosphorylates MAP kinases. Asbestos, working through this mechanism, may induce tumor formation. Asbestos can induce both DNA damage and autophosphorylation of the EGF receptor, which eventually leads to AP-1 expression and cell division.[58] As a result of inactivation of p53, mutations caused by asbestos would not undergo repair at the G1/S checkpoint mediated by p53 through p21. While most DNA alterations will either be of no significance or lead to cell death, a few cells could potentially develop perturbations of key cell cycle regulatory genes,[12] become immortalized and tumorigenic. Evidence in support of this notion comes from experiments with p53 knockout mice, in which p53-deficient animals were shown to be more susceptible to asbestos-induced MMs than wild-type mice.[59]

In summary, there is now a large body of experimental and epidemiological data in support of the assertion that asbestos, or at least amphibole asbestos, causes MM. These data also suggest that exposure to asbestos is usually not sufficient for MM development and that other factors, such as genetic predisposition, may render some individuals more susceptible to asbestos carcinogenicity. Cytogenetic and molecular genetic studies indicate that MM results from the accumulation of numerous somatic genetic events, mainly deletions, suggesting a multistep cascade involving the inactivation of multiple TSGs. To date, several TSGs have been shown to be frequently altered in MMs, and their disruption would be expected to have profound consequences on the growth and behavior of a mesothelial cell. The identification of all of the critical somatic genetic alterations in MM and understanding how each of them contributes to the pathogenesis of this malignancy may ultimately lead to the design of more effective therapeutic strategies.

KEY POINTS

- Cytogenetic analysis has revealed that most human mesotheliomas have complex karyotypes, with the accumulation of extensive aneuploidy and structural rearrangements of multiple chromosomes.
- Despite the great genomic disarray seen in mesotheliomas, a number of recurrent genomic imbalances are found, including deletions of the short (p) arms of chromosomes 1, 3 and 9 and the long (q) arms of chromosomes 6, 13 and 15. Loss of a copy of chromosome 22 is the most common numerical change. Losses of chromosomes 4 and 17 and gains of chromosome 7 and 5p have also been reported in some series.
- Deletion mapping studies have identified a set of commonly deleted sites in several different chromosomes. These sites are thought to represent the locations of putative tumor suppressor genes that contribute to the development and/or progression of mesothelioma.
- Frequent homozygous deletions of chromosome band 9p21 target a set of tumor suppressor genes located there, including the *CDKN2A/ARF* locus, which encodes $p16^{INK4a}$ and $p14^{ARF}$. Inactivation of $p14^{ARF}$ and $p16^{INK4a}$ would collectively disrupt both p53- and pRb-dependent growth regulatory pathways, respectively. The tumor suppressor genes *CDKN2B*, encoding $p15^{INK4b}$, is often co-deleted with the *CDKN2A/ARF* locus in mesotheliomas.

- Biallelic inactivation of the *NF2* tumor suppressor gene, located in chromosome 22q, occurs in approximately 50 percent of mesotheliomas. Inactivation of *NF2* results in increased cell proliferation by promoting Pak-induced cyclin D1. *NF2* inactivation also enhances tumor cell spreading and invasion by augmenting focal adhesion kinase (FAK) activity, suggesting that loss of merlin function is a critical step in the pathogenesis of mesothelioma.
- *Nf2*(+/−) knockout mice treated with asbestos show accelerated formation of mesotheliomas compared with wild-type mice, and the tumors in *Nf2* knockout mice faithfully recapitulate many of the same molecular genetic and signaling perturbations observed in human mesothelioma. Thus, this murine model has significant implications for preclinical testing of novel therapeutic drugs.
- Genetic predisposition may render some individuals more susceptible to mineral fiber carcinogenicity.

ACKNOWLEDGMENTS

This work was supported by NIH grants CA 45745, PO1 CA114047 and CA 06927, and by a gift from the Local 14 Mesothelioma Fund of the International Association of Heat and Frost Insulators and Asbestos Workers, in memory of Hank Vaughan and Alice Haas (to JRT).

REFERENCES

● = Key primary paper
◆ = Major review article

◆1. Antman KH, Pass HI, Schiff PB. Management of mesothelioma. In: DeVita VT, Jr., Hellman S, Rosenberg SA, (eds). *Principles and practice of oncology*, 6th edn. Philadelphia: Lippincott Williams & Wilkins; 2001: 1943–69.

●2. Craighead JE, Mossman BT. The pathogenesis of asbestos-associated diseases. *N Engl J Med.* 1982; **306**: 1446–55.

3. Butel JS, Lednicky JA. Cell and molecular biology of simian virus 40: implications for human infections and disease. *J Natl Cancer Inst.* 1999; **91**: 119–34.

4. Carbone M, Fisher S, Powers A, *et al.* New molecular and epidemiological issues in mesothelioma: role of SV40. *J Cell Physiol* 1999; **180**: 167–72.

5. Mossman BT, Kamp DW, Weitzman SA. Mechanisms of carcinogenesis and clinical features of asbestos-associated cancers. *Cancer Invest* 1996; **14**: 466–80.

6. Pache JC, Janssen YM, Walsh ES, *et al.* Increased epidermal growth factor-receptor protein in a human mesothelial cell line in response to long asbestos fibers. *Am J Pathol* 1998; **152**: 333–40.

7. Ault JG, Cole RW, Jensen CG, *et al.* Behavior of crocidolite asbestos during mitosis in living vertebrate lung epithelial cells. *Cancer Res* 1995; **55**: 792–8.

8. Fung H, Kow YW, Van Houten B, *et al.* Asbestos increases mammalian AP-endonuclease gene expression, protein levels, and enzyme activity in mesothelial cells. *Cancer Res* 1998; **58**: 189–94.

9. Unfried K, Schurkes C, Abel J. Distinct spectrum of mutations induced by crocidolite asbestos: clue for 8-hydroxydeoxyguanosine-dependent mutagenesis *in vivo*. *Cancer Res* 2002; **62**: 99–104.

10. Rosenthal GJ, Simeonova P, Corsini E. Asbestos toxicity: an immunologic perspective. *Rev Environ Health* 1999; **14**: 11–20.

●11. Yang H, Bocchetta M, Kroczynska B, *et al.* TNF-alpha inhibits asbestos-induced cytotoxicity via a NF-kappaB-dependent pathway, a possible mechanism for asbestos-induced oncogenesis. *Proc Natl Acad Sci U S A* 2006; **103**: 10397–402.

12. Murthy SS, Testa JR. Asbestos, chromosomal deletions, and tumor suppressor gene alterations in human malignant mesothelioma. *J Cell Physiol* 1999; **180**: 150–7.

13. Testa JR, Pass HI, Carbone M. Molecular biology of mesothelioma. In: DeVita VT, Jr., Hellman S, Rosenberg SA (eds). *Principles and practice of oncology*, 6th edn. Philadelphia: Lippincott Williams & Wilkins; 2001: 1937–43.

14. Taguchi T, Jhanwar SC, Siegfried JM, *et al.* Recurrent deletions of specific chromosomal sites in 1p, 3p, 6q, and 9p in human malignant mesothelioma. *Cancer Res* 1993; **53**: 4349–55.

15. Balsara BR, Bell DW, Sonoda G, *et al.* Comparative genomic hybridization and loss of heterozygosity analyses identify a common region of deletion at 15q11.1-15 in human malignant mesothelioma. *Cancer Res* 1999; **59**: 450–4.

16. Bjorkqvist AM, Tammilehto L, Anttila S, *et al.* Recurrent DNA copy number changes in 1q, 4q, 6q, 9p, 13q, 14q and 22q detected by comparative genomic hybridization in malignant mesothelioma. *Br J Cancer* 1997; **75**: 523–7.

17. Lee W-C, Balsara B, Liu Z, *et al.* Loss of heterozygosity analysis defines a critical region in chromosome 1p22 commonly deleted in human malignant mesothelioma. *Cancer Res* 1996; **56**: 4297–301.

18. Apostolou S, De Rienzo A, Murthy SS, *et al.* Absence of *BCL10* mutations in human malignant mesothelioma. *Cell* 1999; **97**: 684–6.

19. Apostolou S, Murthy SS, Kolachana P, *et al.* Absence of post-transcriptional RNA modifications of BCL10 in human malignant mesothelioma and colorectal cancer. *Genes, Chromosomes Cancer* 2001; **30**: 96–8.

20. Lu YY, Jhanwar SC, Cheng JQ, Testa JR. Deletion mapping of the short arm of chromosome 3 in human malignant mesothelioma. *Genes Chromosomes Cancer* 1994; **9**: 76–80.

21. Zeiger MA, Gnarra JR, Zbar B, *et al.* Loss of heterozygosity on the short arm of chromosome 3 in mesothelioma cell lines and solid tumors. *Genes Chromosomes Cancer* 1994; **11**: 15–20.

22. Shigemitsu K, Sekido Y, Usami N, *et al.* Genetic alteration of the beta-catenin gene (CTNNB1) in human lung cancer and malignant mesothelioma and identification of a new 3p21.3 homozygous deletion. *Oncogene* 2001; **20**: 4249–57.

23. Bell DW, Jhanwar SC, Testa JR. Multiple regions of allelic loss from chromosome arm 6q in malignant mesothelioma. *Cancer Res* 1997; **57**: 4057–62.

24. Cheng JQ, Jhanwar SC, Lu YY, Testa JR. Homozygous deletions within 9p21-p22 identify a small critical region of chromosomal loss in human malignant mesothelioma. *Cancer Res* 1993; **53**: 4761–3.

25. De Rienzo A, Balsara BR, Apostolou S, *et al.* Loss of heterozygosity analysis defines a 3-cM region of 15q commonly deleted in human malignant mesothelioma. *Oncogene* 2001; **20**: 6245–9.

●26. Kamb A, Gruis NA, Weaver-Feldhaus J, *et al.* A cell cycle regulator potentially involved in genesis of many tumor types. *Science* 1994; **264**: 436–40.

●27. Cheng JQ, Jhanwar SC, Klein WM, *et al.* *p16* alterations and deletion mapping of 9p21-p22 in malignant mesothelioma. *Cancer Res* 1994; **54**: 5547–51.

28. Merlo A, Herman JG, Mao L, *et al.* 5′ CpG island methylation is associated with transcriptional silencing of the tumour suppressor p16/CDKN2/MTS1 in human cancers. *Nat Med* 1995; **1**: 686–92.
●29. Kratzke RA, Otterson GA, Lincoln CE, *et al.* Immunohistochemical analysis of the p16INK4 cyclin-dependent kinase inhibitor in malignant mesothelioma. *J Natl Cancer Inst* 1995; **87**: 1870–5.
30. Palmero I, Pantoja C, Serrano M. p19ARF links the tumour suppressor p53 to Ras. *Nature* 1998; **395**: 125–6.
●31. Altomare DA, Vaslet CA, Skele KL, *et al.* A mouse model recapitulating molecular features of human mesothelioma. *Cancer Res* 2005; **65**: 8090–5.
32. Illei PB, Rusch VW, Zakowski MF, Ladanyi M. Homozygous deletion of CDKN2A and codeletion of the methylthioadenosine phosphorylase gene in the majority of pleural mesotheliomas. *Clin Cancer Res* 2003; **9**: 2108–13.
33. Cote RJ, Jhanwar SC, Novick S, Pellicer A. Genetic alterations of the p53 gene are a feature of malignant mesothelioma. *Cancer Res* 1991; **51**: 5410–6.
34. Metcalf RA, Welsh JA, Bennett WP, *et al.* p53 and Kirstein-*ras* mutations in human mesothelioma cell lines. *Cancer Res* 1992; **52**: 2610–5.
35. Mor O, Yaron P, Huszar M, *et al.* Absence of p53 mutation in malignant mesothelioma. *Am J Respir Cell Mol Biol.* 1997; **16**: 9–13.
●36. Bianchi AB, Hara T, Ramesh V, *et al.* Mutations in transcript isoforms of the neurofibromatosis 2 gene in multiple human tumour types. *Nat Genet* 1994; **6**: 185–92.
●37. Bianchi AB, Mitsunaga S-I, Cheng JQ, *et al.* High frequency of inactivating mutations in the neurofibromatosis type 2 gene (*NF2*) in primary malignant mesotheliomas. *Proc Natl Acad Sci U S A* 1995; **92**: 10854–8.
38. Sekido Y, Pass HI, Bader S, *et al.* Neurofibromatosis type 2 (*NF2*) gene is somatically mutated in mesothelioma but not in lung cancer. *Cancer Res* 1995; **55**: 1227–31.
39. Cheng JQ, Lee WC, Klein MA, *et al.* Frequent mutations of NF2 and allelic loss from chromosome band 22q12 in malignant mesothelioma: evidence for a two-hit mechanism of NF2 inactivation. *Genes Chromosomes Cancer* 1999; **24**: 238–42.
●40. Xiao GH, Gallagher R, Shetler J, *et al.* The NF2 tumor suppressor gene product, merlin, inhibits cell proliferation and cell cycle progression by repressing Rac-induced cyclin D1 expression. *Mol Cell Biol* 2005; **25**: 2384–94.
●41. Shaw RJ, Paez JG, Curto M, *et al.* The Nf2 tumor suppressor, merlin, functions in Rac-dependent signaling. *Dev Cell* 2001; **1**: 63–72.
●42. Xiao GH, Beeser A, Chernoff J, Testa JR. p21-activated kinase links Rac/Cdc42 signaling to merlin. *J Biol Chem* 2002; **277**: 883–6.
●43. Kissil JL, Wilker EW, Johnson KC, *et al.* Merlin, the product of the Nf2 tumor suppressor gene, is an inhibitor of the p21-activated kinase, Pak1. *Mol Cell* 2003; **12**: 841–9.
44. Hirokawa Y, Tikoo A, Huynh J, *et al.* A clue to the therapy of neurofibromatosis type 2: NF2/merlin is a PAK1 inhibitor. *Cancer J* 2004; **10**: 20–6.
45. Sells MA, Boyd JT, Chernoff J. p21-activated kinase 1 (Pak1) regulates cell motility in mammalian fibroblasts. *J Cell Biol* 1999; **145**: 837–49.
46. Poulikakos PI, Xiao GH, Gallagher R, *et al.* Re-expression of the tumor suppressor NF2/merlin inhibits invasiveness in mesothelioma cells and negatively regulates FAK. *Oncogene* 2006; **25**: 5960–8.
●47. Morrison H, Sperka T, Manent J, *et al.* Merlin/neurofibromatosis type 2 suppresses growth by inhibiting the activation of Ras and Rac. *Cancer Res* 2007; **67**: 520–7.
48. Ryu CH, Kim SW, Lee KH, *et al.* The merlin tumor suppressor interacts with Ral guanine nucleotide dissociation stimulator and inhibits its activity. *Oncogene* 2005; **24**: 5355–64.
49. Altomare DA, Wang HQ, Skele KL, *et al.* AKT and mTOR phosphorylation is frequently detected in ovarian cancer and can be targeted to disrupt ovarian tumor cell growth. *Oncogene* 2004; **23**: 5853–7.
50. Baris B, Demir AU, Shehu V, *et al.* Environmental fibrous zeolite (erionite) exposure and malignant tumors other than mesothelioma. *J Environ Pathol Toxicol Oncol* 1996; **15**: 183–9.
◆51. Carbone M, Kratzke RA, Testa JR. The pathogenesis of mesothelioma. *Semin Oncol* 2002; **29**: 2–17.
●52. Roushdy-Hammady I, Siegel J, Emri S, *et al.* Genetic-susceptibility factor and malignant mesothelioma in the Cappadocian region of Turkey. *Lancet* 2001; **357**: 444–5.
53. Dogan AU, Baris YI, Dogan M, *et al.* Genetic predisposition to fiber carcinogenesis causes a mesothelioma epidemic in Turkey. *Cancer Res* 2006; **66**: 5063–8.
●54. Frizelle SP, Grim J, Zhou J, *et al.* Re-expression of p16INK4a in mesothelioma cells results in cell cycle arrest, cell death, tumor suppression and tumor regression. *Oncogene* 1998; **16**: 3087–95.
55. Blaese RM. Gene therapy for cancer. *Sci Am* 1997; **276**: 111–15.
56. Yang CT, You L, Yeh CC, *et al.* Adenovirus-mediated p14(ARF) gene transfer in human mesothelioma cells. *J Natl Cancer Inst* 2000; **92**: 636–41.
57. Batova A, Diccianni MB, Omura-Minamisawa M, *et al.* Use of alanosine as a methylthioadenosine phosphorylase-selective therapy for T-cell acute lymphoblastic leukemia *in vitro. Cancer Res* 1999; **59**: 1492–7.
◆58. Robledo R, Mossman B. Cellular and molecular mechanisms of asbestos-induced fibrosis. *J Cell Physiol* 1999; **180**: 158–66.
59. Marsella JM, Liu BL, Vaslet CA, Kane AB. Susceptibility of *p53*-deficient mice to induction of mesothelioma by crocidolite asbestos fibers. *Environ Health Perspect* 1997; **105**: 1069–72.

12

Proteomics in pleural disease

JOOST HEGMANS, BART LAMBRECHT

PROTEOMICS AND ITS COMPLEXITY

Each cell produces thousands of proteins, each with a specific function. Some proteins are expressed at very low levels, a few copies per cell, while others such as housekeeping gene products are extremely abundant. They may be expressed during short periods during the life of an individual, for example during embryonic development, while others may be continually expressed but with very short half lives. The collection of proteins in a cell is known as the proteome, and, unlike the genome which is constant irrespective of cell type, it differs from cell to cell and is constantly changing through its biochemical interactions with the genome and the environment (Figure 12.1). It changes from moment to moment in response to tens of thousands of intra- and extra-cellular environmental signals, such as other proteins, pH, hypoxia and drug administration, and changes continuously during multigenic processes such as ageing, stress or disease. Proteomics consists not only of the identification and quantification of proteins but also involves the comprehensive study of their structure, localization, modification, interactions, activities and function of all proteins in body fluids, tissues or cell types under given conditions.[1] Proteomics is relatively more challenging than genomics because a single gene can give rise to multiple protein products through alternative splicing, proteolysis of proteins and post-translational modifications (20 000–25 000 different genes versus approximately 1 000 000 different proteins).[2,3] Currently there are more than 300 different types of post-translational modifications known, and new ones are regularly discovered.[4,5] They are often transient and occur *in vivo* only in a small fraction of proteins (<1 percent) and include glycosylation, phosphorylation, acetylation, nitration, ubiquitation and disulfide bond formation.[4–7] Post-translational modifications regulate protein function, determining their activity state, cellular location and dynamic interactions with other proteins or nucleic acids.[6]

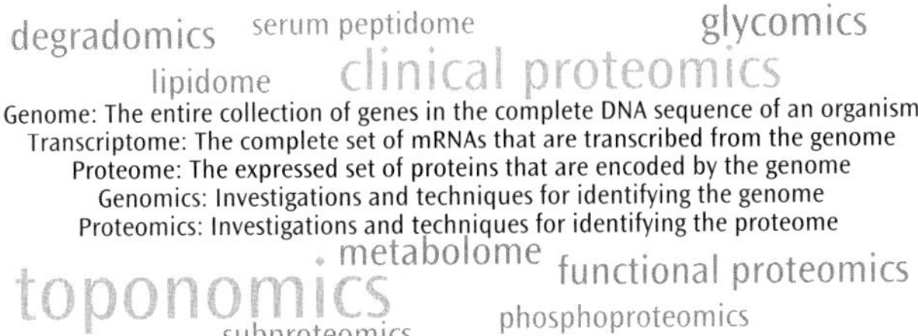

Figure 12.1 The 'omes' and 'omics' era. Because of the success of genomics and proteomics, the suffix '-ome' and 'omics' has now widely migrated to a host of other contexts.

Exploring the structure and activity of proteins is increasingly used to address biomedical questions that may help to elucidate the molecular basis of health and disease and, for example, to address fundamental questions in the progression of a disease from a normal to a pathophysiologic state (clinical proteomics). We will discuss different aspects of proteomics, including new proteomic platforms as well as their limitations. It is of no surprise that none of these proteomic approaches currently come close to detecting all proteins present in complex biological systems. When the obstacles can be overcome, it will enable abundant harvesting of diagnostic biomarkers leading to a new era of personalized clinical medicine.

BIOMARKERS

The levels of particular proteins in tissues, serum and other body fluids have been used extensively to diagnose, monitor or predict disease prognosis using conventional protein quantification techniques, such as immunohistochemistry and enzyme-linked immunosorbent assay (ELISA). These proteins are then called biomarkers and are differentially present in a sample taken from a subject of one phenotypic status (e.g. having a disease) compared with another phenotypic status (e.g. healthy). They can be found (either newly formed, or at increased or decreased amounts) in blood, body fluids or in tissues, and indicate a particular disease state. They are produced and sometimes secreted by transformed cells or they can be the result of the body's response to the development of this disease. Proteinases derived from the diseased tissue microenvironment give rise to peptides within the circulatory system (termed the blood or serum peptidome) and can be a rich source of disease-specific information.[8–10] Examples of characteristic biomarkers that physicians use for diagnosis, prognosis and/or surveillance include: CA 125 (ovarian cancer), estrogen receptor/progesterone receptor, Her2/neu, CA 15-3 and CA 27-29 (breast cancer), PSA (prostate cancer), beta-amyloid and Tau protein (Alzheimer) and CEA (ovarian, lung, breast, pancreas and gastrointestinal tract cancers). These biomarkers can objectively be measured and evaluated as an indicator of normal biological or pathogenic processes or to determine pharmacological responses to a therapeutic intervention. They may support early detection (diagnostic or screening marker), molecular classification, predictor of metastasis in cancer, treatment response, to determine the prognosis, and so forth. The characteristics of an ideal biomarker are specific, sensitive, predictive, robust and preferably easily accessible in a non-invasive way. In the clinical setting, there is a constant need for new biomarkers with improved sensitivity and specificity. The source material for the identification of these new biomarkers is shifting away from tissue-cultured cells to the discovery of proteins that change in actual diseased tissues or body fluids. However, tissues are heterogeneous; they are composed of interacting cell populations. New technology has made it possible to analyze diseased cells in the tissue itself,[11] or to physically separate the desired cells directly from the surrounding cells under microscopic visualization by laser-capture microdissection (Figure 12.2).[12] This technology has been applied to discover dozens of new protein targets that are either a cause or a consequence of the disease process in the actual tissue.[12–19]

Pleural diseases are often accompanied by the presence of pleural fluid in the thoracic cage. Discovering the changes in expression of pleural proteins being overexpressed and/or abnormally shed into the effusion proteome may elucidate the basic molecular mechanisms that either cause, or result from, the diseased state of the patient. For example, cancer cells may release proteins (e.g. various enzymes, cytokines, extracellular matrix molecules, growth factors, degraded products, proteases and cleavage fragments) into the pleural effusion that may have a diagnostic value as biomarkers on their own and will provide further insights into pathological processes. Ultimately, these proteins could become valuable in clinical research, e.g. as targets for the design of drug treatments. However, disease-specific proteins are most often of low abundance and therefore difficult to detect. The low candidate biomarker concentration is caused by high amounts of seemingly non-relevant proteins such as albumin and immunoglobulins (IgG) giving a wide dynamic range (several orders of magnitude) of protein concentrations. It is also apparent that in most diseases, proteins are more subjected to post-translational modifications, different proteolytic cleavage or bound to highly abundant carrier proteins, thereby protecting the bound species from kidney clearance.[20–22] Consequently, the greatest challenge for biomarker discovery is the isolation of these rare candidate biomarkers (proteins or its specific peptide fragments) from the complex pleural effusion of a patient.

As mentioned earlier, pleural diseases may express and probably release proteins into their micro-environment that may have diagnostic value as biomarkers on their own or may provide further insights into the pathological process. Therefore, research into the unique signatures in effusions may yield more information for disease diagnosis, prognosis or the prediction of therapeutic responses in the near future. Pleural effusions are: (i) in close proximity to the site of disease pathology (pleura); (ii) often removed for patient's symptom relief, and (iii) relatively easy to obtain in large amounts. A practical effusion biomarker has certain characteristics, i.e. it is a secreted or shed protein that should be stable (long half-life) and not bound to serum proteins or inhibitors that could interfere with their measurement.

'TRADITIONAL' BIOMARKERS FOR PLEURAL DISEASES

The accumulation of clinically detectable quantities of pleural fluid may indicate the presence of pleural, pulmonary or extrapulmonary disease. In certain cases, the etiology of the fluid is obvious from the clinical picture (e.g. congestive heart failure); in other cases, not. When a patient with a pleural effusion is evaluated, the first question to answer is if the patient's pleural fluid is a transudate or an exudate, usually by applying Light's criteria.[23] Exudates have a much larger differential diagnosis of over 50 causes,[24] predominantly infectious conditions, lymphatic abnormalities, inflammatory processes, and malignant conditions (see also Chapter 17, Pleural fluid analysis). The most frequent etiology of malignant pleural effusion is bronchogenic carcinoma, which causes over one-third of all such cases. Other frequent causes of malignant pleural effusion include metastatic breast

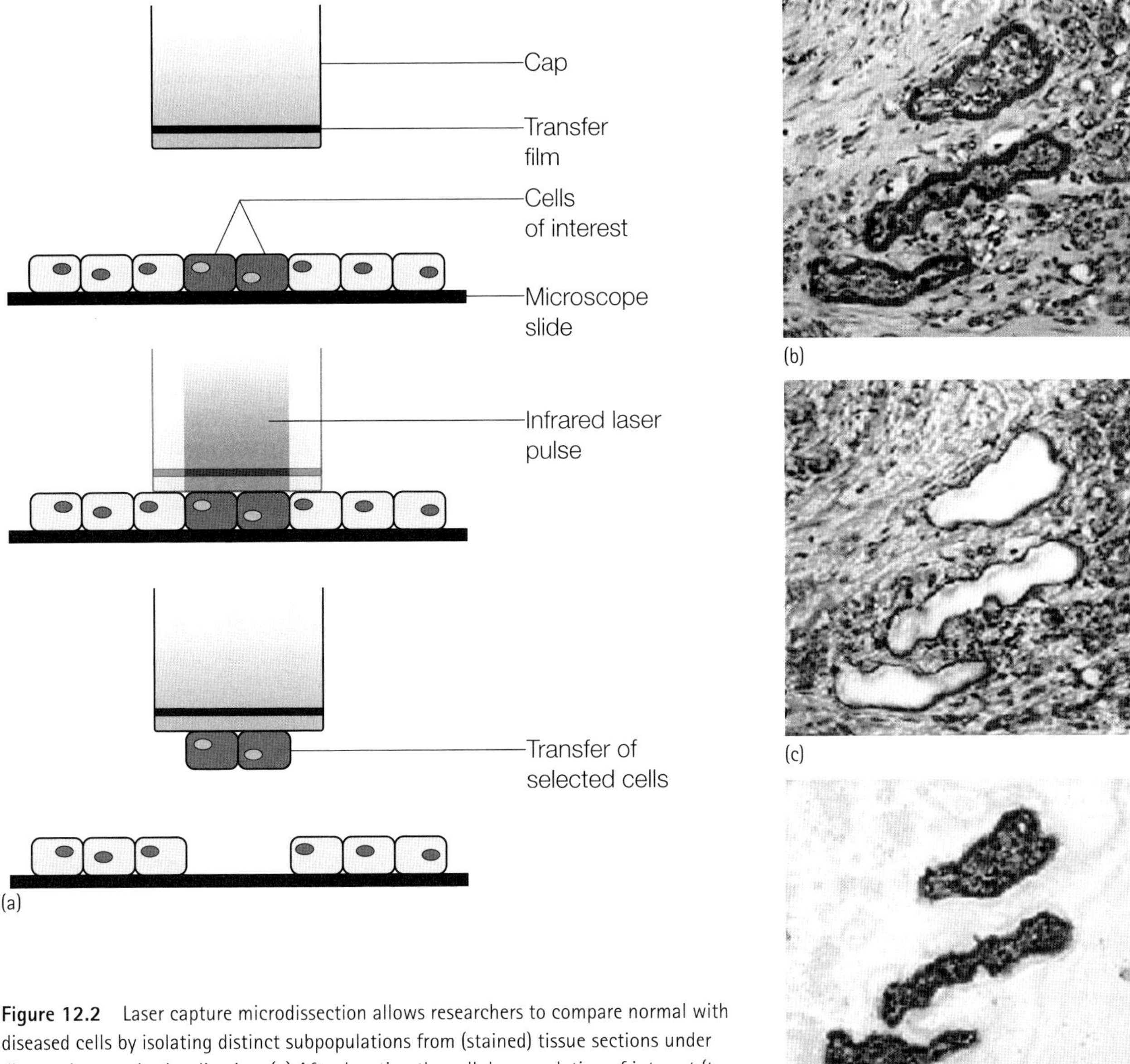

Figure 12.2 Laser capture microdissection allows researchers to compare normal with diseased cells by isolating distinct subpopulations from (stained) tissue sections under direct microscopic visualization. (a) After locating the cellular population of interest (top picture), a cap with film backing is placed over the target area (middle picture). Pulsing the infrared laser locally expands the thermosensitive polymer film to reach down and adhere the target cell(s) beneath the laser pulse. Lifting the cap from the tissue section removes the target cells now attached to the cap (lower picture). The cap holding the captured cells is then transferred to a tube, where an extraction buffer is used to remove the cells for further analysis. An example shows the laser outline of the cells to be collected (b), the remaining cells after laser capture (c), and the cells collected from the outlined area (d). (See also Color Plates 5–7.)

cancer, lymphoma, mesothelioma, gastric or esophageal cancer and ovarian carcinoma. The diagnosis of a malignant pleural effusion is established by demonstrating malignant cells in the pleural fluid or in the pleura itself. Numerous papers have recommended various diagnostic tests, such as cytological and chromosomal analysis of pleural cells, measurement of pH, glucose, amylase, or measurement of proteins as carcinoembryonic antigen (CEA), neuron-specific enolase (NSE), CA125, squamous cell carcinoma antigen, CA19-9, tissue polypeptide antigen (TPA), α-fetoprotein, CYFRA 21-1 or osteopontin in the effusions to discriminate malignant from benign pleural exudates.[25] Although the presence of these tumor markers is highly suggestive when levels are high, it is not very helpful if values are only modestly increased.[26,27] Therefore, diagnosis of a disease based on a pleural effusion is often difficult. Recent advances in proteomics have brought the hope of discovering novel biomarkers that indicate the pathogenic mechanism involved in the production of the effusion.

NOVEL BIOMARKERS FOR PLEURAL DISEASES

Patients with malignancy, pulmonary embolus and infective effusions may have an elevated level of fibrin degradation products in their pleural fluid.[28] Also, elevated β_2-microglobulin levels have been associated with tuberculosis, leukemia, lymphoma and some autoimmune disorders.[29] Distinctive levels of pleural fluid adenosine deaminase isoenzyme 2 (ADA2), specific anti-tuberculous antibodies, lysozyme and interferon-γ are present in the pleural effusion of patients with tuberculous pleuritis compared with patients with effusions of other etiologies.[25] ADA1 isoenzyme is elevated in parapneumonic effusions.[30,31]

Another example of a promising biomarker with diagnostic potential in pleural fluid is soluble mesothelin-related protein (SMRP).[32,33] Pleural and serum levels of SMRP are significantly higher in epithelioid mesothelioma patients than in those with benign pleuritis and pleural metastases.[33] Serum SMRP levels are tumor-size related and decrease upon surgical cytoreduction, suggestive of a role of SMRP in disease monitoring,[34–37] see also Chapter 15, Experimental models: mesothelioma. Efforts are underway to search for biomarkers like SMRP that can be analyzed relatively noninvasively and economically in effusions or serum, for other pleural diseases.

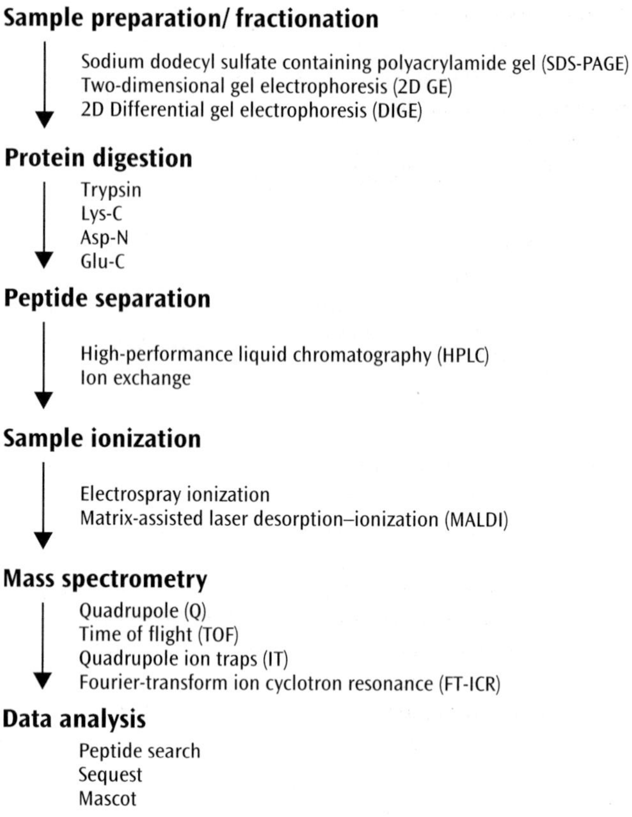

Sample preparation/ fractionation

Sodium dodecyl sulfate containing polyacrylamide gel (SDS-PAGE)
Two-dimensional gel electrophoresis (2D GE)
2D Differential gel electrophoresis (DIGE)

Protein digestion

Trypsin
Lys-C
Asp-N
Glu-C

Peptide separation

High-performance liquid chromatography (HPLC)
Ion exchange

Sample ionization

Electrospray ionization
Matrix-assisted laser desorption–ionization (MALDI)

Mass spectrometry

Quadrupole (Q)
Time of flight (TOF)
Quadrupole ion traps (IT)
Fourier-transform ion cyclotron resonance (FT-ICR)

Data analysis

Peptide search
Sequest
Mascot

Figure 12.3 An outline of a general strategy to perform proteomics. The identification of proteins of interest relies mainly on the separation of a complex protein mixture by electrophoresis, mass measurement of peptides generated after spot proteolysis by mass spectrometry and search in databases.

CURRENT TECHNIQUES FOR PROTEOMIC ANALYSIS TO DISCOVER NOVEL BIOMARKERS

There are a number of options available to profile proteins and identify potential biomarkers. These rely mainly on the separation of a complex mixture of proteins by electrophoresis, mass measurement of peptides generated after spot proteolysis by mass spectrometry (MS) and searches in databases (Figure 12.3), although various other approaches are now used to study differentially expressed proteins. Before starting a proteomics study, the advantages and disadvantages of various methods must be assessed in order to choose the best suitable approach. The choice of an appropriate methodology will depend on the goals of the specific study, amount and number of samples, availability of resources and other factors. Although technical advances have been significant in previous decades, we are still confronted with the challenges of the evaluation and validation of the proteomic technologies, sample preparation and fractionation, understanding the massive volume of data, translating the information to fit clinical contents and incorporating it into clinical studies. We will now summarize some of the available technologies and discuss the limitations that we still face.

Two-dimensional gel electrophoresis

High-resolution one- and two-dimensional gel electrophoresis (1D and 2D GE, respectively) has traditionally been the gold-standard discovery-based tool for proteomics[38,39] and was used for analyzing the proteome of body fluids, for instance for plasma,[40] urine,[41] cerebrospinal fluid[42,43] and pleural fluid.[44–47] Unfortunately, pleural fluids, like most of the body fluids, contain an enormous amount of different proteins and salt ions. Albumin and immunoglobulin fragments are the major protein components, representing 50–70 percent and 10–20 percent of the total pleural proteins, respectively (mg/mL range). Together with transferrin, fibrinogen, haptoglobin, antitrypsin, complement components and a few other proteins, the top 20 proteins are responsible for approximately 99 percent of the protein mass. Pleural effusions contain a tremendous array of very-low-abundance molecules such as signaling and regulatory proteins. For example, comparatively small quantities of cytokines are detected by cytokine arrays and ELISA, such as transforming growth factor-beta (TGF-β), interleukin (IL) (IL-1, IL-6, IL-8, and IL-10) or vascular endothelial growth factor (VEGF), but these are in the ng/mL to pg/mL range, a difference of nine orders of magnitude or more. Therefore, removal of abundantly expressed proteins is a key element of proteome research to allow the visualization of co-migrating proteins on a 1D and 2D gel and to allow a higher sample load for improved visualization of low-abundance proteins.[48–52] A convenient approach to remove high-abundance proteins from body fluids is affinity chromatography with resins carrying highly efficient and specific ligands for these proteins. Removal of these proteins using commercially available kits (e.g. ProteoPrep Blue Albumin Depletion Kit [Sigma-Aldrich, St Louis, MO, USA], or Multiple Affinity Removal System [Agilent Technologies, Santa Clara, CA, USA]) improves the resolution and increases the protein spot count in depleted samples.[52] However, removal may confound the subsequent proteomic analysis because peptides and low molecular weight proteins of interest may be bound to these large carrier proteins.[53]

Samples are normally purified by removal of salts, lipids and other interfering substances and concentrated before applying onto the first dimension (e.g. by using the 2D clean-up kit [GE Healthcare, Fairfield, CT, USA]). In 2D GE, protein mixtures are first separated by isoelectric focusing; on the application of a current, the charged proteins migrate in a gel strip that contains an immobilized pH gradient (IPG) until they reach the pH at which their overall charge is neutral (isoelectric point or pI) in the first dimension.[39] This gel strip is then applied onto a rectangular sodium dodecyl sulfate containing polyacrylamide gel (SDS-PAGE), and the pI focused proteins migrate by electric current into the gel and are separated on the basis of their molecular weights (Figure 12.4a). After electrophoresis, protein spots in a gel can be visualized using a variety of radioactive, chemical stains or fluorescent markers (for example, Coomassie Brilliant Blue or silver). Depending on the type of staining, 200–3000 proteins per gel can be visualized (Figure 12.4b). A large number of spots in a 2D gel result from post-translational or proteolytic modifications of proteins: a protein may, therefore, be present in several locations in the gel. Despite specialized software packages that allow comparisons of multiple gels, the matching of images of different gels can be difficult because they can be distorted by less-defined, less well separated spots, shrinking or swelling of non-backed gels and concentration differences between the gels. There are potentially thousands of intact or cleaved proteins in the human pleural effusion proteome. Finding a single disease-related protein is like searching for a needle in a haystack, requiring the separation and identification of these entities individually. This approach has recently been published for a composite pleural effusion sample from seven lung adenocarcinoma patients. This study revealed at least 472 silver-stained protein spots to be present in a 2D gel map, half of which could be identified by liquid chromatography-tandem MS.[46] Although the results of these studies provide information for a basic understanding of the protein composition of pleural effusions, the value for clinical medicine is limited. Many of the proteins present in pleural fluid are likely to have originated from serum.[46,54–59] Of interest are those proteins that have not previously been reported in the literature to be present in serum. These proteins could then

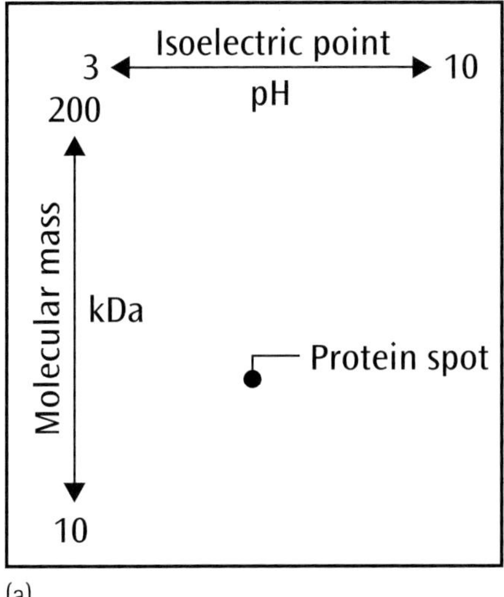

(a)

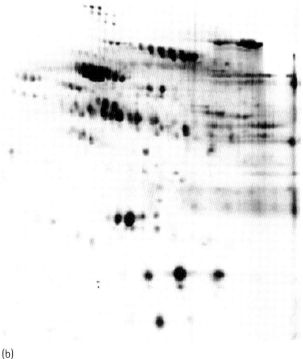

(b)

Figure 12.4 Two-dimensional (2D) electrophoresis is used to separate protein mixtures according to their isoelectric point (first dimension) and to their molecular mass (second dimension) (a). Human pleural effusion was depleted of albumin and immunoglobulin G (IgG) and resolved by 2D gel electrophoresis (b).

originate from diseased cells and may contain disease-specific information and with it represent potential candidates for useful biomarkers concentrated in or only measurable in pleural effusions. To discover these proteins, the development of quantitative proteomics such as differential gel electrophoresis and isotope-coded affinity tags has widened the applicability to detect proteins of interest.

Differential gel electrophoresis

A powerful quantitative technique currently applied is differential gel electrophoresis (DIGE).[60–64] This technology is commercially available (GE Healthcare). It has the potential to overcome many of the limitations of 2D electrophoretic studies by allowing the direct comparison in proteomic profile of different samples at a particular time, under a particular set of conditions.[65] DIGE encompasses a simple strategy involving three molecular weight- and charge-matched cyanine dyes (CyDyes: Cy2, Cy3 and Cy5 [GE Healthcare]) possessing unique absorption and emission spectra.[66,67] The fluorescent dyes bind to the terminal amino group of lysine side chains in proteins with no change in protein charge and add only 0.5 kDa to the mass of the protein, thereby minimizing dye-induced shifting during electrophoresis. Due to a minimal labeling (only 2–5 percent of the total number of lysine residues are labeled), binding of the dye to the protein appears to have no effect on MS analyses. Two different samples are labeled with Cy3 and Cy5 and a third sample, labeled with Cy2, is introduced as an internal control for each gel. The internal control is often a pooled sample comprising equal amounts of each of the samples within the study. This allows normalization and both inter- and intra-gel matching of proteins and is imperative for accurate protein quantification. Once labeled, samples are mixed and isoelectrically focused on an IPG strip and co-electrophoresed on the same 2D gel. The spectrally distinct dyes allow co-separation of different CyDye-labeled samples and ensure that all samples will be subjected to exactly the same 2D GE running conditions. This limits the experimental variation and thus ensures accuracy within gel matching. Each dye is then scanned using different emission filters and images are analyzed with DeCyder Differential In-gel Analysis software (GE Healthcare). This software allows protein alignment and quantification between scanned images. Spots may be directly picked through an automated system. The differential 2D DIGE has been used in the proteomic expression analysis of several cancer cell systems.[68–72] To discover the proteins of interest, we used a strategy of comparative analysis of serum proteome and pleural effusion proteome from the same mesothelioma patient using the DIGE technology (Figure 12.5). Overexpression of proteins by mesothelioma cells can result in their shedding in the pleural effusion and will lead to enhanced intensity spots compared with serum of the same patient. Absence of proteins in the effusion may be caused by specific proteolysis or by specific absorption from the circulation by tumor cells. A protein spot with the approximate molecular mass of 30 kDa and pI of 5.5, significantly expressed in the serum but not in the effusion, was selected for identification and further analyses. Proteins were analyzed by matrix-assisted laser desorption/ionization–time-of-flight (MALDI-TOF) MS analysis using peptide mass fingerprinting and 19 matched peptides with a total coverage of 75 percent are the basis of the identification of the decreased spot in effusions as apolipoprotein A1 (accession number CAA00975), a protein with a molecular mass of 28.061 Da and pI of 5.27. This spot migrated differently from the major apolipoprotein A1 spots and represents a small fraction of the total serum apolipoprotein A1 but is absent in pleural effusion. This directly illustrates the advantage of 2D gel-based approaches in visualizing changes in the molecular weight and pI of a protein. The different pI and slightly different molecular mass reflects biologically significant processing and pI-altering post-translational modifications such as phosphorylation, sulfation or (de-)acetylation. Thus, comparison of the protein spots from serum and effusion by 2D-DIGE provides a very striking quantitative picture of proteins absorbed or shed into body fluids. This truncation product has not been reported previously and it is not known whether the fragmentation was due to *in vivo* biological processing or protease activity. Reductions in the serum levels of apolipoprotein A1 have also been correlated with hepatitis B virus-induced diseases.[73–75] An isoform of apolipoprotein A1 was detected by 2D GE in serum obtained from individuals with high risk for the development of, or those diagnosed with, hepatocellular carcinoma.[76] Apolipoprotein A1 is a potential marker of the aggression in colonic adenocarcinoma[77] and is upregulated in primary carcinoma tissue of the vagina.[78] However, a downregulation of apolipoprotein A1 in serum is described in early stage ovarian cancer.[79,80]

Isotope-coded affinity tagging

Owing to the limitations of these gel-based technologies (Table 12.1), more versatile mass spectrometry-based approaches in conjunction with gel-free protein separations have been developed in recent years. Isotope-coded affinity tags (ICAT) has been the most widely practiced MS-based, non-gel, quantitative approach for biomarker discovery in the last few years but new developments, such as tags for relative and absolute quantification (iTRAQ),[81] metabolic labeling[82] and label-free liquid chromatography MS,[83,84] are emerging. ICAT utilizes stable isotope labeling of cysteine-containing proteins to compare the relative abundance between two comparative reduced protein mixtures.[85] The affinity tags have different masses, but are structurally and chemically identical and covalently bind to all cysteines within a protein. When the light tag (e.g. linker possessing nine carbon-12 atoms) or the heavy tag

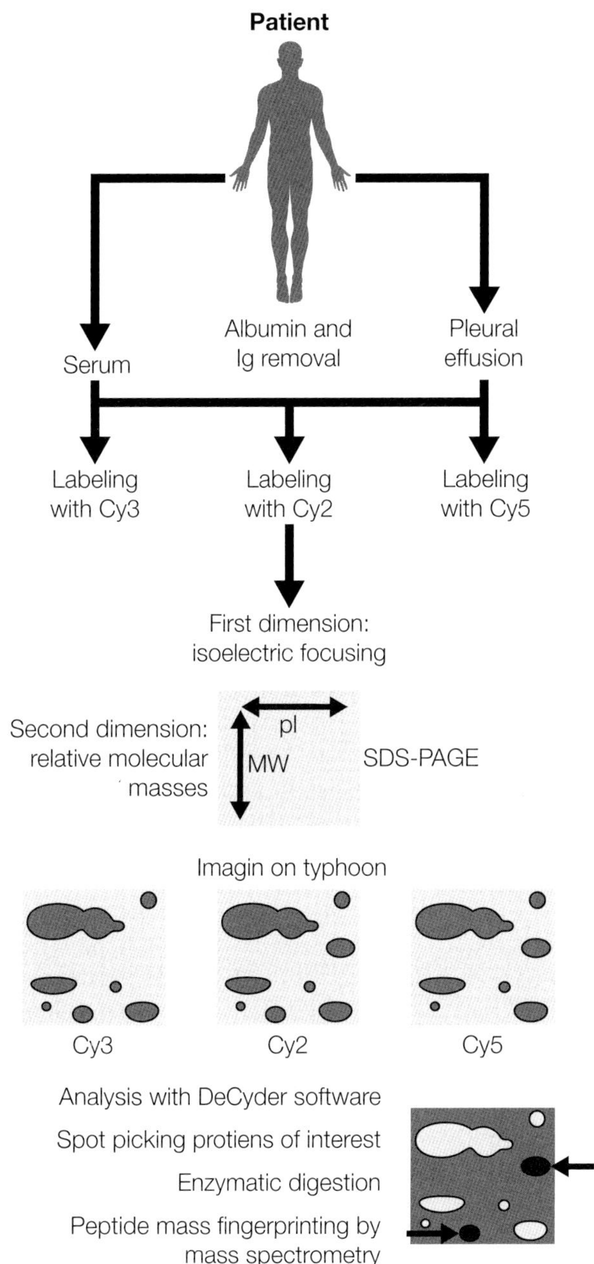

Figure 12.5 Flowchart of differential gel electrophoresis (DIGE) analysis of serum and malignant pleural fluid derived from a patient suffering from malignant mesothelioma. Samples to be compared are labeled with either Cy3 or Cy5, whereas the Cy2 is employed to label a pooled sample comprising equal amounts of serum and effusion within the study. The labeled samples are combined and then run on a single two-dimensional gel. Proteins are detected using a dual laser-scanning device equipped with different excitation/emission filters in order to generate three separate images. The images are matched by a computer-assisted overlay method, signals are normalized using the corresponding Cy2 spot intensities, and spots of interest are excised and analyzed by mass spectrometry. Differentially expressed proteins in serum and pleural effusions of the same patient can be useful to discover proteins that may be the result of the cancer. SDS-PAGE, sodium dodecyl sulfate–polyacrylamide gel electrophoresis.

(linker possessing nine carbon-13 atoms) is bound to the same protein, a concrete mass change of exactly 9.03 Da will be evident when analyzed by MS. One can label a control sample with the light tag, the experimental sample with the heavy tag, for example cells or tissues in two distinct physiological or pathological conditions such as normal or cancerous tissue. The two samples are mixed prior to the proteolytic digestion, and the labeled peptides are separated from bulk using affinity chromatography (Figure 12.6). The captured labeled peptides are separated using ion-exchange chromatography prior to MS, which can resolve these two states (heavy/light) and quantify the relative abundance of the two differentially labeled peptides from the same parent protein.

MALDI-TOF MS

Once proteins are separated by SDS-PAGE and stained, they have to be characterized. MS, and in particular MALDI-TOF MS, is indispensable technology for protein mixture profiling and for the identification of proteins. It was invented in the late 1980s[86,87] and the importance has been recognized by the share of the 2002 Nobel Prize for Chemistry to Koichi Tanaka for its invention.[88]

Spots of interest are excised from the gel, destained and subsequently digested with proteolytic enzymes and/or chemicals. Trypsin is most commonly used in identification studies. Trypsin is a very stable and efficient protease that specifically cleaves at the *C*-terminal side of lysine and

Table 12.1 Advantages and disadvantages of selected proteomic technologies for protein profiling

Technique	Advantages	Disadvantages/limitations
2D GE	Good separation for the larger-molecular mass region of the proteome (between 10 and 150 kDa) Thousands of proteins can be resolved; for each protein the isoelectric point, MW and the relative quantity can be determined Detection of post-translationally modified proteins Proteins can be stored within (dried) gels for months and analyzed at a later date	Low throughput (one sample per gel) Labour intensive Large sample input (>100 μg) Small proteins (<10 kDa) or very large proteins (>150 kDa), extremely acidic or basic proteins, hydrophobic or otherwise insoluble proteins (e.g. membrane proteins) are poorly resolved on gel Low abundance proteins are not detected because of sensitivity limits Gel-to-gel variations confound the analysis process No direct (online) protein identification
DIGE	Direct comparison of up to three samples on one 2D gel Four orders of magnitude dynamic range and good correlation between spot density and protein content Internal standard allows for quantitative comparison of multiple gels	Low throughput (three samples per gel) Labeling dependent on lysine content Mass shift of *c.* 500 Da, impractical for subsequent MS (post-staining required especially for low-molecular-weight proteins) Gel spots only visible under fluorescent light, equipment required for visualization and spot excision
ICAT	Measures the relative abundance of heavy and light peptides simultaneously Relative quantification and direct identification within a single analysis Identification possible for only the differently expressed proteins Does not require metabolic labeling	Low throughput (two samples per run) Large sample input Extensive sample fractionation before MS Involves radioisotope handling by user Targets only cysteine residues (5% of human proteins lack cysteine)
MALDI	High throughput (up to 1536 samples per plate)	Need for (offline) sample fractionation of complex samples Expensive equipment and processing costs Dependent on ionization efficiency
SELDI	High throughput (up to 96 samples per bioprocessor) Direct application of sample ('fast on-chip sample cleanup') Small amount of starting material Unbiased searches	Spectral patterns of masses rather than actual protein identifications are produced Only useful for separating small-molecular-mass proteins (<15 kDa)
Protein array	Relatively high throughput Semi-quantitative measurement of hundreds of proteins in parallel Clinically applicable	Limited availability of antibodies with high specificity and affinity for the proteins of interest Possible cross-reactivity, giving false-positives Different affinities of antibodies on one chip Untargeted proteins will remain undetected Difficult to preserve proteins in their biologically active shape and form

Abbreviations: 2D GE, two-dimensional gel electrophoresis; DIGE, differential gel electrophoresis; ICAT, isotope-coded affinity tag; MALDI, matrix-assisted laser desorption/ionization; MS, mass spectrometry; SELDI, surface-enhanced laser desorption/ionization.

arginine residues into a mixture of peptides. The resulting peptides have, on average, the right size to be usefully detected by MS and are first mixed with UV-absorbing organic acid, also known as matrix solution (e.g. α-cyano-4-hydroxy-*trans*-cinnamic acid) which causes the peptide to form crystals. When irradiated with brief UV laser pulses, the peptide/matrix crystals become detached (i.e. desorption), and gaseous ions are liberated (i.e. ionization). The charged molecules are accelerated through a strong electric field within a high vacuum, and a recording is taken of how long the peptides take to travel a specified distance and strike a detector. The longer the time of flight,

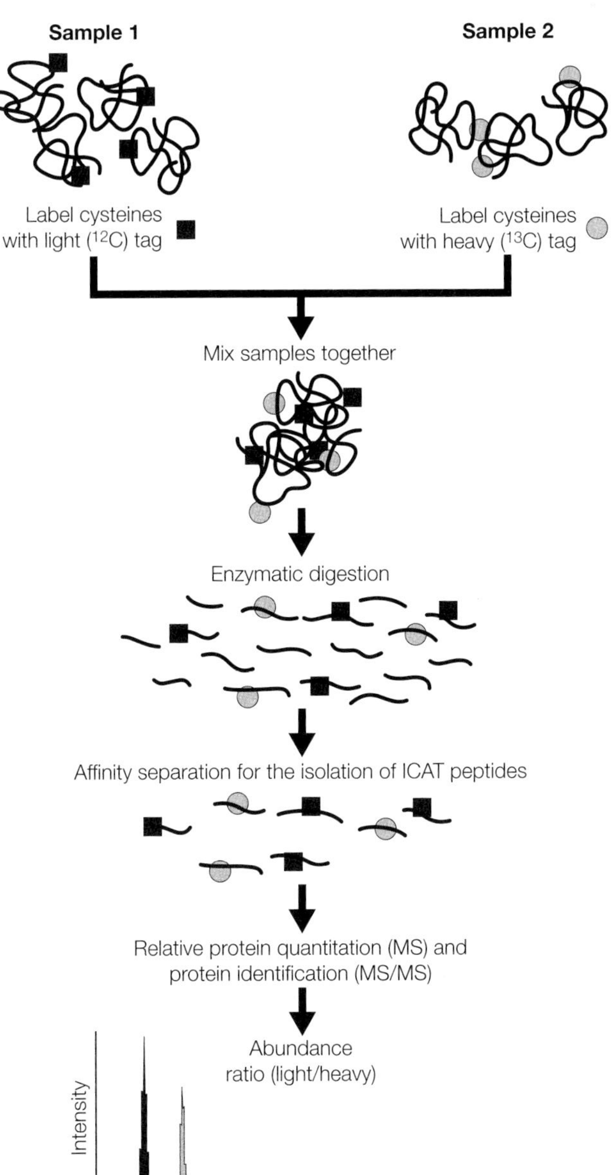

Figure 12.6 Isotope-coded affinity tags (ICAT) utilizes chemical tagging of proteins on cysteine residues with a heavy and light stable isotopic label (for two different samples); after labeling the samples are mixed, proteins digested, and labeled peptides isolated by affinity chromatography and analyzed by mass spectrometry (MS).

the more massive the particle is relative to its charge. Ionized peptides are thus separated on the basis of their mass-to-charge (m/z) ratio. Detected peptides/ions are displayed as a unique series of peaks that are referred to as the peptide mass fingerprint (PMF). This mass mapping spectrum of peptide peaks is then compared with the virtual peptide masses predicted from theoretical digestion of protein sequences currently contained within databases (e.g. UniProt, Swiss-Prot, NCBI) and the protein can be identified, considering the specificity of the protease employed. For further identification, the actual amino acid sequence (primary structure) information for the peptide of interest can be obtained by tandem mass spectrometry (commonly referred to as MS/MS or MS^2), in which the particular peptide ion is isolated and fragmented by collision with an inert gas (such as nitrogen molecules, argon or helium atoms), and complex algorithms are used to correlate the experimental data with data derived from peptide sequences in protein databases (e.g. Peptide Sequence Tags, Sequest or Mascot).

Using the combination of 2D GE followed by MALDI-TOF MS showed, for example, an increase in cyclin D2, XEDAR, p53-binding protein Mdm2, LIM and cysteine-rich domain protein 1, and HSP70-interacting protein and HSPC163 present or increased in lung squamous carcinoma compared with normal bronchial tissue.[89] It also allowed the identification of several individual proteins and specific protein isoforms that were increased in lung adenocarcinomas[90–93] and proteins (e.g. phosphoglycerate kinase 1) that can predict the survival of patients with early-stage lung cancer.[92] This technology was also used to characterize the proteins present in exosomes isolated from malignant pleural effusions from different cancerous origin to gain information on their potential biological function(s).[94]

Surface-enhanced laser desorption/ionization–time-of-flight

Surface-enhanced laser desorption/ionization–time-of-flight (SELDI-TOF, Vermillion [formerly Ciphergen Biosystems], Fremont, CA, USA) MS has been intensely controversial as a tool for quantitative analysis of protein mixtures, mainly because of its methodological shortcomings and bioinformatics artifacts.[95] This technique employs protein biochips, spotted with a protein capture bait such as a chemical affinity resin (i.e. hydrophobic, hydrophilic, metal affinity, cationic or anionic surfaces), receptors and ligands, antibodies, DNA oligonucleotides or enzymes[96] to enrich for the protein or peptide of interest. Microliter quantities of crude protein extracts directly from their 'native' environments are applied to the ProteinChip®, allowing proteins with physical or chemical affinities to the capture molecules to bind to the surface, and then washed to remove impurities or loosely-bound proteins (Figure 12.7). Analytes are laser desorbed and ionized directly from the chip for mass spectral analysis. A SELDI experiment produces a unique sample mass spectral profile (m/z) ranging from small peptides of <1000 Da up to proteins of >300 kDa and can distinguish differences in protein expression levels between samples, which require highly ordered data mining operations for analysis. Artificial intelligence-based systems are uniquely suited for this because it learns, adapts and gains experience over time through constant retraining. It is possible to generate not just one, but multiple combinations of proteomic patterns from a single mass-spectral training set, each pattern combination re-adjusting as the models improve in the adaptive mode. Unlike tandem MS, SELDI alone cannot be used to identify individual proteins in a sample. Other limitations of SELDI are the overall lack of sensitivity and reproducibility, and the potential bias towards certain proteins. It is, however, ideal for high-throughput protein profiling of a large numbers of samples, and is used for biomarker discovery in cancer.[97–103] We studied pleural effusions from patients with confirmed mesothelioma (n = 54) and from patients with effusions due to other causes (n = 54, cancerous and non-cancerous) using SELDI-TOF. All samples were collected, processed and stored in the same way. Samples were fractionated using anion exchange chromatography and then bound to different types of ProteinChip® array surfaces. Peak intensity data were subjected to classification algorithms in order to identify potential classifier peaks that could be used to discriminate between mesothelioma and non-mesothelioma samples. One such protein peak at m/z 6614 was characterized as apolipoprotein (Apo) CI and was decreased in pleural effusions due to mesothelioma. These molecules represent highly abundant proteins produced by the liver, whose concentration may be decreased due to cancer cachexia or malnutrition, rather non-specific effects for many cancer types. In this setting, however, the sensitivity and specificity of this potential biomarker was 76 and 69 percent, respectively. The area under the receiver operating characteristic curve (AUC) for Apo CI was 0.755. We were unable to identify SMRP, probably because of the low sensitivity of the SELDI-TOF approach. External and thorough validation studies are now underway to further investigate a possible role and function of the decrease of Apo CI in the oncogenesis of mesothelioma and to put the SELDI technology into perspective.

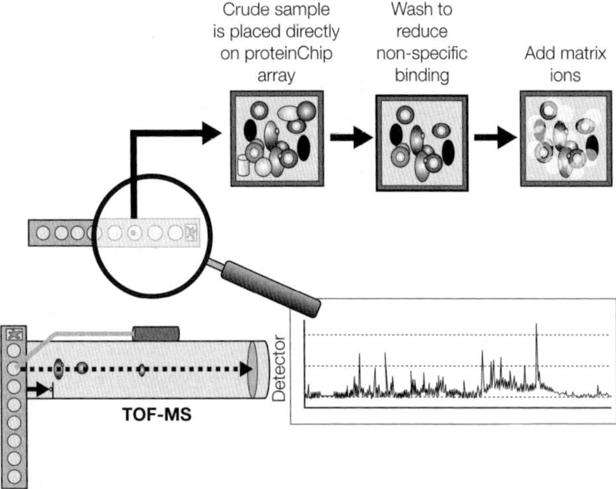

Figure 12.7 Surface-enhanced laser desorption/ionization–time-of-flight (SELDI-TOF) mass spectrometry is a variant of MALDI-TOF in which a selected part of a crude protein mixture is bound to a specific chromatographic surface (ProteinChip array) and the non-binding part is washed away. Retained proteins are treated with an energy-absorbing matrix molecule, ionized by laser, then accelerated through a flight tube, and separated by m/z. As mixtures of proteins are analyzed within different samples, a unique sample fingerprint or signature will result for each sample tested.

Other mass spectrometry technologies

This section provides a rapid view of principles and instrumentation of other mass spectrometric techniques that have seen an amazing rise in popularity in the last decade because they enable rapid access to accurate information on protein identification, sequence and quantification (Figure 12.3).[104] MS instruments consist of at least two basic components: an ionization module and a mass analyzer. There are two so-called 'soft' ionization modules whereby highly polar, nonvolatile molecules with a mass of tens of kDa are transferred into the gas phase without destroying them: MALDI and electrospray ionization (ESI) (Figure 12.8). Earlier we described the principle of MALDI (Figure 12.8a), in which the protein or peptide samples are mixed with matrix molecules and are ionized by a focused laser. Matrix molecules sublime and transfer the embedded non-volatile analyte molecules into the gas phase and these are then accelerated by electric potentials into a mass analyzer of choice. For electrospray ionization

(Figure 12.8b), protein or peptide samples in solution are passed through a fine needle to which high electrical potential (several kV) is applied, which results in a fine spray of highly positively charged sample-containing droplets. Samples are delivered to the mass analyzer after the breakup and evaporation of the solvent, which decreases the size and increases the charge density of the droplets. Electrospray ionization is performed from a liquid sample and liquid-based chromatographic separation (LC) systems, such as low-flow rate LC can be coupled to the needle to allow for protein fractionation of the samples before mass analysis. It separates the samples by eluting from reverse-phase columns using increasing concentrations of organic solvents, which allow separation on the basis of hydrophobicity. Ionized and fragmented protein samples are introduced into a mass analyzer, which separates and detect the ions according to their m/z ratios. Besides the already described time-of-flight device (TOF as in MALDI-TOF and SELDI-TOF), other basic types of mass analyzers are the quadrupole (Q), quadrupole 'ion trap' (IT), and Fourier transform ion cyclotron (FT-ICR-MS or FTMS), each with its own strengths and weaknesses. Each of these instruments generates a mass spectrum, hence the term mass spectrometry.

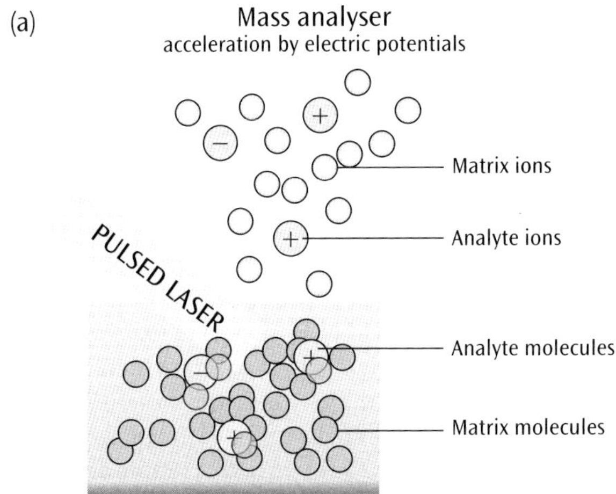

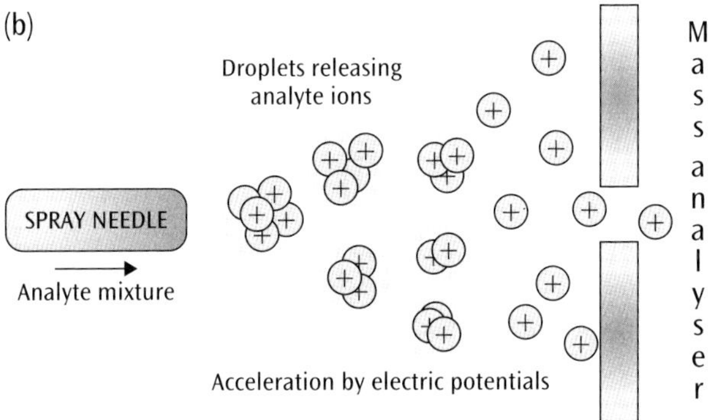

Figure 12.8 'Soft' ionization techniques as matrix-assisted laser desorption/ionization (MALDI) (a) and electrospray ionization (b) are used in biological mass spectrometry to transfer highly polar, non-volatile peptides/proteins into the gas phase without destroying them. (a) Sample and matrix are mixed and allowed to dry forming crystals and in a mass spectrometer ions are formed by irradiating the crystals with a brief laser pulse. (b) The analyte solution is injected via a thin metallized needle on which a potential is applied. A continuous spray forms at the tip of the needle. Under the effect of the potential difference, the spray process forms very small droplets which progressively desolvate, liberating multiply charged ions.

A Q mass filter consists of four parallel rods through which direct current and radio frequency alternate electric fields are applied to sort the introduced ions. For each combination of voltages and frequencies, only ions with a specific m/z ratio pass undeflected through the Q mass filter. Ions of the desired mass are fragmented in a gas collision cell, the masses of these daughter fragments then being measured by a TOF mass analyzer. Precise stepping of the settings allows the quadrupole to be used as a mass analyzer to scan for ions over a large m/z range. In IT mass spectrometry, the ions of a selected mass are first caught (trapped) in a dynamic electric field and are then sequentially – according to their m/z value – ejected onto the detector with the help of another electric field. Trapped ions can also be fragmented by increasing the energy of the trap, with the mass detector measuring the masses of these fragments for peptide identification. In contrast to IT, FTMS keep the ions confined in the high magnetic field of a super-conducting magnet. The ions circle with frequencies that are inversely proportional to their m/z value. This circling induces an alternating current in the metal plates that make up the trap. This time-varying current constitutes a frequency spectrum of the ion motion and is converted by the mathematical operation Fourier transformation – which explains the name – into a mass spectrum with high resolution and mass accuracy.

The number of possible instrumental configurations is large because different analyzers can be coupled with various sources, such as the popular quadrupole-time of flight hybrid (Q-TOF) mass spectrometer. When more accuracy and sensitivity than MALDI or SELDI is needed, for instance for the analysis of post-translational modifications of proteins, high pressure LC is coupled to an ESI source and an FTMS instrument with electron capture dissociation can be used. The LC-ESI-triple quadrupole with multiple ionization sources is the instrument of choice for looking at biomarkers or drug efficacy. However, as there is no single instrument that can do it all, state of the art proteomics facilities need to be equipped with several different types of MS instruments.

Highly complex protein mixtures (e.g. unfractionated cellular lysates) that cannot be efficiently resolved on gel can be reduced, alkylated, digested and fractionated through a strong cationic exchange column, and further separated on a reverse-phase column in a technique known as 'multidimensional protein identification technology'

(MudPIT).[105] This approach, whereby 2D liquid chromatography (cation exchange followed by reverse-phase chromatography) is coupled to tandem MS, was applied to yeast proteomic analysis and a total of 1484 proteins were detected and identified, including the identification of 131 proteins that are membrane localized – a highly problematic class of proteins due to their intrinsic hydrophobic nature. This technique reduces the bias against the detection of basic and hydrophobic proteins and is very sensitive and reproducible.

Protein array system

Protein (micro-)array platforms containing spotted antigens or antibodies have been developed to rapidly screen changes in protein expression or modification on a global scale without much of the specialist and expensive equipment as required by MS-based proteomics.[106,107] Protein microarrays have been prepared by printing the capture proteins on filters or coated microscope slides using purified or recombinant proteins, crude mixtures or antibodies. Although protein microarrays have been anticipated for several years[108] and are predicted to be the 'most likely path to low-cost, routine measurement of large numbers of plasma markers required for an impact on medical practice',[109] the applications of antibody microarrays were limited by a variety of fundamental problems. Among them, cross-reactivity significantly limits the multiplexing ability in parallel sandwich immunoassays, and the limitations to the normalization, sensitivity, robustness and the standardization between experiments.[110] New formats of antibody microarrays are now applied with high throughput and parallel detection for low-abundance proteins in body fluids.[111–115] Proteins arrayed on a flat solid phase were used to simultaneously detect multiple cytokine expression levels from mesothelioma patient's pleural effusions.[116] Angiogenin, VEGF, TGF-β, epithelial neutrophil-activating protein-78 (ENA-78) and several other proteins involved in immune suppression, angiogenesis and plasma extravasation were detected in pleural effusions obtained from mesothelioma patients. Proteins that cause leukocyte infiltration and activation, such as hepatocyte growth factor (HGF), macrophage inflammatory protein (MIP)-1δ, MIP-3α, neutrophil-activating peptide-2 (NAP-2), and pulmonary and activation-regulated chemokine (PARC) were detected.[116] The presence of these cytokines can elucidate the role of the immune system, tumor micro-environment and the potential immunosuppression in mesothelioma.

CURRENT LIMITATIONS OF CLINICAL PROTEOMICS

Clinical proteomics faces several big challenges. One is the biological variability of patients' samples, stemming from differences in (tumor) type, location, size, histology, grade and stage of the disease, and heterogeneity, including differences in genetic background, age, sex, ethnic origin, smoking, alcohol consumption, medication, exercise, diet and many others. Besides this, it is crucial that protein samples are handled and stored consistently throughout the study. Many factors, such as time of collection, containers used, preservatives and other additives, transport to the laboratory, storage and prefractionation, affect the quality of the samples and the stability of the proteins of interest and must be considered at the initial collection stage.

Most discovery platforms require large cellular input samples that are orders of magnitude greater than those procured during a clinical biopsy.[69,105,117–120] Pleural effusions, on the other hand, are relatively easy to obtain in large amounts but there is no single test for exudates that is totally reliable or accurate for the diagnosis of its specific cause as the same results can also be found in other conditions. However, a single biomarker–single disease correlation will be very unlikely. Biomarker discovery is therefore moving away from the idealized single disease-specific biomarker to a panel of many markers to transcend the heterogeneity to reach a higher level of specificity and sensitivity. Thus, bioinformatics tools are required that can extract diagnostic patterns of proteins rather than a single biomarker from complex protein mixtures full of biological noise and individual variability, reliably recognize them in different samples where the patterns may be slightly changed and eventually cross-correlate them with other parameters related to the patients' health and treatment status. Particularly interesting are attempts to use SELDI to identify and combine several potential classifier peaks for a disease profile, however, recent controversy concerning this technology shows the difficulties facing proteomic research.[95] SELDI, like the majority of MS-based methods, primarily identifies smaller abundant peptides with a higher sensitivity and is therefore biased towards a mass range between 1–10 kDa. The other problem is the huge dynamic range of protein concentrations in tissues and body fluids, which exceeds more than 10 orders of magnitude. Components of high molar abundance generally dominate the spectrum and tend to suppress detection of lower abundance proteins. It is clear that significant technological advances will be needed to overcome the huge dynamic range and sensitivity requirements for probing deeper into the proteome. There is no protein equivalent of polymerase chain reaction (PCR) for the amplification of these low-abundance proteins that are more likely to serve as specific biomarkers. Extended analysis to these lower abundance components will therefore require extensive specimen pre-fractionation before analysis, highly specific reagents and sophisticated instrumentation. The different proteomic platforms are expensive and require specialized facilities with skilled staff. Currently, there is no single platform that can provide a complete proteomic coverage to identify the entire effusion proteome (high and low abundance proteins), and each technology has its own specific advantages and limitations (Table 12.1). Clearly, any method used in daily clinical routine must be simple, robust, and technically feasible for use in the clinical setting. (e.g. an ELISA-based colorimetric dipstick).

FUTURE PERSPECTIVES

Due to the aforementioned current limitations, at present, clinical proteomics cannot replace invasive standardized diagnostic procedures such as open pleural biopsy, but holds great promise and potential for future highly improved diagnosis and care of the patient. Many complementary technologies have been developed and are continuously improved, such as DIGE, ICAT, protein arrays and various developments in the field of mass spectrometry. Ongoing rapid developments in separation techniques, automation, sample throughput and bioinformatics will further stimulate the investigation of pleural effusions and will ultimately lead to new insights into the mechanisms of the causative diseases. The identification of pleural biomarkers (single or as a panel) for an earlier diagnosis, prognosis or prediction of therapeutic responses in pleural diseases is still in its infancy. However, recent studies on SMRP in pleural fluid and serum of mesothelioma patients has shown that highly specific biomarkers can be discovered with potential use in a clinical setting, even before the tumor is clinically apparent.

There is still a large gap between the discovery of new pleural disease biomarkers by proteomics and their clinical utility. It can only be overcome by intensive collaboration of teams of research scientists, clinicians and statisticians to conduct large prospective, multicenter clinical trials to validate and standardize these technologies. Recently, a team of 26 authors has attempted to initiate a constructive discussion about the definition of clinical proteomics, study requirements, pitfalls, and (potential) use for clinical proteome analysis.[121] These kinds of initiatives are important for the evaluation and validation of the proteomic technologies. As the different proteomic technologies continues to improve, it will add new dimensions to the analyses of clinically relevant samples and promises to revolutionize the way pleural diseases will be diagnosed, treated and managed in the near future.

KEY POINTS

- Proteomics involves the comprehensive study of the identification, quantification, structure, localization, modification, interactions, activities and function of all proteins in body fluids, tissues or cell types under given conditions.
- The proteome differs from cell to cell and is constantly changing through its biochemical interactions with the genome and the environment.
- Biomarkers are proteins that are differentially present in a sample taken from a subject of one phenotypic status (e.g. having a disease) compared with another phenotypic status (e.g. healthy) and can therefore be used to diagnose, monitor or prognose a particular disease state.
- Potential biomarkers can be identified by the separation of a complex mixture of proteins by electrophoresis, mass measurement of peptides generated after spot proteolysis by mass spectrometry and searching in databases, but various other approaches are now evolving.
- The choice of an appropriate methodology to study novel biomarkers will depend on the goals of the specific study, amount and number of samples, availability of resources and other factors.
- Although technical advances have been significant in previous decades, we are still confronted with the challenges of evaluation and validation of the proteomic technologies, understanding the massive volume of data, translating the information to fit clinical contents and incorporating it into clinical studies.

REFERENCES

● = Key primary paper
◆ = Major review article

1. Fields S. Proteomics. Proteomics in genomeland. *Science* 2001; **291**: 1221–4.
2. Anderson L, Seilhamer J. A comparison of selected mRNA and protein abundances in human liver. *Electrophoresis* 1997; **18**: 533–7.
3. Wilkins MR, Sanchez JC, Williams KL, Hochstrasser DF. Current challenges and future applications for protein maps and post-translational vector maps in proteome projects. *Electrophoresis* 1996; **17**: 830–8.
4. Wold F. *In vivo* chemical modification of proteins (post-translational modification). *Annu Rev Biochem* 1981; **50**: 783–814.
5. Wold F, Moldave K. A short stroll through the posttranslational zoo. *Meth Enzymol* 1984; **107**: xiii–xvi.
6. Mann M, Jensen ON. Proteomic analysis of post-translational modifications. *Nat Biotechnol* 2003; **21**: 255–61.
7. Miklos GL, Maleszka R. Protein functions and biological contexts. *Proteomics* 2001; **1**: 169–78.
8. Selle H, Lamerz J, Buerger K, *et al.* Identification of novel biomarker candidates by differential peptidomics analysis of cerebrospinal fluid in Alzheimer's disease. *Comb Chem High Throughput Screen* 2005; **8**: 801–6.
9. Schulz-Knappe P, Schrader M, Zucht HD. The peptidomics concept. *Comb Chem High Throughput Screen* 2005; **8**: 697–704.
10. Petricoin EF, Ardekani AM, Hitt BA, *et al.* Use of proteomic

patterns in serum to identify ovarian cancer. *Lancet* 2002; **359**: 572–7.

11. Stoeckli M, Chaurand P, Hallahan DE, Caprioli RM. Imaging mass spectrometry: a new technology for the analysis of protein expression in mammalian tissues. *Nat Med* 2001; **7**: 493–6.
12. Emmert-Buck MR, Bonner RF, Smith PD, *et al.* Laser capture microdissection. *Science* 1996; **274**: 998–1001.
13. Emmert-Buck MR, Gillespie JW, Paweletz CP, *et al.* An approach to proteomic analysis of human tumors. *Mol Carcinog* 2000; **27**: 158–65.
14. Craven RA, Totty N, Harnden P, Selby PJ, Banks RE. Laser capture microdissection and two-dimensional polyacrylamide gel electrophoresis: evaluation of tissue preparation and sample limitations. *Am J Pathol* 2002; **160**: 815–22.
15. Ornstein DK, Gillespie JW, Paweletz CP, *et al.* Proteomic analysis of laser capture microdissected human prostate cancer and *in vitro* prostate cell lines. *Electrophoresis* 2000; **21**: 2235–42.
16. Wulfkuhle JD, McLean KC, Paweletz CP, *et al.* New approaches to proteomic analysis of breast cancer. *Proteomics* 2001; **1**: 1205–15.
17. Jones MB, Krutzsch H, Shu H, *et al.* Proteomic analysis and identification of new biomarkers and therapeutic targets for invasive ovarian cancer. *Proteomics* 2002; **2**: 76–84.
18. Knezevic V, Leethanakul C, Bichsel VE, *et al.* Proteomic profiling of the cancer microenvironment by antibody arrays. *Proteomics* 2001; **1**: 1271–8.
19. Nakagawa T, Huang SK, Martinez SR, *et al.* Proteomic profiling of primary breast cancer predicts axillary lymph node metastasis. *Cancer Res* 2006; **66**: 11825–30.
20. Mehta AI, Ross S, Lowenthal MS, *et al.* Biomarker amplification by serum carrier protein binding. *Dis Markers* 2003; **19**: 1–10.
21. Petricoin EF, Belluco C, Araujo RP, Liotta LA. The blood peptidome: a higher dimension of information content for cancer biomarker discovery. *Nat Rev Cancer* 2006; **6**: 961–7.
22. Liotta LA, Petricoin EF. Serum peptidome for cancer detection: spinning biologic trash into diagnostic gold. *J Clin Invest* 2006; **116**: 26–30.
23. Light RW, Macgregor MI, Luchsinger PC, Ball WC, Jr. Pleural effusions: the diagnostic separation of transudates and exudates. *Ann Intern Med* 1972; **77**: 507–13.
24. Bartter T, Santarelli R, Akers SM, Pratter MR. The evaluation of pleural effusion. *Chest* 1994; **106**: 1209–14.
◆25. Burgess LJ. Biochemical analysis of pleural, peritoneal and pericardial effusions. *Clin Chim Acta* 2004; **343**: 61–84.
26. Marel M, Stastny B, Melinova L, Svandova E, Light RW. Diagnosis of pleural effusions. Experience with clinical studies, 1986 to 1990. *Chest* 1995; **107**: 1598–603.
27. San Jose ME, Alvarez D, Valdes L, *et al.* Utility of tumour markers in the diagnosis of neoplastic pleural effusion. *Clin Chim Acta* 1997; **265**: 193–205.
28. Raja OG, Casson IF. Fibrinogen degradation products in pleural effusions. *Br J Dis Chest* 1980; **74**: 164–8.
29. Riska H, Pettersson T, Froseth B, Klockars M. Beta 2 microglobulin in pleural effusions. *Acta Med Scand* 1982; **211**: 45–50.
30. Ungerer JP, Oosthuizen HM, Retief JH, Bissbort SH. Significance of adenosine deaminase activity and its isoenzymes in tuberculous effusions. *Chest* 1994; **106**: 33–7.
31. Carstens ME, Burgess LJ, Maritz FJ, Taljaard JJ. Isoenzymes of adenosine deaminase in pleural effusions: a diagnostic tool? *Int J Tuberc Lung Dis* 1998; **2**: 831–5.
32. Beyer HL, Geschwindt RD, Glover CL, *et al.* MESOMARKTM: A potential test for malignant pleural mesothelioma. *Clin Chem* 2007.
●33. Scherpereel A, Grigoriu B, Conti M, *et al.* Soluble mesothelin-related peptides in the diagnosis of malignant pleural mesothelioma. *Am J Respir Crit Care Med* 2006; **173**: 1155–60.
34. Robinson BW, Creaney J, Lake R, *et al.* Mesothelin-family proteins and diagnosis of mesothelioma. *Lancet* 2003; **362**: 1612–6.
35. Hassan R, Remaley AT, Sampson ML, *et al.* Detection and quantitation of serum mesothelin, a tumor marker for patients with mesothelioma and ovarian cancer. *Clin Cancer Res* 2006; **12**: 447–53.
●36. Robinson BW, Creaney J, Lake R, *et al.* Soluble mesothelin-related protein – a blood test for mesothelioma. *Lung Cancer* 2005; **49**(Suppl 1): S109–11.
37. Creaney J, Robinson BW. Detection of malignant mesothelioma in asbestos-exposed individuals: the potential role of soluble mesothelin-related protein. *Hematol Oncol Clin North Am* 2005; **19**: 1025–40, v.
38. Gorg A, Weiss W, Dunn MJ. Current two-dimensional electrophoresis technology for proteomics. *Proteomics* 2004; **4**: 3665–85.
39. Hanash SM. Biomedical applications of two-dimensional electrophoresis using immobilized pH gradients: current status. *Electrophoresis* 2000; **21**: 1202–9.
40. Anderson L, Anderson NG. High resolution two-dimensional electrophoresis of human plasma proteins. *Proc Natl Acad Sci U S A* 1977; **74**: 5421–5.
41. Anderson NG, Anderson NL, Tollaksen SL, *et al.* Analytical techniques for cell fractions. XXV. Concentration and two-dimensional electrophoretic analysis of human urinary proteins. *Anal Biochem* 1979; **95**: 48–61.
42. Wiederkehr F, Ogilvie A, Vonderschmitt DJ. Cerebrospinal fluid proteins studied by two-dimensional gel electrophoresis and immunoblotting technique. *J Neurochem* 1987; **49**: 363–72.
43. Wildenauer DB, Korschenhausen D, Hoechtlen W, *et al.* Analysis of cerebrospinal fluid from patients with psychiatric and neurological disorders by two-dimensional electrophoresis: identification of disease-associated polypeptides as fibrin fragments. *Electrophoresis* 1991; **12**: 487–92.
44. Felgenhauer K, Hagedorn D. Two-dimensional separation of human body fluid proteins. *Clin Chim Acta* 1980; *100*: 121–32.
45. Giometti CS, Tollaksen SL, Chubb C, Williams C, Huberman E. Analysis of proteins from human breast epithelial cells using two-dimensional gel electrophoresis. *Electrophoresis* 1995; **16**: 1215–24.
46. Tyan YC, Wu HY, Su WC, Chen PW, Liao PC. Proteomic analysis of human pleural effusion. *Proteomics* 2005; **5**: 1062–74.
47. Hsieh WY, Chen MW, Ho HT, You TM, Lu YT. Identification of differentially expressed proteins in human malignant pleural effusions. *Eur Respir J* 2006; **28**: 1178–85.
48. Chromy BA, Gonzales AD, Perkins J, *et al.* Proteomic analysis of human serum by two- dimensional differential gel electrophoresis after depletion of high-abundant proteins. *J Proteome Res* 2004; **3**: 1120–7.
49. Ahmed N, Barker G, Oliva K, *et al.* An approach to remove albumin for the proteomic analysis of low abundance biomarkers in human serum. *Proteomics* 2003; **3**: 1980–7.
50. Fountoulakis M, Juranville JF, Jiang L, *et al.* Depletion of the high-abundance plasma proteins. *Amino Acids* 2004; **27**: 249–59.
51. Fu Q, Bovenkamp DE, Van Eyk JE. A rapid, economical, and reproducible method for human serum delipidation and albumin and IgG removal for proteomic analysis. *Methods Mol Biol* 2007; **357**: 365–71.
52. Darde VM, Barderas MG, Vivanco F. Depletion of high-abundance proteins in plasma by immunoaffinity subtraction for two-dimensional difference gel electrophoresis analysis. *Meth Mol Biol* 2007; **357**: 351–64.
53. Granger J, Siddiqui J, Copeland S, Remick D. Albumin depletion of human plasma also removes low abundance proteins including the cytokines. *Proteomics* 2005; **5**: 4713–8.
54. Pieper R, Gatlin CL, Makusky AJ, *et al.* The human serum proteome: display of nearly 3700 chromatographically separated protein spots on two-dimensional electrophoresis gels and identification of 325 distinct proteins. *Proteomics* 2003; **3**: 1345–64.

55. Sloane AJ, Duff JL, Wilson NL, *et al.* High throughput peptide mass fingerprinting and protein macroarray analysis using chemical printing strategies. *Mol Cell Proteomics* 2002; **1**: 490–9.
56. Wu SL, Amato H, Biringer R, *et al.* Targeted proteomics of low-level proteins in human plasma by LC/MSn: using human growth hormone as a model system. *J Proteome Res* 2002; **1**: 459–65.
57. Choudhary G, Wu SL, Shieh P, Hancock WS. Multiple enzymatic digestion for enhanced sequence coverage of proteins in complex proteomic mixtures using capillary LC with ion trap MS/MS. *J Proteome Res* 2003; **2**: 59–67.
58. Sanchez JC, Appel RD, Golaz O, *et al.* Inside SWISS-2DPAGE database. *Electrophoresis* 1995; **16**: 1131–51.
59. Adkins JN, Varnum SM, Auberry KJ, *et al.* Toward a human blood serum proteome: analysis by multidimensional separation coupled with mass spectrometry. *Mol Cell Proteomics* 2002; **1**: 947–55.
60. Tonge R, Shaw J, Middleton B, *et al.* Validation and development of fluorescence two-dimensional differential gel electrophoresis proteomics technology. *Proteomics* 2001; **1**: 377–96.
61. Von Eggeling F, Gawriljuk A, Fiedler W, *et al.* Fluorescent dual colour 2D-protein gel electrophoresis for rapid detection of differences in protein pattern with standard image analysis software. *Int J Mol Med* 2001; **8**: 373–7.
62. Yan JX, Devenish AT, Wait R, *et al.* Fluorescence two-dimensional difference gel electrophoresis and mass spectrometry based proteomic analysis of Escherichia coli. *Proteomics* 2002; **2**: 1682–98.
63. Nordvarg H, Flensburg J, Ronn O, *et al.* A proteomics approach to the study of absorption, distribution, metabolism, excretion, and toxicity. *J Biomol Tech* 2004; **15**: 265–75.
64. Alban A, David SO, Bjorkesten L, *et al.* A novel experimental design for comparative two-dimensional gel analysis: two-dimensional difference gel electrophoresis incorporating a pooled internal standard. *Proteomics* 2003; **3**: 36–44.
65. Unlu M, Morgan ME, Minden JS. Difference gel electrophoresis: a single gel method for detecting changes in protein extracts. *Electrophoresis* 1997; **18**: 2071–7.
66. Patton WF. Detection technologies in proteome analysis. *J Chromatogr B Analyt Technol Biomed Life Sci* 2002; **771**: 3–31.
67. Lilley KS, Friedman DB. All about DIGE: quantification technology for differential-display 2D-gel proteomics. *Expert Rev Proteomics* 2004; **1**: 401–9.
68. Morita A, Miyagi E, Yasumitsu H, *et al.* Proteomic search for potential diagnostic markers and therapeutic targets for ovarian clear cell adenocarcinoma. *Proteomics* 2006; **6**: 5880–90.
69. Zhou G, Li H, DeCamp D, *et al.* 2D differential in-gel electrophoresis for the identification of esophageal scans cell cancer-specific protein markers. *Mol Cell Proteomics* 2002; **1**: 117–24.
70. Alfonso P, Nunez A, Madoz-Gurpide J, *et al.* Proteomic expression analysis of colorectal cancer by two-dimensional differential gel electrophoresis. *Proteomics* 2005; **5**: 2602–11.
71. Lee IN, Chen CH, Sheu JC, *et al.* Identification of human hepatocellular carcinoma-related biomarkers by two-dimensional difference gel electrophoresis and mass spectrometry. *J Proteome Res* 2005; **4**: 2062–9.
72. Yu KH, Rustgi AK, Blair IA. Characterization of proteins in human pancreatic cancer serum using differential gel electrophoresis and tandem mass spectrometry. *J Proteome Res* 2005; **4**: 1742–51.
73. Nayak SS, Kamath SS, Kundaje GN, Aroor AR. Diagnostic significance of estimation of serum apolipoprotein A along with alpha-fetoprotein in alcoholic cirrhosis and hepatocellular carcinoma patients. *Clin Chim Acta* 1988; **173**: 157–64.
74. Matsuura T, Koga S, Ibayashi H. Increased proportion of proapolipoprotein A-I in HDL from patients with liver cirrhosis and hepatitis. *Gastroenterol Jpn* 1988; **23**: 394–400.
75. Fujii S, Koga S, Shono T, Yamamoto K, Ibayashi H. Serum apoprotein A-I and A-II levels in liver diseases and cholestasis. *Clin Chim Acta* 1981; **115**: 321–31.
76. Steel LF, Shumpert D, Trotter M, *et al.* A strategy for the comparative analysis of serum proteomes for the discovery of biomarkers for hepatocellular carcinoma. *Proteomics* 2003; **3**: 601–9.
77. Tachibana M, Ohkura Y, Kobayashi Y, *et al.* Expression of apolipoprotein A1 in colonic adenocarcinoma. *Anticancer Res* 2003; **23**: 4161–7.
78. Hellman K, Alaiya AA, Schedvins K, *et al.* Protein expression patterns in primary carcinoma of the vagina. *Br J Cancer* 2004; **91**: 319–26.
79. Zhang Z, Bast RC Jr, Yu Y, *et al.* Three biomarkers identified from serum proteomic analysis for the detection of early stage ovarian cancer. *Cancer Res* 2004; **64**: 5882–90.
80. Kuesel AC, Kroft T, Prefontaine M, Smith IC. Lipoprotein(a) and CA125 levels in the plasma of patients with benign and malignant ovarian disease. *Int J Cancer* 1992; **52**: 341–6.
81. Ross PL, Huang YN, Marchese JN, *et al.* Multiplexed protein quantitation in Saccharomyces cerevisiae using amine-reactive isobaric tagging reagents. *Mol Cell Proteomics* 2004; **3**: 1154–69.
82. Ong SE, Blagoev B, Kratchmarova I, *et al.* Stable isotope labeling by amino acids in cell culture, SILAC, as a simple and accurate approach to expression proteomics. *Mol Cell Proteomics* 2002; **1**: 376–86.
83. Higgs RE, Knierman MD, Gelfanova V, Butler JP, Hale JE. Comprehensive label-free method for the relative quantification of proteins from biological samples. *J Proteome Res* 2005; **4**: 1442–50.
84. Wiener MC, Sachs JR, Deyanova EG, Yates NA. Differential mass spectrometry: a label-free LC-MS method for finding significant differences in complex peptide and protein mixtures. *Anal Chem* 2004; **76**: 6085–96.
85. Gygi SP, Rist B, Gerber SA, *et al.* Quantitative analysis of complex protein mixtures using isotope-coded affinity tags. *Nat Biotechnol* 1999; **17**: 994–9.
86. Karas M, Hillenkamp F. Laser desorption ionization of proteins with molecular masses exceeding 10,000 daltons. *Anal Chem* 1988; **60**: 2299–301.
87. Hillenkamp F, Karas M. Mass spectrometry of peptides and proteins by matrix-assisted ultraviolet laser desorption/ionization. *Methods Enzymol* 1990; **193**: 280–95.
88. Cho A, Normile D. Nobel Prize in Chemistry. Mastering macromolecules. *Science* 2002; **298**: 527–8.
89. Li C, Chen Z, Xiao Z, *et al.* Comparative proteomics analysis of human lung squamous carcinoma. *Biochem Biophys Res Commun* 2003; **309**: 253–60.
90. Chen G, Wang H, Gharib TG, *et al.* Overexpression of oncoprotein 18 correlates with poor differentiation in lung adenocarcinomas. *Mol Cell Proteomics* 2003; **2**: 107–16.
91. Chen G, Gharib TG, Thomas DG, *et al.* Proteomic analysis of eIF-5A in lung adenocarcinomas. *Proteomics* 2003; **3**: 496–504.
92. Chen G, Gharib TG, Wang H, *et al.* Protein profiles associated with survival in lung adenocarcinoma. *Proc Natl Acad Sci U S A* 2003; **100**: 13537–42.
93. Chen G, Gharib TG, Huang CC, *et al.* Proteomic analysis of lung adenocarcinoma: identification of a highly expressed set of proteins in tumors. *Clin Cancer Res* 2002; **8**: 2298–305.
94. Bard MP, Hegmans JP, Hemmes A, *et al.* Proteomic analysis of exosomes isolated from human malignant pleural effusions. *Am J Respir Cell Mol Biol* 2004; **31**: 114–21.
95. Diamandis EP. Serum proteomic profiling by matrix-assisted laser desorption-ionization time-of-flight mass spectrometry for cancer diagnosis: next steps. *Cancer Res* 2006; **66**: 5540–1.
96. Merchant M, Weinberger SR. Recent advancements in surface-enhanced laser desorption/ionization-time of flight-mass spectrometry. *Electrophoresis* 2000; **21**: 1164–77.
97. Oh JH, Nandi A, Gurnani P, *et al.* Proteomic biomarker identification for diagnosis of early relapse in ovarian cancer. *J Bioinform Comput Biol* 2006; **4**: 1159–79.

98. Ciordia S, de Los Rios V, Albar JP. Contributions of advanced proteomics technologies to cancer diagnosis. *Clin Transl Oncol* 2006; **8**: 566–80.
99. Oh JH, Gao J, Nandi A, *et al.* Diagnosis of early relapse in ovarian cancer using serum proteomic profiling. *Genome Inform* 2005; **16**: 195–204.
100. Ho DW, Yang ZF, Wong BY, *et al.* Surface-enhanced laser desorption/ionization time-of-flight mass spectrometry serum protein profiling to identify nasopharyngeal carcinoma. *Cancer* 2006; **107**: 99–107.
101. Gourin CG, Xia ZS, Han Y, *et al.* Serum protein profile analysis in patients with head and neck squamous cell carcinoma. *Arch Otolaryngol Head Neck Surg* 2006; **132**: 390–7.
102. Engwegen JY, Gast MC, Schellens JH, Beijnen JH. Clinical proteomics: searching for better tumour markers with SELDI-TOF mass spectrometry. *Trends Pharmacol Sci* 2006; **27**: 251–9.
103. Rubin RB, Merchant M. A rapid protein profiling system that speeds study of cancer and other diseases. *Am Clin Lab* 2000; **19**: 28–9.
104. Aebersold R, Mann M. Mass spectrometry-based proteomics. *Nature* 2003; **422**: 198–207.
105. Washburn MP, Wolters D, Yates JR 3rd. Large-scale analysis of the yeast proteome by multidimensional protein identification technology. *Nat Biotechnol* 2001; **19**: 242–7.
106. Kusnezow W, Hoheisel JD. Antibody microarrays: promises and problems. *Biotechniques* 2002; **Suppl**: 14–23.
107. James P. Chips for proteomics: a new tool or just hype? *Biotechniques* 2002; **Suppl**: 4–10, 12–13.
108. Ekins RP, Chu FW. Multianalyte microspot immunoassay – microanalytical "compact disk" of the future. *Clin Chem* 1991; **37**: 1955–67.
109. Anderson NL, Anderson NG. The human plasma proteome: history, character, and diagnostic prospects. *Mol Cell Proteomics* 2002; **1**: 845–67.
110. Kusnezow W, Syagailo YV, Goychuk I, Hoheisel JD, Wild DG. Antibody microarrays: the crucial impact of mass transport on assay kinetics and sensitivity. *Expert Rev Mol Diagn* 2006; **6**: 111–24.
111. Nitadori J, Ishii G, Tsuta K, *et al.* Immunohistochemical differential diagnosis between large cell neuroendocrine carcinoma and small cell carcinoma by tissue microarray analysis with a large antibody panel. *Am J Clin Pathol* 2006; **125**: 682–92.
112. Song S, Li B, Wang L, *et al.* A cancer protein microarray platform using antibody fragments and its clinical applications. *Mol Biosyst* 2007; **3**: 151–8.
113. Srivastava M, Eidelman O, Jozwik C, *et al.* Serum proteomic signature for cystic fibrosis using an antibody microarray platform. *Mol Genet Metab* 2006; **87**: 303–10.
114. Orchekowski R, Hamelinck D, Li L, *et al.* Antibody microarray profiling reveals individual and combined serum proteins associated with pancreatic cancer. *Cancer Res* 2005; **65**: 11193–202.
115. Gao WM, Kuick R, Orchekowski RP, *et al.* Distinctive serum protein profiles involving abundant proteins in lung cancer patients based upon antibody microarray analysis. *BMC Cancer* 2005; **5**: 110.
116. Hegmans JP, Hemmes A, Hammad H, *et al.* Mesothelioma environment comprises cytokines and T-regulatory cells that suppress immune responses. *Eur Respir J* 2006; **27**: 1086–95.
117. Shen Y, Smith RD, Unger KK, Kumar D, Lubda D. Ultrahigh-throughput proteomics using fast RPLC separations with ESI-MS/MS. *Anal Chem* 2005; **77**: 6692–701.
118. Shen Y, Smith RD. Advanced nanoscale separations and mass spectrometry for sensitive high-throughput proteomics. *Expert Rev Proteomics* 2005; **2**: 431–47.
119. Li J, LeRiche T, Tremblay TL, *et al.* Application of microfluidic devices to proteomics research: identification of trace-level protein digests and affinity capture of target peptides. *Mol Cell Proteomics* 2002; **1**: 157–68.
120. MacBeath G. Proteomics comes to the surface. *Nat Biotechnol* 2001; **19**: 828–9.
◆121. Mischak H, Apweiler R, Banks RE, *et al.* Clinical proteomics: A need to define the field and to begin to set adequate standards. *Proteomics Clin Appl* 2007; **1**: 148–156.

13

Pleural pharmacokinetics

ARYUN KIM, BLAIR CAPITANO, CHARLES H NIGHTINGALE

INTRODUCTION

The main goal in the pharmacotherapeutic treatment of any disease state is relatively simple: to ensure drug delivery to its specific site of action in order to elicit a desired clinical response with minimization of adverse effects. Although the goal of treatment is straightforward, its realization is much more complex. This is due to the fact that the systemic administration of chemotherapeutic agents leads to the diffuse delivery of these agents to vast regions throughout the body in attempt to reach the targeted site(s) of action. If one considers the reverse, direct administration of the drug to a targeted area in the body, the agent must ultimately diffuse throughout the systemic circulation, to some degree, in order to be eliminated. Drug concentration at the intended target site(s) of action may not be easily quantified and exposure of unintended sites will potentially lead to adverse effects. The application of pharmacokinetic principles aids the clinician in determining the necessary dose to achieve drug concentrations within a specific range to maximize therapeutic effect while minimizing adverse effects.

When considering pleural diseases, especially infection and malignancy, the focus of the clinician is drug delivery to the pleural space from systemic administration and the systemic implications of administration of drugs directly to the pleural space. The area of pharmacokinetics dealing specifically with drug delivery to and from the pleural space is not well studied and information is therefore scant. The aim of this chapter is to develop a basic understanding of the pharmacokinetic principles that govern drug delivery to and from the pleural space and explore available data to form conclusions in order to assist the clinician in the optimization of pharmacotherapy.

BASIC PHARMACOKINETIC PRINCIPLES

Introduction to pharmacokinetics

Pharmacokinetics is the study of the movement of the drug throughout the body, which consists of four phases: absorption, distribution, metabolism and elimination (Figure 13.1). A multitude of factors specific to the pharmaceutical agents as well as the patient have the propensity to affect the pharmacokinetics of a particular agent. These factors include, but are not limited to, the chemical structure of the drug, the dosage form, the degree of protein binding, drug interactions, body composition, hepatic and renal functions, as well as the specific disease being treated and any underlying diseases.

While an understanding of basic pharmacokinetic principles is essential for the purposes of this chapter, a

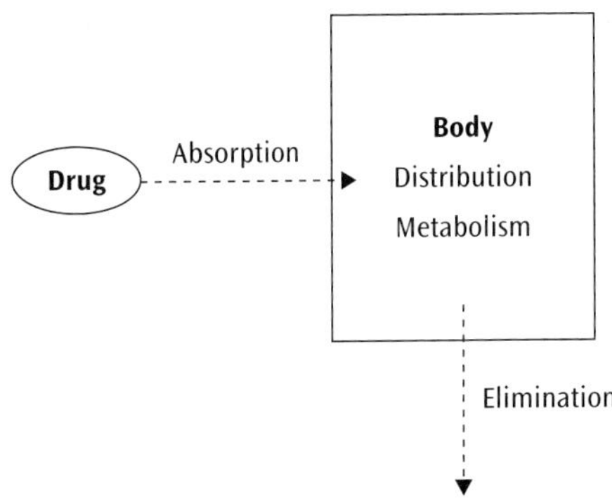

Figure 13.1 Pharmacokinetics: absorption, distribution, metabolism and elimination.

comprehensive discussion is not within its scope. Therefore, this section will only highlight concepts pertinent to discussion of drug delivery to the pleural space. Since intravenous drug administration is most often the approach used when treating pleural disease, the intricacies of the movement of drug from the site of administration to the systemic circulation, known as absorption, will not be addressed. For the purposes of this discussion, it is understood that intravenous administration constitutes immediate placement of the agent into the systemic circulation.

Plasma drug concentration and time

Pharmacokinetics follows the course of a drug in the body over time. The systemic blood circulation is the mode of transport by which the drug reaches the various tissues, spaces and organs throughout the body. In order to depict the movement of drugs throughout the body, it is logical to use concentrations in the systemic circulation as a surrogate marker.

Whole blood contains several components to which the drug may bind, including plasma proteins and cellular components. As a result, the drug concentration within the blood is diverse in that it differs among the plasma, cells, plasma protein and plasma water. Classically, the plasma or serum drug concentration (C_p) is the accepted parameter used to reflect the concentration of drug in the systemic circulation.

The concentration of drug in the plasma may be considered to be in equilibrium with drug concentration in the interstitial fluid that bathes cells and tissues. Plasma concentration, therefore, is the driving force of drug penetration to spaces, tissues and organs throughout the body when considering a systemically administered drug. A concentration gradient is usually the mechanism behind this force. A change in plasma concentration usually reflects, but does not necessarily quantify, changes in drug concentration at the site of action. The degree of correlation of plasma concentration with drug concentration of a specific site such as the pleural space depends on the physiochemical properties of the drug that dictate the efficiency with which it crosses membrane barriers and upon blood perfusion which governs delivery of drug to a specific space.

Once a drug enters the systemic circulation, the processes of distribution and elimination are immediately initiated. The rate of distribution and elimination is determined by characteristics of the drug as well as the patient. The concentration of the drug in the plasma following a dose is not constant, but changes over time as a result of these simultaneous processes. The drug plasma concentration–time curve (Figure 13.2) is used to visualize the time course of drug in the body. The area under the plasma drug concentration–time curve (AUC) represents total drug exposure over the specific time period evaluated.[1–4]

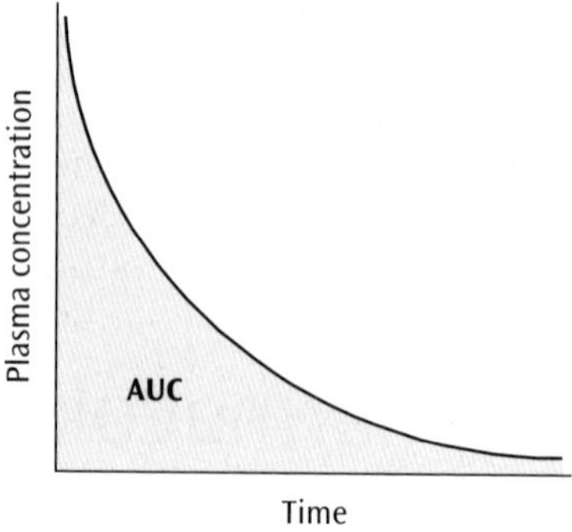

Figure 13.2 Drug concentration–time profile following an intravenous dose. AUC, area under the curve.

Distribution

Distribution refers to the dispersion of the drug from the blood to the extravascular spaces, including organs, tissue and fluids. This process is reversible and may occur rapidly or slowly until distribution equilibrium is reached. The amount of drug that remains in the plasma and that which reaches specific sites in the body, such as the pleural space, at distribution equilibrium depends on a variety of factors. These factors include the physiochemical properties of the agent that affect its ability to permeate membranes, protein- and tissue-binding characteristics of the agent, blood perfusion of the site and the physical condition of the patient. Once distribution equilibrium is reached, the amount of drug at various sites in the body is rarely equal. Depending on the agent and its ability to permeate membranes, the drug concentration in a specific space, tissue or fluid may exceed that of the plasma or may be much lower than plasma.

The apparent volume of distribution (V_d) is a derived pharmacokinetic parameter that allows one to estimate the extent of distribution or the affinity for plasma transfer to tissues of an agent. The V_d is not an actual body volume, but is simply a proportionality constant that relates the amount of drug administered to the resultant plasma concentration. It may be thought of as simply the volume of space needed to account for a total dose given when examining the resultant plasma concentration. The observed decline of plasma concentration over time is due to the fact that drug distribution and elimination commence immediately and simultaneously following administration. The shape and slope of the plasma concentration–time curve reflect the rate of both of these processes. Shortly after intravenous administration, however, the rate of distribution is thought to exceed that of elimination. Immediately following intravenous administration, when the plasma concentration is at its maximum (C_{pmax}), the equation given below may be applied to estimate the dose needed to achieve a specific plasma concentration and characterize the distribution of a particular agent:

$$V_d = Dose/C_{pmax}$$

The V_d is a property that is inherent to each drug. However, it may be affected by disease states that alter total body volume and protein stores that change distribution characteristics of the drug. The V_d may range from one to several liters, depending on the degree of tissue penetration and binding of an individual agent. For example, it may be concluded that the distribution of a drug with a V_d similar to the amount of total body extracellular fluid (15–18 L in a 70 kg person) is limited mainly to the extravascular space. A drug with a V_d that exceeds the total amount of body water is thought to have a large affinity for the tissues and other extravascular spaces.

It follows, therefore, that a drug with a large V_d at distribution equilibrium would be expected to have a small plasma concentration and the reverse is also true. Factors associated with decreased plasma drug concentrations, such as decreased plasma protein binding, would consequently result in a larger V_d. Generally speaking, a drug with a large V_d is thought to have a high degree of distribution to extravascular tissues, spaces and fluids and a smaller plasma concentration. It must be kept in mind, however, that the V_d does not provide insight into the exact distribution sites, it simply estimates the affinity of the drug for extravascular areas of the body.

Compartmental models

The human body is undoubtedly a very complex system composed of a multitude of different tissues, spaces and fluids. Compartment models are used in the area of pharmacokinetics to simplify the complexity of drug distribution and elimination in order to allow the application of mathematical principles to depict and quantify the time-course of drug concentrations in the body. Spaces, tissues and fluids with similar types of drug distribution characteristics are grouped into the same compartment.

The one-compartment model is the most straightforward and holds the underlying assumption that the body behaves as one large container (Figure 13.3). The central compartment or first compartment is thought to be congruent with the systemic circulation and consists of the most highly perfused tissues and organs such as the heart, kidneys and lungs. Since most drugs are metabolized and eliminated via the liver and kidneys, elimination is accepted to occur strictly from the first compartment. Drugs that display one-compartment model behavior are assumed to be distributed and equilibrate very rapidly throughout the body following administration. From another perspective, areas in the body that may be considered as parts of the central compartment contain drug concentrations that equilibrate at a rate that is proportionate to drug concentrations in the plasma. This is not to say that drug concentrations within spaces of a single compartment are identical, simply that the rate at which

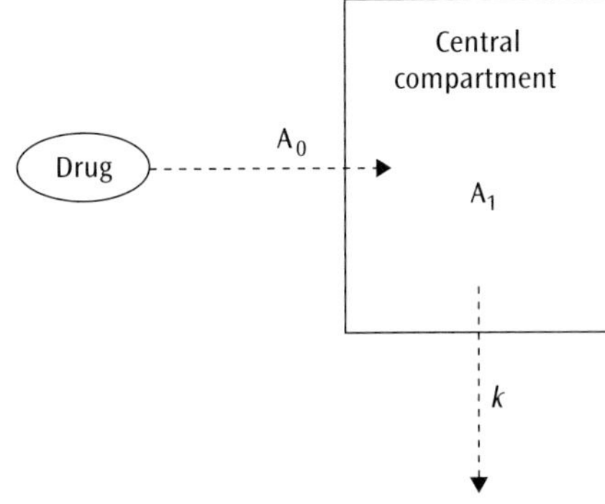

Figure 13.3 A one-compartment model. A_0, amount of drug administered; A_1, amount of drug in body; k, elimination rate constant.

distribution equilibrium is reached in those spaces are similar.

Two-compartment and multi-compartment models are useful when characterizing drugs that equilibrate at different rates to various regions of the body. The peripheral compartment or second compartment, as denoted in a two-compartment model, includes less well-perfused organs, tissues and spaces that are not in rapid equilibrium with the plasma, such as muscle and fat. Membrane penetration, protein binding and other physiochemical properties slow distribution to sites in the second compartment. A three-compartment model represents distribution from the central compartment to two distinct peripheral compartments following administration.

In a two-compartment model, once the drug is distributed throughout the first compartment, the plasma concentration will decline slightly, reflecting a slow and reversible distribution to the second compartment (Figure 13.4). The rate constants, k_{12} and k_{21}, quantify the reversible distribution of the drug from the central compartment to and from the peripheral compartment. As

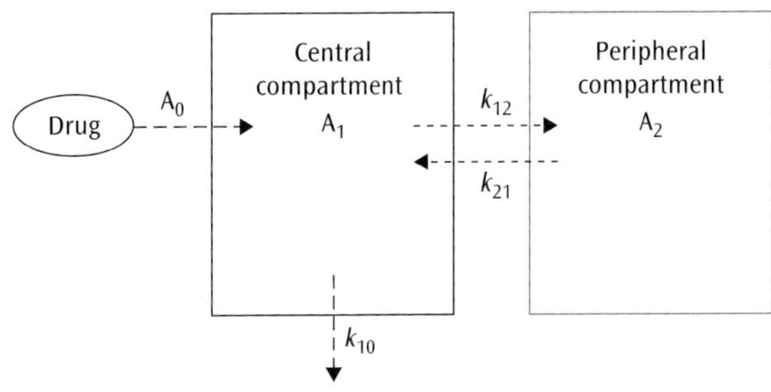

Figure 13.4 A two-compartment model. A_0, amount of drug administered; A_1, amount of drug in body; k_{10}, elimination rate constant from the body; k_{12}, rate constant of transfer from the central compartment to the peripheral compartment; k_{21}, rate constant of transfer from the peripheral compartment to the central compartment.

stated previously, most drugs must be transferred to the central compartment to be eliminated.[1–4]

Examination of the plasma concentration–time profile of drugs that follow multi-compartment pharmacokinetics reveals a curve with varying degrees of slope that correspond to the various rates at which the drug is distributed and eliminated from each compartment (Figure 13.5). The number of compartments required to describe the behavior of a drug is determined by the number of exponential terms that may be applied to the plasma concentration–time data. Three or more compartments may be needed to accurately depict the data generated by some agents in the plasma.

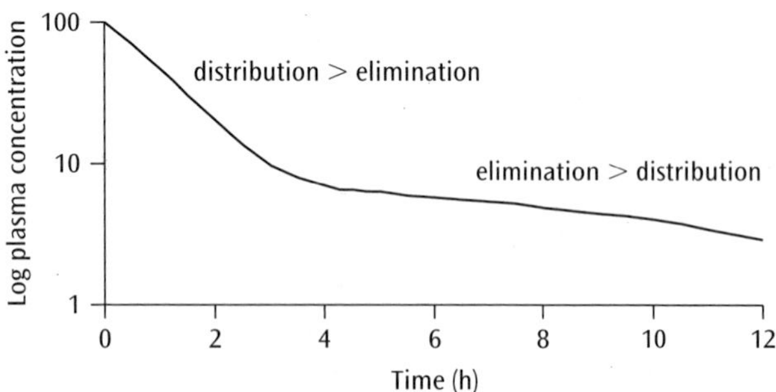

Figure 13.5 The log of the plasma concentration–time profile for a two-compartment drug.

Elimination

Elimination refers to the biochemical conversion of the drug to metabolic products, where appropriate, and the movement of drug and metabolites from the blood to the urine, bile and feces out of the body. Although distribution and elimination immediately and simultaneously occur shortly following intravenous administration, the distribution rate at this point is generally much higher than the rate of elimination. Once distribution is complete, however, elimination predominates and the drug is removed from the body. The initial component of the plasma drug concentration–time curve, for the most part, depicts drug movement within the body and the latter part of the declining curve represents drug movement or elimination from the body.

FIRST-ORDER AND ZERO-ORDER ELIMINATION

The elimination of drugs is classified in the study of pharmacokinetics as a first-order or zero-order process. First-order elimination is characterized by drugs for which the amount of drug eliminated over a certain period is dependent on the amount of drug remaining in the body. Conversely, in a zero-order process, the amount of drug eliminated over time is constant and independent of the amount of drug remaining in the body. When administered in conventional doses, most drugs display first-order elimination and the pharmacokinetic parameters do not change with the size of the dose given.

Although the amount eliminated changes with time in a first-order process, the fraction of drug eliminated over a specific interval remains constant. This fraction of drug eliminated over time is referred to as the elimination rate constant (k). A plot of the drug plasma concentration–time profile for a first-order drug reveals a curve and a plot of the natural log of the plasma concentration–time profile will produce a straight line (Figure 13.6). As a result, available plasma drug concentration data may be used to calculate pharmacokinetic parameters and predict plasma drug concentrations and elimination over time.[1–4]

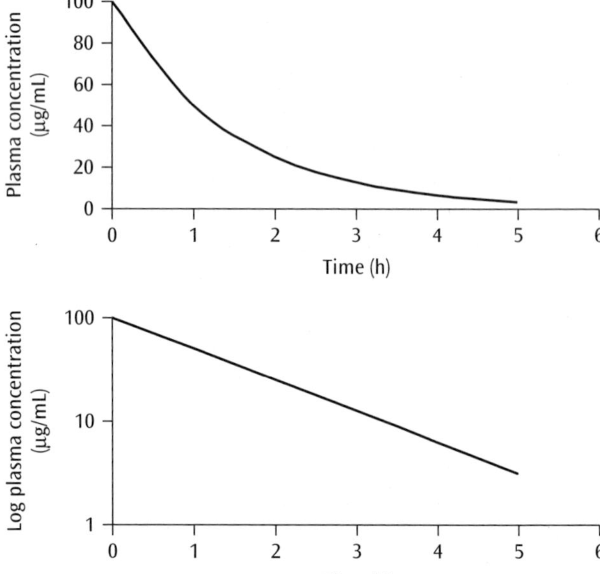

Figure 13.6 Plasma concentration–time plot for first-order elimination.

ELIMINATION RATE CONSTANT AND HALF-LIFE

Pharmacokinetic mathematical models have been developed to assist clinicians in determining proper doses to target specific plasma concentrations based on the fact that a plot of the natural log of the plasma concentration–time profile for a first-order elimination process produces a straight line. The slope of this line yields the elimination rate constant (k) or the percentage of drug eliminated over an interval of time. The formula to find the slope of a straight line is:

$$\text{Slope} = \Delta Y/\Delta X$$

where $\Delta Y = Y_2 - Y_1$ and $\Delta X = X_2 - X_1$. Application of this formula to the straight line of a plot of the natural log of the plasma concentration versus time yields the formula for the elimination rate constant (k) that corresponds to units of inverse time (per hour, per minute). This formula allows for the calculation of k when two plasma concentration timepoints are known for a drug following first-order elimination:

$$k = \ln C_{p2} - \ln Cp_1/t_2 - t_1$$

where $\Delta \ln C_p$ = the natural log of plasma concentration, Δt = the corresponding values for time, and k = the elimination rate constant.

The half-life ($t_{1/2}$) is the time it takes for the plasma concentration to be reduced by 50 percent (Figure 13.7). Practically speaking, it takes five half-lives for the drug to be 97 percent removed from the body. The plasma $t_{1/2}$ may be calculated by the formula:

$$t_{1/2} = 0.693/k$$

Clearance (Cl) refers to the inherent ability of the eliminating organs of the body to remove drug and metabolites from the blood per unit time. It is a function of capacity of organs such as the kidney and liver to process drugs and the degree of blood flow that presents these organs with drugs to eliminate. Clearance does not represent the amount of drug removed but the volume of blood that is cleared of drug over a certain interval of time. The amount of drug cleared depends on the concentration of drug in the plasma as well as the rate of blood flow to eliminating organs. The extraction ratio is the fraction of drug presented to an eliminating organ that is cleared after one pass through that organ. Many factors may affect clearance, such as the extraction ratio, the body surface area of the patient, plasma protein binding, renal and hepatic function and the cardiac output of the patient, which controls blood flow to the eliminating organs. When the rate of administration is equal to the clearance, such as may be the case in continuous infusion, the concentration in the plasma may remain constant or achieve steady-state (C_{pss}). The AUC, which accounts for total drug exposure, may be calculated if the clearance is known.[1–4]

$$\text{AUC} = \text{Dose/Cl}$$

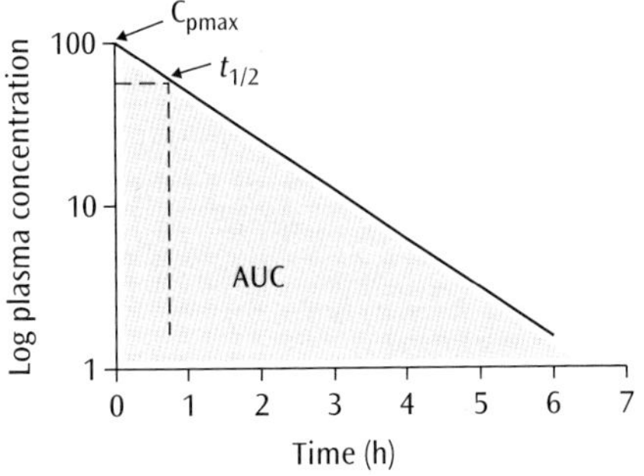

Figure 13.7 First-order elimination of a one-compartment drug. AUC, area under the curve; C_{pmax}, maximum plasma concentration; $t_{1/2}$, half-life (the time it takes for the plasma concentration to be reduced by 50 percent).

PHARMACOKINETICS SPECIFIC TO THE PLEURAL FLUID

Introduction

The pharmacokinetics of drugs in the pleural space is not a well-studied or established topic. Although there are several published studies examining antimicrobial concentrations in pleural fluid and the intrapleural administration of antineoplastic agents, many of these studies are not well controlled and consist of a small number of patients with a wide variety of malignancies and pleural effusion states. In order to best serve the purpose of this chapter, the basic principles of drug permeation through membranes will be considered along with theoretical exploration of drug delivery to the pleura combined with the published data to form educated conclusions.

Exudative effusions associated with infection and malignancy comprise the realm of pleural diseases in which the target site of drug therapy is clearly the pleura/pleural space. Penetration of adequate drug concentrations directly to the pleura/pleural fluid is paramount in the clinical picture of parapneumonic effusions, empyema, malignant effusions and malignant mesothelioma. Hence, our discussion will focus on penetration of antimicrobial and antineoplastic agents to the pleura/pleural fluid and the intrapleural administration of these agents.[3–7]

Drug membrane penetration and protein binding: general considerations

The ability of a drug to ultimately reach the pleura/pleural fluid from the plasma is influenced by several key factors. These factors include, but are not limited to: (1) plasma drug concentration; (2) plasma and tissue protein binding; (3) pleural membrane penetration; (4) blood perfusion of the pleura; and (5) effects of pleural disease on vascular permeability, membrane permeability and protein binding.

Diffusion down a concentration gradient is the mechanism by which most drugs move out of the plasma, into the interstitial fluid and across membranes to the target site of action. The size of the concentration gradient that will power diffusion is dependent on the initial concentration achieved in the plasma. Since distribution and elimination commence simultaneously and immediately following administration, it is imperative that a drug be dosed properly to achieve acceptable initial plasma concentrations. For example, concern should exist about using an antibiotic of which initial plasma concentrations barely exceed the minimum inhibitory concentration (MIC) of a targeted pathogen in the pleural space. Because there may be hindrances of distribution to the site of action and the continuous impact of drug elimination, the concentration that reaches a site of interest may be much lower than that in the plasma.

PROTEIN BINDING

Protein binding usually refers to serum or plasma protein binding. Drugs may bind to tissue proteins but this has not been studied and this section is therefore only concerned with serum or plasma protein binding. Serum drug protein binding is generally not an issue with which the clinician needs to be concerned. Once an agent reaches the market, recommended dosage regimens are based on clinical efficacy with the agent's capacity for protein binding already taken into consideration. However, the implications of protein binding become very relevant when focusing on a specific site of penetration. Biological proteins such as albumin are large and bulky molecules with low lipid solubility. Their size hinders passage through capillaries and low lipophilicity slows transfer across cell membranes. A drug that is protein bound is similarly detained from transfer to tissues. It is widely accepted that the unbound or free drug is the active moiety available for equilibration between intravascular and extravascular sites. Further, it is believed that a drug must dissociate from protein in order to exert any type of pharmacological activity. Protein binding has the propensity to affect three main pharmacokinetic/pharmacodynamic concerns: (1) the propensity of the drug to distribute to body tissues, spaces and fluids; (2) the amount of drug that is available to be eliminated; and (3) interaction of the drug with the site of action.[8]

The plasma contains three proteins that have an affinity for binding drugs including albumin (normal concentration 35–45 g/L), α-1-acid glycoprotein (normal concentration 0.4–1 g/L) and lipoproteins (variable concentrations). Assaying techniques available for most agents generate total plasma drug concentration measurements as opposed to a free drug concentration. Thus, a high peak plasma concentration of a highly protein-bound compound may be deceiving in that it does not accurately reflect the free drug that is readily available for tissue distribution and activity. An inverse relationship exists between plasma protein binding and the V_d. Most body fluids such as lymph, interstitial fluid and the normal pleural fluid contain much lower protein concentrations compared with the plasma and will therefore reflect lower total drug concentrations for highly protein bound drugs.

Protein binding of a drug is rapidly reversible (Figure 13.8). The degree to which an agent is bound depends on the affinity of the protein for the drug and the concentrations of the binding protein compared with the drug. Drug binding to plasma proteins may range from 0 to 99 percent. A fair amount of controversy exists regarding the true impact of plasma protein binding on drug distribution and limitations in the utility of drugs that are highly protein bound. In most cases, the fraction of drug that is free is consistent and does not vary with differing drug concentrations because the number of protein binding sites far exceeds the drug concentrations. A drug must

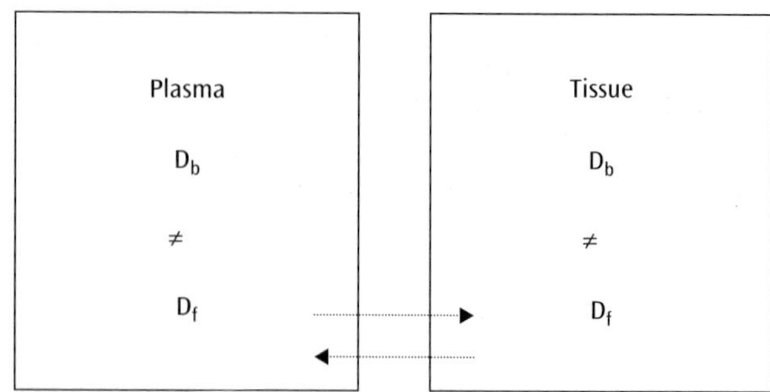

Figure 13.8 Plasma protein binding. D_b, drug bound to protein; D_f, free drug.

have a very high degree of protein binding in order for fluctuating drug concentrations occurring over time to have a direct impact on the fraction bound in the plasma. It has been determined that a drug must exhibit at least 85–90 percent plasma protein binding until a change in plasma concentration leads to a substantial impact in the free drug available for distribution.[5,9,10] Peterson and Gerding[10] found that plasma protein binding in an antibiotic must approach 90 percent in order to have any significant effect on free drug concentration. Once a drug is this highly protein bound, a smaller fraction may be available to move into the tissue with lower plasma concentrations. In other words, a drug must exhibit greater than 85 percent protein binding in order for protein binding to affect the drug pharmacokinetics to any significant degree.

However, the degree of plasma protein binding does not efficiently predict the tissue distribution or half-life of an agent. In fact, it has been found that for drugs that have a relatively short $t_{1/2}$(<2–3 h), a high degree of protein binding (>90 percent) may contribute to persistence in an extravascular space and therefore prolong subsistence periods and enhance tissue distribution.[9]

The implications of a high degree of protein binding may not always be negative when considering protein contained in tissue spaces. Proteins do have the ability to diffuse through tissues, albeit slowly. Although protein binding may hinder drug delivery, this also holds true for clearance. Theoretically, if a pleural effusion contains a large amount of protein, a drug to which protein has a high affinity may become 'trapped' in the effusion, leading to prolonged drug exposure and delayed pleural clearance.

MEMBRANE PENETRATION

Drug molecules must move through a series of spaces and membranes in order to reach a target site of action and conversely, move back into the systemic circulation in order to be cleared from the body. The three modes by which drug molecules accomplish this include: (1) diffusion through the capillary pores; (2) penetration through capillary membranes; and (3) bulk movement through capillary pores.[7] In order to move back into the systemic circulation to be cleared from the body, a drug molecule may do so by diffusion through the capillary pores, penetration of capillary membrane and by bulk flow or diffusion through the lymphatics. The route of drug molecule transfer is determined by the number and size of available pores and by physicochemical properties of the agent. These physicochemical properties include the molecular size and weight, the degree of lipophilicity and the degree of ionization.[1,3,5–7]

Drug molecules with a molecular weight of <1000 will generally move through capillary and lymphatic pores with ease. Large, bulky molecules such as albumin must pass through capillary membranes by endocytosis or pinocytosis and have difficulty crossing lymphatic endothelium. Equilibrium between the plasma and lymph compartment of albumin was found to be realized only after 24 hours.[11] Agents that are bound to albumin are similarly impeded. Small, lipophilic, unionized molecules tend to pass easily through cell membranes, but the larger and more polar the molecule, the greater difficulty of membrane passage.[1,3,5–7]

Ionization of a drug molecule complicates passage through tissue membranes. Most drugs exist in solution as either weak acids or weak bases and equilibrium exists between ionized and unionized fractions. Accumulation of an agent on the side of a membrane with a pH that favors greater ionization may prevent transfer. This is generally not the case as the pH in tissues throughout the body is close to the physiological pH of 7.4. However, the pH associated with an infected area tends to be lower and alkaline antibiotics may become trapped in infected areas.[1,3]

As stated previously, the penetration of a drug molecule to a specific site of action depends largely on the molecular size and weight. Most antibiotics are relatively small with a molecular weight of less than 1000 with the exception of vancomycin (MW 1485.75). The antineoplastic agents that would generally be used in the arena of malignant effusions also have molecular weights of less than 1000. Some agents, however, are larger macromolecules. Antibiotics that are poorly lipid-soluble include the penicillins, cephalosporins, aminoglycosides, vancomycin and clindamycin. Agents such as metronidazole, rifampin, trimethoprim and the quinolones are lipid-soluble and may have the propensity to cross cell membranes with more ease.

Although free drug is believed to be the active moiety and protein binding slows the penetration of drugs through membranes, it must be kept in mind that protein binding is rapidly reversible. Although transfer is slow, protein molecules such as albumin do have the ability to penetrate to the extravascular space and potentially have the capacity to slow diffusion of drug out of a target drug site due to binding within that site. Table 13.1 lists the protein binding characteristics and molecular weights of agents of interest.

Drug penetration to normal pleura cavity: theoretical discussion

From a theoretical perspective, it seems logical that drug delivery and elimination to and from the normal pleural space may follow the same route as the pleural fluid. The pleural space is the cavity that lies between the visceral and parietal pleura and, in healthy humans, contains approximately 0.26 mL/kg of pleural fluid (approximately 18 mL in a 70 kg man) that is relatively low in protein content (approximately 10 mg/mL).[12] The source of pleural fluid is the pulmonary and extrapleural parietal interstitium, with a larger contribution from the latter. The fluid flows down a small pressure gradient at a rate presumed to be approximately 0.02 mL/kg.hour and is drained mainly through the parietal lymphatics back into the systemic circulation.[13–16]

The pleural space may be thought of as an enlarged tissue compartment distinct from the lung parenchyma. Drug delivery to this space may be influenced by five other entities that include the parietal systemic capillaries, the parietal interstitium, the pleural space, the lung interstitium and the visceral systemic capillaries. Because humans have a thick visceral pleura as opposed to the thin visceral pleura found in other animals, the blood supply to both the visceral and parietal pleura is provided by the systemic circulation. Therefore, the proposed route of transfer of drug molecules to the pleural space is directly from the systemic circulation through capillaries and through the visceral and parietal interstitium. Although pleural fluid is thought to enter the pleural space mainly from the parietal pleura, drug may potentially enter from both the visceral and parietal systemic capillaries. The distance of the capillaries from the visceral pleural membrane is approximately 56 μm compared with the shorter distance of 10–12 μm in the parietal pleura. Considering this with the pressure gradient and relative thickness of the visceral pleura, the most direct route giving higher drug delivery is most likely through the parietal pleura.

Adequate penetration of drug molecules into the pleural space requires passage across the first barrier of the capillary endothelium, through the interstitium, then across the second barrier of the mesothelium, which lines the pleural cavity. Drug concentrations in the capillaries are consistent with the plasma and the interstitial fluid is in rapid equilibrium with the plasma. Potential sources of diminishment of drug penetration into the pleural space include the endothelial cell and mesothelial cell membrane barriers and the interstitium.[13–16]

The capillary endothelium is known to be relatively permeable. Water is found to egress from capillaries through interendothelial junctions and albumin must pass through by either endocytosis or pinocytosis. Unbound, lipid-soluble drug may pass directly through the cell membrane and water-soluble drug will easily pass through the inter-endothelial junctions. Protein-bound drug will follow the same, slower route as albumin.

Table 13.1 Protein binding and molecular weight of agents of interest

Agent	Molecular weight	% Protein binding
Aminoglycosides		
Gentamicin	NA	0–30
Amikacin	781.75	4–11
Tobramycin	1425.45	0–30
Penicillins		
Penicillin G potassium	372.48	65
Ampicillin/sulbactam	371.39/255.22	28/38
Piperacillin/tazobactam	539.6/322.3	26–33/26
Carbapenems		
Meropenem	437.52	2
Imipenem/cilastin	317.37/380.43	20/40
Cephalosporins		
Cefazolin	476.48	74–86
Cefoxitin	449.44	65–79
Cefotaxime	477.4	31–50
Cefuroxime	446.37	33–50
Ceftriaxone	661.59	85–90
Ceftazidime	636.6	17
Cefepime	571.5	16–19
Macrolides		
Erythromycin	733.94	75–90
Azithromycin	785	7–50 (concentration dependent)
Clarithromycin	747.96	42–50
Quinolones		
Ciprofloxacin	331.4	16–43
Ofloxacin	361.4	20
Levofloxacin	370.38	50
Moxifloxacin	437.9	50
Gatifloxacin	402.42	20
Miscellaneous		
Vancomycin	1485.75	10–50
Linezolid	337.35	31
Tigecycline	585.65	71–89
Clindamycin	504.96	94
Metronidazole	171.16	<20
Rifampin	822.95	80
Isoniazid	137.14	10–15
Antineoplastics		
Cyclophosphamide	279.1	60[a]
Cisplatin	300.1	Platinum 90[b]
Carboplatin	371.25	0 (platinum 30 irreversible)[c]
Doxorubicin	579.99	74–76
Etoposide	588.58	97
Mitoxantrone	517.41	78
Pemetrexed	597.49	73–81

NA, not applicable.
[a]Refers to the protein binding of cyclophosphamide metabolites including but not limited to 4-hydroxycyclophoshphamide, aldophosphamide, phosphoramide mustard, and acrolein.
[b]At physiologic pH, the predominant species of administered cisplatin are cisplatin and monohydroxymonochloro *cis*-platinum (platinum), the latter of which is 90 percent protein bound.
[c]The platinum form of degraded carboplatin is irreversibly protein-bound up to 30 percent.

The next obstacle is the interstitium, which is basically a meshwork of collagen and fibers combined with glycopolysaccharides and glucosaminoglycans. The interstitium, to all intents and purposes, is similar to a gel through which drug filtration is determined by molecular size, weight and charge. Interestingly, protein-bound drug will pass through the interstitium at a faster rate than unbound drug. The final barrier to pleural drug delivery is the mesothelium. In contrast to earlier reports of the mesothelium as a very 'leaky membrane', Negrini and colleagues[17] determined that the mesothelium in animals is very similar to the endothelium of 'continuous capillaries'. The various sized pores found in the mesothelium have been determined to be larger and more penetrable to albumin than the capillary endothelium. The limit of passage through the mesothelium appears to be the number of pores available, hence the proposed reason given by the investigators for the relatively low protein content of the pleural fluid. If similar properties correspond to human mesothelium, drug passage through this barrier would be similar to that as through the capillary endothelium.[17]

From a pharmacokinetic viewpoint, it seems that the pleural space may be considered to be a part of the peripheral compartment in a two-compartment model. Although the visceral and parietal pleura are well perfused, concentrations of drug in the pleural space may lag behind those of the serum because of the necessity of crossing two membrane barriers and permeating the interstitium.

Stomata are believed to exist in the human parietal pleura that lead to lymphatic lacuna, which provide unidirectional drainage of the pleural space. The maximum capacity of drainage that may be provided for by the parietal lymph is thought to be around 1 mL/kg.hour. The route of drug elimination from the pleural space may also be presumed to be through the parietal lymphatic system, consistent with that of the pleural fluid.[13,16]

Penetration from the plasma to the diseased pleura

The preceding proposed pathway of drug delivery to the pleural space seems logical. The problem with its conception is that the entire topography of the pleural cavity and surrounding tissue changes in the event of an exudative pleural effusion – the type of effusion most often experienced with infection or malignancy. By definition, the permeability characteristics and clearance mechanisms of the pleural cavity are completely altered in this clinical setting. Fluid accumulation in the face of an exudative pleural effusion is thought to be due to increased permeability and either saturated or blocked lymphatic drainage. Inflammation that accompanies either malignancy or infection may potentially increase the vascular permeability and the permeability of the mesothelial cells. Therefore, inflammation may probably lead to greater drug levels achieved in the pleural space. This inflammation, however, may wax and wane and is not predictably consistent. In the case of a parapneumonic effusion, the chemistry of the pleural fluid itself would be expected to change, consisting of higher protein levels, a higher population of cells and, in the case of empyema, a lower pH and lower glucose level. These changes would influence drug pharmacokinetics.[13,16,18,19]

In the case of malignancy, obstructive tumors may block lymphatic drainage of the pleural space. Tumor characteristics that determine the degree and type of blockage cannot be expected to be uniform among patients. Different malignancy in the pleural space will therefore affect the pharmacokinetics of each drug differently for each patient.[13,19]

The pharmacokinetics of agents in the pleural space will be subject to variance based on the drug penetration characteristics as well as the underlying condition of the patient. Penetration and elimination of drugs to and from the pleura would be expected to be markedly different in healthy versus diseased tissue. Inflammation may be expected to increase drug penetration and lymphatic drainage saturation or obstruction would be expected to impede drug clearance. This would result in higher C_{max} levels and prolonged elimination rate constants (k) and half-life ($t_{1/2}$) observed in the diseased pleural space compared with the healthy pleural space.

Intrapleural administration: theoretical discussion

If one considers the intrapleural administration of drug, one must envision administration directly to the peripheral compartment of a multi-compartment model (Figure 13.4). The tendency would be for the drug to equilibrate with other tissues and spaces, including the central compartment. The movement of the agent would follow the basic principles of pharmacokinetics in that the drug would seek to diffuse down a concentration gradient from areas of higher concentration to equilibrate with other spaces of the body that are at lower concentrations. Distribution would be reversible and occur at the rate constants k_{12} and k_{21}.

Elimination from the body would most likely take place strictly from the central compartment. Distribution equilibrium might not be reached since elimination would consistently be taking place from the central compartment, decreasing drug levels in the systemic circulation. A drug would continue to move with this type of behavior until it was fully eliminated from the body.

Since the pleural fluid contains much less protein than the plasma, there is less protein binding that would inhibit transport of drug out of the pleural space. Access to the systemic circulation would be available by two routes. The first route would be through the mesothelium lining of the pleura into the interstitium, followed by transfer across the capillary endothelium into the systemic circulation via either the parietal or visceral pleura. The second route would be through the lymphatics into the systemic circulation. The route, once again, would be expected to be the same as that of the pleural fluid. The rate-limiting factor that would slow drug transfer from the pleural space to the systemic circulation is the number of stomata present on the parietal pleura and the patency of the downstream lymphatic drainage. Fluid is thought to accumulate in the pleural space because of increased fluid formation, as well as obstruction or saturation of the lymphatic drainage of the pleural space. The route to the systemic circulation is through the lymphatics and the main route is through the parietal pleura. It would appear that intrapleural administration of an agent would result in extremely limited clearance from the pleural space because of the limited clearance of pleural fluid. Therefore, drug would be expected to diffuse to a great extent into the visceral and parietal interstitium owing to the high concentration present in the pleura. The levels in the pleura would be expected to consistently exceed those of the plasma in patients with normal hepatic and renal function.

Antimicrobial agents

Since the late 1970s, several studies have examined antimicrobial concentrations obtained in the pleural fluid. Although several studies have been conducted and many reference books and drug package inserts list the degree of pleural penetration of various agents; the data is severely lacking and unsound and reference data should be considered with caution.

The rationale behind this conclusion is that the many studies conducted examined penetration in relatively small, heterogeneous patient groups. The study patients consisted of those that had transudative effusions together with those that had exudative effusions. Many studies included patients that were not infected or combined those that were infected with those that had malignancy.[20–22]

Most studies involved the administration of a single dose of drug as opposed to multiple doses. This is not an ideal condition under which to observe drug pharmacokinetics since the patients' plasma drug levels would not be considered to be at a 'steady-state' distribution equilibrium. Consequently, the pleural fluid levels would not reflect the distribution equilibrium with the plasma and may underestimate drug concentrations. These conditions do not represent those observed in a clinical situation with multiple dosing and possible drug accumulation.

Another limitation to the available literature is that many studies did not follow pleural fluid or plasma drug concentration–time profiles. In many instances, non-simultaneous plasma and pleural fluid levels were taken for each patient. Therefore, it is not known whether the drug levels found in the pleural fluid actually reflect the maximum concentrations attainable. It is clear that antibiotic pharmacokinetics in the pleural space is an area that requires further study.

Despite the limitations of the available data, several conclusions may be made regarding general principles of antibiotic pharmacokinetics in the pleural fluid relative to that of the plasma.

Selected studies will be reviewed to illustrate some key points. Table 13.2 provides a summary of drug penetration and peak pleural fluid to serum ratios.[20,23–34]

LACK OF CORRELATION BETWEEN PLEURAL FLUID AND ASCITIC FLUID PHARMACOKINETICS

Because there are similarities between the pleural and peritoneal cavity with regard to the mesothelium and lymphatic system, an assumption is made by some clinicians that antibiotic characteristics of penetration and elimination from ascitic fluid may be extrapolated to those of the pleural fluid. Although this may be true to a certain extent when considering the permeation of the mesothelium, discriminating conclusions must be made.

Lechi and colleagues[23] examined the pharmacokinetics of cefuroxime, 1 g, administered intravenously to five patients with ascites and six patients with pleural effusion (three transudates, three exudates). Simultaneous serum and ascitic fluid levels were followed over 12 hours and serum and pleural fluid levels were followed at 3-hour intervals for each patient over 6 hours. In other words, continuous data did not exist for all patients in the pleural fluid group.

The average maximum pleural fluid concentration (C_{max}, approximately 8 µg/mL) was reached more quickly in most patients (approximately 1.5–2 hours) compared with that of the ascitic fluid (4–5 hours; approximately 45 µg/mL). The antibiotic penetrated to the ascitic fluid more readily with a mean C_{max} serum–ascitic fluid ratio of 26 percent compared with the mean C_{max} serum–pleural fluid ratio of 8–10 percent ($n = 5$). The pleural fluid concentration never exceeded that of the serum concentration, displaying a maximum average pleural fluid–serum ratio of approximately 50 percent at the end of 6 hours when serum concentrations were at a minimum. Conversely, the cefuroxime ascitic fluid concentration greatly exceeded that of the serum as serum levels declined and at the end of 12 hours, the ascitic fluid–serum ratio was approximately 1.80. The mean elimination $t_{1/2}$ from the pleural fluid was approximately 5.1 hours, two times longer than that of the serum ($n = 4$).

There are many limitations to this study in that continuous data was not supplied for the pleural patients and numerical concentration data was not provided for the ascitic patients. However, two observations may be made. First, it is clear that the pharmacokinetic drug profile in the ascitic fluid contrasted with that of the pleural fluid. The time to C_{max} (T_{max}) and degree of penetration were quite different. Second, it is evident that elimination from the

Table 13.2 Antimicrobial agents in the pleural fluid

Agent	Pleural disease	Levels (*n*)	Dose	Route	C_{max}[a] PF/Serum	AUC[a] PF/Serum	$t_{1/2}$ (h) PF	$t_{1/2}$ (h) Serum	Reference
AMB	Fungal exudative effusion	1	M	IV	0.38	NA	NA	NA	34
AMK	Parapneumonic effusion	1	M	IM	1.00	NA	NA	NA	24
AMK	Post-thoracotomy	10	S	IV	0.43	0.80	4.3	2.62	27
AMK	Post-thoracotomy	10	S	IP	2.39	NA	NA	~2.88	27
AMP	Carcinomatous effusion	1	S	PO	0.60	NA	NA	NA	24
AMP	Carcinomatous effusion	1	M	PO	0.80	NA	NA	NA	24
AMP	Mixed	6	S	IV	0.49	NA	NA	NA	20
CAZ	Carcinomatous effusion	5	S	IV	NA	0.38	NA	NA	28
CFP	Mixed	6	S	IV	0.07	NA	6.96	2.9	29
CIP	Sterile (Group 1)	7	S	IV	0.24	NA	NA	NA	33
CIP	Sterile (Group 2)	3	S	PO	0.50	NA	NA	NA	33
CIP	Sterile (Group 3)	2	S	PO	0.45	NA	NA	NA	33
CIP	Empyema (Group 4)	3	M	PO	2.00	NA	NA	NA	33
CIP	Empyema	5	S	PO	0.70	2.09	NA	NA	31
CIP	Tuberculous/carcinomatous effusion	15	M	PO	0.63	NA	NA	NA	32
CLI	Parapneumonic effusion	1	M	IV	0.80	NA	NA	NA	24
CXM	Uninfected transudative exudative effusion	4	S	IV	NA	NA	~5.10	~2.39	23
GEN	Empyema	1	S	IM	0.20	NA	NA	NA	24
OFX	Tuberculous effusion	21	M	PO	0.82–0.92	2.09	NA	NA	30
OXA	Empyema	1	S	IV	5.10	NA	NA	NA	24
OXA	Empyema	2	M	IV	7.95	NA	NA	NA	24
PEN	Carcinomatous effusion	3	S	PO	0.13	NA	NA	NA	24
PEN	Empyema	2	S	IV	0.75	NA	NA	NA	24
PEN	Empyema	5	M	IV	1.20	NA	NA	NA	24
PEN	Parapneumonic effusion	2	S	IV	0.20	NA	NA	NA	24
PEN	Parapneumonic effusion	3	M	IV	1.10	NA	NA	NA	24
TOB	Parapneumonic effusion	1	M	IM	1.20	NA	NA	NA	24
VAN	Post-thoracotomy	9	M	$IV_{intermittent}$	0.39	0.88 ± 0.07	6.4 ± 1.5	6.3 ± 1.9	25
VAN	Post-thoracotomy	4	M	$IV_{continuous}$	NA	0.86 ± 0.14	NA	NA	25

AMB, amphotericin B; AMK, amikacin; AMP, ampicillin; AUC, area under the drug concentration-time curve; C_{max}, maximum drug concentration; CAP, community-acquired pneumonia; CAZ, ceftazidime; CFP, cefoperazone; CIP, ciprofloxacin; CLI, clindamycin; CXM, cefuroxime; GEN, gentamicin; IM, intramuscular; IP, intrapleural; IV, intravenous; $IV_{continuous}$, continuous intravenous infusion; $IV_{intermittent}$, intermittent intravenous infusion; M, multi-dose; NA, not available; OFX, ofloxacin; OXA, oxacillin; PEN, penicillin; PF, pleural fluid; PO, oral; S, single-dose; $t_{1/2}$, elimination half-life; TOB, tobramycin; VAN, vancomycin.

[a] PF/Serum ratios were determined using mean results.

pleural space lagged behind and was twice as long of that in the serum.

It must be pointed out that these patients received one dose of cefuroxime and were therefore not at steady-state distribution equilibrium. The degree of penetration of cefuroxime into the pleural fluid and ascitic fluid may not be accurately depicted; however, the contrast in pharmacokinetic profiles of the agent in the ascitic compared with the pleural fluid seems accurate.

SELECTED CLINICAL STUDIES

The penetration of a variety of antibiotics, including penicillins, cephalosporins, clindamycin and the aminoglycosides was evaluated in 16 patients with pleural empyema, uncomplicated parapneumonic effusion or carcinomatous effusions, respectively.[24] The mean pleural fluid to serum concentration ratios is displayed in Table 13.2. The penetration for all antibiotics in the case of multiple doses in an infected effusion was very high with a pleural fluid to serum ratio of 0.80 in all cases. Although a small number of patients were studied, the penetration of penicillin, cephalothin and oxacillin appeared to be higher with multiple versus single dosing. Penetration of penicillin in the patients with carcinomatous effusions was found to be lower than that of infected patients. The limitation of the study is that it did not follow simultaneous pleural fluid and plasma drug concentrations over time. However, it illustrates that the penetration of antibiotics into infected pleural effusions was excellent and that penetration into the carcinomatous effusions was less favorable. Further, it hints that greater penetration or accumulation may occur with multiple dosing once steady-state distribution equilibrium is reached.

Another study was conducted in 16 patients with either infected or sterile pleural effusions. The patients were divided into four separate groups and received either single or multiple doses of ciprofloxacin. The study groups were divided as follows. Group 1: seven patients with sterile effusions received a single 200 mg dose of intravenous ciprofloxacin. Group 2: two patients with sterile effusions received a single 750 mg oral dose of ciprofloxacin. Group 3: three patients with sterile effusions received six doses of 750 mg oral ciprofloxacin over 3 days. Group 4: three patients with empyema received 20 doses of oral ciprofloxacin over 10 days. Simultaneous serum and pleural fluid samples were taken from all patients and were obtained after three doses in those that received multiple doses.

This study makes interesting comparisons in that it examines single versus multiple dosing, which may illustrate any potential increase in intrapleural drug levels once a steady state is achieved. It also compares the penetration of uninfected with infected tissue to show any evidence of increased permeability in the face of infection. The results from this study are illustrated in Figure 13.9 and Table 13.2.

The ciprofloxacin peak pleural fluid concentration to serum ratio was the highest and was reached most quickly in patients who were infected and received multiple doses. Drug levels in both the serum and pleural fluid were higher with multiple versus single dosing. The T_{max} of the pleural fluid lagged behind that of the serum by 3–4 hours in Groups 1–3, which consisted of uninfected patients. In the infected group (Group 4), the T_{max} in the pleural fluid was shorter than that of the plasma (1 hour versus 2 hours, respectively), leading to the conclusion that drug penetration may be faster and greater in

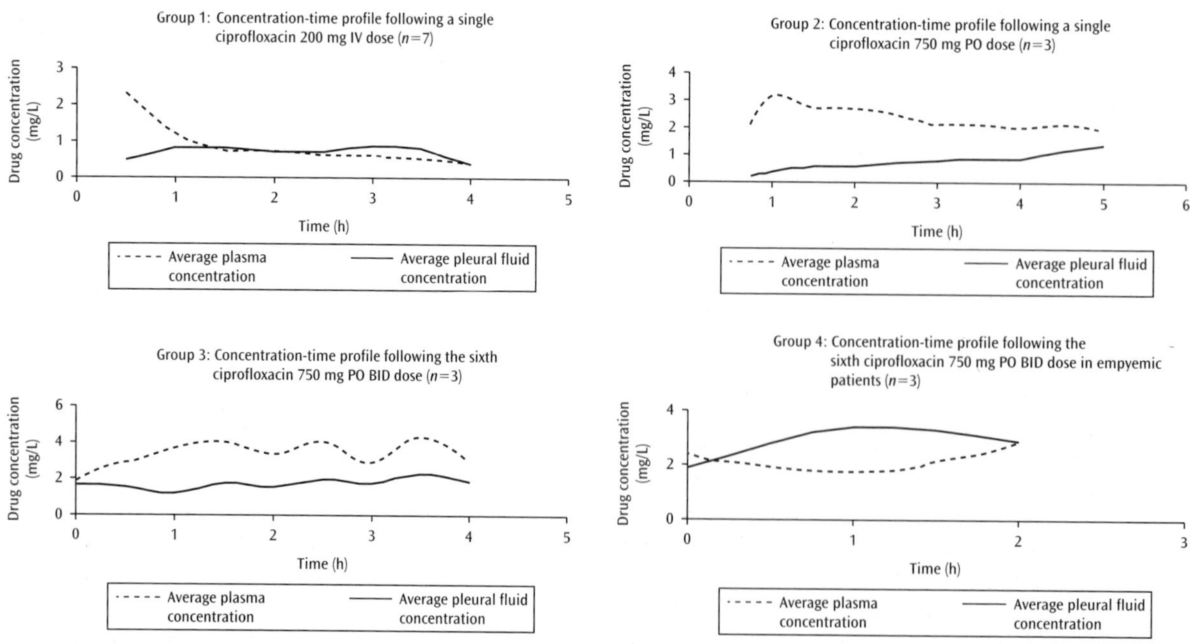

Figure 13.9 Penetration of ciprofloxacin into sterile (Groups 1–3) and empyemic (Group 4) human pleural fluid.[33]

infected patients. Finally, in all patient groups, elimination of drug from the pleural fluid was much slower than that of the plasma.

Vancomycin was found to readily penetrate to the pleural fluid of 16 uninfected patients who underwent thoracotomy for the treatment of bronchial cancer. The patients received vancomycin as either a 15 mg/kg intermittent infusion twice daily ($n = 8$) or a 500 mg loading dose followed by a 30 mg/kg continuous infusion presumably over 24 hours ($n = 8$).[25] The vancomycin AUC_{0-12} pleural fluid–serum ratio exceeded 0.80 in all patients, with an average ratio value of 0.88 ± 0.07 and 0.86 ± 0.14 in the intermittent and continuous infusion groups, respectively. The average vancomycin C_{max} was observed at 1 hour (48.3 ± 14.9 μg/mL) in the serum and at 2 hours (19 ± 4.8 μg/mL) in the pleural fluid, following receipt of intermittent infusion. This indicates a 1-hour lag time for vancomycin penetration from the blood to pleural fluid in these patients. The pleural fluid concentrations ranged from 11.8 ± 2.7 μg/mL at 0 hours to 13.7 ± 3.5 μg/mL at 12 hours, following the start of dose administration in the continuous infusion patient group. An average vancomycin concentration of approximately 14 and 12 μg/mL was maintained in the serum and pleural fluid over 12 hours, respectively, in those patients who received a bolus followed by continuous infusion. The average vancomycin concentration at 12 hours in the intermittent infusion group was 6.6 ± 2.3 μg/mL. It should be noted that blood samples were not obtained beyond the 12-hour timepoint or at steady-state distribution equilibrium. Thus, it would be of interest to know the true lag time for pleural fluid to reach its C_{max} in relation to serum had more samples been obtained once a steady state was achieved.

While the average vancomycin AUC_{0-12} was similar between groups, higher concentrations were achieved more quickly in patients who received the loading dose followed by continuous infusion. As may be expected, higher concentrations were longer sustained in the pleural fluid with administration via continuous infusion. Despite its large molecular size and poor lipid solubility, vancomycin readily reached the pleural fluid in these patients with administration by both intermittent and continuous infusion. A possible explanation of the large degree of pleural fluid penetration may be lung inflammation that may be associated with malignancy.

Pharmacokinetic studies in the pediatric population are infrequent, and even more so when exploring pleural fluid penetration. Giachetto and colleagues[26] reported the pleural fluid and serum concentrations of hospitalized children with community-acquired pneumonia and empyema who received either ampicillin (ages 10 months to 5 years) or penicillin (ages 5–12 years). Blood and pleural fluid samples were collected from the patients after receipt of ampicillin ($n = 9$) 400 mg/kg/day as an intravenous bolus in six divided doses or penicillin ($n = 4$) 200 000 IU/kg.day intravenous infusion over 20 minutes in six divided doses. Drug concentrations were determined in the serum at 0.5 and 3 hours and in the pleural fluid at 1 and 4 hours post antibiotic dose. Although the authors state that many patients were at steady-state distribution equilibrium upon sampling with receipt of greater than six doses, the number of doses received appears to have ranged from one to greater than six and is not reported for individual patients.

The average concentrations of ampicillin were as follows [mean (range)]; serum at 0.5 hours 44.6 μg/mL (17.2–81); pleural fluid at 1 hour 28.4 μg/mL (14.6–41.3); serum at 3 hours ($n = 7$), 14.8 μg/mL (2–33.4); pleural fluid at 4 hours 16.2 μg/mL (25–25.4). The average concentrations of penicillin were as follows [mean (range)]; serum at 0.5 hours 23.8 μg/mL (10.3–34.8); pleural fluid at 1 hour 10.8 μg/mL (9.1–13.1); serum at 3 hours 3.2 μg/mL (1–3.3); pleural fluid at 4 hours 7.7 μg/mL (3.6–11.8). Although an average pleural fluid to serum ratio may not be determined because of the disparity of sampling times, the data indicate substantial penetration of both β-lactam agents into the pleural fluid of these infected pediatric patients.

INTRAPLEURAL ADMINISTRATION OF ANTIBIOTIC

The use of aminoglycosides in parapneumonic effusion or empyema is not recommended as first line therapy. This is because the aminoglycoside antibacterial activity may become compromised in an acidic environment with low oxygen content, as may exist in an infectious locus.

Thys and colleagues[27] conducted a study comparing intrapleural with systemic administration of amikacin, which clarifies several interesting points. A total of 20 post-thoracotomy patients were given a single dose of amikacin either intravenously or intrapleurally. The pleural fluid of these patients was not infected, but contained an increased mean protein level of 3.4 ± 0.2 g/dL. Pleural fluid and serum drug concentrations were simultaneously collected and compared.

The serum C_{max} at 0.5 hours post-dose was 31.2 ± 2.3 μg/mL for systemic administration and 14.1 ± 24.7 μg/mL for intrapleural administration. It is evident that systemic distribution did occur without delay in intrapleural administration, but was half that compared with systemic administration. The peak pleural fluid to serum concentration ratio was 43 percent and occurred within 0.5–2 hours of systemic administration. A significant difference was found in the elimination rate constant, k (serum, 0.28 ± 0.02/hour; pleural fluid, 0.19 ± 0.02/hour; $p < 0.025$) and the $t_{1/2}$ (serum, 2.62 ± 0.22 hours; pleural fluid, 4.3 ± 0.8 hours; $p < 0.0010$) of systemically administered drug. Amikacin was cleared from the pleural fluid at a rate half that for serum.

The mean peak pleural fluid concentration following intrapleural administration was extremely large at 3374 ± 983 μg/mL. The elimination from the pleural fluid in these patients was assisted by suction, so values are misleading; however, the $t_{1/2}$ was approximately 2.88 hours in serum (comparable to the other group) and 1.58 ± 0.23 hours in pleural fluid.

It has become apparent that the clearance of drug from the pleural fluid lags behind that of the plasma. This may be beneficial for agents that display 'time-dependent' versus 'concentration-dependent' activity, but toxicity may become an issue with agents that have a small therapeutic window. Since most studies examine the administration of one dose, the implications of drug accumulation are not known. Intrapleural administration resulted in an exceedingly high peak concentration of amikacin. This suggests that a lower dose may be used in intrapleural administration since toxicity is a concern. Systemic distribution occurred from the pleural space almost immediately, and the elimination rate was unchanged compared with the group that received systemic administration. Since these patients had suction-assisted elimination, the effect of the high pleural concentration compared with serum concentration is unclear over time. Perhaps the serum concentrations would have continued to increase over time as a result of distribution to the systemic circulation from the pleural compartment.

ANIMAL DATA

The main reason why data is lacking regarding the penetration of antimicrobial agents in the setting of infected effusion is the difficulty in performing studies with multiple doses of medication in acutely ill patients over an extended period of time. The pleural empyema rabbit model (Table 13.3) provides us with pertinent information that is difficult to gather in human research trials.[35–40] Although there are undoubtedly differences between the rabbit and human pleural structures and physiology, these studies provide an insight into the relationship between pharmacokinetics of the serum and pleural fluid. These data also provide an insight into the degree of penetration of the mesothelium by antimicrobial agents in the face of infection.

The assumption has been that an empyema is difficult to penetrate because of fibrin encasement and viscous pus content. These data indicate that drug penetration into empyema is actually quite good. Penetration in animals was compared not only by average C_{max} pleural fluid to serum ratios, but also by AUC or total drug exposure. The AUC ratios are higher since the elimination from the pleural space lags behind that of the serum, prolonging drug exposure. The higher the pleural fluid to serum AUC ratio, the more equal the drug exposure between the serum and pleural space. Depending on the pharmacodynamic characteristics of the drug, this may or may not be more important than peak drug concentrations in relation to killing of a pathogen.

CONCLUSIONS REGARDING ANTIBIOTICS

In general, it seems that most antibiotics do attain therapeutic concentrations in the pleural space (Table 13.2) to varying degrees; however, these concentrations lag behind those of the serum. Delayed peak concentration is unlikely

Table 13.3 Antimicrobial agents in the pleural empyema rabbit model

Agent	*n*	C_{max} PF/Serum	AUC PF/Serum	T_{max} PF (hours)	Reference
CLI	2	0.40	0.74	6	36
CLR	3	0.82	1.57	1	39
CRO	2	0.20	0.82	4	36
GEN	2	0.10	0.50	1	36
GEN	10	0.30	NA	3	35
IPM	3	0.08 ± 0.05	0.58 ± 0.17	0.5	40
IPM/CIL	3	0.06 ± 0.02	0.51 ± 0.11	0.5–1	40
LVX	3	0.74	1.13	6	38
MEM	3	0.06 ± 0.02	0.89 ± 0.13	0.5	40
MEM/CIL[a]	3	0.07 ± 0.01	0.79 ± 0.04	0.5	40
MTZ	2	0.70	0.98	0.25	36
MXF	15	0.71	2.01	1.5–2.5	37
MXF	22	0.63	1.17	1.5–2.5	37
MXF	3	0.58	1.37	6	38
PEN	2	0.30	2.31	2	36
VAN	2	0.20	0.61	1	36

AUC, area under the drug concentration-time curve; C_{max}, maximum drug concentration; CLI, clindamycin; CLR, clarithromycin; CRO, ceftriaxone; GEN, gentamicin; IPM, imipenem; IPM/CIL, imipenem/cilastatin; LVX, levofloxacin; MEM, meropenem; MEM/CIL, meropenem/cilastatin; MTZ, metronidazole; MXF, moxifloxacin; NA, not available; PEN, penicillin; PF, pleural fluid; T_{max}, time to maximum drug concentration; VAN, vancomycin.

[a]Meropenem was also studied with cilastatin because although stable in humans, meropenem is easily hydrolyzed by dehydropeptidase in rabbits.

to be an issue with multiple dosing. The quinolones, penicillins and aminoglycosides seem to penetrate the pleural fluid especially well, although the aminoglycosides cannot be recommended. Antibiotic elimination from the pleural space lags behind that of the serum. This may be beneficial to treat infection but accumulation may occur with multiple dosing and caution is advised when administering toxic agents. The lag in clearance of the pleural fluid indicates that AUC pleural fluid to serum ratios will exceed peak pleural fluid to serum ratios for many agents. Therefore, while the pleural fluid peak is lower, total drug exposure may be closer in range. Although unnecessary in the majority of cases, intrapleural administration of antibiotics offers the advantage of achieving higher peak pleural fluid levels and may be considered in special cases. Further, the effects of the extraordinary peaks and the possibility and degree of drug accumulation are not known.

Antineoplastic agents

Since the pharmacological intent of anti-cancer agents is to destroy cells, and these agents effectively do so without discrimination between healthy and malignant cells, antineoplastic agents are undoubtedly the most toxic drugs administered to humans. The greatest challenge in the drug therapy of malignancy lies in the creation of a balance between efficacy and safety. Dosage administration design presents an opportunity to artfully manipulate the balance between efficacy and safety through not only dosage adjustment, but also by route of administration. Intrapleural chemotherapy for treatment of pleural malignancies, especially mesothelioma, has attracted considerable attention. The final focus of this chapter is the pharmacokinetics associated with the intrapleural administration of anti-cancer chemotherapy agents.

INTRAPLEURAL ADMINISTRATION OF ANTI-CANCER CHEMOTHERAPY AGENTS

The rationale for the intrapleural administration of toxic anti-cancer chemotherapy is to maximize drug exposure and the subsequent killing of malignant cells while minimizing systemic exposure of healthy cells to the toxic agents. The main concern with intrapleural administration is the movement of drug into the systemic circulation.

The theoretical movement of intrapleurally administered drug from the pleural space to the systemic circulation is proposed to follow the basic pharmacokinetic principles of a two-compartment model except that drug administration would take place directly to the peripheral compartment (Figure 13.4). These are the same principles set out in the previous section to describe the pharmacokinetics of an intrapleurally administered antibiotic.

High initial pleural drug concentrations in the pleural fluid would drive equilibration with the rest of the body. The reversible movement of drug from the pleural cavity to the systemic circulation may be quantified by the distribution rate constants between compartments, k_{21} and k_{12} (Figure 13.4). This movement would depend on the concentration gradient established between the pleural cavity and the rest of the body as well as the physiochemical properties of the administered agent (molecular weight, protein binding and isoelectric properties). Characteristics specific to the individual patient would also certainly influence the pharmacokinetics to a large degree. It is difficult, therefore, to make generalizations among chemotherapy patients. The pharmacokinetics may potentially be influenced by the local effects of malignant tumor, changes in physiology of the pleura due to surgery/treatment and the underlying renal and hepatic function of the patient. Elimination of drugs from the pleural fluid and the total body will also be influenced by biomedical interventions, such as chest tube drainage of the pleural cavity that is often employed with anti-cancer intrapleural chemotherapy. Inflammation, as in the case of infection, would be expected to increase drug permeability of the mesothelium.

Elimination from the pleural cavity to the systemic circulation, potentially supported mainly from the lymphatics of the parietal pleura, may be blocked by malignancy and might also become saturated. As a result, drug movement out of the pleural cavity may be a very slow process depending on the physiochemical drug properties and the patient. Since total body elimination of drug takes place strictly from the central compartment for most drugs, clearance from the body would be dependent upon transfer from the pleura to the systemic circulation. Although intrapleural administration would diminish systemic drug exposure, concerns still exist over local and systemic toxicity.

Several well-conducted studies have examined the pharmacological effect as well as the pharmacokinetics of intrapleurally administered agents in the treatment of malignancy. Although not all inclusive, examination of the results of these pharmacokinetic studies (Table 13.4) leads to several important conclusions.[41–49]

MAXIMIZATION OF INTRAPLEURAL DRUG EXPOSURE

The area under the drug concentration–time curve reveals total drug exposure. Table 13.4 shows that the direct intrapleural administration of antineoplastic agents maximizes drug exposure of malignant cells located in the pleura or pleural effusion, resulting in very high AUCs and peak (C_{max}) concentrations in the pleural fluid. These concentrations are undoubtedly higher than those achievable with systemic drug administration. Further, while the pleural fluid AUC and C_{max} parameters are large, the plasma or serum levels are lower, indicating a much greater drug exposure in the pleura compared with the plasma. However, with such high concentrations, concern exists about local toxicity in the pleura.

Table 13.4 Antineoplastic agents in the pleural fluid

Agent	N	Dose (mg/m²)	Route	Concentration[a] PF/Serum	C_{max} Serum (mg/L)	AUC[a] PF/Serum	AUC[a] Type	Cl (L/h)[b] PF	Cl (L/h)[b] Serum	Reference
CBDCA	3	270	IP	166 ± 66	3.3 ± 1.1	48	∞	0.13 ± 0.02	5.2 ± 3.0	46
$CDDP_{free}$	3	60	IP	140 ± 19	1.1 ± 0.1	82	∞	0.19 ± 0.0	10.6 ± 1.2	46
CDDP										
total	10	80	IP	59.6	1.8	10.9	24 h	116.9[c]	NA	47
free	10	80	IP	8.38	0.4	104	24 h	10.5[c]	NA	47
CDDP										
total	3	90	IP	NA	1	47.5	4 h	5.68	122	44
free	3	90	IP	NA	2.3	NA	NA	NA	NA	44
CDDP	7	90	IV	NA	2.3	NA	NA	NA	132	44
CDDP										
total	11	100	IP	NA	NA	28.6	4 h	28 ± 14.3	NA	45
free	11	100	IP	NA	NA	47.6	4 h	NA	NA	45
$CDDP_{total}$	14	153–203	IP	129.25	1.5	NA	NA	NA	8.7 ± 6.5	48
CDDP										
total	10	200	IP	NA	2.1	27 ± 4.6	48 h	NA	NA	49
free	10	200	IP	NA	0.8	23 ± 9.2	48 h	NA	NA	49
CDDP										
total	7	200	IP	NA	2.0	25 ± 6.2	48 h	NA	NA	49
free	7	200	IP	NA	0.8	37 ± 7.7	48 h	NA	NA	49
MTC	11	8	IP	NA	NA	195.7	∞	2.3 ± 1.0	5.5 ± 4	45
MTX	12	30	IP	157	NA	NA	NA	2.6	3.9	41
VP-16	10	80	IP	58	3	36.9	24 h	62.5[c]	NA	47
VP-16	1	100	IP	68	2.5	210	∞	NA	NA	42
VP-16	4	100	IP	NA	NA	31	∞	2	NA	43
VP-16	2	150	IP	NA	NA	16	∞	1.5	NA	43
VP-16	2	225	IP	NA	NA	23	∞	2	NA	43

AUC, area under the drug concentration-time curve; C_{max}, maximum drug concentration; CBDCA, carboplatin; CDDP, cisplatin; $CDDP_{free}$, unbound cisplatin; $CDDP_{total}$, unbound and bound cisplatin; Cl, clearance; IP, intrapleural; IV, intravenous; MTC, mitomycin; MTX, methotrexate; NA, not available; PF, pleural fluid; VP-16, etoposide.

[a]PF/Serum ratios were determined using mean results.

[b]Unless otherwise indicated.

[c]Reported as the elimination half-life instead.

SYSTEMIC DRUG DISTRIBUTION AND ELIMINATION

As mentioned previously, in order for the drug to be eliminated from the body, it must first be transferred from the pleural cavity to the systemic circulation through which it may reach the organs of metabolism and elimination, mainly the liver and kidneys. Bogliolo and colleagues[44] administered cisplatin 90 mg/m^2 intrapleurally to four patients and intravenously to seven patients. The drug elimination $t_{1/2}$ from the pleural fluid, representing either transfer to the systemic circulation or tissue binding, was 2.08 ± 0.65 hours for intrapleurally administered drug. The mean platinum AUC of the plasma after 4 hours was 0.27 ± 0.03 mg/minute.mL compared with 12.83 ± 4.06 mg/minute.mL in the pleural fluid. The average total platinum C_{max} drug concentration of those patients that received intravenous cisplatin was two times greater than the average C_{max} plasma concentration of those that received intrapleural cisplatin (2.25 ± 0.58 and 0.96 ± 0.35 mg/L, respectively; $p < 0.01$). The average maximum level of free platinum concentration resulting from intravenous administration (1.45 ± 0.55 mg/L) was more than three times greater than the free peak level achieved with intrapleural administration (0.42 ± 0.18 mg/L).

The administration of 80 mg/m^2 in 10 patients with malignant pleural effusions in another study resulted in an average C_{max} pleural fluid concentration of total platinum of 104.4 mg/L compared with 1.75 mg/L in the plasma which was reached 8 hours following intrapleural administration. The average total drug AUC of the pleural fluid was 1032.99 µg/hour.mL compared with 94.34 µg/hour.mL in the plasma. The free platinum C_{max} was 88 mg/L in the pleural fluid and 0.36 mg/L in the plasma. The average C_{max} of free platinum in the plasma occurred much sooner: only 1 hour after administration and decreased to 0.1 mg/L after approximately 4 hours, with an elimination $t_{1/2}$ of approximately 10.5 hours. The average total platinum concentration in pleural fluid remained at 10 mg/L at 72 hours after administration, revealing a pleural fluid elimination $t_{1/2}$ of 116 hours.[47]

The results of many other studies parallel these in showing that drug administered to the pleural space does move to the systemic circulation. Free drug seems to move at a greater rate than drug that may be protein bound, hence the difference in T_{max} and $t_{1/2}$ between the free and total drug concentrations. Intrapleural administration results in much lower plasma and AUC concentrations than from systemic administration of the same drug, thereby decreasing the potential for toxicity.

The elimination from the plasma or intrapleurally administered drugs is similar to that of systemically administered drugs. The movement and elimination of drug from the pleural fluid is very slow and concentrations may linger for days. Total body drug elimination is dependent on transfer of drug to the systemic circulation, so lagging intrapleural drug concentrations may increase potential nephrotoxicity as well as other toxicities.

CONCLUSIONS REGARDING ANTINEOPLASTIC AGENTS

The intrapleural administration of an anti-cancer chemotherapeutic agent results in much higher intrapleural exposure compared with systemic exposure, as shown by the differences in drug AUC. Drug distributes to the systemic circulation at a very slow rate, prolonging total body elimination and intrapleural exposure. The systemic distribution and prolonged elimination of drug may result in systemic toxicity. Potential toxicity may be combated through the systemic administration of neutralizing agents where appropriate, or facilitated by pleural fluid drug elimination. The lower systemic drug concentration may lead to higher neutralizing agent–toxic agent systemic concentration ratio, resulting in better control of toxicity.[41]

KEY POINTS

- Pharmacokinetic parameters are used to describe the movement of drug through the body over time. Plasma or serum drug concentrations are used to quantify and predict this movement.
- The pharmacokinetics of a drug are dependent on physiochemical properties of the particular agent as well as patient characteristics. The penetration of drug through membranes is dependent on the molecular weight and size of the drug, the degree of protein binding and the isoelectric charge.
- The movement of drug to and from the pleural cavity is dependent on the anatomy of the pleura and characteristics that are subject to change in the face of disease.
- Systemically administered antibiotics appear to penetrate the pleural cavity to an acceptable degree; however, the data in this area are extremely few and further study is needed. The concentrations that reach the pleura are lower than that of the plasma. In order to be effective, the concentrations in the pleural cavity must sufficiently exceed the MIC of the given pathogen.
- The intrapleural administration of anti-cancer chemotherapy agents results in higher direct pleural drug exposure compared with systemic exposure. Transfer of drug from the pleura to the systemic circulation is slow and results in delayed total body drug elimination. As a result of systemic distribution and prolonged drug elimination from the body, toxicity is still an issue.

REFERENCES

● = Key primary paper
◆ = Major review article

◆1. Gibalid M. *Biopharmaceutics and clinical pharmacokinetics*, 3rd edn. Seattle: Lea & Febiger, 1984.
2. Winters M, Koda-Kimble MA (eds.) *Basic clinical pharmacokinetics*, 3rd edn. Vancouver: Applied Therapeutics, 1994.
3. Rowland M, Tozer TN. *Clinical pharmacokinetics: concepts and applications*, 3rd edn. Media: Williams & Wilkins, 1995.
4. Sweeney K, Nightingale CH, Meng X. Methods of pharmacokinetic analysis: theory and principles. In: Kuemmerle HP, Murakawa T, Nightingale CH. (eds.) *Pharmacokinetics of antimicrobial agents: principles, methods, application.* Landsberg/Lech: Ecomed, 1993: 9–17.
◆5. Bergan T. Pharmacokinetics of tissue penetration of antibiotics. *Rev Infect Dis* 1981; **3**: 45–66.
6. Schentag JJ, Gengo FM. Principles of antibiotic tissue penetration and guidelines for pharmacokinetic analysis. *Med Clin North Am* 1982; **66**: 39–49.
◆7. Barza M, Cuchural G. General principles of antibiotic tissue penetration. *J Antimicrob Chemother* 1985; **15** (Suppl A): 59–75.
8. Dudley M, Nightingale CH. Effects of protein binding on the pharmacology of cephalosporins. In: New HC (ed.). *New beta-lactam antibiotics: a review from chemistry to clinical efficacy of new cephalosporins.* Philadelphia: College of Physicians, 1982: 227–39.
9. Bergan T, Engeset A, Olszewski W. Does serum protein binding inhibit tissue penetration in antibiotics? *Rev Infect Dis* 1987; **9**: 713–8.
◆10. Peterson LR, Gerding DN. Influence of protein binding of antibiotics on serum pharmacokinetics and extravascular penetration: clinically useful concepts. *Rev Infect Dis* 1980; **2**: 340–8.
11. Engeset A, Aas M, Olszewski W, Sokolowski J. Time of exchange of 131I-labeled albumin between plasma and peripheral lymph in man. *Lymphology* 1979; **12**: 77–80.

12. Noppen M. Normal volume and cellular contents of pleural fluid. *Curr Opin Pulm Med* 2001; **7**: 180–2.
13. Light RW. Anatomy of the pleura; physiology of the pleural space. In: *Pleural diseases*, 3rd edn. Baltimore: Williams & Wilkins, 1995; 1–17.
14. Lee KF, Olak J. Anatomy and physiology of the pleural space. *Chest Surg Clin N Am* 1994; **4**: 391–403.
15. Wang NS. Anatomy and physiology of the pleural space. *Clin Chest Med* 1985; **6**: 3–16.
◆16. Miserocchi G. Physiology and pathophysiology of pleural fluid turnover. *Eur Respir J* 1997; **10**: 219–25.
17. Negrini D, Venturoli D, Townsley MI, Reed RK. Permeability of parietal pleura to liquid and proteins. *J Appl Physiol* 1994; **76**: 627–33.
18. Hamm H, Light RW. Parapneumonic effusion and empyema. *Eur Respir J* 1997; **10**: 1150–6.
19. Sahn SA. Pleural diseases related to metastatic malignancies. *Eur Respir J* 1997; **10**: 1907–13.
20. Lode H, Dzwillo G. Investigations of the diffusion of antibiotics into the pleural space. *Current Chemotherapy. Proceedings of the 10th International Congress on Chemotherapy.* Washington DC: American Society for Microbiology, 1978: 386–8.
21. Cole DR, Pung J. Penetration of cefazolin into pleural fluid. *Antimicrob Agents Chemother* 1977; **11**: 1003–5.
22. Daschner FD, Gier E, Lentzen H, *et al.* Penetration into the pleural fluid after bacampicillin and amoxycillin. *J Antimicrob Chemother* 1981; **7**: 585–8.
23. Lechi A, Arosio E, Xerri L, *et al.* The kinetics of cefuroxime in ascitic and pleural fluid. *Int J Clin Pharmacol Ther Toxicol* 1982; **20**: 493–6.
●24. Taryle DA, Good JT Jr, Morgan EJ 3rd, *et al.* Antibiotic concentrations in human parapneumonic effusions. *J Antimicrob Chemother* 1981; **7**: 171–7.
●25. Byl B, Jacobs F, Wallemacq P, *et al.* Vancomycin penetration of uninfected pleural fluid exudates after continuous or intermittent infusion. *Antimicrob Agents Chemother* 2003; **47**: 2015–7.
26. Giachetto G, Pirez MC, Nanni L, *et al.* Ampicillin and penicillin concentration in serum and pleural fluid of hospitalized children with community-acquired pneumonia. *Pediatr Infect Dis J* 2004; **23**: 625–9.
27. Thys JP, Serruys-Schoutens E, Rocmans P, *et al.* Amikacin concentrations in uninfected postthoracotomy pleural fluid and in serum after intravenous and intrapleural injection. *Chest* 1984; **85**: 502–5.
28. Walstad RA, Hellum KB, Blika S, *et al.* Pharmacokinetics and tissue penetration of ceftazidime: studies on lymph, aqueous humour, skin blister, cerebrospinal and pleural fluid. *J Antimicrob Chemother* 1983; **12** (Suppl A): 275–82.
29. Yamada H, Iwanaga T, Nakanishi H, *et al.* Penetration and clearance of cefoperazone and moxalactam in pleural fluid. *Antimicrob Agents Chemother* 1985; **27**: 93–5.
30. Yew WW, Lee J, Chan CY, *et al.* Ofloxacin penetration into tuberculous pleural effusion. *Antimicrob Agents Chemother* 1991; **35**: 2159–60.
●31. Morgenroth A, Pfeuffer HP, Seelmann R, Schweisfurth H. Pleural penetration of ciprofloxacin in patients with empyema thoracis. *Chest* 1991; **100**: 406–9.
32. Umut S, Demir T, Akkan G, *et al.* Penetration of ciprofloxacin into pleural fluid. *J Chemother* 1993; **5**: 110–2.
●33. Joseph J, Vaughan LM, Basran GS. Penetration of intravenous and oral ciprofloxacin into sterile and empyemic human pleural fluid. *Ann Pharmacother* 1994; **28**: 313–5.
●34. Kutty K, Neicheril JC. Treatment of pleural blastomycosis: penetration of amphotericin B into the pleural fluid. *J Infect Dis* 1987; **156**: 689–90.
35. Shohet I, Yellin A, Meyerovitch J, Rubinstein E. Pharmacokinetics and therapeutic efficacy of gentamicin in an experimental pleural empyema rabbit model. *Antimicrob Agents Chemother* 1987; **31**: 982–5.
36. Teixeira LR, Sasse SA, Villarino MA, *et al.* Antibiotic levels in empyemic pleural fluid. *Chest* 2000; **117**: 1734–9.
37. Strahilevitz J, Lev A, Levi I, *et al.* Experimental pneumococcal pleural empyema model: the effect of moxifloxacin. *J Antimicrob Chemother* 2003; **51**: 665–9.
38. Liapakis IE, Kottakis I, Tzatzarakis MN, *et al.* Penetration of newer quinolones in the empyema fluid. *Eur Respir J* 2004; **24**: 466–70.
39. Liapakis IE, Light RW, Pitiakoudis MS, *et al.* Penetration of clarithromycin in experimental pleural empyema model fluid. *Respiration* 2005; **72**: 296–300.
40. Niwa T, Nakamura A, Kato T, *et al.* Pharmacokinetic study of pleural fluid penetration of carbapenem antibiotic agents in chemical pleurisy. *Respir Med* 2006; **100**: 324–31.
●41. Howell SB, Chu BB, Wung WE, *et al.* Long-duration intracavitary infusion of methotrexate with systemic leucovorin protection in patients with malignant effusions. *J Clin Invest* 1981; **67**: 1161–70.
42. Jones JM, Olman EA, Egorin MJ, Aisner J. A case report and description of the pharmacokinetic behavior of intrapleurally instilled etoposide. *Cancer Chemother Pharmacol* 1985; **14**: 172–4.
43. Holoye PY, Jeffries DG, Dhingra HM, *et al.* Intrapleural etoposide for malignant effusion. *Cancer Chemother Pharmacol* 1990; **26**: 147–50.
●44. Bogliolo GV, Lerza R, Bottino GB, *et al.* Regional pharmacokinetic selectivity of intrapleural cisplatin. *Eur J Cancer* 1991; **27**: 839–42.
45. Rusch VW, Niedzwiecki D, Tao Y, *et al.* Intrapleural cisplatin and mitomycin for malignant mesothelioma following pleurectomy: pharmacokinetic studies. *J Clin Oncol* 1992; **10**: 1001–6.
46. Lerza R, Vannozzi MO, Tolino G, *et al.* Carboplatin and cisplatin pharmacokinetics after intrapleural combination treatment in patients with malignant pleural effusion. *Ann Oncol* 1997; **8**: 385–91.
●47. Tohda Y, Iwanaga T, Takada M, *et al.* Intrapleural administration of cisplatin and etoposide to treat malignant pleural effusions in patients with non-small cell lung cancer. *Chemotherapy* 1999; **45**: 197–204.
48. Monjanel-Mouterde S, Frenay C, Catalin J, *et al.* Pharmacokinetics of intrapleural cisplatin for the treatment of malignant pleural effusions. *Oncol Rep* 2000; 7:171–5.
49. Shigemura N, Akashi A, Nakagiri T, *et al.* Pleural perfusion thermo-chemotherapy under VATS: a new less invasive modality for advance lung cancer with pleural spread. *Ann Thorac Surg 2004;* 77:1016–22.

14

Experimental models: pleural diseases other than mesothelioma

GEORGIOS T STATHOPOULOS, YC GARY LEE

ANIMAL MODELS FOR PLEURAL DISEASES

Why we need animal models

The pleura is involved in many pulmonary and systemic disorders. As a result, pleural effusions are common clinical presentations. *In vivo* studies have played an invaluable part in enhancing our understanding of the etiology of various pleural diseases. While *in vitro* studies can provide information on isolated cell types, pleural pathologies are inevitably a result of complicated interactions between residential mesothelial cells and infiltrating (e.g. inflammatory, malignant) cells. The pleura is also under close influence of products from the systemic circulation (e.g. cytokines) that cross the vascular and mesothelial barriers. These interactions can only be adequately studied *in vivo*.

Animal studies are also important in evaluating the efficacy and safety of novel therapeutic modalities, information difficult to obtain from humans and *in vitro* experiments. For example, animal studies have assessed the efficacy and adverse effects of various pleurodesing and anti-cancer agents. Animal studies can also provide useful data on the pharmacokinetics of drug delivery into the pleural space, such as antibiotic penetration in empyema, and on physiological responses in health and disease.

The ideal animal model should accurately represent the human disease under investigation; be readily available, affordable, and easy to handle; yield reproducible results and provide adequate biological samples for analysis.[1] While most animal models cannot exactly emulate human disease, a good animal model has sufficient similarity to provide useful insights.

A large number of animal models have been employed in the investigation of pleural diseases. The design of meaningful *in vivo* experiments demands a good understanding of the advantages and limitations of the available models. This chapter outlines the species and methods used in pleural disease studies, as well as the pros and cons of specific models for different pleural diseases.

GENERAL RULES

There is no substitute for careful planning: the objectives and experimental endpoints should be clearly defined in advance. Investigators must attempt to minimize the number of animals sacrificed and the pain or distress to each animal.

Approval from local animal care committees must be obtained before experiments are performed. National and international guidelines on standards of animal use must be strictly adhered to. *The Guide for the Care and Use of Laboratory Animals* is one of the most commonly used reference guides.[2] It is mandatory in many countries that researchers must attend training courses prior to using animals for experiments. The laws and regulations governing laboratory animal research can be found elsewhere.[3] Expert veterinarian advice is invaluable to ensure minimal animal discomfort, optimal surgical approach and efficient specimen collection.

Which animal model to use

CHOICE OF ANIMAL SPECIES

> '... *it is proper to choose certain animals which offer favorable anatomical arrangements or special susceptibility to certain influences. ... the proper choice of animals is so important that the solution of a physiological or pathological problem often depends solely on the appropriate choice of the animal for the experiment so as to make the result clear and searching.*'

Claude Bernard (1813–1878) – for many the founder of experimental medicine – so stated in 1865.[4]

Many animal species are used in pleural disease investigations. Rabbits, mice, rats and sheep are the most common. Several factors govern the choice of species for experimentation, including size of animals, their anatomy, costs, availability of reagents suitable for the species, possibility of genetic manipulation, etc.

Smaller animals (e.g. mice) cost less and are easier to handle. Small size, however, makes intrapleural injections difficult and provides a limited amount of biological material for examination. Larger animals are costly, but provide larger sample quantities.

Investigators must realize two important anatomical characteristics of the species they use. First, many animals (e.g. mice, dogs), have incomplete mediastina and the two pleural cavities communicate freely, prohibiting the use of the contralateral pleura as a control.[5] Second, larger animals (e.g. sheep) have a thick visceral pleura resembling that of humans, whereas smaller animals (e.g. rabbits, mice) have a thin visceral membrane. This difference bears implications on fluid and particulate transport across the pleura.

The choice of species may also be dictated by the availability of reagents to process the experimental samples. Commercial enzyme-linked immunosorbent assays (ELISA) are commonly used for measurement of cytokines, but are usually available only against humans and mice.

The choice of species for experimentation is often influenced by the knowledge of the genomic sequence of the species and by the availability of research tools to manipulate gene expression in animals. The mouse (*Mus musculus*) has emerged as the most popular choice and genetically engineered mice are increasingly used in pleural disease investigations, providing valuable insights into the molecular pathogenesis of pleural diseases. Murine models have several advantages:[6–8] (i) The mouse genome shares sufficient homology with that of humans; (ii) a wide array of genetically engineered mice are available; (iii) the large litter size of *Mus musculus* makes breeding timelier and easier; (iv) high-throughput genotyping methods (e.g. using genomic DNA from tail fragments) have been developed for the mouse; (v) many inbred strains of *Mus musculus* have been isolated over the years. Inbred animals share a great degree of genetic identity, reducing experimental variability. Moreover, differences between inbred mouse strains can be exploited to discover mechanisms of disease.

The use of novel molecular biology technologies in the mouse has greatly enhanced research into the pathogenesis of pleural diseases. The pleura has been used for overexpression of gene products using various vectors.[9,10] Several constitutive and conditional gene knockout and knockin mice have been used in pleural disease investigations,[11–13] and the development of systems that facilitate conditional gene overexpression or silencing in the adult mouse, such as the tetracycline on–off models, is expected to greatly enhance research in this area.[14,15] Recently, methods to silence gene expression *in vivo* using RNA interference were introduced, which are anticipated to further boost pleural disease investigations.[16,17]

ACCESS TO PLEURAL SPACE

The next question is how to deliver the experimental agent to the pleural space. Direct intrapleural injection with a fine needle is the least invasive; a small injection volume is adequate. Using Tc-99 labeled fluid, it has been shown that an injection volume as low as 0.5 mL is enough to allow the injectate to be distributed throughout the whole pleural surface of rabbits. Rotation of the animals is unnecessary for distribution of the injectate throughout the pleural space.[18]

Alternatively, small plastic 'chest tubes' can be inserted into the pleural space (see Appendix 14.1). This has the advantage of allowing repeat intrapleural administration of reagents, pleural fluid sampling or lavage of the pleural cavity. This provides longitudinal data on the biological changes within the pleural space, helping reduce the number of animals required in time-course studies. Chest tubes can induce mild inflammation,[19] which in our experience is insignificant. In studies of pleurodesis, the insertion of chest tubes more closely resembles the procedure performed in clinical practice.

Thoracotomy[20] and thoracoscopy[21] have also been used to deliver material into the pleural space, but are more invasive. Systemic delivery of substances can be achieved by intravenous injections. For repeated blood sampling, central venous access can be established.

EXPERIMENTAL END-POINTS

Several parameters are commonly used as endpoints in animal pleural studies. In lethal models, survival is the definitive endpoint. Pleural tissues can be collected at autopsy for macroscopic and/or microscopic examination and semi-quantitative assessment for inflammatory or malignant changes. For pleural fibrosis studies, the pleura can be macroscopically graded for adhesions (see Table 14.1), which correlates well with histological measurements of collagen deposition and pleural thickening.[22] The

Table 14.1 Pleurodesis grading scheme[22–24]

Pleurodesis grading scale of 1 to 8:	
1	No adhesions between the visceral and parietal pleura
2	Rare adhesions between the visceral and parietal pleura with no symphysis
3	A few scattered adhesions between the visceral and parietal pleura with no symphysis
4	Many adhesions between the visceral and parietal pleura with no symphysis
5	Many adhesions between the visceral and parietal pleura with symphysis involving <5% of the hemithorax
6	Many adhesions between the visceral and parietal pleura with symphysis involving 5–25% of the hemithorax
7	Many adhesions between the visceral and parietal pleura with symphysis involving 25–50% of the hemithorax
8	Many adhesions between the visceral and parietal pleura with symphysis involving >50% of the hemithorax

Adhesions are defined as fibrous connections between the visceral and parietal pleura.
Symphysis is present if the visceral and parietal pleura are difficult to separate as a result of adhesions.

volume of pleural fluid produced, as well as its cellular and protein contents, may serve as surrogate markers for inflammation or tumor progression. Pleural vascular permeability can be determined by measurement of the pleural fluid levels of an albumin-binding substance after intravenous injection (e.g. Evans' blue, H^3-labeled albumin). Blood samples can be obtained to compare with the intrapleural levels of mediators, to evaluate systemic responses and to study the pharmacokinetics of drugs delivered via the pleural space.

Advanced imaging techniques (e.g. magnetic resonance imaging [MRI]) are increasingly applied to animal research to allow longitudinal monitoring of pathophysiologic processes. Recently, transthoracic ultrasonography has been shown to be useful in detecting and grading pleurodesis in rabbits,[23,24] without sacrificing the animals. It is anticipated that more imaging modalities will be adopted for pleural research in coming years.

Specific pleural disease models

MODELS FOR PLEURAL FIBROSIS/PLEURODESIS

The study of pleural fibrosis (pleurodesis), frequently employed to treat recurrent pleural effusions and pneumothoraces, represents one of the most common uses of animal studies in pleural disease research. There is active ongoing research for better pleurodesing agents, as currently available compounds either have suboptimal efficacy or carry significant adverse effects[25] (see Chapter 46, Pleurodesis).

The rabbit model is most commonly used in pleurodesis studies,[22,26] though mice,[27] sheep[28] (see Appendix 14.2), rats,[29] dogs[21] and pigs[30] have been employed. The results of common pleurodesing agents applied to different species appear similar; hence the choice of species depends mainly on experience and cost.

With New Zealand white rabbits, the pleurodesing agent is injected either directly or via a chest tube, the method of delivery having little effect on the outcome.[31] Likewise, the pH of the pleurodesing agent does not affect its effectiveness.[32,33] Conventional agents, e.g. talc, doxycycline and bleomycin, induce acute pleural inflammation and denudement of mesothelial cells.[23,34,35] Inflammation may resolve (failed pleurodesis) or, if sufficiently intense, will persist and lead to collagen deposition, fibrosis and symphysis.[36] Pleurodesis is usually evident 14 to 28 days after administration of the pleurodesing agent. However, with pro-fibrotic transforming growth factor beta (TGF-β), significant adhesions can be seen as soon as after 24 hours.[22]

Pleural fibrosis can be graded macroscopically at autopsy (Table 14.1). In addition, pleural thickening and collagen deposition can be measured microscopically using multiple samples from different lung regions to avoid sampling bias, and the contralateral pleural space as the control.[22,37] In our experience, chest tube insertion and saline or albumin injections do not result in significant adhesions. Hemothoraces, however, either from trauma or the experimental agent, can induce adhesions. Recently, a pleurodesis grading system based on transthoracic ultrasound findings, specifically the disappearance of the normal pleural gliding sign, was developed in rabbits and was validated against pleurodesis grading at autopsy[23,24] (Table 14.2). Whether this system is applicable to other species, including humans, remains to be tested.

One concern of the published pleurodesis studies is that they were performed in animals with normal pleura, whereas human pleurodesis is usually applied to patients with abnormal pleurae (especially malignant pleural metastases). However, pleurodesis results from animal models are similar to those from clinical investigations. For example, talc was effective in producing pleurodesis,

Table 14.2 Ultrasound pleurodesis grading scheme[23,24]

Grade	Gliding sign
0	Definitely present
1	Questionable
2	Definitely absent

Score 0–2 is determined at three sites as far away from the diaphragm as possible: midclavicular line (anterior chest wall); midaxillary line (lateral chest wall); midscapular line (posterior chest wall).
Total score = sum of scores for each of the three sites.
Range = 0–6 (Score 0 represents a normal appearing pleura, while score 6 represents greater likelihood of effective pleurodesis, e.g. definitely absent pleural gliding sign at all three sites tested).

and was significantly more so than bleomycin in both rabbit[38] and sheep pleurodesis studies[39] – the same as in randomized clinical trials.[40]

There are no available models for pleurodesis in malignant pleural effusions. Most models for malignant effusions are created in mice (see below), which are too small for adequate assessment of pleurodesis. On the other hand, attempts have been made to mimic the setting of pleurodesis for pneumothorax, where chemical pleurodesis remained effective despite the presence of air in the pleural space or active air leaks.[38,41]

MODELS FOR MALIGNANT PLEURAL EFFUSION

Malignant pleural effusions, most commonly resulting from adenocarcinomas of the lung and breast, affect about 200 000 patients each year in the USA alone, causing significant morbidity and mortality.[42–45] The pathogenesis of malignant effusions and their best management are still unclear. Animal studies can shed light on the mechanisms of effusion formation, as in recent studies on vascular endothelial growth factor (VEGF),[46–48] and on the proinflammatory axes of interleukin (IL)-6/Stat3[49] and of tumor necrosis factor (TNF)-α/nuclear factor (NF)-κB.[50]

Most animal studies on malignant pleural effusions have been performed using mice. Athymic nude mice are commonly used as they allow the development of pleural metastases by xenogenic (e.g. human) tumor cells. Various human cancer cell lines have been successfully introduced into the pleural space of immunodeficient mice, which give rise to malignant effusions.[47,48] Among the different tumor cell types used, adenocarcinomas produce the highest rate of effusions, similar to clinical presentations where adenocarcinomas tend to produce pleural metastases.[51] The shortcoming of these models is the need for immunodeficient (e.g. severe combined immunodeficient [SCID] or recombination activation gene-RAG-2 null) mice, which have impaired immunogenic responses to malignancies.

Stathopoulos *et al.*[50] recently described a murine model of adenocarcinoma-induced malignant effusion in immunocompetent mice, which will allow better elucidation of the mechanism of malignant effusion formation and its treatment.

Malignant cells can be implanted into the pleural space directly (by surgery or intrapleural injection) or indirectly from metastases from tumors deposited in the lungs. Orthotopic implantation of freshly isolated human adenocarcinoma tissues into nude mice can produce a high takeup rate of the cancer[52] but requires thoracotomy and tying of tumor tissues into the visceral and parietal pleurae. This method is more invasive and does not provide additional information compared with intrapleural or intravenous injection of tumor cells. In the latter cases, commercially available cancer cell lines grown in cell culture conditions are titrated before injection to standardize the tumor load per mouse. Intravenous injection of human adenocarcinoma (e.g. A549) cells produces numerous lung lesions, pleural metastases and effusions, in contrast with human squamous or large cell carcinoma cell lines, where malignant effusions are uncommon.[47,51] Transfection of antisense VEGF gene reduced VEGF expression, tumor vascularity, pleural metastases and effusions induced by adenocarcinoma cells.[47]

Tumors can also be injected directly into the pleural space, which is best performed by a left lateral subdiaphragmatic approach aimed cephalically. Extra-fine needles (28G) should be used. Up to 1.0 mL of fluid can be injected into an adult mouse, but small volumes (e.g. 50–100 μL) usually suffice. Accurate intrathoracic delivery is confirmed by transient chest expansion and dyspnea. Alternatively, a small skin incision (~5 mm) can be made, preferably on the left hemithorax, and tumor cells can be injected into the pleural space under direct vision. This method requires minimal surgery and has the advantages of on-site confirmation of orthotopic tumor cell delivery to the pleura and is reliably reproducible.[50]

Intrapleural injections of tumor cells (usually 10^5–10^6 per mice) result in local implantations in the chest wall, mediastinum, lungs and diaphragm by 1–2 weeks (Figure 14.1a). Pleural effusions (usually bloody exudates) develop approximately 2–3 weeks after inoculation.[50,51] At later stages, ascites may accumulate. When immunocompetent mice are used with syngeneic tumor cells (e.g. C57BL/6 mice – Lewis lung adenocarcinoma cells), the effusions are rich in inflammatory cells (Figure 14.1b).[50] Most mice eventually develop respiratory distress and weight loss, and die from local effects of the effusion, cachexia, and distant metastases.

Weight loss and survival are commonly used endpoints. The volume of pleural effusion, tumor load (number, size and weight), and the presence of distant metastases are other parameters useful for assessing therapeutic response. Pleural fluid and tissue collected allow the study of pathological mediators. Effusion-associated vascular permeability can be easily determined by intravenous injection of an albumin-binding dye (see 'Models for the study of pleural vascular permeability' and Figure 14.1c).[50]

Using these models, the role of important mediators and biological pathways (e.g. VEGF/VEGFR, IL-6/Stat3 and TNF-α/NF-κB) in effusion formation have been uncovered.[47–50] Other studies have assessed novel anticancer therapies, such as IL-12 and IL-15,[53] and inhibitors of topoisomerase II[51] and of VEGF receptor tyrosine kinase.[48] The intrapleural injection model has also been successfully applied to transgenic mice, such as nitric oxide synthase knockouts.[11]

MODELS FOR PLEURAL INFLAMMATION

The pleural cavity is regarded by some as 'the ideal site for the induction of inflammatory reactions'.[54] In the clinical setting, inflammation is often assessed histologically, which is subject to sampling error and can only provide

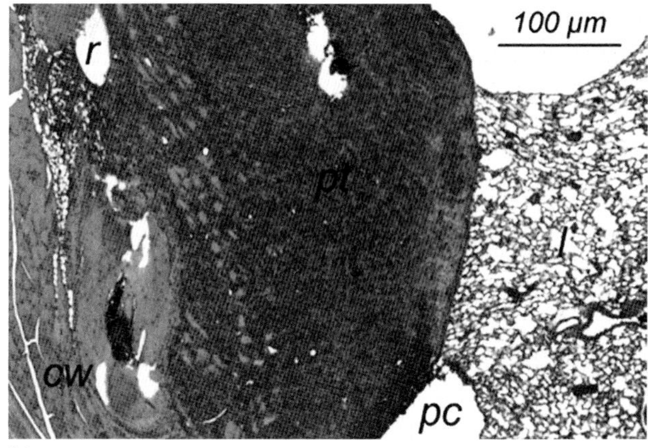

(a)

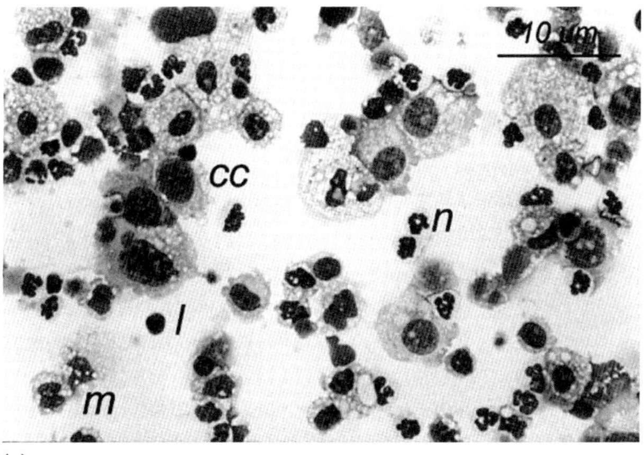

(b)

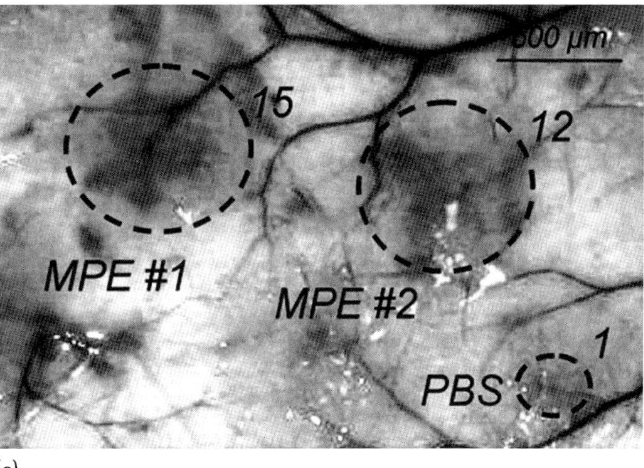

(c)

Figure 14.1 (a) Histological section through a Lewis lung adenocarcinoma (LLC)-induced pleural tumor in a C57BL/6 mouse, stained with hematoxylin and eosin (× 40). Note that the tumor bridges the parietal and visceral pleurae. cw, chest wall; l, lung; r, rib; pt, pleural tumor; pc, pleural cavity. (b) Cytocentrifugal preparation of malignant pleural effusion cells from the LLC-C57BL/6 model, stained with May-Grünwald-Giemsa (× 400). Alien adenocarcinoma cells are mixed with host inflammatory cells. cc, cancer cell; m, mononuclear cell; l, lymphocyte; n, neutrophil polymorphonuclear cell. (c) Vascular hyperpermeability induced in the skin of a C57BL/6 mouse by malignant pleural fluids from the LLC-C57BL/6 model, compared with PBS (negative control). After intradermal injection of 50 μL pleural fluid or PBS, the mouse received 0.8 mg Evans' blue in 200 μL normal saline. The mouse was killed and the skin inverted and photographed after 30 minutes. Circles represent areas of dye extravasation, and numbers relative surface area in respect to PBS (control). Evans' blue avidly binds to albumin; hence its extravasation indicates vascular hyperpermeability. (See also Color Plates 8–10.)

qualitative rather than quantitative data. Also, if inflammatory mediators are to be investigated, they have to be extracted from histology tissues. *In vitro* studies of inflammatory cells fail to provide knowledge on the complex interactions between various cells and mediators. Therefore, investigators often employ animal models of pleural inflammation that allow the study of cells and fluids accumulated during inflammation.[55]

Pleural models of inflammation offer several advantages. The pleural cavity provides a confined compartment lined by mesothelial cells in close contact with the systemic circulation where inflammatory cells and mediators collect. These can be monitored in a dynamic fashion by assaying the pleural fluid. The histological changes of inflammation can be assessed in pleural tissues and effects of pro- or anti-inflammatory agents can be investigated following their intrapleural administration.

Various methods have been used to induce pleural inflammation (Table 14.3), and each yields an inflammatory reaction characterized by a distinct profile of cell and mediator accumulation. Depending on the predominant inflammatory cell type recruited to the pleural cavity, the various animal models have been coined models of neutrophilic, mononuclear or eosinophilic pleural inflammation. For example, intrapleural lipopolysaccharide (LPS) results in mainly neutrophilic, but also, to a lesser extent, mononuclear, and eosinophilic pleural inflammation.[56–58]

The most widely used pleural inflammation model is the carrageenan pleurisy model.[55] Carrageenan can be administered intrapleurally by a needle injection, causing dose-dependent inflammation.[55] The detailed onset, progression and resolution of carrageenan pleurisy have been extensively studied and validated.[59] In brief, pleural exudation begins within an hour of injection, and is characterized by neutrophil followed by monocytic influx, followed by vascular hyperpermeability and pleural exudation.[55] Pleural fluids and serum can be serially collected for analysis, and pleural tissues can be obtained at necropsy. Numerous studies have utilized this model successfully in mice, rats and rabbits.[60] For example, mice that do not express IL-6[12] or nitric oxide synthase[61] exhibit significantly reduced pleural inflammation, confirming the

Table 14.3 A large variety of agents have been used to induce pleural inflammation. This table outlines the common and some of the uncommon agents used. Interested readers can refer to the references for individual agents for details

Agent to induce pleural inflammation	Representative reference
Most common	
Carrageenan	Bliven *et al.*[55]
	Vinegar *et al.*[59]
Common	
Endotoxin or lipopolysaccharide	Broaddus *et al.*[65]
	Fukumoto *et al.*[66]
Reverse Passive Arthur Reaction	Yamamoto *et al.*[54]
	Berkenkopf *et al.*[167]
Zymosan	Utsunomiya *et al.*[168]
Uncommon	
Azoles	Hanada *et al.*[169]
Bradykinin	Saleh *et al.*[170]
Calcium pyrophosphate crystals	Perianin *et al.*[171]
Ionophore A23187	Wang *et al.*[172]
Kaolin	Kawamura *et al.*[173]
Phorbol myristate acetate	Oh-ishi *et al.*[174]
Platelet activating factor	Tarayre *et al.*[175]
Substance P	Frode-Saleh *et al.*[176]

essential roles of these compounds in the inflammatory process.

Using the carrageenan model in conditional macrophage-deficient mice, the important role of resident pleural macrophages in neutrophil recruitment to the inflamed pleura was elucidated.[62] This probably occurs via production of 15-deoxy-prostaglandin (PG)J2 that induces transcription factor Nrf2, to facilitate recruitment of neutrophils to the pleura, to switch off neutrophilic and switch on monocytic inflammation.[63]

Several authors have injected LPS into the pleural cavity of rats and mice to generate inflammation. LPS induces influx of neutrophils within 4 hours, followed by monocytes, lymphocytes and eosinophils.[56–58] These studies have yielded interesting results on the differential role of the various selectins (L-, P- and E-) and of IL-8 in inflammatory neutrophil and eosinophil recruitment to the pleura.[64–66]

The reverse passive Arthus reaction has also been studied, particularly in rats.[54] Intravenous bovine serum albumin (BSA), followed by an intrapleural injection of purified anti-BSA 20 minutes later, induces pleural inflammation characterized by fluid extravasation (peak at 6 hours), neutrophil (peak at 6 hours) and mononuclear (peak at 12–24 hours) influx.

MODELS FOR EOSINOPHILIC (ALLERGIC) PLEURITIS

While allergic pleuritis is uncommon in humans, the pleural cavities of rats and mice have been used as surrogate systems for the study of the mechanisms of allergic responses. The pleural responses have been extrapolated to explain the pathophysiology of other allergic diseases, such as asthma and atopic dermatitis.

In these models, mice or rats are sensitized with ovalbumin adsorbed to $Al(OH)_3$ gel injected subcutaneously 14 days prior to the experiment. This sensitization process elicits peripheral and pleural eosinophilia. The experiment is then performed with an intrapleural injection of ovalbumin (10 μg per pleural cavity), which induces mast cell degranulation, immunoglobulin E (IgE) accumulation and eosinophil chemotaxis.[67,68] The role of mediators in eosinophilic recruitment and the efficacy of anti-allergy therapies can then be evaluated.[67–70] Pleural lavage can be performed to quantify eosinophil influx and allergic mediators, such as leukotrienes and platelet-activating factor. Using ovalbumin allergic pleurisy in nuclear factor of activated T cells (NFAT)1-gene-defficient mice, the role of NFAT1 in the suppression of T-helper type 2 immune-responses was elucidated.[71] In addition to ovalbumin, direct intrapleural delivery of biological mediators has been used to provoke eosinophilic inflammation. Intrapleural injection of chemokine ligand (CCL) 22, macrophage inflammatory protein (MIP)-1α, RANTES (regulated upon activation, normally T-cell expressed and secreted) and eotaxin resulted in dose- and time-dependent recruitment of eosinophils.[72,73]

Another mouse model of eosinophilic pleural inflammation exploits the pleural eosinophilia observed in patients with pneumothoraces. In this model, large numbers of eosinophils, among other inflammatory cells, are retrieved from the pleural lavage of mice after transthoracic injection of air.[74] Using IL-5- and IL-13-gene-deficient mice, investigators revealed that pleural recruitment of eosinophils is dependent on IL-5 but not IL-13.

As described above, intrapleural injection of LPS in rats and mice results in recruitment of eosinophils, along with other cell types.[56–58,64,65] Eosinophil levels rise significantly after 24 hours and their recruitment appears to be mediated by T lymphocytes.[58] LPS-induced pleural eosinophilia is mediated by P-selectin and IL-8 and is inhibited by corticosteroids.[56,64,65] The clinical value of this model remains unclear.

MODELS FOR PLEURAL INFECTION BY COMMON PATHOGENS (EMPYEMA)

Thoracic empyema remains a common disease with significant morbidity and mortality.[75,76] Animal experiments on empyema are most commonly performed using New Zealand white rabbits, though mice and sheep have been used.

Developing an adequate empyema model is difficult. Direct introduction of bacteria (such as *Streptococcus* or *Peptostreptococcus* species) into the pleural space usually results in their complete clearance.[77] To successfully initiate pleural infection, prior injury to the pleura may be required. However, under such situations, overwhelming sepsis and death can occur if too large a pathogen load is administered.

Sahn *et al.*[78] used an intrapleural injection of turpentine in rabbits, resulting in inflammation and an exudative neutrophilic pleural effusion by 72 hours.[79] At that point, bacteria (e.g. *Streptococcus pneumonia*,[78] *Escherichia coli*, *Peptostreptococcus anaerobius*, *Bacillus fragilis*[79] or their combinations) were introduced by thoracentesis into the effusion to create an empyema. Turpentine, however, may impose artifacts, and the authors reported that a high percentage of animals did not develop an exudative effusion to allow bacterial inoculation.[79]

Alternatively, Sasse *et al.*[77] showed that intrapleural injection of a potent rabbit pathogen, *Pasteurella multocida*, in brain–heart infusion agar could produce empyema without prior administration of turpentine. In this model, rabbits required daily intramuscular penicillin injections, to prevent death from sepsis. One drawback of this model is that *P. multocida* is a rabbit pathogen but rarely infects humans.[80] Hence, this model is not suitable for certain investigations, such as studies of antimicrobial treatment of empyema.

These models are well validated and exhibit pleural changes similar to that of human empyemas. In the models of Sahn *et al.*[78] and Sasse *et al.*[77] the induced pleural fluids showed significant increases in leukocytes and inflammatory indices, as well as markedly reduced pH and glucose. Pleural adhesions and macroscopic suppurative changes were evident at necropsy.

Another interesting model of pleural infection by *Staphylococcus aureus* was developed using a common mouse strain, C57BL/6.[13] Although intrapleural inoculation of the microorganism did not result in frank empyema, inflammatory cell influx and local cytokine and chemokine production was observed. This model is interesting for two reasons. First, it can be applied to genetically engineered animals. In the aforementioned study, CD4 knockout mice showed reduced inflammatory response and retarded pathogen clearance compared with wild-type mice.[13] Second, *S. aureus* is also pathogenic to humans, making these data more readily applicable to humans. Other methods to introduce empyema in guinea pigs and sheep have been published, but did not gain popularity.[81–83]

There is one important limitation of all these models. In humans, empyema occurs usually as a complication of pneumonia, while isolated pleural infection is uncommon. The animal models used in the literature all involve direct introduction of microbes into the pleural cavity and development of isolated pleural infection without pneumonia. Hence, the results of these experiments may not be directly extrapolated to humans.

Animal models of empyema have facilitated the study of the pathogenesis of the disease. Studies on rabbits and mice have revealed the important role of CD4+ lymphocytes in empyema-associated inflammation and bacterial clearance[13] and of TGF-β1 in empyema-associated pleural fibrosis.[84] Other studies have provided valuable information on the optimal treatment of empyema. Animal studies have lent support to repeated early thoracentesis,[85] early chest tube insertion[86] and intrapleural (single or combined) fibrinolytics for empyema.[79,87] Finally, the penetration of antibiotics into the pleural space has been studied using rabbit models of empyema.[88–90]

MODELS FOR PLEURAL INFECTION BY MYCOBACTERIA (TUBERCULOUS PLEURITIS)

Tuberculosis (TB) pleuritis continues to be a common clinical challenge in the new millennium. Our understanding of its pathogenesis and best management strategies remain limited. Animal models were used to study TB pleuritis as early as 1917 when Patterson investigated the disease using guinea pigs.[91] Rabbits and mice have also been used subsequently.

In the guinea pig model modified by Widstrom *et al.*[92,93] outbred guinea pigs are first vaccinated with intradermal 0.1–0.4 mg Bacille Calmette–Guerin (BCG). A higher dose of either BCG or heat killed *Mycobacterium tuberculosis* is injected intrapleurally 10–15 weeks later using a blunt needle connected to a manometer[93] or a 20G needle directed subdiaphragmatically into the pleural space.[94] With prior vaccination, most guinea pigs remain clinically well after intrapleural mycobacteria injection, despite the development of TB pleuritis.[92] Vaccination is successful in >90 percent of cases and can be confirmed by purified protein derivative (PPD) testing 3 weeks later. Shorter time gaps between vaccination and intrapleural infection produced inconsistent results and higher incidence of hemothoraces.[92] Antony *et al.*[95,96] applied similar strategies on New Zealand white rabbits to induce a TB pleuritis, rabbits being relatively resistant to *M. tuberculosis*, but susceptible to BCG. They also induced neutropenia in the rabbits by pretreatment with nitrogen-mustard, a modification that can allow the study of TB pleuritis in immunocompromised hosts.[96]

Several important points concerning these models deserve mention. It is believed that the dose of organisms, but not their virulence, is important for short-term TB pleuritis models. In the guinea pig model, both heat-inactivated *M. tuberculosis*[94] and BCG[92] induce TB pleuritis. Unilateral injections of mycobacteria in guinea pigs often result in bilateral pleural reactions.[92] Whether this is due to incomplete mediastinal separation of the pleural cavities or represents bacterial dissemination is unknown. Nonetheless, the contralateral pleural cavity should not be used as a control.

Tuberculosis pleuritis induced using these animal models closely represents the disease in humans. Exudative pleural effusions develop following intrapleural BCG injections, characterized by early neutrophilic, intermediate monocytic and late lymphocytic influx.[92,93,95] Similar to humans, lymphocytes in guinea pig TB pleuritis are mainly CD2+ T-lymphocytes.[94] However, while TB pleural effusions in humans are sometimes characterized by low pH and glucose, this is not the case in animal models, presumably due to lower levels of infection and inflammation. Histologically, the pleura of infected animals shows caseating granulomata, multi-nucleated giant cells and late pleural fibrosis.[92,94,95] Regional lymph nodes can also be affected. If live mycobacteria are used, they can be recovered from cultures of the pleural fluid or lymph nodes.[92]

Smaller animals such as mice (either Balb/c or C57BL/6 strains) have been used to investigate the early inflammation accompanying TB pleuritis.[97,98] Without prior vaccination, intrathoracic injection of BCG can effectively induce pleuritis while inactivated *Mycobacterium leprae* (isolated from livers of armadillo) cannot.[97] While the pleural fluid cellular composition in mouse TB pleurisy appeared similar to that in humans, the histological changes with this model have not been described.

Investigators should be aware of certain limitations of existing models. In these models, isolated TB pleuritis is induced by transthoracic mycobacterial inoculation, while human TB pleuritis usually develops as a result of pleural spread from adjacent lung parenchymal infection. Also, only BCG or heat-killed *M. tuberculosis*, rather than live *M. tuberculosis* (the most common pathogen in humans), are used in these models. Thus, it is difficult to determine if results of therapeutic interventions using these models can be directly applied to humans.[95]

Despite their limitations, the guinea pig and rabbit models of tuberculous pleuritis have provided valuable insights into the pathogenesis of the disease. Using rabbits, Antony *et al.*[96] have shown the importance of neutrophils in recruiting mononuclear cells into the TB-infected pleural space. Using guinea pigs, Allen *et al.*[99,100] have charted the time-course of pleural fluid accumulation, leukocyte influx and mediator expression after intrapleural injection of heat-inactivated *M. tuberculosis*, and reported continual increase of TGF-β1, even during the resolution phase of the pleuritis.

MODELS FOR BENIGN ASBESTOS-INDUCED PLEURAL DISEASES

Asbestos is a recognized cause for various pleural diseases, such as circumscribed (plaque) and diffuse pleural thickening, benign asbestos pleural effusion (BAPE), rounded atelectasis and malignant mesothelioma.[101–103] Mesothelial cells appear sensitive to the toxic effects of asbestos fibers, either by direct injury or via indirect effects from other asbestos-exposed cells[104] (see Chapter 10, Pleural reaction to mineral dusts). Extensive research has been conducted in the pathogenesis and treatment for malignant mesothelioma (See Chapter 15, Experimental models: Mesothelioma), but relatively little work has been invested in the study of benign asbestos-induced pleural diseases, despite their much higher prevalence. In addition to the pleura, asbestos damages the lung parenchyma causing fibrosis (asbestosis) and increasing lung cancer risk. Experimental models for the study of these conditions are outside the scope of this chapter.

Route of delivery

To study the effect of asbestos on the animal pleura, fibers can be introduced either via the respiratory tract or by direct intrapleural injection.[104,105] The former resembles human exposure to asbestos and fibers can be delivered by intratracheal instillation,[106–109], by direct delivery to a lobar bronchus[110] or by inhalation of aerosolized fibers in a closed chamber.[111–114] The resulting pleural and pulmonary inflammatory and fibroproliferative reactions have a dose–response relationship with the amount of fibers delivered.[111,112]

Both the inhalation and the intrapleural injection methods have drawbacks. Administered by inhalation, fiber deposition in the peripheral lung, and hence their toxic effects to the pleura, varies. In addition, pleural changes in animals may take months to years to develop, similar to humans.[115,116] By contrast, direct intrapleural injection can ensure immediate delivery of a known amount of fibers into the pleural cavity and accurate identification of time zero of pleural injury. It also facilitates the study of isolated fiber effects on the pleura without the influence by other lung parenchymal changes. However, this method of delivery differs significantly from how fibers reach the pleura in humans. Wagner *et al.*[117] compared intrapleural and inhalation delivery of chrysotile to rats. Mesotheliomas developed more frequently with intrapleural injections, whereas malignant lung tumors were much more common than mesotheliomas if fibers were delivered by inhalation.

Choice of species

Rats, mice and hamsters are most commonly used. Larger animals, such as rabbits, guinea pigs and dogs, have also been used, especially if direct intrapleural injection is employed. It is important to note that intra- and inter-species differences in susceptibility to asbestos-induced damage exist.[118] The propensity of mice to develop pulmonary fibrosis in response to asbestos varies significantly among strains, in accord with fibrotic susceptibility to radiation or bleomycin. Mice of the 129 strain respond to asbestos with lower TNF-α and TGF-β expression and minimal fibroproliferative lung lesions, compared with C57BL/6 mice.[119] Balb/c mice, another commonly used strain, have also been found to develop lung changes similar to human asbestosis after exposure to aerosolized chrysotile.[114] Although no studies have compared murine strain susceptibility with asbestos-induced pleural fibrosis, investigators should be aware that variation is likely to exist. Interspecies comparison is an important issue, particularly regarding extrapolation of animal study results to humans. Several reviews concurred that the rat model is most appropriate for extrapolation of toxicological data to humans.[118,120,121] Maxim and McConnell[118] found a significant difference in relative incidence of mesothelioma and lung cancer between rats and hamsters and concluded that the rat is a better model than hamsters for human risk evaluation. They also reported that cells of humans and rodents have comparable sensitivity to asbestos exposure, in terms of cytotoxicity and production of mediators. The deposition rate of respirable fibers is lower in humans than in rats, but so is the clearance rate. Hence, humans and rats develop fibrosis at comparable normalized fiber burdens.[118]

Fiber types

The potency of different types of asbestos fibers to induce fibrosis and malignancies differs and appears to be related to their physical properties, especially fiber length and biopersistence.[118] Long, but not short, crocidolite fibers were able to induce fibrotic reactions in the lung and pleura.[106,122,123] However, no fiber type should be considered harmless.[107] Also, contamination of the asbestos fiber preparation with other mineral dusts is common and can make the results of studies difficult to interpret. It is therefore crucial that investigators analyze and document the physical characteristics of the asbestos preparation used in their experiments. Chrysotile, crocidolite and amosite are the commonly used fibers in experimental models. In most studies, administration of the vehicle in which the fibers were suspended served as the control. Alternatively, woolastonite, a relatively non-pathogenic calcium silicate fiber, has been used as control and is known to induce significantly less mesothelial cell damage than crocidolite.[104] Recently, models for asbestos-induced pleural disease have been extended to investigate the effects of man-made fibers, especially fibreglass.[112,124]

Endpoints

Ideally, development of the asbestos-induced pleural diseases, such as pleural fibrosis, BAPE or mesothelioma, should be the experimental endpoint. However, since the lag time for development of such disease is long, many studies focused on the more immediate/early effects of fibers upon the lung and pleura. Pleural lavage can be analyzed for mediators induced after fiber exposure of the pleura. Mesothelial cells can be harvested for assessment of proliferative responses, apoptosis or other immunohistochemical analyses.

Animal studies of asbestos exposure have been invaluable in revealing the mechanisms of asbestos-induced lung and pleural injury. After asbestos inhalation, the pleura can be assaulted via direct or indirect mechanisms. Using scanning electron microscopy, inhaled asbestos has been shown to produce cystic degradation of the pleural surface, allowing penetration of single fibers through the visceral pleura.[125] Inhaled chrysotile fibers have been detected in pleural cells of rats by electron microscopy within varying time intervals, ranging from 1 week to 3 years after exposure.[110,115,126]

Rodent studies have shown morphological changes in mesothelial cells within 2 hours of intratracheal amosite instillation, followed by early mesothelial proliferation and macrophage influx within 24 hours.[108,127] In addition, asbestos has been shown to stimulate intracellular signalling cascades such as mitogen-activated protein kinases (MAPK) and extracellular signal-regulated kinases (ERK) in mesothelial cells.[128,129] These acute changes occur in the absence of direct penetration of amosite fibers into the pleural space, supporting the view that pleural reactions result from pleural migration of mediators induced by asbestos in the airways and lung parenchyma.[106] In fact, antibodies to keratinocyte growth factor (but not to platelet-derived growth factor) reduce crocidolite-induced mesothelial proliferation.[130]

The pleural inflammatory reaction to asbestos is multifactorial. Pleural macrophages produce large quantities of proinflammatory nitric oxide and TNF-α after inhaled chrysotile.[126] Reactive nitrogen species and nitrotyrosine were also found in both visceral and parietal pleurae and are likely to play a role in pleural injury.[113] Intrapleural crocidolite in rabbits also resulted in significant elevation of IL-8 synthesis and neutrophil influx.[105] These inflammatory changes are usually accompanied by mesothelial cell proliferation.[111] Knockout mice deficient in both the 55 and 75 kDa TNF-α receptors are protected from the pulmonary fibroproliferative changes induced by chrysotile,[131] further confirmation of the essential role of TNF-α.

Although BAPE is a common asbestos-induced pleural condition that precedes diffuse pleural thickening (fibrosis), it has only occasionally been studied in experimental settings. Shore *et al.*[132] injected crocidolite intrapleurally into rabbits and showed the development of a neutrophilic exudative effusion within 4 hours of injection. When the fluid was reinjected into another rabbit, a polymorphonuclear neutrophil (PMN) response was also elicited.[132]

Asbestos-related lung and pleural diseases are likely to continue to increase. While legislation has been implemented in most developed countries to minimize occupational and environmental asbestos exposure since the early 1970s, the long lag time between exposure and clinical presentation means there is still a large population at risk of developing disease. Also, chrysotile now constitutes 99 percent of current global asbestos production and sales remain strong in developing nations despite the recent conclusion of the International Program on Chemical Safety of the World Health Organization that 'exposure to chrysotile poses increased risks for asbestosis, lung cancer and mesothelioma in a dose-dependent manner'.[101] Hence, it is anticipated that animal studies will remain important in the ongoing effort to understand the pathogenesis of asbestos pleural damage and to design new treatment strategies.

MODELS FOR CHYLOTHORAX

Chylothorax, the accumulation of chyle in the pleural space, results from impaired lymphatic drainage due to various causes, such as surgery or trauma to the thoracic duct and malignancy (see Chapter 29, Effusions from lymphatic disruptions). Surgical ligation or interruption of the thoracic duct has been performed in a canine model. Mongrel dogs were fed milk fat prior to surgery to increase lymphatic drainage and allow easy identification and transection of the thoracic duct, leaving chest tubes in place for drainage. Using this model, octreotide has been shown to enhance closure of the fistula and reduce chyle leak.[133]

Congenital defects of the lymphatic duct and lymphangiectasia are uncommon causes of chylothoraces. Recently, mice homozygous for a null mutation of the gene encoding the $\alpha9$ subunit of the $\alpha9\beta1$ integrin were bred to examine the roles of the $\alpha9$ integrins. Unexpectedly, these mice had genetic defects in their lymphatic system resulting in bilateral chylothoraces by 6–12 days after birth, and died eventually of respiratory failure.[134] The role of the $\alpha9\beta1$ integrin in lymphatic development appears to be mediated via binding to lymphangiogenic VEGF-C and -D.[135] This model may be useful for further investigation of the mechanism of chylothorax development.

MODELS FOR PLEURAL EFFUSIONS FROM ESOPHAGEAL RUPTURE

Esophageal perforation is an uncommon cause of pleural effusion. Only one model has been developed using insertion and overinflation of a 16F Foley catheter into the esophagus of anesthetized New Zealand white rabbits.[136,137] Pleural effusions developed 2 hours later and were bilateral in half of the rabbits. Serial thoracenteses revealed exudative effusions with progressively increasing acidity and leukocytosis, rising levels of protein, very high amylase and low glucose, and positive bacterial cultures, consistent with the classical pleural fluid findings in patients with ruptured esophagus.[136] Interestingly, when the animals were rendered neutropenic by pretreatment with nitrogen mustard, no reduction in pleural fluid pH was observed, suggesting that the reduced pH results from neutrophil metabolism rather than anaerobic bacterial infection.[137]

MODELS FOR PLEURAL EFFUSIONS FROM FLUID OVERLOADS

Human transudative pleural effusions, commonly caused by congestive cardiac failure, renal failure or hepatic cirrhosis, are not easily recapitulated in animal models. A sheep model of intravenous oleic acid infusion has been used to induce pulmonary edema and bilateral pleural effusions.[138] Oleic acid resulted in reduced cardiac contractility, raised pulmonary arterial pressures, alveolar edema and pleural transudation. The biochemical composition of the pleural fluid was similar to that of the alveolar fluid. While this model is useful, it is not entirely similar to pleural effusion from cardiac failure. First, oleic acid infusion causes alveolar damage. Second, the pleural fluid to plasma protein ratio was 0.6–0.7, classifying the pleural fluid as an exudate.

A murine model of renal failure and fluid overload has been described by Song *et al.*[139] Renal failure is generated by bilateral renal vessel ligation and fluid overload by intraperitoneal delivery of isotonic saline of 40 percent body weight. After 3 hours, the mice develop bilateral pleural effusions (approximately 100 µL).[139] This model was developed to study the role of aquaporin water channels in pleural fluid homeostasis, but can be used to study other aspects of pleural effusion secondary to renal failure.

MODELS FOR PLEURAL PHYSIOLOGY STUDIES

Numerous animal models have been employed for the investigation of pleural physiology in health and disease. The main areas of interest are mechanisms of pleural fluid formation and absorption and pleural pressure changes in the presence of effusion or pneumothorax.

To study the transfer of lung water into the pleural space through the visceral pleura, Broaddus *et al.*[140] subjected anesthetized ventilated sheep to volume overload. The chest was open and a bag was wrapped around the exposed lung to collect the fluid leak from lung parenchyma into the pleural space. Their experiments confirmed that the pleural space provided an important route of clearance of pulmonary edema. Similar methods have been used in mongrel dogs to study the factors that alter the permeability of the visceral pleura.[141,142]

Different animal models have been used to study the removal of pleural fluid and proteins from the pleural space. Many studies have been performed in sheep[143] and rabbits,[144] and occasionally dogs.[145] Labeled particles, such as I^{125}-albumin[146] or florescent isothiocyanate-labeled dextran,[147] can be used as a tracer to follow the efflux and reabsorption of protein in the pleural space.

Readers should beware of potential drawbacks when extrapolating the results of these animal studies to human physiology. First, fluid exchange mechanisms in animals may not always parallel those of humans, as humans (and sheep) have thick visceral pleurae in contrast to the thin visceral pleural membranes of rabbits: thus, the results of rabbit fluid absorption studies may not represent human conditions. Second, in humans, pleural fluid often accumulates in pathologic conditions with abnormal (e.g. inflammed or malignant) pleura, and the pathophysiology of fluid formation and regression may well differ from studies performed in animals with normal pleurae. Third, respiratory patterns may affect pleural fluid absorption, making sedated animals not ideal representatives of 'real life' situations. In rabbits, the rate of pleural absorption of particles can be influenced by their molecular weight.[148] Whether this applies to other animals remains to be tested.

Animal studies have also been used to assess cardiorespiratory impairment induced by pleural effusion or pneumothorax. Fluid or air can be introduced intrapleurally and physiological changes (e.g. electrocardiogram, hemodynamic changes, arterial oxygenation, lung function) measured.[149–152] Large pleural effusions affect the dynamic elastance and resistance of the respiratory system, and produce hypoxemia in a dose-dependent fashion. It is noteworthy that in animal experiments effusions are produced acutely, whereas most human effusions (e.g. malignant) accumulate over time. Chronic measurement of the effects of artificially induced effusion is difficult, but has been reported by Murphy *et al.*[153] who surgically inserted catheters in the serosal layer of the rat esophagus, allowing measurement of pleural pressures for up to 14 weeks.

MODELS FOR THE STUDY OF PLEURAL VASCULAR PERMEABILITY

Leakage of protein-rich exudate from blood capillaries in the lung interstitium, and beneath the mesothelium into the pleural space, has been implicated in the pathogenesis of various pleural effusions and has been demonstrated in human disease and animal models.[47–50,154–156] Albumin is the most abundant protein contained in exudative pleural effusions and is, as a result, most commonly used to determine vascular permeability. Studies of pleural vascular permeability are feasible in any species, but mice have been used preferentially.

Pleural vascular permeability can be assessed using two mutually complementary methods. Permeability can be determined using an albumin tracer (e.g. Evans' blue, fluoro-isothiocyanate or radioisotope-labeled albumin) introduced intravenously into animals bearing pleural effusion or inflammation.[47–50] Shortly thereafter (e.g. 5–30 minutes), the levels of the tracer in the pleural fluid or lavage can be determined (e.g. measuring absorbance, fluorescence or scintillation), and reflects the rate of albumin leakage into the pleural space.

Another experimental approach, the Miles vascular permeability assay, determines the effects of mediators contained in pleural fluid on vascular permeability in the mouse or rat skin (Figure 14.1c),[48,49,155,156] Cell-free pleural fluid supernatants are injected intradermally and Evans' blue is administered intravenously. After a predetermined time interval, extravasation of the dye into the mouse dermis is determined by measuring Evans' blue levels in tissue extracts or by morphometry. Vascular permeability induced by the fluid under examination can be compared with saline (negative control) or VEGF solutions (positive control), and the contribution of individual mediators to overall vascular permeability can be assessed after their neutralization in the pleural fluid prior to injection into the skin.

Using these methods, the contribution of VEGF,[47,48,156] IL-6[49] and TNF-α (Stathopoulos *et al.*, unpublished observations) to the induction of vascular hyperpermeability in malignant pleural effusions has been established.

OTHER MODELS

Various other models have been published over the years. For example, the turpentine model (see Models for pleural infection) has been used to mimic effusions from rheumatoid arthritis.[157]

Intrapleural gene therapy for replacement therapy or for mesothelioma has been studied in animal models. In our experience, mesothelial cells can be easily transfected *in vitro* and *in vivo*. Plasmids delivered intrapleurally can transfect the mesothelial cells and the protein product can be recovered from pleural fluids and from plasma.[158]

Rabbits have also been used to study the pharmacokinetics of intrapleurally administered drugs.[159,160] This may be relevant to intrapleural chemotherapy, which has been increasingly used in clinical trials for control of malignant mesothelioma.

IN VITRO STUDIES OF MESOTHELIAL CELLS AND *IN SITU* STUDIES OF MESOTHELIAL MONOLAYERS

While *in vitro* studies have limitations, the study of cultured mesothelial cells in isolation can provide information supplemental to animal studies. Mesothelial cell lines are commercially available but are transformed by viral infection or transformation. Mesothelial cells from the pleura or the peritoneum can be harvested for primary culture. While their biological behaviors are likely to be similar, this has seldom been compared or confirmed. However, when *in vitro* studies of mesothelial cells are undertaken to address the pathophysiology of pleural diseases, it would be ideal to use pleural and not peritoneal mesothelial cells.

Normal human pleural mesothelial cells are difficult to obtain, and have most commonly been isolated from pleural effusions caused by heart failure. Culture methods of human and animal mesothelial cells are similar.[104,161] However, mesothelial cells from human effusions, even from transudative ones, have likely been exposed to mediators and may not truly represent 'normal' mesothelial cells. For that reason, studies often employ primary culture of pleural mesothelial cells from animals, e.g. rabbits or mice. Principles of harvesting the cells and points of caution are summarized in Appendix 14.3. In our experience, primary rabbit mesothelial cells grow rapidly and maintain their biological activities up to seven or eight passages. In contrast, murine mesothelial cells divide very slowly (the initial growth rate increases with density of seeded cells), and rarely survive a third passage.

To overcome the limitations of human mesothelial cell culture outlined above, Kim *et al.* devised a new *in vitro* system for culture of mesothelioma tissues in the form of spheroids, based on a technique previously developed for culture of intact bronchial mucosa.[162,163] Using this method, mesothelioma tissue retained many of its *in vivo* characteristics. This model closely emulates intrapleural mesothelioma growth and is expected to greatly facilitate studies on mesothelioma apoptotic resistance to novel therapies. Such techniques can be adopted for experiments on non-malignant pleural tissue cultured *ex vivo*.

Other studies have been performed on isolated mesothelial barriers *in situ*, most commonly obtained from sheep.[164–166] Ussing chambers, special devices that function as voltage clamps, have been used to measure the transpleural resistance in pleura stripped from animals, before and after an intervention. The resistance measured supposedly reflects the permeability of the pleural barrier. This model has its limitations: pleural fluid formation is governed largely by vascular (rather than mesothelial) permeability, and the findings of these studies of normal pleura may not be applicable to pleural structures in disease states.

CONCLUSIONS

> *'If we look carefully enough we will eventually find an animal model for every disease.'*

Leader (1969) at the Federation of American Societies for Experimental Biology.

Animal experimentation represents one of the fundamental approaches in the long arduous path towards the understanding of the pathogenesis of various pleural diseases. *In vivo* studies are essential in the evaluation of novel therapeutic approaches in pleural diseases, in the study of pharmacokinetics of drug delivery in the pleural space and in the investigation of pleural physiological changes in both normal and disease states.

No animal model is ideal. Investigators should understand the advantages and limitations of the use of different animal species and models. Only through doing so would they be able to choose or design the most suitable *in vivo* model or *in vitro* experiment that provides the best chance of answering the scientific question(s) raised. Animal studies should be planned, conducted and supervised with a similar degree of scrutiny as that applied to clinical trials. The ultimate aim should always be to provide better care to patients with pleural diseases.

Advances in other areas of biomedical sciences, especially animal imaging techniques, should allow the design of more sophisticated animal models that will improve our understanding and clinical management of pleural diseases.

KEY POINTS

- Animal models have been invaluable in the study of the pathogenesis of pleural diseases. *In vivo* studies are essential in evaluating new therapeutic options for pleural diseases, in assessing the pharmacokinetics of drug delivery to the pleura and in examining physiological changes in the pleural space in health and disease.
- It is critical for researchers to understand the characteristics and limitations of experimental models available in order to use the most appropriate method that can best answer the scientific question asked.
- Researchers must adhere to standard guidelines for animal care and gain approval from local ethics committees. Every effort should be made to minimize animal discomfort and the number of animals required.
- *In vitro* studies allow the study of mesothelial and other cells that may engage in the pathogenesis of pleural diseases in isolation. *In vitro* experiments can help explain pathologies observed in animal or human studies. Conversely, novel information derived from cell culture experiments can be tested *in vivo* using appropriate animal models.
- Animal models exist for common types of pleural diseases (e.g. pleural effusion due to malignancy, infection and inflammation), as well as for pleural pathologies that are uncommonly encountered in clinical practice (e.g. chylothorax, esophageal rupture).
- Advancement in biomedical technology, e.g. novel methods for gene transfer and further development of genetically engineered mice, will allow the design of increasingly sophisticated models to provide further significant insights into pleural diseases.

REFERENCES

● = Key primary paper
◆ = Major review article

◆1. Migaki G, Capen CC. Animal models in biomedical research. In: Fox JG, Cohen BJ, Loew FM (eds). *Laboratory animal medicine*. New York: Academic Press Inc., 1984: 667–98.

◆2. Institute for Laboratory Animal Research, Commission on Life Sciences, National Research Council. *Guide for the care and use of laboratory animals*. Washington DC: National Academy Press, 1996.

◆3. McPherson CW. Laws, regulations, and policies affecting the use of laboratory animals. In: Fox JG, Cohen BJ, Loew FM (eds). *Laboratory animal medicine*. New York: Academic Press Inc., 1984: 19–30.

4. Cohen BJ, Loew FM. Laboratory animal medicine: Historical perspectives. In: Fox JG, Cohen BJ, Loew FM (eds). *Laboratory animal medicine*. New York: Academic Press Inc., 1984: 1–18.

5. Dechman G, Mishima M, Bates JH. Assessment of acute pleural effusion in dogs by computed tomography. *J Appl Physiol* 1994; 76: 1993–8.

◆6. Silver LM. *Mouse genetics*. New York/Oxford: Oxford University Press, 1995.

◆7. Bockamp E, Maringer M, Spangenberg C, *et al*. Of mice and models: improved animal models for biomedical research. *Physiol Genomics* 2002; **11**: 115–32.

◆8. Wade CM, Daly MJ. Genetic variation in laboratory mice. *Nat Genet* 2005; **37**: 1175–80.

9. van der Most RG, Robinson BWS, Nelson DJ. Gene therapy for malignant mesothelioma: beyond the infant years. *Cancer Gene Ther* 2006; **13**: 897–904.

10. Mae M, Crystal RG. Gene transfer to the pleural mesothelium as a strategy to deliver proteins to the lung parenchyma. *Hum Gene Ther* 2002; **13**: 1471–82.

11. Wang B, Xiong Q, Shi Q, *et al*. Genetic disruption of host nitric oxide synthase II gene impairs melanoma-induced angiogenesis and suppresses pleural effusion. *Int J Cancer* 2001; **91**: 607–11.

12. Cuzzocrea S, Sautebin L, De Sarro G, *et al*. Role of IL-6 in the pleurisy and lung injury caused by carrageenan. *J Immunol* 1999; **163**: 5094–104.

13. Mohammed KA, Nasreen N, Ward MJ, Antony VB. Induction of acute pleural inflammation by Staphylococcus aureus. I. CD4+ T cells play a critical role in experimental empyema. *J Infect Dis* 2000; **181**: 1693–9.

●14. Gossen M, Bujard H. Tight control of gene expression in mammalian cells by tetracycline-responsive promoters. *Proc Natl Acad Sci U S A* 1992; **89**: 5547–51.

◆15. Lewandoski M. Conditional control of gene expression in the mouse. *Nature Rev Genet* 2001; **2**: 743–55.

●16. Elbashir SM, Harborth J, Lendeckel W, *et al*. Duplexes of 21-nucleotide RNAs mediate RNA interference in cultured mammalian cells. *Nature* 2001; **411**: 494–8.

◆17. Engels BM, Hutvagner G. Principles and effects of microRNA-mediated post-transcriptional gene regulation. *Oncogene* 2006; **25**: 6163–9.

18. Vargas FS, Teixeira LR, Coelho IJ, *et al*. Distribution of pleural injectate. Effect of volume of injectate and animal rotation. *Chest* 1994; **106**: 1246–9.

19. Carvalho P, Kirk W, Butler J, Charan NB. Effects of tube thoracostomy on pleural fluid characteristics in sheep. *J Appl Physiol* 1993; **74**: 2782–7.

20. Bresticker MA, Oba J, LoCicero Jr, Greene R. Optimal pleurodesis: a comparison study. *Ann Thorac Surg* 1993; **55**: 364–6.

21. Colt HG, Russack V, Chiu Y, *et al*. A comparison of thoracoscopic talc insufflation, slurry, and mechanical abrasion pleurodesis. *Chest* 1997; **111**: 442–8.

●22. Lee YCG, Teixeira LR, Devin CJ, *et al*. Transforming growth factor-β2 induces pleurodesis significantly faster than talc. *Am J Respir Crit Care Med* 2001; **163**: 640–4.

23. Dikensoy O, Zhu Z, Donnelly E, *et al*. Combination therapy with intrapleural doxycycline and talc in reduced doses is effective in producing pleurodesis in rabbits. *Chest* 2005; **128**: 3735–42.

●24. Zhu Z, Donnelly E, Dikensoy O, *et al*. Efficacy of ultrasound in the diagnosis of pleurodesis in rabbits. *Chest* 2005; **128**: 934–9.

◆25. Lee YCG, Light RW. Management of malignant pleural effusions. *Respirology* 2004; **9**: 148–56.

●26. Light RW, Cheng DS, Lee YCG, *et al*. A single intrapleural injection of transforming growth factor beta-2 produces an excellent pleurodesis in rabbits. *Am J Respir Crit Care Med* 2000; **162**: 98–104.

27. Marchi E, Vargas FS, Acencio MMP, *et al*. Pleurodesis: a novel experimental model. *Respirology* 2007; **12**: 500–4.

●28. Lee YCG, Lane KB, Parker RE, *et al*. Transforming growth factor beta-2 (TGFβ2) produces effective pleurodesis in sheep with no systemic complications. *Thorax* 2000; **55**: 1058–62.

29. Werebe EC, Pazetti R, Milanez de Campos JR, *et al*. Systemic distribution of talc after intrapleural administration in rats. *Chest* 1999; **115**: 190–3.

30. Cohen RG, Shely WW, Thompson SE, *et al*. Talc pleurodesis: Talc slurry versus thoracoscopic talc insufflation in porcine model. *Ann Thorac Surg* 1996; **62**: 1000–2.

31. Wu W, Teixeira LR, Light RW. Doxycycline pleurodesis in rabbits: comparison of results with and without chest tube. *Chest* 1998; **114**: 563–8.

32. Sahn SA, Good JT, Jr. The effect of common sclerosing agents on the rabbit pleural space. *Am Rev Respir Dis* 1981; **124**: 65–7.

33. Hurewitz AN, Lidonicci K, Wu CL, Reim D, Zucker S. Histologic changes of doxycycline pleurodesis in rabbits. Effect of concentration and pH. *Chest* 1994; **106**: 1241–5.

34. Kennedy L, Harley RA, Sahn SA, Strange C. Talc slurry pleurodesis. Pleural fluid and histologic analysis. *Chest* 1995; **107**: 1707–12.

35. Bilaceroglu S, Guo Y, Hawthorne ML, *et al*. Oral forms of tetracycline and doxycycline are effective in producing pleurodesis. *Chest* 2005; **128**: 3750–6.

◆36. Mutsaers SE, Kalomenidis I, Wilson NA, Lee YCG. Growth factors in pleural fibrosis. *Curr Opin Pulm Med* 2006; **12**: 251–8.

37. Lee YCG, Devin CJ, Teixeira LR, *et al*. Transforming growth factor beta-2 induced pleurodesis is not inhibited by corticosteroids. *Thorax* 2001; **56**: 643–8.

38. Xie C, Teixeira LR, McGovern JP, Light RW. Effect of pneumothorax on pleurodesis induced with talc in rabbits. *Chest* 1998; **114**: 1143–6.

39. Lee YCG, Yasay JR, Johnson JE, *et al*. Comparing transforming growth factor (TGF)-β_2, talc and bleomycin as pleurodesing agents in sheep. *Respirology* 2002; **7**: 209–16.

40. Diacon AH, Wyser C, Bollinger CT, *et al*. Prospective randomized comparison of thoracoscopic talc poudrage under local anaethesia versus bleomycin instillation for pleurodesis in malignant pleural effusions. *Am J Respir Crit Care Med* 2000; **162**: 1445–9.

41. Macoviak JA, Stephenson LW, Ochs R, Edmunds LHJ. Tetracycline pleurodesis during active pulmonary-pleural air leak for prevention of recurrent pneumothorax. *Chest* 1982; **81**: 78–81.

42. Antony VB, Loddenkemper R, Astoul P, *et al*. Management of malignant pleural effusions. *Eur Respir J* 2001;**18**: 402–19.

43. Antunes G, Neville E, Duffy J, Ali N. Pleural Diseases Group, Standards of Care Committee, British Thoracic Society. BTS guidelines for the management of malignant pleural effusions. *Thorax* 2003; **58**: ii29–38.

44. Sugiura S, Ando Y, Minami H, *et al*. Prognostic value of pleural effusion in patients with non-small cell lung cancer. *Clin Cancer Res* 1997; **3**: 47–50.

45. Naito T, Satoh H, Ishikawa H, *et al*. Pleural effusion as a significant prognostic factor in non-small cell lung cancer. *Anticancer Res* 1997; **17**: 4743–6.

◆46. Lee YCG, Malkerneker D, Thompson PJ, Light RW, Lane KB. Transforming growth factor-β induces vascular endothelial growth factor elaboration from pleural mesothelial cells *in vivo* and *in vitro*. *Am J Respir Crit Care Med* 2002; **165**: 88–94.

●47. Yano S, Shinohara H, Herbst RS, *et al.* Production of experimental malignant pleural effusions is dependent on invasion of the pleura and expression of vascular endothelial growth factor/vascular permeability factor by human lung cancer cells. *Am J Pathol* 2000; **157**: 1893–1903.

48. Yano S, Herbst RS, Shinohara H, *et al.* Treatment for malignant pleural effusion of human lung adenocarcinoma by inhibition of vascular endothelial growth factor receptor tyrosine kinase phosphorylation. *Clin Cancer Res* 2000; **6**: 957–65.

49. Yeh HH, Lai WW, Chen HH, Liu HS, Su WC. Autocrine IL-6-induced Stat3 activation contributes to the pathogenesis of lung adenocarcinoma and malignant pleural effusion. *Oncogene* 2006; **25**: 4300–9.

●50. Stathopoulos GT, Zhu Z, Everhart MB, *et al.* Nuclear factor-kappaB affects tumor progression in a mouse model of malignant pleural effusion. *Am J Respir Cell Mol Biol* 2006; **34**: 142–50.

51. Kraus-Berthier L, Jan M, Guilbaud N, *et al.* Histology and sensitivity to anticancer drugs of two human non-small cell lung carcinomas implanted in the pleural cavity of nude mice. *Clin Cancer Res* 2000; **6**: 297–304.

52. Astoul P, Colt HG, Wang X, Hoffman RM. Metastatic human pleura ovarian cancer model constructed by orthotopic implantation of fresh histologically intact patient carcinoma in nude mice. *Anticancer Res* 1993; **13**: 1999–2002.

53. Kimura K, Nishimura H, Matsuzaki T, *et al.* Synergistic effect of interleukin-15 and interleukin-12 on antitumor activity in a murine malignant pleurisy model. *Cancer Immunol Immunother* 2000; **49**: 71–7.

54. Yamamoto S, Dunn CJ, Deporter DA, *et al.* A model for the quantitative study of Arthus (immunologic) hypersensitivity in rats. *Agents Actions* 1975; **5**: 374–7.

55. Bliven ML, Otterness IG. Carrageenan pleurisy. *Meth Enzymol* 1988; **162**: 334–9.

56. Bozza PT, Castro-Faria-Neto HC, Martins MA, *et al.* Pharmacological modulation of lipopolysaccharide-induced pleural eosinophil in the rat: a role for a newly generated protein. *Eur J Pharmacol* 1993; **248**: 41–7.

57. Bozza PT, Castro-Faria-Neto HC, Penido C, *et al.* Requirement for lymphocytes and resident macrophages in LPS-induced pleural eosinophil accumulation. *J Leukoc Biol* 1994; **56**: 151–8.

58. Penido C, Castro-Faria-Neto HC, Larangeira AP, *et al.* The role of gammadelta T lymphocytes in lipopolysaccharide-induced eosinophil accumulation into the mouse pleural cavity. *J Immunol* 1997; **159**: 853–60.

◆59. Vinegar R, Truax JF, Selph JL, Voelker FA. Pathway of onset, development and decay of carrageenan pleurisy in the rat. *Fed Proc* 1982; **41**: 2588–95.

60. Strange C, Tomlinson JR, Wilson C, *et al.* The histology of experimental pleural injury with tetracycline, empyema and carrageenan. *Exp Mol Pathol* 1989; **51**: 205–19.

●61. Cuzzocrea S, Mazzon E, Calabro G, *et al.* Inducible nitric oxide synthase-knockout mice exhibit resistance to pleurisy and lung injury caused by carrageenan. *Am J Respir Crit Care Med* 2000; **162**: 1859–66.

●62. Cailhier JF, Sawatzky DA, Kipari T, *et al.* Resident pleural macrophages are key orchestrators of neutrophil recruitment in pleural inflammation. *Am J Respir Crit Care Med* 2006; **173**: 540–47.

●63. Itoh K, Mochizuki M, Ishii Y, *et al.* Transcription factor Nrf2 regulates inflammation by mediating the effect of 15-deoxy-$\Delta^{12,14}$-prostaglandin J2. *Mol Cell Biol* 2004; **24**: 36–45.

64. Henriques GMO, Miotla JM, Cordeiro RSB, *et al.* Selectins mediate eosinophil recruitment in vivo: a comparison with their role in neutrophil influx. *Blood* 1996; 187: 5297–304.

65. Broaddus VC, Boylan AM, Hoeffel JM, *et al.* Neutralization of IL-8 inhibits neutrophil influx in a rabbit model of endotoxin-induced pleurisy. *J Immunol* 1994; **152**: 2960–7.

66. Fukumoto T, Matsukawa A, Yoshimura T, *et al.* IL-8 is an essential mediator of the increased delayed-phase vascular permeability in LPS-induced rabbit pleurisy. *J Leukoc Biol* 1998; **63**: 584–90.

67. Klein A, Talvani A, Cara DC, *et al.* Stem cell factor plays a major role in the recruitment of eosinophils in allergic pleurisy in mice via the production of leukotriene B4. *J Immunol* 2000; **164**: 4271–6.

68. Pasquale CP, e Silva PM, Lima MC, *et al.* Suppression by cetirizine of pleurisy triggered by antigen in actively sensitized rats. *Eur J Pharmacol* 1992; **223**: 9–14.

69. Martins MA, Castro-Faria-Neto HC, Bozza PT, *et al.* Role of PAF in the allergic pleurisy caused by ovalbumin in actively sensitized rats. *J Leukoc Biol* 1993; **53**: 104–11.

70. Martins MA, Pasquale CP, e Silva PM, Cordeiro RS, Vargaftig BB. Eosinophil accumulation in the rat pleural cavity after mast cell stimulation with compound 48/80 involves protein synthesis and is selectively suppressed by dexamethasone. *Int Arch Allergy Appl Immunol* 1990; **92**: 416–24.

●71. Viola JPB, Kiani A, Bozza PT, Rao A. Regulation of allergic inflammation and eosinophil recruitment in mice lacking the transcription factor NFAT1: Role of interleukin-4 (IL-4) and IL-5. *Blood* 1998; **91**: 2223–30.

72. Pinho V, Oliveira SH, Souza DG, *et al.* The role of CCL22 (MDC) for the recruitment of eosinophils during allergic pleurisy in mice. *J Leukoc Biol* 2003;**73**: 356–62.

73. Klein A, Talvani A, Silva PMR, *et al.* Stem cell factor-induced leukotriene B4 production cooperates with eotaxin to mediate the recruitment of eosinophils during allergic pleurisy in mice1. *J Immunol* 2001; **167**: 524–31.

74. Kalomenidis I, Guo Y, Peebles RS, *et al.* Pneumothorax-associated pleural eosinophilia in mice is interleukin-5 but not interleukin-13 dependent. *Chest* 2005; **128**: 2978–83.

75. Light RW, Girard WM, Jenkinson SG. The incidence and significance of parapneumonic effusions. *Am J Med* 1980; **69**: 507–12.

76. Strange C, Sahn SA. Management of paraneumonic pleural effusions and empyema. *Infect Dis Clin North Am* 1991; **5**: 539–59.

●77. Sasse SA, Causing LA, Mulligan ME, Light RW. Serial pleural fluid analysis in a new experimental model of empyema. *Chest* 1996; **109**: 1043–48.

78. Sahn SA, Reller LB, Taryle DA, Antony VB, Good JT Jr. The contribution of leukocytes and bacteria to the low pH of empyema fluid. *Am Rev Respir Dis* 1983; **128**: 811–15.

79. Strange C, Allen ML, Harley R, Lazarchick J, Sahn SA. Intrapleural streptokinase in experimental empyema. *Am Rev Respir Dis* 1993; **147**: 962–6.

80. Boyce JM. *Pasteurella multocida*. In: Mandell GL (ed.). *Principles and practice of infectious diseases.* New York: Churchill Livingstone, 1990: 1746–8.

81. Mavroudis C, Gamzel BL, Katzmark S, *et al.* Effect of hemothorax on experimental empyema in the guinea pig. *J Thorac Cardiovasc Surg* 1985; **89**: 42–49.

82. Mavroudis C, Gamzel BL, Cox SK, *et al.* Experimental aerobic-anaerobic thoracic empyema in the guinea pig. *Ann Thorac Surg* 1987; **43**: 298–302.

83. Pfeffer A, Rogers KM, O'Keeffe L, Osborn PJ. Acute phase protein response, food intake, live weight change and lesions following intrathoracic injection of yeast in sheep. *Res Vet Sci* 1993; **55**: 360–6.

84. Sasse SA, Jadus MR, Kukes GD. Pleural fluid transforming growth factor-beta1 correlates with pleural fibrosis in experimental empyema. *Am J Respir Crit Care Med* 2003; **168**: 700–5.

85. Sasse S, Nguyen T, Texeira LR, Light RW. The utility of daily therapeutic thoracentecis for the treatment of early empyema. *Chest* 1999; **116**: 1703–8.

86. Sasse S, Nguyen TK, Mulligan M, *et al.* The effects of early chest tube placement on empyema resolution. *Chest* 1997; **111**: 1679–83.
87. Zhu Z, Hawthorne ML, Guo Y, *et al.* Tissue plasminogen activator combined with human recombinant deoxyribonuclease is effective therapy for empyema in a rabbit model. *Chest* 2006; 129: 1577–83.
88. Strahilevitz J, Lev A, Levi I, Fridman E, Rubinstein E. Experimental pneumococcal pleural empyema model: the effect of moxifloxacin. *J Antimicrob Chemother* 2003; **51**: 665–9.
89. Teixeira LR, Sasse SA, Villarino MA, *et al.* Antibiotic levels in empyemic pleural fluid. *Chest* 2000; **117**: 1734–9.
90. Liapakis IE, Light RW, Pitiakoudis MS, *et al.* Penetration of clarithromycin in experimental pleural empyema model fluid. *Respiration* 2005; **72**: 296–300.
91. Patterson RC. The pleural reaction to innoculation with tubercle bacilli in vaccinated and normal guinea pigs. *Am Rev Tuberc* 1917; **1**: 353–71.
92. Widstrom O, Nillsson BS. Pleurisy induced by intrapleural BCG in immunized guinea pigs. *Eur Respir J* 1982; **63**: 425–34.
93. Widstrom O, Egberg N, Chmielewska J, Blomback M. Fibrinolytic and coagulation mechanisms in stages of inflammation: a study of BCG-induced pleural exudate in guinea pig. *Thromb Res* 1983; **29**: 511–19.
●94. Phalen SW, McMurray DN. T-lymphocyte response in a guinea pig model of tuberculous pleuritis. *Infect Immun* 1993; **61**: 142–5.
95. Antony VB, Repine JE, Harada RN, Good JT Jr, Sahn SA. Inflammatory responses in experimental tuberculosis pleurisy. *Acta Cytol* 1983; **27**: 355–61.
●96. Antony VB, Sahn SA, Antony AC, Repine JE. Bacillus Calmette-Guerin-stimulated neutrophils release chemotaxins for monocytes in rabbit pleural spaces and *in vitro*. *J Clin Invest* 1985; **76**: 1514–21.
97. Moura AC, Leonardo PS, Henriques MG, Cordeiro RS. Opposite effects of M. leprae or M. bovis BCG delipidation on cellular accumulation into mouse pleural cavity. Distinct accomplishment of mycobacterial lipids *in vivo*. *Inflamm Res* 1999; **48**: 308–13.
98. Menezes-de-Lima-Junior O, Werneck-Barroso E, Cordeiro RS, Henriques MG. Effects of inhibitors of inflammatory mediators and cytokines on eosinophil and neutrophil accumulation induced by *Mycobacterium bovis* bacillus Calmette-Guerin in mouse pleurisy. *J Leukoc Biol* 1997; **62**: 778–85.
●99. Allen SS, McMurray DN. Coordinate cytokine gene expression in vivo following induction of tuberculous pleurisy in guinea pigs. *Infect Immun* 2003; **71**: 4271–7.
●100. Allen SS, Cassone L, Lasco TM, McMurray DN. Effect of neutralizing transforming growth factor β1 on the immune response against *Mycobacterium tuberculosis* in guinea pigs. *Infect Immun* 2004; **72**: 1358–63.
♦101. Lee YCG, De Klerk NH, Henderson DW, Musk AW. Malignant mesothelioma. In: Hendrick DJ, Burge PS, Beckett WS, Churg A (eds). *Occupational disorders of the lung. Recognition, management and prevention.* London, UK: W B Saunders & Co., 2002: 359–379.
102. Chapman SJ, Cookson WO, Musk AW, Lee YC. Benign asbestos pleural diseases. *Curr Opin Pulm Med* 2003; **9**: 266–71.
103. Stathopoulos GT, Karamessini M, Sotiriadi AE, Pastromas VG. Rounded atelectasis of the lung. *Respir Med* 2005; **99**: 615–23.
●104. Marchi E, Liu W, Broaddus VC. Mesothelial cell apoptosis is confirmed in vivo by morphological change in cytokeratin distribution. *Am J Physiol Lung Cell Mol Physiol* 2000; **278**: L528–35.
●105. Boylan AM, Ruegg C, Kim KJ, *et al.* Evidence of a role for mesothelial cell-derived interleukin-8 in the pathogenesis of asbestos-induced pleurisy in rabbits. *J Clin Invest* 1992; **89**: 1257–67.
106. Adamson IYR, Bakowska J, Bowden DH. Mesothelial cell proliferation after instillation of long or short asbestos fibers into mouse lung. *Am J Pathol* 1993; **142**: 1209–16.
107. Dodson RF, Atkinson MAL, Levin JL. Asbestos fiber length as related to potential pathogenicity: a critical review. *Am J Ind Med* 2003; **44**: 291–7.
108. Dodson RF, Ford JO. Early response of the visceral pleura following asbestos exposure: an ultrastructural study. *J Toxicol Environ Health* 1985; **15**: 673–86.
109. Viallat JR, Raybuad F, Passarel M, Boutin C. Pleural migration of chrysotile fibers after intratracheal injection in rats. *Arch Environ Health* 1986; **41**: 282–6.
110. Fasske E. Pathogenesis of pulmonary fibrosis induced by chrysotile asbestos. Longitudinal light and electron microscopic studies on the rat model. *Virchows Arch A Pathol Anat Histopathol* 1986; **408**: 329–46.
111. Coin PG, Osornio-Vargas AR, Roggli VL, Brody AR. Pulmonary fibrogenesis after three consecutive inhalation exposures to chrysotile asbestos. *Am J Respir Crit Care Med* 1996; **154**: 1511–19.
112. McConnell EE, Axten C, Hesterberg TW, *et al.* Studies on the inhalation toxicology of two fiberglasses and amosite asbestos in the Syrian golden hamster. Part II. Results of chronic exposure. *Inhal Toxicol* 1999; **11**: 785–835.
●113. Tanaka S, Choe N, Hemenway DR, *et al.* Asbestos inhalation induces reactive nitrogen species and nitrotyrosine formation in the lungs and pleura of the rat. *J Clin Invest* 1998; **102**: 445–54.
114. Bozelka BE, Sestini P, Gaumer HR, *et al.* A murine model of asbestosis. *Am J Pathol* 1983; **112**: 326–37.
115. Fasske E. Experimental lung tumors following specific intrabronchial application of chrysotile asbestos. Longitudinal light and electron microscopic investigations in rats. *Respiration* 1988; **53**: 111–27.
116. Humphrey EW, Ewing SL, Wrigley JV, *et al.* The production of malignant tumors of the lung and pleura in dogs from intratracheal asbestos instillation and cigarette smoking. *Cancer* 1981; **47**: 1994–9.
117. Wagner JC, Berry G, Skidmore JW, Pooley FD. The comparative effects of three chrysotiles by injection and inhalation in rats. *IARC Sci Publ* 1980; **30**: 362–72.
♦118. Maxim LD, McConnell EE. Interspecies comparisons of the toxicity of asbestos and synthetic vitreous fibers: A weight-of-the-evidence approach. *Regul Toxicol Pharmacol* 2001; **33**: 319–42.
119. Brass DM, Hoyle GW, Poovey HG, Liu J-Y, Brody AR. Reduced tumor necrosis factor-a and transforming growth factor-b1 expression in the lungs of inbred mice that fail to develop fibroproliferative lesions consequent to asbestos exposure. *Am J Pathol* 1999; **154**: 853–62.
120. National Research Council. In: Council NR (ed.). *Review of the US Navy's exposure standard for manufactured vitreous fibers.* Washington DC: National Academies Press, 2000: 1–63.
121. Warheit D, Hartsky MA. Influence of gender, species and strain differences in pulmonary toxicological assessments of inhaled particles and/or fibers. In: Mohr U, Dungworth DL, Mauderly JL, Oberdorster G (eds). *Toxic and carcinogenic effects of solid particles in the respiratory tract.* Washington DC: ILSI Press, 1994.
122. Adamson IYR, Bowden DH. Response of mouse lung to crocidolite asbestos. 1. Minimal fibrotic reaction to short fibres. *J Pathol* 1987; **152**: 99–107.
123. Adamson IYR, Bowden DH. Response of mouse lung to crocidolite asbestos. 2. Pulmonary fibrosis after long fibres. *J Pathol* 1987; **152**: 109–17.
124. Hesterberg TW, Axten C, McConnell EE, *et al.* Studies on the inhalation toxicology of two fiberglasses and amosite asbestos in the syrian golden hamster. Part I. Results of a subchronic study and dose selection for a chronic study. *Inhal Toxicol* 1999; **11**: 747–84.
125. Voss B, Kerenyi T, Muller KM, Wilhelm M. Scanning electron microscopical investigations of broncho-alveolar casts after intratracheal asbestos fibre instillation. *Int J Hyg Environ Health* 2000; **203**: 127–34.

126. Choe N, Tanaka S, Xia W, *et al.* Pleural macrophage recruitment and activation in asbestos-induced pleural injury. *Environ Health Perspect* 1997; **105** (Suppl 5): 1257–60.
127. Oberdoerster G, Ferin J, Marcello NL, Meinhold SH. Effect of intrabronchially instilled amosite on lavagable lung and pleural cells. *Environ Health Perspect* 1983; **51**: 41–8.
●128. Zanella CL, Posada J, Tritton TR, Mossman BT. Asbestos causes stimulation of the extracellular signal-related kinase 1 mitogen-activated protein kinase cascade after phosphorylation of the epidermal growth factor receptor. *Cancer Res* 1996; **56**: 5334–8.
129. Robledo RF, Buder-Hoffman SA, Cummins AB, *et al.* Increased phosphorylated extracellular signal-regulated kinase immunoreactivity associated with proliferative and morphologic lung alterations after chrysotile asbestos inhalation in mice. *Am J Pathol* 2000; **156**: 1307–16.
130. Adamson IYR, Prieditis H, Young L. Lung mesothelial cell and fibroblast responses to pleural and alveolar macrophage supernatants and to lavage fluids from crocidolite-exposed rats. *Am J Respir Cell Mol Biol* 1997; **16**: 650–6.
131. Liu J-Y, Brass DM, Hoyle GW, Brody AR. TNF-a receptor knockout mice are protected from the fibroproliferative effects of inhaled asbestos fibers. *Am J Pathol* 1998; **153**: 1839–47.
●132. Shore BL, Daughaday CC, Spilberg I. Benign asbestos pleurisy in the rabbit. A model for the study of pathogenesis. *Am Rev Respir Dis* 1983; **128**: 481–5.
133. Markham KM, Glover JL, Welsh RJ, Lucas RJ, Bendick PJ. Octreotide in the treatment of thoracic duct injuries. *Am Surg* 2000; **66**: 1165–7.
●134. Huang XZ, Wu JF, Ferrando R, *et al.* Fatal bilateral chylothorax in mice lacking the integrin a9b1. *Mol Cell Biol* 2000; **20**: 5208–15.
135. Vlahakis NE, Young BA, Atakilit A, Sheppard D. The lymphangiogenic vascular endothelial growth factors VEGF-C and -D are ligands for the integrin $\alpha 9\beta 1$. *J Biol Chem* 2005; **280**: 4544–52.
136. Maulitz R, Good JT, Kaplan RL, Reller LB, Sahn SA. The pleuropulmonary consequences of esophageal rupture: An experimental model. *Am Rev Respir Dis* 1979; **120**: 363–7.
137. Good JTJ, Antony VB, Reller B, Maulitz R, Sahn SA. The pathogenesis of the low pleural fluid pH in esophageal rupture. *Am Rev Respir Dis* 1983; **127**: 702–4.
●138. Wiener-Kronish JP, Broaddus VC, Albertine KH, *et al.* Relationship of pleural effusions to increased permeability pulmonary edema in anesthetized sheep. *J Clin Invest* 1988; **82**: 1422–9.
●139. Song Y, Yang B, Matthay MA, Ma T, Verkman AS. Role of aquaporin water channels in pleural fluid dynamics. *Am J Physiol Cell Physiol* 2000; **279**: C1744–50.
●140. Broaddus VC, Wiener-Kronish JP, Staub NC. Clearance of lung edema into the pleural space of volume-loaded anesthetized sheep. *J Appl Physiol* 1990; **68**: 2623–30.
141. Kinasewitz GT, Groome LJ, Marshall RP, Leslie WK, Diana JN. Effect of hypoxia on permeability of pulmonary endothelium of canine visceral pleura. *J Appl Physiol* 1986; **61**: 554–60.
142. Ashino Y, Tanita T, Ono S, *et al.* Roles of the visceral pleura in the production of pleural effusion in permeability pulmonary edema. *Tohoku J Exp Med* 1997; **182**: 283–96.
143. Broaddus VC, Wiener-Kronish JP, Berthiauma Y, Staub NC. Removal of pleural liquid and protein by lymphatics in awake sheep. *J Appl Physiol* 1988; **64**: 384–90.
144. Agostoni E, Zocchi L. Solute-coupled liquid absorption from the pleural space. *Respir Physiol* 1990; **81**: 19–27.
145. Nakamura T, Tanaka Y, Fukabori T, *et al.* The role of lymphatics in removing pleural liquid in discrete hydrothorax. *Eur Respir J* 1988; **1**: 826–31.
146. Broaddus VC, Araya M. Liquid and protein dynamics using a new minimally invasive pleural catheter in rabbits. *J Appl Physiol* 1992; **72**: 851–7.
147. Wang PM, Lai-Fook SJ. Effect of mechanical ventilation on regional variation of pleural liquid thickness in rabbits. *Lung* 1997; **175**: 165–73.
148. Stashenko GJ, Robichaux A, Lee YCG, *et al.* Pleural fluid exchange in rabbits. *Respirol*, in press.
149. Nishida O, Arellano R, Cheng DC, DeMajo W, Kavanagh BP. Gas exchange and hemodynamics in experimental pleural effusion. *Crit Care Med* 1999; **27**: 583–7.
150. Sousa AS, Moll RJ, Pontes CF, Saldiva PH, Zin WA. Mechanical and morphometrical changes in progressive bilateral pneumothorax and pleural effusion in normal rats. *Eur Respir J* 1995; **8**: 99–104.
151. Dechman G, Sato J, Bates JH. Effect of pleural effusion on respiratory mechanics, and the influence of deep inflation, in dogs. *Eur Respir J* 1993; **6**: 219–24.
152. Rush JE, Hamlin RL. Effects of graded pleural effusion on QRS in the dog. *Am J Vet Res* 1985; **46**: 1887–91.
153. Murphy DJ, Renninger JP, Gossett KA. A novel method for chronic measurement of pleural pressure in conscious rats. *J Pharmacol Toxicol Methods* 1998; **39**: 137–41.
154. Wilkinson PD, Keegan J, Davies SW, Bailey J, Rudd RM. Changes in pulmonary microvascular permeability accompanying re-expansion oedema: evidence from dual isotope scintigraphy. *Thorax* 1990; **45**: 456–9.
●155. Clauss M, Sunderkoetter C, Sveinbjoernsson B, *et al.* A permissive role for tumor necrosis factor in vascular endothelial growth factor–induced vascular permeability. Blood 2001; **97**: 1321–9.
156. Zebrowski BK, Yano S, Liu W, *et al.* Vascular endothelial growth factor levels and induction of permeability in malignant pleural effusions. *Clin Cancer Res* 1999; **5**: 3364–8.
157. Faurschou P, Grunnet N, Winding O, Dirksen A, Faarup P. Rheumatoid arthritis cells and biological changes in turpentine-induced pleuritis in rabbits. *APMIS* 1989; **97**: 413–18.
158. Devin CJ, Lee YCG, Light RW, Lane KB. Pleural space as a site of ectopic gene delivery: Transfection of pleural mesothelial cells with systemic distribution of gene product. *Chest* 2003; **123**: 202–8.
159. Katano K, Tsujitani S, Saito H, *et al.* Hypotonic intrapleural cisplatin chemotherapy as treatment for pleural carcinomatosis in an experimental model. *Anticancer Res* 1997; **17**: 4547–52.
160. Rosenfeldt FL, Glover JR, Marossy D. Systemic absorption of noxythiolin from the pleural cavity in man and in the rabbit. *Thorax* 1981; **36**: 278–81.
●161. Antony VB, Owen CL, Hadley KJ. Pleural mesothelial cells stimulated by asbestos release chemotactic activity for neutrophils in vitro. *Am Rev Respir Dis* 1989; **139**: 199–206.
162. Fjellbirkeland L, Bjerkvig R, Steinsvag SK, Laerum OD. Nonadhesive stationary organ culture of human bronchial mucosa. *Am J Respir Cell Mol Biol* 1996; **15**: 197–206.
●163. Kim K-U, Wilson SM, Abayasiriwardana KS, *et al.* A novel *in vitro* model of human mesothelioma for studying tumor biology and apoptotic resistance. *Am J Respir Cell Mol Biol* 2005; **33**: 541–8.
164. Zarogiannis S, Hatzoglou C, Stefanidis I, *et al.* Adrenergic influence on the permeability of sheep diaphragmatic parietal pleura. *Respiration* 2007; **74**: 118–20.
165. Zarogiannis S, Hatzoglou C, Stefanidis I, *et al.* Effect of adrenaline on transmesothelial resistance of isolated sheep pleura. *Respir Physiol Neurobiol* 2006; **150**: 165–72.
166. Vogiatzidis K, Hatzoglou C, Zarogiannis S, *et al.* mu-Opioid influence on transmesothelial resistance of isolated sheep pleura and parietal pericardium. Eur J Pharmacol 2006; **530**: 276–80.
167. Berkenkopf JW, Weichman BM. Comparison of several new 5-lipoxygenase inhibitors in a rat Arthus pleurisy model. *Eur J Pharmacol* 1991; **193**: 29–34.
168. Utsunomiya I, Ito M, Oh-ishi S. Generation of inflammatory cytokines in zymosan-induced pleurisy in rats: TNF induces IL-6 and cytokine-induced neutrophil chemoattractant (CINC) *in vivo*. *Cytokine* 1998; **10**: 956–63.
169. Hanada S, Oga S, Hirano MT. Some characteristics of econazole-induced pleurisy in rats. *Gen Pharmacol* 1985; **16**: 637–40.

170. Saleh TS, Calixto JB, Medeiros YS. Pro-inflammatory effects induced by bradykinin in a murine model of pleurisy. *Eur J Pharmacol* 1997; **331**: 43–52.
171. Perianin A, Roch-Arveiller M, Giroud JP, Hakim J. *In vivo* interaction of nonsteroidal anti-inflammatory drugs on the locomotion of neutrophils elicited by acute non-specific inflammations in the rat – effect of indomethacin, ibuprofen and flurbiprofen. *Biochem Pharmacol* 1984; **33**: 2239–43.
172. Wang JP, Ho TF, Lin CN, Teng CM. Effect of norathyriol, isolated from *Tripterospermum lanceolatum*, on A23187-induced pleurisy and analgesia in mice. *Naunyn Schmiedebergs Arch Pharmacol* 1994; **350**: 90–5.
173. Kawamura K, Oh-ishi S. Rat pleurisy induced by kaolin or croton oil: time course of fluid accumulation and white cell migration. *Int J Tissue React* 1985; **7**: 381–6.
174. Oh-ishi S, Hayashi I, Hayashi M, Yamaki K, Utsunomiya I. Pharmacological demonstration of inflammatory mediators using experimental inflammatory models: rat pleurisy induced by carrageenan and phorbol myristate acetate. *Dermatologica* 1989; **179** (Suppl 1): 68–71.
175. Tarayre JP, Delhon A, Bruniquel F, *et al.* Exudative, cellular and humoral reactions to platelet-activating factor (PAF-acether) in the pleural cavity of rats. *Eur J Pharmacol* 1986; **124**: 317–23.
176. Frode-Saleh TS, Calixto JB, Medeiros YS. Analysis of the inflammatory response induced by substance P in the mouse pleurisy model. *Peptides* 1999; **20**: 259–65.

APPENDIX 14.1: RABBIT CHEST TUBE INSERTION[22]

1 New Zealand white rabbits (>1.5 kg) are anesthetized with an intramuscular injection of ketamine hydrochloride (35 mg/kg) and xylazine hydrochloride (5 mg/kg). The chest is shaven and the skin sterilized with 10 percent povidone iodine.*
2 The rabbit is placed in the lateral decubitus position and a small (<3 cm) skin incision is made midway between the tip of the scapula and the sternum approximately 2 cm above the costal margin. Chest tubes are made from intravenous solution set tubes with three extra openings near the distal end of the tube to enhance drainage.
3 The chest tube is inserted by blunt dissection into the right pleural cavity and secured at the muscle layers with purse-string sutures (3.0 ethilon). The proximal end of the chest tube is then tunneled underneath the skin and drawn out through the skin posteriorly and superiorly between the two scapulae. The exterior end of the chest tube is sealed with a one-way valve with cap via an adapter and sutured to the skin using a 2.0 silk suture.

* An alternative method of pleural catheter placement has been described by Broaddus *et* al.[65] Rabbits were anesthetized with halothane and ventilated via tracheotomy. The upper abdomen was opened and the diaphragm was punctured through which a fine catheter was passed into the pleural space, and secured with sutures. This method is more invasive but is effective and can avoid any potential lung trauma from blunt dissection into the pleura.

4 A three-way stopcock is attached to the end of the chest tube through which any aspirated air is immediately evacuated from the pleural space.
5 Reagents can be administered intrapleurally via the chest tube, followed by the instillation of 1.0 mL of 0.9 percent sodium chloride solution or sterile phosphate-buffered saline (PBS) to clear the dead space.
6 The chest tubes can be aspirated for pleural fluid. Alternatively, pleural lavage can be performed by the administration of 5–10 mL of sterile PBS via the chest tube. The rabbit is then rotated and the PBS aspirated back from the chest tube.
7 The chest tube should be removed under light sedation as soon as it is no longer required in order to minimize risks of infection and discomfort.
8 At time of sacrifice, the rabbits are sedated and killed with carbon dioxide. The thorax is removed *en bloc*. The lungs are expanded by the injection of 50 mL of 10 percent neutral-buffered formalin into the exposed trachea via a plastic catheter. The trachea is then ligated and the entire thorax submerged in 10 percent neutral-buffered formalin solution for at least 48 hours.

APPENDIX 14.2: SHEEP PLEURODESIS MODEL[28]

1 Yearling sheep of mixed breeds can be anesthetized with an intravenous injection of 2.5 percent sodium thiopental at 20 mg/kg.
2 The chest should be shaven and the skin sterilized with 2 percent chlorhexidine and then with 10 percent povidone iodine.
3 Using a laryngoscope, an endotracheal tube (8.5 mm internal diameter) is inserted with an attached plastic 'bite block' and secured with tape. Anesthesia is maintained with a gaseous mixture of room air, oxygen, and 1.5–2.5 percent halothane at a ventilation rate of 10 breath cycles/minute with a volume of 15 mL/kg per breath cycle. The sheep is placed on its side on a surgical table and the feet secured to the table.
4 A 5 cm incision is made in the lateral chest wall at the 7th intercostal space. By blunt dissection, an 18G French Foley ballooned-catheter with 30 mL balloon volume is inserted into the pleural space under aseptic conditions, tunneled underneath the skin and brought to the surface just lateral to the vertebrae. The tube is secured at the skin with purse-string sutures.
5 The sheep is then ventilated with a positive end expiratory pressure of 15 cmH_2O. A three-way stopcock is attached to the end of the Foley catheter through which all air is evacuated from the pleural space immediately after the chest tube insertion.
6 Intrapleural injection of agents can be made via the chest tube. The buffer or vehicle can be injected to the contralateral side and serve as the control.

7 The chest tube is aspirated (with the Foley catheter balloon inflated) regularly for any pleural fluid produced. To minimize discomfort and risk of infection, we recommend that the chest tubes be removed as soon as no further intrapleural injections or pleural sample collections is needed.

For pleural fibrosis/pleurodesis studies, the sheep are killed 14 days after the chest tube insertion with an intravenous injection of sodium phenobarbital solution.

APPENDIX 14.3: METHODS FOR HARVESTING RABBIT AND MICE MESOTHELIAL CELLS[22,161]

1 Pleural mesothelial cells are obtained from mice of adult size or from New Zealand white rabbits (commonly 2 kg).
2 After the animals are killed, the abdomen is opened to expose the diaphragm. Hank's Balanced Salt Solution (HBSS) is injected into the pleural cavity from beneath the hemi-diaphragms under direct vision and then aspirated out after 2 minutes. This is to remove surface proteolytic enzymes to allow greater efficacy of trypsin (see below). In mice, there is no mediastinal separation and a single injection of 1mL of HBSS is sufficient to rinse the pleural surface in the left and right chest.* In rabbits, 10 mL is injected into *each* pleural cavity.
3 Trypsin-EDTA (ethylenediamine tetraacetic acid) (0.25 percent) is injected into the pleural cavity and left *in situ* for 10 minutes during which the animal should be rotated. The solution, with the mesothelial cells, is then aspirated and put into fetal calf serum (FCS) or culture media (e.g. DMEM [Dulbecco's modified Eagles medium] with 10 percent FCS) on ice. The serum contains tryptase that will terminate the action of, and any potential damage from, the injected trypsin. An injectate volume of 1 mL is used in mice, and 10 mL (for each side) in rabbits.
4 The FCS is centrifuged at 1000 rpm for 5 minutes. The cell pellet is washed and resuspended in DMEM with 1 percent (v/v) L-glutamine, 1 percent (v/v) penicillin–streptomycin and 10 percent (v/v) FCS.
5 The cells can be plated in standard cell culture flasks, and incubated at 37°C with 95 percent of air and 5 percent of CO_2. Initial cell population will consist of a large number of erythrocytes and leukocytes as well as the mesothelial cells.
6 The media should be changed after overnight incubation. Mesothelial cells should adhere to the culture flasks, and contaminating cells can usually be removed with the media.
7 The cells can be stained for mesothelial markers to confirm the epithelial origin of the cells. Fibroblasts that may have adhered to the culture flasks are cytokeratin negative. Most investigators are able to achieve a 95 percent purity of mesothelial cells using this technique.

* In our experience, very fine needles (28G) should be used in mice pleural injections.

15

Experimental models: mesothelioma

DELIA NELSON, BRUCE WS ROBINSON

REASONS FOR ESTABLISHING MODELS OF MALIGNANT MESOTHELIOMA

Malignant mesothelioma (MM) is often diagnosed late in disease progression and, at this stage, is associated with a rapid decline in health and death within a short period of time; the average period of survival being 9 months post-diagnosis. Additionally, in the absence of reliable specific tumor markers that could be utilized for early diagnosis, MM will remain undetectable until characteristic clinical symptoms manifest, which then require rigorous histopathological confirmation of disease. As a result, the tumor cell biology, as well as the specific and non-specific immune responses to MM, are difficult to monitor in humans. Hence, experimental models of MM remain the only option available to facilitate a deeper understanding of (i) how this cancer progresses *in vivo*, (ii) how the immune system is responding, and (iii) how we can alter tumor growth with varying single and combination therapies. This chapter will explore the experimental approaches that have been, or are being, undertaken to address features of MM development. These approaches are divided into models that utilize human-derived MM tumor cells, and environmentally (asbestos or glass fibers and/or *Simian virus 40* [SV40]) induced animal MM tumor systems. Examples of the experimental models used and their outcomes are discussed.

HUMAN MALIGNANT MESOTHELIOMA AS EXPERIMENTAL MODELS

Generating cell lines from human MM primary tumors

Examination of samples of excised tumors reveals useful information, however this approach is limited to a few technologies such as histopathology, although microarray analysis is now providing additional important data. Therefore, to gain further insights, cell lines that have been generated from human tumors and prepared as single-cell suspensions, cloned and their phenotypes, soluble factor secretion and responses to numerous agents including chemotherapeutics and gene transfer vectors, have been studied in detail. Much of this work has provided the basis of clinical trials and is the foundation for animal experimental models that are discussed in detail below.

Identifying the cellular effects of asbestos injury and modeling the transformation process

In 1960, Wagner *et al.*[1] reported an association between asbestos and both pleural and peritoneal malignant mesothelioma in a case series from the North Western Cape Province of South Africa where blue asbestos (crocidolite) was mined. Since then, many reports from all parts of the world have confirmed the relationship between exposure to asbestos and the development of MM. Once epidemiological studies had identified a clear association between asbestos fibers and the subsequent development of MM in humans, a number of studies were undertaken to examine the effects that exposure to asbestos fibers has on cell types located within the site 'injured' by these fibrous particles; i.e. serosal tissue consisting of a surface mesothelial layer and subsurface spindled connective tissue cells. Mesothelial cells were shown to be inherently susceptible to asbestos fibers; they are actively phagocytic in culture and ingest asbestos fibers.[2] Mesothelial cells are up to 10 times more susceptible than bronchial epithelial cells to the direct cytotoxic effects of asbestos fibers.[3] However, *in vitro* responses were different depending on fiber types (chrysotile versus amphiboles) as well as the chemical state of these fibers.[4,5]

The presence of asbestos fibers leads to the formation of reactive oxygen metabolites which are directly toxic causing DNA point mutations, as well as strand and chromosomal breaks in mesothelial cells.[6] These abnormalities usually result in cellular apoptosis. However, particular mutations in combination with direct mitotic damage[7] and increased cell division may result in cell survival, despite their profound genetic abnormalities, thereby increasing the risk of neoplastic transformation. Studies exposing fibroblasts to chrysotile fibers demonstrated distinctive morphological changes within the first 12 hours of exposure. Continued serial passage was associated with further changes, including increasing cell size and loss of control of directional growth, indicating the beginning of transformation.[4]

Understanding the molecular changes of mesothelial cells as they differentiate into MM is a topic of ongoing research. These include studies demonstrating that asbestos-transformed cells expressed transforming growth factor (TGF)-α transcripts, whilst spontaneously transformed cells do not. In addition, TGF-α inhibited only the growth of spontaneously transformed mesothelial cells, indicating that TGF-α acts as an autocrine growth factor for asbestos-transformed rat mesothelial cells.[8] Similarly, we have demonstrated clear inhibition of MM cell growth using antisense oligonucleotides which block TGF-β and platelet-derived growth factor (PDGF)-A chain, indicating key roles for these factors in MM proliferation.[9,10] Differences in mesothelioma etiology may be reflected in differences in the molecular alterations present in these tumors.[8] Others have recently shown that proteoglycan (PG) expression is closely associated with the morphology and biological behavior of tumor cells, and that MM has a different PG profile from epithelial tumors.[11]

The role of Simian virus in the development of MM

The transformation process may not be as simple as a direct relationship between asbestos fiber exposure and mesothelial cells. Many humans were accidentally exposed to this small double-stranded DNA monkey virus via contaminated polio vaccines (produced in monkey cells) in the 1950s and 1960s. SV40 DNA sequences have been found in a defined group of human cancers, of which MM has been reported to have the highest frequency of detection;[12–14] although the latter is currently the subject of controversy.

The biology of SV40 has been well studied. Following infection of a host cell, SV40 expresses two proteins, small t (transforming) antigen (tag) and large T antigen (TAg), which interact with host cell proteins to cause cell proliferation and DNA replication and hence the production of more viral particles. Tag is the replicase of SV40 and its expression can lead to cellular transformation, principally through inhibition of cellular p53 and retinoblastoma (Rb) family proteins.[15] SV40 infects cells from different species: it causes lytic infection in the cells of its natural primate host where it does not induce tumors. In contrast, it is non-lytic and highly oncogenic in rodents.[16] Crucially, infection is semi-permissive in human cell lines and, in some reports, up to 60 percent of human mesotheliomas contain SV40 DNA.[14,17] According to microdissection experiments, SV40 is present in the malignant cells and sometimes in reactive mesothelial cells but not in normal adjacent tissues; neither is it found in lung cancers.[18,19] It should be noted that although many different laboratories have reported the presence of SV40 in human MM and other cancers, there is still uncertainty over the prevalence of SV40 in mesothelioma. The most common method used to detect SV40 sequences has been by polymerase chain reaction (PCR). The potential risk of false positives from contamination by the SV40 DNA contained in commonly used laboratory plasmids led to a lack of confidence in the data. However, SV40 has been detected using other technical approaches and strains of SV40 never used in laboratories have been rescued from human biopsies. Nonetheless, this issue remains controversial.

Fibroblasts are transformed by SV40 at a low rate, whereas mesothelial cells are uniformly infected, but not lysed, leading to a high rate of transformation and immortalization.[20] Crocidolite asbestos increases the rate of transformation, though the increment is not huge, perhaps suggesting that asbestos and SV40 may be co-carcinogens. It is feasible that asbestos has a more profound effect *in vivo* because it is immunosuppressive, or because it causes the production of mutagenic free radicals from activated macrophages. Taken together, these results suggest that mesothelial cells might be unusually susceptible to SV40 infection and transformation. Why this is so and how the infected cells interact with asbestos is not fully understood.

Hahn and colleagues[21] have shown that epithelial cells can be transformed and become tumorigenic upon combined transfection with TAg, H-ras and the catalytic subunit of telomerase. Given the fact that SV40 TAg inhibits both Rb and p53 proteins, they suggested that a minimum of four distinct signaling pathways need to be affected to transform normal human cells. It would not be surprising then if SV40-infected mesothelial cells still need a strong proliferation-driving signal such as H-ras for tumorigenicity; mutations of ras are not a feature of mesotheliomas, but the pathway is functional.

It should be noted that epidemiological studies have been unable to link increased incidence of mesothelioma or other cancers with the contaminated vaccines; nonetheless, concern has been raised that vaccinated people worldwide may have been inadvertently exposed to an oncogenic virus. A thorough assessment of all the relevant epidemiological data was investigated by the Institute of Medicine; they concluded that the current evidence was insufficient and inadequate to accept or reject a direct causal relationship between SV40-containing vaccines and cancer.

To develop a useful model and explore the role of SV40 one approach was to transfect normal human mesothelial cells with a plasmid containing SV40 early region DNA, and select cells for their longevity; i.e. passaged continuously for more than 2 years.[12] These cells expressed SV40 large T antigen, exhibited features of mesothelial cells, including sensitivity to the cytotoxic effects of asbestos fibers, but failed to develop into tumors when injected subcutaneously or intraperitoneally into nude mice, suggesting that other co-factors (such as asbestos fibers) were a prerequisite for malignancy to develop. Thus, these cells may represent an ideal model to assess the role of SV40 as an MM co-factor. More recently, SV40 transgenic animal models have been developed and are discussed below.

ANIMAL MALIGNANT MESOTHELIOMA MODELS

Faithful animal models (experimentally reproducing the human disease) remain necessary to study the natural history of MM, and to test standard or novel treatments.

Using human tumors in animals

Experimental models were often constructed by inoculating human tumors into immunologically deficient mice, such as the athymic bald mouse (nude mouse) or severe combined immunologically deficient (SCID) mice to avoid immunological rejection. These murine models often employ subcutaneous injection of cloned human MM cells, or subcutaneous implantation of tumor fragments, as well as pleural implantation of intact human tumors; the latter attempting to more closely conserve the biological characteristics of the original tumor. Examples include studies such as those undertaken by Chahinian *et al.*[22] and Reale *et al.*[23] who transplanted human pleural MM from patients into nude mice. Tumors grew as a solid neoplastic mass. Light and electron microscopy, as well as immunocytochemistry, demonstrated a similarity of the transplanted solid and fluid malignancies with the human primary MM. Both groups concluded that their models mimicked the clinical behavior of human MM.

Uncontrolled environmentally induced animal models

Animals share man's domicile environment, yet do not indulge in activities (e.g. smoking and working environments) which confound interpretation of epidemiological studies. Glickman *et al.*[24] used pet dogs with spontaneous (histologically confirmed) MM to identify environmental exposures that might increase their owner's risk of asbestos-related disease. An asbestos-related occupation, or hobby, of a household member and use of flea repellents on the dog were significantly associated with MM. In addition, there was an increased risk of MM within an urban residence. Lung tissue from dogs with MM had higher levels of chrysotile asbestos fibers than lung tissue from control dogs. The authors argued that these findings suggest that well-designed epidemiological studies of spontaneous tumors in pet animals may provide insight into the role of environmental factors in human cancers and serve as a valuable sentinel model to identify environmental health hazards for humans

Controlled environmentally induced tumors

A number of studies have examined the effects exposure to asbestos fibers has in animal models. As early as 1969, rats were inoculated with asbestos fibers and the incidence of MM determined.[25] Detailed studies of pulmonary deposition, biodurability, biopersistence and carcinogenicity after asbestos fiber inhalation in rats, mice and hamsters were conducted.[26–29] Animals were examined for the presence of benign and malignant lung tumors and MM. The MM tumors usually occurred at intervals between 12 and 31 months after asbestos exposure. Whilst these models confirmed a direct association between inhalation of asbestos fibers and MM, some concern has been expressed that rodent inhalation models may not be sensitive enough to predict the cancer risk posed by varying fiber types for humans.

Hesterberg *et al.*[30] exposed hamsters and rats to a range of man-made fibers and confirmed that exposure to crocidolite or chrysotile asbestos induced pulmonary fibrosis, lung tumors and MM in rats. Interestingly, however, they also demonstrated that exposure to refractory ceramic fibers (RCF) resulted in significant increases in lung tumors and MM. In contrast, inhalation of fiber-glass (MMVF [man-made vitreous fiber] 10 or 11), slag wool (MMVF 22) and rock wool (stone wool: MMVF 21) was not associated with MM. These studies support the argument that chemical composition and the surface physicochemical properties of the fibers may play an important role in MM development.[4,5,31]

Kucharczuk *et al.*[32] established a pleural-based model of MM in immune-competent Fischer rats. This was achieved by placing a syngeneic MM cell line (II-45) into the pleural cavity via a modified left anterior lateral thorocotomy. Pleural MM that closely resembles the human disease was seen with animals dying within 1 month. However, this is an invasive and labor-intensive model and is restricted in its experimental applicability. An alternative approach involved exposing rat pleural mesothelial cells to chrysotile fibers *in vitro*, and then prior to their transformation into MM, transplanting them into nude mice.[33] Interestingly, tumors arose even from untreated rat mesothelial cells, but the delay between cell injection and tumor formation was 22 weeks, whereas only 2 weeks were needed with asbestos-treated cells.

Similar studies have been conducted in rodents using the intraperitoneal route to inject asbestos and other fibers. The intraperitoneal model may be more sensitive for testing the carcinogenicity of inorganic fibers than the inhalation model.[31] Murine MM tumor cell lines have been established after intraperitoneal inoculation of asbestos fibers into the major strains of mice, including CBA, BALB/c and C57BL/6, and are diagnostically similar to human MM tumors.[31,34–36] Similar to human mesothelial cells, growth of the murine MM cell lines can be stimulated by epidermal growth factor.[36] Upon subcutaneous injection of these murine MM cell lines into mice, solid tumors form and grow rapidly. There is minimal lymphocytic infiltration and the most prominent infiltrating leukocyte is the macrophage that makes up 50 percent of the tumor mass. These murine models allow evaluation of different aspects of immune responsiveness and biological diversity (due to genetic or strain differences) and are the basis for experimental models designed to answer specific questions (discussed below) (Table 15.1).

SV40 MODELS

The role of SV40 in the development of mesotheliomas has been explored in animal models in a variety of ways and SV40 alone induces mesotheliomas in hamsters. However, we recently used the mesothelin promoter to construct four mouse lines that express SV40 TAg in mesothelial cells at different levels.[37] All of these mice show a relatively

Table 15.1 Comparison of human and murine malignant mesothelioma (MM)

	Human MM	Murine MM
Asbestos induced	+	+
Variable latency	+	+
Effusion	+	+
Histology:		
Epithelial	+	+
Sarcomatous	+	+
Mixed	+	+
Ultrastructure:		
Microvilli	+	+
Glycogen granules	+	+
Tight junctions	+	+
Growth in culture	± (approx. 12%)	+ (86%)
Variable morphology in culture	+	+
MHC surface expression:		
Class I	+	±
Class II	–	–
Tumorigenicity	± (nude mice)	+ (syngeneic mice)
Tumor suppressor expression:		
p53	+	+
Soluble factor secretion:		
TGF-β	+	+
VEGF	+	+
PDGF-A chain	+	+
IL-6	+	+

MHC, major histocompatibility complex; TGF-β, transforming growth factor beta; VEGF, vascular endothelial growth factor; PDGF, platelet-derived growth factor; IL-6, interleukin 6.

low level of spontaneous tumor development. When exposed to asbestos fibers, high-copy mice rapidly developed faster growing and more invasive mesotheliomas than those developing in wild-type or single-copy mice. These data support the concept of co-carcinogenicity between SV40 and asbestos. This model is ideal for *in vivo* mesothelioma studies as it provides spontaneous tumors that occur in response to asbestos and does not employ transplantable tumor cell lines.

USES OF EXPERIMENTAL MODELS OF MALIGNANT MESOTHELIOMA

Use of MM cell lines to identify genetic alterations arising from asbestos fiber injury: oncogenes and tumor suppressor genes

Neoplastic transformation leads to genomic damage which should be detected and repaired by normal cellular processes. Tumor suppressor (TS) genes are involved in these processes and arrest the cell cycle to allow repair of genetic abnormalities; if these are not repaired cells enter programmed cell death (apoptosis). Mutation or loss of a TS gene encourages unrestricted growth and proliferation of an altered cell. The best-described TS gene is p53 which is mutated in the majority of human cancers.[38] Mutations in p53 have been identified in 75 percent of murine MM cell lines.[39]. However, p53 may overexpressed in most human MM cell lines and in human MM primary tumors.[40–43] Similarly, the retinoblastoma gene was shown to be expressed normally in a number of human MM cell lines.[44] However, use of monoclonal antibodies directed against two different epitopes of the retinoblastoma gene product, and immunohistochemistry of primary tumors, revealed differing reaction patterns in neoplastic and non-neoplastic mesothelial cells,[44] suggesting that the expressed retinoblastoma gene product may be abnormal in MM.

The Wilm's tumor gene (WT-1) is another interesting TS gene which is often mutated in Wilm's tumor and is expressed in mesothelium during embryogenesis. Expression of this gene has been detected in both human MM cell lines and in primary tumors.[45,46] One of the actions of the WT-1 protein is to control the transcription of genes such as PDGF-A,[47] insulin-like growth factor (IGF)-II[48] and TGF-β.[49] These agents have been described as potential autocrine growth factors in MM and the deletion of WT-1 could lead to their de-regulated production. However, it has recently been shown that there is no inverse correlation in expression of WT-1, IGF-II or PDGF-A in MM.[50]

Specific oncogenes contribute directly to the progression of malignancy and the v-src gene has been shown to cause MM in chickens,[51] whilst transfection of the EJ-ras gene into mesothelial cells causes neoplastic transformation.[52] When rat pleural mesothelial cells are exposed to asbestos the levels of both c-fos and c-jun mRNA become upregulated.[53] However, no consistent association of these particular oncogenes to human MM has been demonstrated.[54,55]

To assess the role of SV40 in the evolution of mesothelioma

An important link between mesothelioma and SV40 was made in 1993 when injection of wild-type SV40 into the pleural space of hamsters resulted in development of pericardial or pleural mesothelioma in 100 percent of cases.[16] Interestingly, the presence of antisense IGF-1 receptor DNA inhibited the tumorigenicity of SV40 in these hamsters[56] suggesting that SV40 uses the IGF signaling pathway to induce MM.

Simian virus 40 is highly immunogenic and has a number of mapped immunodominant epitopes which are recognized by cytotoxic T lymphocytes in mice.[57] Thus, Imperiale *et al.*[58] speculated that the unique properties of the SV40 virus could be exploited to treat patients with SV40-positive MM. A modified SV40 T antigen, from which the transforming domains were removed but immunogenicity preserved, was cloned into a vaccinia virus vector and shown, in an animal tumor model, to be effective against SV40 Tag expressing pre-existing tumors and subsequent tumor challenge. Survival duration was increased when pre-existing tumors were treated with the SV40 vaccinia virus construct in combination with immunotherapy. Plans to investigate the potential of this construct in a human trial are in progress.

To assess the efficiency of varying single or multi-modality therapeutic approaches

Much of the early work (often employing *in vitro* models) examining a single therapy (such as chemotherapy, discussed below) indicated doses and sensitivities for use in clinical trials however, the results of these trials have generally been disappointing. It is becoming increasingly clear in human studies, as well as in animal models, that single-modality therapy is unlikely to result in long-term survival. Hence, relatively new techniques, particularly those that offer an adjuvant setting, are being considered for use in combination with other treatments. Gene therapies are under active investigation employing either established animal models or constructing new ones, and these are described in more detail below.

To assess the efficiency of chemotherapeutic drugs

Standard chemotherapy drugs result in response rates that are usually less than 20 percent and with little evidence of any meaningful increased response using combination chemotherapy.[59] A large number of new chemotherapy agents have been developed in the last decade. Many of these have shown activity against a wide range of solid tumors and some are now being tried in MM. It would be desirable to trial each of these drugs alone and in combination in MM; unfortunately, this is difficult given the small numbers of patients who are eligible for such trials in any one center. One extensively used alternative to assess the clinical potential of single and combination chemotherapeutic drugs is to examine their *in vitro* effects on MM cell lines.[60,61] Similarly, much of the work involving human tumors transplanted into immunocompromised mice was established primarily to examine the chemosensitivity of these tumors *in vivo*.[22,62] Based on the results, several clinical trials have been conducted. For example, after a combination of mitomycin C and cisplatin was described as the most effective regimen for xenografted human MM, a clinical trial using the same chemotherapeutic agents reported that four of 12 patients showed objective responses (one complete and three partial).[63]

However, the benefits of chemotherapy should not be exclusively assessed by measuring response rates as determined by tumor shrinkage. Where a cancer is not curable, the aim of treatment can be prolongation of life or palliation of symptoms. Mesothelioma patients often exhibit severe systemic features and it is thought that one of the major mediators is the cytokine interleukin (IL)-6. IL-6 is a pro-inflammatory cytokine and its blockade with anti-IL-6 antibodies has been shown to reduce cachexia and improve clinical status in mice with mesothelioma. Using *in vitro* analysis, we have shown that irinotecan and gemcitabine are not only more likely to be active against mesothelioma than other chemotherapy agents, but may also produce a palliative effect in non-responders to these agents by decreasing IL-6 secretion.[64]

To assess the efficiency of new forms of therapy

Bacterial products such as diphtheria toxin and mycobacterial heat shock protein 65 (HSP65)[65,66] have been assessed for their *in vivo* tumoricidal effects in animal models. A single intraperitoneal or IV dose of diphtheria toxin consistently and rapidly cured athymic mice of advanced stage experimental human MM. The complete and direct tumoricidal effect without an associated immune response implies that toxin readily reached, entered and preferentially killed human cancer cells. Similarly, long-term survival was seen in immunocompetent mice bearing intraperitoneal progressing syngeneic MM cells (AC29 or AB12) that had been treated with cationic lipid complexed with plasmid DNA (pDNA) containing hsp65.[66] Interestingly, survivors were also observed in groups treated with lipid complexed with any pDNA, although lipid alone or DNA alone provided no demonstrable survival advantage. Re-challenging long-term survivors in both murine models with the parental tumor cell line demonstrated the generation of specific, long-lasting systemic immunity mediated by cytolytic CD8+ T cells and natural killer (NK) cells.

Immunotoxins, constructed by linking ricin to murine monoclonal antibodies reactive with the human transferrin receptor, were shown to be potent *in vitro* cytotoxins against human MM cell lines. Their *in vivo* potential was evaluated in a nude mouse model of human MM.[67] The survival of tumor-bearing mice was significantly extended but no long-term cure was reported.

Identifying molecular targets for pharmacological therapies

Methionine aminopeptidase-2 (MetAP2) is the molecular target of the angiogenesis inhibitor fumagillin which can also inhibit cancer cell proliferation. MM cells express higher MetAP2 mRNA levels than primary normal mesothelial cells and fumagillin induced apoptosis that was restricted to the malignant cells, suggesting that MetAP2 inhibition may represent a potential target for therapeutic intervention in human mesothelioma.[68]

Non-immunological gene therapy

The nature and accessibility of MM tumors in humans means that they are suitable candidates for direct cytokine and gene-transfer therapeutic approaches. Gene therapy represents the introduction of a gene of interest into a site where it should be most effective. The methods of gene delivery vary greatly in terms of complexity, and are often determined by the ultimate experimental or therapeutic aims. For example, the aim might be to understand the role of a gene as a therapeutic agent, or it might be to determine whether or not this gene is significant in the natural progression of MM. The latter approach was often employed to understand which immunologically active molecules were important to induce or maintain an effective immune response and involved transfecting cDNA coding for these molecules into MM cell lines and determining their *in vivo* tumorigenicity (see below). The cytokine gene therapy approaches are described elsewhere.

Gene therapy using adenovirus to deliver *Herpes simplex virus* (HSV) thymidine kinase (Ad.HSVtk) was evaluated in immunocompetent mice with established abdominal MM tumor.[69] Mice were treated with multiple intraperitoneal injections of Ad.HSVtk followed by daily administration of the pro-drug ganciclovir, and showed significantly improved survival versus singly injected animals and control animals. However, the response was significantly improved in immunosuppressed mice, therefore immunosuppression may be a useful adjunct.[70] Similarly, a modified, non-neurovirulent HSV effectively treated a localized intraperitoneal malignancy (human MM cells) in SCID mice.[71]

Pleural models of MM demonstrated a widespread distribution of infectious virus particles throughout the thorax after intrapleural treatment with adenovirus vectors that resulted in tumor growth inhibition.[32,72] The use of these models led to a number of clinical trials.

EXPERIMENTAL MODELS DESIGNED TO CHARACTERIZE THE ROLE OF THE IMMUNE SYSTEM IN MALIGNANT MESOTHELIOMA

Many experimental models were established to understand the role of the (innate and adaptive) immune system as the MM tumors naturally progress, and to identify which, if any, therapies that act as immune adjuvants could be successfully translated into a clinical trial. More recently, exquisitely sensitive models using T cell receptor (TCR) transgenic mice have been constructed and the power of these experimental systems is described below.

Use of transfection/transgenic models to understand tumor-specific immune responses to MM

Dissecting out the critical components involved in a specific immune response directed against MM has been hampered by the current lack of known MM tumor antigens. Whilst identifying MM-specific tumor antigens represents work-in-progress, one experimental approach that has been employed to overcome this obstacle is the construction of defined model systems using mouse MM tumor cell lines transfected with nominal antigens such as influenza hemagglutinin (HA)[73] and ovalbumin (OVA),[74] to which TCR transgenic mice are available. Importantly, expression of either HA or OVA as neo tumor antigens does facilitate tumor rejection in syngeneic, immunologically intact animals. In both systems the class I and class II peptide reactivities are well defined and, anti-HA as well as anti-OVA, TCR transgenic mice are available with class I and II specificities. The advantage of using these TCR transgenic mice is that they provide a virtually monoclonal source of cells of known specificity where the respective roles of tumor-specific CD8+ and CD4+ T cells can be evaluated. Thus, it is possible to investigate when and where MM-associated tumor antigens are presented *in vivo* during tumor progression, how the frequency of tumor-specific T cells influences tumor immunity, and the role that specific CD4+ T cells play in modulating the immune response.

The pathobiology and immunobiology of MM

Murine models for MM have been used to gain insight into the mechanism(s) whereby MM might escape immune surveillance. We have shown that numerous immune cell types infiltrate MM tumors including T cells, B cells, NK cells and large numbers of macrophages (our unpublished data).[75,76] There is contradictory evidence regarding their local regulation although downregulation of some lymphocyte surface markers, known to be involved in T cell activation, has been demonstrated in tumor infiltrating lymphocytes (TIL).[77] Similarly, expression of MHC class II antigen and integrins was weak on tumor infiltrating macrophages (TIM), suggesting altered functional activity. Significant amounts of TGF-β, IL-6, IL-1 and tumor necrosis factor (TNF) were produced during the course of MM tumor development which may contribute both to derangement of anti-tumor effector mechanisms and to the clinical and pathological manifestations of this disease.[78,79]

Although MM tumor cells have abundant MHC class I molecules, they do not express the co-stimulatory molecules necessary to ensure that CD8+ T cells will become effector cells. Hence, MM tumor cells are not able to induce a class I-restricted response by directly presenting their own antigens to CD8+ T cells. Furthermore, MM cell lines express little or no MHC class II molecules and are therefore are unable to directly activate CD4+ helper T cells. Thus, the only possible mechanism through which MM-specific immune responses can be generated is via a third party antigen presenting cell (APC) that has collected MM tumor antigens after trafficking through the tumor on its way to draining lymph nodes – a process referred to as cross-presentation. Use of the transfection/transgenic models showed that MM tumor growth in normal inbred mice is associated with constitutive tumor antigen cross-presentation.[79] Interestingly, in the odd instance when a mouse did not develop a solid tumor, *in vivo* tumor antigen presentation was detectable for up 6 months after tumor cell inoculation, implying that either the immune system kept tumor growth in check or that the tumor antigen was somehow trapped within the draining lymph nodes.

Adoptive transfer of both tumor-specific CD4+ and CD8+ T cells together offered complete protection from tumor growth,[81] and induced regression in MM tumor-bearing mice. Tumor-specific CD4+ T cells were required for the prolonged survival or 'maintenance' of functional tumor-specific CD8+ T cells, as well as their emigration into the tumor mass itself. It was only in the presence of CD4+ T cells that MM tumors exhibited upregulation of major histocompatibility complex (MHC) class II and intercellular adhesion molecule (ICAM) expression which may be necessary to generate an effective anti-tumor immune response.

More recently, potent regulatory T cells (Treg) that can be identified by their co-expression of CD4, CD25 and the transcription factor FoxP3 have been demonstrated in murine and human MM tumors.[82,83] Treg cells play a major role in the maintenance of self-tolerance, the control of autoimmune and, more deleteriously, in anti-tumor immune responses. Depletion of Treg cells significantly reduced tumor growth underlining their regulatory capacity. These data suggest that combining therapies with Treg depletion may be clinically beneficial.

Susceptibility of MM tumor cells to lymphoid effector cells

Early work involved using experimental models to determine the susceptibility of MM tumor cells to lysis by effector cells from the innate (e.g. NK cells) and/or adaptive compartments of the immune system. Human peripheral blood lymphocytes (PBL) incubated with IL-2 generated lymphokine activated killer (LAK) cells that lysed non-cultured, NK cell resistant tumor cells. Both human and murine MM cell lines are susceptible to non-MHC restricted lysis *in vitro* by LAK cells, some gamma-delta ($\gamma\delta$) T lymphocytes, but not by NK cell lysis.[34,84,85] There is also evidence that MM tumor cells can be lysed by CD8+ CTL, particularly if the tumor cells have been exposed to interferon (IFN)-γ.[81] These studies suggest that selected immunotherapeutic strategies involving the use of IL-2 may be successful in the control of MM via stimulation of LAK cells and CD8+ CTL.

Cytokine and growth factor production

Human and murine MM tumor cell lines have been intensively studied for their soluble factor secreting profiles. Several cytokines and growth factors are produced by MM cells including PDGF-A and -B, insulin-like growth factor (IGF)-I and -II, TGF-α and -β, granulocyte-macrophage colony stimulating factor (GM-CSF), IL-6, leukemia inhibitory factor (LIF) and other mitogenic factors that have not yet been defined.[9,10,86–91]

Transforming growth factor-β is a powerful immunosuppressant, which can inhibit T cell responses. Most MM cell lines secrete significant amounts of various isoforms of TGF-β[77,87] and these may act locally to inhibit T cell activity. This conclusion is supported by *in vivo* studies showing that tumor cells transfected with an inducible TGF-β antisense construct, thereby blocking TGF-β activity, promote increased numbers of tumor-infiltrating T lymphocytes.[77]

Interleukin-6 has pro-inflammatory, immunoregulatory and hemopoietic effects, is produced by the majority of MM cell lines[79,91] and can be isolated in large amounts from MM pleural effusions.[92] Its role in the pathogenesis of human MM is unclear, but it is likely to be involved in the development of MM-associated fever, thrombocytosis and cachexia.

The influence of these factors on tumor progression, and on the development of an anti-MM immune response, is yet to be fully elucidated. The role of the potent immuno-modulatory factors, particularly those that are released systemically, can only be realistically evaluated using *in vivo* models.

Immunotherapies using cytokines and cytokine gene therapy

Experiments utilizing murine MM models with syngeneic tumor cell lines show that whilst unmanipulated MM tumors cannot induce an effective anti-tumor response, they are susceptible to eradication by the immune system when immune stimulating transfectants are used. The murine MM cell line, AC29, derived from tumors induced by crocidolite asbestos injected intraperitoneally into a CBA mouse, was transfected with genes coding for IL-4, GM-CSF, B7-1, allogeneic MHC and IL-2.[93–96] All are immunogenic, i.e. they either fail to grow (those expressing B7.1, allogeneic class I MHC and IL-4) or grow slowly (those expressing IL-2 and GM-CSF) compared with the parental AC29 cell line, and they all induce some protection against rechallenge suggesting that any, or all, of these molecules may be useful in generating an anti-MM response.

A BALB/c MM tumor cell line (AB-1) transfected with the IL-12 gene cannot grow in syngeneic mice[97,98] due to an immune mediated response. IL-12 is associated with the differentiation of T-cell mediated CD8+ T-cell cytolytic responses that are critical for tumor destruction. Both CD4+ and CD8+ T cells are required to infiltrate the site of tumor inoculation before complete tumor eradication is seen. Furthermore, immunization with the transfectant induced long-term immunity that was effective at reducing the incidence of parental MM tumors.[97] However, when IL-12 was given systemically to mice with established tumor, it only delayed tumor growth during the treatment period.

In vivo studies in a murine MM model (AB22) reported that detectable serum IL-6 levels preceded macroscopically detectable tumor growth, clinical signs (cachexia, abdominal distension, diarrhoea) and changes in the peripheral lymphoid organs (cell depletion and functional depression). Treatment with either anti-IL-6 antibody or with recombinant (r) IFN-α curtailed clinical symptoms. The latter treatment attenuated IL-6 mRNA expression in tumors and serum IL-6 levels, ameliorated the depression of lymphocyte activities and enhanced the number of tumor-infiltrating lymphocytes and macrophages, implying a palliative role for combination therapy using rIFN-α and anti-IL-6 for MM patients.[79,99]

Intra-tumoral administration of rIL-2 into a murine MM cell line derived after asbestos inoculation into the peritoneum of C57BL/6 mice (AE17) exhibited delayed or static tumor growth, and in some cases tumor regression in a dose-dependent manner.[74] Tumor size at the commencement of IL-2 treatment proved critical for a successful outcome. Mice with small tumors when treatment began exhibited objective responses including complete and permanent tumor regression. This response was associated with tumor infiltrating CD8+ T cells and reduced tumor-associated vascularity. Tumor progression inevitably occurred in mice with large tumors when treatment was commenced. It was evident that there was only a small time-frame in which IL-2 treatment could be effective.

Use of agonist anti-CD40 antibody therapy in mesothelioma

CD40 is an M_r 40 000 type I glycoprotein and a member of the tumor necrosis factor receptor superfamily, which was initially identified on bladder carcinoma cells and later on normal and malignant B cells. It is expressed on a range of immune and non-immune cells, the most important immune cell being dendritic cells (DCs). Its ligand, CD40L (CD154), is expressed on CD4 T cells shortly after TCR triggering. CD40–CD154 interactions have an important role in cytotoxic lymphocyte (CTL) priming and their interaction is central to the decision whether CTLs become primed or tolerized. Thus, use of an activating (agonist) anti-CD40 antibody can replace or augment CD4 help in priming DCs to activate CD8 T cells. Systemic treatment with an activating anti-CD40 antibody, FGK45, in our murine MM models causes transient tumor regression over the treatment period, followed by rapid tumor outgrowth.[100] In contrast, intra-tumoral anti-CD40 antibody can completely cure small but not large MM tumors (our unpublished data). These data suggest that CD40 triggering can only be effective when combined with other therapeutic modalities.

Chemotherapy and anti-MM immunity

Cytotoxic chemotherapy is generally considered immunosuppressive, with neutropenia and lymphopenia being common adverse side effects. However, we have shown that whilst the cytidine analogue gemcitabine abolishes humoral responses, it in fact augments antigen-specific cellular anti-tumor immunity.[101] This augmentation occurs in the context of increased antigen cross-presentation, T lymphocyte expansion and tumor infiltration. Combining gemcitabine with a CD40-triggering immunotherapy resulted in synergistic, leading to long-term, protective cure when applied to small tumors. Thus, chemotherapy has the capacity to augment cellular antitumor immunity.

Combination immune therapy with debulking surgery in murine MM

We have previously shown that debulking surgery is rarely permanently effective as resected MM tumors eventually re-emerge. However, when debulking surgery was performed in conjunction with vaccination using syngeneic MM tumor cells transfected with genes encoding for B7-1 or high levels of GM-CSF, there was a statistically significant delay of tumor growth.[96] Debulking surgery appeared to play a pivotal role in promoting an anti-tumor immune response induced by immunological gene therapy.

More recently, we have shown that partial and complete debulking surgery was highly effective in eradicating MM tumors when combined with chemotherapy and a CD40-based immunotherapy.[102] However, only those mice with partially debulked tumors plus the combination regimen generated long-term, tumor-specific, protective memory. We postulate that chemotherapy induced apoptosis of residual tumor cells following incomplete resection is absolutely required for the induction of long-term immunological memory. These data are the basis of a current clinical trial.

In conclusion, experimental models of MM continue to offer meaningful information for direct clinical translation.

KEY POINTS

- Mesothelioma models are generally similar to human mesothelioma – this is unusual for mouse tumor models.
- Sarcomoatoid rather than epithelial mesothelioma are more commonly seen in mice, in contrast to human mesothelioma.
- New transgenic models have added powerful tools to the existing repertoire of mesothelioma models of transplantable or asbestos-induced *in situ* models.
- These models are proving useful for the analysis of biological events in mesothelioma.
- These models are also useful for preclinical screening of potential therapies.

REFERENCES

● = Key primary paper
◆ = Major review article

◆1. Wagner J, Sleggs C, Marchand P. Diffuse pleural mesothelioma and asbestos exposure in the North Western Cape Province. *Br J Ind Med* 1960; **17**: 260–71.
2. Jaurand M, Kaplan H, Thiollet J, *et al.* Phagocytosis of chrysotile fibers by pleural mesothelial cells in culture. *Am J Pathol* 1979; **94**: 529–38.
3. Lechner J, Tokiwa T, LaVeck M, *et al.* Asbestos-associated chromosomal changes in human mesothelial cells. *Proc Natl Acad Sci U S A* 1985; **82**: 3884–8.
4. Joseph L, Stephens R, Ottolenghi A, *et al.* Morphological transformation *in vitro* of normal human fibroblasts by chrysotile. *Environ Health Perspect* 1983; **51**: 17–22.

5. Bignon J, Jaurand M. Biological *in vitro* and *in vivo* responses of chrysotile versus amphiboles. *Environ Health Perspect* 1983; **51**: 73–80.
6. Walker C, Everitt J, Barrett J. Possible cellular and molecular mechanisms for asbestos carcinogenicity. *Am J Ind Med* 1992; **21**: 253–73.
7. Yegles M, Saint-Etienne L, Renier A, *et al.* Induction of metaphase and anaphase/telophase abnormalities by asbestos fibers in rat pleural mesothelial cells *in vitro*. *Am J Respir Cell Mol Biol* 1993; **9**: 186–91.
8. Walker C, Everitt J, Ferriola P, *et al.* Autocrine growth stimulation by transforming growth factor alpha in asbestos-transformed rat mesothelial cells. *Cancer Res* 1995; **55**: 530–6.
9. Garlepp M, Christmas T, Manning L, *et al.* The role of platelet-derived growth factor in the growth of human malignant mesothelioma. *Eur Respir Rev* 1993; **3**: 189–91.
10. Garlepp M, Christmas T, Mutsaers S, *et al.* Platelet-derived growth factor as an autocrine factor in murine malignant mesothelioma. *Eur Resp Rev* 1993; **3**: 192–4.
11. Dobra K, Andang M, Syrokou A, *et al.* Differentiation of mesothelioma cells is influenced by the expression of proteoglycans. *Exp Cell Res* 2000; **258**: 12–22.
12. Ke Y, Reddel R, Gerwin B, *et al.* Establishment of a human *in vitro* mesothelial cell model system for investigating mechanisms of asbestos-induced mesothelioma. *Am J Pathol* 1989; **134**: 979–91.
●13. Procopio A, Strizzi L, Vianale G, *et al.* Simian virus-40 sequences are a negative prognostic cofactor in patients with malignant pleural mesothelioma. *Genes Chromosomes Cancer* 2000; **29**: 173–9.
14. McLaren B, Haenel T, Stevenson, *et al.* RA. SV40 like sequences in cell lines and tumour biopsies from Australian malignant mesotheliomas. *Aust NZ J Med* 2000; **30**: 450–6.
15. Bryan T, Reddel R. SV40-induced immortalization of human cells. *Crit Rev Oncog* 1994; **5**: 331–57.
16. Cicala C, Pompetti F, Carbone M. SV40 induces mesotheliomas in hamsters. *Am J Pathol* 1993; **142**: 1524–33.
17. Butel J, Lednicky J. Cell and molecular biology of simian virus 40: Implications for human infections and disease. *J Natl Cancer Inst* 1999; **91**: 119–134.
18. Carbone M. Simian virus 40 and human tumours: It is time to study mechanisms. *J Cell Biochem* 1999; **76**: 189–93.
19. Shivapurkar N, Wiethege T, Wistuba I, *et al.* Presence of simian virus 40 sequences in malignant mesotheliomas and mesothelial cell proliferations. *J Cell Biochem* 1999; **76**: 181–8.
20. Bocchetta M, Di Resta I, Powers A, *et al.* Human mesothelial cells are unusually susceptible to simian virus 40-mediated transformation and asbestos cocarcinogenicity. *Proc Nat Am Soc* 2000; **97**: 10214–19.
21. Hahn W, Counter C, Lundberg A, *et al.* Creation of human tumour cells with defined genetic elements. *Nature* 1999; **400**: 464–8.
22. Chahinian A, Beranek J, Suzuki Y, *et al.* Transplantation of human malignant mesothelioma into nude mice. *Cancer Res* 1980; **40**: 181–5.
23. Reale F, Griffin T, Compton J, *et al.* Characterization of a human malignant mesothelioma cell line (H-MESO-1): a biphasic solid and ascitic tumor model. *Cancer Res* 1987; **47**: 3199–205.
24. Glickman L, Domanski L, Maguire T, *et al.* Mesothelioma in pet dogs associated with exposure of their owners to asbestos. *Environ Res* 1983; **32**: 305–13.
◆25. Berry G, Wagner J. The application of a mathematical model describing the times of occurrence of mesotheliomas in rats following inoculation with asbestos. *Br J Cancer* 1969; **23**: 582–6.
26. Fasske E. Experimental lung tumors following specific intrabronchial application of chrysotile asbestos. Longitudinal light and electron microscopic investigations in rats. *Respiration* 1988; **53**: 111–27.
27. Smith W, Hubert D, Holiat S, *et al.* An experimental model for treatment of mesothelioma. *Cancer* 1981; **47**: 658–63.
28. Miller B, Jones A, Searl A, *et al.* Influence of characteristics of inhaled fibers on development of tumours in the rat lung. *Ann Occup Hyg* 1999; **43**: 167–79.
29. Muhle H, Pott F. Asbestos as reference material for fiber-induced cancer. *Int Arch Occup Environ Health* 2000; **73** (Suppl): S53–9.
●30. Hesterberg T, Miller W, Thevenaz P, Anderson R. Chronic inhalation studies of man-made vitreous fibers: characterization of fibers in the exposure aerosol and lungs. *Ann Occup Hyg* 1995; **39**: 637–53.
31. Pott F. Detection of mineral fiber carcinogenicity with the intraperitoneal test: recent results and their validity. *Ann Occup Hyg* 1995; **39**: 771–9.
◆32. Kucharczuk J, Elshami A, Zhang H, *et al.* Pleural-based mesothelioma in immune competent rats: a model to study adenoviral gene transfer. *Ann Thorac Surg* 1995; **60**: 593–7.
33. Fleury-Feith J, Nebut M, Saint-Etienne L, *et al.* Occurrence and morphology of tumors induced in nude mice transplanted with chrysotile-transformed rat pleural mesothelial cells. *Biol Cell* 1989; **65**: 45–50.
◆34. Christmas T, Manning L, Davis MR, *et al.* HLA antigen expression and malignant mesothelioma. *Am J Respir Cell Mol Biol* 1991; **5**: 213–20.
35. Davis M, Manning L, Whitaker D, *et al.* Establishment of a murine model of malignant mesothelioma. *Int J Cancer* 1992; **52**: 881–6.
36. Goodglick L, Vaslet C, Messier N, Kane A. Growth factor responses and protooncogene expression of murine mesothelial cell lines derived from asbestos-induced mesotheliomas. *Toxicol Pathol* 1997; **25**: 565–73.
37. Robinson C, van Bruggen I, Segal A, *et al.* A novel SV40 TAg transgenic model of asbestos-induced mesothelioma: malignant transformation is dose dependent. *Cancer Res* 2006; **66**: 10786–94.
38. Hollstein M, Sidransky D, Vogelstein B, Harris C. p53 mutations in human cancers. *Science* 1991; **253**: 49–53.
39. Cora E, Kane A. Alterations in a tumour suppressor gene, p53, in mouse mesotheliomas induced by crocidolite asbestos. *Eur Resp Rev* 1993; **3**: 148–150.
40. Metcalf R, Welsh J, Bennett W, *et al.* p53 and Kirsten-ras mutations in human mesothelioma cell lines. *Cancer Res* 1992; **52**: 2610–15.
41. Mor O, Yaron P, Huszar M, *et al.* Absence of p53 mutations in malignant mesotheliomas. *Am J Respir Cell Mol Biol* 1997; **16**: 9–13.
42. Creaney J, McLaren B, Stevenson S, *et al.* p53 autoantibodies in patients with malignant mesothelioma: stability through disease progression. *Br J Cancer* 2001; **84**: 52–6.
43. Van der Meeren A, Seddon M, Betsholtz C, *et al.* Tumorigenic conversion of human mesothelial cells as a consequence of platelet-derived growth factor-A chain overexpression. *Am J Respir Cell Mol Biol* 1993; **8**: 214–21.
44. Ramael M, Segers K, Van Marck E. Differential immunohistochemical staining of the retinoblastoma protein with the antibodies C15 and IF8 in malignant mesothelioma. *Pathol Res Pract* 1994; **190**: 138–41.
45. Walker C, Rutten F, Yuan X, *et al.* Wilms' tumor suppressor gene expression in rat and human mesothelioma. *Cancer Res* 1994; **54**: 3101–6.
46. Amin K, Litzky L, Smythe W, *et al.* Wilms' tumor 1 susceptibility (WT1) gene products are selectively expressed in malignant mesothelioma. *Am J Pathol* 1995; **146**: 344–56.
47. Wang Z, Madden S, Deuel T, Rauscher F. The Wilms' tumor gene product, WT1, represses transcription of the platelet-derived growth factor A-chain gene. *J Biol Chem* 1992; **267**: 21999–2002.
48. Drummond I, Madden S, Rohwer-Nutter P, *et al.* Repression of the insulin-like growth factor II gene by the Wilms tumor suppressor WT1. *Science* 1992; **257**: 674–8.
49. Dey B, Sukhatme V, Roberts A, *et al.* Repression of the transforming growth factor-beta 1 gene by the Wilms' tumor suppressor WT1 gene product. *Mol Endocrinol* 1994; **8**: 595–602.

50. Langerak A, Williamson K, Miyagawa K, *et al.* Expression of the Wilms' tumor gene WT1 in human malignant mesothelioma cell lines and relationship to platelet-derived growth factor A and insulin-like growth factor 2 expression. *Genes Chromosomes Cancer* 1995; **12**: 87–96.
51. England J, Panella M, Ewert D, Halpern S. Induction of a diffuse mesothelioma in chickens by intraperitoneal inoculation of v-src DNA. *Virology* 1991; **182**: 423–9.
52. Reddel R, Malan-Shibley L, Gerwin B, *et al.* Tumorigenicity of human mesothelial cell line transfected with EJ-ras oncogene. *J Natl Cancer Inst* 1989; **81**: 945–8.
53. Heintz N, Janssen Y, Mossman B. Persistent induction of c-fos and c-jun expression by asbestos. *Proc Natl Acad Sci U S A* 1993; **90**: 3299–303.
54. Fung H, Quinlan T, Janssen Y, *et al.* Inhibition of protein kinase C prevents asbestos-induced c-fos and c- jun proto-oncogene expression in mesothelial cells. *Cancer Res* 1997; **57**: 3101–5.
55. Suzuki Y, Weston A. Immunocytochemical analysis of oncoproteins and growth factors in human malignant mesothelioma. *Oncol Rep* 1995; **12**: 897–902.
56. Pass H, Mew, D. Carbone, M. Inhibition of hamster mesothelioma tumorigenesis by an antisense expression plasmid to the insulin-like growth factor-1 receptor. *Cancer Res* 1996; **50**: 4044–8.
57. Tevethia S. Recognition of simian virus 40 T antigen by cytotoxic T lymphocytes. *Mol Biol Med* 1990; **7**: 83–96.
58. Imperiale M, Pass H, Sanda M. Prospects for an SV40 vaccine. *Semin Cancer Biol* 2001; **11**: 81–5.
59. Ong S, Vogelzang N. Chemotherapy in malignant pleural mesothelioma. A review. *J Clin Oncol* 1996; **14**: 1007–17.
60. Goodman G, Yen Y, Cox T, Crowley J. Effect of verapamil on *in vitro* cytotoxicity of adriamycin and vinblastine in human tumor cells. *Cancer Res* 1987; **47**: 2295–304.
61. Bowman R, Manning L, Davis M. Chemosensitivity and cytokine sensitivity of malignant mesothelioma. *Cancer Chemother Pharmacol* 1991; **28**: 420–6.
62. Arnold W, Tanneberger S, Nowak C, Naundorf H. Recent results with clinically used antineoplastic drugs and drug combinations *in vivo*. *Oncology* 1980; **37** (Suppl 1): 34–41.
63. Chahinian A, Norton L, Holland J, *et al.* Experimental and clinical activity of mitomycin C and cis- diamminedichloroplatinum in malignant mesothelioma. *Cancer Res* 1984; **44**: 1688–92.
64. McLaren BR, Robinson BWS, Lake RA. New chemotherapeutics in malignant mesothelioma: Effects on cell growth and IL6 production. *Cancer Chemother Pharmacol* 2000; **45**: 502–8.
65. Raso V, McGrath J. Cure of experimental human malignant mesothelioma in athymic mice by diphtheria toxin. *J Natl Cancer Inst* 1989; **81**: 622–7.
66. Lanuti M, Rudginsky S, Force S, *et al.* Cationic lipid:bacterial DNA complexes elicit adaptive cellular immunity in murine intraperitoneal tumor models. *Cancer Res* 2000; **60**: 2955–63.
67. Griffin T, Richardson C, Houston L, *et al.* Antitumor activity of intraperitoneal immunotoxins in a nude mouse model of human malignant mesothelioma. *Cancer Res* 1987; **47**: 4266–70.
68. Catalano A, Romano M, Robuffo I, *et al.* Methionine aminopeptidase-2 regulates human mesothelioma cell survival : role of bcl-2 expression and telomerase activity. *Am J Pathol* 2001; **159**: 721–31.
69. Lambright E, Force S, Lanuti M, *et al.* Efficacy of repeated adenoviral suicide gene therapy in a localized murine tumor model. *Ann Thorac Surg* 2000; **70**: 1865–70.
70. Elshami A, Kucharczuk J, Sterman D, *et al.* The role of immunosuppression in the efficacy of cancer gene therapy using adenovirus transfer of the herpes simplex thymidine kinase gene. *Ann Surg* 1995; **222**: 298–307.
•71. Kucharczuk J, Randazzo B, Chang M, *et al.* Use of a 'replication-restricted' herpes virus to treat experimental human malignant mesothelioma. *Cancer Res* 1997; **57**: 466–71.
72. Esandi M, van Someren G, Vincent A, *et al.* Gene therapy of experimental malignant mesothelioma using adenovirus vectors encoding the HSVtk gene. *Gene Ther* 1997; **4**: 280–7.
73. Marzo A, Kinnear B, Lake R, *et al.* Tumor-specific CD4+ T cells have a major 'post-licensing' role in CTL mediated anti-tumor immunity. *J Immunol* 2000; **165**: 6047–55.
•74. Jackaman C, Bundell C, Kinnear B, *et al.* IL-2 intratumoral immunotherapy enhances CD8$^+$ T cells that mediate destruction of tumor cells and tumor-associated vasculature: a novel mechanism for IL-2. *J Immunol* 2003; **171**: 5051–63.
75. Garlepp M, Leong C, Biological and immunological aspects of malignant mesothelioma. *Eur Respir J* 1995; **8**: 643–50.
76. Bielefeldt-Ohmann H, Fitzpatrick D, Marzo A, *et al.* Patho- and immunobiology of malignant mesothelioma: characterisation of tumour infiltrating leucocytes and cytokine production in a murine model. *Cancer Immunol Immunother* 1994; **39**: 347–59.
77. Fitzpatrick D, Bielefeldt-Ohmann H, Himbeck R, *et al.* Transforming growth factor-beta: antisense RNA-mediated inhibition affects anchorage-independent growth, tumorigenicity and tumor-infiltrating T-cells in malignant mesothelioma. *Growth Factors* 1994; **11**: 29–44.
78. Fitzpatrick D, Peroni D, Bielefeldt-Ohmann H. The role of growth factors and cytokines in the tumorigenesis and immunobiology of malignant mesothelioma. *Am J Respir Cell Mol Biol* 1995; **12**: 455–60.
79. Bielefeldt-Ohmann H, Marzo A, Himbeck R, *et al.* Interleukin-6 involvement in mesothelioma pathobiology: inhibition by interferon alpha immunotherapy. *Cancer Immunol Immunother* 1995; **40**: 241–50.
80. Marzo A, Lake R, Lo D, *et al.* Tumor antigens are constitutively presented in the draining lymph nodes. *J Immunol* 1999; **162**: 5838–45.
81. Marzo A, Lake R, Robinson B, Scott B. T-cell receptor transgenic analysis of tumor-specific CD8 and CD4 responses in the eradication of solid tumors. *Cancer Res* 1999; **59**: 1071–9.
82. Meloni F, Morosini M, Solari N, *et al.* Foxp3 expressing CD4+ CD25+ and CD8+CD28– T regulatory cells in the peripheral blood of patients with lung cancer and pleural mesothelioma. *Hum Immunol* 2006; **67**: 1–12
83. Needham D, Lee J, Beilharz M. Intra-tumoural regulatory T cells: a potential new target in cancer immunotherapy. *Biochem Biophys Res Commun* 2006; **343**: 684–91
84. Manning L, Bowman R, Darby S, Robinson B. Lysis of human malignant mesothelioma cells by natural killer (NK) and lymphokine-activated killer (LAK) cells. *Am Rev Respir Dis* 1989; **139**: 1369–1374.
85. Mavaddat N, Robinson B, Rose A, *et al.* An analysis of the relationship between gamma delta T cell receptor V gene usage and non-major histocompatibility complex-restricted cytotoxicity. *Immunol Cell Biol* 1993; **71**: 27–37.
86. Versnel M, Hagemeijer A, Bouts M, *et al.* Expression of c-sis (PDGF B-chain) and PDGF A-chain genes in ten human malignant mesothelioma cell lines derived from primary and metastatic tumors. *Oncogene* 1988; **2**: 601–5.
87. Gerwin B, Lechner J, Reddel R, *et al.* Comparison of production of transforming growth factor-beta and platelet-derived growth factor by normal human mesothelial cells and mesothelioma cell lines. *Cancer Res* 1987; **47**: 6180–4.
88. Demetri G, Zenzie B, Rheinwald J, Griffin J. Expression of colony-stimulating factor genes by normal human mesothelial cells and human malignant mesothelioma cells lines *in vitro*. *Blood* 1989; **74**: 940–6.
89. Lee TC, Zhang Y, Aston C, *et al.* Normal human mesothelial cells and mesothelioma cell lines express insulin-like growth factor I and associated molecules. *Cancer Res* 1993; **53**: 2858–64.
90. Lauber B, Leuthold M, Schmitter D, *et al.* An autocrine mitogenic activity produced by a pleural human mesothelioma cell line. *Int J Cancer* 1992; **50**: 943–50.
91. Schmitter D, Lauber B, Fagg B, Stahel RA. Hematopoietic growth

factors secreted by seven human pleural mesothelioma cell lines: interleukin-6 production as a common feature. *Int J Cancer* 1992; **51**: 296–301.

92. Monti G, Jaurand M, Monnet I, *et al.* Intrapleural production of interleukin 6 during mesothelioma and its modulation by gamma-interferon treatment. *Cancer Res* 1994; **54**: 4419–23.
93. Leong C, Marley J, Loh S, *et al.* Transfection of the gene for B7-1 but not B7-2 can induce immunity to murine malignant mesothelioma. *Int J Cancer* 1997; **71**: 476–82.
94. Leong C, Robinson B, Garlepp M. Generation of an antitumour immune response to a murine mesothelioma cell line by the transfection of allogeneic MHC genes. *Int J Cancer* 1994; **59**: 212–16.
95. Mukherjee S, Nelson D, Loh S, *et al.* The immune anti-tumor effects of GM-CSF and B7-1 gene transfection are enhanced by surgical debulking of tumor. *Cancer Gene Ther* 2001; **8**: 580–8
96. Leong C, Marley J, Loh S, *et al.* The induction of immune responses to murine malignant mesothelioma by IL-2 gene transfer. *Immunol Cell Biol* 1997; **75**: 356–9.
97. Caminschi I, Venetsanakos E, Leong C, *et al.* Cytokine gene therapy of mesothelioma. Immune and antitumor effects of transfected interleukin-12. *Am J Respir Cell Mol Biol* 1999; **21**: 347–56.
98. Caminschi I, Venetsanakos E, Leong C, *et al.* Interleukin-12 induces an effective antitumor response in malignant mesothelioma. *Am J Respir Cell Mol Biol* 1998; **19**: 738–46.
99. Bielefeldt-Ohmann H, Fitzpatrick D, Marzo A, *et al.* Potential for interferon-alpha-based therapy in mesothelioma: assessment in a murine model. *J Interferon Cytokine Res* 1995; **15**: 213–23
100. Stumbles P, Himbeck R, Frelinger J, *et al.* Cutting edge: tumor-specific CTL are constitutively cross-armed in draining lymph nodes and transiently disseminate to mediate tumor regression following systemic CD40 activation. *J Immunol* 2004; **173**: 5923–8.

◆101. Nowak, A, Robinson B, Lake R. Synergy between chemotherapy and immunotherapy in the treatment of established murine solid tumors. *Cancer Res* 2003; **63**: 4490–6.

●102. Broomfield S, Currie A, van der Most R. Partial, but not complete, tumor-debulking surgery promotes protective antitumor memory when combined with chemotherapy and adjuvant immunotherapy. *Cancer Res* 2005; **65**: 7580–4.

PART 2

CLINICAL SCIENCE

16

Approach to patients with pleural diseases

STEVEN A SAHN

Patients with pleural effusions may present with symptoms, such as pleuritic chest pain, dyspnea or cough, or the effusion may be suspected on physical examination or observed on chest radiograph. The diagnosis of a pleural effusion signifies that the physiologic balance between normal pleural fluid formation and removal has been disturbed, resulting in pleural fluid accumulation. Since a pleural effusion can be a manifestation of disease in virtually any organ in the body, its presence provides the clinician with the opportunity to support or confirm their clinical diagnosis. Awareness that not only disease in the thorax can cause a pleural effusion, but abnormalities of organs juxtaposed to the diaphragm, such as the liver or spleen, can lead to earlier diagnosis.[1] In addition, systemic diseases, such as systemic lupus erythematosus and rheumatoid arthritis, and diseases of the lymphatic system, such as yellow nail syndrome, may also cause pleural effusions. Therefore, the evaluation of a patient with a pleural effusion starts with, and requires, a thorough history and physical examination in conjunction with pertinent laboratory tests to allow the clinician to formulate a prethoracentesis diagnosis. Pleural fluid analysis can provide a confident diagnosis when the likelihood of a clinical diagnosis is high.

HISTORY

Patients presenting with a pleural effusion may be asymptomatic, such as with benign asbestos pleural effusions (BAPE)[2] or rheumatoid pleurisy[3] (Table 16.1) or have symptoms as with lupus pleuritis[4] or bacterial pneumonia (Table 16.2). Patients with small pleural effusions and without underlying cardiopulmonary disease may be asymptomatic at presentation and the effusion discovered

Table 16.1 Patients presenting with a pleural effusion who are commonly asymptomatic

Commonly asymptomatic patients presenting with a pleural effusion
• Benign asbestos pleural effusion (BAPE)
• Hypoalbuminemia
• Nephrotic syndrome
• Peritoneal dialysis
• Rheumatoid pleurisy
• Trapped lung
• Urinothorax
• Yellow nail syndrome

Table 16.2 Patients presenting with a pleural effusion who are typically symptomatic

Typically symptomatic patients presenting with a pleural effusion
• Bacterial pneumonia
• Carcinomatous pleural effusion
• Congestive heart failure
• Lupus pleuritis
• Malignant mesothelioma
• Postcardiac injury syndrome (PCIS)
• Pulmonary embolism
• Tuberculous pleural effusion
• Viral pleurisy

on a routine chest radiograph. Dyspnea and chest pain are the two most common presenting symptoms of a pleural effusion. The patient may complain of dyspnea with a massive (occupying the entire hemithorax) or large (occupying >50 percent of the hemithorax) pleural effusion and normal lungs, a moderate (one-third to <50 percent) effusion with underlying lung disease, or a small (less than one-third of the hemithorax) effusion in patients with severe underlying lung disease. A large or massive effusion causes contralateral mediastinal shift, depression of the ipsilateral hemidiaphragm, outward movement of the ipsilateral chest wall, and lung compression, in the absence of an endobronchial lesion causing atelectasis or a fixed mediastinum. It is postulated that dyspnea perceived by these patients results from decreased compliance of the chest wall and lung modulated by the input of neurogenic receptors from these structures.[5] While lung compression is caused by large to massive effusions, a small to moderate effusion tends to cause lung displacement and generally has minimal or no effect on pulmonary function.[6] The major cause of dyspnea in patients with a small to moderate pleural effusion may be related to chest pain with splinting and atelectasis or a primary parenchymal process, such as pneumonia.

Pleuritic chest pain is associated with pleural inflammation and is typically accompanied by a pleural effusion.[7] Pleuritic chest pain varies with the intensity of the pleural inflammation. Patients have described pleuritic chest pain as 'stabbing' or 'shooting' in quality and as having a 'stitch in the side'. Pleuritic chest pain is typically exacerbated by a deep inspiration, coughing or sneezing. Manual pressure over the chest wall, which results in splinting, will minimize the pain; however, a splinting maneuver cannot differentiate pleural inflammation from other causes of chest pain, such as a rib fracture.

Pleuritic chest pain may be focused over the precise location of the inflammation or it may be referred. With costal pleural inflammation, the pain tends to be localized directly over the site of pleural involvement and is often associated with tenderness on pressure and cutaneous hypersensitivity; abdominal pain is absent. When the lateral, anterior and portions of the posterior diaphragm are inflamed, pain is perceived diffusely over the lower thorax, back and abdomen, associated with cutaneous hyperesthesia, and exacerbated by pressure over the site with muscle rigidity. In contrast, inflammation of the central portion of the diaphragmatic pleura does not result in local pain, as pain is referred to the ipsilateral posterior neck, shoulder and trapezius muscle; this referred pain is associated with tenderness, hyperesthesia, hyperalgesia and muscle spasm. Central diaphragmatic pleural inflammation causes referred pain because the sensory fibers of the phrenic nerve enter the spinal cord at the C4 level, which is the usual entry point of sensation from the shoulder.[7]

Because the primary symptoms of a pleural effusion, chest pain and dyspnea, are nonspecific, a more detailed history is critical in narrowing the differential diagnosis prior to pleural fluid analysis. Orthopnea, paroxysmal nocturnal dyspnea, peripheral edema and decreased exercise tolerance suggest that the patient's effusions are the result of congestive heart failure (CHF). A history of loss of consciousness in an alcoholic, 14 days prior, who presents with fever and fatigue suggests that the patient has an anaerobic empyema. The onset of dyspnea in a patient with a recent leg fracture that required a cast suggests the effusion was caused by pulmonary thromboembolic disease. A unilateral pleural effusion in a man who has worked in a shipyard for 20 years should raise the suspicion of BAPE. The postcardiac injury syndrome (PCIS) should be suspected in a patient who underwent cardiac surgery 3 weeks previously and presents with fever, dyspnea, and left pleuritic chest pain.[8] Esophageal rupture should be considered in a patient who had recent esophageal dilatation, presents with a history of severe retching and upper abdominal or lower chest pain, or has sustained severe chest trauma.[9] Procainamide use for the past 12 months or a known diagnosis of systemic lupus erythematosus should suggest lupus pleuritis.[10] A history of Stage II or III sarcoidosis, rheumatoid disease or chronic hemodialysis (uremic pleural effusion, tuberculous pleurisy) should suggest diagnostic possibilities. Although the number of drugs associated with pleural disease is significantly less than those that are presumed to cause parenchymal lung disease, drugs should always be considered as a possible cause of pleural effusion or fibrosis. Some of the drugs that have been associated with a pleural effusion in more than a single report include bromocriptine, dantrolene, nitrofurantoin, mitomycin, practolol, procarbazine, methotrexate, mesalamine and isotretinoin[11] (see Chapter 33, Effusions caused by drugs).

PHYSICAL EXAMINATION

Pleural fluid interferes with sound transmission from the lung to the stethoscope because it separates the lung from the chest wall. The physical signs of a pleural effusion depend upon the volume of pleural fluid and the degree of lung compression. The status of the underlying lung and the patency of the bronchial tree will modulate the physical findings.

When only 250–300 cm^3 of pleural fluid is present, detection by physical examination will be problematic.[12] At a pleural fluid volume of approximately 500 cm^3, the typical physical findings are: (1) dullness to percussion; (2) decreased fremitus; and (3) normal vesicular breath sounds of decreased intensity compared with the contralateral side.[12] At a pleural fluid volume exceeding 1000 cm^3, there usually is: (1) absence of inspiratory retraction and mild bulging of the intercostal spaces; (2) decreased expansion of the ipsilateral chest wall; (3) dullness to percussion up to the level of the scapula and axilla; (4) decreased or absent fremitus posteriorly and laterally; (5) bronchovesicular breath sounds, which may be of decreased intensity at the upper level of the effusion; and (6) egophony (E to A change) at the upper level of the effusion. With more marked lung compression, auscultation may elicit bronchial breath sounds.[12] When the effusion fills the entire hemithorax (massive), physical examination will show: (1) bulging of the intracostal spaces; (2) minimal to no expansion of the ipsilateral chest wall; (3) a dull or flat percussion note over the entire hemithorax; (4) absent breath sounds over the majority of the chest with possible bronchovesicular bronchial breath sounds at the apex; (5) egophony at the upper level of the pleural effusion; and (6) a palpable liver or spleen due to significant diaphragmatic depression.[12]

DIAGNOSTIC TESTS

Radiology

The chest radiograph can provide further diagnostic insight. Specific diseases should be considered if the only abnormal radiographic finding is a pleural effusion or if the effusion is associated with other abnormalities. For example, when the only abnormality on the chest radiograph is a pleural effusion, infectious causes such as a tuberculous pleural effusion,[13] viral pleurisy[14] or a small bacterial pneumonia are possibilities. An isolated pleural effusion is more commonly observed with lupus pleuritis[4] and rheumatoid pleurisy[15] than with another thoracic manifestation of these diseases. Metastatic cancer, non-Hodgkin lymphoma, and leukemia can also present as a solitary pleural effusion. Other diseases where a pleural effusion is typically the only radiographic abnormality include BAPE,[2] pulmonary embolism,[16] drug-induced pleural disease,[11] yellow nail syndrome,[17] hypothyroidism,[18] uremic pleuritis,[19] chylothorax[20] and constrictive pericarditis.[21] When a massive effusion is present that causes contralateral mediastinal shift, the most likely diagnosis is carcinoma, usually a non-lung primary.[22] With a large or massive pleural effusion without contralateral shift, lung cancer[23] and malignant pleural mesothelioma[24] are most likely.

Solitary pleural effusions may also be associated with disease below the diaphragm.[1] Transudates from hepatic hydrothorax,[25] nephrotic syndrome,[26] urinothorax[27] and peritoneal dialysis[28] can cause this radiographic pattern. Exudates from acute[29] and chronic pancreatitis,[30] Meigs syndrome,[31] chylous ascites[32] and subphrenic,[33] hepatic[34] and splenic abscesses[35] or splenic hematomas[36] can also be causative.

Bilateral pleural effusions are most commonly transudates, as seen with congestive heart failure, nephrotic syndrome, hypoalbuminemia, peritoneal dialysis and constrictive pericarditis. The cardiac silhouette is virtually always enlarged in congestive heart failure but may be of normal size with nephrotic syndrome, other causes of hypoalbuminemia and constrictive pericarditis.[37] Bilateral exudative effusions with a normal heart size are most commonly malignant but can also be seen with lupus pleuritis and rheumatoid pleurisy.[37]

When a chest radiograph shows a pleural effusion(s) with interstitial infiltrates, the differential diagnosis includes congestive heart failure, rheumatoid disease,[15] asbestos pleuropulmonary disease,[2] lymphangitic carcinomatosis,[38] lymphangioleiomyomatosis (LAM),[39] viral and mycoplasma pneumonia,[40] sarcoidosis[41] and *Pneumocystis jiroveci* pneumonia.[42]

Pleural effusions associated with multiple nodules suggest cancer (most common), Wegener's granulomatosis,[43] rheumatoid disease,[2] septic pulmonary emboli,[44] sarcoidosis[41] and tularemia.[45]

Pleural fluid analysis

Virtually all patients with a newly discovered pleural effusion should undergo thoracentesis to assist in diagnosis and management. Exceptions would be a secure clinical diagnosis, such as typical congestive heart failure or a very small pleural effusion in a patient with presumed viral pleurisy. Observation is warranted in the above examples; however, if the clinical situation worsens or is atypical, a thoracentesis should be performed without delay. For example, if the patient with CHF has pleuritic chest pain, fever, a unilateral pleural effusion, a normal cardiac silhouette or an oxygen tension out of proportion to the clinical situation, a thoracentesis should be performed promptly.

In a prospective study of 129 patients with pleural effusions, thoracenteses provided a definitive diagnosis (i.e. malignancy) in only 18 percent of patients and a presumptive diagnosis (i.e. CHF) in 55 percent of patients.[46] In the remaining 27 percent of patients, the pleural fluid findings were not helpful diagnostically because the values were compatible with two or more clinical possibilities; however, in a number of these patients, the findings were useful in excluding possible diagnoses, such as empyema. Therefore, the clinician must assess the history and physical examination, radiological evaluation and ancillary blood tests in establishing a pre-thoracentesis diagnosis so that the pleural fluid findings can provide a confident, clinical diagnosis if the results are not definitive. With a more complete knowledge of pleural fluid analysis, the cases of undiagnosed pleural effusions should continue to decrease.

A definitive diagnosis can only be established by pleural fluid analysis in a limited number of diseases that include empyema, malignancy, chylothorax, rheumatoid pleurisy, and others[47] (Table 16.3).

If the pleural effusion is clearly a transudate (see Chapter 17, Pleural fluid analysis), with low protein and lactate dehydrogenase (LDH) values, the diagnosis is limited and usually easily discernible from the patient's clinical presentation. Most transudates are due to CHF with the next most common (but much less frequent)

Table 16.3 Diagnoses that can be established definitively by pleural fluid analysis

Diseases	Diagnostic pleural fluid tests
Empyema	Observation (pus, putrid odor); culture
Malignancy	Positive cytology
Lupus pleuritis	LE cells present
Tuberculous pleural effusion	Positive AFB stain, culture; ADA >40–60 U/L
Esophageal rupture	High salivary amylase, pleural fluid acidosis (often as low as 6.00); presence of food particles or squamous epithelial cells
Fungal pleurisy	Positive KOH stain, culture
Cholesterol effusion	Cholesterol >300 mg/dL; cholesterol/triglyceride >1.0; cholesterol crystals
Chylothorax	Triglycerides >110 mg/dL; chylomicrons present
Hemothorax	Hematocrit (pleural fluid/blood ratio >0.5)
Urinothorax	Creatinine (pleural fluid/serum ratio >1.0)
Peritoneal dialysis	Protein <1.0 g/dL; glucose >300 mg/dL
Extravascular migration of a central venous catheter	Observation (milky if lipids are infused) pleural fluid/serum glucose substantially >1.0 (glucose infusion)
Rheumatoid pleurisy	Characteristic cytology diagnostic (pH <7.00, glucose <30 mg/dL; LDH >1000 IU/L)
Duro-pleural fistula	Presence of β_2-transferrin

LE, lupus erythematosus; AFB, acid-fast bacilli; ADA, adenosine deaminase; LDH, lactate dehydrogenase.
From Sahn SA.[47]

cause being hepatic hydrothorax. An exudative pleural effusion, in contrast, has a much larger differential diagnosis of over 50 causes (see Chapter 17). Transudative effusions are caused by imbalances in hydrostatic and oncotic pressures with normal pleurae, while exudative effusions are the result of inflammatory processes, malignancy and lymphatic abnormalities.

The differential diagnosis of the exudate may be further narrowed by complete pleural fluid analysis. If the pleural fluid pH is <7.30 with a normal blood pH, the exudative effusion essentially can be limited to six diagnoses[48,49] (see Chapter 17). These include a complicated parapneumonic effusion or empyema (most common), malignancy, esophageal rupture, rheumatoid pleurisy, lupus pleuritis and tuberculous pleural effusion. Rare causes of a low pH exudative pleural effusion are herniated bowel with infarction[50] and a large hemothorax with an abnormal pleura.[48] The only singular cause of a transudate with a low pH is urinothorax, which is associated with ipsilateral obstructive uropathy.[51] The same differential associated with a low pleural fluid pH is found with a low pleural fluid glucose (<60 mg/dL or a pleural fluid/serum ratio of <0.5)[52] (see Chapter 17).

The presence of ≥80 percent lymphocytes or ≥10 percent eosinophils of the total pleural fluid nucleated cell count is found with a limited number of diseases[47] (see Chapter 17); a tuberculous pleural effusion is the most common diagnosis associated with marked lymphocytosis and hemothorax is most prevalent with eosinophilia.

It has been suggested that if the clinical likelihood of a transudative effusion is high, only total protein and LDH should initially be measured and fluid for other chemistries and cell counts saved by the laboratory.[53] If the protein and LDH are low (total protein <3.0 gm/dL or pleural fluid/serum ratio <0.5,[54–56] or pleural fluid LDH <0.67[54,55] or <0.82[56] of the upper limits of normal of the serum LDH), further testing is unnecessary. If the fluid is exudative, additional tests can be performed on the pleural fluid saved by the laboratory. Using this algorithm, there can be significant savings for the patient. If the preclinical diagnosis suggests an exudative effusion, most commonly from pneumonia, malignancy or pulmonary embolism, total cell count with differential and pH or glucose should be determined. If pancreatic disease or malignancy is in the differential, amylase concentration should be determined. If there is clinical suspicion of rheumatoid pleurisy or lupus pleuritis, rheumatoid factor and a search for lupus erythematosus (LE) cells, respectively, should be assessed. If chylothorax or a cholesteroal effusion is a consideration or the fluid is milky or turbid, the fluid should be centrifuged; if the supernatant remains milky or cloudy, cholesterol and triglycerides should be measured. Since it is rare for a malignant effusion to be transudative, cytology does not need to be ordered routinely unless, for example, the patient is elderly and has concomitant CHF. Cytology should be ordered in most patients with unilateral and those with bilateral exudative effusions and a normal heart size, if they are over 40 years of age, have a history of cancer or the diagnosis is uncertain. Gram, fungal and acid-fast bacilli (AFB) stains and corresponding cultures should be obtained in all exudates where infection is likely based on the clinical presentation.

TIME TO RESOLUTION

Knowledge of the time of resolution, either spontaneous or with therapy, of pleural effusions can be helpful diagnostically[57] (Table 16.4). For example, an effusion from a pulmonary embolism rarely persists for more than 1 month,[16] BAPE may not resolve for 2–6 months,[58–60] tuberculous pleural effusions resolve over 1–4 months[61] and effusions from yellow nail syndrome[62] and trapped lung are persistent.[63]

UNDIAGNOSED EFFUSIONS

In the patient with an undiagnosed exudative pleural effusion following the initial pleural fluid analysis including cytology and cultures, the options include observation, repeat thoracentesis with or without percutaneous pleural biopsy and medical or video-assisted thoracic surgery (VATS). The most likely causes of an undiagnosed effusion are early-stage malignancy (cancer and lymphoma (usually Hodgkin's lymphoma) and mesothelioma), less commonly tuberculosis, and benign persistent effusions from yellow nail syndrome, trapped lung, constrictive pericarditis or drug-induced pleural effusions.

Whether or not the patient with a tuberculous pleural effusion is treated with anti-tuberculosis medications, the effusion will resolve in 4–16 weeks, unless lung entrapment develops; however, the untreated patient has a 65 percent chance of developing active pulmonary or extrapulmonary tuberculosis within the next 5 years.[61] Culture of pleural fluid and tissue from pleural biopsy and pleural tissue histology should establish the diagnosis of tuberculosis in 75–80 percent of cases.[64] If the aforementioned studies are negative and the pleural fluid is a lymphocytic (usually >80 percent) exudate and the patient is PPD (purified protein derivative) positive, the patient should be treated for tuberculosis. If the patient has a negative PPD skin test, it should be repeated in 6–8 weeks; if positive, treatment should be given. With a negative repeat skin test, the pleural fluid should be studied with flow cytometry to evaluate for lymphoma.

If the patient has a pleural malignancy, a repeat thoracentesis a few weeks later will increase the yield of a positive cytology, as the disease has become more advanced. Pleural fluid carcinoembryonic antigen (CEA) has a high (85 percent) diagnostic accuracy in diagnosing a carcinomatous pleural effusion.[65] If the patient or physician wants to establish the diagnosis sooner, an experienced thoracoscopist will be able to diagnose malignancy in 95 percent of cases.

The pleural fluid from pulmonary embolism is present on admission to the hospital, is small in volume (less than one-third of the hemithorax), peaks at 72 hours and resolves within 7–10 days when radiographic infarction is not present.[16] When radiographic infarction (consolidation) is visualized, the effusion will also peak by 72 hours but will not resolve completely for 2–3 weeks.[16]

If an undiagnosed effusion is persistent and relatively unchanged for several months or years, malignancy is less likely and trapped lung, yellow nail syndrome, other lymphatic abnormalities or a cholesterol effusion should be considered. A trapped lung is a unilateral effusion of variable size that, following thoracentesis, will return to its pre-procedure volume within a few days. The initial pleural liquid pressure is typically negative and the pleural space elastance is increased (>15 cmH_2O/L of fluid removed).[63] Pleural fluid analysis with trapped lung typically reveals a serous lymphocyte-predominant transudate; however, the protein concentration may be >3.0 g/dL if the initial pleural injury is not completely resolved. The pleural fluid from yellow nail syndrome is a lymphocyte-predominant (≥80 percent) exudate and may be associated with slow-growing yellow nails and lymphedema or may

Table 16.4 Resolution of pleural effusions by time intervals

<2 months	2–6 months	6 months to 1 year	Benign persistent
Acute pancreatitis	BAPE	BAPE	Cholesterol effusion (lung entrapment)
CABG surgery	CABG surgery	Rheumatoid pleurisy	LAM (chylothorax)
CHF	Chronic pancreatic effusion		Lymphangiectasia
Lupus pleuritis	PCIS		Noonan's syndrome (chylothorax)
Parapneumonic effusion	Rheumatoid pleurisy		Trapped lung
PCIS	Sarcoidosis		YNS
Post lung/heart/liver transplant	Tuberculous effusion		
Pulmonary embolism			
Sarcoidosis			
Traumatic chylothorax			
Uremic pleural effusion			

BAPE, benign asbestos pleural effusion; CABG, coronary artery bypass graft; LAM, lymphangioleiomyomatosis; CHF, congestive heart failure; PCIS, postcardiac injury syndrome; YNS, yellow nail syndrome.
From Cohen M, Sahn SA.[57]

be the initial manifestation.[62] The pleural fluid in yellow nail syndrome is often a discordant exudate with a consistently high protein concentration and a variable (low or high) LDH.

By utilizing all available information from the history, physical examination, chest radiograph and computed tomography (CT) scan, initial pleural fluid analysis and time to resolution, a diagnosis should be established either definitively or presumptively in over 95 percent of cases. In the remaining patients, an experienced thoracoscopist can make the diagnosis of malignancy in more than 95 percent of cases.[66] Tuberculous pleural effusion can also be diagnosed readily by thoracoscopy, but the diagnosis can usually be established by pleural fluid and tissue culture and histology following percutaneous pleural biopsy. A pleural fluid adenosine deaminase (ADA) >40–60 U/L[67] supports the diagnosis if empyema and rheumatoid pleurisy have been excluded.

FUTURE DIRECTIONS

With a more comprehensive knowledge of pleural fluid analysis in conjunction with all available clinical information to formulate a pre-test diagnosis, the number of patients with an undiagnosed effusion should continue to diminish. As new biochemical, cytological and molecular biological tests are developed and incorporated into analysis of pleural effusions, the frequency of undiagnosed pleural effusions should decrease further. Large, prospective studies of pleural fluid analysis in patients with clearly established diagnoses should enhance the presumptive diagnostic value of pleural fluid analysis and thereby avoid the necessity of repeat thoracentesis or thoracoscopy. As more pulmonologists develop expertise in thoracoscopy, enhanced by improved instrumentation, it should be a rare occurrence to encounter a patient with an unexplained pleural effusion.

KEY POINTS

- A definitive diagnosis can be established by pleural fluid analysis in a limited number of disease states.
- Pleural fluid analysis is most helpful when the likelihood of a clinical diagnosis is high, based on the history, physical examination, chest radiograph and laboratory tests.
- On chest radiograph, finding a solitary pleural effusion, massive effusion, bilateral effusions or associated interstitial disease or nodules narrows the pre-thoracentesis diagnosis.
- Finding a transudative effusion limits the differential diagnosis, which is easily discernible from the clinical presentation.
- The differential diagnosis of the exudative effusion can be narrowed by finding a pleural fluid pH <7.30 or a pleural fluid/serum glucose ratio <0.5, a pleural fluid lymphocytosis >80 percent or pleural fluid eosinophilia.
- Non-malignant pleural effusions that persist for more than 1 year are found with trapped lung, yellow nail syndrome, lymphangiectasia and cholesterol effusion (a form of lung entrapment).
- The most likely causes of undiagnosed pleural effusions are early-stage malignancy and chronic benign persistent effusions, particularly yellow nail syndrome, trapped lung and drug-induced pleural effusion.

REFERENCES

● = Key primary paper
◆ = Major review article

1. Lorch DG, Sahn SA. Pleural effusions due to diseases below the diaphragm. *Sem Respir Med* 1987; **9**: 75–85.
●2. Epler GR, McLoud TC, Gaensler EA. Prevalence and incidence of benign asbestos pleural effusion in a working population. *J Am Med Assoc* 1982; **247**: 617–22.
3. Carr DT, Mayne JG. Pleurisy with effusion in rheumatoid arthritis, with reference to the low concentration of glucose in pleural fluid. *Am Rev Respir Dis* 1962; **85**: 345–50.
●4. Good JT Jr, King TE, Antony VB, Sahn SA. Lupus pleuritis: clinical features and pleural fluid characteristics with special reference to pleural fluid antinuclear antibody titers. *Chest* 1983; **84**: 714–18.
5. Estenne M, Yernault JC, Detroyer A. Mechanism of relief of dyspnea after thoracentesis in patients with large pleural effusions. *Am J Med* 1983; **74**: 813–19.
6. Anthonisen NR, Martin RR. Regional lung function in pleural effusion. *Am Rev Respir Dis* 1977; **116**: 201–7.
7. Sahn SA, Heffner JE. Approach to the patient with pleurisy. In: Kelley WN (ed). *Textbook of internal medicine*. Philadelphia: JB Lippincott Co, 1991: 1887–90.
●8. Stelzner TJ, King TE, Antony VB, Sahn SA. The pleuropulmonary manifestations of the postcardiac injury syndrome. *Chest* 1983; **84**: 383–7.
9. Triggiani E, Belsey R. Oesophageal trauma: incidence, diagnosis, and management. *Thorax* 1977; **32**: 241–9.
10. Henningsen NC, Cederberg A, Hanson A, *et al.* Effects of long-term treatment with procainamide: a prospective study with special regard to ANF and SLE in fast and slow acetylators. *Acta Med Scand* 1975; **198**: 475–82.
◆11. Sahn SA. Drug-induced pleural disease. In: Camus P, Rosenau E (eds). *Drug-induced and iatrogenic lung disease*. London: Hodder Arnold; 2009, in press.
12. Hopkins HU. *Principles and methods of physical diagnosis*, 3rd ed. Philadelphia: W.B. Saunders, 1965.
◆13. Gopi A, Madhavan SM, Sharma SK, Sahn SA. Diagnosis and treatment of tuberculous pleural effusion in 2006. *Chest* 2007; **131**: 874–9.
14. Alptekin F. An epidemic of pleurisy with effusion in Bitlis, Turkey: a study of 559 cases. *US Arm Forces Med J* 1958; **9**: 1–11.
●15. Walker WC, Wright V. Pulmonary lesions in rheumatoid arthritis. *Medicine* 1968; **47**: 501–19.
●16. Bynum LJ, Wilson JE III. Radiographic features of pleural effusions in pulmonary embolism. *Am Rev Respir Dis* 1978; **117**: 829–34.

17. Hiller E, Rosenow E, Olsen A. Pulmonary manifestations of the yellow nail syndrome. *Chest* 1972; **61**: 452–8.
18. Gottehrer A, Roa J, Stanford GG, *et al.* Hypothyroidism and pleural effusions. *Chest* 1990; **98**: 1130–2.
●19. Berger HW, Rammohan G, Neff MS, Buhain WJ. Uremic pleural effusion. A study in 14 patients on chronic dialysis. *Ann Intern Med* 1975; **82**: 362–4.
20. Reeder MM, Felson B. *Gamuts in radiology.* Cincinnati: Audiovisual Radiology, 1975.
●21. Tomasilli G, Gamsu G, Stulbarg MS. Constrictive pericarditis presenting as pleural effusion of unknown origin. *Arch Intern Med* 1989; **149**: 201–3.
22. Maher GG, Berger HW. Massive pleural effusions: malignant and non-malignant causes in 46 patients. *Am Rev Respir Dis* 1972; **105**: 458–60.
23. Lieberson M. Diagnostic significance of the mediastinal profile in massive unilateral pleural effusions. *Am Rev Respir Dis* 1963; **88**: 176–80.
24. Heller RM, Janower ML, Weber AL. The radiological manifestations of malignant pleural mesothelioma. *Am J Roentgenol* 1971; **108**: 53–9.
●25. Lieberman FL, Hidemura R, Peters RL, Reynolds TB. Pathogenesis in treatment of hydrothorax complicating cirrhosis with ascites. *Ann Intern Med* 1966; **64**: 341–51.
26. Cavina C, Vichi G. Radiological aspects of pleural effusions in medical nephropathy in children. *Ann Radiol Diagn* 1958; **31**: 163–202.
●27. Stark DD, Shanes JG, Baron RL, Roach DD. Biochemical features of urinothorax. *Arch Intern Med* 1982; **42**: 1505–11.
28. Bargman JM. Complications of peritoneal dialysis related to increased intra-abdominal pressure. *Kidney Intl* 1993; **43**: S75–80.
29. Kaye MD. Pleuropulmonary complications of pancreatitis. *Thorax* 1968; **23**: 297–306.
30. Anderson WJ, Skinner DB, Zuidema GD, *et al.* A chronic pancreatic pleural effusion. *Surg Gynecol Obstet* 1973; **137**: 827–30.
31. Majzlin G, Stevens FL. Meigs' syndrome: case report and review of literature. *J Int Coll Surg* 1964; **42**: 623–30.
32. Press OW, Press NO, Kaufman SD. Evaluation and management of chylous ascites. *Ann Intern Med* 1982; **96**: 358–64.
33. De Cosse JJ, Poulin TL, Fox PS, Condon RE. Subphrenic abscess. *Surg Gynecol Obstet* 1974; **138**: 841–6.
34. Rubin RH, Swartz MN, Malt R. Hepatic abscess: changes in clinical, biologic, and therapeutic aspects. *Am J Med* 1974; **57**: 601–10.
35. Chun CH, Raff MF, Contreras L, *et al.* Splenic abscess. *Medicine* 1980; **59**: 50–64.
36. Koehler PR, Jones R. Association of left-sided pleural effusions in splenic hematomas. *AJR Am J Roentgenol* 1980; **135**: 851–3.
●37. Rabin CB, Blackman NS. Bilateral plerual effusions. Its significance in association with a heart of normal size. *J Mt Sinai Hosp* 1957; **24**: 45–53.
38. Janower ML, Blennerhassett JB. Lymphangetic spread of metastatic cancer to the lung: a radiologic–pathologic classification. *Radiology* 1971; **101**: 267–73.
●39. Taylor JR, Ryu J, Colby TV, Raffin TA. Lymphangioleiomyomatosis. Clinical course in 32 patients. *N Engl J Med* 1990; **323**: 1254–60.
40. Fine NL, Smith LR, Sheedy PF. Frequency of pleural effusions in mycoplasma and viral pneumonias. *N Engl J Med* 1970; **283**: 790–3.
41. Huggins JT, Doelken P, Sahn SA, *et al.* Pleural effusions in a series of 181 outpatients with sarcoidosis. *Chest* 2006; **129**: 1599–604.
42. Horowitz ML, Schiff M, Samuels J, *et al. Pneumocystis carinii* pleural effusion. Pathogenesis and pleural fluid analysis. *Am Rev Respir Dis* 1993; **148**: 232–4.
43. Maguire R, Fauci AS, Doppman JL, *et al.* Unusual radiographic features of Wegener's granulomatosis. *AJR Am J Roentgenol* 1978; **130**: 233–8.
44. Gumbs RV, McCauley DI. Hilar and mediastinal adenopathy in septic pulmonary embolic disease. *Radiology* 1982; **142**: 313–15.
45. Rubin SA. Radiographic spectrum of pleuropulmonary tularemia. *AJR Am J Roentgenol* 1978; **131**: 277–81.
●46. Collins TR, Sahn SA. Thoracentesis: complications, patient experience and diagnostic value. *Chest* 1987; **91**: 817–22.
47. Sahn SA. Diagnostic value of pleural fluid analysis. *Sem Respir Crit Care Med* 1995; **16**: 269–78.
●48. Good JT, Taryle DA, Maulitz RM, *et al.* The diagnostic value of pleural fluid pH. *Chest* 1980; **78**: 55–59.
◆49. Sahn SA. Pleural fluid pH in the normal state and in diseases affecting the pleural space. In: Chritein J, Bignon J, Hirsch A (eds). *The pleura in health and disease.* New York: Marcel Dekker, 1985: 253–66.
50. Sahn SA, Collins DD. Pleural fluid acidosis and diagphragmatic hernia. *Ann Intern Med* 1982; **96**: 380–1.
51. Miller KS, Wooten S, Sahn SA. Urinothorax: a cause of a low pH transudate. *Am J Med* 1988; **85**: 448–9.
◆52. Sahn SA. Pathogenesis and clinical features of diseases associated with a low pleural fluid glucose. In: Chretein J, Bignon J, Hirsch A (eds). *The pleura in health and disease.* New York: Marcel Dekker, 1985: 267–85.
53. Peterman TA, Speicher CE. Evaluating pleural effusions. A two-stage laboratory approach. *J Am Med Assoc* 1984; **252**: 1051–3.
●54. Light RW, MacGregor I, Luchsinger PC, Ball WC Jr. Pleural effusion: the diagnostic separation of transudates and exudates. *Ann Intern Med* 1972; **77**: 507–13.
●55. Heffner JE, Brown LK, Barbieri C. Diagnostic value of tests that discriminate between exudative and transudative pleural effusions. *Chest* 1997; **111**: 970–9.
56. Joseph J, Badrinath P, Basran G, Sahn SA. Is the pleural fluid transudate or exudate? A revisit of the diagnostic criteria. *Thorax* 2001; **56**: 867–70.
●57. Cohen M, Sahn SA. Resolution of pleural effusions. *Chest* 2001; **119**: 1547–62.
58. Hillerdal G, Ozesmi M. Benign asbestos pleural effusion: 73 exudates in 60 patients. *Eur J Respir Dis* 1987; **71**: 113–21.
59. Mattson SB. Monosymptomatic exudative pleurisy in persons exposed to asbestos dust. *Scand J Respir Dis* 1997; **56**: 263–72.
60. Robinson BWS, Musk AW. Benign asbestos pleural effusion: diagnosis and course. *Thorax* 1981; **36**: 896–900.
●61. Roper WH, Waring JJ. Primary serofibrinous pleural effusion in military personnel. *Am Rev Tuberc* 1955; **71**: 616–35.
●62. Nordkild P, Kromann-Andersen H, Struve-Christsen E. Yellow nail syndrome – the triad of yellow nails, lymph edema, and pleural effusions. *Acta Med Scand* 1986; **219**: 221–27.
63. Huggins JT, Sahn SA, Heidecker J, *et al.* Characteristics of trapped lung: Pleural fluid analysis, manometry, and air-contrast CT. *Chest* 2007; **131**: 206–13.
64. Ferrer J. Pleural tuberculosis. *Eur Respir J* 1997; **10**: 942–7.
65. Shitrit D, Zingerman B, Shitrit A, *et al.* Diagnostic value of CYFRA-21, CEA, CA 19-9, CA 15-3 and CA 125 assays in pleural effusions: Analysis of 116 cases and review of the literature. *Oncologist* 2007; **10**: 501–7.
◆66. Loddenkemper R. Thoracoscopy – State of the art. *Eur Respir J* 1998; **11**: 213–21.
67. Kataria YP, Khurshid I. Adenosine deaminase in the diagnosis of tuberculous pleural effusion. *Chest* 2001; **120**: 334–6.

17

Pleural fluid analysis

STEVEN A SAHN, JOHN E HEFFNER

Because pleural effusions can be caused by diseases in the chest, organ dysfunction or infections below the diaphragm, drugs[1] and systemic disease, it is not surprising that there is an estimated 1.3 million new cases of pleural effusions annually in the USA.[2] Approximately two-thirds of these effusions result from congestive heart failure (CHF), pneumonia, malignancy and pulmonary embolism.

Clinicians may first suspect a pleural effusion on physical examination or become aware of its presence on a standard chest radiograph. If a standard radiograph is only suggestive of a pleural effusion, a lateral decubitus film or pleural ultrasound may be confirmatory. Once the presence of a pleural effusion is established, in most instances a diagnostic thoracentesis should be performed to assess the characteristics and cause of the pleural fluid. If the fluid is free flowing and at least of moderate size, the physical examination can safely guide thoracentesis. If uncertainty exists, ultrasound-guided thoracentesis should be carried out, which will increase the safety of the procedure.[3]

Not all patients with pleural effusions require a diagnostic thoracentesis. For example, if the patient has the classic presentation of CHF, appropriate treatment can be instituted and the patient's course closely observed. However, if the patient presents with atypical features for CHF, such as fever and pleuritic chest pain, or unusual radiographic findings, such as a unilateral effusion, bilateral effusions of disparate size, left effusion greater than right effusion, or a normal heart size, diagnostic thoracentesis should be performed without delay. Another example of appropriate watchful waiting is in a patient with a viral syndrome with pleuritic chest pain and a small pleural effusion that can only be demonstrated clearly on a lateral decubitus radiograph or ultrasonography. Observation is also warranted in any clinically stable patient with a very small pleural effusion; if the patient's clinical condition progresses, the effusion usually will increase in volume and thoracentesis can be performed safely.

APPEARANCE

A diagnosis can be established at the bedside by visual examination of the pleural fluid as it is aspirated from the pleural space. The color, character and odor of the fluid may be either diagnostic or helpful in diagnosis (Table 17.1) A clear, straw-colored fluid suggests a transudate but also may be seen in pauci-cellular exudates. A serosanguinous appearance typically signifies a pleural fluid hematocrit <1 percent and is diagnostically unhelpful. However, a grossly bloody effusion narrows the differential diagnosis to malignancy, benign asbestos pleural effusion (BAPE), post-cardiac injury syndrome (PCIS), pulmonary infarction and trauma. A hemothorax, which is most commonly due to trauma,[4] may also occur with invasive procedures,[5] metastatic disease to the pleura, anticoagulation in the setting of a pulmonary infarction[6] and catamenial hemothorax.[7] To diagnose a hemothorax, the pleural fluid hematocrit should be compared with the blood hematocrit; if the pleural fluid hematocrit is at least 50 percent of the peripheral blood hematocrit, a

Table 17.1 Observations of pleural fluid helpful in diagnosis

	Suggested diagnosis
Color of fluid	
Pale yellow (straw)	Transudate, pauci-cellular exudate
Red (bloody)	
Hematocrit <5%	Malignancy, BAPE, PCIS, pulmonary infarction
Hematocrit PF/S ≥0.5	Trauma
White (milky)	Chylothorax or cholesterol effusion
Brown	Long-standing bloody effusion; rupture of amebic liver abscess into pleural space
Black	Spores of *Aspergillus niger*
Yellow-green	Rheumatoid pleurisy
Color of enteral tube	
Feeding or central	
Venous line infusate	Feeding tube has entered pleural space; extravascular catheter migration into mediastinum/pleural space
Character of fluid	
Pus	Empyema
Viscous	Mesothelioma
Debris	Rheumatoid pleurisy
Turbid	Inflammatory exudate or lipid effusion
Anchovy paste	Amebic liver abscess rupture
Odor of fluid	
Putrid	Anaerobic empyema
Ammonia	Urinothorax

BAPE, benign asbestos pleural effusion; PCIS, post-cardiac injury syndrome; PF, pleural fluid; S, serum.

hemothorax is defined and chest tube drainage should be performed without delay.

Withdrawing a white or milky fluid from the pleural space diagnoses either a chylothorax or a cholesterol effusion; occasionally an empyema may simulate this appearance. Centrifugation of the fluid will separate a lipid effusion from an empyema; in the lipid effusion, the supernatant will remain white while with empyema suspended cells settle and the supernatant clears.

A pleural effusion that appears brown usually represents a long-standing bloody effusion, while brownish fluid that is viscous in nature may represent an amebic liver abscess that has ruptured into the pleural space;[8] the fluid of amebiasis represents a combination of blood, small pieces of liver parenchyma and cytolysed liver tissue. Black pleural fluid suggests *Aspergillus niger* infection,[9] while a yellow-green tint has been observed in some patients with rheumatoid pleural effusion.[10] If an enteral feeding tube has entered the pleural space, the pleural fluid color will mirror that of the feeding solution.[11] Likewise, if a central venous catheter has migrated out of the vasculature and into the mediastinum, the pleural fluid will be similar in color and composition to the infusate (white if lipid is infused).[12]

The character of the fluid will also suggest a diagnosis. If pus is aspirated, an empyema is established. Pus is best described as a thick, viscous, yellow-white, opaque fluid. If the pus has a putrid odor, anaerobic organisms are usually present. When the pleural fluid appears to contain debris, rheumatoid pleurisy with exfoliation of portions of rheumatoid nodules from the visceral pleural surface into the pleural space is likely causative.[13] Anchovy-paste appearing pleural fluid is virtually diagnostic of an amebic liver abscess that has ruptured into the pleural space. When pleural fluid smells of ammonia, the diagnosis of urinothorax, which is caused by obstructive uropathy, is established.[14]

EXUDATIVE VERSUS TRANSUDATIVE

After gross inspection of pleural fluid obtained by thoracentesis, classification of a pleural effusion as a transudate or exudate by chemical testing represents the initial step in determining the cause of an effusion.[15] A broad array of underlying conditions cause exudative effusions (Table 17.2), while a limited number of disorders cause transudates (Table 17.3). It is important to categorize effusions accurately because exudates and transudates present different diagnostic and therapeutic implications. The presence of an exudative effusion, for instance, may warrant

Table 17.2 Causes of exudative pleural effusions

Causes		
Infectious	**Malignancy**	**Connective tissue disease**
Bacterial pneumonia	Carcinoma	Lupus pleuritis
Tuberculous effusion	Lymphoma	Rheumatoid pleurisy
Fungal disease	Mesothelioma	Mixed connective tissue disease
Atypical pneumonias	Leukemia	Sjögren syndrome
Nocardia, Actinomyces	Chylothorax	
Subphrenic abscess		
Hepatic abscess	**Other inflammatory**	**Endocrine dysfunction**
Splenic abscess	Pancreatitis	Hypothyroidism
Hepatitis	BAPE	Ovarian hyperstimulation syndrome
Spontaneous esophageal rupture	Pulmonary infarction	
Parasites	**Radiation therapy**	**Lymphatic abnormalities**
	Sarcoidosis	Malignancy
Iatrogenic	PCIS	Chylothorax
Drug-induced	Hemothorax	Yellow nail syndrome
Esophageal perforation	ARDS	Lymphangiomyomatosis (chylothorax)
Esophageal sclerotherapy	Cholesterol effusion	Lymphangiectasis
Central venous catheter misplacement/migration		
Enteral feeding tube in pleural space	**Increased negative intrapleural pressure**	**Movement of fluid from abdomen to pleural space**
	Atelectasis	Acute pancreatitis
Vasculitis	Trapped lung	Pancreatic pseudocyst
Wegener granulomatosis		Meigs syndrome
Churg–Strauss syndrome		Carcinoma
Familial Mediterranean fever		Chylous ascites

ARDS, acute respiratory distress syndrome; BAPE, benign asbestos pleural effusion; PCIS, post-cardiac injury syndrome.

Table 17.3 Causes of transudative pleural effusions

Diagnosis	Comment
Congestive heart failure	Acute diuresis can increase pleural fluid protein and LDH concentrations
Cirrhosis	Uncommon without clinical ascites
Nephrotic syndrome	Typically small and bilateral; unilateral, larger effusion may be due to pulmonary embolism
Peritoneal dialysis	Large right effusion may develop within 48 hours of initiating dialysis
Hypoalbuminemia	Edema fluid rarely isolated to pleural space; small bilateral effusions
Urinothorax	Unilateral effusion caused by ipsilateral obstructive uropathy
Atelectasis	Small effusion caused by increased intrapleural negative pressure; common in ICU patients
Constrictive pericarditis	Bilateral effusions with normal heart size
Trapped lung	Unilateral effusion from imbalance in hydrostatic pressures from a remote inflammatory process
Superior vena caval obstruction	Due to acute systemic venous hypertension or acute obstruction of lymphatics
Duropleural fistula	Cerebrospinal fluid in pleural space; β_2-transferrin diagnostic

ICU, intensive care unit; LDH, lactate dehydrogenase.

pleural biopsy or pleural space drainage because of the high incidence of underlying malignant and infectious conditions. In contrast, most patients with transudates have clinically apparent systemic disorders as the cause of their effusions, which frequently resolve with treatment of these conditions, such as with diuretic therapy for heart failure.

Pleural fluid tests that discriminate exudates from transudates measure the concentration of large molecular weight constituents in pleural fluid (Table 17.3). Because exudative effusions typically result from increased permeability and passage between mesothelial cells, these large molecules can enter the pleural space or undergo release from intrapleural inflammatory or neoplastic cells. In contrast, transudative effusions result from hydrostatic mechanisms and have lower concentrations of large molecular weight constituents because intact pleural membranes act as a diffusion barrier to these compounds.

Various pleural fluid testing strategies reported in the literature recommend either a single pleural fluid test result or multiple tests combined in diagnostic rules to establish the presence of an exudate. The multi-test strategies combine test results in 'or' rules, which means that any one of multiple test results can diagnose an exudative effusion if the single result exceeds a certain limit. As with any diagnostic test, combining multiple tests in an 'or-rule,' increases sensitivity with the inevitable consequence of decreasing specificity.[16,17] Single test results, therefore, should be used when the goal is to increase specificity and thereby 'rule in' an exudative effusion. Multiple tests combined with in 'or-rules' increase sensitivity and help clinicians to 'rule out' an exudative effusion if the test result is negative for an exudate. A positive result of a multiple test strategy, however, has a decreased positive predictive value for identifying exudative effusions. In most circumstances, clinicians would favor an initial multi-test screening strategy with a high sensitivity for evaluating patients with new onset pleural effusions because of the importance of not missing an exudative effusion, which carries important prognostic considerations.

Light's criteria comprise a three-test strategy that screens patients for exudates by measuring pleural fluid and concurrent serum concentrations of protein and lactate dehydrogenase (LDH). Test results are combined into three criteria: (1) pleural fluid to serum protein ratio; (2) pleural fluid to serum LDH ratio; and (3) pleural fluid LDH concentration relative to the laboratory's upper limit of normal for serum LDH.[18] An exudative effusion is defined by the presence of any one of the following criteria: a pleural fluid to serum protein ratio >0.5, pleural fluid to serum LDH ratio >0.6 or a pleural fluid LDH concentration > two-thirds the laboratory's upper limit of normal for serum. Aggregate data from a meta-analysis of multiple studies demonstrates that Light's criteria has a sensitivity of 98 percent and specificity of 74 percent in identifying exudative effusions.[19]

Other tests have been reported to have good discriminating properties for identifying exudative versus transudative effusions (Table 17.4). These tests include pleural fluid cholesterol,[20–25] albumin,[26] protein[27,28] and adenosine deaminase [29] used as single tests or combined with serum results to calculate a ratio or gradient. Although multiple reports have compared these single tests with the Light's criteria multi-test strategy to determine their relative diagnostic performance, the inevitable effects of test combinations to increase sensitivity and decrease specificity have been largely overlooked. As would be expected, most of these studies with Light's criteria report a higher sensitivity and lower specificity compared with each of the individual test strategies.

A meta-analysis was used to examine the comparative diagnostic accuracies of the available individual tests and multi-test strategies commonly used in clinical practice for discriminating between exudates and transudates.[19] This analysis reported that all of the individual pleural fluid tests, except for pleural fluid bilirubin, had similar diagnostic operating characteristics (Table 17.5). Other investigators have recently confirmed the similar performance of individual tests commonly used in clinical practice.[28,30] This result would be expected because the evaluated pleural tests share a common approach for detecting exudates, which is the measurement of large molecular weight pleural fluid constituents.

Because all of the individual pleural fluid tests, except for bilirubin, had similar operating characteristics in the meta-analysis by Heffner and colleagues,[19] their combination in various multi-test combination 'or-rules' had similar overall diagnostic accuracy compared with Light's

Table 17.4 Cut-off points derived from a meta-analysis of pooled data and cut-off points commonly recommended by individual studies

Pleural fluid test	Meta-analysis ROC cutoff point[5]	Previously reported cutoff points
P-PF	>2.9 g/dL	>3 g/dL[42]
P-R	>0.5	>0.5[18]
LDH-PF	>0.45% of upper limits of serum normal	>2/3 of upper limits of serum normal[41]
		>81% upper limits of serum normal [30]
LDH-R	>0.6	>0.6 [18]
C-PF	>45 mg/dL	>45 mg/dL[20]
		>54 mg/dL[23]
		>55 mg dL[43]
		>60 mg/dL[21,22]
C-R	>0.3	>0.3 [21–24]
A-G	≤1.2 g/dL	≤1.2 g/dL[44, 45]
P-G	Not assessed	≤3.1 g/dL[27,28]

P-PF, pleural fluid protein; P-R, pleural fluid to serum protein ratio; LDH-PF, pleural fluid LDH; LDH-R, pleural fluid to serum LDH ratio; C-PF, pleural fluid cholesterol; C-R, pleural fluid to serum cholesterol ratio; A-G, serum to pleural fluid albumin gradient;[19] P-G, serum to pleural protein gradient.[27,28]

Table 17.5 Operating characteristics of tests that identify exudates

Pleural fluid test	Sensitivity, % (95% CI)	Specificity, % (95% CI)	AUC (95% CI)
P-PF	91.5	83.0	94.2
n = 1187 (19)	(89.3 to 93.7)	(77.6 to 88.4)	(92.6 to 95.9)
P-R	89.5	90.9	95.4
n = 1393 (19)	(87.4 to 91.6)	(87.4 to 94.5)	(94.3 to 96.7)
LDH-PF	88.0	81.8	93.3
n = 1438 (19)	(85.8 to 90.3)	(77.1 to 86.6)	(91.8 to 94.8)
LDH-R	91.4	85.0	94.7
n = 1388 (19)	(89.4 to 93.3)	(80.6 to 89.4)	(93.4 to 96.0)
C-PF	89.0	81.4	93.3
n = 1348 (19)	(86.8 to 91.2)	(76.6 to 86.2)	(91.7 to 94.8)
C-R	92.0	81.4	94.1
n = 1123 (19)	(90.1 to 93.9)	(76.6 to 86.2)	(92.5 to 95.7)
A-G	86.8	91.8	94.0
n = 386 (19)	(82.2 to 91.4)	(86.4 to 97.3)	(91.3 to 96.6)
P-G	83.8	90.6	Not available
n = 249 (2A)	(77.5 to 88.6)	(80.1 to 96.1)	

AUC, area under the receiver operating characteristic curve; CI, confidence interval; P-PF, pleural fluid protein; P-R, pleural fluid to serum protein ratio; LDH-PF, pleural fluid LDH; LDH-R, pleural fluid to serum LDH ratio; C-PF, pleural fluid cholesterol; C-R, pleural fluid to serum cholesterol ratio; A-G, serum to pleural fluid albumin gradient; P-G, pleural fluid to serum protein gradient. Data extracted from references 19 and 28.

criteria. As expected, sensitivity increased and specificity decreased compared with the individual test performance as these tests are combined into two-test and three-test strategies.

Advantages exist for using multi-test strategies other than Light's criteria, which requires concurrent serum samples for LDH and protein assay and drives up the cost and discomfort of pleural fluid analysis. The combination diagnostic rule of pleural fluid LDH (> two-thirds the upper limits of normal for serum LDH) and pleural fluid cholesterol (>45 mg/dL) and the three-test combination of pleural fluid protein (>2.9 mg/dL), pleural fluid LDH (> two-thirds the upper limits of normal for serum LDH), and pleural fluid cholesterol (>45 mg/dL) have a sensitivity and specificity equal to the three-test Light's criteria.[19]

When combining tests into multi-test combinations, a basic principle directs that each test used is independently of the other and does not measure the same patient attribute. Tests that depend on a common patient attribute would be expected to correlate highly with each other and degrade the performance of the multi-test strategy. Note that Light's criteria include the pleural fluid to serum LDH ratio and the absolute value of pleural fluid LDH relative to laboratory normal values; both of these criteria include the same factor of pleural fluid LDH. Because these two LDH criteria were found in the metanalysis by Heffner and coworkers[19] to be highly correlated (Pearson product-moment correlation 0.84), one or the other can be omitted from Light's criteria without significantly altering diagnostic performance. The sensitivity and specificity of the three-component Light's criteria is 97.9 and 74.3 percent, respectively, compared with 97.3 and 80.3 percent with the two-test 'Abbreviated Light's criteria' that contains pleural fluid to serum protein and pleural fluid to serum LDH.[19] The abbreviated Light's criteria rule has been confirmed to have similar diagnostic accuracy compared with the three-criteria Light's criteria in independent data sets.[31,32]

In evaluating patients for exudative pleural effusions, clinicians should recognize that considerable uncertainty exists in categorization when pleural fluid tests return results near cut-off points. For example, pleural fluid from patients with CHF treated with diuretic therapy has an increased incidence of misclassification as exudate when evaluated by the three-test Light's criteria.[33] These misclassifications represent false-positives for exudative effusions, and most such patients have borderline pleural fluid test results. Light's criteria has an overall diagnostic accuracy greater than 90 percent, but its accuracy decreases below 70–80 percent when any one of its three criteria returns a borderline test result (Figure 17.1).[34]

Evaluation of an additional single pleural fluid test in certain settings may improve diagnostic accuracy when an initial screening multi-test strategy, such as Light's criteria, returns a borderline result. In the case of patients with CHF undergoing diuresis, one study reported the serum to pleural fluid albumin gradient >1.2 g/dL correctly identified 96 percent of transudates among patients incorrectly classified as having exudates by Light's criteria.[31] The overall diagnostic accuracy of the albumin gradient for patients with and without heart failure in this study was only 75 percent. Another study demonstrated that neither the serum to pleural fluid albumin gradient nor the serum

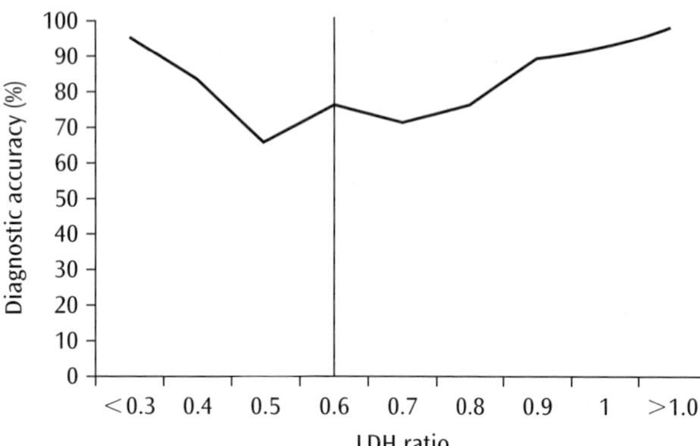

Figure 17.1 Diagnostic accuracy of Light's criteria for identifying an exudate when one of the three criteria, shown here is the pleural fluid to serum LDH ratio, varies across its range. Note that the accuracy of the three-test rule decreases markedly when the LDH ratios is near its cut-off point (vertical line). (Adapted from reference 32.)

to pleural protein gradient improved discrimination when applied to patients with congestive heart failure who were misclassified after diuretic therapy as exudates by Light's criteria.[28] Also, recent studies indicate that measurement of pleural fluid B-type natriuretic peptides (BNP) correctly categorizes effusions as transudates in the setting of chronic CHF by establishing the presence of acute cardiac decompensation.[35–38] Variable performance of pleural fluid BNP tests between studies, however, complicates determination of the most accurate BNP cut-off point. Moreover, the incremental diagnostic value of pleural fluid BNP compared with other clinical tests for detecting decompensated heart failure, such as echocardiogram, among patients with pleural effusions has not been sufficiently evaluated. The added value of pleural fluid BNP compared with serum BNP in this setting also has not been determined considering that pleural fluid BNP concentrations correlate closely with serum results,[38] and serum BNP levels are elevated in patients with pleural effusions caused by heart failure.[39] For these reasons, the role of pleural fluid BNP assay remains unclear as a follow-up examination for patients undergoing evaluation of pleural effusions.

A more general approach requires clinicians to recall that all existing tests and strategies for classifying exudative effusions are imperfect, and that test results cannot substitute for clinical judgment. A classification as an exudate or transudate that does not correlate with the clinical impression – especially when test results are borderline – warrants continued patient evaluation or observation.

A quantitative approach integrating clinical impressions with test results and clinical decision-making uses the Bayesian theorem.[40] This approach recognizes that a diagnostic result only increases or decreases a clinician's pretest clinical suspicion that a target condition exists. In the example of evaluating free-flowing pleural fluid in a patient with CHF who is undergoing diuresis, the physician would have a low 'pretest' clinical suspicion of an exudative effusion in the absence of clinical signs of a coexisting clinical condition. Findings of Light's criteria being slightly in the exudative range would not sufficiently increase the clinician's initial low pretest suspicion of an exudative effusion to justify a post-test diagnosis of an exudative effusion. The clinician should conclude that the patient has a transudative effusion with exudative characteristics by Light's criteria as a result of diuresis (i.e. false positive test result).

This approach to pleural fluid analysis relies on knowledge of the likelihood ratio associated with an individual pleural fluid test result.[17, 40] A likelihood ratio is the likelihood that a given test result would be expected in a patient with the target disorder compared with the likelihood that the same result would be expected in a patient without that disorder, in this case, an exudative pleural effusion. The clinician then estimates the pretest that an exudate probably exists based on their clinical experience and other relevant laboratory results, converts the probability to pretest odds and multiplies the odds by the likelihood ratio to calculate the post-test odds, which is then re-converted to a post-test probability.

Binary likelihood ratios that provide single likelihood ratio values for test results above and below the cut-off point overestimate the probability of an exudative effusion if test results return slightly above the cut-off point and severely underestimate the probability of an exudate when results return extremely high values (Figure 17.2). Multilevel and continuous likelihood ratios provide more precise likelihood values for specific pleural fluid test results. Both multilevel and continuous likelihood ratios have been reported for pleural fluid tests that discriminate between exudates and transudates for pooled[34, 41] and single-center patient series data.[30] Their application has been reviewed recently elsewhere.[15] Although seemingly cumbersome, these calculations are quickly performed by pre-programmed computer systems integrated with laboratory reporting software. Whether used in regular clinical practice or not, the application of likelihood ratios to selected patients demonstrates that tests used for discriminating between transudates and exudates have less clinical value, compared with a physician's clinical impressions, than what is commonly believed.

In summary, Light's criteria have served well for three decades in assisting clinicians in discriminating between exudative and transudative effusions. Because two of the criteria in Light's criteria (pleural fluid LDH and pleural fluid-to-serum LDH) are highly correlated, one or the other should be excluded from the model (Abbreviated Light's criteria) to improve the rule's diagnostic performance.[19,31,32] Because most of the individual pleural fluid tests reported in the literature have similar diagnostic properties, as compared with each criterion within Light's criteria,[19,30,31] multi-test strategies that avoid venipuncture may have clinical utility. The two-test diagnostic combina-

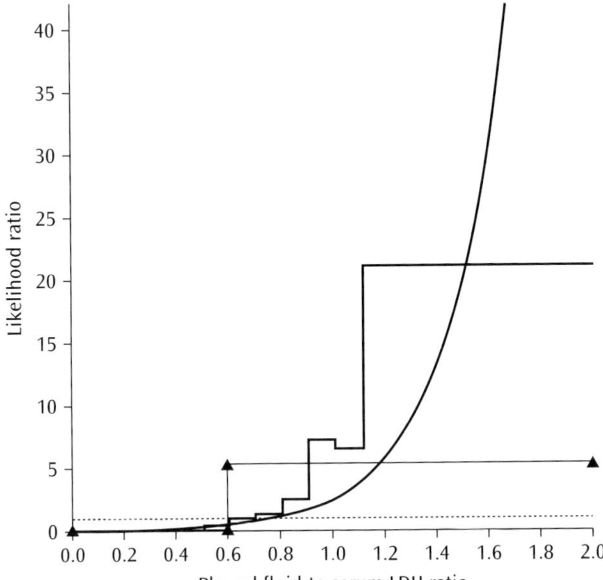

Figure 17.2 Likelihood ratios for pleural fluid to serum LDH ratio using a single cut-off point (lines with triangles – binary likelihood ratios), multiple discrete cut-off points (staggered staircase line – multilevel likelihood ratios) and cut-off points for every discrete test result (curved line – continuous likelihood ratio). Note how the single cut-off point under- and over-estimates the likelihood of an exudate at values close to and extremely above its cut-off point. (Adapted from reference 32.)

tion of pleural fluid LDH and pleural fluid cholesterol and the three-test combination of pleural fluid protein, pleural fluid LDH and pleural fluid cholesterol used as 'or' rules have similar diagnostic accuracy compared with Light's criteria. Clinicians should recognize that results of pleural fluid tests only increase or decrease their pretest suspicion that an exudative effusion exists. A high or low clinical suspicion should not be altered by borderline test results. In difficult cases, applying likelihood ratios demonstrate the quantitative effects of test results on this pretest suspicion, which helps to avoid overly inflating the value of a pleural fluid test and thereby preventing misclassification of pleural effusions.[15]

PROTEIN AND LACTATE DEHYDROGENASE

Knowledge of the total protein pleural fluid concentration may be helpful. Tuberculous pleural effusions are almost never associated with total protein concentrations <4.0 gm/dL,[46] while protein concentrations show a wide range of values in malignancy and parapneumonic effusions.[18] Finding a total protein concentration of >7.0 gm/dL suggests Waldenström's macroglobulinemia[47] or multiple myeloma.[48]

When the pleural fluid LDH is in the exudative range, but the total protein measurement suggests a transudate, malignancy,[18] parapneumonic effusions[18] and *Pneumocystis carinii* pneumonia should be considered.[49] A pleural fluid LDH concentration greater than three times the upper limits of normal for serum LDH is typically seen only in a complicated parapneumonic effusion or empyema,[50,51] rheumatoid pleurisy[52] or pleural paragonimiasis[53]; it is less often observed with malignancy and rarely with a tuberculous pleural effusion.[18]

NUCLEATED CELLS

The total nucleated cell count is rarely diagnostic but may provide useful information. Most exudates have >1000 nucleated cells/μL, while transudates usually contain <1000 nucleated cells/μL.[1,54] When the pleural fluid nucleated cell count exceeds 10 000/μL, the differential diagnosis includes parapneumonic effusions, acute pancreatitis, subdiaphragmatic abscess, liver, hepatic and splenic abscess, and splenic infarction.[1,43,54] Nucleated counts >10 000/μL are less common with pulmonary infarction, malignancy, tuberculosis, post-cardiac injury syndrome and lupus pleuritis.[1,43,54] Nucleated cell counts >50 000/μL are usually seen only in complicated parapneumonic effusions and empyema but, occasionally, can occur with acute pancreatitis and pulmonary infarction.[1,43,54] Chronic exudates typically have nucleated cell counts <5000/μL, as with a tuberculous pleural effusion and malignancy.[54–56] When pus is aspirated from the pleural space (empyema), the nucleated cell count may be as low as a few hundred cells because the majority of the neutrophils have undergone autolysis due to pleural fluid acidosis and low oxygen tension.

The predominant cellular population is determined by the type of pleural injury and the timing of thoracentesis in relation to the acute pleural injury. The acute response to any pleural injury, whether infectious, immunological or inflammatory, attracts neutrophils to the pleural space.[57] One of the major chemotaxins for neutrophils in the pleural space is interleukin-8 (IL-8).[58,59] Absolute neutrophil counts have been correlated with IL-8 levels, with the highest IL-8 levels found in empyema.[59] Within 48–72 hours following the cessation of acute pleural injury, mononuclear cells enter the pleural space from the peripheral blood and become the predominant cell type.[60] This macrophage predominance is eventually replaced by lymphocytes, which become the predominant cell in effusions that persist for more than 2 weeks. A neutrophil-predominant, exudative effusion would be the rule when the patient presents shortly after the onset of symptoms. Therefore, acute bacterial pneumonia, acute pulmonary embolism with infarction and acute pancreatitis are typically neutrophil predominant. When the disease has an insidious onset, as with malignancy and tuberculosis, the fluid will be lymphocyte predominant. Transudative effusions are never neutrophil predominant and should suggest a secondary diagnosis (such as pneumonia) when

Table 17.6 Pleural fluid lymphocyte predominant (≥80%) exudates

Disease	Comment
Tuberculous effusion	most common cause of lymphocyte predominant exudate; usually 90–95% lymphocytes
Chylothorax	400–6800 lymphocytes/μL; lymphoma most common cause
Lymphoma	Often 100% of nucleated cells are lymphocytes; diagnostic yield on cytology or pleural biopsy higher with non-Hodgkin lymphoma
Yellow nail syndrome	A cause of a persistent effusion
Rheumatoid pleurisy (chronic)	Usually associated with lung entrapment
Sarcoidosis	Usually >90% lymphocytes; prevalence <2%
Acute lung rejection	New or increased effusion 2–6 weeks after transplant
CABG surgery	Occurs >2 months following surgery; not associated with unexpandable lung
Uremic pleuritis	Renal failure present for 1–2 years; most effusion resolve with continued dialysis in 4–6 weeks

CABG, coronary artery bypass graft.

the pretest diagnosis is a transudate. Transudative effusions are mononuclear cell predominant, a combination of lymphocytes, macrophages and mesothelial cells.

When the lymphocyte population is 80 percent or greater of the total nucleated cells, the differential diagnosis of the exudative effusion is narrowed to the following diagnoses (Table 17.6).[61] The most common of these diagnoses is a tuberculous effusion.[62] Lymphoma,[62] yellow nail syndrome,[63] chronic rheumatoid pleurisy,[56,64] uremic pleuritis,[65] sarcoidosis,[66,67] chylothorax,[68] acute lung rejection[69] and post-coronary artery by-pass surgery (CABG surgery)[70] are also causes of >80 percent of lymphocytes in pleural fluid. All of the aforementioned diagnoses can occur with a lymphocyte population of <80 percent; however, a lymphocyte population of <50 percent is rarely found. In contrast to lymphoma, only about 60 percent of patients with metastatic carcinoma to the pleura have a majority of lymphocytes (usually 50–75 percent of total nucleated cells).[62] An undiagnosed, lymphocyte-predominant, exudative effusion is the most appropriate indication for percutaneous pleural biopsy and the most sensitive diagnostic procedure in tuberculous pleural effusion with the exception of thoracoscopy.[71,72] Lymphoma, carcinoma, sarcoidosis and occasionally rheumatoid pleurisy may be diagnosed by percutaneous pleural biopsy.

Pleural fluid eosinophilia (PFE) is defined as a pleural fluid eosinophil count ≥10 percent of the total nucleated cell count. It appears that eosinophils, produced in the bone marrow, are attracted to the pleural space by the chemotactic factor, IL-5.[73] Causes of PFE are shown in Table 17.7. Pneumothorax and hemothorax are the most common causes of PFE. It had been thought that the finding of PFE virtually excluded the diagnosis of malignancy. However, recent studies have shown that the prevalence of malignancy is similar in both eosinophilic and non-eosinophilic pleural effusions.[74,75] Eosinophilic pleuritis is a common early finding in patients who require thoracotomy or thoracoscopy for spontaneous pneumothorax. In contrast to the rapid movement of eosinophils into pleural tissue and pleural fluid in pneumothorax,[76] following hemothorax eosinophils do not appear in the pleural space for 7–14 days.[77] Furthermore, PFE is associated with peripheral blood eosinophilia following trauma that does not clear until the pleural fluid completely resolves.[78,79] Approximately 30 percent of individuals with BAPE have been noted to have PFE with eosinophil percentages sometimes reaching 50 percent.[80,81] These asbestos related effusions are often hemorrhagic. Other causes of PFE, such as pulmonary embolism with infarction and carcinoma, are also associated with pleural space hemorrhage. Fungal disease, particularly coccidioidomycosis and histoplasmosis, drug-induced pleurisy, Churg–Strauss syndrome, lymphoma, particularly Hodgkin

Table 17.7 Diseases associated with pleural fluid eosinophilia[a]

Disease	Comment
Pneumothorax	Effusion in 10–20%; tissue eosinophilia and PFE occurs early and is a common finding
Hemothorax	PFE occurs 1–2 weeks following a hemothorax
Benign asbestos	30% incidence of PFE; up to 50% eosinophils/total nucleated cells
Pulmonary embolism	Associated with infarction and pleural space hemorrhage
Parasitic disease	Paragonimiasis, hydatid disease, amebiasis, ascariasis
Fungal disease	Histoplasmosis, coccidioidomycosis
Drug-induced	Dantrolene, bromocriptine, nitrofurantoin, valproic acid
Lymphoma	Hodgkin disease
Carcinoma	5–8% with PFE
Churg–Strauss Syndrome	High pleural fluid eosinophil counts; associated with blood eosinophilia
Tuberculous pleurisy	Rare
Sarcoid pleurisy	Rare

[a]PFE, pleural fluid eosinophils/total nucleated pleural fluid cells ≥10%.

lymphoma, and parasitic diseases are also associated with PFE.[61,74,75] A tuberculous effusion has rarely been reported as a cause of PFE; it is unclear from the literature whether a previous thoracentesis resulting in air or blood entering the pleural space was the cause of the PFE.

Pleural fluid macrophages, which originate from blood monocytes, are not diagnostic.[77] Mesothelial cells are exfoliated into normal pleural fluid in small numbers.[77] Although common in transudative effusions and some exudates, mesothelial cells are rarely found in a tuberculous effusion, most likely due to the extensive pleural involvement by the hypersensitivity reaction to tuberculin protein, which inhibits mesothelial shedding.[77,82] A paucity of mesothelial cells is the typical finding in other inflammatory processes, such as empyema, chemical pleurodesis, rheumatoid pleuritis and chronic malignant effusions.[77]

A large number of plasma cells in pleural fluid suggest pleural involvement with multiple myeloma,[77] while a small number of plasma cells is non-diagnostic and has been observed in several non-malignant diseases.[77] A few basophils, occasionally found in pleural fluid, are of no clinical significance. However, when basophils represent >10 percent of the nucleated cells, leukemic involvement of the pleura is likely.[77]

The separation of T and B lymphocytes in lymphocyte predominant effusions has not been of diagnostic value. The T lymphocyte represents about 70 percent of the pleural fluid lymphocyte population.[83,84] However, if a high percentage of B lymphocytes are found in pleural fluid, lymphoma or chronic lymphatic leukemia should be suspected.[85]

pH

Pathogenesis

A limited number of pleural effusions are associated with a low pleural fluid pH (<7.30) (Table 17.8).[86,87] Pleural fluid pH should only be measured with a blood gas analyzer. Pleural fluid pH decreases as a result of high metabolic activity of intrapleural cellular constituents or by an abnormal pleural membrane that blocks the efflux of protons and organic acids from the pleural space into the circulation.[87] Urinothorax is a rare cause of a low pleural fluid pH in patients with acidic urine and is the only transudate associated with pleural fluid acidosis.[88] The extravasated urine from the capsule of the kidney moves retroperitoneally across the diaphragm into the ipsilateral pleural space.

The presence of a low pleural fluid pH provides diagnostic and prognostic information in various clinical settings. A low pH may also confound pleural fluid analysis by suggesting an alternative diagnosis, such as pleural space infection, when it occurs in the setting of a less common condition associated with a low pH effusion, such as rheumatoid pleurisy.

In the only study of acid–base characteristics of normal human pleural fluid, the pH was measured at 7.64, 0.23 pH

Table 17.8 Diagnoses associated with pleural fluid acidosis (pH <7.30)

Disease	Estimated incidence of pH <7.30 (%)	Range of pH	Comments
Parapneumonic effusion			
Uncomplicated	0–5	7.45–7.20	Nonpurulent, nonloculated fluid with negative bacteriology; resolves with antibiotics only
Complicated or empyema	~100	7.29–5.00	Requires pleural space drainage for resolution
Esophageal rupture	~100	6.80–5.00	pH 6.00 and high salivary amylase
Rheumatoid pleurisy (chronic)	~100	7.15–6.80	Associated with glucose < 30 mg/dL and LDH >1000 IU/L
Malignant effusion	30–40	7.50–6.90	pH <7.30: worse survival, increased yield on cytology and pleural biopsy, poorer response to pleurodesis
Lupus pleuritis	15–20	7.40–6.85	Associated with low glucose; diagnosis by LE cells in PF
Tuberculous effusion	10–20	7.40–6.95	Associated with low glucose; when pH low, usually between 7.29 and 7.10
Hemothorax	<10	7.50–7.17	Occurs when PF hematocrit approaches blood hematocrit and associated pleural injury
Pancreatic effusion	Rare	7.50–7.28	Occurs with very high amylase and severe pleural injury
Pulmonary infarction	Rare	7.52–7.29	Occurs with grossly bloody PF and extensive pleural injury
Diaphragmatic hernia with bowel infarction	Single report	7.15	Acid products of dead bowel overwhelm efflux capacity of pleural space

LDH, lactate dehydrogenase; LE, lupus erythematosus; PF, pleural fluid.

units greater than the simultaneously measured blood pH.[89] We and others have measured an alkaline pH (>7.60) in normal animals.[90,91] As the partial pressure of CO_2 (PCO_2) in pleural fluid was equivalent to arterial PCO_2, a bicarbonate gradient between pleural fluid and blood explains the alkaline pH of normal pleural fluid.[89,90] Human transudative effusions have a pleural fluid pH ranging from 7.45 to 7.55. The vast majority of exudative effusions have pH values that range from 7.45 to 7.30. However, only a small number of exudates are associated with pleural fluid acidosis (pH <7.30) and are the result of a substantial accumulation of hydrogen ions in the pleural space.[86,87]

The pleural fluid pH is determined by hydrogen ion production by pleural fluid and pleural tissue, efflux of hydrogen ions from the pleural space and the buffering capacity of pleural fluid.[87,92] Since the pleural fluid protein concentration of inflammatory pleural effusions approaches that of plasma, a poor buffering capacity probably plays a minor role in determination of the pleural fluid pH.[92] Furthermore, since a low pleural fluid pH is found with diagnoses as diverse as empyema, malignancy, lupus pleuritis and rheumatoid pleurisy, the pathogenesis of the low pleural fluid pH in each of these diseases probably differs. We have shown that, after incubating human pleural fluid anaerobically, the rate of change of pH in most effusions is similar whether or not the pH is <7.30 or >7.30.[92] Thus, the acid generating capacity of pleural fluid is not the sole determinant of pleural fluid pH. However, some low pH fluids generate a substantial amount of acid (empyema), while other low pH effusions have minimal metabolic activity (chronic rheumatoid pleurisy).[92] Malignant pleural effusions have an acid generation capacity intermediate between empyema and rheumatoid pleural fluid.[92] Therefore, in a low pH rheumatoid effusion, where the fluid has minimal acid generating capacity, impaired hydrogen ion efflux must play a major role in determining the low pH of the effusion. In malignancy, there appears to be a contribution from both acid generation of the fluid and pleural tissue and impaired hydrogen ion efflux from the pleural space.

In an experimental empyema model, we have shown that pleural fluid pH decreases within hours following the injection of bacteria into pleural fluid.[93] The decrease in pH is associated with an increase in pleural fluid PCO_2 and lactate concentration and a concomitant fall in pleural fluid glucose. We subsequently demonstrated, in *in vivo* and *in vitro* experiments, that both leukocyte/phagocytosis and bacterial metabolism contributes to the low pH of empyema fluid.[94]

Patients with low pleural fluid pH malignant effusions have a lower pleural fluid glucose concentration and oxygen tension and higher PCO_2 and lactate concentration than patients with normal pH malignant effusions.[95] In glucose transfer experiments, we demonstrated that patients with low pH malignant effusions had a block in both transfer of glucose from blood to pleural fluid and from pleural fluid to blood; those with normal pH malignant effusions did not show impaired glucose transfer.[95] Following 2 minutes of hyperventilation, patients with low pH malignant effusions did not lower their pleural fluid PCO_2, while those with normal pH malignant effusions had a significant fall in pleural fluid PCO_2.[95] We also demonstrated a block in oxygen transfer from blood to pleural fluid in low pH malignant effusions. Following 100 percent oxygen administration for 20 minutes, those with low pH malignant effusions had no change in the partial pressure of O_2 (PO_2) in pleural fluid, while those with normal pH malignant effusions had a significant increase in pleural fluid PO_2.[95]

Therefore, in patients with low pH malignant effusions, the pleural fluid glucose is low because, in addition to the metabolism of glucose from cells in pleural fluid and pleural tissue, there is a block of transfer of glucose from blood to the pleural space. Furthermore, the CO_2 and lactate from glycolysis accumulate in the pleural space because of a relative efflux block, which is due to tumor and associated fibrosis on the pleural surface. Similarly, the oxygen tension of a malignant pleural effusion is typically low as oxygen is utilized by malignant cells in pleural fluid and pleural tissue, and there is a block of oxygen transfer from blood to pleural fluid.

Parapneumonic effusions

Some experts categorize parapneumonic effusions as uncomplicated or complicated. Uncomplicated parapneumonic effusions resolve with antibiotic therapy alone. Complicated effusions require pleural fluid drainage to accelerate patient recovery and avoid progression to an empyema or lung entrapment. Because these categorizations require knowledge of a patient's subsequent clinical course, various strategies have been investigated to estimate the likely course of a parapneumonic effusion upon initial presentation. Pleural fluid pH has been found to be lower in patients who follow a complicated rather than an uncomplicated course.[50,51,86,96–99]

A meta-analysis examined the prognostic performance of pleural fluid pH in patients with parapneumonic effusions.[100] This study combined patient-level data from seven primary investigations that measured pleural fluid pH in samples from patients with non-purulent parapneumonic effusions.[50,51,86,96–99] Receiver operating characteristics were used to determine the diagnostic accuracy of pleural fluid pH, which was reported as the area under the receiver operating characteristic curve (AUC).[101] The met-analysis found that pleural fluid pH was lower in pleural fluid samples from patients who followed a complicated rather than an uncomplicated course and that the AUC for pH was 0.89.[100] This value for AUC indicated that pleural fluid pH had good discriminative properties for differentiating between complicated and uncomplicated parapneumonic effusions.

Published primary studies recommend various cutpoints below which a complicated effusion can be defined;[46,51,86,96–99] these range between pH 7.10 and pH 7.30. The metanalysis of pleural fluid pH recommended a Bayesian approach for using pleural fluid pH by considering the likelihood that the patient had a complicated parapneumonic effusion and the risk to the patient of misclassifying the effusion.[100] A high-risk patient might be identified by a clinical presentation that suggests a complicated course and a poor ability to tolerate misclassification of an effusion as uncomplicated. Such a patient might have a large effusion, radiographic evidence of thickened pleural membranes, pleural loculations and a Gram-negative pneumonia, all of which are associated with a complicated course. The patient might also be elderly with poor host responses to infection, which would decrease the patient's ability to tolerate misclassification of the effusion as uncomplicated and a delay in pleural fluid drainage. A pleural fluid pH <7.30 would warrant pleural fluid drainage in this high-risk patient. Conversely, a young, relatively well-appearing patient with pneumococcal pneumonia (good tolerance of a misclassification of the parapneumonic effusion) who has a small, free-flowing effusion (low pretest suspicion for a complicated course) would require drainage of the pleural space only if the pH were below 7.10.

The Bayesian approach to using pleural fluid pH described above recognizes that no single pH value can accurately dichotomize patients into complicated and uncomplicated categories. Pleural fluid pH, therefore, serves as adjunctive information that should be combined with the clinician's general impression as to the utility of pleural fluid drainage. This adjunctive role of pleural fluid pH was recommended by the recent American College of Chest Physicians consensus statement on the management of empyema.[102]

Malignant pleural effusions

Pleural fluid pH has been examined for its clinical utility in selecting patients with malignant effusions to undergo pleurodesis.[103–109] Low pleural fluid pH values have been observed in patients who fail pleurodesis, and pleural fluid pH correlates with survival among patients with malignant effusions, with shorter survivals being associated with lower pleural pH values.[103–109] It has been suggested that a low pH may identify patients who should be spared pleurodesis because of a low likelihood of benefit.[110]

Two recent meta-analyses,[111,112] however, collected primary patient-level data from seven investigators in 11 data sources and found pleural fluid pH alone had insufficient prognostic accuracy to be useful in clinical practice. The studies found a highly statistically significant direct correlation of pH with both survival and failure of pleurodesis, but pH by itself was a weak explanatory variable for these outcomes. The sensitivity and specificity of a pleural pH <7.28 for identifying pleurodesis failure were 56 and 78 percent, respectively.[111] Kaplan–Meier estimates of the 3-month survival were 39 percent (95 percent confidence interval [CI], 31.1 to 46.8) for patients with pleural fluid pH values ≤7.28 compared with 62 percent (95 percent CI, 55.7 to 67.4) patients with pleural fluid pH values >7.28 ($n = 268$) ($p < 0.0001$).[112] Unfortunately, patients with the lowest pH values still had a 65 percent probability of a successful pleurodesis. Similarly, pH corresponded with survival but patients with the lowest pH values still had nearly a 45 percent likelihood of survival for greater than 3 months, thereby, warranting efforts for pleurodesis to manage symptoms. At present, pleural fluid pH may have an adjunctive value in determining potential for benefit from pleurodesis, but it requires further examination in clinical practice.

GLUCOSE

In the normal physiological state, blood and fluid glucose concentration should be equivalent because glucose is of low molecular weight and should be transported from blood to pleural fluid by simple diffusion across the endothelial and mesothelial membranes. It is unlikely that a carrier transport system for glucose exists between blood and pleural fluid, as is postulated between blood and cerebrospinal fluid,[113] because all transudative effusions and most exudative effusions have a pleural glucose that mirrors blood glucose. A small group of exudative pleural effusions, the same as those with a low pleural fluid pH, may present with a low pleural fluid glucose concentration.[114] A low pleural fluid glucose concentration has been defined as <60 mg/dL or a pleural fluid to serum glucose ratio of <0.5 (Table 17.9). Post-pneumonic empyema and the anaerobic empyema associated with esophageal rupture have low pleural fluid glucose concentrations that tend to increase towards normal with treatment. In experimental empyema, the glucose falls rapidly following penetration of bacteria into the pleural space.[93] Glucose concentration correlates inversely with pleural fluid lactate and pCO_2, both *in vivo* and *in vitro*, suggesting that the accumulation of these glucose end-products is responsible for the decrease of pleural fluid pH in empyema.[93] Glucose utilization is increased by neutrophil phagocytosis and bacterial metabolism and exceeds the replacement of glucose from blood to pleural fluid.[94] While increased glucose utilization is the primary mechanism for low glucose in empyema, an abnormal pleural membrane produced by the rheumatoid state is the cause of low glucose concentration in rheumatoid pleurisy.[115,116] A pleural fluid glucose concentration of zero is found almost exclusively in patients with empyema and rheumatoid pleurisy.[114]

Like rheumatoid effusions, the major mechanism of the low glucose concentration in malignancy is an abnormal pleura, which is due to tumor infiltration that decreases glucose movement into the pleural space. In some cases, free cancer cells contribute to increased glucose utilization and an increase in the end-products of glucose metabolism, CO_2 and lactate acid, which accumulate due to

Table 17.9 Diagnoses associated with low pleural fluid glucose concentration (glucose <60 mg/dL or PF/S <0.5)

Disease	Estimated incidence of glucose pleural fluid/serum <0.5	Range of glucose concentration (mg/dL)	Comments
Rheumatoid pleurisy	85–90%	0–118	Glucose <30 mg/dL in 75%; PF triad of glucose <30 mg/dL, pH 7.00 and LDH >1000 IU/L; may precede articular manifestations by 3 years
Empyema	80–90%	0–145	Low glucose not as sensitive marker as low pH but correlation of glucose and pH is strong
Esophageal rupture	40–50%	15–120	Characteristic pH of 6.00 and high pleural fluid amylase (salivary)
Malignant effusion	30–40%	15–167	Low glucose concentration with chronic effusion in far-advanced pleural malignancy
Lupus pleuritis	20–30%	32–160	Transient; associated with severe pleural inflammation; LE cells diagnostic
Tuberculous effusion	20–30%	10–140	No correlation between low glucose and clinical course or pleural bacteriology

PF/S, pleural fluid/serum; LDH, lactate dehydrogenase; LE, lupus erythematosus.

impaired efflux and cause pleural fluid acidosis.[117] We have previously demonstrated that patients with carcinomatous pleurisy have pleural fluid acid generation intermediate between empyema fluids and rheumatoid effusions.[92]

The literature in the pre-chemotherapy era suggested that a low pleural fluid glucose was a common finding in a tuberculous pleural effusion. It is probable that many of these patients had tuberculous empyema or a markedly abnormal pleural membrane responsible for this finding. However, in the post-chemotherapy era, a low pleural fluid glucose is found in only approximately 20 percent of patients with a tuberculous pleural effusion.[46,118] In three patients who had glucose transport studies, two showed no impairment of glucose movement from blood to pleural fluid and one, with a markedly thick pleura and encapsulated effusion, showed no change in pleural fluid glucose concentration.[119] It is likely that the cause of low pleural fluid glucose concentration in tuberculous effusion is increased glycolysis by metabolically active cells in the pleural fluid or pleural membrane. In an acute tuberculous pleural effusion, impaired glucose transfer from blood to pleural fluid appears unlikely.

The low glucose in lupus pleuritis tends to be transient. All three patients in one study with lupus pleuritis and a low pleural fluid glucose ratio had low pleural fluid nucleated cell counts, suggesting that pleural fluid cellular metabolism is not a major contributor to the low glucose concentration.[120] Therefore, it is likely that active glycolysis by an inflamed pleura, in addition to impaired glucose transport across this abnormal membrane, play important roles in the low glucose concentration in lupus pleuritis. When patients are treated with corticosteroids and the pleural fluid inflammation resolves, pleural fluid glucose concentration returns to a concentration similar to serum glucose.

In an experimental model of esophageal rupture, we demonstrated that pleural fluid glucose concentration began to decrease within 2 hours following rupture and decreased below 60 mg/dL by 12 hours.[121] The lowest pleural fluid glucose concentrations were associated with the highest pleural fluid leukocyte counts. Furthermore, the pleural fluid glucose concentration correlated directly with pleural fluid pH and inversely with pleural fluid PCO_2 and lactate. It appears that the low pleural fluid glucose concentration in esophageal rupture results from the same mechanisms as in post-pneumonic empyema – increased glucose metabolism by constituents in pleural fluid, leukocytes and bacteria. It is doubtful that there is a marked decrease in glucose transfer from blood to pleural fluid following esophageal rupture, as at least initially only the mediastinal pleura is affected. The lag in the decrease in pleural fluid glucose and pH following esophageal rupture probably reflects the time required for the pleural space to become contaminated with microorganisms and for leukocytes to move into the pleural space. A high pleural fluid amylase concentration is the earliest marker of esophageal rupture and represents a direct communication between the oral cavity and the pleural space.[121]

AMYLASE

An increased pleural fluid amylase, defined as either a value greater than the upper limits of normal of the serum or a pleural fluid amylase ratio >1.0, is found in pancreatic disease,[118,122–124] esophageal rupture[110,111,121,125,126] and malignancy.[111,112,123,127,128] Rarely, an amylase-rich pleural effusion has been reported in pneumonia, ruptured ectopic pregnancy, hydronephrosis and cirrhosis.[123] Both acute and chronic pancreatitis can cause an amylase-rich pleural effusion. In acute pancreatitis, the effusion appears to result from direct contact of the pancreatic enzymes with the diaphragmatic pleura and movement of pancreatic fluid into the pleural space through diaphragmatic defects.[129,130] Pleural fluid amylase increases in concentration because it is not cleared rapidly by the pleural lymphatics, while amylase is cleared quickly from the blood by the kidney resulting in an increased pleural fluid to serum amylase ratio. In early pancreatitis, pleural fluid amylase may be normal but increases to a high level a few days following the onset of the pleural effusion.[118] In chronic pancreatitis, fluid moves via a fistulous track from a pseudocyst, either directly into the pleural space or into the mediastinum with eventual rupture of the mediastinal parietal pleura.[124] In chronic pancreatitis, pleural fluid amylase is always elevated and may reach extremely high levels of over 100 000 IU/L.[127] Serum amylase may be elevated in chronic pancreatitis due to back-diffusion from the pleural space or it may be normal.[131]

An increased pleural fluid amylase concentration occurs in 10 to 14 percent of patients with a malignant pleural effusion.[118,123,128,132] By isoenzyme analysis, the amylase is virtually all salivary type.[118,123,128] Adenocarcinoma of the lung is the most common malignancy associated with a salivary amylase-rich pleural effusion,[123,128] followed by adenocarcinoma of the ovary.[128] Lymphoma, leukemia and other types of lung cancer have also been reported with a salivary isoamylase-rich pleural effusion.[123,128] When a salivary isoamylase-rich pleural effusion is found in a patient who clinically does not have esophageal rupture (status post-endoscopy or Boerhaave syndrome), there is a high likelihood that the effusion is malignant and, most commonly, from adenocarcinoma of the lung. While it has been documented that tumor tissue can produce a salivary-like isoamylase,[127] this has rarely been shown with mesothelioma. The amylase in esophageal rupture has its origin in the salivary glands in the mouth, and the enzyme enters the pleural space through a rent in the esophagus and mediastinum. If the diagnosis is not established early, an anaerobic empyema will ensue. In an experimental model, we have shown that amylase is increased within 2 hours following the esophageal tear.[121]

In contrast to patients with acute pancreatitis who typically have symptoms of abdominal pain, fever and chest pain, patients with chronic pancreatic pleural effusions present predominantly with dyspnea and without evidence of acute pancreatitis. The pleural fluid amylase level is highest in chronic pancreatitis, moderately elevated in acute pancreatitis, and lowest in amylase-rich effusions secondary to malignancy.[123]

The routine measurement of pleural fluid amylase does not appear to be clinically indicated or cost effective. Pleural fluid amylase should be measured only if there is a pretest suspicion of pancreatic disease, esophageal rupture or malignancy.[133]

TRIGLYCERIDES AND CHOLESTEROL

When the supernatant of a milky or whitish pleural effusion remains opaque after centrifugation, excluding a large number of leukocytes, the differentiation between a chylous (chylothorax) and a cholesterol effusion (chyliform effusion or pseudochylothorax) needs to be established. Therefore, the first test that should be ordered is a pleural fluid triglyceride concentration. A diagnosis of chylothorax can be made presumptively if the triglyceride concentration exceeds 110 mg/dL;[134] if the triglyceride concentration is <50 mg/dL, it is highly unlikely that the patient has a chylothorax. When the triglyceride concentration is between 50 and 110 mg/dL, the presence of chylomicrons should be determined; if chylomicrons are present, the diagnosis of a chylothorax is established.[134] Importantly, in many cases of chylothorax, the pleural effusion will not appear milky. Blood can mask the milky appearance and, at times, the fluid is serous or turbid if the patient has not eaten recently.[130,131,134,135] Lymphocytes are the primary cells in chyle with counts ranging from 400 to 6800/μL;[68] the percentage of lymphocytes usually exceeds 80 percent.[68]

In the patient with a milky effusion and a low triglyceride concentration, pleural fluid cholesterol should be measured and the sediment evaluated microscopically. On observation, the pleural fluid may appear to have a satin-like sheen, which is distinctive from any other pleural effusion. Under the microscope, cholesterol crystals can be recognized as large, polyhydric crystals. When pleural fluid cholesterol exceeds 200 mg/dL, it most likely represents a cholesterol pleural effusion.[136] However, it should be recognized that high cholesterol levels may also be found in some chylous effusions.[134] In addition, some cholesterol pleural effusions have triglyceride levels of >250 mg/dL.[137] If there is clinical uncertainty about the diagnosis, the presence of chylomicrons should be determined.

Patients with chylothorax tend to have an acute or subacute onset of dyspnea with exertion and may have contralateral mediastinal shift on chest radiograph; patients with a cholesterol pleural effusion have long-standing pleural effusions associated with lung entrapment and an absence of mediastinal shift.[137]

IMMUNOLOGICAL STUDIES

Approximately half of the patients with systemic lupus erythematosus will develop pleuritic chest pain or a pleural effusion during the course of their disease and, in 5 percent of patients, pleuritis may be the presenting manifestation.[138] Approximately 5 percent of patients, mostly men with active rheumatoid disease, will develop pleurisy.[139,140]

In patients with these two diseases, immunology studies are appropriate. We previously reported that pleural fluid anti-nuclear antibodies (ANA) titer ≥1:160 in conjunction with a pleural fluid to serum ANA ratio of ≥1 was suggestive of lupus pleuritis.[120] We further showed that pleural fluid ANA titers were negative in a large number of patients with pleural effusion of other etiologies.[120] In a small number of patients with systemic lupus erythematosus (SLE) and an effusion of another cause, the pleural fluid to serum ANA ratio was <1.[120] Others have also found elevated titers of pleural fluid ANA in patients who do not have lupus pleuritis, but when ANA titers exceed 1:320, lupus pleuritis was likely.[141] However, while the ANA titer and pleural fluid to serum ratios are suggestive of lupus pleuritis, only finding LE cells in pleural fluid is diagnostic. Although most clinical laboratories do not perform LE tests because there is better immunological testing for SLE, a simple Wright stain of pleural fluid sediment that has remained at room temperature for several hours will increase the likelihood of finding LE cells and confirm the diagnosis of lupus pleuritis.

When rheumatoid pleurisy is considered, a rheumatoid factor should be measured in pleural fluid. If the pleural fluid rheumatoid factor titer is ≥1:320 and equal to or greater than the serum rheumatoid factor, it is likely that the effusion is caused by rheumatoid arthritis.[142] Lower titers of pleural fluid rheumatoid factor are non-diagnostic and have been documented in patients with parapneumonic effusions and malignancy.[143] Pleural fluid complement levels, whether CH_{50}, C3 or C4, are typically are low in patients with lupus pleuritis and rheumatoid pleurisy.[142,144–146] However, levels may be low in other exudates. CH_{50} levels below 10 U/mL[144] or C4 levels below 10×10^{-5} U/g protein[142] are rarely seen with exudates other than lupus pleuritis or rheumatoid pleurisy.[142] Nevertheless, a rheumatoid effusion has a diagnostic cytological picture of a background of degenerative cells and large, elongated tadpole-shaped cells representing exfoliation from visceral pleural rheumatoid nodules.[13]

CYTOLOGICAL EXAMINATION

Pleural fluid cytology has a widely variable diagnostic yield, ranging from 40 to 90 percent of patients with pleural malignancy.[143,144,147,148] There are several reasons for this variability. One important consideration is that the effusion may be paramalignant, which is defined as a pleural effusion associated with a known malignancy but the pleura is not involved with tumor.[149] These paramalignant effusions result from local effects of the tumor, such as obstructive atelectasis or pneumonia, systemic effects such as pulmonary embolism, and complications of therapy, such as radiation pleuritis or drug-induced pleurisy. Other explanations for the variable cytological diagnosis include the type of tumor (high positivity with adenocarcinoma[150] and low in Hodgkin lymphoma),[151] the number of specimens submitted (yields tend to increase with additional specimens due to exfoliation of fresher cells),[151] the stage of pleural involvement (the more advanced the stage, the higher the diagnostic yield), and, lastly, the interest and expertise of the cytopathologist. At times, the pleural effusion is unrelated to the malignant process, such as CHF or non-obstructive pneumonia.

FLOW CYTOMETRY

While flow cytometry should not be routinely used to differentiate benign and malignant pleural effusions, it can be helpful in the diagnosis of lymphoma involving the pleura. Flow cytometry can specifically define lymphocyte surface markers.[152] Therefore, it can define clonality of a population of lymphocytes to determine whether the cells are from T- or B-cell lineage. Therefore, flow cytometry is most helpful in patients with a lymphocyte predominant pleural effusion when lymphoma is in the differential diagnosis.

ADENOSINE DEAMINASE

Adenosine deaminase (ADA) is an enzyme found in most cells and is important in the degradation of purines. It is required for lymphoid cell differentiation and is also involved in monocyte–macrophage maturation. The assay for ADA is easily and rapidly performed, is of relatively low cost and has been used in areas of high tuberculosis prevalence to aid in the diagnosis of tuberculosis.[153,154] Pleural fluid/serum ADA ratios of >1 have been observed, not only in tuberculous effusions, but in rheumatoid disease and empyema, while other exudates have similar ADA levels in pleural fluid and serum.[151,155] Furthermore, patients with tuberculous effusions, rheumatoid pleurisy, empyema and malignancy have higher ADA activity in pleural fluid than other exudates and CHF.[156] The diagnostic cut-off points for ADA have been reported from 40 to 60 U/L.[157–161] Selecting a cut-off point of 40 U/L will increase the sensitivity of ADA but decrease its specificity, while choosing a cut-off point of 60 U/L will increase specificity but decrease sensitivity.

Some authors have suggested that determination of ADA isoenzymes will enhance its diagnostic utility. In a tuberculous effusion, ADA-2 is the predominant isoform accounting for over 80 percent of ADA activity, whereas ADA-1 accounts for approximately 70 percent of the activity of the total ADA activity in empyema.[158] ADA-2 probably reflects monocyte/macrophage origin, while ADA-1 originates from lymphocyte or neutrophil turnover. However, measurement of ADA-2 is substantially more expensive than measurement of total ADA and, currently, is not available clinically in the USA.[153] The decline in the number of cases of tuberculous pleural effusions in the USA may have contributed to the relative unavailability of

ADA assay commercially. However, total ADA has a high negative predictive value for tuberculosis and should be measured in the 15–20 percent of patients who are suspected of having tuberculosis but have negative cultures from pleural fluid and pleural tissue, and pleural tissue that does not show granulomas.

FUTURE DIRECTIONS

Pleural fluid analysis provides a safe and accessible means for diagnosing conditions that affect the pleural space. Most tests of pleural fluid, however, have not been evaluated in large patient populations to determine their operating characteristics. More specifically, likelihood ratios do not exist for any pleural fluid test results except for those that discriminate between exudative and transudative effusions. In the future, investigators will be asked to present their results in a manner that allows calculation of likelihood ratios across the range of test values. Such investigations will allow a Bayesian approach to pleural fluid analysis by which clinicians will use test results to quantitatively increase or decrease their pretest suspicion of disease. Also, more rigorous studies are needed of pleural fluid tests that adhere to published standards for evaluating diagnostic test performance. These studies will rely on improved diagnostic 'gold standards', such as thoracoscopy, advanced imaging modalities and comprehensive patient follow-up that will provide more accurate reference standards. Such studies will improve the accuracy and precision of pleural fluid analysis.

KEY POINTS

- A diagnosis can be established definitively or presumptively or the differential narrowed by observing the color, character or odor of pleural fluid.
- Exudates are caused by a myriad of diseases, predominantly by inflammatory, infectious and malignant conditions; in contrast, a limited number of conditions cause transudates from hydrostatic mechanisms.
- The results of pleural fluid tests increase or decrease the pretest suspicion that an exudate exists; a high or low clinical suspicion should not be altered by borderline test results.
- Acute pleural exudates are neutrophil predominant, while chronic exudates are lymphocyte predominant. Pleural fluid lymphocytosis ≥80 percent and pleural fluid eosinophilia limit the differential of the exudate.
- A low pleural fluid pH (<7.30) or glucose (pleural fluid/serum <0.5) narrows the differential of the exudate to complicated parapneumonic effusion/empyema, malignancy, rheumatoid pleurisy, tuberculosis, esophageal rupture and lupus pleuritis.
- Amylase should be measured on pleural fluid only if there is a pretest suspicion of pancreatic disease, esophageal rupture or malignancy.
- Chylothorax can be diagnosed presumptively if the triglyceride concentration exceeds 110 mg/dL and is highly unlikely if the triglyceride concentration is <50 mg/dL. Chylomicron determination should be carried out for triglyceride levels between 50 and 110 mg/dL; its presence confirms a chylothorax.
- Rheumatoid pleurisy can be diagnosed by characteristic cytological findings that include a background of granular material, large elongated cells and giant round or oval multinucleated cells.

REFERENCES

● = Key primary paper
◆ = Major review article

◆1. Sahn SA. Drug-induced pleural disease. In: Camus P, Rosenow E (eds). *Drug-induced and iatrogenic lung disease*. London: Hodder Arnold; 2009, in press.
◆2. Light RW. *Pleural diseases*, 4th edn. Baltimore: Williams & Wilkins, 1995: 87–95.
3. Mayo P, Doelken P. Pleural ultrasonography. *Clin Chest Med* 2006; **27**: 215–28.
4. Shorr RM, Crittenden M, Indeck M, *et al.* Blunt thoracic trauma. Analysis of 515 patients. *Ann Surg* 1987; **206**: 200–5.
5. Krauss D, Schmidt GA. Cardiac tamponade and contralateral hemothorax after subclavian vein catheterization. *Chest* 1991; **99**: 517–18.
6. Rostand RA, Feldman RI, Block ER. Massive hemothorax complicating heparin anticoagulation for pulmonary embolus. *Am Med J* 1977; **70**: 1128–30.
◆7. Joseph J, Sahn SA. Thoracic endometriosis syndrome: new observations from an analysis of 110 cases. *Am J Med* 1996; **100**: 164–70.
◆8. Roberts PP. Parasitic infections of the pleural space. *Semin Respir Infect* 1988; **3**: 362–82.
9. Metzger JB, Garagusi VF, Kerwan DM. Pulmonary oxalosis caused by *Aspergillus niger*. *Am Rev Respir Dis* 1984; **129**: 501–2.
10. Lillington GA, Carr DT, Mayne JG. Rheumatoid pleurisy with effusion. *Arch Intern Med* 1971; **128**: 764–8.
11. Miller KS, Tomlinson JR, Sahn SA. Pleuropulmonary complications of enteral tube feedings. Two reports, review of the literature, and recommendations. *Chest* 1985; **88**: 230–3.
12. Ellis LM, Vogal SB, Copeland EM. Central venous catheter vascular erosions. Diagnosis and clinical course. *Ann Surg* 1989; **209**: 475–8.
●13. Nosanchuk JS, Naylor B. A unique cytologic picture in pleural fluid from patients with rheumatoid arthritis. *Am J Clin Pathol* 1968; **50**: 330–5.

●14. Stark DD, Shanes JG, Baron RL, Roach DD. Biochemical features of urinothorax. *Arch Intern Med* 1982; **42**: 1505–11.
15. Heffner JE. Discriminating between transudates and exudates. *Clin Chest Med* 2006; **27**: 241–52.
16. Heffner JE, Feinstein D, Barbieri C. Methodologic standards for diagnostic test research in pulmonary medicine. *Chest* 1998; **114**: 877–85.
17. Heffner JE. Evaluating diagnostic tests in the pleural space. Differentiating transudates from exudates as a model. *Clin Chest Med* 1998; **19**: 277–93.
●18. Light RW, MacGregor I, Luchsinger PC, Ball WC. Pleural effusion: the diagnostic separation of transudates and exudates. *Ann Intern Med* 1972; **77**: 507–13.
19. Heffner JE, Brown LK, Barbieri C. Diagnostic value of tests that discriminate between exudative and transudative pleural effusions. *Chest* 1997; **111**: 970–9.
20. Costa M, Quiroga T, Cruz E. Measurement of pleural fluid cholesterol and lactate dehydrogenase. A simple and accurate set of indicators for separating exudates from transudates. *Chest* 1995; **108**: 1260–3.
21. Hamm H, Brohan U, Bohmer R, Missmahl H-P. Cholesterol in pleural effusions. A diagnostic aid. *Chest* 1987; **92**: 296–302.
22. Romero S, Candela A, Martín C, *et al.* Evaluation of different criteria for the separation of pleural transudates from exudates. Chest 1993; **104**: 399–04.
23. Suay VG, Moragón EM, Viedma EC, *et al.* Pleural cholesterol in differentiating transudates and exudates. A prospective study of 232 cases. *Respiration* 1995; 62: 57–63.
24. Valdés L, Pose A, Suàrez J, *et al.* Cholesterol: a useful parameter for distinguishing between pleural exudates and transudates. *Chest* 1991; **99**: 1097–102.
25. Chibante A, Neves D, Miranda S, Dias R. [Cholesterol as a diferential parameter to separate pleural transudates from exsudates.]. *Rev Port Pneumol* 2006; **12** (6 Suppl 1): 25.
26. Roth BJ, O'Meara TF, Cragun WH. The serum-effusion albumin gradient in the evaluation of pleural effusions. *Chest* 1990; **98**: 546–9.
27. Romero-Candeira S, Fernandez C, Martin C, Sanchez-Paya J, Hernandez L. Influence of diuretics on the concentration of proteins and other components of pleural transudates in patients with heart failure. *Am J Med* 2001; **110**: 681–6.
28. Romero-Candeira S, Hernandez L, Romero-Brufao S, *et al.* Is it meaningful to use biochemical parameters to discriminate between transudative and exudative pleural effusions? *Chest* 2002; **122**: 1524–9.
29. Atalay F, Ernam D, Hasanoglu HC, Karalezli A, Kaplan O. Pleural adenosine deaminase in the separation of transudative and exudative pleural effusions. *Clin Biochem* 2005; **38**: 1066–70.
30. Porcel JM, Pena JM, Vicente de Vera C, *et al.* Bayesian analysis using continuous likelihood ratios for identifying pleural exudates. *Respir Med* 2006; **100**: 1960–5.
31. Gonlugur U, Gonlugur TE. The distinction between transudates and exudates. *J Biomed Sci* 2005; **12**: 985–90.
32. Joseph J, Badrinath P, Basran GS, Sahn SA. Is the pleural fluid transudate or exudate? A revisit of the diagnostic criteria. *Thorax* 2001; **56**: 867–70.
33. Chakko SC, Caldwell SH, Sforza PP. Treatment of congestive heart failure. Its effect on pleural fluid chemistry. *Chest* 1989; **95**: 798–802.
34. Heffner JE, Highland K, Brown LK. A meta-analysis derivation of continuous likelihood ratios for diagnosing pleural fluid exudates. *Am J Respir Crit Care Med* 2003; **167**: 1591–9.
35. Tomcsanyi J, Nagy E, Somloi M, *et al.* NT-brain natriuretic peptide levels in pleural fluid distinguish between pleural transudates and exudates. *Eur J Heart Fail* 2004; **6**: 753–6.
36. Porcel JM. The use of probrain natriuretic peptide in pleural fluid for the diagnosis of pleural effusions resulting from heart failure. *Curr Opin Pulm Med* 2005; **11**: 329–33.
37. Light RW. The undiagnosed pleural effusion. *Clin Chest Med* 2006; **27**: 309–19.
38. Kolditz M, Halank M, Schiemanck CS, Schmeisser A, Hoffken G. High diagnostic accuracy of NT-proBNP for cardiac origin of pleural effusions. *Eur Respir J* 2006; **28**: 144–50.
39. Gegenhuber A, Mueller T, Dieplinger B, *et al.* Plasma B-type natriuretic peptide in patients with pleural effusions: preliminary observations. *Chest* 2005; **12**: 1003–9.
40. Sackett DL, Straus SE, Richardson WS, Rosenberg W, Haynes RB. *Evidence-based medicine. How to practice and teach EBM*, 2nd edn. Edinburgh: Churchill Livingstone, 2000.
●41. Heffner JE, Sahn SA, Brown LK. Multilevel likelihood ratios for identifying exudative pleural effusions. *Chest* 2002; **121**: 1916–20.
42. Leuallen EC, Carr DT. Pleural effusion, a statistical study of 436 patients. *N Engl J Med* 1955; **252**: 79–83.
43. Light RW. *Pleural diseases*. Baltimore: Williams & Wilkins, 1995: 36–74.
44. Meisel S, Shamiss A, Thaler M, *et al.* Pleural fluid to serum bilirubin concentration for the separation of transudates and exudates. *Chest* 1990; **98**: 141–4.
45. Burgess L, Maritz FJ, Taljaard JJF. Comparative analysis of the biochemical parameters used to distinguish between pleural transudates and exudates. *Chest* 1995; **107**: 1604–9.
◆46. Sahn SA. State of the art. The pleura. *Am Rev Respir Dis* 1988; **138**: 184–234.
47. Winterbauer RH, Riggins RCK, Griesman FA, Bauermeister DE. Pleuropulmonary manifestions of Waldenstrom's macroglobulinemia. *Chest* 1974; **66**: 368–75.
48. Rodriguez JN, Pereira A, Martinez JC, *et al.* Pleural effusion in multiple myeloma. *Chest* 1994; **105**: 622–4.
49. Horwitz ML, Schiff M, Samuels J, *et al. Pneumocystis carinii* pleural effusion. Pathogenesis and pleural fluid analysis. *Am Rev Respir Dis* 1993; **148**: 232–4.
●50. Light RW, Girard WM, Jenkinson SG, George RB. Parapneumonic effusions. *Am J Med* 1980; **69**: 507–11.
●51. Potts DE, Levin DC, Sahn SA. Pleural fluid pH in parapneumonic effusions. *Chest* 1976; **70**: 328–31.
52. Pettersson T, Klockars M, Helmstrom PE. Chemical and immunological features of pleural effusions: comparison between rheumatoid arthritis and other diseases. *Thorax* 1982; **37**: 354–61.
53. Johnson JR, Falk A, Iber C, Davies S. Paragonimiasis in the United States. A report of 9 cases in Hmong immigrants. *Chest* 1982; **82**: 168–71.
●54. Light RW, Erozan YS, Ball WC Jr. Cells in pleural fluid: their value and differential diagnosis. *Arch Intern Med* 1973; **132**: 854–60.
55. Berger HW, Mejiia E. Tuberculous pleurisy. *Chest* 1973; **63**: 88–92.
56. Pettersson T, Riska H. Diagnostic value of total and differential leukocyte counts in pleural effusions. *Acta Med Scand* 1981; **210**: 129–35.
57. Antony VB, Repine JE, Sahn SA. Experimental models of inflammation in the pleural space. In: Chretein J, Bignon J, Hirsch A (eds). *The pleural in health and disease*. New York: Marcel Dekker, 1985: 387–400.
58. Antony VB, Godbey SW, Kunkel SL, *et al.* Recruitment of inflammatory cells to the pleural space. Chemotactic cytokines, IL-8, and monocyte chemotactic peptide-1 in human pleural fluids. *J Immunol* 1993; **151**: 7216–23.
59. Broaddus VA, Hebert CA, Vitangcol RV, *et al.* Interleukin-8 is a major neutrophil chemotactic factor in pleural liquid of patients with empyema. *Am Rev Respir Dis* 1992; **146**: 825–30.
60. Antony VB, Sahn SA, Antony AC, Repine JE. Bacillus Calmette-Guerin-stimulated neutrophils release chemotaxins for monocytes in rabbit pleural spaces and *in vitro*. *J Clin Invest* 1985; **76**: 1514–21.
●61. Sahn SA. Diagnostic value of pleural fluid analysis. *Semin Respir Crit Care Med* 1995; **16**: 269–78.

●62. Yam LT. Diagnostic significance of lymphocytes in pleural effusion. *Ann Intern Med* 1967; **66**: 972–82.

●63. Nordkild P, Kromann-Andersen H, Struve-Christsen E. Yellow nail syndrome – the triad of yellow nails, lymph edema, and pleural effusions. *Acta Med Scand* 1986; **219**: 221–7.

64. Sahn SA, Kaplan RL, Maulitz RM, Good JT Jr. Rheumatoid pleurisy. Observation on the development of low pleural fluid pH and glucose levels. *Arch Intern Med* 1980; **140**: 1237–8.

●65. Berger HW, Rammohan G, Neff MS, Buhain WJ. Uremic pleural effusion. A study in 14 patients on chronic dialysis. *Ann Intern Med* 1975; **82**: 362–4.

66. Nicholls AJ, Friend JAR, Legge JS. Sarcoid pleural effusions: three cases and review of the literature. *Thorax* 1980; **35**: 277–81.

67. Huggins JT, Doelken P, Sahn SA, *et al.* Pleural effusions in a series of 181 outpatients with sarcoidosis. *Chest* 2006; **129**: 1599–1604.

68. Miller JJ. Anatomy of the thoracic duct and chylothorax. In: Shields T, Locicero J, Ponn R (eds). *General thoracic surgery*, 6th edn. Philadelphia: Lippincott, Williams and Wilkins; 2005: 879–88.

●69. Judson MA, Handy JR, Sahn SA. Pleural effusion from acute lung rejection. *Chest* 1997; **111**: 1128–30.

●70. Lee Y, Vaz M, Ely K, *et al.* Symtomatic persistent post-coronary artery bypass graft pleural effusions requiring operative treatment. *Chest* 2001; **119**: 795–800.

71. Scharer L, McClement JH. Isolation of tubercle bacilli from needle biopsy specimens of parietal pleura. *Am Rev Respir Dis* 1968; **97**: 466–8.

72. Levine H, Metzger W, Lacera D, Kay L. Diagnosis of tuberculous pleurisy by culture or pleural biopsy specimen. *Arch Intern Med* 1970; **126**: 269–71.

73. Nakamura Y, Ozaki T, Kamei T, *et al.* Factors that stimulate the proliferation and survival of eosinophils in eosinophilic pleural effusion: relationship to granulocytes/macrophage colony-stimulating factor, interleukin-5 and interleukin-3. *Am Rev Cell Mol Biol* 1993; **8**: 605–11.

●74. Rubins JB, Rubins HB. Etiology and prognostic signifcance of eosinophilic pleural effusions. A prospective study. *Chest* 1996; **110**: 1271–4.

●75. Martinez-Garcia MA, Cases-Viedma E, Cordero-Rodriguez PJ, *et al.* Diagnostic utility of eosinophils in the pleural fluid. *Eur Respir J* 2000; **15**: 166–9.

76. Askin FB, McCann BG, Kuhn C. Reactive eosinophilic pleuritis. *Arch Path Lab Med* 1997; **101**: 187–91.

77. Spriggs AI, Boddington MM. *The cytology of effusions*, 2nd edn. New York: Grune & Stratton, 1968: 5–17.

78. Maltais F, Laberge F, Cormier Y. Blood hypereosinophilia in the course of posttraumatic pleural effusion. *Chest* 1990; **98**: 348–51.

79. Heidecker J, Sahn SA. The four faces of a parapneumonic effusion. *Respirology* 2007; **12**: 610–13.

80. Mattson SB. Monosymptomatic exudative pleurisy in persons exposed to asbestos dust. *Scand J Respir Dis* 1997; **56**: 263–72.

●81. Hillerdal G, Ozesmi M. Benign asbestos pleural effusion: 73 exudates in 60 patients. *Eur J Respir Dis* 1987; **71**: 113–21.

82. Hurwitz S, Leiman G, Shapiro C. Mesothelial cells in pleural fluid: TB or not TB? *S Afr Med J* 1980; **57**: 937–9.

83. Potrykus AM, Steinmann G, Stein E, Mertelsmann R. T- and B-cell responses in patients with malignant pleural effusions. *Br J Cancer* 1981; **43**: 471–7.

84. Pettersson T, Klockars M, Hellstrom PE, *et al.* T and B lymphocytes in pleural effusions. *Chest* 1978; **73**: 49–51.

85. Domagala W, Emeson EE, Kos LG. T and B lymphocyte enumeration in the diagnosis of lymphocyte-rich pleural fluids. *Acta Cytol* 1981; **25**: 108–10.

●86. Good JT, Taryle DA, Maulitz RM, *et al.* The diagnostic value of pleural fluid pH. *Chest* 1980; **78**: 55–9.

◆87. Sahn SA. Pleural fluid pH in the normal state and in diseases affecting the pleural space. In: Chretien J, Bignon J, Hirsch A (eds). *The pleura in health and disease.* New York: Marcel Dekker, 1985: 253–66.

88. Miller KS, Wooten S, Sahn SA. Urinothorax: a cause of a low pH transudate. *Am J Med* 1988; **85**: 448–9.

89. Yamada S. Uber die serose Flussigkeit in der Plerachohle der gesunden menschen. *Z Ges Exp Med* 1993; 90: 343–8.

90. Sahn SA, Willcox ML, Good JT Jr, *et al.* Characteristics of normal rabbit pleural fluid: physiologic and biochemical implications. *Lung* 1979; **156**: 63–9.

91. Rolf LL, Travis DM. Pleural fluid-plasma bicarbonate gradients in oxygen-toxic and normal rats. *Am J Physiol* 1973; **224**: 857–61.

92. Taryle DA, Good JT Jr, Sahn SA. Acid generation by pleural fluid: possible role in the determination of pleural fluid pH. *J Lab Clin Med* 1979; **93**: 1041–6.

93. Sahn SA, Taryle DA, Good JT Jr. Experimental empyema: time course and pathogenesis of pleural fluid acidosis and low pleural fluid glucose. *Am Rev Respir Dis* 1979; **120**: 355–61.

●94. Sahn SA, Reller LB, Taryle DA, *et al.* The contribution of leukocytes and bacteria to the low pH of empyema fluid. *Am Rev Respir Dis* 1983; **128**: 811–5.

●95. Good JT Jr, Taryle DA, Sahn SA. The pathogenesis of low glucose, low pH malignant effusions. *Am Rev Respir Dis* 1985; **131**: 737–41.

96. Poe RH, Marin MG, Israel RH, Kallay MC. Utility of pleural fluid analysis in predicting tube thoracostomy/decortication in parapneumonic effusions. *Chest* 1991; **100**: 963–7.

97. Potts DE, Taryle DA, Sahn SA. The glucose-pH relationship in parapneumonic effusions. *Arch Intern Med* 1978; **138**: 1378–80.

98. Limthongkul S, Charoenlap P, Nuchprayoon C, Songkhla YN. Diagnostic and prognostic significance of pleural fluid pH and pCO2 in the exudative phase of parapneumonic effusions. *J Med Assoc Thailand* 1983; **66**: 762–8.

99. Light R, MacGregor M, Ball WC Jr, Luchsinger PC. Diagnostic significance of pleural fluid pH and PCO2. *Chest* 1973; **64**: 591–6.

●100. Heffner JE, Brown LK, Barbieri C. Pleural fluid chemical analysis in parapneumonic effusions. A meta-analysis. *Am J Respir Crit Care Med* 1995; **151**: 1700–8.

101. Hanley JA, McNeil BJ. The meaning and use of the area under the receiving operating characteristic (ROC) curve. *Radiology* 1982; **143**: 29–36.

◆102. Colice GL, Curtis A, Deslauriers J, *et al.* Medical and surgical treatment of parapneumonic effusions : an evidence-based guideline. *Chest* 2000; **118**: 1158–71.

●103. Sahn SA, Good JT. Pleural fluid pH in malignant effusions. Diagnostic, prognostic, and therapeutic implications. *Ann Intern Med* 1988; 108: 345–9.

104. Sanchez-Armengol A, Rodriguez-Panadero F. Survival and talc pleurodesis in metastatic pleural carcinoma revisited. Report of 125 cases. *Chest* 1993; **104**: 1317–19.

105. Martinez-Moragon E, Aparicio J, Sanchis J, *et al.* Malignant pleural effusion: prognostic factors for survival and response to chemical pleurodesis in a series of 120 cases. *Respiration* 1998; **65**: 108–13.

106. Lan RS, Lo SK, Chuang ML, *et al.* Elastance of the pleural space: a predictor for the outcome of pleurodesis in patients with malignant pleural effusion. *Ann Intern Med* 1997; **126**: 768–74.

107. Rodriguez-Panadero F, Segado A, Martin Juan J, *et al.* Failure of talc pleurodesis is associated with increased pleural fibrinolysis. *Am J Respir Crit Care Med* 1995; **151**: 785–90.

108. Rodriguez-Panadero F, Lopez Mejias J. Low glucose and pH levels in malignant pleural effusions. Diagnostic significance and prognostic value in respect to pleurodesis. *Am Rev Respir Dis* 1989; **139**: 663–7.

109. Salomaa ER, Pulkki K, Helenius H. Pleurodesis with doxycycline or *Corynebacterium parvum* in malignant pleural effusion. *Acta Oncol* 1995; **34**: 117–21.

110. Rodriguez-Panadero F, Antony VB. Pleurodesis: state of the art. *Eur Respir J* 1997; **10**: 1648–54.

●111. Heffner JE, Nietert PJ, Barbieri C. Pleural fluid pH as a predictor of pleurodesis failure: analysis of primary data. *Chest* 2000; **117**: 87–95.

●112. Heffner JE, Nietert PJ, Barbieri C. Pleural fluid pH as a predictor of survival for patients with malignant pleural effusions. *Chest* 2000; **117**: 79–86.
113. Fishman RA. Carrier transport and concentration of glucose in cerebrospinal fluid in meningeal diseases. *Ann Intern Med* 1965; **63**: 153–5.
◆114. Sahn SA. Pathogenesis and clinical features of diseases associated with a low pleural fluid glucose. In: Chretien J, Bignon J, Hirsch A (eds). *The pleura in health and disease.* New York: Marcel Dekker, 1985: 267–85.
115. Dodson WH, Hollingsworth JW. Pleural effusion in rheumatoid arthritis. Impaired transport of glucose. *N Engl J Med* 1966; **275**: 1337–42.
●116. Carr DT, McGuckin WF. Pleural fluid glucose. Serial observations of its concentration following oral administration of glucose in the patient with rheumatoid pleural effusions and malignant effusions. *Am Rev Respir Dis* 1968; **97**: 302–5.
117. Clarkson B. Relationship between cell type, glucose concentration, and response to treatment in neoplastic effusions. *Cancer* 1964; **17**: 914–28.
●118. Light RW, Ball WC Jr. Glucose and amylase in pleural effusions. *J Am Med Assoc* 1973; **225**: 257–60.
119. Russakoff AH, le Maistre CA, Dewlett HJ. An evaluation of the pleural fluid glucose determination. *Am Rev Respir Dis* 1962; **85**: 220–3.
●120. Good JT Jr, King TE, Antony VB, Sahn SA. Lupus pleuritis: clinical features and pleural fluid characteristics with special reference to pleural fluid antinuclear antibody titers. *Chest* 1983; **84**: 714–8.
121. Maulitz RM, Good JT Jr, Kaplan RL, *et al.* The pleuropulmonary consequences of esophageal rupture in an experimental model. *Am Rev Respir Dis* 1979; **120**: 363–7.
122. Kaye MD. Pleuropulmonary complications of pancreatitis. *Thorax* 1968; **23**: 297–306.
123. Joseph J, Viney S, Beck P, *et al.* A prospective study of amylase-rich pleural effusion with special reference to amylase isoenzyme analysis. *Chest* 1992; **102**: 1455–9.
124. Rockey DC, Cello JP. Pancreaticopleural fistula: a report of 7 cases and review of the literature. *Medicine* 1990; **69**: 332–4.
125. Abbott OA, Mansour KA, Logan WD Jr, *et al.* Atraumatic so-called 'spontaneous' rupture of the esophagus. A review of 47 personal cases with comments on a new method of surgical therapy. *J Thorac Cardiovasc Surg* 1970; **59**: 67–83.
126. Sherr HP, Light RW, Merson MH, *et al.* Origin of pleural fluid amylase in esophageal rupture. *Ann Intern Med* 1972; **76**: 785–6.
127. Ende N. Studies of amylase activity in pleural effusions and ascites. *Cancer* 1960; **13**: 283–7.
◆128. Kramer MR, Sepero RJ, Pitchenik AE. High amylase in neoplasm-related pleural effusions. *Ann Intern Med* 1989; **110**: 567–9.
129. Perry TT. Role of lymphatic vessels in the transmission of lipase in deceminated pancreatic lymphatic necrosis. *Arch Pathol* 1947; **43**: 456–65.
130. Dumont AE, Doubilet H, Mulholind JH. Lymphatic pathways of pancreatic secretion in man. *Ann Surg* 1960; **153**: 403–9.
131. Lueng KC. Pancreatic pleural effusion with normal serum amylase levels. *J R Soc Med* 1985; **78**: 698.
132. Buckler H, Honeybourne D. Raised pleural fluid amylase level as an aid in the diagnosis of adenocarcinoma of the lung. *Br J Clin Pract* 1984; **38**: 359–61, 371.
133. Rodriguez BP, Rogers JT, Ayo DS, *et al.* Routine measurement of pleural fluid amylase is not indicated. *Arch Intern Med* 2001; **161**: 228–32.
●134. Staats BA, Ellefson RD, Budahn LL, *et al.* The lipoprotein profile of chylous and nonchylous pleural effusions. *Mayo Clin Proc* 1980; **55**: 700–4.
135. Teba L, Dedhia AT, Bowen R, Alexander JC. Chylothorax review. *Crit Care Med* 1985; **13**: 49–52.
136. Hamm H, Pfalzer B, Fabel H. Lipoprotein analysis in a chyliform pelural effusion: implications for pathogenesis and diagnosis. *Respiration* 1991; **58**: 294–300.
●137. Coe JE, Aikawa JK. Cholesterol pleural effusion. *Arch Intern Med* 1961; **108**: 763–74.
138. Harvey AM, Shulman LE, Tumulty PA, *et al.* Systemic lupus erythematosis: review of the literature and clinical analysis of 138 cases. *Medicine* 1954; **33**: 291–437.
139. Walker WC, Wright V. Rheumatoid pleuritis. *Ann Rheum Dis* 1967; **26**: 467–74.
140. Horler AR, Thompson M. The pleural and pulmonary complications of rheumatoid arthritis. *Ann Intern Med* 1959; **50**: 1179–1203.
141. Khare V, Baethge B, Lang S, *et al.* Antinuclear antibodies in pleural fluid. *Chest* 1994; **106**: 866–71.
142. Halla JT, Schrohenloher RE, Volanakis JE. Immune complexes and other laboratory features of pleural effusions. *Ann Intern Med* 1980; **92**: 748–52.
143. Levine H, Szanto M, Grieble HG, *et al.* Rheumatoid factor in non-rheumatoid pleural effusions. *Ann Intern Med* 1968; **69**: 487–92.
144. Hunder GG, McDufie FC, Heppern GG. Pleural fluid complement in systemic lupus erythematosus in rheumatoid arthritis. *Ann Intern Med* 1972; **76**: 357–62.
145. Glovsky MM, Louie JS, Pitts WH Jr, Alenty A. Reduction of pleural fluid complement activity in patients with systemic lupus erythematosus and rheumatoid arthritis. *Clin Immunol Immunopathol* 1976; **6**: 31–41).
146. Andrews BS, Arora NS, Shadforth MF, *et al.* The role of immune complexes in the pathogenesis of pleural effusions. *Am Rev Respir Dis* 1981; **125**: 115–20.
147. Grunze H. The comparative diagnostic accuracy, efficiency, and specificity of cytologic techniques used in the diagnosis of malignant neoplasm and serous effusions of the pleuroperitoneal cavities. *Acta Cytol* 1964; **8**: 150–64.
148. Jarvi OH, Kunnas RJ, Laitio MT, Tyrkko JES. The accuracy and significance of cytologic cancer diagnosis of pleural effusions. *Acta Cytol* 1972; **16**: 152–7.
149. Sahn SA. Malignant pleural effusions. *Sem Respir Med* 1987; **9**: 43–53.
150. Naylor B, Schmidt RW. The case for exfoliative cytology of serous effusions. *Lancet* 1964; i: 711–2.
151. Melamed MR. The cytologic presentation of malignant lymphomas in related diseases and effusions. *Cancer* 1963; **16**: 413–31.
152. Moriarty AT, Wiersema L, Snyder W, *et al.* Immunophenotyping of cytologic specimens by flow cytometry. *Diagn Cytopathol* 1993; **9**: 252–8.
153. Kataria YP, Khurshid I. Adenosine deaminase in the diagnosis of tuberculous pleural effusion. *Chest* 2001; **120**: 334–6.
154. Roth BJ. Searching for tuberculosis in the pleural space. *Chest* 1999; **116**: 3–5.
155. Pettersson T, Kaarina O, Weber TH. Adenosine deaminase in the diagnosis of pleural effusions. *Acta Med Scand* 1984; **215**: 299–304.
156. Lee YCG, Rogers JT, Rodriguez RM, *et al.* Adenosine deaminase levels in nontuberculous lymphocytic pleural effusions. *Chest* 2001; **120**: 356–61.
157. Valdes L, San Jose E, Alvares D, *et al.* Diagnosis of tuberculous pleurisy using the biologic parameters adenosine deaminase, lysozyme, and interferon-gamma. *Chest* 1993; **103**: 458–65.
158. Ungerer JPJ, Oosthuizen HM, Retief JH, Bissbort SH. Significance of adenosine deaminase and its isoenzymes in tuberculous effusions. *Chest* 1994; **106**: 33–7.
159. Burgess LJ, Maritz FJ, Roux IL, Taljaard JJ. Use of adenosine deaminase as a diagnostic tool for tuberculous pleurisy. *Thorax* 1995; **50**: 672–4.
●160. Valdes L, Alvarez D, San Jose E, *et al.* Tuberculous pleurisy: a study of 254 patients. *Arch Intern Med* 1998; **158**: 2017–21.
161. Valdes L, Alvares D, San Jose E, *et al.* Value of adenosine deaminase in the diagnosis of tuberculous pleural effusions in young patients in a region of high prevalence of tuberculosis. *Thorax* 1995; **50**: 600–3.

18

Pleural manometry

DAVID FELLER-KOPMAN, ARMIN ERNST

INTRODUCTION

The first measurements of intrapleural pressure (Ppl) during the removal of pleural fluid were made by the German internist Heinrich Quincke in 1878.[1] The clinical use of pleural manometry gained favor in the early twentieth century, when physicians would measure pleural pressure to confirm entry into the pleural space while inducing pneumothorax for the treatment of tuberculosis. It was also noted at that time that approximately 5 percent of patients would develop 'unexpandable lung' due to parenchymal or visceral pleural scarring, with the formation of a pleural effusion *ex vacuo*.[2] The monitoring of pleural pressure, though interesting from a physiological standpoint in and of itself, can be used clinically to minimize the pressure-related complications associated with thoracentesis including the development of symptoms, such as chest discomfort[3] and re-expansion pulmonary edema, as well as to predict the success of pleurodesis in patients with malignant effusions.[4] Though the last three decades have seen a resurgence of using pleural manometry in the care of patients, it remains an underutilized technique. This chapter will review the pressure physiology of the pleural space, and discuss the clinical application of manometry.

NORMAL PLEURAL PRESSURE PHYSIOLOGY

At functional residual capacity (FRC) Ppl is slightly subatmospheric, approximately –3 to –5 cmH_2O.[5] This results from the equilibrium achieved by the elastic recoil forces of the lung and the tendency of the chest wall to expand. Pleural pressure actually consists of pleural liquid pressure and pleural surface pressure. The difference between these two pressures relates to deformation forces created by areas of parietal and visceral pleural contact. These deformation forces result in a pleural liquid pressure that is slightly more subatmospheric than one would expect, based solely on the recoil pressures of the lung and chest wall.[6]

When fluid accumulates in the pleural space, the deformation forces are in part released, and three distinct pressure zones are created. In the upper zone, the thickness of the pleural liquid is normal and the pleural liquid pressure remains lower than the pleural surface pressure. In the middle zone, where pleural liquid thickness starts to increase, to where pleural liquid pressure becomes zero, pleural liquid pressure is equal to pleural surface pressure. In the lower zone, the pressure of pleural liquid is positive, and the lung and chest wall are pushed apart.[6,7] These concepts, however, represent only one school of thought, based upon the 'hydrostatic theory' that pleural liquid is in a hydrostatic equilibrium maintained by a vertical gradient in pleural pressure of 1 cmH_2O/cm height.[8]

Another model maintains that pleural liquid pressure is always equal to pleural surface pressure. This concept suggests that pressure gradients due to gravity and regional differences in pleural surface pressure drive a small viscous flow of fluid in the pleural space, and requires the presence of a small continuous pleural fluid space with no contact between the lung and chest wall.[8] As pleural fluid accumulates, the viscous resistance to flow falls rapidly and the gradient in the pleural pressure approaches that of the hydrostatic pressure gradient.[8–10]

Measurement of pleural liquid and surface pressure in the normal pleural space is technically challenging due to the fact that the normal pleural space is only approximately 20 μm thick, and the insertion of any device into the pleural space will create deformation forces not present prior to the insertion of the device.[10] Though there continues to be great debate between the two dominant theories of normal pleural pressure physiology,[10,11] these conceptual differences may only be of practical importance at the termination of a thoracentesis, when there is only a physiological amount (5–8 mL) of pleural fluid present. In the presence of even a small effusion (several hundred milliliters), one can measure Ppl with a variety of techniques as the viscous resistance to flow becomes negligible. The pressure measured, therefore, is an accurate representation of the hydrostatic pressure in the effusion at the level of the catheter/transducer.

There has been some suggestion that when measuring Ppl, the height of the manometer relative to the effusion is insignificant.[12] The reason for this was assumed to be that as Pascal's law states, in an enclosed system such as the chest, pressure is transmitted equally in all directions and will exert the same force equally on the lung, chest wall and manometer, regardless of where the needle is inserted. This is in contrast to an open system, where the only force is that of gravity.[12]

More realistically, in a hydrothorax, a hydrostatic pressure gradient of 1 cmH_2O/cm height is present, and so the pressure read by the manometer represents the pressure at a specific level, and not the pressure thoughout the hydrothorax. With the removal of pleural fluid and a reduction in the height of the fluid column above the catheter, the influence of the hydrostatic pressure gradient becomes less. The measured Ppl therefore does depend on where in the effusion the catheter is placed. Placing the catheter at the most dependent part of the effusion has the potential benefits of (1) maximizing the amount of fluid that is able to be removed, and (2) minimizing the creation of deformation forces from the contact of the catheter with the lung. With this approach, the pressure measured at the level of the catheter will reflect the pressure in the pleural space, and hence the pressure exerted on the lung and chest wall, at that level (Figure 18.1).

Depending on the cause of the effusion, as fluid builds up in the pleural space, Ppl typically rises. As fluid is removed, one expects the lung to expand, the chest wall contract and the Ppl reach its steady state at FRC. Pleural pressure, however, can be negative, as in the case of trapped lung, or start out positive and drop rapidly, as is the case with lung entrapment.

DEFINITIONS: LUNG ENTRAPMENT VERSUS TRAPPED LUNG

Though confusing terms, 'lung entrapment' and 'trapped lung' describe different pathophysiology and are thought to represent a spectrum of pleural inflammation and repair. Lung entrapment describes an inability of the lung to re-expand due to visceral pleural thickening, endobronchial obstruction or diseases that lead to an increase in the elastic recoil of the lung such as interstitial lung disease and lymphangitic carcinomatosis. Patients often present with dyspnea related to the effusion as well as with signs and symptoms related to the underlying disease. Chest discomfort or other signs of pleural inflammation may also be present. The effusion associated with lung entrapment is typically exudative, representing an active inflammation. With normal healing of the underlying process, the effusion may completely resolve.

Trapped lung, on the other hand, is the sequelae of prior pleural inflammation resulting in visceral pleural scarring.[13,14] This creates negative pressure in the pleural space and results in an 'effusion *ex-vacuo*'. Since there is no active pleural inflammation, patients typically present with a chronic, and asymptomatic, effusion that is identified on routine physical examination or chest X-ray. As the pleural fluid formation results from an excess of negative pleural pressure, it is rare to see contralateral mediastinal shift on a chest radiograph, even in the presence of a moderate to large effusion. Likewise, as the effusion is due to an

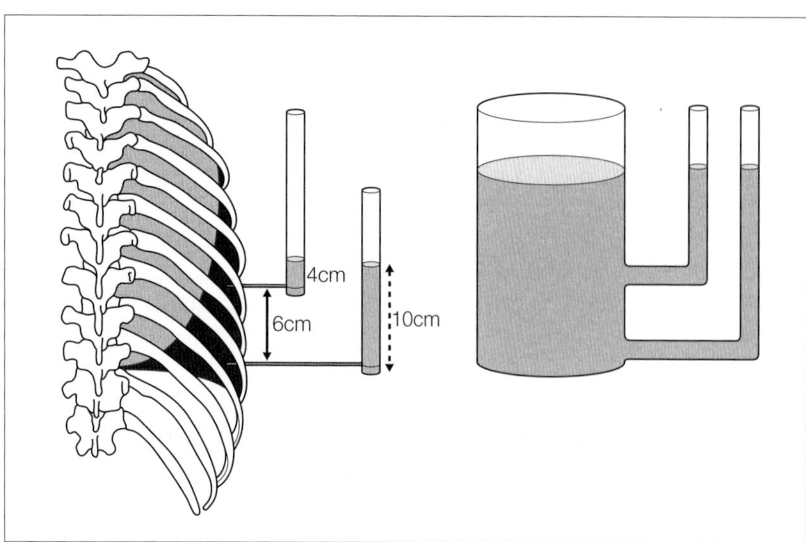

Figure 18.1 Hydrostatic pressures in an open and closed system (from Feller-Kopman, D. Therapeutic thoracentesis: The role of ultrasound and pleural manometry. *Curr Opin Pulm Med* 2007; **13**: 312–18 [modified from: Bernstein A, White FZ. Unusual physical findings in pleural effusion: intrathoracic manometric studies. *Ann Intern Med* 1952; **37**: 733-8)].

imbalance of hydrostatic forces, it is always transudative in nature. Since the large majority of these patients are asymptomatic, therapy aimed at the pleural effusion is usually not required. Should the patient have exertional dyspnea resulting from a restrictive ventilatory defect due to the effusion, decortication will likely be required to expand the underlying lung.

As mentioned above, lung entrapment and trapped lung are part of a continuum of the natural healing process of the underlying disease and, as such, one may occasionally obtain pleural fluid results that fall in the exudative range, even in the setting of trapped lung physiology, depending on when the thoracentesis is performed in the healing process.[15]

TECHNIQUE

Pleural pressure can be measured via several techniques. These include using a U-shaped water manometer,[16] an 'overdamped' water manometer[17] or sophisticated electronic transducer systems that allow sampling several times a second as well as the ability to store data for further analysis. A benefit of the U-shaped manometer is the fact that it is relatively inexpensive. A disadvantage, however, is the fact that it may be difficult to accurately record values due to the inspiratory and expiratory pleural pressure swings. Electronic transducer systems can be configured to standard monitors in the intensive care unit (ICU), however, one needs to calibrate an 'offset' as these monitors are not calibrated to measure negative pressure. Additionally, ICU hemodynamic transducers report data in mmHg, instead of the standard cmH_2O typically used for Ppl measurements. This problem is easily resolved by adding the conversion factor of 1 mmHg = 1.36 cmH_2O. A distinct advantage of using an electronic transducer system is the ability to examine the Ppl curves after the data has been collected. This allows one to measure end inspiratory and end expiratory, as well as mean Ppl. Though it is unclear at this time which of these pressures is clinically most important, it is likely that future studies will clarify this issue. Most authors currently report mean or end-expiratory (i.e. FRC) Ppl. It may be, however, that end inspiratory pressure is most related to the development of complications such as re-expansion pulmonary edema (RPE). Doelken *et al.*[17] have recently described their use of an overdamped water manometer that uses a 22ga needle as a resistor, and have shown excellent correlation to the electronic system ($r = 0.97$). The benefits of this system are that it is relatively easy to set up and it also provides real-time mean Ppl without the large respirophasic swings that are encountered with systems that are not damped.

MANOMETRY IN THE CLINICAL SETTING

In 1980, Light and colleagues[16] used a water-filled U-shaped manometer connected to an Abram's needle to measure mean pleural pressure during thoracenteses in 52 patients with the goal of determining the clinical utility of pleural manometry, and to evaluate the safety of large-volume thoracentesis. Pleural fluid was removed until either the mean Ppl fell to less than −20 cmH_2O, no more fluid could be obtained or patients developed symptoms described as more than minimal in severity. Though the initial Ppl varied widely (−21 cmH_2O to +8 cmH_2O) an initial pressure of less than −5 cmH_2O was only seen in patients with malignant effusions or trapped lung. They also measured pleural elastance (change in pressure divided by change in volume) and described three distinct pleural elastance curves: (1) removal of a large amount of fluid with minimal change in pressure (as can be seen in patients with hepatic hydrothorax); (2) a relatively normal initial curve followed by a sharp drop in pressure; and (3) a negative initial pressure with a rapid drop in pressure (Figure 18.2). They felt that the first curve (open circles) represented a normal pleural elastance, the second curve (closed circles) that of lung entrapment, and the third curve (x marks) was consistent with trapped lung. A pleural elastance >25 cmH_2O/L was seen in patients with malignancy or trapped lung.

Light's group later investigated the relationship between changes in Ppl during thoracentesis and improvement in lung function.[18] They found that although the improvement in mean forced vital capacity (FVC) following thoracentesis was related to the volume of fluid removed (approximately 21 mL for each 100 mL removed), the correlation coefficient was only 0.49. Interestingly, the improvement in FVC was most closely related to Ppl after the removal of 800 mL of fluid ($r = -0.57$, $p < 0.01$). Improvement in FVC was also significantly (and negatively) related to initial Ppl, as well as the change in Ppl after removal of 400 and 800 mL of pleural fluid. The negative correlation indicates that the larger pressure changes were associated with smaller improve-

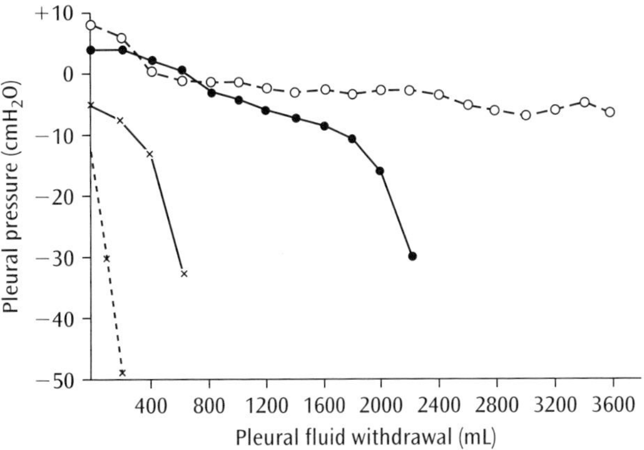

Figure 18.2 Pleural elastance curves (from Light RW, Jenkinson SG, Minh VD, George RB. Observations on pleural fluid pressures as fluid is withdrawn during thoracentesis. *Am Rev Respir Dis* 1980; **121**: 799–804.

ments in FVC, consistent with the physiology of unexpandable lung. That is to say, the lack of increase in lung volume correlates with more negative pleural pressure.

Huggins and colleagues[15] have recently described their use of an 'air-contrast' computed tomography (CT) scan to visualize visceral pleural thickening and help define the cause of unexpandable lung in a group of 247 consecutive patients undergoing pleural manometry during thoracentesis. They identified 11 patients with a clinical diagnosis of trapped lung. All of these patients developed a mean Ppl of less than –25 cmH_2O and had prior pleural fluid analysis that was not suggestive of malignancy or pleural inflammation. At the termination of the therapeutic thoracentesis, they instilled atmospheric air, a 'diagnostic pneumothorax' with the goal of raising the Ppl to a more physiological mean of –5 cmH_2O. A subsequent CT scan confirmed visceral pleural thickening in all 11 patients. As expected, all of these patients had a high pleural elastance (Eps >19 cmH_2O/L). The authors favor using the air-contrast CT as part of the diagnostic approach to patients with trapped lung as a way of minimizing additional pleural interventions that will be of little value, and in fact have incorporated the 'diagnostic pneumothorax' as part of their routine protocol should patients develop significantly low Ppl and pleural fluid is still present.

RE-EXPANSION PULMONARY EDEMA

During a thoracentesis, one would ideally like to remove as much fluid as is safely possible. The goals of completely draining the pleural space include maximizing symptomatic relief, sparing the patient multiple procedures, increasing the yield of other diagnostic tests, such as a post-thoracentesis CT scan, and documenting lung re-expansion prior to attempts at pleurodesis. In Light's original study, they showed that if thoracenteses were terminated when the Ppl dropped to less than –20 cmH_2O, re-expansion pulmonary edema was avoided despite removing large quantities of fluid.[16] They conclude that, 'as the operator cannot easily estimate pleural pressure... therapeutic thoracentesis should be limited to 1000 mL unless pleural pressures are monitored'. A pressure of –20 cmH_2O was arbitrarily chosen based on prior animal studies[19,20] that showed a minimal risk of re-expansion pulmonary edema if Ppl was kept above –20 mmHg (approximately –27 cmH_2O), but a significant risk was present with Ppl of –40 mmHg (approximately –54 cmH_2O). The above quote has led to the majority of clinicians terminating thoracentesis after removing 1000–1500 mL without regard to the amount of remaining pleural fluid, the potential benefit of removing that fluid or consideration of pleural pressure.

Pleural manometry allows for the safe drainage of large volumes of fluid as well as avoiding the pressure-related consequences of thoracentesis such as RPE. In a study of 61 patients, Villena and colleagues[21] used manometry to define the relationships of Ppl to underlying diagnosis as well as complications of therapeutic thoracentesis. Although there was no significance to a negative initial Ppl, all patients with an initial Ppl of less than –4 cmH_2O and an elastance of the pleural space (Eps) >33 cmH_2O/L had trapped lung. There were no cases of re-expansion pulmonary edema, despite a mean removal of 1.45 L of pleural fluid. We routinely use pleural manometry during therapeutic thoracentesis, and terminate the tap if patients develop chest discomfort, end-expiratory Ppl is less than –20 cmH_2O, or when there is no more fluid. In our recent series of over 185 large volume (>1 L) thoracenteses (mean 1.67 L, range 1000–6550 mL), only one patient developed clinically significant RPE.[22] There was no relationship to the volume of pleural fluid removed, Ppl, Eps or symptoms during the thoracentesis, suggesting that RPE is a rare event, and that large effusions can be drained completely, provided that patients do not develop chest discomfort (see below) or Ppl is less than –20 cmH_2O.

PLEURODESIS

For pleurodesis to be successful, the pleural surfaces need to appose each other. If the lung is entrapped and does not re-expand during thoracentesis, the odds of successful pleurodesis are reduced. This fact is likely the single largest confounder in the multiple studies comparing pleurodesis agents, as documentation of lung re-expansion was used as a criteria prior to randomization in only two studies.[23,24] Lan and colleagues[4] used pleural manometry to predict lung re-expansion and found that a pleural space elastance of ≥19 cmH_2O after the removal of 500 mL of pleural fluid predicted pleurodesis failure. This is clinically important, as patients with lung entrapment can still achieve pleural palliation with a significant reduction in their dyspnea with the placement of a chronic indwelling (PleurX™) catheter,[25] and one should not attempt pleurodesis prior to documenting full lung expansion by either manometry or imaging after complete removal of pleural fluid.

SYMPTOMS

The development of symptoms such as cough and chest pain/discomfort is quite common during therapeutic thoracentesis. As most physicians do not currently perform pleural manometry during thoracentesis, we investigated the relationship of Ppl to patient symptoms as pleural fluid is removed.[3] We measured end expiratory Ppl during therapeutic thoracentesis in 169 consecutive patients undergoing therapeutic thoracentesis. Symptoms developed in 17 percent of patients (cough in 6 percent and chest discomfort in 11 percent). We distinguished between the sensations of a sharp, ipsilateral pain that is typically felt over the ipsilateral shoulder/scapula and another, more vague chest discomfort that is often felt anteriorly. The former sensation was felt to be due to catheter irritation of the diaphragm, whereas the latter could be related to the development of significantly negative Ppl. If patients developed sharp pain, the catheter was repositioned, whereas if patients developed persistent chest discomfort, the procedure was terminated. There was no relationship between the volume of fluid removed or opening Ppl to symptom development. Closing Ppl and the change in Ppl, however, were both significantly lower in the patients who developed chest discomfort. Interestingly, there was a trend toward a lower pleural elastance in the patients who developed cough, possibly suggesting that cough is due to normal expansion of the lung as the pleural fluid is removed. Additionally, nearly 9 percent of patients were asymptomatic despite potentially dangerous drops in Ppl.

CONCLUSION

In conclusion, pleural manometry provides a better understanding of the underlying pleural pathophysiology and aids the physician in both diagnostic and therapeutic decisions. Measurement of Ppl can distinguish between lung entrapment and trapped lung, allows for the safe removal of large effusions and is a useful tool to select appropriate patients with malignant pleural effusions for pleurodesis. If formal manometry is not performed during thoracentesis, the symptom of a vague chest discomfort can be used as a surrogate for potentially dangerous drops in pleural pressure.

KEY POINTS

- In the presence of a pleural effusion, the pressure in the pleural space is dependent on the cause of the effusion as well as the ability of the lung to re-expand with removal of the fluid.
- Trapped lung and lung entrapment represent distinct entities of unexpandable lung.
- The majority of patients with trapped lung do not require specific therapy aimed at the pleural space.
- Pleural manometry should be used to best select patients with malignant pleural effusions for palliation by pleurodesis or PleurX™ catheter placement.
- If formal manometry is not performed during thoracentesis, the development of chest discomfort should raise the suspicion of unexpandable lung.
- Introduction of air into the pleural space, a diagnostic pneumothorax, can be used to help visualize visceral pleural thickening in patients with unexpandable lung.

REFERENCES

● = Key primary paper
◆ = Major review article

1. Otis AB. History of respiratory mechanics. In: Fishman AP, Macklem PT, Mead J, Geiger SR (eds.). *Handbook of respiratory physiology: A critical, comprehensive presentation of physiological knowledge and concepts*. Bethesda: American Physiologic Society, 1986: 1–12.
2. Farber JE, Lincoln NS. The unexpandable lung. *Am Rev Tuberc* 1939; **40**: 704–9.
●3. Feller-Kopman D, Walkey A, Berkowitz D, Ernst A. The relationship of pleural pressure to symptom development during therapeutic thoracentesis. *Chest* 2006; **129**: 1556–60.
●4. Lan RS, Lo SK, Chuang ML, *et al*. Elastance of the pleural space: a predictor for the outcome of pleurodesis in patients with malignant pleural effusion. *Ann Intern Med* 1997; **126**: 768–74.
5. Broaddus VC, Light RW. Disorders of the pleura: General principles and diagnostic approach. In: Murray JF, Nadel JA (eds). *Textbook of respiratory medicine*. Philadelphia: WB Saunders Company, 1994: 2145–2163.
6. Agostoni E. Mechanics of the pleural space. *Physiol Rev* 1972; **52**: 57–128.
7. Agostoni E, D'Angelo E. Thickness and pressure of the pleural liquid at various heights and with various hydrothoraces. *Respir Physiol* 1969; **6**: 330–42.
8. Lai-Fook SJ. Mechanics of the pleural space: fundamental concepts. *Lung* 1987; **165**: 249–67.
9. Boggs DS, Kinasewitz GT. Review: pathophysiology of the pleural space. *Am J Med Sci* 1995; **309**: 53–9.
◆10. Lai-Fook SJ. Pleural mechanics and fluid exchange. *Physiol Rev* 2004; **84**: 385–410.
◆11. Agostoni E, D'Angelo E. Pleural liquid pressure. *J Appl Physiol* 1991; **71**: 393–403.
12. Bernstein A, White FZ. Unusual physical findings in pleural effusion: intrathoracic manometric studies. *Ann Intern Med* 1952; **37**: 733–8.
◆13. Doelken P, Sahn SA. Trapped lung. *Semin Respir Crit Care Med* 2001; **22**: 631–5.
14. Moore PJ, Thomas PA. The trapped lung with chronic pleural space, a cause of recurring pleural effusion. *Mil Med* 1967; **132**: 998–1002.
●15. Huggins JT, Sahn SA, Heidecker J, *et al*. Characteristics of trapped lung: Pleural fluid analysis, manometry, and air-contrast chest CT. *Chest* 2007; **131**: 206–13.
●16. Light RW, Jenkinson SG, Minh VD, George RB. Observations on pleural fluid pressures as fluid is withdrawn during thoracentesis. *Am Rev Respir Dis* 1980; **121**: 799–804.
●17. Doelken P, Huggins JT, Pastis NJ, Sahn SA. Pleural manometry: technique and clinical implications. *Chest* 2004; **126**: 1764–9.
●18. Light RW, Stansbury DW, Brown SE. The relationship between pleural pressures and changes in pulmonary function after therapeutic thoracentesis. *Am Rev Respir Dis* 1986; **133**: 658–61.
19. Pavlin J, Cheney FW, Jr. Unilateral pulmonary edema in rabbits after reexpansion of collapsed lung. *J Appl Physiol* 1979; **46**: 31–5.
20. Miller WC, Toon R, Palat H, Lacroix J. Experimental pulmonary edema following re-expansion of pneumothorax. *Am Rev Respir Dis* 1973; **108**: 654–6.
21. Villena V, Lopez-Encuentra A, Pozo F, *et al*. Measurement of pleural pressure during therapeutic thoracentesis. *Am J Respir Crit Care Med* 2000; **162**: 1534–8.
●22. Feller-Kopman D, Berkowitz D, Boiselle P, Ernst A. Large volume thoracentesis and the risk of re-expansion pulmonary edema. *Ann Thorac Surg* 2007; **84**: 1656–62.

23. Diacon AH, Wyser C, Bolliger CT, *et al.* Prospective randomized comparison of thoracoscopic talc poudrage under local anesthesia versus bleomycin instillation for pleurodesis in malignant pleural effusions. *Am J Respir Crit Care Med* 2000; **162**: 1445–9.
24. Dresler CM, Olak J, Herndon JE, *et al.* Phase III intergroup study of talc poudrage vs talc slurry sclerosis for malignant pleural effusion. *Chest* 2005; **127**: 909–15.
25. Tremblay A, Michaud G. Single-center experience with 250 tunnelled pleural catheter insertions for malignant pleural effusion. *Chest* 2006; **129**: 362–8.

19

Radiology: diagnostic

FERGUS V GLEESON

TECHNIQUES

Chest radiography (CXR), ultrasound (US), computed tomography (CT), multislice computed tomography (MSCT), high-resolution computed tomography (HRCT), magnetic resonance imaging (MRI) and positron emission tomography combined with computed tomography (PET-CT) may all be used to investigate pleural diseases. Interestingly, except for MRI, all techniques are also able to demonstrate normal pleural surfaces.

Chest radiography

Whenever possible, both posterior–anterior (PA) and lateral CXRs should be performed to assess the pleura. Conventional high-kilovoltage and digital CXR may be used. Additional films may be of value, for example a lateral decubitus CXR to demonstrate small volumes of fluid,[1] a shoot-through lateral supine CXR to detect a pneumothorax in patients in the intensive care unit (ICU)[2] and oblique films to confirm pleural thickening. However, oblique views have mostly been replaced by CT and HRCT for this purpose,[3] and the increasing use of CT and US is replacing the lateral supine CXR in the ICU. Supine CXRs are commonly performed in critically ill patients but are of less value than an erect film in the detection of fluid and air.[4]

Ultrasound

Ultrasound, because of its low cost, ease of use and portability, is commonly performed to assess pleural disease detected on CXR. It can be performed on inpatients and outpatients, and is of great value in the critically ill, such as ICU patients. A small-footprint probe enables the easiest intercostal access. Higher-frequency linear array transducers (7.5 MHz) provide the greatest spatial resolution, particularly of the normal pleural surfaces,[5] but may not provide enough penetration in larger patients or those with large-volume pleural disease. In general, a variable frequency 3.5–5.0 MHz sector transducer with a small footprint provides excellent images in most patients, and can also be used to aid interventional procedures.[2,6] Although currently only a research tool, contrast enhanced ultrasound (CEUS) has been used to evaluate pleural disease and may be relatively specific in the identification of benign and malignant disease.[7]

Computed tomography and high-resolution computed tomography

Computed tomography is an excellent means of further assessing pleural disease detected on CXR or US. Whenever possible, CT should be performed using spiral sequences, single or multislice, enabling overlapping and multiplanar reconstruction. Unless HRCT alone is being performed, intravenous contrast should be administered prior to scanning, and a delay of 20–60 seconds used to enable maximum soft tissue enhancement.[8] Spiral CT should be performed with a slice thickness of 5 mm and at a pitch that allows overlapping reconstructions in the coronal and sagittal planes to be performed.[9]

High-resolution computed tomography is of value in determining whether possible pleural thickening/plaques detected on a CXR are genuine, and should be performed with thin sections of less than 2 mm and a high spatial resolution reconstruction algorithm.[9] CT has also been shown to be of value in the quantification of pleural disease and to correlate with functional measures in patients with impaired lung function secondary to pleural thickening.[10]

Magnetic resonance imaging

Magnetic resonance imaging has a limited role in the investigation of pleural disease. It has been shown to be of value in assessing tumor extension through the pleura and in the detection of pleural malignancy. For MR chest imaging, respiratory compensation and cardiac gating should be routinely used.[10–13] A body coil is initially used to obtain the large field-of-view scout images. Specialized coils may then be used if further dedicated images are required. The pulse sequences and imaging planes must be tailored to the individual examination. Typical sequences are T1-weighted spin echo, proton-density and T2-weighted spin echo or fast spin echo with fat saturation, STIR (short T1 inversion recovery) and gradient-recalled acquisition in the steady state. The slice thickness and intersection gap depend on the area to be scanned and should be adjusted accordingly.

T1-weighted images show excellent contrast between abnormalities in the pleural space and extrapleural fat, and are also excellent for anatomic resolution.[6] T2-weighted images offer more tissue-specific information and may show increased tumor to muscle contrast,[6] and T1 post-intravenous gadolinium may also be of value in detecting pleural enhancement in malignancy.[14] Dynamic contrast enhanced MRI (DCEMRI) may be used to assess malignant pleural vascularity and predict chemotherapy disease response in patients with mesothelioma (see later).[15]

Positron emission tomography combined with computed tomography

The development of combined PET and CT scanners (PET-CT) has expanded the use of PET imaging throughout the body, and the chest is no exception, although its cost, limited availability and the length of examination times relative to the other imaging modalities persist as constraints on its use. The low spatial resolution of PET scanners has now been overcome to a certain extent by co-registration using combined CT and PET scanners.[16] 18-fluorodeoxyglucose (^{18}FDG) is the only commercially available radioisotope for the investigation of pleural malignancy.[17] Malignant cells are more metabolically active than non-malignant cells and therefore concentrate ^{18}FDG more avidly than normal tissue. Consequently, the greater positron emission from such areas may enable the detection and differentiation of malignant from benign pleural disease. One study of 98 patients showed ^{18}FDG activity in 61 of 63 patients with pleural malignancy compared to an absence of activity in 31 of 35 patients with benign disease. ^{18}FDG activity was intense in 51 of the patients with malignant pleural thickening and moderate in 10.[18]

NORMAL ANATOMY

Chest radiography

On a standard radiograph, the normal pleura is visualized only where the visceral pleura invaginates into the lung to form the fissures,[19–24] and where the two lungs contact one another at the junctional lines.[25,26] The oblique and horizontal fissures consist of a double layer of infolded visceral pleura,[24] and are only seen on a chest radiograph when they are tangential to the X-ray beam. They are often incomplete and thus do not extend all the way to the hilum.[21,25]

The normal visceral pleura may also be identified in patients with a pneumothorax; it is normally less than 1 mm thick. The normal parietal pleura is never visualized.

Ultrasound

Normal pleura is seen as an echogenic stripe, the ‘pleural stripe’ (Figure 19.1), comprising both the opposing visceral and parietal layers, associated with distal reverberation echoes, because the pleura reflects most of the acoustic energy of the ultrasound beam. These distal reverberation artifacts, often described as ‘comet tails’, are produced by any small, highly reflective object in the scanning plane[27] and manifest as an echogenic band extending from the object into the deeper portions of the image.[28] A ‘comet tail’ can be produced by different structures at the pleural surface, such as small foreign bodies, foci of calcification and discrete air collections.

During respiration, small hypoechoic inhomogeneities are seen to move at the pleural stripe, producing a shimmering movement described as the ‘lung sliding’ sign.[29] The ‘comet tail’ and ‘lung sliding’ signs disappear in the presence of a pneumothorax.[29–31]

Ultrasound is also able to assess the pleural surface of the diaphragm in the normal individual.[32] It is best assessed in the right or left intercostal spaces between the anteroaxillary and midaxillary lines to observe the zone of apposition of the diaphragm 0.5–2 cm below the costophrenic recess. On ultrasound, the diaphragm is seen to consist of five layers: two outer bright parallel lines representing the pleural and peritoneal membranes separated from the bright layer of the diaphragm muscular layer by hypoechoic layers of connective tissue on either side.[32,33]

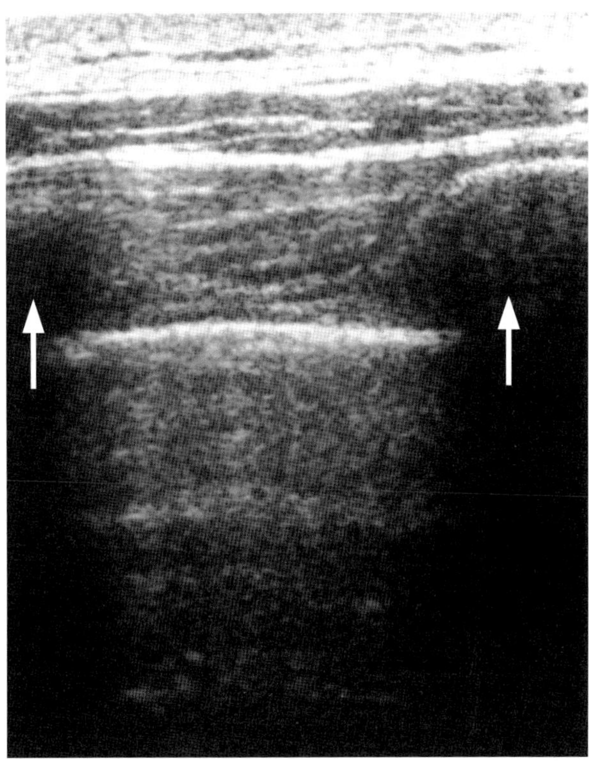

Figure 19.1 The normal pleural surfaces (parietal and visceral) seen as a bright stripe on ultrasound. Note the position of the ribs (arrows).

Computed tomography

VISCERAL PLEURA: FISSURES AND JUNCTION LINES

The fissures are not directly visualized on thick section (5 mm) CT. The oblique fissures are visualized in approximately 80–95 percent of patients as curvilinear avascular bands extending from the hilum to the chest wall.[34,35] The horizontal fissure, detected less often than the oblique fissure, is also seen as an avascular band extending from the major fissure to the chest wall, and is usually best visualized on a section between the origins of the upper and middle lobe bronchi.

High-resolution computed tomography

In contrast to the avascular band-like densities seen on conventional CT, on HRCT the fissures are seen as smooth, linear opacities (Figure 19.2). The normal fissure is less than 1 mm thick and sharply defined.[36] In a normal individual the visceral pleura, subpleural interstitium, and parietal pleura along the costal and mediastinal surfaces of the lung are not visualized on HRCT.[36]

Along the costal pleural surface adjacent to the parietal pleura is a thin layer of extrapleural fat, separating the pleura from the endothoracic fascia.[37] It is this combination of tissues plus the innermost intercostal muscle that is

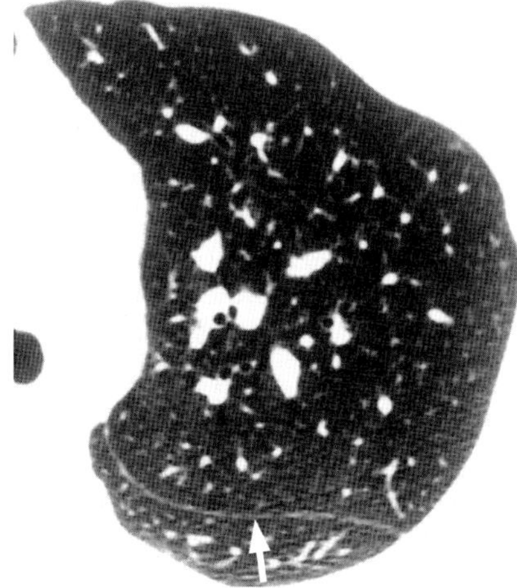

Figure 19.2 Left oblique fissure visualized as sharply defined thin line on 1-mm high-resolution computed tomography section (arrow).

visualized as the normal intercostal stripe on HRCT (Figure 19.3). This is visible as a 1–2 mm thick stripe in the anterolateral and posterolateral intercostal spaces, at the point of contact between lung and chest wall.[36,37] On HRCT, the innermost intercostal muscle can also be seen internal to the tapering edges of the visible rib segments, thus mimicking pleural thickening.[37] However, it is seen to be continuous with the normal innermost muscle in the adjacent interspaces and is not seen internal to the entire rib segment, both of which distinguish it from pleural thickening.[37]

The normal stripe can be seen internal to the entire length of the visible rib segment when the rib is horizontal, as is common posteriorly. Again, this may mimic pleural thickening. The visible rib segment should appear thinner than usual.[37]

Occasionally, normal soft tissue may be seen internal to a rib: the layer of fatty tissue located between the parietal

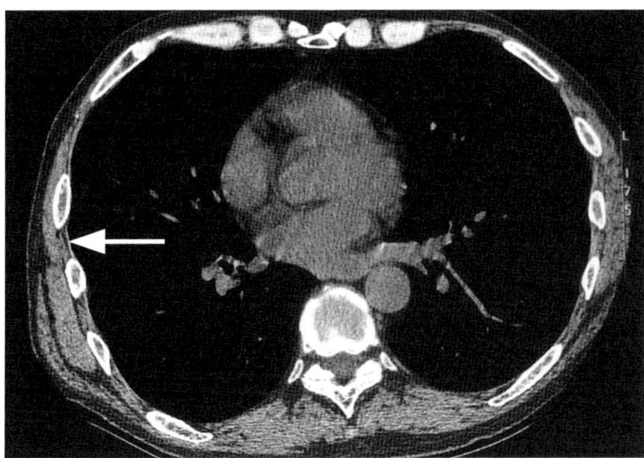

Figure 19.3 High-resolution computed tomography demonstrating the intercostal stripe (arrow).

pleura and the endothoracic fascia thickens adjacent to the lateral ribs, producing fat pads several millimeters thick, especially over the fourth to eighth ribs which can extend into the intercostal spaces or fissures.[38,39]

The transverse thoracic and subcostal muscles may be visible internal to the end of a rib or costal cartilage, the former at the level of the heart adjacent to the lower sternum or xiphoid process and the latter posteriorly at the same level. They should be smooth, uniform in thickness and bilaterally symmetrical.[37]

In a paravertebral location, the pleura and fascia combine to produce a thinner line than that seen laterally. The innermost muscle is absent. Occasionally, the paravertebral line is thicker than expected, which may reflect segments of the intercostal vessels.[37,40]

Magnetic resonance imaging

As a result of their sub-1 mm thickness and consequent lack of signal, the normal pleural surfaces including fissures and junctional lines are not visualized on MRI.

PLEURAL FLUID

Chest radiography

POSTERIOR–ANTERIOR AND LATERAL RADIOGRAPHS

Pleural fluid tends to collect along dependent surfaces. As the amount of fluid increases, the diaphragm appears flattened and blunting of the lateral costophrenic angle is seen on the PA radiograph.[41] Accumulation of 200 mL or more of fluid leads to blunting of the lateral costophrenic sulcus, although up to 500 mL may be present without blunting.[42] The lateral decubitus view is far more sensitive in the detection of pleural fluid than the erect PA CXR and can demonstrate as little as 5 mL of fluid.[1]

As the amount of fluid increases, a typical 'meniscus' sign is seen on a standard PA CXR.[25] This is demonstrated by a homogeneous lower zone opacity with a concave upward sloping at the costophrenic angle that extends higher laterally than medially. This meniscus sign is explained by the fact that the X-ray beam traverses a greater thickness of fluid at the periphery.[43,44] If fluid collects at the point of contact of the fissures with the chest wall, then a 'tongue-like' intrusion of fluid into the fissures is seen more superiorly and peripherally.[25] A small amount of fluid in the horizontal fissure may produce a similar appearance.[45]

If fluid extends into the fissures in a step-like manner laterally below the horizontal fissure, then the appearance of the 'middle lobe step' is seen. This appearance can be explained by overlapping fluid intrusion into incomplete oblique and horizontal fissures.[21,46]

A massive effusion leads to complete or near-complete opacification of the hemithorax with mediastinal shift to the contralateral side.[47] A centrally located mediastinum in the presence of a large effusion suggests that either the mediastinum is fixed or there is associated pulmonary collapse.[48]

Inversion of the diaphragm may occur, especially with large effusions (see Chapter 6, Physiology: changes with pleural effusion and pneumothorax). This occurs most commonly on the left owing to the protective effect of the liver on the right (Figure 19.4).[49,50] An inverted diaphragm, which has reverted to a normal position, is one explanation for an apparent failure of a pleural effusion to decrease on a CXR post thoracentesis.

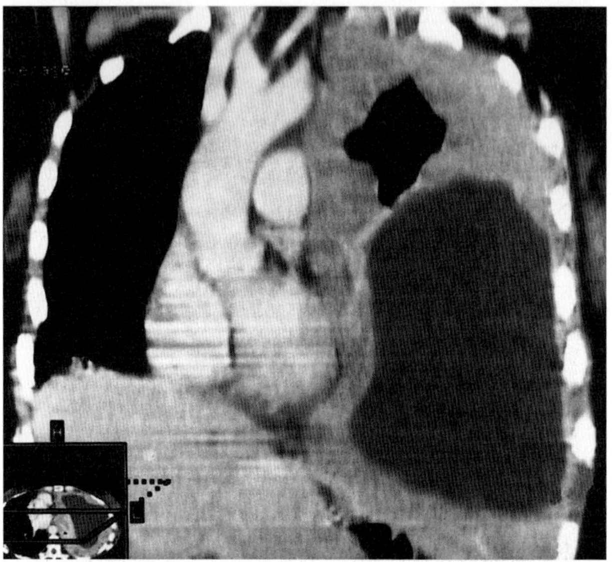

Figure 19.4 Multislice computed tomography coronal reconstruction demonstrating a large left pleural effusion and thickening. The large-volume disease has inverted the left hemidiaphragm.

Free fluid may collect within the interlobar fissures, simulating a mass, pulmonary abscess or loculated effusion (Figure 19.5), and fluid collecting along the mediastinum may be mistaken for a mediastinal mass.[21] These appearances can be differentiated by obtaining radiographs in different positions as free fluid shifts while masses and loculated collections do not.

Loculated effusions do not move freely in the pleural space and occur when there are adhesions between the visceral and parietal pleura. They are most commonly seen with exudative effusions such as empyemas and hemothoraces.[40] They tend to have a sharp medial margin and a hazy lateral margin, with the margins making an obtuse angle with the chest wall.[25] Occasionally, they may be indistinguishable from chest wall or pleural masses which tend to have their greatest depth opposite the pleural point

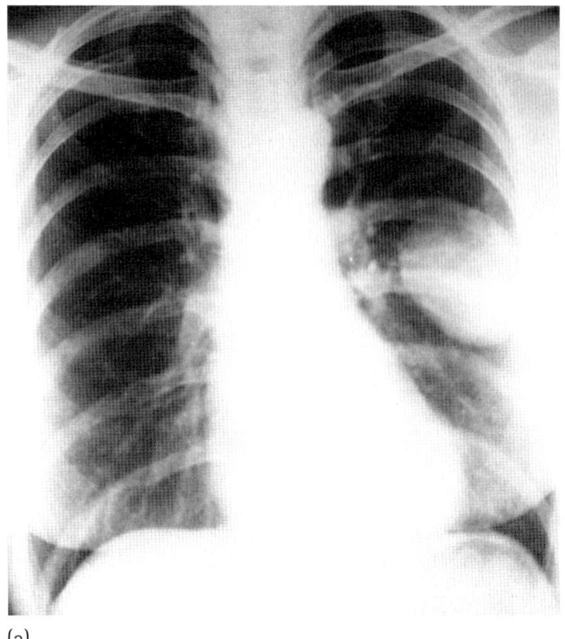

(a)

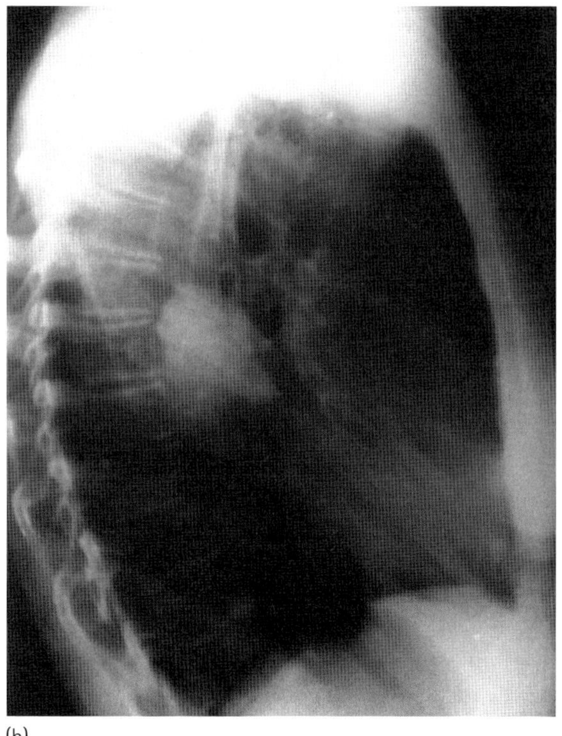

(b)

Figure 19.5 Fluid in the left oblique fissure simulating a mass on both posterior–anterior (a) and lateral chest radiography (b).

of attachment and, if malignant, may involve the underlying rib. If a loculated effusion is suspected, a decubitus film may demonstrate fluid movement enabling differentiation between a mass and fluid. In addition, loculated effusions may simulate a mass if they collect in the interlobar fissures or along the mediastinum. These are more frequently right-sided and in the horizontal rather than the oblique fissure. On a PA radiograph the appearance of a loculated effusion in the horizontal fissure is that of a round or oval density, while on a lateral radiograph it takes on a lentiform shape with a characteristic tail extending along the fissure. If a loculated effusion occurs in the oblique fissure then the appearances can resemble middle lobe collapse or consolidation. Features that favor the former are: identification of a separate horizontal fissure; one or more convex margins on the lateral radiograph; no effacement of the right heart border; and both ends of the effusion tapering on the lateral film.[25]

Lamellar pleural effusions are those that collect in the connective tissue beneath the visceral pleura and are frequently seen with cardiac failure. It is the lamellar shape with the shadow outlining the pleural boundary that suggests pulmonary rather than pleural fluid.

SUPINE RADIOGRAPHS

Large amounts of fluid can be missed on a supine radiograph as the pleural fluid layers posteriorly.[40] On a supine radiograph, approximately 175–525 mL of fluid is required to cause blunting of the costophrenic angle and this amount of fluid may also cause a general increased haziness over the lower pulmonary zones or a density over the apex.[44] The presence of an apical cap occurs because the apex is dependent in the supine position and so fluid tends to pool in this area.[21] A normal supine radiograph does not exclude an effusion. Several radiographic signs suggest the presence of fluid: increased homogeneous density over the lung, an apical cap, blunting of the costophrenic sulcus, elevation of the hemidiaphragm, accentuation of the horizontal fissure and reduced lower lobe vasculature.[51]

SUBPULMONARY EFFUSION

Pleural fluid may also collect in a subpulmonary location.[40] These effusions are often transudates associated with cardiac, renal and hepatic failure. They can be unilateral or bilateral and tend to occur on the right side if unilateral.[52] The main findings include elevation of the ipsilateral hemidiaphragm, flattening of its medial aspect and displacement of the peak of the diaphragm laterally, with the contour on either side of the peak being straighter than usual. The medial slope is gradual and the lateral one is steep. These appearances are accentuated on expiration. The costophrenic angle is often ill-defined, while both the lateral and posterior angles may be well-defined. A further way of distinguishing a subpulmonic effusion from a normal effusion is by the apparent absence of vessels below the hemidiaphragm owing to the absence of parenchymal tissue passing below the hemidiaphragm on the PA radiograph.[53] A subpulmonic effusion is more easily recognized on the left because of separation of the stomach bubble from the apparent left hemidiaphragm. Occasionally, a diaphragmatic spur will be seen if fluid enters the inferior accessory fissure. If fluid extends into a paramediastinal distribution then a triangular retrocardiac shadow may be produced.[25]

Ultrasound

Ultrasound is commonly used to further assess a pleural effusion detected on a CXR.[54,55] In addition to confirming the presence or absence of suspected pleural fluid, it may be used to guide aspiration or chest-drain insertion.[56,57] On ultrasound, fluid is most frequently seen as an anechoic or hypoechoic collection, often delineated by the echogenic line of visceral pleura and/or lung (Figure 19.6). In addition to confirming an effusion, it may be possible to distinguish between a transudative and exudative effusion.[57,58] The internal echogenicity of pleural effusions can be anechoic (non-complex), or echoic (complex) and non-septated or septated, such that pleural fluid appearances can range from anechoic to echoic and septated (complex septated) (Figure 19.7).[57] Transudates are always anechoic, whereas an anechoic effusion can either be a transudate or an exudate.[58] Pleural effusions that are complex septated, complex non-septated or homogeneously echogenic are always exudates. Thickened pleura, a pleural nodule or an associated parenchymal lesion detected in adjacent consolidated or atelectatic lung are also indicative of an exudate.[58] The detection of a pleural nodule, commonly positioned on the diaphragm, is strongly suggestive of malignancy (Figure 19.8); homogeneous echogenic effusions are mostly caused by a hemorrhagic effusion or an empyema.[58]

Other signs that may occur in patients with an effusion include dynamic 'flap' or 'swirl' signs, often caused by consolidated or collapsed lung, debris attached to the chest wall, or by movement of a septa within a loculated collection.[59] Malignant pleural effusions are more likely to have an echogenic swirling pattern secondary to respiratory movement or cardiac pulsation than benign disease, but neither this finding nor the echotexture of the effusion is specific enough for clinical use.[60] Pleural fluid can be readily distinguished from a solid mass if fibrin strands and septae are seen within the visualized hypoechoic space.[61] These fibrin strands occur in exudates rich in protein and are often associated with infected or malignant effusions.[61,62] Sometimes they are so profuse that they resemble a honeycomb appearance (Figure 19.9).

Ultrasound is now also being used to aid in decisions on whether and how to treat patients with pleural effusions. The size of the effusion and its character has been shown to be of value in determining whether to drain the very commonly seen pleural effusions present in ICU patients.[63] Echogenic, complex and hyperechoic effusions may warrant drainage. Ultrasound has also been used to stratify patients with parapneumonic effusions and

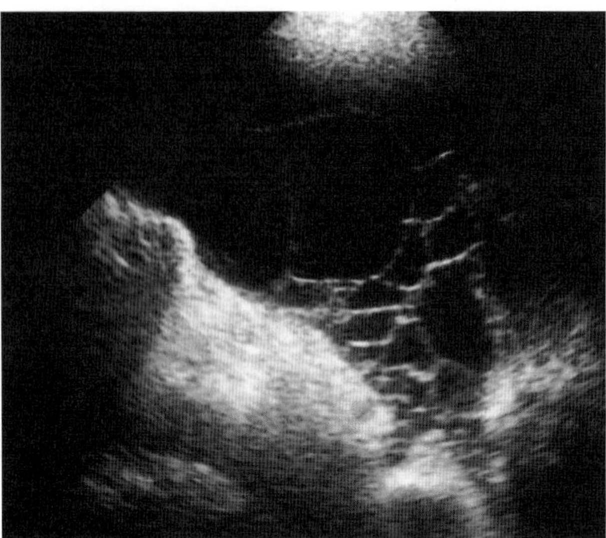

Figure 19.7 Multiple septations seen on ultrasound in a patient with empyema.

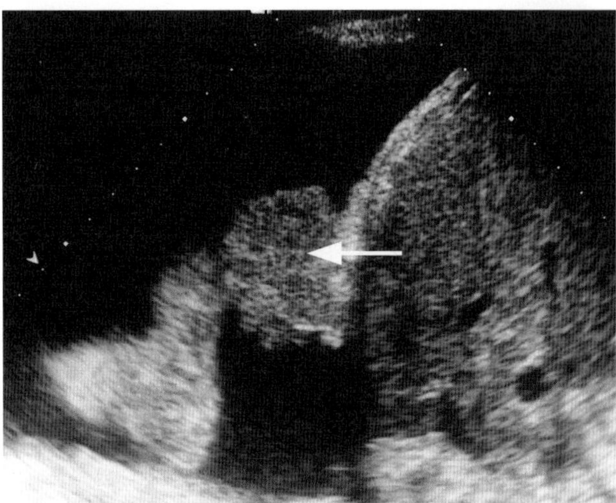

Figure 19.8 Malignant nodule seen on the diaphragm (arrow) in a patient with a malignant pleural effusion.

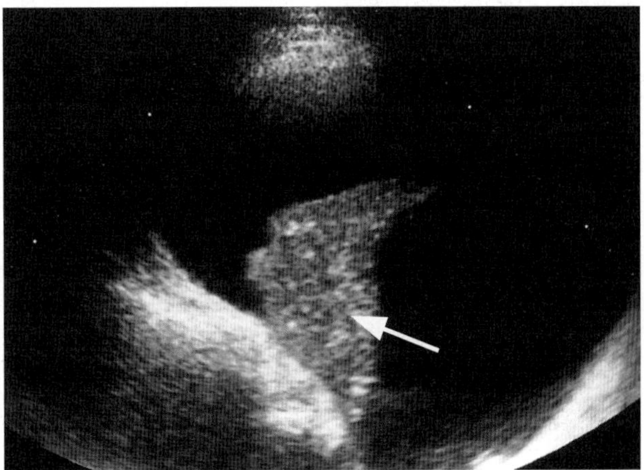

Figure 19.6 Anechoic pleural effusion and collapsed lung (arrow) seen on ultrasound.

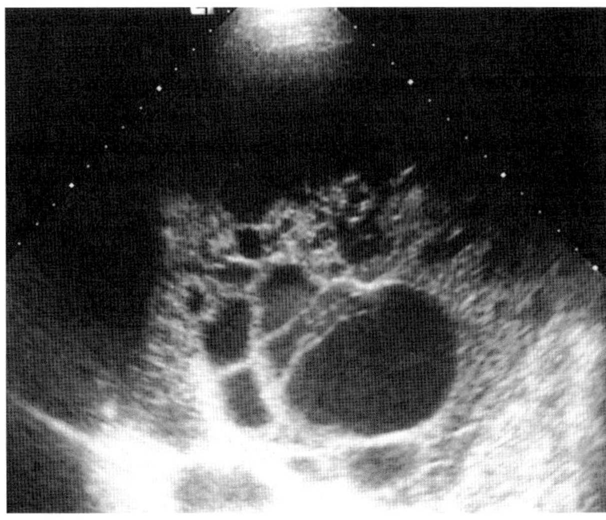

Figure 19.9 Honeycomb appearance on ultrasound in a patient with empyema.

empyema into treatment by chest drain or medical thoracoscopy.[64]

Pleural thickening may sometimes be difficult to distinguish from pleural fluid, as both may be anechoic or hypoechoic. Color Doppler in this instance can be used to help differentiate between the two. Pleural thickening provides little or no color Doppler signal, whereas movement in pleural fluid induced by respiratory or cardiac motion produces a significant color Doppler signal.[65,66]

The combination of ultrasound and CXR enables the confirmation of an effusion and the differentiation of this from thickening or tumor in virtually all patients.[56] Ultrasound may also be used to estimate the volume of the effusion.[67] This may be a simple subjective assessment based on the opinion and experience of the operator, and reported as small, moderate or large. Other approaches such as measuring the pleural effusion depth, or more complex strategies to account for the complex shape of the chest have been used, but are probably not of practical use in clinical practice.[68,69]

Ultrasound has recently also been used experimentally to assess the efficacy of pleurodesis and in one study in rabbits, the absence of the gliding sign strongly correlated with a successful pleurodesis.[70]

Computed tomography

The majority of patients with transudative or parapneumonic effusions can be managed with CXR and US. Non-infective exudative effusions such as those caused by malignancy frequently require contrast-enhanced CT either to aid in diagnosis or to help in clinical management and follow-up.

Identification of pleural fluid and its etiology is readily performed with contrast-enhanced CT.[71] When scanned supine, fluid is seen to collect initially in the deep lateral and posterior pleural recesses.[40] Occasionally, particularly in patients with inverted hemidiaphragms, it may be difficult to distinguish pleural fluid from abdominal fluid.[40] As such, a sharp interface between the fluid and the liver or spleen is characteristic of ascitic fluid; whereas a hazy or unsharp fluid interface with the liver or spleen is indicative of a right or left pleural effusion due to the interposition of the diaphragm between fluid and liver or spleen.[72] Furthermore, as the lungs and pleura lie adjacent and peripheral to the convexity of the hemidiaphragm, pleural fluid will lie peripherally to the diaphragm while ascitic fluid will lie internal to the hemidiaphragm.[40]

Sometimes, patients with an inverted hemidiaphragm caused by a pleural effusion may appear to have fluid lying central to the diaphragm, although this is readily determined both by viewing all the CT images and the crura, as pleural fluid displaces the crus of the diaphragm anteriorly when it is interposed between the crus and the vertebral column.[73]

It may be difficult to distinguish a small effusion from pleural thickening, although contrast enhancement enables this in the vast majority of patients.[40] The internal character of the pleural effusion is less readily assessed on CT than on US. Only very thick septations are visualized on CT, although their presence may be inferred by air or gas, if present, collecting as multiple small pockets (Figure 19.10).[74]

The presence of pleural enhancement enables the identification of exudative effusions from transudates (Figure 19.11).[75,76] There may be additional features on the CT scan, such as pleural thickening, nodules or disease elsewhere, that enable further characterization as to the cause of the effusion (Figure 19.12).[77]

Computed tomography is also good at assessing loculated effusions, which may have simulated a mass on CXR.

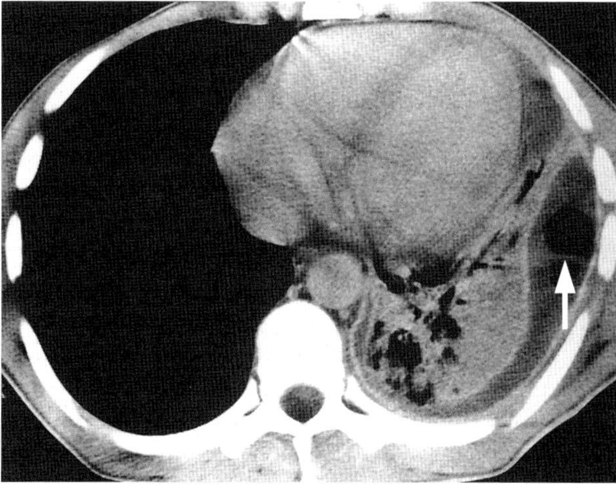

Figure 19.10 Septation (arrow) demonstrated on contrast enhanced computed tomography by the separation of pockets of air within a left pleural effusion.

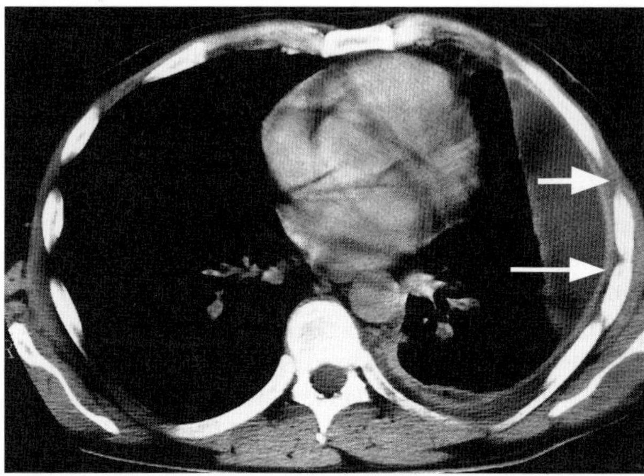

Figure 19.11 Pleural enhancement (long arrow) and increase in attenuation of extrapleural fat (short arrow) in keeping with a parapneumonic effusion.

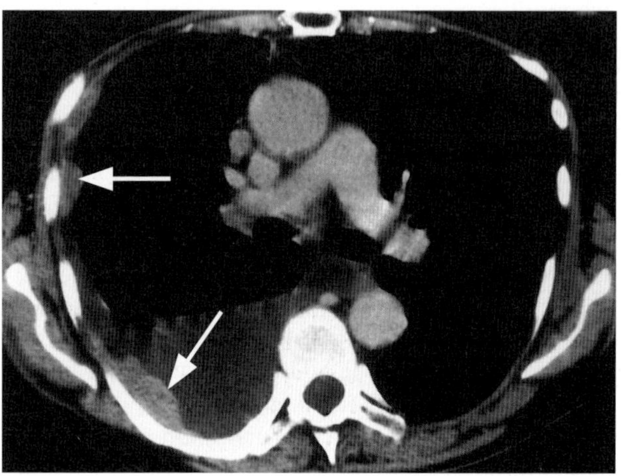

Figure 19.12 Pleural nodules seen laterally and posteriorly on the right (arrows) in a patient with a pleural effusion.

On CT they have a lentiform configuration, smooth margins, are of homogeneous attenuation and displace the adjacent parenchyma.[44]

Magnetic resonance imaging

Pleural fluid returns low signal intensity on T1-weighted images and a relatively high signal intensity on T2-weighted images (Figure 19.13). Magnetic resonance may be superior to CT in the differentiation of transudates and exudates.[78] Using a triple-echo pulse sequence and normalized MRI intensities, complex exudates have greater signal intensity than simple exudates, which in turn are brighter than transudates.[40,78] Magnetic resonance also allows differentiation of pleural effusion from parenchymal disease and from pleural tumor. Subacute and chronic hemorrhage into the pleural space can also be recognized on MR images by very high signal intensity on both T1- and T2-weighted images. In subacute or chronic hematomas a concentric ring sign may be seen. This is composed of an outer dark rim due to hemosiderin and a bright center as a result of the shortening effects of methemoglobin.[79]

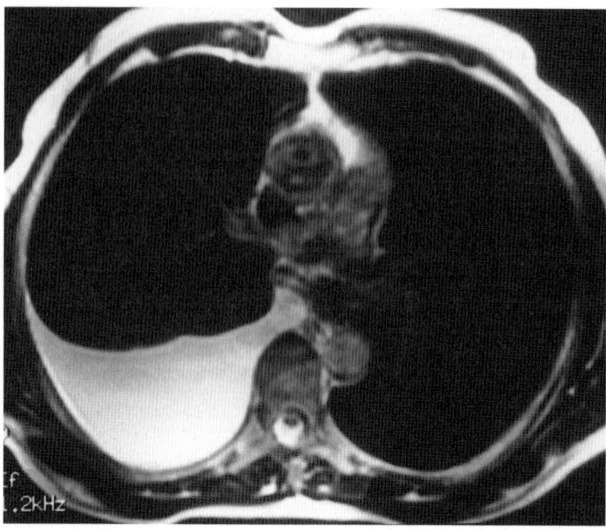

Figure 19.13 A T2-weighted magnetic resonance imaging sequence demonstrating high signal intensity pleural fluid.

EMPYEMA

The imaging features of parapneumonic effusion and empyema depend to a degree upon the state of evolution of the effusion, and the underlying etiology, such as post-traumatic or community-acquired infection. In addition, the imaging required will be very much circumstance led; often a PA and lateral CXR plus ultrasound enables diagnosis and management, with contrast-enhanced CT only required for ill patients such as those on ICU.

Chest radiography

An erect PA and lateral CXR should be performed in all patients with suspected parapneumonic effusion or empyema. If clinico-radiological doubt remains, then either a lateral decubitus film or US may be required. In general, a pleural effusion is demonstrated often in association with consolidation. The effusion is commonly unilateral, but if bilateral the infected side is usually the larger.[80] If the effusion is uncomplicated, it behaves like other non-infected sterile effusions with a normal meniscus sign and changes position and appearance when a decubitus film is performed, unless there has been prior scarring of the pleural cavity.[40]

If the effusion presents at a later stage or evolves from presentation, it may be loculated. This loculated effusion will then have the characteristic appearance of a lentiform, pleural-based opacity. If the collection is fissural it will have the previously described appearance of a 'pseudotumor'. Suspicion that the patient may have a pulmonary abscess rather than an empyema may arise either from the clinical history or CXR.[44] Although the differentiation may be difficult, a pulmonary abscess tends to be smaller and rounder, with similar dimensions on both the PA and lateral CXR;[81] it forms acute angles with the chest wall and has thicker, irregular walls if cavitation is present.[82,83] CT may be used to confirm the diagnosis.

It was previously thought that empyema size on a CXR correlated with the need for surgery.[84] More recently, the ability to predict outcome and requirement for surgery assessed on the size of the effusion on CXR has been questioned, perhaps owing to more aggressive medical management.[74]

Ultrasound

If further imaging is required, US should be performed. The majority of parapneumonic effusions and empyemas requiring US will be septated and may be hyperechoic, although anechoic effusions may be frank pus on aspiration.[58,59] Whereas septations are readily visualized on US, pleural thickening is poorly visualized and if confirmation of this is required, contrast-enhanced CT should be performed.[75,76] Unfortunately, there is no apparent correlation between US appearance and the stage of evolution of the effusion, neither can it be used as a predictor of treatment outcome.[74] As mentioned earlier, US may be used to help determine the need for drainage and the use of tube drainage or video assisted thoracoscopy.[64,65]

Computed tomography

Critically ill patients and those who for other reasons are unsuitable for assessment by US may be imaged by contrast-enhanced CT. As with other exudative effusions, pleural enhancement is seen.[75,76] Parietal pleural enhancement and thickening is readily visualized, although visceral pleural enhancement, often adjacent to consolidated or atelectatic lung, may not be appreciated.[71,76,81] There is also an increase in thickening and attenuation of the adjacent extraparietal pleural fat (Figure 19.11).[76] There is a trend for CT-detected pleural thickening to increase with the stage of the effusion but it is unfortunately not possible to predict outcome in this regard.[74] It has also been shown that marked pleural thickening or 'pleural peel' may completely resolve on long-term follow-up.[85]

If a lung abscess is suspected from the CXR, then CT may be used to confirm the diagnosis (Figure 19.14).[43] As on the CXR, pulmonary abscesses tend to be rounder than empyemas and often make an acute angle with the chest wall compared with the obtuse angle commonly seen in an empyema on CT.[81] In addition, the 'passive' atelectasis seen adjacent to the empyema, as a result of reduction in hemithorax space, is not seen in patients with a pulmonary abscess as these replace lung rather than displace it. Pulmonary abscesses also tend to have significantly thicker walls than empyemas.

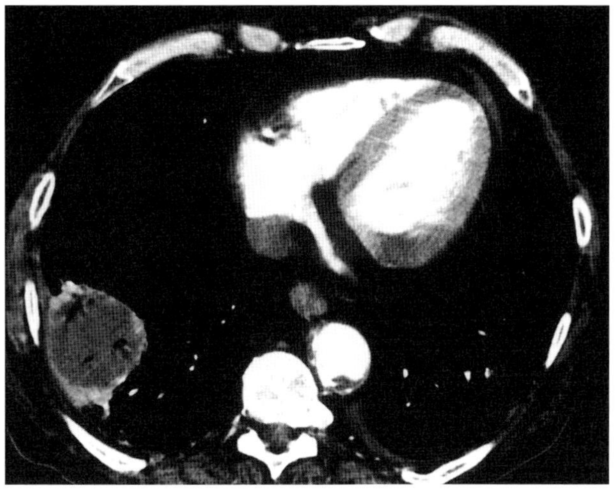

(a)

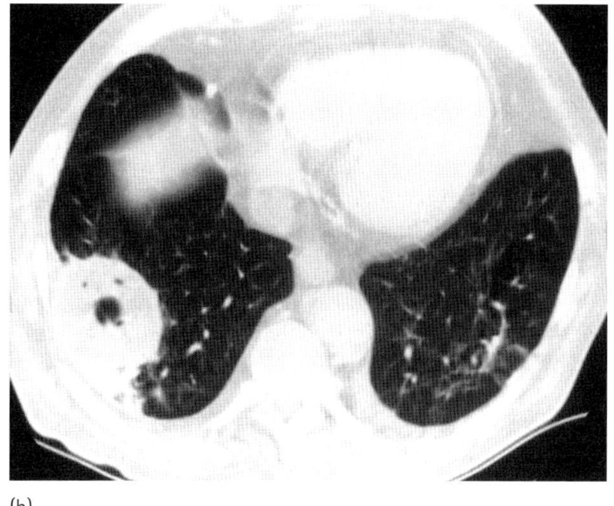

(b)

Figure 19.14 Characteristic pulmonary abscess on computed tomography forming an acute angle with the right chest wall. (a) The abscess on mediastinal windows. (b) The abscess on lung windows. Note the absence of significant 'passive' atelectasis.

TUBERCULOUS EMPYEMA

In patients with a tuberculous empyema, the pleural appearance may be significantly different from those described previously. In this instance the typical findings are those of a moderate to large loculated pleural effusion with pleural calcification and often enlargement of the overlying ribs.[86]

Computed tomography scanning shows a thick calcific pleural rind with rib thickening surrounding a loculated pleural effusion.[87] Complications associated with a tuberculous empyema include a bronchopleural fistula and empyema necessitans.[88,89] The latter is seen on CT as a thick-walled, well-encapsulated calcific pleural mass. The differential diagnoses of this appearance include bacterial empyema, lung abscess, blastomycosis and actinomycosis.[86]

MALIGNANT PLEURAL EFFUSIONS

Not all patients with pleural metastases have an associated pleural effusion. Imaging of pleural thickening without an effusion is discussed later. The majority of malignant pleural effusions (see Chapter 25, Effusions from malignancy) are secondary to lung or breast carcinoma and these patients are likely to have an appropriate clinical history and radiology.[90,91] Most patients presenting with pleural metastases have large volume effusions, with up to 10 percent of patients having massive effusions causing complete hemithorax opacification;[92] the majority of massive effusions are, in turn, secondary to malignancy.[47] It should also be remembered that pleural effusions in patients with known malignancy may be non-malignant in etiology (i.e. associated with pulmonary thromboembolic disease). In most instances these effusions tend to be small and are often asymptomatic.

If the primary malignancy is bronchogenic then the effusion is likely to be ipsilateral, otherwise there is no ipsilateral predilection and the effusions may on occasion be bilateral.

Chest radiography

The appearance of malignant pleural effusions ranges from an isolated non-loculated effusion of varying size to an effusion with an associated pulmonary or mediastinal mass. The presence of associated abnormalities on the CXR will direct appropriate further investigation which, in most instances, is contrast-enhanced CT. In the absence of an abnormality other than the effusion, further imaging will be directed by clinical history and examination, and the results of aspiration cytology.

Ultrasound

As with parapneumonic effusions and empyema, malignant pleural effusions may be anechoic, echoic or complex septated.[58] The detection of a pleural or diaphragmatic nodule appears specific for malignancy[93,94] and if US is used as an aid to thoracentesis, the assessment of the diaphragmatic pleural surface is of value since the majority of patients with malignant effusions have associated diaphragmatic pleural thickening that is detectable on US (Figure 19.15).[95] Pleural thickening outside the diaphragmatic surface may be difficult to detect on US.

Computed tomography

In patients with suspected malignant pleural effusion and negative cytology on aspiration, contrast-enhanced CT is the next most commonly performed investigation. As with other causes of exudative effusions, pleural enhancement is commonly seen in patients with malignant effusions.[75,92] This is commonly nodular or irregular, or has a pleural thickness of >1 cm (Figure 19.16).[95] Using these criteria for assessment, contrast-enhanced CT has been shown to have a sensitivity of >80 per cent and to be highly specific in the evaluation of patients with suspected malignant effusions.[77,95] In addition, confirmation that there is no apparent malignant cause for the effusion appears reliable with CT.[77] Further information such as bone or liver metastases may also be apparent on scanning.[77,90] The distribution of malignant pleural thickening detected with CT appears to correlate with that seen at thoracoscopy. The majority of patients have thickening, which is either solely or maximally posteriorly and basally. A secondary role for CT is the ability to either directly or indirectly guide biopsy of a detected abnormality (Figure 19.17).[96]

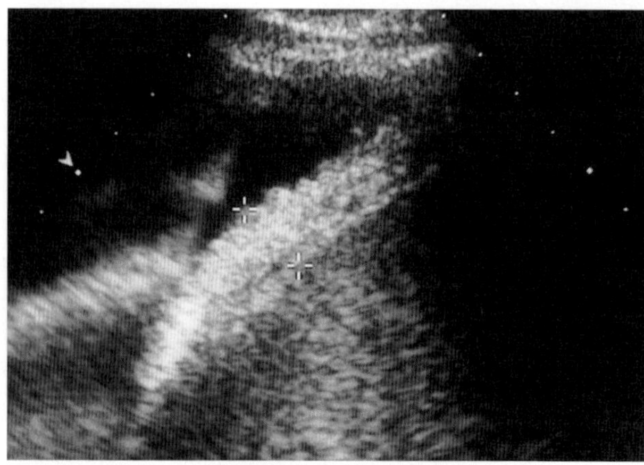

Figure 19.15 Diaphragmatic pleural thickening on ultrasound in patients with a malignant pleural effusion.

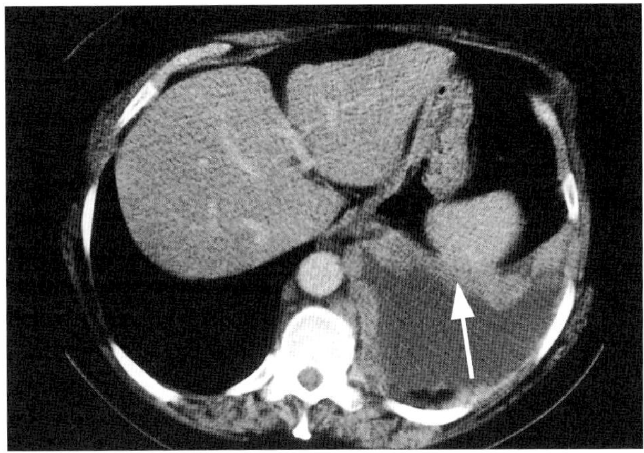

Figure 19.16 Nodular left pleural thickening (arrow) and effusion suggestive of malignancy on computed tomography.

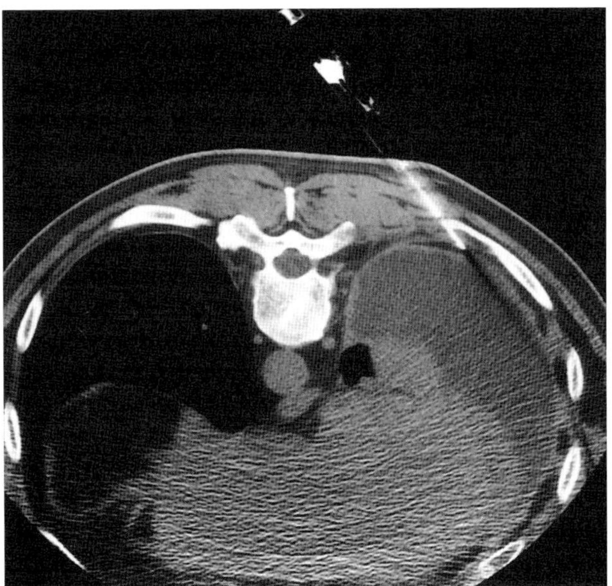

Figure 19.17 Computed tomography-guided pleural biopsy. The patient is in the prone position for biopsy.

Magnetic resonance imaging

The role of MRI in the investigation of suspected pleural effusion is, at present, not clearly defined since there have only been a few non-randomized studies. Because of its very high contrast resolution, the ability to detect small pleural nodules against the background of an effusion is likely to be superior to contrast enhanced CT (Figure 19.18). However, this superior contrast resolution will be offset by inferior spatial resolution and increased respiratory and cardiac motion artifact. In addition to routinely using cardiac and respiratory gating, T2-weighted and post-contrast T1-weighted sagittal and axial sequences should be performed.

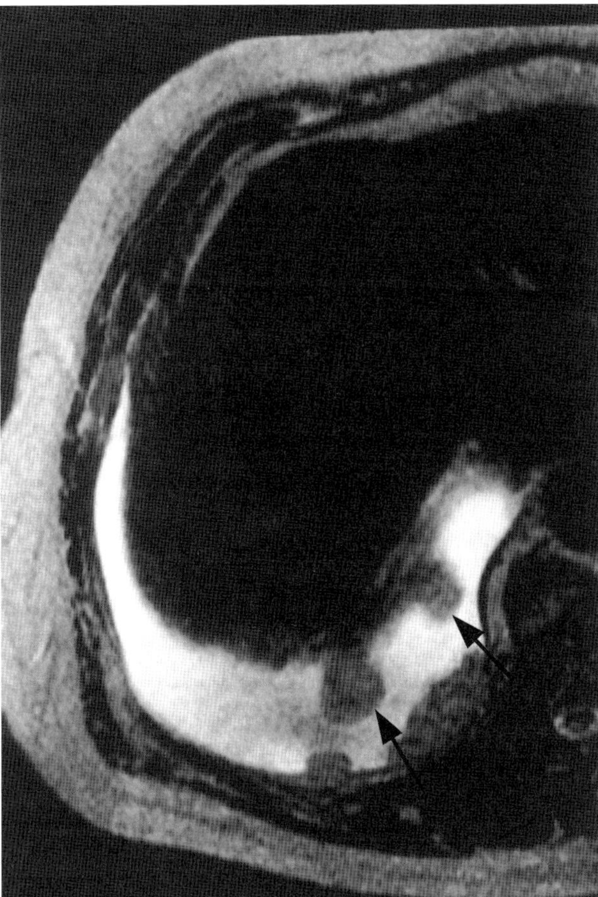

Figure 19.18 A T2-weighted magnetic resonance imaging sequence showing multiple pleural nodules (arrows), easily seen against the high T2 signal of pleural fluid.

Positron emission tomography combined with CT

Positron emission CT is now being evaluated in patients with suspected malignant pleural effusions.[97–99] Unfortunately, it is likely to be a poor discriminator between infective and malignant causes,[100] and potentially in patients with low-grade or relatively indolent malignancy such as fibrous mesothelioma. There may also be difficulty in detecting small-volume disease such as 'studding' of the pleural surface by tumor, commonly seen at thoracoscopy.

CHYLOTHORAX AND PSEUDOCHYLOTHORAX

Chest radiography

Unless associated with lymphangioleiomyomatosis, chylothoraces (see Chapter 29, Effusions from lymphatic disruptions) cannot be distinguished from other effusions on a standard radiograph. They can be unilateral or bilateral and can range in size from small to massive. A chylothorax is usually right-sided, but if secondary to damage or obstruction at the level of the aorta, a left-sided effusion is seen.

Pseudochylothorax is a fairly common finding in patients with large pleural peel. In the majority of cases the cause is benign and, again, there are no specific CXR determinants.

Computed tomography

Computed tomography may help to define the cause of the chylothorax that is not apparent on the CXR, such as tumor compressing the thoracic duct.[101] However, the CT attenuation of the chyle is often indistinguishable from other effusions because it is protein rich.

Magnetic resonance imaging

Although not commonly performed, it is possible to distinguish a chylothorax from other causes of a pleural effusion on MRI because of its fatty content. On a T1-weighted image the chyle is bright and on a T2-weighted image the fatty component shows T2 shortening, with a signal intensity similar to subcutaneous fat.[79]

Lymphoscintigraphy

This technique uses ^{99m}Tc-sulphur microcolloid, antimony sulfide colloid, stannous phytate, rhenium sulfur colloid, human serum albumin or dextran injected subcutaneously between the toes and scanning 2–6 hours later. Its use in investigating chylothorax has been limited to a few case reports. It is able to demonstrate abnormal lymphatic drainage in the cases of chylothorax.[102] It may be possible to distinguish between lymphatic drainage and transdiaphragmatic movement of chylous peritoneal fluid through the pleuroperitoneal canal by radioisotope migration speed. Overall, lymphoscintigraphy may be useful in selecting those patients that would be suitable for surgery and to assess the effects of surgery.[102]

HEMOTHORAX

Hemothorax usually results from trauma, although several other conditions may be causative.[103] On a standard radiograph the presence of rib fractures and a known clinical history of trauma may help to distinguish a hemothorax from a pleural effusion. A CT scan may also show areas of active bleeding as foci of high attenuation (Figure 19.19).[104] Loculation is frequently seen and fibrin bodies may also form. The end stage of a hemothorax may result in massive pleural thickening.

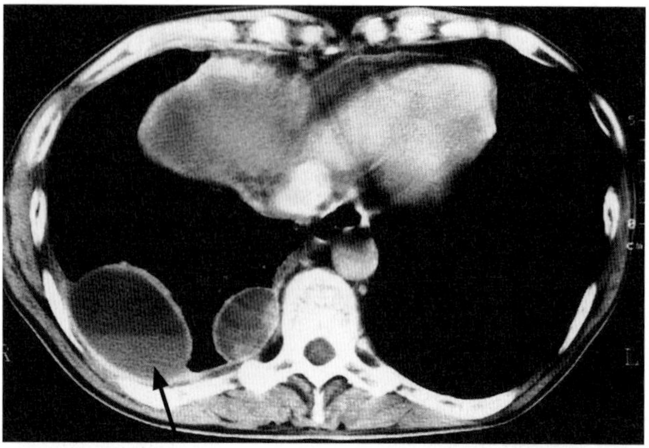

Figure 19.19 Computed tomography demonstrating recent hemorrhage into two pleural locules with the development of fluid–fluid levels, the heme is the more dependent high-attenuation material (arrow).

FOCAL PLEURAL DISEASE

Pleural plaques

CHEST RADIOGRAPHY

A PA and lateral CXR should always be performed as the initial investigation in detecting asbestos related disease (see Chapter 40, Asbestos-related pleural diseases). The criteria set by the International Labour Office[105] suggest that the sensitivity of a CXR in the detection of plaques ranges from 30 to 80 percent and the specificity ranges from 60 to 80 percent. Their detection is dependent on the number, size, shape, position, degree of calcification and technical quality of the CXR (Figure 19.20).[106]

Pleural plaques almost always involve the parietal pleura alone, although rarely they may involve the visceral interlobular fissures, and may simulate a pulmonary nodule.[107] Oblique views are helpful in the diagnosis of the plaques, although CT and HRCT are now more commonly performed.[108,109] *En face* imaging may cause problems because of the difficulty in distinguishing between plaques and the normal muscle and fat companion shadows of the chest wall.[24] Extrapleural fat is suggested by a bilateral and symmetric distribution along the midlateral chest wall. Plaques are unilateral on a CXR in approximately 25 percent of cases, more frequently on the left, and if bilateral are asymmetrical.[110]

As they calcify they produce a white line on the tangential views that parallels the chest wall, diaphragm or cardiac border. If these calcifications are seen *en face*, they produce irregular linear or stippled calcifications with an uneven density.

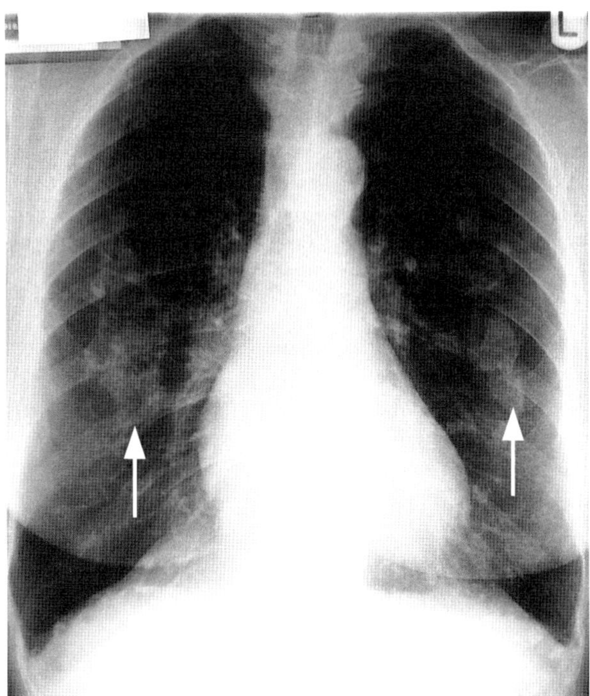

Figure 19.20 Characteristic appearance of bilateral calcified pleural plaques on chest radiography (arrows).

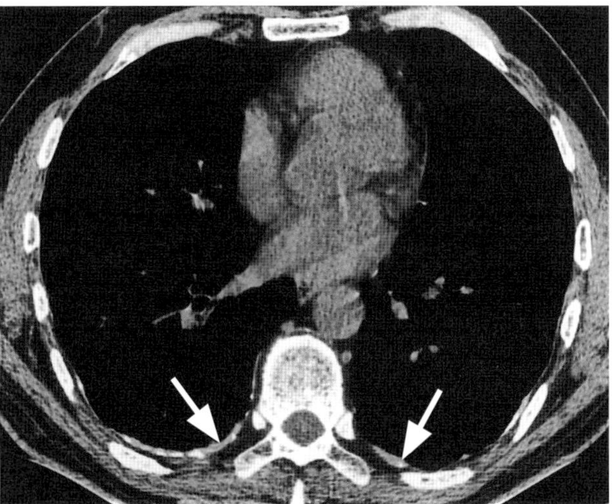

Figure 19.21 Characteristic high-resolution computed tomography appearance of partly calcified pleural plaques positioned predominantly posteriorly and in a paravertebral distribution (arrows).

COMPUTED RADIOGRAPHY

The advent of multislice CT scanning has brought into question the use of HRCT in the detection of suspected pleural plaques on the CXR or in differentiating plaques from extrapleural fat shadows or other causes of increased radio-opacity.[111] Patients should be scanned prone, enabling comment on possible pulmonary parenchymal asbestos-related disease that may also be present.[112] Both HRCT and MSCT are far more sensitive than the CXR in differentiating subpleural fat from pleural plaques[113,114]

Pleural plaques on MSCT and HRCT appear as circumscribed areas of pleural thickening separated from the underlying rib and extrapleural soft tissues by a thin layer of fat (Figure 19.21). Any soft tissue internal to a rib (remembering the comment describing the innermost intercostal muscle) or paravertebral region is regarded as abnormal.[37] Both techniques are also able to detect small foci of calcification within the plaques.[115] Pleural plaques may be classified according to their CT appearance:[116]

1 minimal pleural plaques – less than 1 mm thick, 1–3 cm long, and few in number;
2 moderate pleural plaques – 1–3 mm thick, 2–5 cm long and multiple;
3 severe pleural plaques – thicker than 3 mm, clearly indenting adjacent lung, up to 8 cm in craniocaudal dimension and extensive in width.

MAGNETIC RESONANCE IMAGING

The detection of pleural plaques is possible with MRI, but the sensitivity is inferior to HRCT. They appear as areas of low signal on both T1- and T2-weighted sequences. Calcification within plaques is seen as a signal void.

Localized fibrous tumor of the pleura

CHEST RADIOGRAPHY

Localized fibrous tumors are smooth rounded or oval homogeneous masses on CXR (Figure 19.22). They have a sharply delineated contour that forms an obtuse angle with the pleural surface in 74–94 percent of cases.[24,91] They are seen more frequently in the lower half of the chest on either side. The location may be in a fissure (30 percent), along the mediastinal pleura (18 percent), the thoracic pleura (46 percent) or adjacent to the hemidiaphragm (6 percent).[91] Those on pedicles have a tendency to change position with respiration or posture.[117]

COMPUTED TOMOGRAPHY

On unenhanced CT scans, localized fibrous tumors are homogeneous and sharply marginated, calcification is rarely seen and, in larger tumors, the adjacent lung parenchyma may be displaced with atelectasis and bowing of the bronchi and pulmonary vessels around the mass and a smooth tapering margin at the junction of the mass with the pleura.[117]

Enhancement is variable after intravenous contrast; it is always equal to or greater than that of other soft tissues, and is most commonly homogeneous but may be hetero-

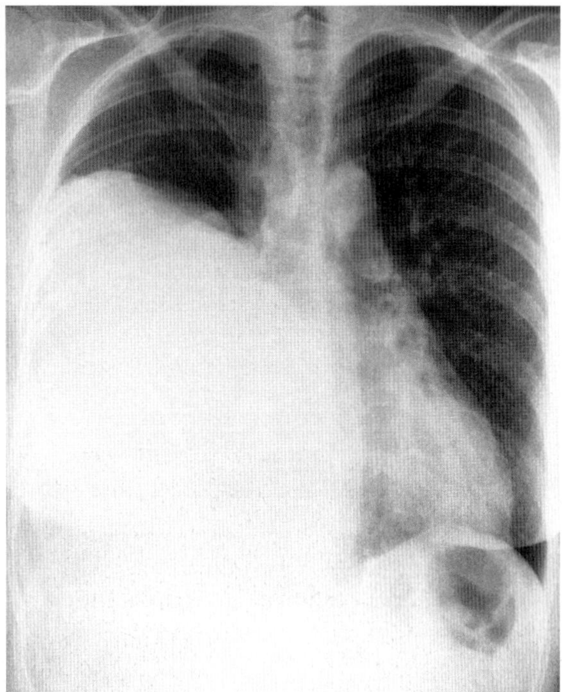

Figure 19.22 Large right lower lobe fibroma mimicking a large right pleural effusion.

geneous in up to 40 percent of cases (Figure 19.23).[118] The intense enhancement reflects the rich vascular supply, with heterogeneous enhancement occurring owing to myxoid or cystic degeneration or hemorrhage into the lesion.[119] If malignant change has occurred, central necrosis may be demonstrated on CT scans.[120] A pedunculated tumor can show changes in position and shape on CT in the supine and prone positions, although the pedicle is seldom visualized.

The absence of fat excludes a diaphragmatic hernia or a pleural lipoma. CT may rarely show invasion of the chest wall or infradiaphragmatic structures that occasionally occur.

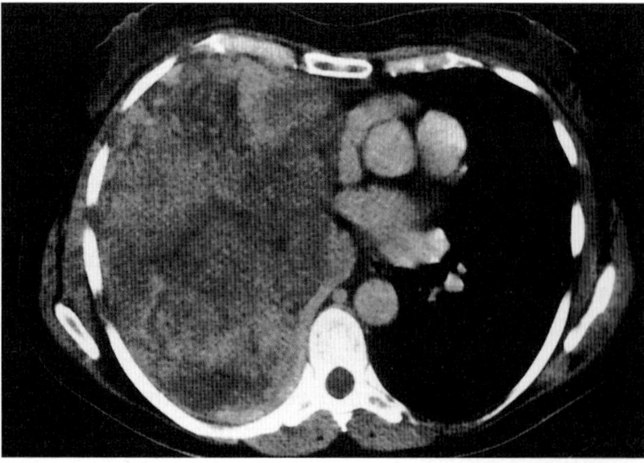

Figure 19.23 Characteristically heterogeneously enhancing right pleural fibroma on contrast enhanced computed tomography.

If the tumor fills the hemithorax, then ultrasound is a useful adjuvant in the diagnosis, although there is no pathognomonic radiological feature for a localized fibrous tumor. If the tumor has been inadequately excised there may be recurrence locally or elsewhere along the pleural surface, demonstrated by local or distal pleural nodularity.

MAGNETIC RESONANCE IMAGING

Magnetic resonance imaging demonstrates the contour of a well-defined mass in contact with the pleural space, whose largest dimension is in the longitudinal plane.[91] The MR features of a fibrous tumor include low-signal on T1-weighted images and heterogeneous high-signal on T2-weighted images.[91,121] Sometimes a peripheral rim of low intensity is seen on the T1-weighted images. As with contrast-enhanced CT, T1-weighted images post-gadolinium may demonstrate homogeneous or heterogeneous enhancement. MR is more often able to show the origin of the mass from the pleura than CXR or CT. Sagittal images are useful if the mass is located close to the diaphragm or superior sulcus. Imaging in the coronal plane demonstrates a soft, sloping angle in continuity with the chest wall.

Pleural lipoma and liposarcoma

On CXR these may be poorly demonstrated, or appear similar to other soft tissue masses or collections abutting the pleural surface (Figure 19.24a). On CT scans they appear as a well-defined mass of homogeneous fat density forming obtuse angles with the chest wall and displacing the adjacent parenchyma.[40] If the attenuation values are greater than 250 HU and the tumor is heterogeneous, then a liposarcoma should be considered.[122] On MR scans, they are of bright signal intensity on T1-weighted images (Figure 19.24b) and can be moderately bright on T2-weighted images.

Lymphoma

Lymphomatous pleural masses are rare, with the more usual manifestation of pleural disease being pleural effusion with pleural thickening or nodules in association with disease elsewhere.

CHEST RADIOGRAPHY

A pleural effusion is usually accompanied by mediastinal lymphadenopathy visible on a CXR; pulmonary involvement is less commonly present.[123] Pleural effusions are commonly unilateral, and may be of considerable size.

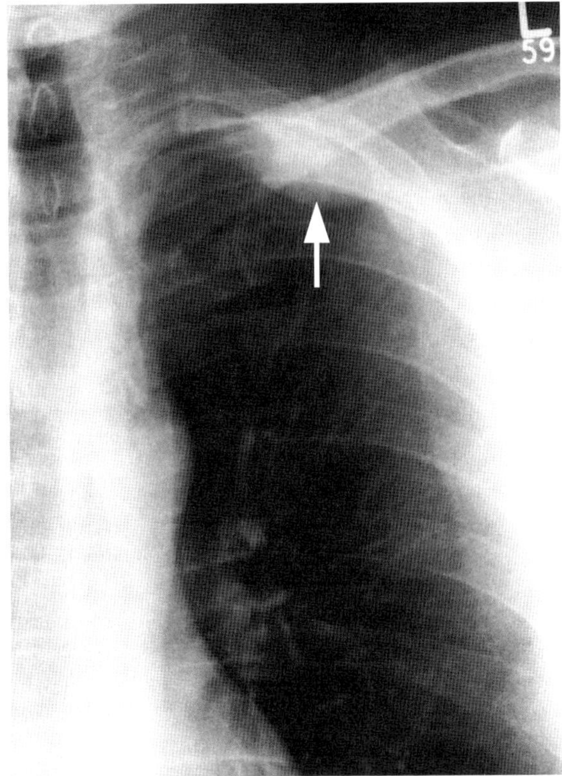

(a)

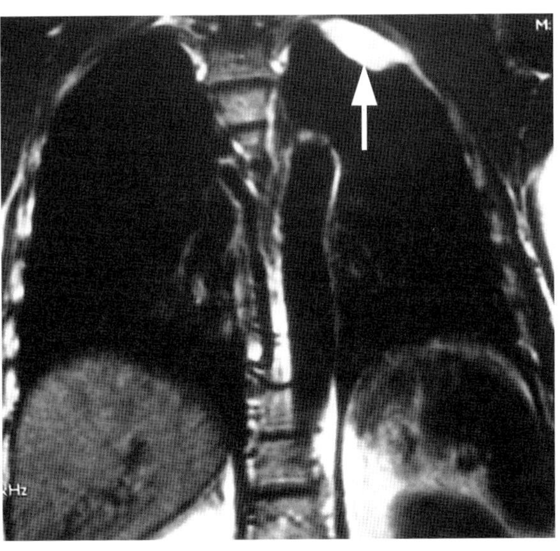

(b)

Figure 19.24 Localized view of a chest radiography showing a left apical lobulated mass (arrow) (a), which, on coronal magnetic resonance imaging, is of a high T2 signal in keeping with a pleural lipoma (arrow) (b).

Discrete pleural nodules or diffuse pleural thickening are very infrequently demonstrated.[124,125]

COMPUTED TOMOGRAPHY AND MAGNETIC RESONANCE IMAGING

Both imaging modalities more clearly demonstrate the almost invariable mediastinal lymphadenopathy present in patients with pleural involvement, particularly in Hodgkin's disease (Figure 19.25).[126] Contrast enhancement is required to demonstrate pleural thickening associated with pleural effusions if the effusions are not secondary to venous and lymphatic obstruction from mediastinal lymphadenopathy, the more common cause of an effusion.[127] The majority of effusions are moderate in size and are commonly bilateral.[128] MRI appears to detect the presence and extent of pleural disease more accurately than CT,[129,130] with similar appearances to other causes of pleural malignancy in association with an effusion (see earlier).

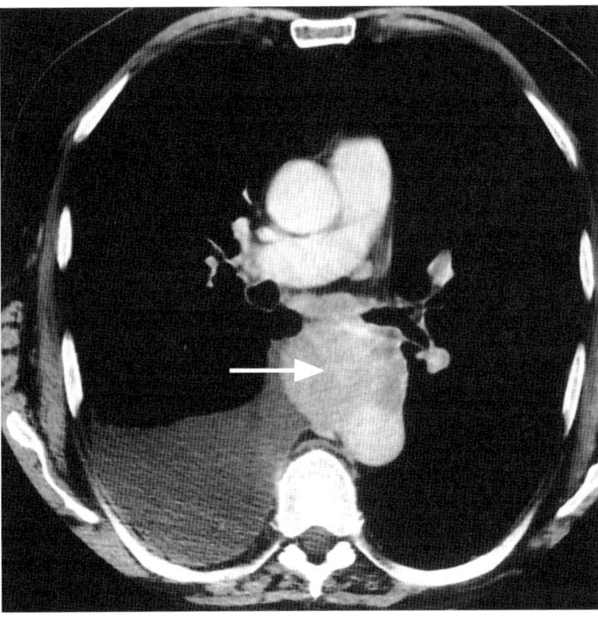

Figure 19.25 Moderate right pleural effusion with large subcarinal node (arrow) in patient with Hodgkin's disease.

DIFFUSE PLEURAL DISEASE

Diffuse benign pleural thickening – asbestos related

CHEST RADIOGRAPHY

The radiographic appearance is of a smooth, uninterrupted pleural density extending over at least one-fourth of the chest wall, often as a subtle increase in radiographic density, with or without costophrenic angle obliteration.[131]

COMPUTED TOMOGRAPHY

Appearance on CT is of a continuous sheet of pleural thickening more than 5 cm wide, more than 8 cm in craniocaudal extent and more than 3 mm thick. It affects the posterior and posteromedial pleura over the lower lobes and is often associated with rounded atelectasis.[116] Thickening of the visceral pleura may be identified on HRCT as an extension of subpleural fibrosis and appears irregular in outline. As mentioned earlier in this chapter, the degree of pleural thickening seen on CT has been shown to correlate with the restrictive defect measured on pulmonary function testing. In addition, it is possible to assess the degree of impairment in lung function secondary to both the pleural thickening and the emphysema very commonly seen in these patients.[132]

Diffuse benign pleural thickening – non-asbestos related

CHEST RADIOGRAPHY

The radiographic appearance often reflects the underlying etiology, such as post-thoracotomy or post-traumatic. Patients with prior tuberculous empyema may well have extensive unilateral pleural calcification, thickening and evidence of prior pulmonary parenchymal disease. In general, the CXR changes are unilateral, characteristically affect the lateral and posterior costophrenic recesses, and appear as smooth, often angular thickening compared with the more gentle curvilinear appearance of pleural fluid (Figure 16.26a). Decubitus CXRs and ultrasound may help to confirm pleural thickening. *En face* extensive pleural thickening produces a veil-like increase in radio-opacity, often with poorly defined margins and extending across fissures. In profile, a thickened pleural rim may be identified.

Post-pleurodesis, the CXR may demonstrate varying degrees of pleural thickening and pleural fluid dependent on the agent used, the success of the procedure and the underlying disease process requiring pleurodesis.

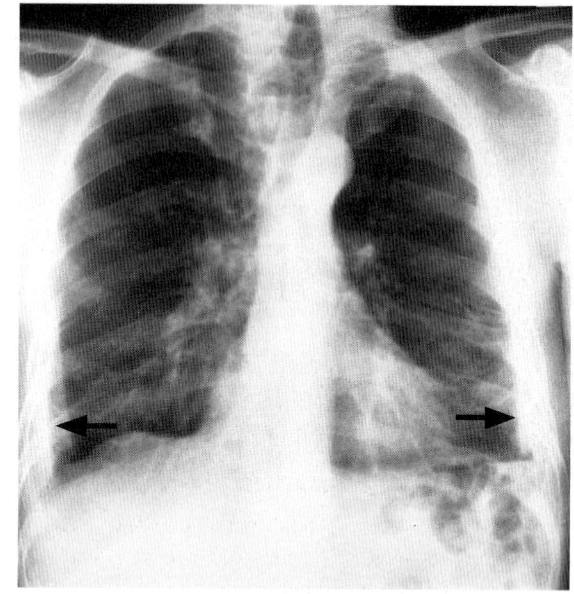

(a)

(b)

Figure 19.26 Diffuse bilateral angular pleural thickening on chest radiography (a) (arrows). Diffuse extensive pleural thickening on computed tomography extending up to the posterior mediastinal surfaces bilaterally but not onto them (b) (arrows).

ULTRASOUND

Pleural thickening is poorly identified on US, and cannot be reliably identified until greater than 1 cm in depth.[6] The thickening may be echogenic, indistinguishable from extrapleural fat and not identified because of the normally bright lung–pleural interfaces.

COMPUTED TOMOGRAPHY

High-resolution CT or spiral CT may be used to assess pleural thickening (Figure 19.26b). Contrast enhancement in the absence of pleural fluid is not necessary. The HRCT should be performed in assessing asbestos related disease (see earlier), and may also be required to clarify equivocal findings on conventional CT. The pleural thickening is seen as an increase in soft tissue at the lung–pleural interface. As with pleural plaques, pleural thickening is best assessed inside the ribs, where there should be no discernible soft tissue, and in the paravertebral space.[37]

Post pleurodesis, the CT appearance will again reflect the agent used, as with the CXR appearance. If performed using talc and for malignancy, CT demonstrates a characteristic talc 'sandwich', with soft tissue parietal pleural thickening, high attenuation talc and then increased soft tissue visceral pleural thickening (Figure 19.27).[133] Post-talc pleurodesis has also been reported to be responsible for false positive results on PET scanning[134,135] (see later).

Diffuse pleural thickening – apical pleural cap

Apical pleural thickening is a frequent finding on CXR and is often idiopathic. It is usually a homogeneous soft tissue opacity, which extends to the lung apex. The caudal

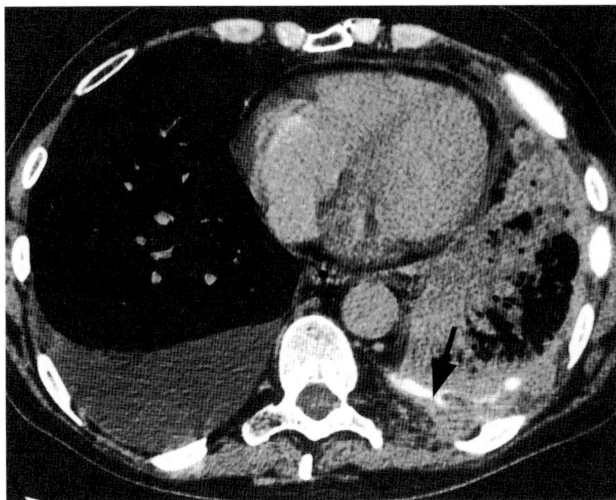

Figure 19.27 High-resolution talc shown post pleurodesis on computed tomography to be sandwiched between visceral and parietal pleural thickening (arrow).

margin is clearly defined but may be smooth, curvilinear or undulating, often with a minor amount of adjacent parenchymal distortion. Apical pleural thickening may be unilateral or bilateral and, if bilateral, often asymmetric. Its frequency increases with age, occurring in approximately 5 percent of adults up to 45 years of age, and 15 percent over 45 years of age.[136] CT demonstrates that the majority of the cap, if associated with prior tuberculosis, is secondary to an increase in apical extrapleural fat.[137]

It is important to distinguish benign apical pleural thickening from a Pancoast tumor.[138] Malignant thickening is asymmetrical, usually of greater thickness than benign disease, may have associated bone destruction and is commonly associated with pain. CT of malignant apical disease demonstrates soft tissue, possibly with extrapleural extension and/or bone destruction. MRI is of value in detecting subtle extrapleural extension; the apical tissue may enhance post gadolinium, and have increased T2 or STIR signal. PET-CT scanning may be used to detect either residual disease or tumor relapse in an area of apical pleural thickening post radiotherapy.[16]

Diffuse malignant pleural thickening

CHEST RADIOGRAPHY

Patients presenting with unilateral pleural thickening may give a clear clinical history suggestive of malignancy. In most instances this will correspond to a CXR appearance of lobular or nodular pleural thickening that may extend into the adjacent fissures and may have adjacent parenchymal distortion. The appearance of a decrease in size of the hemithorax is characteristic but not diagnostic for mesothelioma (see Chapter 41, Malignant mesothelioma) (Figure 19.28).[139] The differentiation of malignant mesothelioma from other malignant cases may also be suggested on clinical grounds or from associated radiographic features such as pleural plaques or asbestosis.[91]

COMPUTED TOMOGRAPHY AND MAGNETIC RESONANCE IMAGING

Spiral CT should be performed to assess the pleural thickening and also to assess the lungs and mediastinum. In differentiating malignant from benign pleural thickening the most useful CT signs are: circumferential thickening (100 percent specificity); nodularity (94 percent specificity); parietal pleural thickening >1 cm (94 percent specificity); and mediastinal pleural involvement (88 percent specificity) (Figure 19.29).[95] Using these CT features and cutting needle biopsy provided a positive and negative predictive value of 100 percent.[140] It has, however, been shown that the presence of circumferential pleural thickening in the presence of a pleural effusion is less specific for malignancy.[77] Two reports suggest that MRI may be of value in helping differentiate benign from malignant disease (Figure 19.30).[13,141] The use of contrast-enhanced fat-saturated T1 sequences appears helpful in differentiating disease etiology in particular, by assessing focal thickening and enhancement of interlobar fissures.

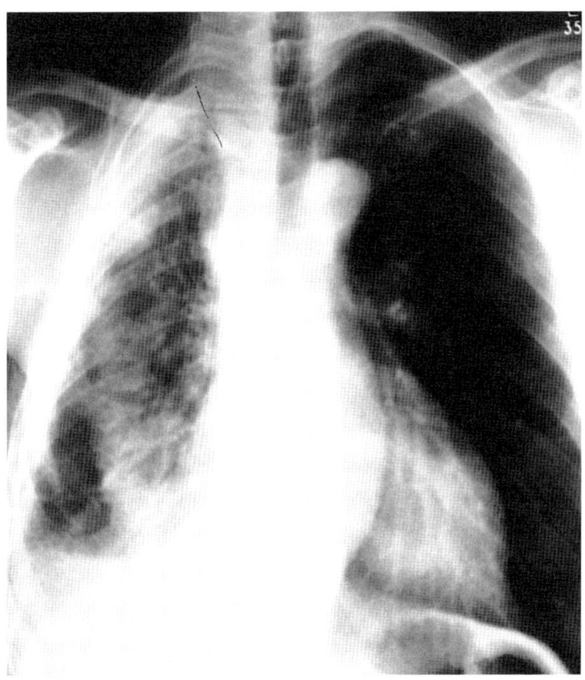

Figure 19.28 Chest radiography demonstrating characteristic decrease in size of right hemithorax due to extensive mesothelioma.

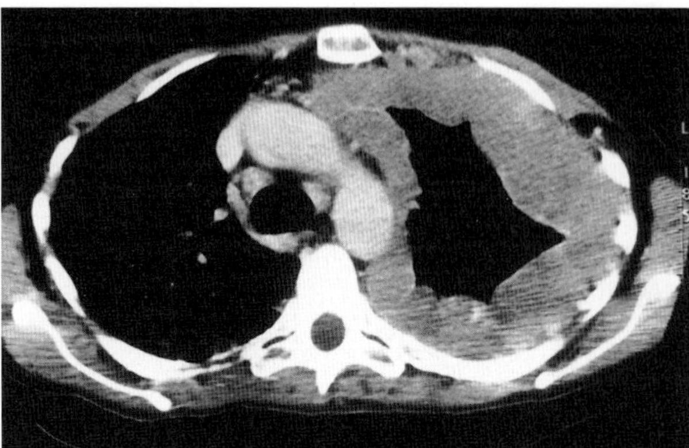

Figure 19.29 Markedly thickened, >1 cm, circumferential malignant pleural thickening on contrast enhanced computed tomography.

POSITRON EMISSION TOMOGRAPHY

There are increasing numbers of reports on the use of ^{18}FDG PET in the assessment of pleural malignancy (see earlier). PET may be of value in this since it correctly identified all 16 cases of malignancy in one series with only two false positives[97] and had an accuracy of 92 percent in another series.[102] It is worth remembering that any cause of significantly metabolically active disease may result in increased ^{18}FDG activity and this is perhaps best illustrated in the increased activity seen in patients post talc pleurodesis.[134,135]

Malignant mesothelioma

CHEST RADIOGRAPHY

The most common findings of diffuse malignant mesothelioma (see Chapter 41, Malignant mesothelioma) are irregular, nodular opacities around the periphery of the lung with or without an associated pleural effusion.[142,143] The effusion is usually unilateral and is present in 60 percent of patients, with only 5 percent of patients having bilateral disease.[144] The effusion may obscure underlying pleural masses until thoracentesis is performed. The effusion is characteristically not associated with contralateral shift of the mediastinum because of lung encasement by the pleural tumor. The mediastinum is either centrally located or may be shifted towards the affected side.[139] However, large effusions may be associated with contralateral shift of the mediastinum. Volume loss on the affected side may be demonstrated by narrowing of the intercostal spaces, elevation of the hemidiaphragm or ipsilateral shift of the mediastinum. Pleural masses without an associated effusion are seen in less than 25 per cent of patients on their initial radiograph.[95]

Evidence of previous asbestos exposure may also be apparent on the radiograph, especially the presence of benign calcified or noncalcified pleural plaques. However,

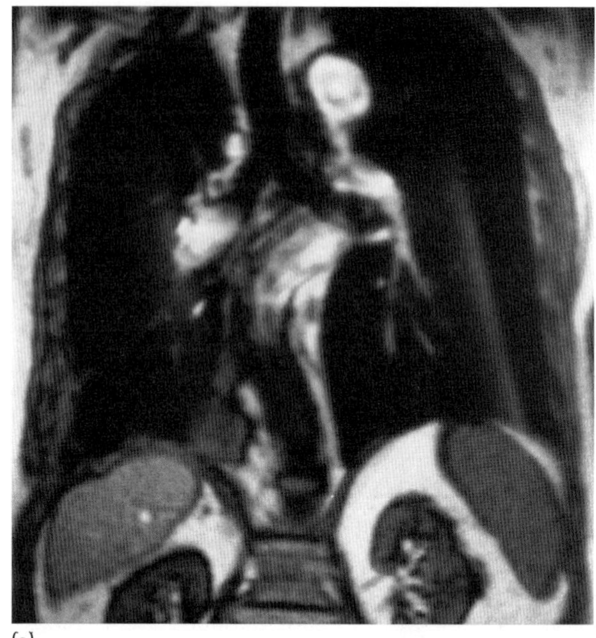

(a)

POST CONTRAST

(b)

Figure 19.30 Coronal magnetic resonance imaging sequences pre-(T1) (a) and post-gadolinium (fat-saturated T1) (b), demonstrating the avid enhancement of right-sided pleural malignancy (arrow).

only 20 percent of patients have radiographic evidence of interstitial disease or asbestosis.[144] Rib destruction is uncommon and mostly only seen in the advanced stages of the disease.[142]

COMPUTED TOMOGRAPHY

Several studies have shown that CT is superior to radiography in the assessment of the presence and extent of mesothelioma. The CT findings of mesothelioma include pleural thickening in 90 percent, extending into the interlobular fissures in 90 percent, pleural effusion in 70 percent, loss of volume of the affected hemithorax in 40 percent, pleural calcification in 20 percent and invasion of the chest wall in up to 20 percent of patients.[145]

The CT features suggestive of mesothelioma are similar to other causes of pleural malignancy described earlier. However, the presence of calcification within the pleural thickening suggests a benign process, with 10 percent of patients with mesothelioma having evidence of pleural calcification compared with up to 50 per cent of patients with benign pleural thickening.[95,146]

Although volume loss is often seen in mesothelioma it is a relatively non-specific finding, since it is seen in both benign and malignant disease.[142,145]

A benign pleural effusion (see Chapter 40, Asbestos-related pleural diseases) may also occur in up to 3 percent of the asbestos exposed population. The effusion is usually unilateral and other manifestations of asbestos-related disease may be present. Differentiation of a benign asbestos effusion and asbestos-related mesothelioma can be difficult, but benign asbestos-related disease tends to be a symmetrical process and, on CT, pleural involvement is bilateral in most patients.[95] Also, as previously described, malignant pleural disease tends to involve the entire pleural surface whereas benign disease does not involve the mediastinal pleura.[95]

Differentiation of mesothelioma from metastatic disease is limited radiologically. The presence of hilar adenopathy is more common in metastatic disease.[95,147] True hilar involvement with no mediastinal involvement is rare in metastatic pleural disease except for bronchogenic carcinoma, lymphoma and renal cell carcinoma. Unfortunately, the tendency for mesothelioma to involve the inferior hemithorax appears non-specific.[95] Rib destruction and chest wall invasion are also good indicators of malignancy. Although rarely seen, infections such as actinomycosis, tuberculosis and nocardiosis may cause rib destruction but often at a single site rather than the multiple sites often seen in malignancy.

Computed tomography not only has an important role in diagnosis and staging but also in follow up.[148] The advent of new effective chemotherapeutic agents means that the assessment of tumor response is now an important criteria for both continuing chemotherapy and the evaluation of new therapies. Tumor response is assessed using contrast enhanced CT and may be evaluated using either the World Health Organisation (WHO)[149] assessment criteria or now more commonly the Response Evaluation Criteria in Solid Tumors (RECIST) guidelines.[150,151] Difficulties in accurate measurement of pleural thickening on CT, and in accurately measuring the same area of thickening on sequential scans, make the measurements less reliable than in other organs. Interobserver variability is a further confounding factor and the use of automated or semi-automated software may produce more consistent methods for measurement in the future.[148]

MAGNETIC RESONANCE IMAGING

Along with CT, MRI allows clear visualization of the circumferential pleural thickening, fissural thickening, pleural effusion and diaphragmatic invasion. The full extent of the tumor may be readily assessed on coronal and sagittal images. Mesothelioma returns an intermediate signal on T1-weighted images and an increased signal relative to the chest wall musculature on T2-weighted images;[13] it may also show avid pleural enhancement on T1-weighted sequences post gadolinium, and this may be of value in differentiating benign from malignant disease.[13,141] Additional fissural and diaphragmatic invasion detected by MRI appears reliable in differentiating mesothelioma from other causes of malignant pleural thickening.[141] Although MRI offers no apparent advantages over contrast-enhanced MSCT in staging disease,[91,152] when performed as a dynamic contrast enhanced examination it may be of value in predicting response to chemotherapy, although PET-CT may also be of value in this regard (see below).[15]

POSITRON EMISSION TOMOGRAPHY COMBINED WITH CT

Although PET-CT is not routinely used in the investigation of mesothelioma, it has been shown to be of value in providing prognostic information and assessing response to chemotherapy in patients with mesothelioma (Figure 19.31).[153] Tumours with a low standardized uptake value are more likely to be epithelioid and to have a better prognosis. A reduction in metabolic activity post chemotherapy correlates with an increased time to progression and increased survival. The pattern and measurement of metabolic activity may also correlate with the surgical stage. It may also be more accurate than the other imaging modalities in detecting distant metastatic disease.[154] In a study of 29 patients, PET-CT detected additional metastatic disease not identified on clinical examination and CT scanning in 7 of 29 patients.[154]

Staging of mesothelioma

Using the recent international TNM staging system proposed by the International Mesothelioma Interest Group, the CT and MR criteria for RESECTABILITY are as follows:

1. Preserved extrapleural fat planes.
2. Normal CT attenuation values and MR signal intensity characteristic of structures adjacent to the tumor.
3. Absence of extrapleural soft tissue masses.
4. Smooth inferior diaphragmatic surface.

The imaging criteria for UNRESECTABILITY are as follows:

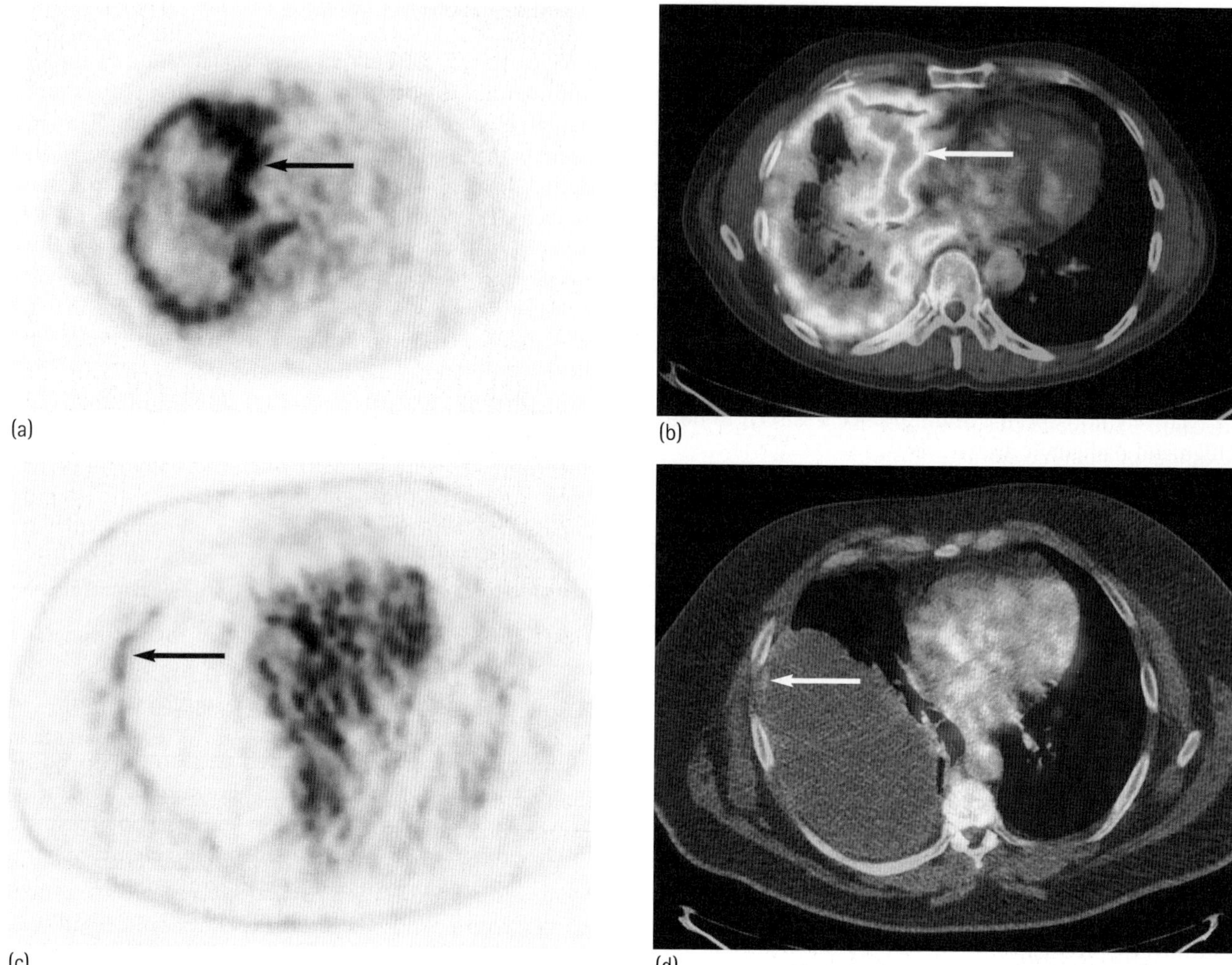

(a) (b) (c) (d)

Figure 19.31 (a) Positron emission tomography (PET) scan and (b) PET-computed tomography (CT) scan demonstrating high grade FDG activity (arrowed) in sarcomatoid mesothelioma, with circumferential pleural thickening. (c) PET scan and (d) integrated PET-CT scan demonstrating epithelioid mesothelioma (arrowed), with low grade fluorodeoxyglucose (FDG) activity, associated with pleural effusion. (For (b) and (d), see also Color Plates 11 and 12.)

1 Tumor encasement of the diaphragm.
2 Invasion of the extrapleural fat or soft tissues.
3 Involvement of the ribs or bone destruction.
4 Invasion of mediastinal structures.

Computed tomography and MR cannot easily distinguish between stages T1a, T1b and T2 as they cannot easily distinguish the parietal and visceral pleura or detect diaphragmatic muscle invasion. They can, however, enable distinction of stage 3 from stage 4.[91,155,156]

AIR

Pneumothorax

CHEST RADIOGRAPHY

The majority of pneumothoraces are identified on a standard PA CXR taken on inspiration.[157,158] Routinely, only inspiratory radiographs are recommended for the initial examination. If, however, the pneumothorax is not definitely seen on the inspiratory film, then an expiratory film may help to confirm it,[159] as the constant volume of the pneumothorax is accentuated by an overall reduction in the size of the hemithorax on expiration.

The radiographic diagnosis of a pneumothorax is based on the identification of a visceral pleural line separated from the parietal pleura by a radiolucent airspace, demonstrated by the absence of pulmonary vessels beyond the visceral line. Free air moves preferentially to the less dependent pleural spaces, and in the upright patient tends to accumulate in an apicolateral location.[24] The underlying etiology of primary spontaneous pneumothorax is demonstrated in the minority (15 percent) of patients.[160] The etiology of secondary spontaneous pneumothorax is more frequently demonstrated.

Curvilinear opacities projected over the chest from gowns, skinfolds or hair may mimic the visceral pleural surface. Following such a line outside the bony thorax is helpful to elucidate the cause, as is looking for vessels lateral to it. Visceral pleura tends to be well delineated and very thin, whereas skinfolds are more band-like, with a slight increase in attenuation medially, and have a well-defined lateral border.[161] The translucency adjacent to a skin fold is due to a visual phenomenon known as the Mach effect.[162] Care must be taken not to mistake a bulla or cyst for a pneumothorax (Figure 19.32). These tend to have medially concave surfaces and may be clearly limited to a lobe.[163] A lateral film is often helpful in confirming this.

Pneumothoraces are less readily demonstrated on a lateral film, and usually manifest as an anterior or posterior line.[164] Supine chest radiographs are insensitive in the detection of pneumothorax and detection depends to a great extent on the size of the pneumothorax.[165,166] Various features have been described to aid the detection of a pneumothorax in the supine patient (Figure 19.33).[167–170] The air is most often seen in an anteromedial and sub-pulmonary location. It is often seen as a lucent focus adjacent to the diaphragm, along the juxtacardiac region and extending into the lateral costophrenic recess: the 'deep sulcus' sign.[171] The hemithorax, or part of it, may appear of increased translucency and the mediastinal margin may appear sharp.

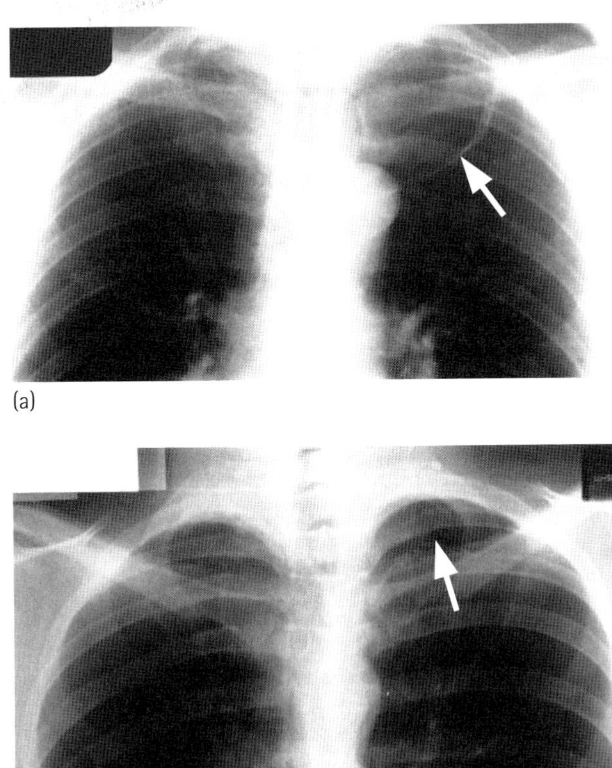

Figure 19.32 Left upper lobe bulla on chest radiography (arrow), (a) readily differentiated from an apical left pneumothorax with abnormal lung (arrow) by its concave surface (b).

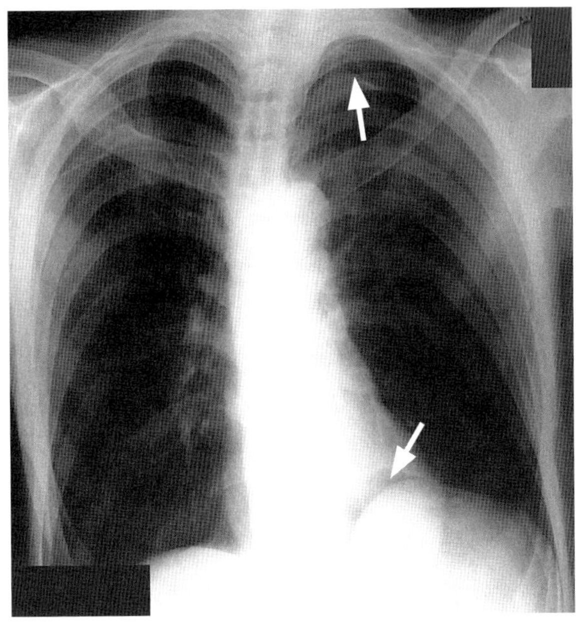

Figure 19.33 Supine left pneumothorax on chest radiography, seen lying in an apical and anteromedial location (arrows).

If fluid as well as air is present in the pleural space, then an air–fluid level is produced (Figure 19.34). This is clearly seen on an erect film. If the patient is supine the diagnosis is more difficult.

A pneumothorax is considered to be under tension when the pressure in the pleural space exceeds atmospheric pressure. The signs of a tension pneumothorax include diaphragmatic inversion, displacement of the anterior junctional line to the contralateral side, or

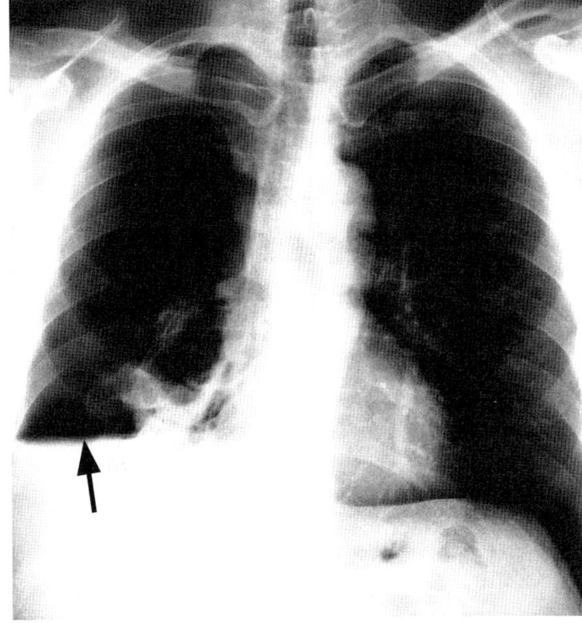

Figure 19.34 Large right hydropneumothorax identified on chest radiography by the straight line of the air–fluid level (arrow).

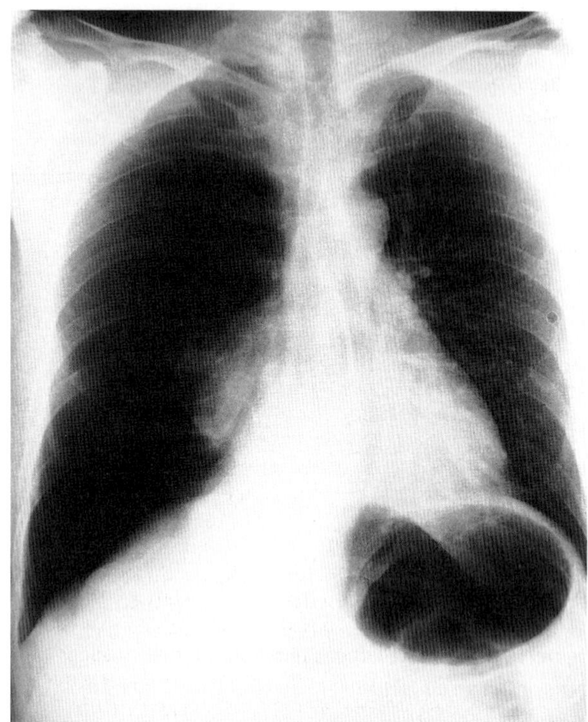

Figure 19.35 Right-sided tension pneumothorax on chest radiography with mediastinal shift and depression of the hemidiaphragm.

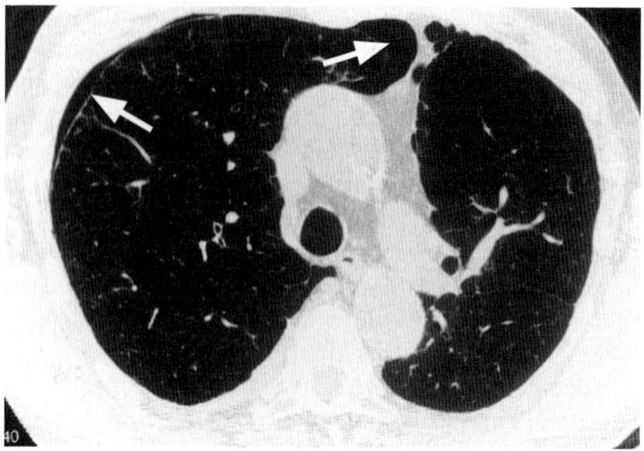

Figure 19.36 Small right-sided pneumothorax seen on computed tomography (arrows) but not visible on chest radiography.

displacement of the azygoesophageal recess (Figure 19.35). In addition, the heart border and other vascular structures are seen to be flattened.[172]

ULTRASOUND

As described in the section on normal US of the pleura, 'comet tails' and the 'lung sliding' sign are seen in the normal patient.[5,27] The presence of a pneumothorax is characterized by a lack of respiratory motion and a strongly echogenic interface lacking the 'comet tail' artifacts. Using post-lung-biopsy patients, US has been shown to be more sensitive than CXR in the detection of a pneumothorax.[27,28] It has also been shown to be false positive in patients with impaired lung function, in particular in patients with chronic obstructive pulmonary disease.[173] The false positive rate, inability to determine the volume of the pneumothorax and the necessity to scan the whole chest clearly limit the use of this technique.

Patients in the ICU are at an increased risk of developing a pneumothorax, which can rapidly become a tension pneumothorax. In these patients, pneumothorax detection is difficult on a supine radiograph and most accurate on a CT scan.[165,166]

COMPUTED TOMOGRAPHY

Computed tomography is significantly more sensitive than CXR in the detection of pneumothoraces, with between 25 and 40 percent of patients with a pneumothorax post lung-biopsy not detected by CXR but present on CT (Figure 19.36).[158] Several studies have also shown that CT is superior to a supine radiograph in the detection of a pneumothorax, with up to 50 percent of pneumothoraces detected only by CT.[158,165,174] In those patients where the pneumothorax is secondary to trauma, CT scanning may also demonstrate other signs such as parenchymal contusion, infiltrates, pneumatoceles and pericardial effusion.

Bronchopleural fistula

CHEST RADIOGRAPHY

The radiographic features commonly reflect the underlying etiology (e.g. post pneumonectomy, empyema, etc.). If a bronchopleural fistula arises as a complication following a recent pneumonectomy, several signs are demonstrated on the CXR. These include an increase in the amount of air in the operated hemithorax, a decreased amount of fluid, loss of the normal mediastinal shift toward the operated side and, occasionally, an aspiration pneumonitis. The clinico-radiographic features usually enable a diagnosis. If clinical doubt persists, then CT[175] or ventilation scanning may be diagnostic (Figure 19.37).[176]

COMPUTED TOMOGRAPHY

Computed tomography is the optimal way of demonstrating the communication between the lung or airway and the pleural space. Thin-section CT may be required to determine the location, size and number of fistulas.[175] In addition to demonstrating fistulas, CT may provide additional diagnostic information such as tumor recurrence.

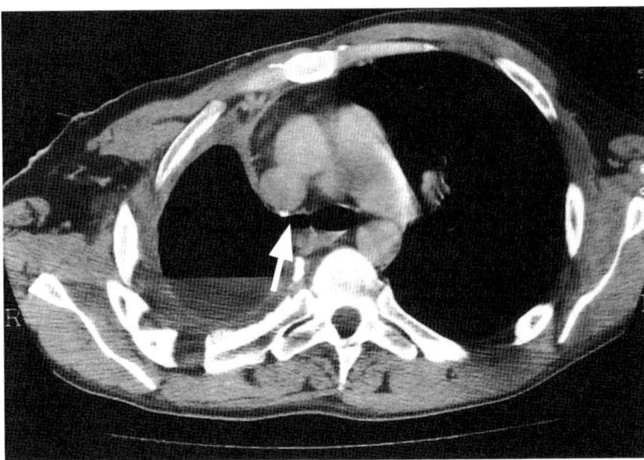

Figure 19.37 Post pneumonectomy right-bronchopleural fistula shown on computed tomography (arrow).

FUTURE DIRECTIONS

The proven value of US and CT in the assessment of patients with pleural disease has inevitably led to an increase in their clinical use. The decreased cost of portable US machines has led to an explosion in its use and a move away from its provision by radiologists. The advent of MSCT has also enabled CT scans to be performed on patients previously thought unfit to scan. The advent of PET-CT has also opened the door to the use of PET scanning in patients with pleural malignancy. Increasingly these tests are being used not only in diagnosis and staging, but also to guide therapeutic decisions and are being investigated as surrogate markers of function and morphology. It is perhaps their role as surrogate biomarkers of disease that is the next and most exciting step in their use.

KEY POINTS

- The majority of pleural effusions are reliably diagnosed on CXR.
- Ultrasound may be used to confirm the presence of a pleural effusion, assess features specific for exudative effusions such as a septations and pleural nodularity, and to aid drain placement.
- Multislice CT is accurate in the diagnosis of benign and malignant pleural thickening.
- Image-guided biopsy is of value in the diagnosis of malignant pleural disease, including malignant mesothelioma.
- Multislice CT is significantly more sensitive than CXR in the detection of pneumothorax, and is of particular use in trauma and intensive care patients.
- MSCT, DCEMRI and PET-CT may be used as correlates of function and morphology and act as surrogate biomarkers of disease processes.

REFERENCES

● = Key primary paper
◆ = Major review article

1. Moskowitz H, Platt RT, Schacher R, Mellins H. Roentgen visualization of minute pleural effusion. *Radiology* 1973; **109**: 33–5.
◆2. Patel MC, Flower CDR. Radiology in the management of pleural disease. *Eur Radiol* 1997; **7**: 1454–62.
◆3. Sahn SA. The pleura. *Am Rev Respir Dis* 1988; **138**: 184–234.
4. Woodring JH. Recognition of pleural effusion on supine radiographs. *Am J Roentgenol* 1984; **142**: 59–64.
◆5. Wernecke K. Sonographic features of pleural disease. *Am J Roentgenol* 1997; **168**: 1061–6.
◆6. McLoud TC, Flower CDR. Imaging the pleura: sonography, CT, and MR imaging. *Am J Roentgenol* 1991; **156**: 1145–53.
7. Gorg C, Bert T, Gorg K. Contrast-enhanced sonography for differential diagnosis of pleurisy and focal pleural lesions of unknown cause. *Chest* 2005;**128**: 3894–99.
8. Fishman EK, Jeffrey RB. *Spiral CT. Principles, techniques and clinical applications.* Philadelphia: Lippincott-Raven, 1996.
◆9. Knisely BL, Kuhlman JE. Radiographic and CT imaging of complex pleural disease. *Crit Rev Diagn Imaging* 1997; **38**: 1–58.
10. Copley SJ, Well AU, Rubens MB, *et al.* Functional consequences of pleural disease evaluated with chest radiography and CT. *Radiology* 2001; **220**: 237–43.
◆11. Knisely BL, Broderick LS, Kuhlman JE. MR imaging of the pleura and chest wall. *MRI Clin North Am* 2000; **8**: 125–41.
◆12. White CS. Magnetic resonance imaging of the chest. *Respir Care* 2001; **46**: 922–31.
◆13. Schmutz GR, Fisch-Ponsot C, Regent D, Sylvestre J. Computed tomography and magnetic resonance imaging of pleural masses. *Crit Rev Diagn Imaging* 1993; **34**: 309–83.
●14. Falaschi F, Battolla L, Mascalchi M, *et al.* Usefulness of MR signal intensity in distinguishing benign from malignant pleural disease. *Am J Roentgenol* 1996; **166**: 963–8.
15. Giesel FL, Bischoff H, von Tengg-Kobligk H, *et al.* Dynamic contrast-enhanced MRI of malignant pleural mesothelioma: A feasibility study of noninvasive assessment, therapeutic follow-up, and possible predictor of improved outcome. *Chest* 2006; **129**: 1570–76.
16. Von Schulthess GK, Steinert HC, Hany TF. Integrated PET/CT: Current applications and future directions. *Radiology* 2006; **238**: 405–22.
◆17. Goldsmith SJ, Kostakoglu L. Nuclear medicine imaging of lung cancer. *Radiol Clin North Am* 2000; **38**: 511–24.
18. Duysinx B, Nguyen D, Louis R, *et al.* Evaluation of pleural disease with 18-fluorodeoxyglucose positron emission tomography imaging. *Chest* 2004; **125**: 489–493.
19. Speckman JM, Gamsu G, Webb WR. Alterations in CT mediastinal anatomy produced by an azygos lobe. *Am J Roentgenol* 1981; **137**: 47–50.
20. Godwin JD, Tarver RD. Accessory fissures of the lung. *Am J Roentgenol* 1985; **144**: 39–47.
21. Raasch BN, Carsky EW, Lane EJ, O'Callaghan JP, Heitzman ER. Pleural effusion: explanation of some typical appearances. *Am J Roentgenol* 1982; **139**: 899–904.
22. Proto AV, Ball JB. The superolateral major fissures. *Am J Roentgenol* 1983; **140**: 431–7.
23. Austin JHM. The left minor fissure. *Radiology* 1986; **161**: 433–6.
24. Fraser RG, Muller NL, Colman N, Pare PDL. *Diagnosis of diseases of the chest*, 4th edn. Philadelphia: WB Saunders Co, 1999.
25. Armstrong P, Wilson AG, Dee P, *et al. Imaging of diseases of the chest*, 3rd edn. London: Mosby, 2000.
26. Cimmono CV. The oesophageal-pleural stripe: an update. *Radiology* 1981; **140**: 607–13.

27. Goodman TR, Traill ZC, Phillips AJ, Berger J, Gleeson FV. Ultrasound detection of pneumothorax. *Clin Radiol* 1999; **54**: 736–9.
28. Sistrom CL, Reiheld CT, Gay SB, Wallace KK. Detection and estimation of the volume of pneumothorax using real-time sonography: efficacy determined by receiver operating characteristic analysis. *Am J Roentgenol* 1996; **166**: 317–21.
29. Lichtenstein DA, Menu Y. A bedside ultrasound sign ruling out pneumothorax in the critically ill. Lung sliding. *Chest* 1995; **108**: 1345–8.
●30. Wernecke K, Galanski M, Peters PE, *et al.* Pneumothorax: evaluation by ultrasound-preliminary results. *Thorac Imaging* 1987; **2**: 76–8.
31. Targhetta R, Bourgeois JM, Chavagneux R, *et al.* Ultrasonic signs of pneumothorax: preliminary work. *J Clin Ultrasound* 1993; **21**: 245–50.
32. Ueki J, De Bruin PF, Pride NB. *In vivo* assessment of diaphragm contraction by ultrasound in normal subjects. *Thorax* 1995; **50**: 1157–61.
33. McCool FD, Benditt JO, Conomos P, *et al.* Variability of diaphragm structure among healthy individuals. *Am J Respir Crit Care Med* 1997; **155**: 1323–8.
34. Proto AV, Ball JB. Computed tomography of the major and minor fissures. *Am J Roentgenol* 1983; **140**: 439–48.
35. Marks BW, Kuhns LR. Identification of the pleural fissures with computed tomography. *Radiology* 1982; **143**: 139–41.
36. Webb RW, Muller NL, Naidich DP. *High resolution CT of the lung*, 2nd edn. Philadelphia: Lippincott, Williams and Williams, 1996.
37. Im J-G, Webb WR, Rosen A, Gamsu G. Costal pleura: appearances at high-resolution CT. *Radiology* 1989; **171**: 125–31.
38. Vix VA. Extrapleural costal fat. *Radiology* 1974; **112**: 563–5.
39. Sargent EN, Boswell WD, Ralls PW, Markovitz A. Subpleural fat pads in patients exposed to asbestos: distinction from non-calcified pleural plaques. *Radiology* 1984; **152**: 273–7.
◆40. Mueller NL. Imaging of the pleura. *Radiology* 1993; **186**: 297–309.
41. Collins JD, Burwell D, Furmanski S, Lorber P, Steckel RJ. Minimal detectable pleural effusions. *Radiology* 1972; **105**: 51–3.
42. Blackmore CC, Black WC, Dallas RV, Crow HC. Pleural fluid volume estimation: a chest radiograph prediction rule. *Acad Radiol* 1996; **3**: 103–9.
43. Davis S, Gardner Q. The shape of a pleural effusion. *Br Med J* 1963; **26**: 436–7.
◆44. Henschke CI, Davis SD, Romano PM, Yankelevitz DF. Pleural effusions: pathogenesis, radiologic evaluation, and therapy. *J Thorac Imag* 1989; **4**: 49–60.
45. Oestreich AE, Haley C. Pleural effusion: the thorn sign. *Chest* 1981; **79**: 365–6.
◆46. Fleischner FG. Atypical arrangement of free pleural effusion. *Radiol Clin North Am* 1963; **1**: 347–62.
47. Maher GG, Berger HW. Massive pleural effusion: malignant and non-malignant causes in 46 patients. *Am Rev Respir Dis* 1972; **105**: 458–60.
48. Liberson M. Diagnostic significance of the mediastinal profile in massive unilateral pleural effusions. *Am Rev Respir Dis* 1963; **88**: 176–80.
49. Mulvey RB. The effect of pleural fluid on the diaphragm. *Am J Roentgenol* 1965; **84**: 1080–5.
50. Yousef MMA. Case of the fall season. *Semin Roentgenol* 1980; **15**: 269–71.
51. Ruskin JA, Gurney JW, Thorsen MK, Goodman LR. Detection of pleural effusions on supine chest radiographs. *Am J Roentgenol* 1987; **148**: 681–3.
52. Petersen JA. Recognition of infrapulmonary pleural effusion. *Radiology* 1960; **74**: 34–41.
53. Schwartz MI, Marmorstein BL. A new radiologic sign of subpulmonic effusion. *Chest* 1975; **67**: 176–8.
54. Eibenberger KL, Dock WI, Ammann ME, *et al.* Quantification of pleural effusions: sonography versus radiography. *Radiology* 1994; **191**: 681–4.
55. Gryminski J, Krakowka P, Lypacewicz G. The diagnosis of pleural effusion by ultrasonic and radiologic techniques. *Chest* 1976; **70**: 33–7.
56. Lipscomb DJ, Flower CDR, Hadfield JW. Ultrasound of the pleura: an assessment of its clinical value. *Clin Radiol* 1981; **32**: 289–90.
57. Hirsch JH, Rogers JV, Mack LA. Real-time sonography of pleural opacities. *Am J Roentgenol* 1981; **136**: 297–301.
58. Yang P-C, Luh K-T, Chang D-B, Wu C-J, Kuo S-H. Value of sonography in determining the nature of pleural effusion: analysis of 320 cases. *Am J Roentgenol* 1992; **159**: 29–33.
59. Lomas DJ, Padley SG, Flower CDR. The sonographic appearances of pleural fluid. *Br J Radiol* 1993; **66**: 619–24.
60. Chian CF, Su WL, Soh LH, *et al.* Echogenic swirling pattern as a predictor of malignant pleural effusions in patients with malignancies. *Chest* 2004; **126**: 129–34.
61. Marks WM, Filly RA, Callen PW. Real-time evaluation of pleural lesions: new observations regarding the probability of obtaining free fluid. *Radiology* 1982; **142**: 163–4.
62. Rosenberg ER. Ultrasound in the assessment of pleural densities. *Chest* 1983; **84**: 283–5.
63. Tu CY, Hsu WH, Hsia TC, *et al.* Pleural effusions in febrile medical ICU patients: Chest ultrasound study. *Chest* 2004; **126**: 1274–80.
64. Brutsche MH, Tassi GF, Gyorik S, *et al.* Treatment of sonographically stratified multiloculated thoracic empyema by medical thoracoscopy. *Chest* 2005; **128**: 3303–9.
65. Wu RG, Yang PC, Kuo SH, Luh KT. 'Fluid color' sign: a useful indicator for discrimination between pleural thickening and pleural effusion. *J Ultrasound Med* 1995; **14**: 767–9.
66. Wu RG, Yuan A, Liaw YS, *et al.* Image comparison of real-time gray-scale ultrasound and color doppler ultrasound for use in diagnosis of minimal pleural effusion. *Am J Respir Crit Care Med* 1994; **150**: 510–14.
67. Mayo PH, Dolken P. Pleural ultrasonography. *Clin Chest Med* 2006; **27**: 215–27.
68. Eibenberger KL, Dock WI, Ammann ME, *et al.* Quantification of pleural effusions: sonography versus radiography. *Radiology* 1994; **191**: 681–4.
69. Roch A, Bojan M, Michelet P, *et al.* Usefulness of ultrasonography in predicting pleural effusions >500 mL in patients receiving mechanical ventilation. *Chest* 2005; **127**: 224–32.
70. Zhu Z, Donnelly E, Dikensoy O, *et al.* Efficacy of ultrasound in the diagnosis of pleurodesis in rabbits. *Chest* 2005; **128**: 934–39.
71. Bressler EL, Francis IR, Glazer GM, Gross BH. Bolus contrast medium enhancement for distinguishing pleural from parenchymal lung disease: CT features. *J Comput Assist Tomogr* 1987; **11**: 436–40.
72. Teplick JG, Teplick SK, Goodman L, Haskin ME. The interface sign: a computed tomographic sign for distinguishing pleural and intra-abdominal fluid. *Radiology* 1982; **144**: 359–62.
73. Dwyer A. The displaced crus: a sign for distinguishing between pleural fluid and ascites on computed tomography. *J Comput Assist Tomogr* 1978; **2**: 598–9.
74. Kearney SE, Davies CWH, Davies RJO, Gleeson FV. Computed tomography and ultrasound in parapneumonic effusions and empyema. *Clin Radiol* 2000; **55**: 542–7.
75. Aquino SL, Webb WR, Gushiken BJ. Pleural exudates and transudates: diagnosis with contrast-enhanced CT. *Radiology* 1994; **192**: 803–8.
76. Waite RJ, Carbonneau RJ, Balikian JP, *et al.* Parietal pleural changes in empyema: appearances at CT. *Radiology* 1990; **175**: 145–50.
77. Traill ZC, Davies RJO, Gleeson FV. Thoracic computed tomography in patients with suspected malignant pleural effusions. *Clin Radiol* 2001; **56**: 193–6.
78. Davis SD, Henschke CI, Yankelevitz DF, Cahill PT, Yi Y. MR imaging of pleural effusions. *J Comput Assist Tomogr* 1990; **14**: 192–8.
◆79. McLoud TC. CT and MR in pleural disease. *Clin Chest Med* 1998; **19**: 261–76.

80. Hanna JW, Reed JC, Choplin RH. Pleural infections: a clinical-radiologic review. *J Thorac Imaging* 1991; **6**: 68–79.
81. Stark DD, Federle MP, Goodman PC, Podrasky AE, Webb WR. Differentiating lung abscess and empyema: radiography and computed tomography. *Am J Roentgenol* 1983; **141**: 163–7.
82. Friedman PJ, Hellekant AG. Radiologic recognition of bronchopleural fistula. *Radiology* 1977; **124**: 289–95.
83. Hsu JT, Bennett GM, Wolff E. Radiologic assessment of bronchopleural fistula with empyema. *Radiology* 1972; **103**: 41–5.
84. Ferguson AD, Prescott RJ, Selkon JB, Watson D, Swinburn CR. Empyema subcommittee of the Research Committee of the British Thoracic Society. The clinical course and management of thoracic empyema. *QJM* 1996; **89**: 285–9.
85. Neff CC, van Sonnenberg E, Lawson DW, Patton AS. CT follow-up of empyemas: pleural peels resolve after percutaneous catheter drainage. *Radiology* 1990; **176**: 195–7.
86. Sahn SA, Iseman MD. Tuberculous empyema. *Semin Respir Infect* 1999; **14**: 82–7.
87. Hulnick DH, Naidich DP, McCauley DI. Pleural tuberculosis evaluated by computed tomography. *Radiology* 1983; **149**: 759–65.
88. Bhatt GM, Austin HM. CT demonstration of empyema necessitatis. *J Comp Assist Tomogr* 1985; **9**: 1108–9.
89. Glicklich M, Mendelson DS, Gendal ES, *et al.* Tuberculous empyema necessitatis. Computed tomography findings. *Clin Imaging* 1990; **14**: 23–5.
90. American Thoracic Society. Management of malignant pleural effusions. *Am J Respir Crit Care Med* 2000; **162**: 1987–2001.
◆91. Bonomo L, Feragalli B, Sacco R, Merlino B, Storto ML. Malignant pleural disease. *Eur J Radiol* 2000; **34**: 98–118.
◆92. Sahn SA. Pleural diseases related to metastatic malignancies. *Eur Respir J* 1997; **10**: 1907–13.
93. Goerg C, Schwerk WB, Goerg K, Walters E. Pleural effusion: an 'acoustic window' for sonography of pleural metastases. *J Clin Ultrasound* 1991; **19**: 93–7.
◆94. Goerg C, Restrepo I, Schwerk WB. Sonography of malignant pleural effusion. *Eur Radiol* 1997; **7**: 1195–8.
●95. Leung AN, Muller NL, Miller RR. CT in differential diagnosis of diffuse pleural disease. *Am J Roentgenol* 1990; **154**: 487–92.
96. Adams R, Gleeson FV. Percutaneous image guided cutting needle biopsy of the pleura in the presence of a suspected malignant effusion. *Radiology* 2001; **219**: 510–14.
97. Bury TH, Paulus P, Dowlati A, *et al.* Evaluation of pleural diseases with FDG-PET imaging – preliminary report. *Thorax* 1997; **52**: 187–9.
98. Schaffler GJ, Wolf G, Schoellnast H, *et al.* Non-small cell lung cancer: Evaluation of pleural abnormalities on CT scans with ^{18}F FDG PET. *Radiology* 2004; **231**: 858–65.
99. Gupta NC, Rogers JS, Graeber GM, *et al.* Clinical role of F-18 fluorodeoxyglucose positron emission tomography imaging in patients with lung cancer and suspected malignant pleural effusion. *Chest* 2002; **122**: 1918–24.
100. Erasmus JJ, McAdams HP, Rossi SE, *et al.* FDG PET of pleural effusions in patients with non-small cell lung cancer. *Am J Roentgenol* 2000; **175**: 245–9.
101. Hillerdal G. Chylothorax and pseudochylothorax. *Eur Respir J* 1997; **10**: 1157–62.
102. Pui MH, Yueh T-C. Lymphoscintigraphy in chyluria, chyloperitoneum and chylothorax. *J Nucl Med* 1998; **39**: 1292–6.
103. Groskin SA. Selected topics in chest trauma. *Radiology* 1992; **183**: 605–17.
104. Wolverson MK, Crepps LF, Sundaram M, *et al.* Hyperdensity of recurrent haemorrhage at body computed tomography: incidence and morphologic variation. *Radiology* 1983; **148**: 779–84.
105. International Labour Office. *Guidelines for the use of the ILO international classification of radiographs of pneumoconiosis.* Revised edition. Occupational Health and Safety Series, No. 22 (Rev. 80). Geneva: International Labour Office,1980.
◆106. Peacock C, Copley SJ, Hansell DM. Asbestos-related benign pleural disease. *Clin Radiol* 2000; **55**: 422–32.
107. Rockoff SD, Kagan E, Schwartz A, *et al.* Visceral pleural thickening in asbestos exposure: the occurrence and implications of thickened interlobar fissures. *J Thorac Imaging* 1987; **2**: 58–66.
◆108. McLoud TC. Conventional radiography in the diagnosis of asbestos-related disease. *Radiol Clin North Am* 1992; **30**: 1177–89.
109. Sargent EN, Gordonson J, Jacobson G, Birnbaum W, Shaub M. Bilateral pleural thickening: a manifestation of asbestos dust exposure. *Am J Roentgenol* 1978; **131**: 579–85.
110. Proto AV. Conventional chest radiographs: anatomic understanding of newer observations. *Radiology* 1992; **183**: 593–603.
111. Remy-Jardin M, Sobaszek A, Duhamel A, *et al.* Asbestos-related pleuropulmonary diseases: Evaluation with low-dose four-detector row spiral CT. *Radiology* 2004; **233**: 182–90.
◆112. Staples CA. Computed tomography in the evaluation of benign asbestos-related disorders. *Radiol Clin North Am* 1992; **30**: 1191–207.
113. Friedman AC, Fiel SB, Fisher MS, *et al.* Asbestos-related pleural disease and asbestosis: a comparison of CT and chest radiography. *Am J Roentgenol* 1988; **150**: 269–75.
114. Aberle DR, Gamsu G, Roy CS. High resolution CT of benign asbestos-related disorders: clinical and radiographic correlation. *Am J Roentgenol* 1988; **151**: 883–91.
◆115. Gefter WB, Epstein DM, Miller WT. Radiographic evaluation of asbestos-related chest disorders. *Crit Rev Diagn Imaging* 1984; **21**: 133–81.
◆116. Lynch DA, Gamsu G, Aberle DR. Conventional and high resolution computed tomography in the diagnosis of asbestos-related diseases. *Radiographics* 1989; **9**: 523–51.
117. Dedrick CG, McLoud TC, Shepard JO, Shipley RT. Computed tomography of localized pleural mesothelioma. *Am J Roentgenol* 1985; **144**: 275–80.
118. Mendelson DS, Meary E, Buy JN, Pigeau I, Kirschner PA. Localized fibrous pleural mesothelioma: CT findings. *Clin Imaging* 1991; **15**: 105–8.
119. Lee KS, Im JG, Choe KO, Kim CJ, Lee BH. CT findings in benign fibrous mesothelioma of the pleura: pathologic correlation in nine patients. *Am J Roentgenol* 1992; **158**: 983–6.
120. Saifuddin A, Da Costa P, Chalmers AG, Carey BM, Robertson RJH. Primary malignant localized fibrous tumors of the pleura: clinical, radiological, and pathological features. *Clin Radiol* 1992; **45**: 13–17.
◆121. Dynes MC, White EM, Fry WA, Ghahremani GG. Imaging manifestations of pleural tumors. *Radiographics* 1992; **12**: 1191–201.
122. Epler GR, McLoud TC, Munn CS, Colby TV. Pleural lipoma: diagnosis by computed tomography. *Chest* 1986; **90**: 265–8.
123. Filly R, Blank N, Castellino RA. Radiographic distribution of intrathoracic disease in previously untreated patients with Hodgkin's disease and non-Hodgkin's lymphoma. *Radiology* 1976; **120**: 277–81.
124. Burgener FH, Hamlin DJ. Intrathoracic histiocytic lymphoma. *Am J Roentgenol* 1981; **136**: 499–504.
125. Balikian JP, Herman PG. Non-Hodgkin lymphoma of the lungs. *Radiology* 1979; **132**: 569–76.
126. Castellino RA, Blank N, Hoppe RT, *et al.* Hodgkin disease: contributions of chest CT in initial staging evaluation. *Radiology* 1986; **160**: 603–5.
127. Shuman LS, Libshitz HI. Solid pleural manifestations of lymphoma. *Am J Roentgenol* 1984; **142**: 269–73.
128. Okada F, Ando Y, Kondo Y, *et al.* Thoracic CT Findings of Adult T-Cell Leukaemia or Lymphoma. *Am J Roentgenol* 2006; **182**: 761–7.
129. Carlsen SE, Bergin CJ, Hoppe RT. MR imaging to detect chest wall and pleural involvement in patients with lymphoma: effect on radiation therapy planning. *Am J Roentgenol* 1993; **160**: 1191–5.

130. Negendank WG, Alkatib AM, Karanes C, Smith MR. Lymphomas: MR imaging contrast characteristics with clinico-pathologic correlations. *Radiology* 1990; **177**: 209–16.
131. McLoud TC, Woods BO, Carrington CB, Epler GR, Gaensler EA. Diffuse pleural thickening in an asbestos-exposed population: prevalence and causes. *Am J Roentgenol* 1985; **144**: 9–18.
132. Copley SJ, Lee YCG, Hansell DM, *et al.* Asbestos-induced and smoking-related disease: Apportioning pulmonary function deficit by using thin-section CT. *Radiology* 2007; **242**: 258–66.
133. Murray JG, Patz EF Jr, Eramus JJ, Gilkeson RC. CT appearance of the pleural space after talc pleurodesis. *Am J Roentgenol* 1997; **169**: 89–91.
134. Murray JG, Eramus JJ, Bahtiarian EA, Goodman PC. Talc pleurodesis simulating pleural metastases on 18F-fluoro-deoxygenase positron emission tomography. *Am J Roentgenol* 1997; **168**: 359–60.
135. Kwek BH, Aquino SL, Fischman AJ. Fluorodeoxyglucose positron emission tomography and CT after talc pleurodesis. *Chest* 2004; **125**: 2356–60.
136. Renner RR, Pernice NJ. The apical cap. *Semin Roentgenol* 1977; **12**: 299–302.
137. Im JG, Webb WR, Han MC, *et al.* Apical opacity associated with pulmonary tuberculosis: high resolution CT findings. *Radiology* 1991; **178**: 727–31.
138. McLoud TC, Isler RJ, Novelline RA, *et al.* The apical cap, review. *Am J Roentgenol* 1981; **137**: 299–306.
139. Miller BH, Rosado-de-Christenson ML, Mason AC, *et al.* Malignant pleural mesothelioma: radiologic-pathologic correlation. *Radiographics* 1996; **16**: 613–44.
140. Scott EM, Marshall TJ, Flower CD, Stewart S. Diffuse pleural thickening: percutaneous CT-guided cutting needle biopsy. *Radiology* 1995; **194:** 867–70.
141. Knuuttila A, Kivisaari L, Kivisaari A, *et al.* Evaluation of pleural disease using MR and CT with special reference to malignant pleural mesothelioma. *Acta Radiol* 2001; **42**: 502–7.
142. Ng CS, Munden RF, Libshitz HI. Malignant pleural mesothelioma: the spectrum of manifestations on CT in 70 cases. *Clin Radiol* 1999; **54**: 415–21.
143. Boylan AM. Mesothelioma: new concepts in diagnosis and management. *Curr Opin Pulm Med* 2000; **6**: 157–63.
◆144. Astoul P. Pleural mesothelioma. *Curr Opin Pulm Med* 1999; **5**: 259–68.
145. Kawashima A, Libshitz HI. Malignant pleural mesothelioma: CT manifestations in 50 cases. *Am J Roentgenol* 1990; **155**: 965–9.
146. Hierholzer J, Luo L, Bittner RC, *et al.* MRI and CT in the differential diagnosis of pleural disease. *Chest* 2000; **118**: 604–9.
147. Adams VI, Unni KK, Muhm JR, *et al.* Diffuse malignant mesothelioma of pleura: diagnosis and survival in 92 cases. *Cancer* 1986; **58**: 1540–51.
148. Armato III SG, Ogarek JL, Starkey A, *et al.* Variability in mesothelioma tumor response classification. *Am J Roentgenol* 2006;**186**: 1000–6.
149. Miller AB, Hogestraeten B, Staquet M, Winkler A. Reporting results of cancer treatment. *Cancer* 1981; **47**: 207–14.
150. James K, Eisenhauer EA, Christian M, *et al.* Measuring response in solid tumors: Unidimensional versus bidimensional measurement. *J Natl Cancer Inst* 1999; **91**: 523–8.
151. Therasse P, Arbuck SG, Eisenhauer EA, *et al.* New guidelines to evaluate the response to treatment in solid tumors. *J Natl Cancer Inst* 2000; **92**: 205–16.
152. Patz EF, Shaffer K, Piwnica-Worms DR, *et al.* Malignant pleural mesothelioma: value of CT and MR imaging in predicting resectability. *Am J Roentgenol* 1992; **159**: 961–6.
153. Gerbaudo VH, Britz-Cunningam S, Sugarbaker DJ, Treves ST. Metabolic significance of the pattern, intensity and kinetics of 18F-FDG uptake in malignant pleural mesothelioma. *Thorax* 2003; **58**: 1077–82.
154. Erasmus JJ, Truong MT, Smythe WR, *et al.* Integrated computed tomography-positron emission tomography in patients with potentially respectable malignant pleural mesothelioma: Staging implications. *J Thorac Cardiovasc Surg* 2005; **129**: 1364–70.
155. Heelan RT, Rusch VW, Begg CB, *et al.* Staging of malignant pleural mesothelioma: comparison of CT and MR imaging. *Am J Roentgenol* 1999; **172**: 1039–46.
156. Patz EF, Rusch VW, Heelan R. The proposed new international TNM staging system for malignant pleural mesothelioma: application to imaging. *Am J Roentgenol* 1996; **166**: 323–7.
157. Bradley M, Williams C, Walshaw MJ. The value of routine expiratory films in the diagnosis of pneumothorax. *Arch Emerg Med* 1991; **8**: 115–16.
158. Bungay HK, Berger J, Traill ZC, Gleeson FV. Pneumothorax post CT-guided lung biopsy: a comparison between detection on chest radiographs and CT. *Br J Radiology* 1999; **72**: 1160–3.
159. Seow A, Kazerooni EA, Cascade PN, *et al.* Comparison of upright inspiratory and expiratory chest radiographs for detecting pneumothoraces. *Am J Roentgenol* 1996; **166**: 313–16.
160. Killen DA, Gobbel WG. *Spontaneous pneumothorax.* Boston: Little, Brown & Company, 1968.
161. Fisher JK. Skinfold versus pneumothorax. *Am J Roentgenol* 1978; **130**: 791–2.
162. Lane EJ, Proto AV, Phillips JW. Machbands and density perception. *Radiology* 1976; **121**: 9–17.
163. Greene R, McLoud TC, Stark P. Pneumothorax. *Semin Roentgenol* 1977; **12**: 313–25.
164. Glazer HS, Anderson DJ, Wilson BS, *et al.* Pneumothorax: appearance on lateral chest radiographs. *Radiology* 1989; **173**: 701–11.
165. Tocino IM, Miller MH, Frederick PR, Bahr AL, Thomas F. CT detection of occult pneumothorax in head trauma. *Am J Roentgenol* 1984; **143**: 987–90.
166. Wall SD, Federle MP, Jeffrey RB, Brett CM. CT diagnosis of unsuspected pneumothorax after blunt abdominal trauma. *Am J Roentgenol* 1983; **141**: 919–21.
167. Tocino IM, Miller MH, Fairfax WR. Distribution of pneumothorax in the supine and semirecumbent critically ill adult. *Am J Roentgenol* 1985; **144**: 901–5.
168. Rhea JT, vanSonnenberg E, McLoud TC. Basilar pneumothorax in the supine adult. *Radiology* 1979; **133**: 593–5.
169. Ziter FMH, Westcott JL. Supine subpulmonary pneumothorax. *Am J Roentgenol* 1981; **137**: 699–701.
170. Moskowitz PS, Griscom NT. The medial pneumothorax. *Radiology* 1976; **120**: 143–7.
171. Gordon R. The deep sulcus sign. *Radiology* 1980; **13**: 25–7.
◆172. Gallardo X, Castaner E, Mata JM. Benign pleural diseases. *Eur J Radiol* 2000; **34**: 87–97.
173. Slater A, Goodwin M, Anderson K, Gleeson FV. COPD can mimic the appearances of pneumothorax on ultrasound. *Chest* 2006; **129**: 545–50.
174. vanSonnenberg E, Casola G, Ho M, *et al.* Difficult thoracic lesions: CT-guided biopsy experience in 150 cases. *Radiology* 1988; **167**: 457–61.
175. Westcott JL, Valpe JP. Peripheral bronchopleural fistula: CT evaluation in 20 patients with pneumonia, empyema, or post operative air leak. *Radiology* 1995; **196**: 175–91.
176. Zelefski MN, Freeman LM, Stern H. A simple approach to the diagnosis of bronchopleural fistula. *Radiology* 1977; **124**: 843–4.

20

Radiology: interventional

EDITH M MAROM, JEREMY J ERASMUS, EDWARD F PATZ JR

INTRODUCTION

Abnormalities of the pleura and pleural space are caused by a variety of disorders including infection, trauma, inflammation and neoplasms. Although some patients can be managed conservatively, interventional procedures including pleural fluid aspiration with or without placement of a drainage catheter, or pleural biopsies are frequently performed for either diagnostic or therapeutic purposes. The type of intervention depends on a spectrum of clinical and imaging features including symptoms, extent of disease and the etiology of the pleural abnormality. This review discusses the more common transthoracic interventional procedures that are used to diagnose and treat pleural disease, including thoracentesis, pleural catheter placement and pleural biopsy.

PRE-PROCEDURE PREPARATION

Before any procedure is performed, the indications, contraindications, management issues including goals and risks of the procedure should be reviewed. These risks and benefits should be explained in detail to the patient and informed consent obtained. Although laboratory blood work including platelet count, prothrombin time and international normalization ratio (INR) are typically performed, in the absence of a known bleeding diathesis or blood dyscrasia, the true utility of such tests has not been clearly determined. Most institutions suggest a relative contraindication to pleural intervention are patients with a platelet count <50 000, prothrombin time >3 seconds above control or an INR of >1.5.

Prior to beginning most procedures, an intravenous catheter is placed so that sedatives and analgesics may be administered if required. Continuous electrocardiographic, blood pressure and blood oxygen saturation monitoring is typically performed throughout the procedure, although this is not always required.

SELECTION OF IMAGING GUIDANCE

The type of interventional procedure, user preference and presumed etiology of the pleural abnormality will determine whether ultrasound, computed tomography (CT) or fluoroscopy will be used. Because ultrasound is accurate in detecting small fluid collections and can image the patient in any position (thus facilitating access to small effusions), it is the most commonly used imaging modality in patients with uncomplicated pleural collections. Its disadvantage is its inability to image through normal lung or bone.

Computed tomography is most commonly used to assist in transthoracic catheter placement into loculated or complex pleural fluid collections. CT allows one to identify other thoracic abnormalities such as lymphadenopathy, obstructing endobronchial disease or thick diffuse pleural disease, which may alter patient management. Disadvantages of CT include the inability to continuously monitor the procedure (even with the use of fluoroscopic CT), radiation exposure and limitations of patient positioning that can complicate drainage of a small effusion or biopsy of a pleural abnormality. At this time, fluoroscopic guidance is typically limited to chest tube placement for pneumothorax, as the air within the pleural space adjacent to the collapsed lung can be easily identified. Only brief periods of radiation exposure are needed for imaging localization and guidance for tube placement.

Additional factors influencing the choice of imaging modality used to assist pleural interventional procedures include the type, size, position and accessibility of the pleural abnormality. In most practices, ultrasound is usually used to assist the placement of a drainage catheter into uncomplicated effusions. CT is preferred for small loculated or medially placed fluid collections or for biopsy of pleural masses. Fluoroscopy is used for pneumothorax and chest tube placement.

THORACENTESIS

Patients presenting with a pleural effusion usually have a thoracentesis as the initial diagnostic procedure to determine the etiology, so that the appropriate treatment strategy can be determined. Thoracentesis of pleural effusions can be performed at the bedside without imaging-assisted guidance.[1,2] However, thoracentesis without the use of imaging-assisted guidance has been reported to be unsuccessful in approximately 12–15 percent of patients and serious complications occur in up to one-third.[3–6] The use of imaging-assisted guidance increases the success of thoracentesis and decreases serious complications to 0–3 percent.[3,5,7] A common practice is to determine the site for optimal needle placement with imaging and then perform the procedure later at the bedside. It should be noted that some have suggested that this management strategy results in complication and failure rates that are the same as if thoracentesis was performed without imaging-assisted guidance.[3,8]

Once the optimal site for needle placement has been determined (usually the shortest route that avoids traversing lung or diaphragm), the patients should be prepped and draped in sterile fashion and the site anesthetized to the pleural surface using 2 percent lidocaine. The needle selected to perform the aspiration varies, but is usually a 20 to 22G (Precision Glide Needle or Spinal Needle; Becton Dickinson & Co., Franklin Lakes, NJ, USA). The size of needle is determined according to the anticipated fluid to be drained. Thicker fluids (pus, blood collections) usually require at least a 20 gauge needle whereas transudates can be drained with smaller gauge needles.

The amount of fluid removed for a diagnostic tap depends on the clinical scenario. If the collection is suspected to be infected, and a diagnostic tap is requested, then only a small amount (approximately 10 cm^3) is necessary for cultures. If the fluid is purulent, as much fluid as possible should be drained and a tube should be placed. If malignancy is suspected, then larger amounts (no more than 1 L at presentation) should be drained, as the yield of cytology appears to increase with increasing amounts of fluid sent for analysis. The yield of cytology for malignant pleural effusions also improves with repeated pleural fluid cytologic specimens and when combined with a percutaneous pleural biopsy.[9]

TUBE THORACOSTOMY

Catheter thoracostomy is usually used to manage patients with malignant pleural effusions, parapneumonic effusions or empyemas, and pneumothoraces.

Malignant pleural effusions

Malignant pleural effusions are common in cancer patients with metastatic disease. Approximately 50 percent of patients with breast carcinoma, 25 percent of patients with lung carcinoma and 35 percent of patients with lymphoma develop a malignant effusion during the course of their disease. These three tumors and ovarian carcinoma account for over 75 percent of all malignant effusions.[10–14]

Treatment of malignant effusions is palliative and is typically performed to improve symptoms of dyspnea, cough and chest pain.[11,14–16] Most malignant effusions, with the exception of lymphoma and small cell lung cancer, are not controlled by systemic chemotherapy, and treatment options include repeated thoracentesis, catheter thoracostomy and sclerotherapy, video-assisted sclerotherapy, pleuroperitoneal shunts and long-term indwelling pleural catheters. Traditionally, treatment of malignant effusions has been performed with large-bore thoracostomy catheters (greater than 24 French)[17,18] as repeated thoracentesis has a 97 percent recurrence rate and pleuro-peritoneal shunts tend to malfunction with malignant effusions.[19] Because large-bore catheters are associated with moderate discomfort and wound infection in up to 16 percent of patients,[20] small-bore catheters placed using imaging-assisted guidance are being used more frequently. The small-bore catheters are associated with less discomfort and response rates (70–90 percent) are equal to those obtained with large-bore catheters.[17,18,21–27]

It must be recognized that the rationale for tube placement in these patients is to improve symptomatology, i.e. dyspnea and cough. This is purely a palliative, quality of life procedure with good results if patient selection is appropriate. Because a high Karnofsky's performance status score correlates with good outcome of the pleurodesis, ideally patients should have an expected survival of a few months.[28] Otherwise, repeat thoracenteses should be considered. Patients with a thick pleural rind or a central endobronchial lesion obstructing the airway, precluding lung re-expansion and improved aeration, usually will not benefit from short-term pleural fluid drainage and alternative treatment options such as a long-term indwelling pleural catheter, should be considered.

TECHNIQUE

Small-bore catheters are ideally placed in the mid-axillary line in the sixth or seventh intercostal space so that the patient can lie supine comfortably. Patients are prepped and draped using aseptic technique and after imaging has localized the optimal needle placement site, this region is anesthetized to the pleural surface using 2 percent lidocaine (up to 10 cm^3 or 200 mg). Because the tube traverses the parietal pleura and patients can still experience pain after local anesthetic administration, intravenous analgesia or conscious sedation is used routinely. A skin incision large enough to accommodate a 14 F all-purpose drainage (APD) catheter (Flexima, APD; Medi-Tech, Inc., MA, USA) is made. An 18-gauge Trocar needle is then placed into the pleural space and a small amount of fluid aspirated to assure adequate placement. A 100-cm 0.38 floppy-tipped wire (Cook, Bloomington, IN, USA), is then advanced into the pleural space and sequential dilators (usually 8, 10, 12 F) are passed along the guide wire to enlarge the catheter tract. The 14 F pigtail chest drainage catheter is then advanced over the wire into the pleural fluid. The pigtail catheter is curled and locked, and up to 1 L of fluid is aspirated at the time of the initial procedure. It has been suggested that rapid removal of larger amounts of fluid increases the risk for re-expansion pulmonary edema.[29] If the patient begins to cough before 1 L has been removed, aspiration is discontinued as this is usually indicative of poor re-expansion of the lung due to a decrease in compliance. Catheters are secured to the skin using an adhesive disc arrangement (Molnar external retention disc; Cook, Inc., Bloomington, IN, USA, or Hollister, Inc., IL, USA).

A post-procedure chest radiograph is obtained to assure proper catheter placement and assess the amount of remaining fluid. It should be recognized that up to 30 percent of patients may have air within the pleural space on this chest film. This *ex vacuo* pneumothorax does not require additional therapy and is thought to occur because the lung is relatively non-compliant and incapable of immediate re-expansion.[30]

The catheter is connected via a three-way stopcock to a drainage system such as a Pleur-evac (DeKnatel Division, Pfizer Hospital Products Group, Fall River, MA, USA) with continuous wall suction at 20–30 cm H_2O. To prevent catheter occlusion, the tube should be flushed with 10 mL of normal saline every 8 hours. Daily chest radiographs are not essential when drainage continues without difficulty. When drainage decreases to approximately 150 mL in a 24-hour period, a chest radiograph is performed to exclude loculated fluid and to confirm complete lung re-expansion. Patients with decreased drainage but radiographically evident fluid should have their catheters flushed to determine patency. Heparin or streptokinase, or occasionally insertion of a guide wire, is required to open a clogged catheter.

Because successful pleurodesis requires close contact between the visceral and parietal pleural surface, it is important that the pleural fluid be adequately drained. If the fluid becomes loculated, instillation of streptokinase (250 000 units in 100 mL of normal saline) may be used to break down adhesions and improve drainage.[31,32] After the streptokinase is instilled, the tube is clamped, and patients are instructed to rotate so as to distribute the lytic solution. Two hours later the tube is reopened and placed back to wall suction. Streptokinase instillation can be repeated on subsequent days if necessary.

Once the pleural space has been completely drained (usually 2–5 days), a sclerosant is instilled into the pleural space in an effort to prevent reaccumulation of fluid. The sclerosant causes local pleural injury and healing leads to adherence of the visceral and parietal pleura.[33] Sclerosing agents that can be instilled into the pleural space include talc, biological substances, antibiotics, anti-neoplastic agents and radioisotopes.[13,18,20,23,34–64] Currently, talc is preferred for pleurodesis because of its low cost and high success and low complication rate.[26]

After the sclerosing agent is introduced, the catheter is closed and the patient is instructed to change position (roll from side to side) every 15 minutes for 2 hours in an effort to uniformly distribute the sclerosant throughout the pleural space. The catheter is then reopened to suction for 24 hours at which time if the drainage remains less than 200 mL the catheter is removed. A second dose of sclerosant is usually administered if drainage exceeds 200 mL.

An alternative option to performing pleurodesis as an inpatient procedure is ambulatory drainage and sclerotherapy in patients with a reasonable performance status.[65] The technique is similar to that used with in-patients. The only difference is that instead of using continuous wall suction, the catheter is connected to a Tru-Close 600 mL bag (UreSil, L.P. Skokie, IL, USA) for gravity drainage. The design of the bag allows it to be emptied by the patient without backflow of air into the pleural space. Patients are provided with home care instructions and told that when drainage falls below 200 mL per day, to return to the hospital or outpatient clinic for sclerotherapy. Once the patient returns to the hospital the sclerosant is introduced and the catheter is clamped for 2 hours after which time the catheter is reopened to gravity drainage. The patient is then sent home and returns the following day for catheter removal.

A further option that is increasingly being used to curtail hospitalization is to manage patients with malignant effusions with long-term indwelling pleural silicone catheters (Pleurx; Surgimedics, Denver Biomaterials, Denver, CO, USA) (Figure 20.1).[66–73] These drainage catheters are also useful in the management of recurrent malignant pleural effusions and in patients with a malignant effusion and trapped lung when pleurodesis is not an option. Because Pleurx catheters have fenestrations that extend from the tip over 24 cm, they are usually used to manage moderate to large pleural effusions rather than small effusions.[70] The catheters can be inserted with or without the use of image guidance and are left in the pleural space indefinitely or

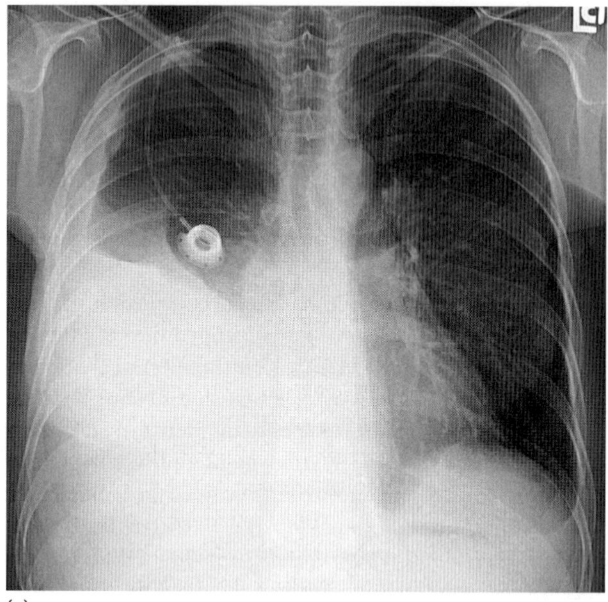

(a)

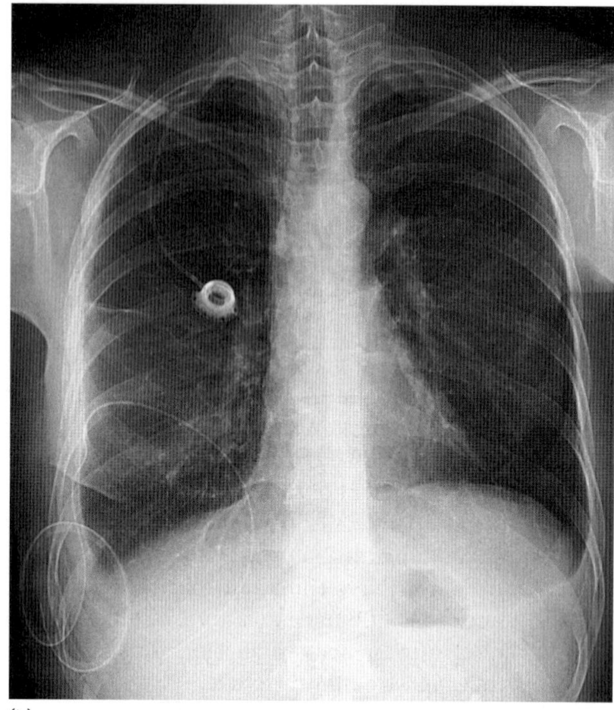

(b)

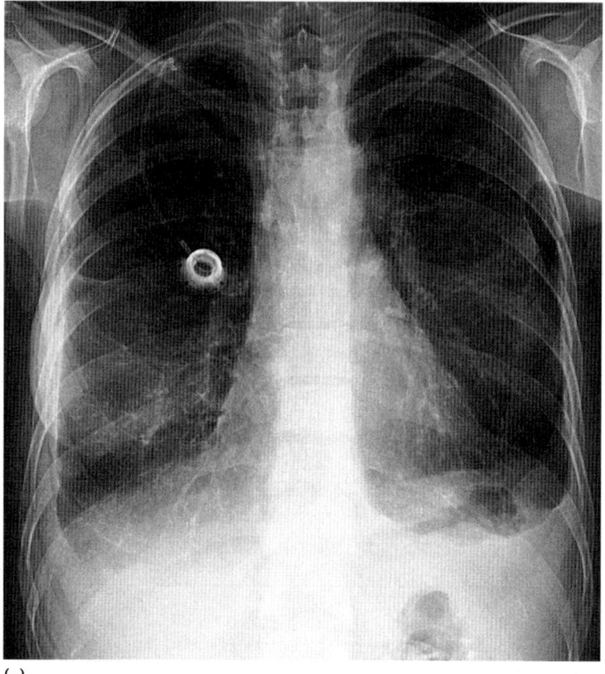

(c)

Figure 20.1 Fifty-one-year old woman with metastatic breast cancer presents with 2 weeks of shortness of breath. (a) Frontal chest radiograph shows a large right pleural effusion. At the time of this film, a Pleurx catheter was placed into the right pleural effusion. (b) Frontal chest radiograph obtained 3 months later shows the Pleurx catheter in the small pleural effusion. The Pleurx catheter was removed at that time. (c) Frontal chest radiograph 16 months after removal of the Pleurx catheter shows that the right pleural effusion remains small. Patient's shortness of breath did not recur.

until fluid drainage ceases. Similar to the approach described above for pigtail catheter insertion, a guidewire is placed into the pleural fluid, a 1-cm incision is made approximately 5–8 cm posterior to the entrance site of the guidewire and a subcutaneous chest wall tunnel is created. The catheter is pulled through this tunnel to the entrance skin incision of the guidewire. The wire tract is then dilated with a Teflon 'peel away' sheath. These tubes are soft and may kink during placement. The advantage of using imaging guidance for their placement is to gain control over the tube by inserting a guidewire or a dilator through one of the side holes of the indwelling catheter to stiffen it, prevent it kinking and guide it to the correct location under fluoroscopic guidance. Pleural fluid is then drained periodically into 600 mL vacuum bottles by placing the firm dilator on the preconnected tube into the valve at the distal end of the Pleurx catheter.

In patients with long-term indwelling catheters, the degree of symptomatic improvement in dyspnea is comparable to pleurodesis.[66,67,70–73] Additionally, in patients with trapped lung syndrome, most have symptomatic benefit with a decrease in dyspnea and improved exercise tolerance.[68,70] Late recurrence of effusions is uncommon (<15 percent) and approximately 50 percent of patients will have spontaneous pleurodesis, usually within a month.[70] Tube malfunction is uncommon and the catheters usually remain in place until the patient's demise (mean duration 56–115 days).[66,68,72] However, because of their long-term use, catheter infection with localized skin breakdown as well as tumor seeding along the tract has been reported as a complication.[68,70]

Parapneumonic effusion and empyema

Patients with parapneumonic effusions have a high risk of morbidity and mortality and approximately 15–40 percent require drainage and prolonged hospitalization.[74,75] There are sequential stages in the evolution of a parapneumonic effusion and development of an empyema and the clinical determination as to which pleural effusions require drainage to avoid progression to an empyema can be difficult.[76–80] To assist in this decision, the American College of Chest Physicians (ACCP) has published recommendations on the clinical management of patients with parapneumonic effusions based on the categorization of the effusion according to size, chemistry and bacteriology.[76]

Thoracentesis and the categorization of parapneumonic effusions is recommended in all patients except if the effusion is minimal (<1 cm on decubitus radiograph) and free-flowing (Category 1). Category 2 (small to moderate [>1 cm less than 50 percent of hemithorax], free-flowing effusions with pleural pH >7.2, glucose >60 mg/dL, lactate dehydrogenase [LDH] <3× the upper limit of serum and Gram stain and culture negative) usually do not require drainage as most patients respond to antibiotic therapy. Category 3 (large [>50 percent of hemithorax], free-flowing effusions, loculated effusions or effusions with thickened parietal pleura and/or pleural pH <7.2, and/or pleural glucose <60 mg/dL, and/or Gram stain and culture positive) and Category 4 (frank pus in the pleural space), require drainage.

In a retrospective study, the value of the ACCP recommendations as well as the British Thoracic Society guidelines to predict which patients with non-purulent parapneumonic effusions warranted chest tube drainage were evaluated.[80] A pleural fluid pH <7.20, a pleural glucose <60 mg/dL or a large pleural effusion size predicted with a likelihood of >5 ratio that the effusion would not resolve unless drainage was instituted. Overall, the ACCP guidelines had a sensitivity of 97 percent and specificity of 56 percent in distinguishing which non-purulent parapneumonic effusion warranted drainage. In contradistinction, there is no correlation between the CT and sonographic appearance of parapneumonic effusions and the severity of infection as determined by established microbiological and biochemical indicators.[81] Furthermore, neither imaging modality can predict those patients who will subsequently require surgical intervention after failed management by chest tube drainage and intrapleural fibrinolytics.[81]

Traditionally, complicated parapneumonic effusions and empyemas have been treated by large-bore catheter thoracostomy[82–87] followed, if needed, by rib resection and open drainage,[88–91] video-assisted thoracoscopic surgery[92,93] or decortication.[75,94,95] However, studies have shown that these collections may be adequately treated by imaging-assisted placement of small-bore catheters (8–16 F) rather than using the standard 22–34 F catheters. In fact, the insertion of small-bore catheters under imaging-assisted guidance (CT or sonography), is strongly recommended: the procedure is safe, whereas conventional trocar placement can be hazardous,[96] the mean duration of approximately 6 days for image-guided thoracostomy is shorter than for traditional catheter thoracostomy,[32,97–99] and the success rate is higher than traditional catheter thoracostomy (81 versus 47 percent, respectively)[100,101] (Figure 20.2). In our experience, small-bore catheter placement under image guidance is highly effective for the treatment of parapneumonic effusions. These patients are always treated with intravenous antibiotics and typically show clinical improvement within 24–48 hours. If patients do not respond to therapy within several days then management changes including alternative antibiotics, additional catheters, and sometimes surgical drainage may be required.

TECHNIQUE

The catheter insertion site is determined by the location of the effusion. If there are multiple loculations, more than one drainage catheter may be required. CT is preferred over ultrasound to more accurately assess the location and extent of loculated fluid. Additionally, CT better demonstrates the presence of a thick pleural rind that can preclude chest catheter placement as an initial treatment option and other anatomic abnormalities within the thorax. Following insertion, the catheter is connected via a three-way stopcock to an underwater drainage system such as a Pleur-evac (DeKnatel Division, Pfizer Hospital Products Group, Fall River, MA, USA) with continuous wall suction at 20–30 cmH_2O. To prevent catheter occlusion, the catheter is flushed with 10 mL of normal saline every eight hours.

Patients with a persistent complex pleural collection or a decrease in fluid drainage but radiographically evident collection may benefit from the installation of a fibrinolytic agent into the pleural space through the drainage catheter. Specifically, intrapleural fibrinolytics, if used early in the fibrinopurulent stage of a parapneumonic effusion, may dissolve fibrinous adhesions, improve pleural fluid drainage, prevent pleural fluid loculation and decrease the rate of surgical intervention and length of hospitalization. The rational for this management, which is included in the guidelines of the ACCP, is based on small studies although clinical evidence from high-quality trials is not available.[76,102–105] The consensus in favor of the use of intrapleural fibrinolytics in the management of complex

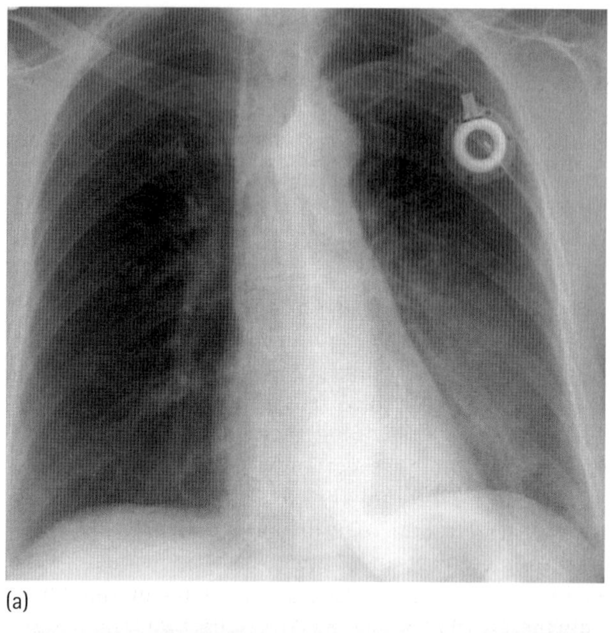
(a)

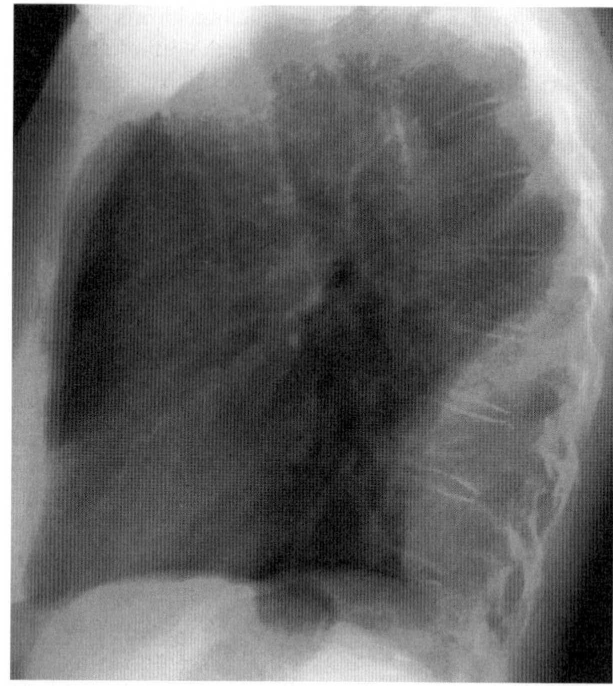
(b)

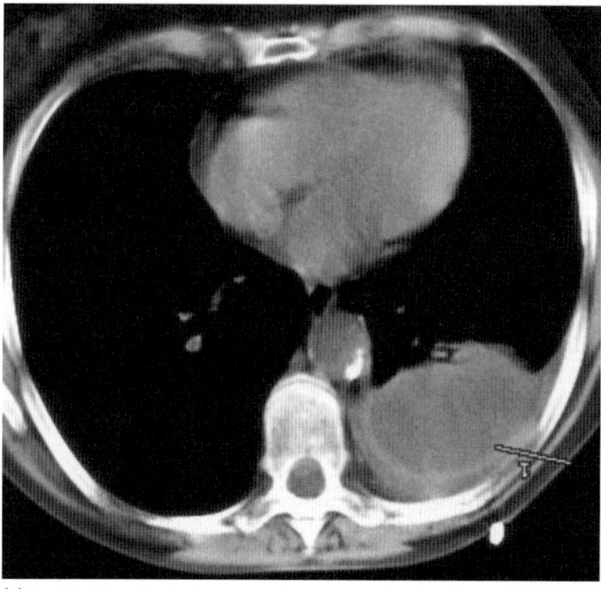
(c)

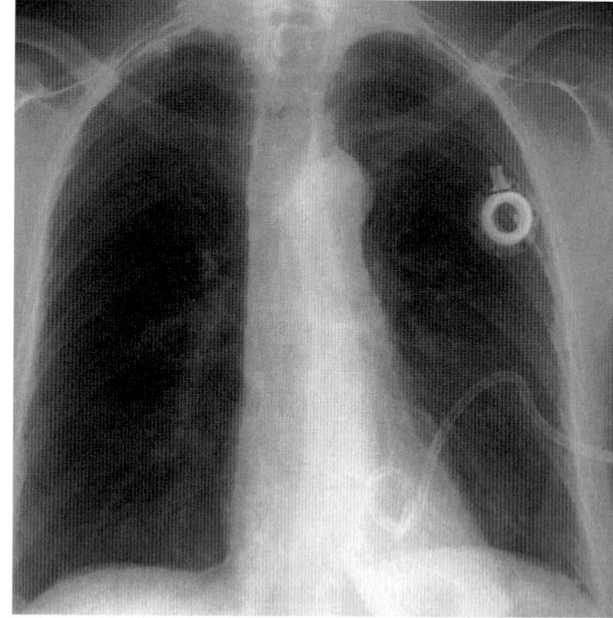
(d)

Figure 20.2 Forty-two-year-old woman presents with cough and fever. (a) Frontal chest radiograph demonstrates a poorly defined opacity in the left base. (b) Lateral radiograph suggests this posterior opacity is in the pleural space. (c) Axial computed tomography image confirms a posterior fluid collection. (d) Follow-up chest radiograph 2 days after the pig-tail chest tube shows almost complete resolution of the infected collection.

parapneumonic pleural effusions is, to a large extent, based on increased drainage volume/radiologic improvement although the effect on duration of hospitalization, need for surgery and long-term clinical outcome is controversial.[104–107] In a recent small randomized study by Diacon *et al.*,[104] 9 percent of patients with empyemas who received intrapleural streptokinase required surgical drainage compared with 45 percent of patients who received intrapleural saline.[104] In contradistinction, a recent randomized trial of 454 patients by Maskell *et al.*[107] showed that the use of intrapleural fibrinolytics did not affect length of hospitalization, rate of surgery or mortality.

Although the overall available evidence suggests that fibrinolytics are useful in patients with parapneumonic effusions, the choice of fibrinolytic agent remains controversial. Different agents available for instillation into the pleural space include streptokinase, urokinase, alteplase and tissue plasminogen activator (tPA). Streptokinase is more commonly used because it is much cheaper than the other agents but it may be antigenic and can cause fever in up to 28 percent of patients. Urokinase is non-antigenic, does not usually cause fever and may be slightly more effective than streptokinase. Although temporarily withdrawn from the USA because of the associated risks of viral disease transmission, urokinase is now available for clinical use. Alteplase and tPA are less commonly used, have been proven to be effective but are more expensive than streptokinase. In addition, some preliminary results suggest that tPA may be associated with an increased risk of intrapleural bleeding in patients simultaneously receiving therapeutic levels of systemic anticoagulation

When streptokinase is chosen as the fibrinolytic agent, it is common to begin by instilling 250 000 U of streptokinase mixed in 100 cm^3 of normal saline through the tube directly into the pleural space. The catheter is then closed for 2 hours to allow the agent to distribute throughout the pleural space and to dissolve the fibrin membranes. It is then reopened to continuous suction. Instillation is repeated on a daily basis as needed, sometimes up to five consecutive days if the results improve drainage. Patients are evaluated daily to assure proper catheter function and to record catheter output. Daily chest radiographs are not required when drainage continues without difficulty and the patient's fever and clinical symptoms continue to improve. When drainage is minimal or ceases and the patient's temperature has returned to normal, a chest radiograph is performed to exclude loculated fluid, and to confirm complete lung re-expansion. The catheter is removed when the output is less than 50 cm^3 a day, the patient is afebrile, leukocytosis has resolved and the patient is ready to be placed on oral antibiotics.

Pneumothorax

Imaging can be used to place a chest catheter in patients with a symptomatic pneumothorax, or in high-risk patients with a small, but expanding pneumothorax. It is very useful in patients with lung or pleural disease and a loculated pneumothorax that requires a chest tube. Although pneumothoraces are not uncommon after transthoracic needle aspiration biopsies of the lung (up to 61 percent),[108–118] or transbronchial biopsy, chest catheter placement is typically only performed when patients are symptomatic or when the pneumothorax is increasing in size[96,112,119,120] (Figure 20.3). Success rates of small-bore catheters (7–10 F) is high (87–97 percent) with most pneumothoraces resolving within 24–72 hours following catheter insertion.[112,121,122] The treatment of a pneumothorax with a small-bore catheter has a similar success rate to that of large-bore chest tube drainage. Lack of response is usually due to technical factors (catheter malposition and occlusion) or a very large air leak.[112,121,123,124]

TECHNIQUE

Imaging-assisted guidance is chosen according to availability and the clinical scenario: if the pneumothorax

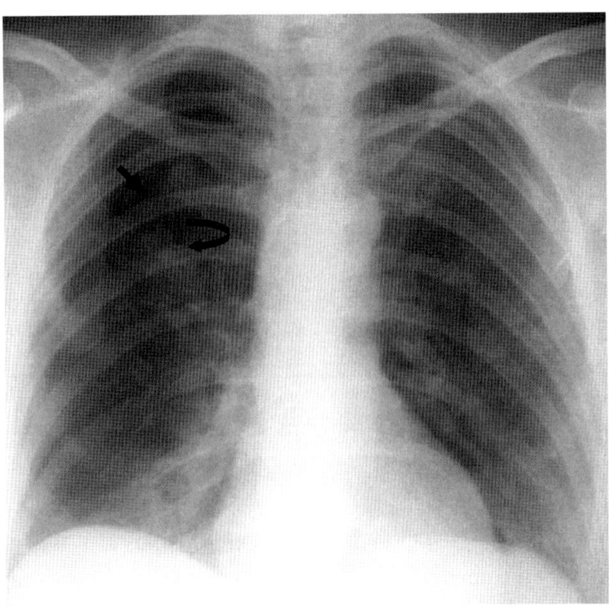

(a)

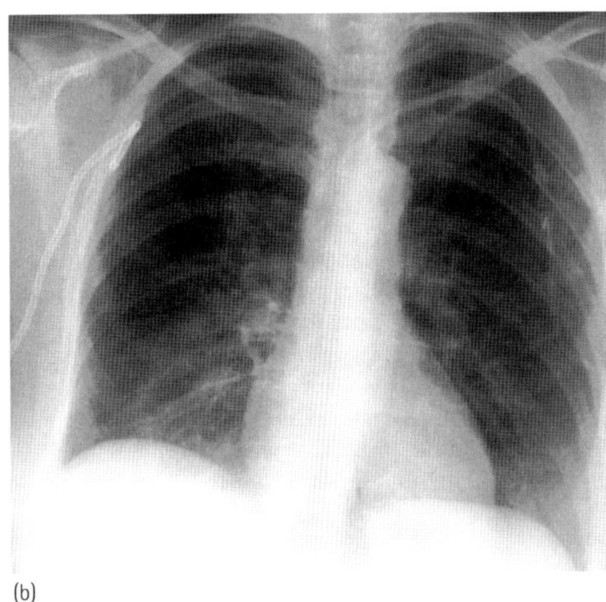

(b)

Figure 20.3 Fifty-seven-year-old man with a right upper lobe nodule presents for percutaneous biopsy. (a) Chest film immediately following the biopsy shows the poorly defined right nodule (curved arrow) and a right pneumothorax (straight arrow). (b) Follow-up chest film after the pig-tail catheter shows almost complete resolution of the pneumothorax.

occurs during a biopsy, a chest catheter is inserted using the imaging modality used to perform the biopsy, while those that occur later are usually performed using fluoroscopic guidance. CT guidance is used for small or loculated pneumothoraces in ventilated patient as it helps to prevent intraparenchymal catheter placement. The entry site depends on the location and size of the pneumothorax. The catheter is usually inserted in the sixth intercostal space in the region of the mid-axillary line and the tip positioned in the upper, anterior aspect of the hemithorax.[125] However, there is a tendency for the tip of small-bore catheters to be displaced posteriorly with this approach. Small-bore catheters can also be placed through the third or fourth anterior intercostal space. This placement results in more constant positioning of the catheter tip in the apex of the pleural space.[112,126]

The choice of drainage catheter depends on physician preference and whether there is fluid within the pleural space. An 8–10 F straight catheter can be used for rapid placement in a single-step procedure but is usually not recommended if there is an accompanying pleural effusion. The Seldinger technique can be used to place a guide-wire into the pleural space prior to placement of an 8–10 F pigtail catheter. Although this prolongs the procedure by a few minutes, using a pigtail catheter is advantageous as it effectively drains any accompanying pleural fluid and rarely dislodges (a common problem of the straight catheter).[124]

The catheter/trocar system is angled in a cranial direction adjacent to the superior aspect of the rib to avoid injury to the intercostal neurovascular bundle and advanced into the pleural space. A gush of air occurs when the catheters tip transverses the parietal pleura. The trocar is then held in position and the catheter advanced to the lung apex. Once the tip is in a satisfactory position the trocar is removed. Straight catheters are secured to the skin with sutures, while pigtail catheters are secured to an adhesive disc. The catheter is then connected to a one-way Heimlich valve. Patients with a large air leak and non-expansion of the lung may have the catheter connected to an underwater drainage system such as a Pleur-evac with continuous suction (approximately 20 cmH_2O).

Upright posterior–anterior and lateral chest radiographs are obtained after the procedure to determine the size of any residual pneumothorax and to confirm the position of the drainage catheter. A repeat radiograph is performed after 18–24 hours of drainage. If the pneumothorax has resolved, the catheter is clamped for approximately 4 hours after which a repeat chest film is obtained. If the lung remains completely expanded the catheter is removed. If a pneumothorax persists and there is no pressure variation in the water-seal chamber of the Pleur-evac with breathing, the catheter is either malpositioned or occluded.[112] However, there may also be a persistent tear in the visceral pleura. In these cases drainage should continue for several days, which may be sufficient time to allow the air leak to seal. If the leak persists, patients may require chemical pleurodesis using sclerosing agents such as doxycycline, talc or bleomycin, or placement of a large-bore tube may be necessary.[127–130]

PLEURAL BIOPSY

Infections, inflammation and neoplasms of the pleura can manifest as diffuse or focal pleural abnormalities. When there is an accompanying effusion, thoracentesis may be diagnostic. However, a pleural biopsy is often required to establish a diagnosis as the yield from thoracentesis in some diseases, including tuberculosis or malignancy, is less than optimal.[131] In some cases, cytological evaluation of specimens obtained from transthoracic needle aspiration may be ambiguous, such as seen with benign disease, or it may be difficult to distinguish reactive mesothelial cell hyperplasia from metastatic adenocarcinoma and mesothelioma.[132–135] Thus, depending on the clinical scenario, a core-needle biopsy that can obtain larger tissue samples may be required.[133] These larger core specimens can be obtained using Cope or Abrams biopsy needles without imaging-assisted guidance, although imaging-assisted biopsy has a higher diagnostic yield. For instance, by using ultrasound guidance, the confirmation of tuberculous pleural involvement increases from 20 to 86 percent when compared with procedures performed without imaging-assisted guidance. Similarly, for patients with either primary or metastatic pleural disease, the use of ultrasound or CT increases the diagnostic rate.[136,137] In rare cases, additional tissue is needed for special pathology stains and analysis, and video-assisted thoracoscopic surgery (VATS) may be necessary.[138] In one comparative study, the diagnostic sensitivity of VATS for mesothelioma was 94 percent, compared with 86 percent for image guided core needle biopsy, but the procedure requires that the visceral and parietal pleurae not be adherent.[139] A further disadvantage is that chest wall seeding occurs in 22 percent of surgical biopsies as compared with only 4 percent in image guided core needle biopsy.[139] This seeding along the needle tract can be eliminated by treating the region of biopsy with radiotherapy.[140]

Technique

Large pleural masses can usually be biopsied under fluoroscopic guidance, but ultrasound and CT are usually used. The needle insertion site should be selected to avoid traversing lung or vessels. In this regard, it is best to place the needle parallel to a small pleural abnormality (rather than perpendicular), to enable adequate needle manipulation at the time of biopsy without violation of the visceral pleura. A coaxial biopsy needle may be used so that multiple specimens can be obtained if necessary. The outer sheath is introduced to the level of the parietal pleural. Multiple specimens are then obtained with an automated cutting needle device such as the Temno II Scalpel Tip Biopsy Device (Allegiance Healthcare Corporation, McGraw Park, IL, USA) or Achieve Biopsy System (Bauer Medical, Inc., Clearwater, FL, USA) as the diagnostic yield is increased with two or more specimens.[141] Using a biopsy needle with a diameter of 18 gauge or larger can also increase diagnostic yield.[142,143] If no acute complication occurs, the patient is observed for two hours. If the patient remains asymptomatic and there are no acute abnormalities on the follow-up radiograph, the patient is discharged.

CONCLUSIONS AND FUTURE DIRECTION

Improvements in percutaneous interventional techniques now allow patients to undergo image-guided diagnostic and therapeutic pleural procedures with less morbidity and mortality than surgical intervention. The use of ultrasound, CT or fluoroscopy permits optimal needle or catheter placement and safe and effective percutaneous evacuation of pleural air and fluid collections. Image-guided percutaneous intervention should be considered the initial procedure performed to treat malignant effusions, parapneumonic effusions and pneumothoraces. At present, novel chemotherapeutic agents such as vascular endothelial growth factor (VEGF) tyrosine kinase inhibitors are being tested for instillation through pleural catheters. VEGF is over-expressed in several tumors, including non-small cell lung cancer, and treatment with a VEGF inhibitor has been shown to control malignant pleural effusions caused by non-small-cell lung cancer.[144] We anticipate that in the future new diagnostic capabilities, refinements in chest tubes and novel biologic sclerosing agents should result in even further improvements in patient care.

KEY POINTS

- Imaging provides an accurate assessment of the pleural space.
- Imaging is extremely useful in directing interventional procedures for pleural abnormalities.
- Image-guided drainage procedures are effective in treating patients with malignant effusions, parapneumonic effusions, empyemas and pneumothoraces.

REFERENCES

1. Mathisen DJ. A surgeon's view of interventional radiology in general thoracic surgery patients. *Semin Intervent Radiol* 1991; **8**: 85–7.
2. Light RW. *Pleural diseses*, 3rd ed. Baltimore: Williams and Wilkins, 1995.
3. Raptopoulos V, Davis LM, Lee G, *et al.* Factors affecting the development of pneumothorax associated with thoracentesis. *AJR Am J Roentgenol* 1991; **156**: 917–20.
4. Seneff MG, Corwin RW, Gold LH, Irwin RS. Complications associated with thoracocentesis. *Chest* 1986; **90**: 97–100.
5. Grogan DR, Irwin RS, Channick R, *et al.* Complications associated with thoracentesis. A prospective, randomized study comparing three different methods. *Arch Intern Med* 1990; **150**: 873–7.
6. Collins TR, Sahn SA. Thoracocentesis. Clinical value, complications, technical problems, and patient experience. *Chest* 1987; **91**: 817–22.
7. Jones PW, Moyers JP, Rogers JT, *et al.* Ultrasound-guided thoracentesis: is it a safer method? *Chest* 2003; **123**: 418–23.
8. Kohan JM, Poe RH, Israel RH, *et al.* Value of chest ultrasonography versus decubitus roentgenography for thoracentesis. *Am Rev Respir Dis* 1986; **133**: 1124–6.
9. Ong KC, Indumathi V, Poh WT, Ong YY. The diagnostic yield of pleural fluid cytology in malignant pleural effusions. *Singapore Med J* 2000; **41**: 19–23.
10. Anderson CB, Philpott GW, Ferguson TB. The treatment of malignant pleural effusions. *Cancer* 1974; **33**: 916–22.
11. Bruneau R, Rubin P. The management of pleural effusions and chylothorax in lymphoma. *Radiology* 1965; **85**: 1085–92.
12. Fracchia AA, Knapper WH, Carey JT, Farrow JH. Intrapleural chemotherapy for effusion from metastatic breast carcinoma. *Cancer* 1970; **26**: 626–9.
13. Johnston WW. The malignant pleural effusion. A review of cytopathologic diagnoses of 584 specimens from 472 consecutive patients. *Cancer* 1985; **56**: 905–9.
14. Sahn SA. Pleural effusion in lung cancer. *Clin Chest Med* 1993; **14**: 189–200.
15. Chernow B, Sahn SA. Carcinomatous involvement of the pleura: an analysis of 96 patients. *Am J Med* 1977; **63**: 695–702.
16. Tattersall M. Pleural effusions. *Curr Opin Oncol* 1992; **4**: 642–6.
17. Hausheer FH, Yarbro JW. Diagnosis and treatment of malignant pleural effusion. *Semin Oncol* 1985; **12**: 54–75.
18. Seaton KG, Patz EF Jr, Goodman PC. Palliative treatment of malignant pleural effusions: value of small-bore catheter thoracostomy and doxycycline sclerotherapy. *AJR Am J Roentgenol* 1995; **164**: 589–91.
19. Andrews CO, Gora ML. Pleural effusions: pathophysiology and management. *Ann Pharmacother* 1994; **28**: 894–903.
20. Kennedy L, Sahn SA. Talc pleurodesis for the treatment of pneumothorax and pleural effusion. *Chest* 1994; **106**: 1215–22.
21. Clementsen P, Evald T, Grode G, *et al.* Treatment of malignant pleural effusion: pleurodesis using a small percutaneous catheter. A prospective randomized study. *Respir Med* 1998; **92**: 593–6.
22. Parulekar W, Di Primio G, Matzinger F, Dennie C, Bociek G. Use of small-bore vs large-bore chest tubes for treatment of malignant pleural effusions. *Chest* 2001; **120**: 19–25.
23. Goff BA, Mueller PR, Muntz HG, Rice LW. Small chest-tube drainage followed by bleomycin sclerosis for malignant pleural effusions. *Obstet Gynecol* 1993; **81**: 993–6.
24. Morrison MC, Mueller PR, Lee MJ, *et al.* Sclerotherapy of malignant pleural effusion through sonographically placed small-bore catheters. *AJR Am J Roentgenol* 1992; **158**: 41–3.
25. O'Moore PV, Mueller PR, Simeone JF, *et al.* Sonographic guidance in diagnostic and therapeutic interventions in the pleural space. *AJR Am J Roentgenol* 1987; **149**: 1–5.
26. Marom EM, Patz EF Jr, Erasmus JJ, *et al.* Malignant pleural effusions: treatment with small-bore-catheter thoracostomy and talc pleurodesis. *Radiology* 1999; **210**: 277–81.
27. Parker LA, Charnock GC, Delany DJ. Small bore catheter drainage and sclerotherapy for malignant pleural effusions. *Cancer* 1989; **64**: 1218–21.

28. Barbetakis N, Antoniadis T, Tsilikas C. Results of chemical pleurodesis with mitoxantrone in malignant pleural effusion from breast cancer. *World J Surg Oncol* 2004; **2**: 16.
29. Light RW, Jenkinson SG, Minh VD, George RB. Observations on pleural fluid pressures as fluid is withdrawn during thoracentesis. *Am Rev Respir Dis* 1980; **121**: 799–804.
30. Chang YC, Patz EF Jr, Goodman PC. Pneumothorax after small-bore catheter placement for malignant pleural effusions. *AJR Am J Roentgenol* 1996; **166**: 1049–51.
31. Bouros D, Schiza S, Patsourakis G, *et al.* Intrapleural streptokinase versus urokinase in the treatment of complicated parapneumonic effusions: a prospective, double-blind study. *Am J Respir Crit Care Med* 1997; **155**: 291–5.
32. Moulton JS, Benkert RE, Weisiger KH, Chambers JA. Treatment of complicated pleural fluid collections with image-guided drainage and intracavitary urokinase. *Chest* 1995; **108**: 1252–9.
33. Kennedy L, Harley RA, Sahn SA, Strange C. Talc slurry pleurodesis. Pleural fluid and histologic analysis. *Chest* 1995; **107**: 1707–12.
34. Bethune N. Pleural poudrage: a new technique for deliberate production of pleural adhesions as preliminary to lobectomy. *J Thorac Surg* 1935; **4**: 251–61.
35. Card RY, Cole DR, Henscke UK. Summary of ten years of the use of radioactive colloids in intracavitary therapy. *J Nucl Med* 1960; **1**: 195–8.
36. Casali A, Gionfra T, Rinaldi M, *et al.* Treatment of malignant pleural effusions with intracavitary *Corynebacterium parvum*. *Cancer* 1988; **62**: 806–11.
37. Colt HG, Russack V, Chiu Y, *et al.* A comparison of thoracoscopic talc insufflation, slurry, and mechanical abrasion pleurodesis. *Chest* 1997; **111**: 442–8.
38. Cunningham TJ, Olson KB, Horton J, *et al.* A clinical trial of intravenous and intracavitary bleomycin. *Cancer* 1972; **29**: 1413–19.
39. Davis M, Williford S, Muss HB, *et al.* A phase I-II study of recombinant intrapleural alpha interferon in malignant pleural effusions. *Am J Clin Oncol* 1992; **15**: 328–30.
40. Fentiman IS, Rubens RD, Hayward JL. A comparison of intracavitary talc and tetracycline for the control of pleural effusions secondary to breast cancer. *Eur J Cancer Clin Oncol* 1986; **22**: 1079–81.
41. Fingar BL. Sclerosing agents used to control malignant pleural effusions. *Hosp Pharm* 1992; **27**: 622–8.
42. Gupta N, Opfell RW, Podova J, *et al.* Intrapleural bleomycin vs tetracycline for control of malignant pleural effusion: a randomized study. *Proc Am Assoc Cancer Res* 1980; **21**: 366.
43. Holoye PY, Jeffries DG, Dhingra HM, *et al.* Intrapleural etoposide for malignant effusion. *Cancer Chemother Pharmacol* 1990; **26**: 147–50.
44. Ike O, Shimizu Y, Hitomi S, Wada R, Ikada Y. Treatment of malignant pleural effusions with doxorubicin hydrochloride-containing poly(L-lactic acid) microspheres. *Chest* 1991; **99**: 911–15.
45. Kitamura S, Sugiyama Y, Izumi T, Hayashi R, Kosaka K. Intrapleural doxycycline for control of malignant pleural effusion. *Curr Ther Res* 1981; **30**: 515–21.
46. Liu X. Effectiveness of treatment with transfer of autologous or allogenic LAK cells combined with rIL-2 in 121 patients with malignant pleural effusion. *Chinese Med J* 1993; **15**: 205–8.
47. Maiche AG, Virkkunen P, Kontkanen T, Moykkynen K, Porkka K. Bleomycin and mitoxantrone in the treatment of malignant pleural effusions. A comparative study. *Am J Clin Oncol* 1993; **16**: 50–3.
48. Mansson T. Treatment of malignant pleural effusion with doxycycline. *Scand J Infect Dis Suppl* 1988; **53**: 29–34.
49. Markman M, Cleary S, King ME, Howell SB. Cisplatin and cytarabine administered intrapleurally as treatment of malignant pleural effusions. *Med Pediatr Oncol* 1985; **13**: 191–3.
50. McLeod DT, Calverley PM, Millar JW, Horne NW. Further experience of *Corynebacterium parvum* in malignant pleural effusion. *Thorax* 1985; **40**: 515–18.
51. Millar JW, Hunter AM, Horne NW. Intrapleural immunotherapy with *Corynebacterium parvum* in recurrent malignant pleural effusions. *Thorax* 1980; **35**: 856–8.
52. Moffett MJ, Ruckdeschel JC. Bleomycin and tetracycline in malignant pleural effusions: a review. *Semin Oncol* 1992; **19**(2 Suppl 5): 59–62; discussion 62–3.
53. Ostrowski MJ, Halsall GM. Intracavitary bleomycin in the management of malignant effusions: a multicenter study. *Cancer Treat Rep* 1982; **66**: 1903–7.
54. Ostrowski MJ. An assessment of the long-term results of controlling the reaccumulation of malignant effusions using intracavity bleomycin. *Cancer* 1986; **57**: 721–7.
55. Paladine W, Cunningham TJ, Sponzo R, *et al.* Intracavitary bleomycin in the management of malignant effusions. *Cancer* 1976; **38**: 1903–8.
56. Pearson FG, MacGregor DC. Talc poudrage for malignant pleural effusion. *J Thorac Cardiovasc Surg* 1966; **51**: 732–8.
57. Robinson LA, Fleming WH, Galbraith TA. Intrapleural doxycycline control of malignant pleural effusions. *Ann Thorac Surg* 1993; **55**: 1115–21; discussion 21–2.
58. Ruckdeschel JC, Moores D, Lee JY, *et al.* Intrapleural therapy for malignant pleural effusions. A randomized comparison of bleomycin and tetracycline. *Chest* 1991; **100**: 1528–35.
59. Rusch VW, Figlin R, Godwin D, Piantadosi S. Intrapleural cisplatin and cytarabine in the management of malignant pleural effusions: a Lung Cancer Study Group trial. *J Clin Oncol* 1991; **9**: 313–19.
60. Sorensen PG, Svendsen TL, Enk B. Treatment of malignant pleural effusion with drainage, with and without instillation of talc. *Eur J Respir Dis* 1984; **65**: 131–5.
61. Trotter JM, Stuart JFB, McBeth F, *et al.* The management of malignant effusions with bleomycin. *Br J Cancer* 1979; **40**: 310.
62. Webb HE, Oaten SW, Pike CP. Treatment of malignant ascitic and pleural effusion with *Corynebacterium parvum*. *Br Med J* 1978; **1**: 338–40.
63. Yasumoto K, Ogura T. Intrapleural application of recombinant interleukin-2 in patients with malignant pleurisy due to lung cancer. A multi-institutional cooperative study. *Biotherapy* 1991; **3**: 345–9.
64. Zimmer PW, Hill M, Casey K, Harvey E, Low DE. Prospective randomized trial of talc slurry vs bleomycin in pleurodesis for symptomatic malignant pleural effusions. *Chest* 1997; **112**: 430–4.
65. Patz EF Jr, McAdams HP, Goodman PC, Blackwell S, Crawford J. Ambulatory sclerotherapy for malignant pleural effusions. *Radiology* 1996; **199**: 133–5.
66. van den Toorn LM, Schaap E, Surmont VF, *et al.* Management of recurrent malignant pleural effusions with a chronic indwelling pleural catheter. *Lung Cancer* 2005; **50**: 123–7.
67. Pollak JS, Burdge CM, Rosenblatt M, *et al.* Treatment of malignant pleural effusions with tunneled long-term drainage catheters. *J Vasc Interv Radiol* 2001; **12**: 201–8.
68. Pien GW, Gant MJ, Washam CL, Sterman DH. Use of an implantable pleural catheter for trapped lung syndrome in patients with malignant pleural effusion. *Chest* 2001; **119**: 1641–6.
69. Putnam JB Jr, Walsh GL, Swisher SG, *et al.* Outpatient management of malignant pleural effusion by a chronic indwelling pleural catheter. *Ann Thorac Surg* 2000; **69**: 369–75.
70. Putnam JB Jr, Light RW, Rodriguez RM, *et al.* A randomized comparison of indwelling pleural catheter and doxycycline pleurodesis in the management of malignant pleural effusions. *Cancer* 1999; **86**: 1992–9.
71. Musani AI, Haas AR, Seijo L, Wilby M, Sterman DH. Outpatient management of malignant pleural effusions with small-bore, tunneled pleural catheters. *Respiration* 2004; **71**: 559–66.
72. Tremblay A, Michaud G. Single-center experience with 250

tunnelled pleural catheter insertions for malignant pleural effusion. *Chest* 2006; **129**: 362–8.
73. Ohm C, Park D, Vogen M, *et al.* Use of an indwelling pleural catheter compared with thorascopic talc pleurodesis in the management of malignant pleural effusions. *Am Surg* 2003; **69**: 198–202.
74. Davies CW, Kearney SE, Gleeson FV, Davies RJ. Predictors of outcome and long-term survival in patients with pleural infection. *Am J Respir Crit Care Med* 1999; **160**: 1682–7.
75. Ferguson AD, Prescott RJ, Selkon JB, Watson D, Swinburn CR. The clinical course and management of thoracic empyema. *QJM* 1996; **89**: 285–9.
76. Colice GL, Curtis A, Deslauriers J, *et al.* Medical and surgical treatment of parapneumonic effusions: an evidence-based guideline. *Chest* 2000; **118**: 1158–71.
77. Barnes NP, Hull J, Thomson AH. Medical management of parapneumonic pleural disease. *Pediatr Pulmonol* 2005; **39**: 127–34.
78. Davies CW, Gleeson FV, Davies RJ. BTS guidelines for the management of pleural infection. *Thorax* 2003; **58** (Suppl 2): ii18–28.
79. Light RW. Parapneumonic effusions and empyema. *Proc Am Thorac Soc* 2006; **3**: 75–80.
80. Manuel Porcel J, Vives M, Esquerda A, Ruiz A. Usefulness of the British Thoracic Society and the American College of Chest Physicians guidelines in predicting pleural drainage of non-purulent parapneumonic effusions. *Respir Med* 2006; **100**: 933–7.
81. Kearney SE, Davies CW, Davies RJ, Gleeson FV. Computed tomography and ultrasound in parapneumonic effusions and empyema. *Clin Radiol* 2000; **55**: 542–7.
82. Vianna NJ. Nontuberculous bacterial empyema in patients with and without underlying diseases. *J Am Med Assoc* 1971; **215**: 69–75.
83. Smith JA, Mullerworth MH, Westlake GW, Tatoulis J. Empyema thoracis: 14-year experience in a teaching center. *Ann Thorac Surg* 1991; **51**: 39–42.
84. Ali I, Unruh H. Management of empyema thoracis. *Ann Thorac Surg* 1990; **50**: 355–9.
85. LeBlanc KA, Tucker WY. Empyema of the thorax. *Surg Gynecol Obstet* 1984; **158**: 66–70.
86. Pothula V, Krellenstein DJ. Early aggressive surgical management of parapneumonic empyemas. *Chest* 1994; **105**: 832–6.
87. Wehr CJ, Adkins RB Jr. Empyema thoracis: a ten-year experience. *South Med J* 1986; **79**: 171–6.
88. Refaely Y, Weissberg D. Gangrene of the lung: treatment in two stages. *Ann Thorac Surg* 1997; **64**: 970–3; discussion 3–4.
89. Serletti JM, Feins RH, Carras AJ, *et al.* Obliteration of empyema tract with deepithelialized unipedicle transverse rectus abdominis myocutaneous flap. *J Thorac Cardiovasc Surg* 1996; **112**: 631–6.
90. Weissberg D, Refaely Y. Pleural empyema: 24-year experience. *Ann Thorac Surg* 1996; **62**: 1026–9.
91. Garcia-Yuste M, Ramos G, Duque JL, *et al.* Open-window thoracostomy and thoracomyoplasty to manage chronic pleural empyema. *Ann Thorac Surg* 1998; **65**: 818–22.
92. Striffeler H, Gugger M, Im Hof V, *et al.* Video-assisted thoracoscopic surgery for fibrinopurulent pleural empyema in 67 patients. *Ann Thorac Surg* 1998; **65**: 319–23.
93. Cassina PC, Hauser M, Hillejan L, Greschuchna D, Stamatis G. Video-assisted thoracoscopy in the treatment of pleural empyema: stage-based management and outcome. *J Thorac Cardiovasc Surg* 1999; **117**: 234–8.
94. Renner H, Gabor S, Pinter H, *et al.* Is aggressive surgery in pleural empyema justified? *Eur J Cardiothorac Surg* 1998; **14**: 117–22.
95. Thourani VH, Brady KM, Mansour KA, Miller JI Jr, Lee RB. Evaluation of treatment modalities for thoracic empyema: a cost-effectiveness analysis. *Ann Thorac Surg* 1998; **66**: 1121–7.
96. Klein JS, Schultz S, Heffner JE. Interventional radiology of the chest: image-guided percutaneous drainage of pleural effusions, lung abscess, and pneumothorax. *AJR Am J Roentgenol* 1995; **164**: 581–8.
97. Bouros D, Schiza S, Panagou P, Drositis J, Siafakas N. Role of streptokinase in the treatment of acute loculated parapneumonic pleural effusions and empyema. *Thorax* 1994; **49**: 852–5.
98. Lee KS, Im JG, Kim YH, *et al.* Treatment of thoracic multiloculated empyemas with intracavitary urokinase: a prospective study. *Radiology* 1991; **179**: 771–5.
99. Pollak JS, Passik CS. Intrapleural urokinase in the treatment of loculated pleural effusions. *Chest* 1994; **105**: 868–73.
100. Merriam MA, Cronan JJ, Dorfman GS, Lambiase RE, Haas RA. Radiographically guided percutaneous catheter drainage of pleural fluid collections. *AJR Am J Roentgenol* 1988; **151**: 1113–6.
101. Ulmer JL, Choplin RH, Reed JC. Image-guided catheter drainage of the infected pleural space. *J Thorac Imaging* 1991; **6**: 65–73.
102. Misthos P, Sepsas E, Konstantinou M, *et al.* Early use of intrapleural fibrinolytics in the management of postpneumonic empyema. A prospective study. *Eur J Cardiothorac Surg* 2005; **28**: 599–603.
103. Bouros D, Schiza S, Patsourakis G, *et al.* Intrapleural streptokinase versus urokinase in the treatment of complicated parapneumonic effusions: a prospective, double-blind study. *Am J Respir Crit Care Med* 1997; **155**: 291–5.
104. Diacon AH, Theron J, Schuurmans MM, Van de Wal BW, Bolliger CT. Intrapleural streptokinase for empyema and complicated parapneumonic effusions. *Am J Respir Crit Care Med* 2004; **170**: 49–53.
105. Davies RJ, Traill ZC, Gleeson FV. Randomised controlled trial of intrapleural streptokinase in community acquired pleural infection. *Thorax* 1997; **52**: 416–21.
106. Ozol D, Oktem S, Erdinc E. Complicated parapneumonic effusion and empyema thoracis: microbiologic and therapeutic aspects. *Respir Med* 2006; **100**: 286–91.
107. Maskell NA, Davies CW, Nunn AJ, *et al.* U.K. Controlled trial of intrapleural streptokinase for pleural infection. *N Engl J Med* 2005; **352**: 865–74.
108. Anderson CL, Crespo JC, Lie TH. Risk of pneumothorax not increased by obstructive lung disease in percutaneous needle biopsy. *Chest* 1994; **105**: 1705–8.
109. Berger R. Iatrogenous pneumothorax. *Chest* 1994; **105**: 980–2.
110. Berger R. Pleurodesis for spontaneous pneumothorax. Will the procedure of choice please stand up? *Chest* 1994; **106**: 992–4.
111. Berger R, Smith D. Efficacy of the lateral decubitus position in preventing pneumothorax after needle biopsy of the lung. *South Med J* 1988; **81**: 1140–3.
112. Klein JS, Schultz S. Interventional chest radiology. *Curr Probl Diagn Radiol* 1992; **21**: 219–77.
113. Westcott JL. Percutaneous transthoracic needle biopsy. *Radiology* 1988; **169**: 593–601.
114. vanSonnenberg E, Casola G, Ho M, *et al.* Difficult thoracic lesions: CT-guided biopsy experience in 150 cases. *Radiology* 1988; **167**: 457–61.
115. Fish GD, Stanley JH, Miller KS, Schabel SI, Sutherland SE. Postbiopsy pneumothorax: estimating the risk by chest radiography and pulmonary function tests. *AJR Am J Roentgenol* 1988; **150**: 71–4.
116. Harter LP, Moss AA, Goldberg HI, Gross BH. CT-guided fine-needle aspirations for diagnosis of benign and malignant disease. *AJR Am J Roentgenol* 1983; **140**: 363–7.
117. Miller KS, Fish GB, Stanley JH, Schabel SI. Prediction of pneumothorax rate in percutaneous needle aspiration of the lung. *Chest* 1988; **93**: 742–5.
118. Poe RH, Kallay MC, Wicks CM, Odoroff CL. Predicting risk of pneumothorax in needle biopsy of the lung. *Chest* 1984; **85**: 232–5.
119. Lindskog GE, Halasz NA. Spontaneous pneumothorax: a consideration of pathogenesis and management with review of seventy-two hospitalized cases. *Arch Surg* 1957; **75**: 693–8.

120. Rhea JT, DeLuca SA, Greene RE. Determining the size of pneumothorax in the upright patient. *Radiology* 1982; **144**: 733–6.
121. Conces DJ Jr, Tarver RD, Gray WC, Pearcy EA. Treatment of pneumothoraces utilizing small caliber chest tubes. *Chest* 1988; **94**: 55–7.
122. Casola G, vanSonnenberg E, Keightley A, *et al.* Pneumothorax: radiologic treatment with small catheters. *Radiology* 1988; **166**: 89–91.
123. Reinhold C, Illescas FF, Atri M, Bret PM. Treatment of pleural effusions and pneumothorax with catheters placed percutaneously under imaging guidance. *AJR Am J Roentgenol* 1989; **152**: 1189–91.
124. Peters J, Kubitschek KR. Clinical evaluation of a percutaneous pneumothorax catheter. *Chest* 1984; **86**: 714–17.
125. Erasmus JJ, Goodman PC, Patz EF Jr. Management of malignant pleural effusions and pneumothorax. *Radiol Clin North Am* 2000; **38**: 375–83.
126. Tarver RD, Conces DJ Jr. Chest intervention: drainage and biopsies. In: Castaneda-Zuniga WR, Tadavarthy SM (eds). *Interventional radiology*, 2nd ed. Baltimore: Williams & Wilkins; 1997: 1357–81.
127. Alfageme I, Moreno L, Huertas C, *et al.* Spontaneous pneumothorax. Long-term results with tetracycline pleurodesis. *Chest* 1994; **106**: 347–50.
128. Janzing HM, Derom A, Derom E, *et al.* Intrapleural quinacrine instillation for recurrent pneumothorax or persistent air leak. *Ann Thorac Surg* 1993; **55**: 368–71.
129. Milanez JR, Vargas FS, Filomeno LT, *et al.* Intrapleural talc for the prevention of recurrent pneumothorax. *Chest* 1994; **106**: 1162–5.
130. Perlmutt LM, Braun SD, Newman GE, *et al.* Transthoracic needle aspiration: use of a small chest tube to treat pneumothorax. *AJR Am J Roentgenol* 1987; **148**: 849–51.
131. Jay SJ. Diagnostic procedures for pleural disease. *Clin Chest Med* 1985; **6**: 33–48.
132. Diacon AH, Theron J, Schubert P, *et al.* Ultrasound-assisted transthoracic biopsy: fine-needle aspiration or cutting-needle biopsy? *Eur Respir J* 2007; **29**: 357–62.
133. Miller BH, Rosado-de-Christenson ML, Mason AC, *et al.* From the archives of the AFIP. Malignant pleural mesothelioma: radiologic–pathologic correlation. *Radiographics* 1996; **16**: 613–44.
134. McCaughey WT, Al-Jabi M. Differentiation of serosal hyperplasia and neoplasia in biopsies. *Pathol Annu* 1986; **21**: 271–93.
135. Chan JK, Loo KT, Yau BK, Lam SY. Nodular histiocytic/mesothelial hyperplasia: a lesion potentially mistaken for a neoplasm in transbronchial biopsy. *Am J Surg Pathol* 1997; **21**: 658–63.
136. Heilo A, Stenwig AE, Solheim OP. Malignant pleural mesothelioma: US-guided histologic core-needle biopsy. *Radiology* 1999; **211**: 657–9.
137. Metintas M, Ozdemir N, Isiksoy S, *et al.* CT-guided pleural needle biopsy in the diagnosis of malignant mesothelioma. *J Comput Assist Tomogr* 1995; **19**: 370–4.
138. Boutin C, Rey F. Thoracoscopy in pleural malignant mesothelioma: a prospective study of 188 consecutive patients. Part 1: Diagnosis. *Cancer* 1993; **72**: 389–93.
139. Agarwal PP, Seely JM, Matzinger FR, *et al.* Pleural mesothelioma: sensitivity and incidence of needle track seeding after image-guided biopsy versus surgical biopsy. *Radiology* 2006; **241**: 589–94.
140. West SD, Foord T, Davies RJ. Needle-track metastases and prophylactic radiotherapy for mesothelioma. *Respir Med* 2006; **100**: 1037–40.
141. Scott EM, Marshall TJ, Flower CD, Stewart S. Diffuse pleural thickening: percutaneous CT-guided cutting needle biopsy. *Radiology* 1995; **194**: 867–70.
142. Andriole JG, Haaga JR, Adams RB, Nunez C. Biopsy needle characteristics assessed in the laboratory. *Radiology* 1983; **148**: 659–62.
143. Haaga JR, LiPuma JP, Bryan PJ, Balsara VJ, Cohen AM. Clinical comparison of small-and large-caliber cutting needles for biopsy. *Radiology* 1983; **146**: 665–7.
144. Matsumori Y, Yano S, Goto H, *et al.* ZD6474, an inhibitor of vascular endothelial growth factor receptor tyrosine kinase, inhibits growth of experimental lung metastasis and production of malignant pleural effusions in a non-small cell lung cancer model. *Oncol Res* 2006; **16**: 15–26.

21

Radiology: pleural ultrasound

COENRAAD FN KOEGELENBERG, CHRIS T BOLLIGER, ANDREAS DIACON

INTRODUCTION

Although the introduction of diagnostic sonography of the abdomen dates back to the late 1940s, ultrasonography of the thorax lagged behind by many decades. The inability of ultrasound (US) to penetrate aerated tissue has diverted chest physicians from recognizing its excellent ability to visualize the chest wall, pleura and pathology of lung abutting the pleura. The major advantages of thoracic US include its dynamic properties, low cost, lack of radiation, mobility and short examination time.[1–6] It is also well suited for use in intensive care units, where suboptimal conditions for radiography make the diagnosis of clinically significant thoracic abnormalities difficult.[3] Furthermore, US of the chest is increasingly being used to guide interventional procedures, such as thoracentesis, biopsies of the chest wall, pleura or abutting lung and the placement of intercostal drains. The indications for pleural and chest wall US are summarized in Table 21.1. The main aim of this chapter is to demystify ultrasonography for the chest physician by reviewing the basic principles and techniques from the perspective of the non-radiologist.

Table 21.1 The indications for pleural and chest wall ultrasound[a]

Indications	
1	To detect a pleural effusion and guide thoracentesis and drainage, especially in small or loculated effusions
2	To differentiate a subpulmonary effusion from a subphrenic fluid accumulation and diaphragm paralysis in radiographically elevated hemidiaphragms
3	To localize pleural tumors, pleural thickening and lung tumors that abut the pleural surface and to guide needle aspiration and/or biopsies thereof
4	To assist the evaluation of patients with pleuritic chest pain
5	To clarify the nature of unknown pleural densities
6	To recognize pneumothorax, especially for emergency situations, or when radiographic equipment is unavailable
7	To localize pleural fluid prior to a thoracoscopy
8	To evaluate empyema and a parapneumonic pleural effusion in order to detect loculations and septae, and to guide aspiration with or without tube drainage

[a]Adapted with permission from: Tsai TH, Yang PC. Ultrasound in the diagnosis and management of pleural disease. *Curr Opin Pulm Med* 2003; 9: 282–90.

AN APPROACH TO THORACIC ULTRASONOGRAPHY

Technical principles

'Ultrasounds' are acoustic waves with a frequency above human hearing. Most US scanners operate in the frequency range of 2–15 megahertz (MHz). A very basic understanding of how the US scanner employs these ultrasounds to generate an image is paramount in order to comprehend its uses and limitations.

The US unit produces sound by means of a piezoelectric transducer encased in a handheld probe that is attached to the processing unit with an electric cable. This sound is focused in the transducer and is efficiently transmitted into the thorax. Ultrasound waves are propagated in liquid media (e.g. pleural effusions) or in tissues with a high water content (e.g. muscle, liver, consolidated lung or tumors), but are reflected off interfaces between dissimilar densities (e.g. gas or bone). If the US encounters gas (e.g. normal aerated lungs or a pneumothorax) or solids (e.g. ribs), the density difference is so great that most of the acoustic energy is reflected. This phenomenon is known as acoustical impedance and explains why structures deeper than the visceral pleura are invisible by means of ultrasonography in the non-diseased state.

The reflected part of the sound waves is detected as an echo. The time delay between emitted US and the received echo is used to calculate the depth of the structure causing the reflection. Furthermore, the greater the difference between acoustic impedances, the larger the echo will be. The transducer captures sound waves returning to the probe and converts these echoes into electrical pulses, which are ultimately processed and transformed into a digital image. The intensity and distribution of the pixels appearing on the screen is determined by three characteristics of the echo, namely (1) its direction, (2) its intensity and (3) the time elapsed from emission to capture. Images may contain 'hyperechoic' or white areas caused by high-amplitude echoes and 'hypoechoic' or dark areas from low-amplitude echoes.

The ultrasound unit

Adequate pleural and chest wall ultrasonography can be performed by means of the most basic, entry-level, two-dimensional black-and-white US equipment. Doppler and color flow echo are not required for routine pleural examination. For documentation of still images, a basic thermal printer is sufficient. Most modern scanners also allow for the transferral of images to data storage devices and can capture dynamic information in video format, which is preferable.

The US scanner is adorned by a confusing array of controls and options. It is imperative that the occasional sonographer familiarizes themself with the scanner and its most important function keys. It is helpful to differentiate between settings to optimize the machine for thoracic US in general, and controls for fine tuning the scanning for the individual case. For occasional thoracic scanning, basic settings programmed for abdominal sonography will suffice. However, if a machine is to be used mainly for thoracic US, we recommend calling upon an expert to assist with the basic setting up of the machine, which includes contrast and brightness of the monitor as well as default settings of depth and gain when using different probes.

Thoracic US is best performed with two transducers. A 3.7 MHz (range: 2–5 MHz) curvilinear probe is compulsory, and an 8 MHz (range: 5–10 MHz) linear probe is a very helpful addition. As a rule, higher frequency gives better resolution closer to the probe, but at the cost of lower penetration. A lower frequency probe (e.g. 3.5 MHz) with curvilinear shape for covering a large area is therefore suitable for initial screening of superficial and deeper structures, while the high frequency probe (e.g. 8 MHz) with a linear shape is used for refined assessment of an abnormal chest wall or pleural area.

The three most important controls on a standard keyboard are 'depth', 'gain' and 'freeze'. The depth function is a digital zoom that defines what portion of the scanned image is displayed on the monitor at what magnification. The scale is displayed on a vertical axis. Obese subjects or patients with a large effusion or intrathoracic tumors may require a depth setting of up to 12 cm. High frequency scanning is performed at a maximum depth of around 3–4 cm. The gain is, in essence, a measure for the amplification of the echoes and determines the brightness of the image. The freeze function allows for the capturing of still images, and to perform measurements with the appropriate keys and the trackball. Only experienced users should change advanced parameters, such as the frequency of a particular probe.

Patient positioning

The optimal patient position for scanning is a paramount but under-appreciated aspect. Sonographic access to the chest can be achieved via the abdomen, intercostal spaces or the upper thoracic aperture (supraclavicular fossa). It is important to review a patient's chest radiograph and computed tomography (CT) scan prior to performing a chest US examination. This will not only identify the area of interest, but will also guide the positioning of the patient. The posterior chest is best scanned with the patient in the sitting position using a bedside table as an armrest (Figure 21.1a,b), whereas the lateral and anterior chest wall can be examined with the patient in either the lateral decubitus or even supine position (Figure 21.1c). Maximum visualization of the lung and pleura is achieved by examining along the intercostal spaces. Raising the arm above the patient's head increases the intercostal space distance and facilitates scanning in erect or recumbent positions. A patient can fold the arms across the chest in order to displace the scapulae when surveying the upper posterior thorax. Superior sulcus pathology can be visualized apically with the patient in the supine or sitting position.

Scanning

Once the patient is adequately positioned and the area of interest is identified, liberal application of gel is the final step before scanning. It is advisable to hold the probe like a pen for writing on paper, and not like chalk for writing on a blackboard (Figure 21.1b). Experienced sonographers keep their eyes on the screen while their hand moves the probe across the area of interest and provides the posi-

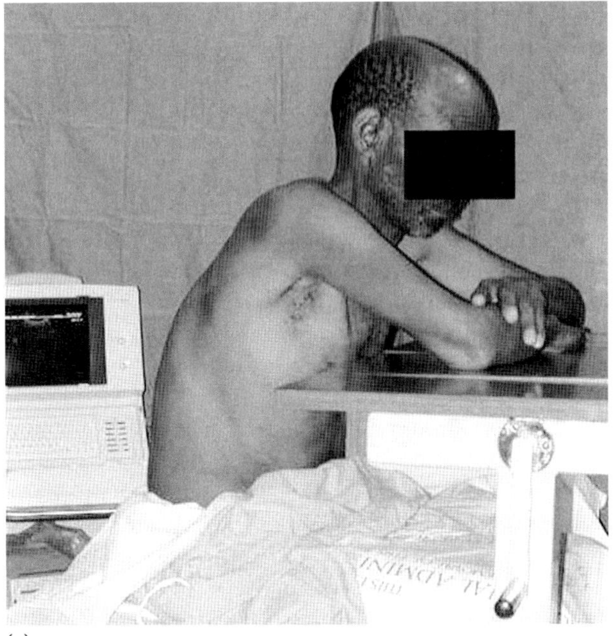

(a)

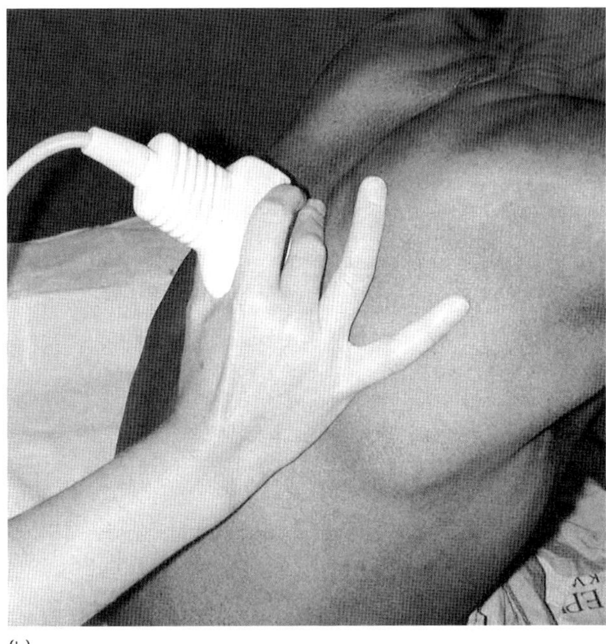

(b)

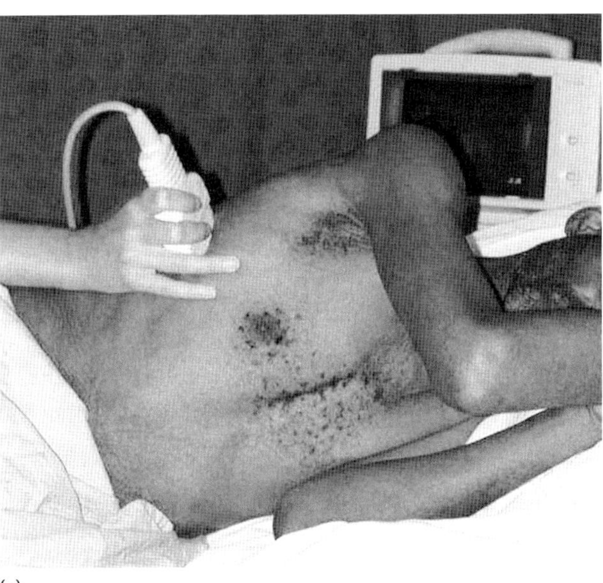

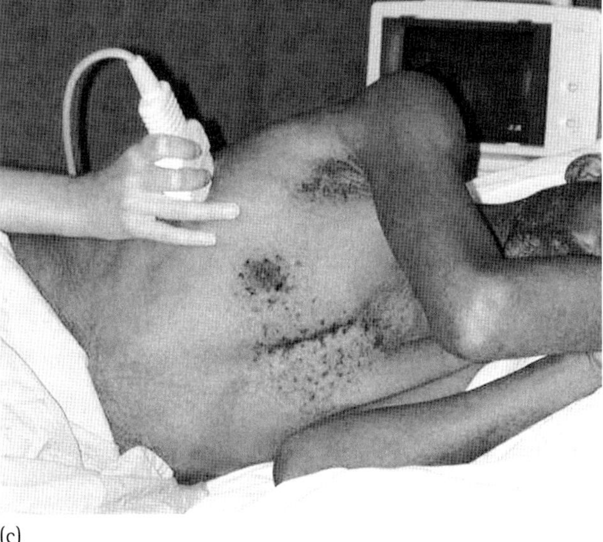

(c)

Figure 21.1 Scanning positions for chest ultrasound. (a) The posterior chest is best scanned with the patient in the sitting position using a bedside table as an armrest. (b) Note the way in which the probe is held. It is important to ask the patient to fold their arms across the chest when surveying the superior posterior chest. (c) The lateral chest wall can be examined with the patient in the lateral decubitus position with the arm raised, and the anterior chest wall with the patient supine (not shown).

tional information. The probe is moved slowly, preferably along intercostal spaces, which are oblique and not horizontal. Frequent pauses are needed for observing the spontaneous movement of structures with respiration. Unclear findings can be compared with the contralateral side.

DIAGNOSTIC THORACIC ULTRASONOGRAPHY

Normal chest wall and pleura

The initial surveillance of a normal chest with the low frequency probe will yield a series of echogenic layers of muscles and fascia planes (Figure 21.2a). The ribs appear as curvilinear structures on transverse scans, associated with posterior acoustic shadowing (Figure 21.2b). When the ribs are scanned along the longitudinal, the anterior cortex appears as a continuous echogenic line.

The visceral and parietal pleura can normally not be differentiated by means of a low-frequency probe, which instead displays one highly echogenic line representing the pleura and pleuropulmonary surface. With a high-resolution linear probe (e.g. 8 MHz), the visceral and parietal portions of the pleura can be seen as two distinct echogenic lines, with the latter seemingly thinner in appearance. The two layers can be seen to slide over each other with respiratory motion. The respiratory movement of the lung relative to the chest wall is visible with both probes and is called the 'lung sliding' sign. Its presence on real-time US is strong evidence against a pneumothorax.[7]

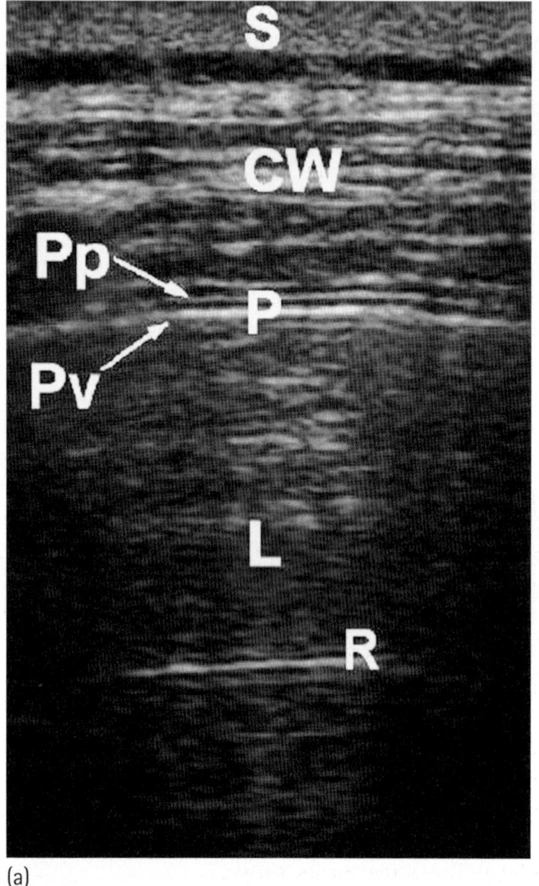

(a)

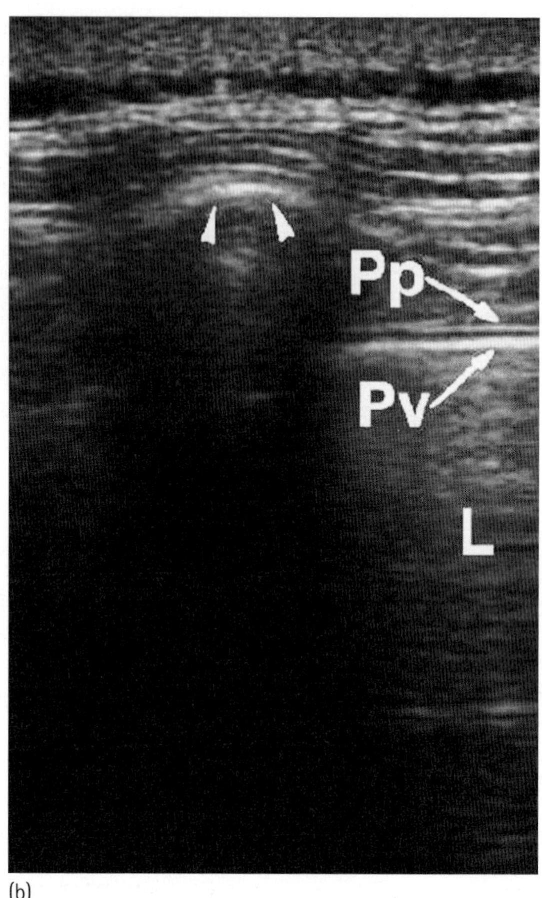

(b)

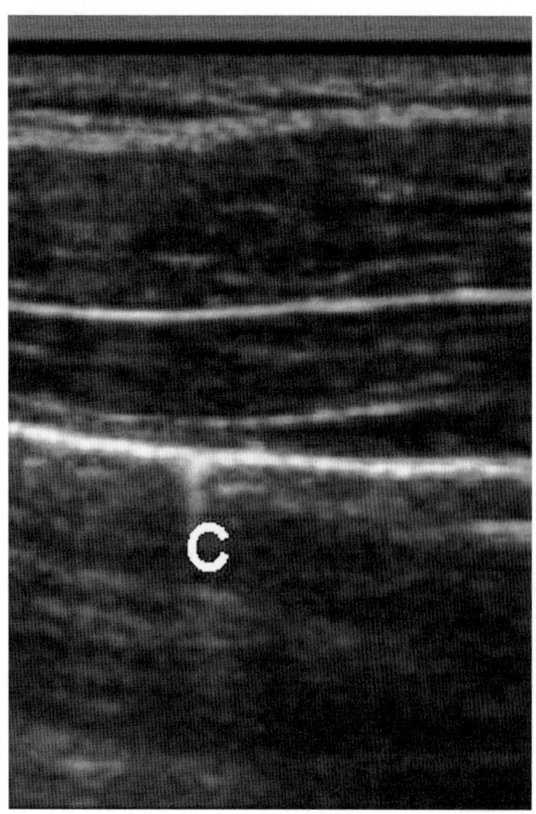

(c)

Figure 21.2 The typical appearance of a normal chest on ultrasound. (a) Transverse image through the intercostal space. The chest wall is visualized as multiple layers of echogenicity representing muscles and fascia. The visceral and parietal pleura appear as echogenic bright lines that slide during respiration (sliding sign). Reverberation artifacts beneath the pleural lines imply an underlying air-filled lung. S, skin; CW chest wall; P, pleura; Pp, parietal pleura; Pv, visceral pleura; L, lung; R, reverberation artifact. (b) Longitudinal image across the ribs. Normal ribs are seen as hyperechoic chambered surfaces (arrowheads) with prominent acoustic shadows beneath the ribs. Pp, parietal pleura; Pv, visceral pleura. (c) An example of a comet tail artifact observed in an otherwise normal subject. C, comet-tail artifact. Reproduced with permission from: Tsai TH, Yang PC. Ultrasound in the diagnosis and management of pleural disease. *Curr Opin Pulm Med* 2003; **9**: 282–90.

The 'curtain-sign' describes the variable obscuring of underlying structures by air containing tissue. In normal subjects, the curtain-sign is seen in the costophrenic angle. The upper abdominal organs are easily visible on expiration, but during inspiration the normal air-filled lung is moved downwards in front of the probe and temporarily obscures the sonographic window.

The parenchyma of normal aerated lungs is invisible by means of US. The large change in acoustic impedance at the pleura–lung interface causes horizontal artifacts that are seen as a series of echogenic parallel lines equidistant from one another below the pleura. These bright but formless lines are known as reverberation artifacts and diminish in intensity with increasing distance from the pleura (Figure 21.2a). Vertical 'comet-tail' artifacts (Figure 21.2c), caused by fluid-filled subpleural interlobular septae, can also be seen originating at the pleura–lung interface. The normal diaphragm is best seen through the lower intercostal spaces or via the liver or spleen. It is seen as an echogenic 1 mm thick line which contracts with inspiration.

Pleural effusions

SONOGRAPHIC DIAGNOSIS

The value of ultrasonography for detection and quantification of pleural effusions is uncontested. Ultrasound is particularly helpful in determining the nature of localized or diffuse pleural opacities, and is more sensitive than decubitus expiratory films in identifying minimal or loculated effusions.[8] Sonographically, a pleural effusion appears as an anechoic, homogeneous space between parietal and visceral pleura (Figure 21.3). This space may change in shape with respiration, and the atelectatic lung inside a large effusion may appear as a tongue-like structure within the effusion. In inflammatory effusions, adhesions between the two pleural surfaces may result in the absence of lung motion above the effusion. If an abnormal elevation of a hemidiaphragm is noted on the chest radiograph, subpulmonary effusion can be differentiated from a subphrenic fluid collection or diaphragm paralysis.[9]

DETERMINING THE NATURE OF A PLEURAL EFFUSION

The sonographic appearance of a pleural effusion depends on its nature, cause and chronicity. Four appearances are recognized based on the internal echogenicity: anechoic; complex but non-septated; complex and septated; and homogenously echogenic. Transudates are invariably anechoic, unseptated and free flowing, whereas complex, septated or echogenic effusions are usually exudates.[10,11] Malignant effusions are often anechoic. Nodular pleural thickening is apparent in the minority of malignant effusions, and echogenic swirling patterns have recently been linked to these effusions.[12] Inflammatory effusions are often associated with strands of echogenic material and septations which show more or less mobility with respiration and the cardiac cycle. The presence of septae has several implications. Chen *et al.*[13] demonstrated that patients with septated effusions needed longer chest tube drainage, longer hospital care and were more likely to require fibrinolytic therapy or surgery compared with those with unseptated effusions. Tu *et al.*[14] recently confirmed some of these findings in medical intensive care unit patients. Empyema may cause a strongly echogenic effusion that may be mistaken for a solid pleural lesion.

ESTIMATING THE VOLUME OF A PLEURAL EFFUSION BY ULTRASOUND

Several studies have shown reasonable correlation between the volume of an effusion estimated with planimetric measurements and its square dimensions.[15–17] Such geometric calculations are hampered by the uneven distribution of fluid in the presence of pleuropulmonary adhesions. We suggest the following practical way to classify the volume of an effusion: minimal, if the echo-free space is confined to the costophrenic angle; small, if the space is greater than the costophrenic angle but still within the range of the area covered with a 3.5 MHz curvilinear probe; moderate, if the space is greater than a one-probe range but within a two-probe range; and large, if the space is bigger than a two-probe range.

DIFFERENTIATION OF EFFUSION FROM PLEURAL THICKENING

To distinguish small effusions from anechoic pleural thickening can be challenging. Both may appear as anechoic on US. Nearly 20 percent of echo-free pleural lesions will not yield free fluid, whereas a significant percentage of complex-appearing lesions will do so. Mobility is a good sign for effusion. Marks *et al.*[18] found that if a lesion changed shape with respiratory excursion and if it contained movable strands or echo densities, the lesion was an effusion. If a color Doppler is available, the fluid color sign is the most sensitive and specific ultrasonographic evidence of a small effusion. The sign refers to the presence of a color signal within the fluid collection that is believed to arise from transmitted motion during respiratory or cardiac cycles. This sign has a sensitivity of 89.2 percent and specificity of 100 percent in detecting minimal fluid collections.[19]

Pleural thickening

Pleural thickening is defined as focal lesions arising from the visceral or parietal pleura that is greater than 3 mm in width with or without an irregular margin (Figure 21.4). It appears as broadening of the pleura and does not exhibit a fluid color sign or display movement relative to the chest wall. Pleural thickening most often appears hypoechoic,

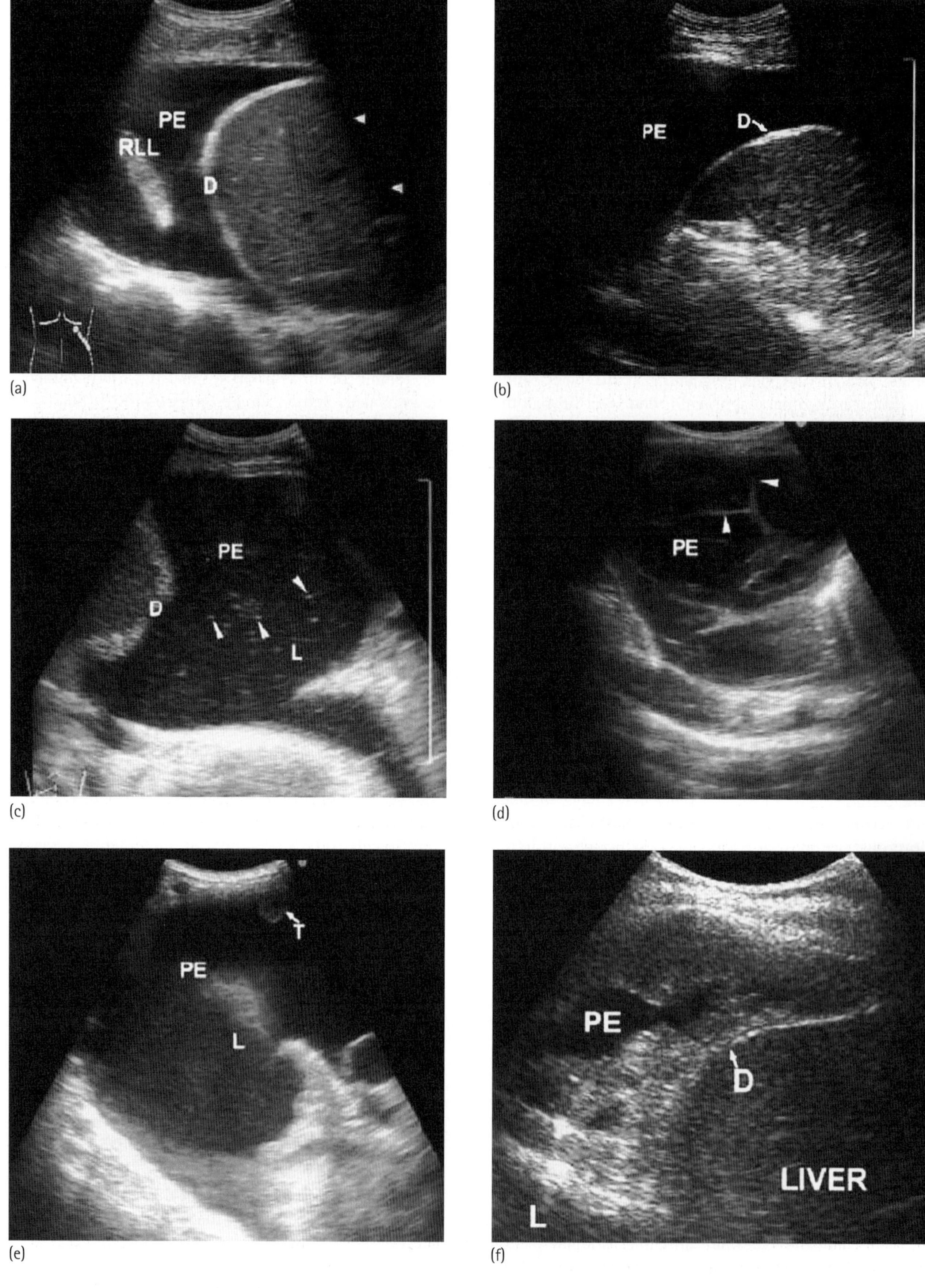

(a) (b) (c) (d) (e) (f)

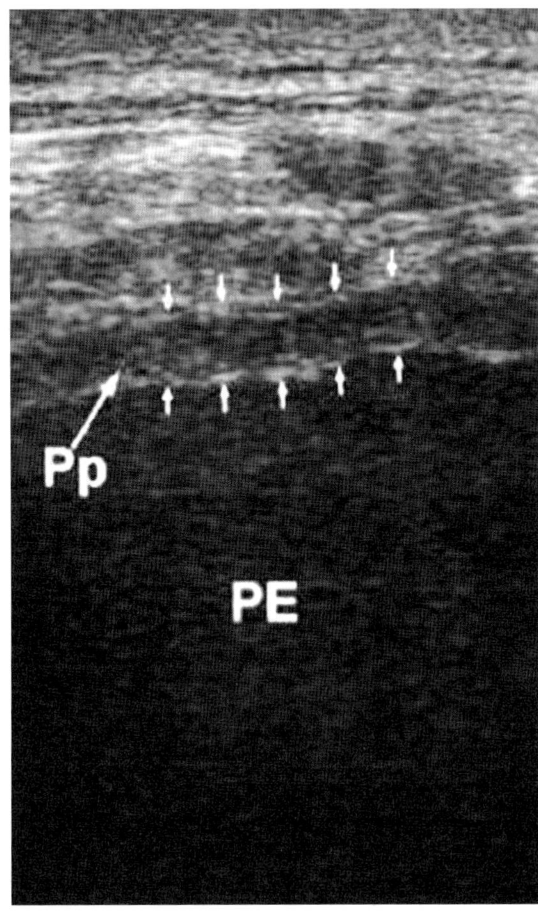

Figure 21.4 Pleural thickening: The arrows indicate sheetlike pleural thickening. Pp, parietal pleura; PE, pleural effusion. Reproduced with permission from: Tsai TH, Yang PC. Ultrasound in the diagnosis and management of pleural disease. *Curr Opin Pulm Med* 2003; 9: 282–90.

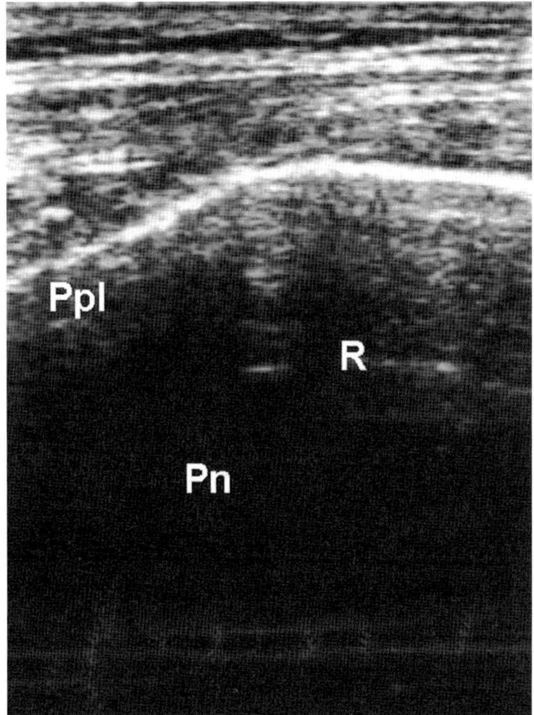

Figure 21.5 A pneumothorax. It should be appreciated that the most specific sign, namely the absence of the sliding sign (see text), can only observed in real time. Note the broadened pleural line, reverberation artifact and absence of comet-tail artifacts. Ppl, parietal pleura; Pn, pneumothorax; R, reverberation artifact.

but increased echogenicity with focal shadowing is sometimes observed and is indicative of calcification.

Pneumothorax and hydropneumothorax

Pneumothorax detection requires more skill and experience than the investigation of pleural fluid. A pneumothorax (Figure 21.5) can be diagnosed by means of the absence of normal lung sliding, exaggerated horizontal reverberation artifacts and the loss of comet-tail artifacts, provided that no diaphragmatic paralysis, prior pleurodesis, pleural adhesions or adult respiratory distress syndrome are present.[20–22] Chronic obstructive pulmonary disease (COPD) can mimic the sonographic sings of pneumothorax. This allows the exclusion, but not the confirmation of pneumothorax in such patients with US.[23] Despite these limitations, ultrasonography is particularly useful in intensive care units and in other situations where radiographic equipment is unavailable. Herth *et al.*[24] have recently shown that a pneumothorax following transbronchial biopsy can be reliably excluded with US (sensitivity 100 percent; specificity 83 percent). This is likely to reduce costs for chest radiographs, increase patient comfort and offers an excellent opportunity to acquire and practice pneumothorax detection.

Hydropneumothorax can also be identified with US by means of the visualization of air–fluid boundary.[25] The sliding sign above the air–fluid level will be absent. A mobile air–fluid level will generate a 'curtain sign' with respiration, because the air within the pleura obscures the underlying effusion during inspiration.

Figure 21.3 (opposite) (a) Pleural effusion is presented as an echo-free space between the visceral and parietal pleura. Compressive atelectasis of the lung may be seen in a large effusion. The effusion can be subclassified as anechoic (b), complex non-septated (c), complex septated (d), or homogenously echogenic (e). Note the movable echogenic spots within the complex non-septated effusion, and the floating strands and septa within the complex septated effusion (arrowheads). (f) Pleural effusion associated with pleural nodules or nodular thickenings is characteristic of malignant effusion. PE, pleural effusion; D, diaphragm; RLL, right lower lobe; L, lung; T, pleural tumor. Reproduced with permission from: Tsai TH, Yang PC. Ultrasound in the diagnosis and management of pleural disease. *Curr Opin Pulm Med* 2003; 9: 282–90.

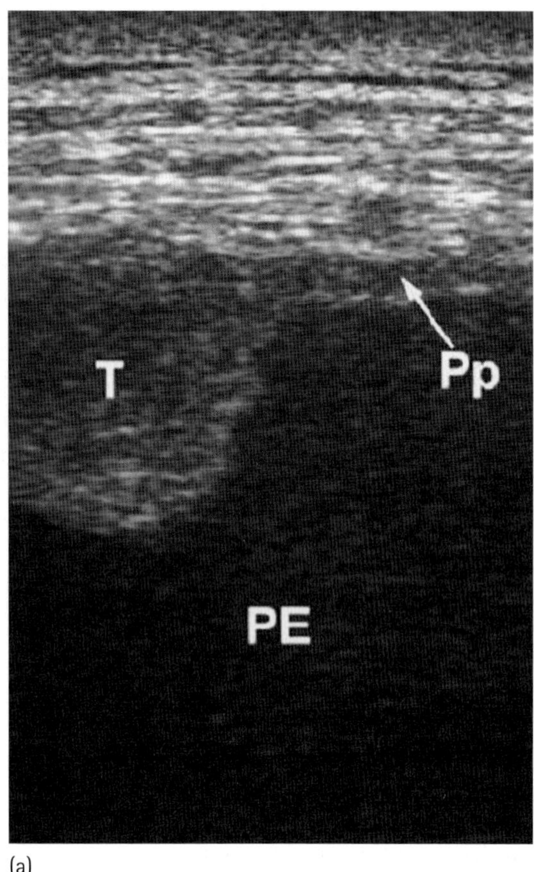

(a)

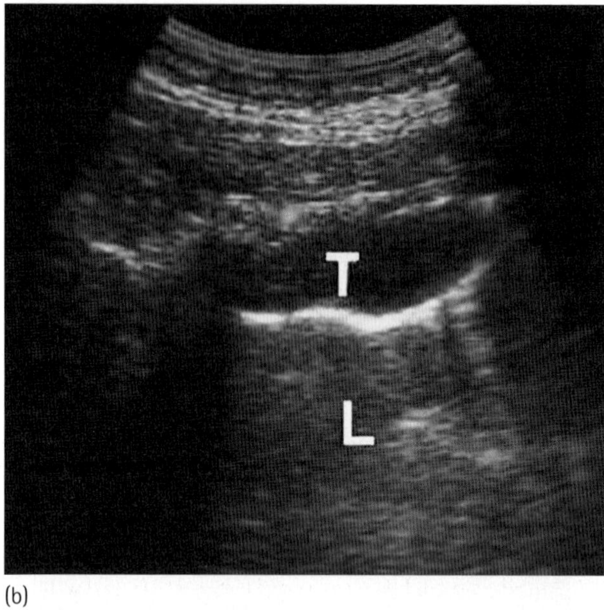

(b)

Figure 21.6 Pleural tumors: Two examples of the ultrasound appearance of pleural tumors, one with a large pleural effusion (a) and one without (b). Note the posterior echo enhancement. PE, pleural effusion; T, pleural tumor; Pp, parietal pleura; L, lung. Reproduced with permission from: Tsai TH, Yang PC. Ultrasound in the diagnosis and management of pleural disease. *Curr Opin Pulm Med* 2003; **9**: 282–90.

Pleural tumors

Benign pleural tumors appear on US as well-defined rounded masses of variable echogenicity on either the parietal or visceral pleura. Both metastatic pleural tumors and malignant mesothelioma appear as polypoid pleural nodules or irregular sheetlike pleural thickening,[26] often with large pleural effusions (Figure 21.6).Tumors with low echogenicity can exhibit posterior echo enhancement.

Lung tumors abutting or invading the pleura and chest wall

A peripheral lung tumor will be detectable by US provided that pleural contact is present (Figure 21.7). Visceral pleura or chest wall invasion has important implications for lung tumor staging (T2 or T3 staging, respectively). Although CT is routinely used for determining the extent of invasion, high-resolution real-time US scanning has been found to be superior to routine chest CT in evaluating tumor invasion of the pleura and chest wall.[27,28] When a tumor abutted to the chest wall is visualized with US, all layers of the chest wall, i.e. muscle, fascia, parietal pleura and visceral pleura, can be examined and the extent of tumor invasion can be accurately determined (Figure 21.8).

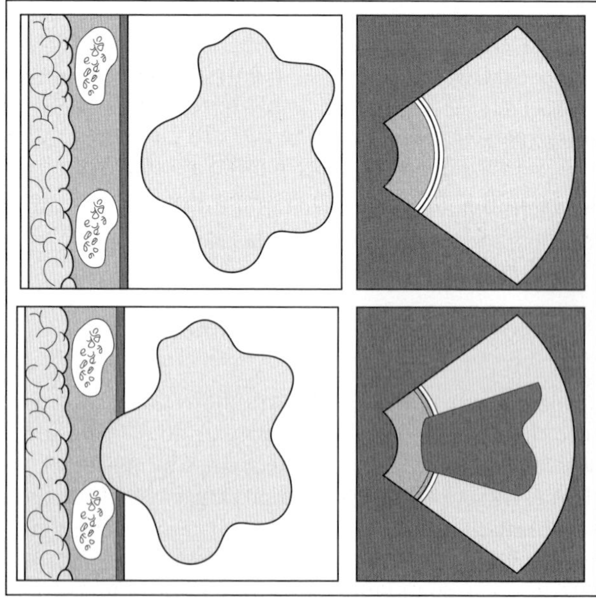

Figure 21.7 A peripheral lung lesion is shown schematically on the left without (top) and with (bottom) pleural contact. The corresponding sonar images recorded with a sector scanner are shown on the right. Only the lesion with pleural contact is visible on ultrasound. Note that the acoustic window is too narrow to demonstrate the whole circumference of the lesion, but it allows determination of its full depth. Reproduced with permission from: Diacon AH, Theron J, Bolliger CT. Transthoracic ultrasound for the pulmonologist. *Curr Opin Pulm Med* 2005; **11**: 307–12.

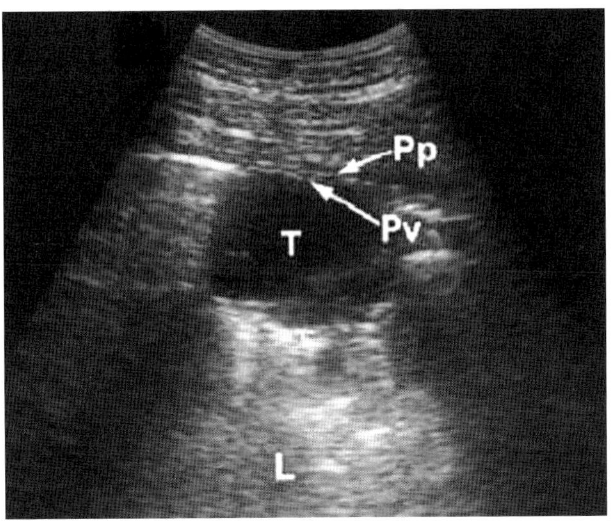

(a)

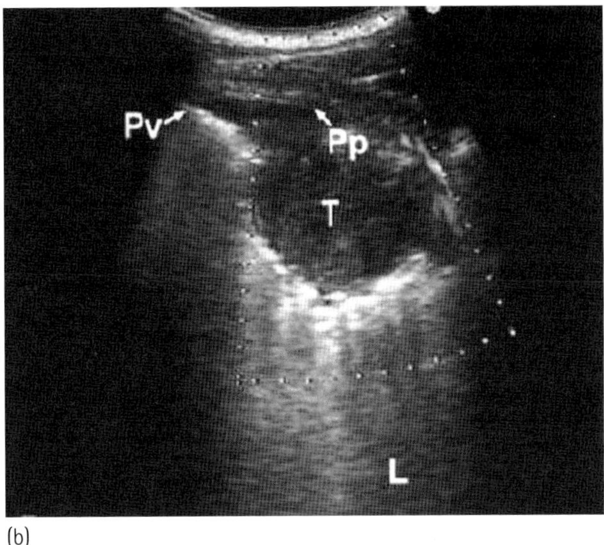

(b)

Figure 21.8 (a) An ultrasound (US) image showing a lung tumor with posterior echo enhancement. Note that both of the visceral and parietal pleural lines are intact. (b) This US shows tumor extension beyond the pleura. The visceral pleural line is interrupted, and the respiratory movement of the tumor is disturbed in real-time US. Invasion of the pleural cavity by the tumor is evident. L, lung; T, tumor; Pv, visceral pleural; Pp, parietal pleura. Reproduced with permission from: Diacon AH, Theron J, Bolliger CT. Transthoracic ultrasound for the pulmonologist. *Curr Opin Pulm Med* 2005; **11**: 307–12.

Chest wall pathology

Soft-tissue masses such as lipomas can readily be detected by high-frequency US. Supraclavicular and axillary lymph nodes with malignant infiltration appear bulky, rounded and hypoechoic.[29] Extracapsular spread is suggested by irregular borders. Sonography can detect bony metastases to the ribs, which appear as hypoechoic masses in place of the normal echogenicity of the rib with disruption of the cortical line. US is also reported to be more sensitive than radiography in the detection of rib fracture, which appears as a breach or displacement of the cortex of the rib with or without localized swelling or haematoma.

Diaphragmatic paralysis

The diaphragm is best visualized at the costophrenic angle or through the liver or spleen. Sonographic examination of a paralyzed diaphragm will yield paradoxical movement of the diaphragm with respiration.[30] This can be accentuated with forced inspiration ('sniff' test). Long-term paralysis causes muscle atrophy.[30]

Diverse pulmonary pathology

Apart from solid tumors, numerous pathological processes can replace the air within lung tissue and thereby become detectable with US, provided that the pleura is abutted.

PNEUMONIA AND LUNG ABSCESSES

Pleural based pneumonic consolidation is detectable by means of US, although the extent of disease appears smaller on US than on chest radiographs. In the early phase of consolidation the lung appears diffusely echogenic, resembling the sonographic texture of the liver. Air bronchograms appear as echogenic branches. Fluid bronchograms are sometimes observed. They appear as anechoic tubular structures, representing fluid-filled airways, and are typically seen in bronchial obstruction. Their presence should alert the clinician to the possibility of a post-obstructive pneumonitis, secondary to a proximal tumor. Sonographically observed consolidation is not indicative of an infective etiology. Pulmonary infarction, hemorrhage and bronchoalveolar carcinoma are three examples of non-infective consolidation that is similar in appearance on US. US may guide transthoracic needle aspirations or biopsies of peripheral pulmonary infiltrates in cases with diagnostic uncertainty regarding the aetiology.[31]

A lung abscess abutting the pleura appears sonographically as a hypoechoic lesion with a well-defined or irregular wall (Figure 21.9). The centre of the abscess is most often anechoic, but may reveal internal echoes and septations. Abscesses with air fluid levels on chest radiograph are more inhomogeneous and will display the curtain sign.

PULMONARY EMBOLISM

Ultrasound can serve for the acute bedside assessment of patients presenting with possible pulmonary embolism.[32] Pulmonary infarction is recognized as a peripheral wedge-

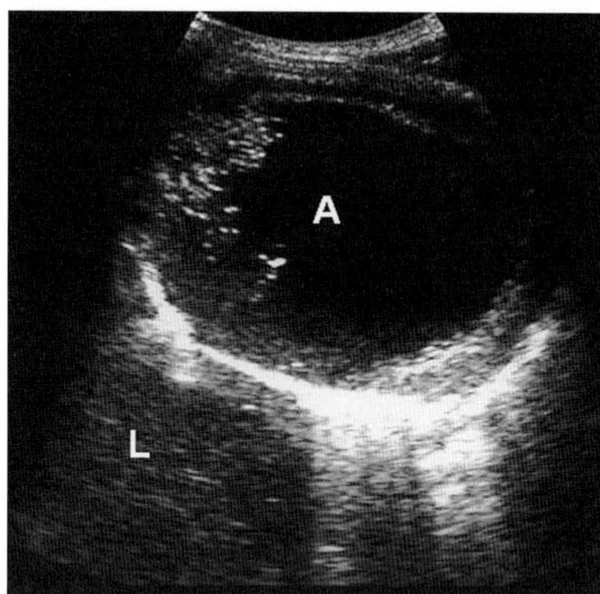

Figure 21.9 A peripheral lung abscess. Note the hypoechoic centre and irregular wall. A, abscess cavity; L, lung.

shaped consolidation, often accompanied by a pleural effusion. US is also useful to diagnose venous thrombosis as well as the sequelae of thromboembolic disease such as right ventricular overload and dilated hepatic veins. This indication of US is currently still reserved for experienced physicians with a keen interest in US, as pulmonary spiral CT angiography remains the investigation of choice.

PULMONARY EDEMA

In the setting of patients with acute dyspnea it has been reported that the presence of bilateral, widespread comet-tail artifacts is a reliable sign to differentiate patients with pulmonary edema from those with chronic obstructive airway disease in the intensive care unit (ICU).[33] Comet-tail artifacts were absent in 92 percent of patients with chronic obstructive airway disease.

ULTRASOUND-GUIDED INTERVENTIONS

Principles

Ultrasound is particularly well suited for assisting pleural and chest wall interventions, including diagnostic thoracentesis, closed tube drainage, chest wall and pleural biopsies and biopsies of lung tumors abutting or invading the pleura. The use of US for these procedures increases the success rate and minimizes risk compared with procedures carried out blindly.

With regard to needle biopsies, specific reusable probes for real-time US guidance of needle biopsies are commercially available. Many prefer the so-called 'freehand' technique for its simplicity. Following adequate patient positioning, the intended site of needle insertion is sonographically identified and marked, while the direction, the depth of interest and the safety range for the procedure are memorized. The patient must not change position in order to prevent a positional shift of the area of interest relative to the skin mark. It is occasionally even necessary to ask the patient to hold their breath for the duration of the aspiration. The practice of identifying a puncture site at a radiology department prior to transporting a patient elsewhere for thoracentesis should be discouraged, particularly in the case of small effusions, as both the fluid collection and the skin mark might shift considerably with minor changes in body position.

Thoracentesis

Sonography is superior to chest radiographs in detecting pleural effusions and identifying the optimal site for diagnostic thoracentesis.[34] The largest and most accessible area of fluid accumulation can be identified, and an aspiration can easily be performed by means of the 'freehand' technique. The success rate of US-guided thoracentesis can be as high as 97 percent.[35] US guided thoracentesis improves the diagnostic yield and decreases the risk of complications in all patients, but is particularly helpful when a safe procedure is mandatory, e.g. in patients with bleeding diathesis or the critically ill patient.

Closed tube drainage

Ultrasound is ideal for identifying the optimal site for effective and safe pleural drainage. This is particularly relevant in an ICU setting and in patients with loculated parapneumonic effusions and empyemas with septations. Depending on operator experience, US may also guide further decisions regarding the need for subsequent intrapleural fibrinolytics or for surgical intervention in addition to drainage and antibiotics.[36]

Effusions can also be accessed by means of an 18- or 16-gauge needle under direct (real-time) US visualization. This allows direct thoracentesis followed by an insertion of a guide wire, which is used to guide serial incremental dilatation of a tract and deployment of a pigtail small-bore catheter (8–14 F). These tubes are better tolerated than large bore (20–24 F) intercostal drains.[37]

Closed pleural biopsy in the presence of a pleural effusion

Sonography is an extremely useful guide for biopsies of the pleura. Focal pleural abnormalities (thickening or tumors) can be identified with US, and biopsy can be aimed at these areas of interest. The ability to estimate the size of an associated effusion decreases the risk of visceral pleural lacerations, which is particularly relevant in cases with minimal pleural effusion.

Conventionally, closed pleural biopsies (e.g. with the Abrams needle) could only safely be performed in the presence of a sizeable pleural effusion or pneumothorax determined clinically or on chest radiography. However, US can demonstrate small fluid collections and facilitate the use of devices that were not primarily designed for fluid aspiration (e.g. Tru-cut needles). Numerous studies have concluded that US-guided Tru-cut needle biopsies have higher sensitivity and specificity in the diagnosis of pleural malignancy and tuberculosis than unaided Abrams needle biopsies.[38–41]

Transthoracic fine needle aspirations and needle biopsies of solid tumors

Ultrasound-guided fine needle aspiration or cutting biopsy performed under local anesthesia is safe and has a high diagnostic yield.[42] Chest wall and anterior mediastinal masses, pleural tumors or thickening, as well as peripheral lung tumors that either abut or invade the pleura or chest wall, are ideally suited for US-guided biopsy procedures. The risk of pneumothorax is low as no air-containing tissue needs to be transversed with the biopsy device. US-guided biopsies can be performed at the bedside, which offers advantages in distressed patients with advanced disease. The shortened procedure time is also particularly helpful in less cooperative patients.

Transthoracic fine needle aspirations (TTFNA) are performed under local anaesthesia, preferably with a 22-gauge injection-type or spinal needle. A recent prospective study found that TTFNA and closed needle biopsies corresponded well in the diagnosis of epithelial lung carcinoma and in the distinction of small cell and non-small cell lung cancer. TTFNA alone seems sufficient for the diagnosis of epithelial lung carcinoma, while closed needle biopsies have a higher yield in non-carcinomatous lesions and pleural tumors.[43]

Cutting needle biopsies follow the same principles as TTFNA, but such devices are more invasive and carry the risk of vascular trauma if the anatomical locations of subclavian, brachial, intercostal and mammarian arteries are not respected. Chang *et al.*[38] found that US-guided Tru-cut had a sensitivity of 61.5 percent and specificity of 100 percent. Tru-Cut biopsy is particularly helpful for diagnosing malignant mesothelioma without open surgical biopsy. A recent study of cutting needle biopsies under CT-guidance in diffuse pleural thickening showed a sensitivity and specificity for mesothelioma of 88 and 100 percent, respectively.[44] In a study employing US for tumors greater than 3 cm in diameter, the sensitivity and specificity for mesothelioma was 100 percent.[42]

Cytopathological support for rapid on-site evaluation (ROSE) of TTFNA smears is extremely helpful in deciding whether a histological specimen obtained via cutting needle biopsy is needed or not.[43] In the absence of ROSE, cutting biopsies should be performed in all cases where cytology is non-contributory and in cases where a diagnosis other than lung cancer is suspected. Conveniently, US is a good tool for exclusion of a pneumothorax post-aspiration or biopsy. If the lesion remains visible on US and is unchanged in location, shape and size, it implies that no free air is present between the sampled lesion and the visceral pleura, and that a clinically relevant pneumothorax is unlikely. US-guided biopsies are safe procedures, with an overall complication rate of only 1–2 percent.[42,43]

Aspiration and biopsy of diffuse pulmonary infiltrates, consolidations and lung abscesses

The indications for US-assisted TTFNA and biopsies are by no means limited to solid tumors. Yang *et al.*[31] found US-guided biopsy of pulmonary consolidation helpful in determining its cause, and reported a diagnostic yield of as high as 93 percent. This procedure is particularly useful in the immunocompromised patient, given the extensive differential diagnosis. The same author was able to sonographically demonstrate abscess cavities in 94 percent of 35 patients with radiologically confirmed lung abscesses.[45] By US, lung abscesses were depicted as hypoechoic lesions with irregular outer margins and an abscess cavity that was manifested as a hyperechoic ring. More than 90 percent of all aspirates of these abscesses yielded pathogens, whereas less than 10 percent of patients had positive blood cultures.

CONCLUSION

The usefulness of US for chest physicians is firmly established. Basic thoracic ultrasonography is an elegant and low-cost investigation that extends the physicians' diagnostic and interventional potential at the bedside in peripheral lung, pleural and chest wall disease. It has the potential to replace CT-guided fine needle aspirations or biopsies of all lesions involving the pleura and chest wall, as well as lung masses or consolidations abutting the pleura. Basic thoracic sonography is fairly simple and easy to learn. Academic institutions should strive to have a basic formal training program in ultrasonography in place in order to ensure that all aspiring chest physicians are familiar with chest ultrasonography.

ACKNOWLEDGEMENTS

We would like to thank Carol Lochner and Belinda Muller for technical assistance with this manuscript. We are indebted to the Holland-Stellenbosch Medical Foundation, Veldhoven, The Netherlands for continued support.

KEY POINTS

- Thoracic ultrasonography can be performed by means of the most basic ultrasound equipment.
- In healthy individuals, ultrasound can visualize the chest wall, the diaphragm and the pleura, but not the lung parenchyma.
- The main domain of thoracic ultrasound is the investigation of chest wall abnormalities, pleural thickening and pleural tumors, and the qualitative and quantitative description of pleural effusions.
- Ultrasound can visualize lung tumors and other parenchymal pulmonary processes provided that they abut the pleura.
- Ultrasound is the ideal tool to assist with thoracentesis and drainage of effusions.
- Ultrasound-assisted fine needle aspiration and cutting needle biopsy of lesions arising from the chest wall, pleura and lung are safe and have a high yield in the hands of chest physicians.
- New applications of ultrasound include the diagnosis of pneumothorax and pulmonary embolism.

REFERENCES

● = Key primary paper
◆ = Major review article

◆1. Tsai TH, Yang PC. Ultrasound in the diagnosis and management of pleural disease. *Curr Opin Pulm Med* 2003; **9**: 282–90.
◆2. Diacon AH, Theron J, Bolliger CT. Transthoracic ultrasound for the pulmonologist. *Curr Opin Pulm Med* 2005; **11**: 307–12.
◆3. Yu CJ, Yang PC, Chang DB, Luh KT. Diagnostic and therapeutic use of chest sonography: value in critically ill patients. *Am J Roentgenol* 1992; **159**: 695–701.
◆4. Koh DM, Burke S, Davies N, *et al.* Transthoracic US of the chest: clinical uses and applications. Radiographics 2002; 22: E1. Available: http://radiographics.rsnajnls.org/cgi/content/full/22/1/e1
◆5. Mayo PH, Doelken P. Pleural ultrasonography. *Clin Chest Med* 2006; **27**: 215–17.
◆6. Evans AL, Gleeson FV. Radiology in pleural disease: state of the art. *Respirology* 2004; **9**: 300–12.
●7. Lichtenstein DA, Menu Y. A bedside ultrasound sign ruling out pneumothorax in the critically ill. *Chest* 1995; **108**: 1345–8.
8. Kocijancic I, Kocijancic K, Cufer T. Imaging of pleural fluid in healthy individuals. *Clin Radiol* 2004; **59**: 826–9.
9. Ko JC, Yang PC, Chang DB, *et al.* Ultrasonographic evaluation of peridiaphragmatic lesions: a prospective study. *J Med Ultrasound* 1994; **2**: 84–92.
10. Yang PC, Luh KT, Chang DB, *et al.* Value of sonography in determining the nature of pleural effusion: analysis of 320 cases. *AJR Am J Roentgenol* 1992; **159**: 29–33.
11. Hirsch JH, Rogers JV, Mack LA. Real-time sonography of pleural opacities. *Am J Roentgenol* 1981; **136**: 297–301.
12. Chian CF, Su WL, Soh LH, *et al.* Echogenic swirling pattern as a predictor of malignant pleural effusions in patients with malignancies. *Chest* 2004; **126**: 129–34.
13. Chen KY, Liaw YS, Wang HC, *et al.* Sonographic septation: a useful prognostic indicator of acute thoracic empyema. *J Ultrasound Med* 2000; **19**: 837–43.
14. Tu CY, Hsu WH, Hsia TC, *et al.* Pleural effusions in febrile medical ICU patients: chest ultrasound study. *Chest* 2004; **126**: 1274–80.
15. Eibenberger KL, Dock WI, Ammann ME, *et al.* Quantification of pleural effusions: sonography versus radiography. *Radiology* 1994; **191**: 681–4.
16. Lorenz J, Borner N, Nikolaus HP. Sonographic volumetry of pleural effusions. *Ultraschall Med* 1988; **9**: 212–15.
17. Balik M, Plasil P, Waldauf P, *et al.* Ultrasound estimation of volume of pleural fluid in mechanically ventilated patients. *Intensive Care Med* 2006; **32**: 318–21.
18. Marks WM, Filly RA, Callen PW. Real-time evaluation of pleural lesions: new observations regarding the probability of obtaining free fluid. *Radiology* 1982; **142**: 163–4.
19. Wu RG, Yang PC, Kuo SH, Luh KT. 'Fluid color' sign: a useful indicator for discrimination between pleural thickening and pleural effusion. *J Ultrasound Med* 1995; **14**: 767–9.
●20. Chan SS. Emergency bedside ultrasound to detect pneumothorax. *Acad Emerg Med* 2003; **10**: 91–4.
21. Chan SS. The comet tail artifact in the diagnosis of pneumothorax. *J Ultrasound Med* 2002; **21**: 1060.
22. Simon BC, Paolinetti L. Two cases where bedside ultrasound was able to distinguish pulmonary bleb from pneumothorax. *J Emerg Med* 2005; **29**: 201–5.
23. Slater A, Goodwin M, Anderson KE, Gleeson FV. COPD can mimic the appearance of pneumothorax on thoracic ultrasound. *Chest* 2006; **129**: 545–50.
●24. Herth FJ, Eberhardt R, Ernst A, *et al.* Diagnosis of pneumothorax by means of transthoracic ultrasound: a prospective trial. *Eur Respir J* 2004; **24**: S491.
25. Targhetta R, Bourgeois JM, Chavagneux R, *et al.* Ultrasonographic approach to diagnosing hydropneumothorax. *Chest* 1992; **101**: 931–4.
26. Gorg C, Restrepo I, Schwerk WB: Sonography of malignant pleural effusion. *Eur Radiol* 1997; **7**: 1195–8.
●27. Sugama Y, Tamaki S, Kitamura S, *et al.* Ultrasonographic evaluation of pleural and chest wall invasion of lung cancer. *Chest* 1988; **93**: 275–9.
28. Suzuki N, Saitoh T, Kitamura S: Tumor invasion of the chest wall in lung cancer: diagnosis with US. *Radiology* 1993; **187**: 39–42.
29. Bruneton JN, Caramella E, Hery M *et al.* Axillary lymph node metastases in breast cancer: preoperative detection with US. *Radiology* 1986; **158**: 325–6.
30. Gottesman E, McCool MD. Ultrasound evaluation of the paralyzed diaphragm. *Am J Resp Crit Care Med* 1997; **155**: 1570–4.
●31. Yang PC, Chang DB, Yu CJ, *et al.* Ultrasound guided percutaneous cutting biopsy for the diagnosis of pulmonary consolidation of unknown aetiology. *Thorax* 1992; **47**: 457–60.
●32. Reissig A, Kroegel C. Transthoracic ultrasound of lung and pleura in the diagnosis of pulmonary embolism: a novel non-invasive bedside approach. *Respiration* 2003; **70**: 441–52.
33. Lichtenstein D, Meziere G. A lung ultrasound signs allowing bedside distinction between pulmonary edema and COPD: the comet-tail artifact. *Intensive Care Med* 1998; **24**: 1331–4.
34. Diacon AH, Brutsche MH, Soler M. Accuracy of pleural puncture sites: a prospective comparison of clinical examination with ultrasound. *Chest* 2003; **123**: 436–41.
●35. Yang PC, Kuo SH, Luh KT: Ultrasonography and ultrasound-guided needle biopsy of chest diseases: indications, techniques, diagnostic yields and complications. *J Med Ultrasound* 1993; **1**: 53–63.
36. Chen KY, Liaw YS, Wang HC, *et al.* Sonographic septation: a useful prognostic indicator of acute thoracic empyema. *J Ultrasound Med* 2000; **19**: 837–43.
37. Tatersall DJ, Traill ZC, Gleeson FV. Chest drains: does size matter? *Clin Radiol* 2000; **55**: 415–21.

●38. Chang DB, Yang PC, Luh KT, Kuo SH, Yu CJ. Ultrasound guided pleural biopsy with Tru-cut needle. *Chest* 1991; **100**: 1328–33.

39. Heilo A, Stenwig AE, Solheim OP. Malignant pleural mesothelioma: US-guided histologic core needle biopsy. *Radiology* 1999; **211**: 657–9.

40. McLeod DT, Ternouth I, Nkanza N. Comparison of the Tru-cut biopsy needle with the Abrams punch for pleural biopsy. *Thorax* 1989; **44**: 794–6.

41. Theron J, Diacon AH, Williams Z, Walzl G, Bolliger CT. Abrams versus TruCut needle in tuberculous pleuritis: a pilot study. *Eur Respir J* 2004; **24**: 73s.

●42. Diacon AH, Schuurmans MM, Theron J, *et al.* Safety and yield of ultrasound assisted transthoracic biopsy performed by pulmonologists. *Respiration* 2004; **71**: 519–22.

43. Diacon AH, Theron J, Schubert P, *et al.* Ultrasound-assisted transthoracic biopsy: fine-needle aspiration or cutting-needle biopsy? *Eur Respir J* 2007; **29**: 357–362.

44. Maskell NA, Gleeson FV, Davies RJ. Standard pleural biopsy versus CT-guided cutting-needle biopsy for diagnosis of malignant disease in pleural effusions: a randomised controlled trial. *Lancet* 2003; **361**: 1326–30.

45. Yang PC, Luh KT, Lee YC, *et al.* Lung abscesses: US examination and US-guided transthoracic aspiration. *Radiology* 1991; **180**: 171–75.

22

Pathology: histology

TIMOTHY C ALLEN, PHILIP T CAGLE

INTRODUCTION

Since neoplastic and non-neoplastic diseases of the pleura may produce very similar clinical, radiographic and gross findings, histopathology of pleural biopsies often has a crucial role in patient care. Surgical samples of pleural tissue may range from tiny needle biopsies to larger open or thoracoscopic biopsies to decortication specimens to extrapleural pneumonectomies.

Interpretation of pleural biopsies can be one of the most challenging areas in surgical pathology because of overlapping histopathological features of benign and malignant diseases, as well as among different types of malignancy. Sampling error, sample size and artifacts may impact on the ability to arrive at a diagnosis. Immunohistochemical stains are often used for problematic pleural biopsies and special panels of expert pleural pathologists, for example, the United States and Canadian Mesothelioma Reference Panel, have been set up for biopsy referrals.

NON-NEOPLASTIC LESIONS OF THE PLEURA

Fibrinous and fibrous pleuritis

Causes of fibrinous and fibrous pleuritis are discussed in detail elsewhere but include the following categories: (1) infections, including bacterial, viral, tuberculosis (TB), fungal and parasitic; (2) underlying pulmonary diseases, for example, pneumonias, abscesses, non-infectious inflammatory processes and malignancies; (3) leakage of air or blood from the lung; (4) collagen vascular diseases; (5) drug reactions; (6) asbestos exposure; (7) surgery and trauma; and (8) non-specific.[1]

Fibrinous pleuritis is characterized by fibrin deposits along the pleural surface, in the pleural cavity and in the superficial pleural tissue. Hemorrhage may be present in some biopsies, but may represent a procedural artifact. Fibrous pleuritis typically follows fibrinous pleuritis with in-growth of granulation tissue consisting of capillaries, fibroblasts and loose connective tissue stroma. Some biopsies will show a mixture of fibrinous and fibrous pleuritis as the exudative process begins to organize.

The number of inflammatory cell infiltrates in fibrinous and fibrous pleuritis may vary from essentially none to profuse. The type of inflammatory cells may be helpful in making a diagnosis. In infection and empyema especially, inflammatory cell infiltrates may be the dominant component of pleuritis and leukocytic (dirty) necrosis may be observed. Necrosis is not common in non-infectious pleuritis. Varying amounts of pleural effusion are also present in many cases of pleuritis and may provide important diagnostic information. Mesothelial cell hyperplasia is often seen in pleuritis and these cells shed into the pleural fluid. The mesothelial cells acquire a cuboidal shape with more abundant and denser cytoplasm. They may demonstrate features of increased cellularity, reactive cytological atypia, mitoses and immunoreactivity for keratin, calretinin and other mesothelial cell markers.

The typical histopathological findings in chronic pleuritis are mild to moderate lymphoplasmacytic infiltrates, possibly lymphoid aggregates with or without germinal centers and mild pleural fibrosis. Findings of a more specific diagnosis or more active fibrinous/fibrous pleuritis may occasionally be present elsewhere in the same biopsy and may surpass the findings of chronic pleuritis. Clinically, patients with these findings may have recurrent or persistent pleuritis accompanied by recurrent or persistent pleural effusions. Underlying lung tissue or parietal pleura included in a biopsy may provide clues to the cause of pleuritis; for example, pneumonia observed in subpleural lung tissue.

Eosinophilic pleuritis

In eosinophilic pleuritis there is an increased number of eosinophils, sometimes strikingly so, in the inflammatory infiltrate which otherwise may show features of fibrinous or fibrous pleuritis, mesothelial hyperplasia, etc. Since eosinophilic pleuritis is often associated with some distinctive clinical situations, there may be accompanying histopathological findings in any underlying lung tissue that may be sampled. A classic etiology of eosinophilic pleuritis is spontaneous pneumothorax, which occurs generally in young adults. In these cases, the eosinophilic pleuritis may be associated with focal blebs, bullae or focal honeycombing of the underlying lung tissue. Pneumothorax or hemothorax from a wide variety of causes can potentially result in eosinophilic pleuritis and lymphangioleiomyomatosis may be seen in the underlying lung tissue in women of childbearing age. Eosinophilic pleuritis may also be associated with certain drug reactions and infections which may also produce characteristic findings in the underlying lung tissue.

Granulomatous pleuritis

Granulomatous pleuritis is characterized by the presence of granulomatous inflammation, which may consist of well-formed granulomas or less circumscribed areas of granulomatous inflammation depending on the etiology. Granulomatous pleuritis is often accompanied by features of chronic pleuritis (i.e. chronic inflammation and fibrosis).

Infections, such as TB or fungal infections, that involve the pleura classically produce well-formed granulomas with or without central necrosis, but may occasionally form less circumscribed areas of granulomatous inflammation. It is important to remember that special stains for organisms, for example the acid-fast stain for tuberculosis or the Grocott's methenamine silver (GMS) stain for fungus, are very helpful when positive, but a negative special stain can occur even when infection is present. Therefore, cultures are always recommended even when special stains are negative.

Sarcoidosis is characterized by well-formed, compact granulomas in a lymphangitic distribution that includes the pleura. Significant necrosis is not a usual feature of sarcoidosis granulomas, although small punctate areas of necrosis may be present in some granulomas. Sarcoidosis granulomas may be surrounded by chronic inflammatory infiltrates or by fibrosis. Endogenous materials, for example, Schaumann bodies or calcium oxalate crystals, are often seen in the histiocytes of sarcoidosis, but are not pathognomonic and may be seen in other types of granulomas. These should not be mistaken for foreign material.

Wegener's granulomatosis (see Chapter 32, Effusions from connective tissue diseases) may involve the pleura and causes a less circumscribed type of granulomatous inflammation rather than well-formed granulomas. The classic histopathology picture is one of palisading histiocytes mixed with multinucleated giant cells, other inflammatory cells and fibroblasts surrounding a central area of necrosis. The necrosis begins as micro-abscesses with neutrophils and leukocytoclastic necrosis that coalesce and enlarge into so-called 'geographic' areas of basophilic necrosis. While these features and those of vasculitis can be seen in the pleura, Wegener's granulomatosis is usually diagnosed on a biopsy of lung tissue.

Foreign body granulomatous reactions may occur in the pleura. Most of these are the result of deliberate pleurodesis or iatrogenic instillation of foreign material into the pleural cavity to cause its obliteration for the purpose of treating recurrent pleural effusions.

Localized pleural fibrosis

Apical caps which also involve the subpleural tissue are often associated with emphysema. Apical caps consist of elastotic scars with thick fragments of elastic tissue with a grayish tint on hematoxylin and eosin (H&E) staining reminiscent of solar elastosis in the skin. An ischemic origin has been suggested for apical caps and these lesions do have a resemblance to scars from pulmonary infarcts.[2]

Pleural plaques show a histopathological pattern of dense, acellular collagen arranged in a distinctive basketweave pattern. Additional findings may include calcifications and ossification. Pleural plaques result from organized pleuritis and thus can result from many causes, including occupational levels of exposure to asbestos, chest surgery and trauma, and infections involving the pleura. Examination of the pleural plaques themselves for asbestos bodies is virtually always non-productive, even when the plaques are caused by asbestos exposure. The possible association of a pleural plaque with asbestos exposure is based on (1) observation of increased asbestos bodies in lung tissue sections and/or (2) the finding of elevated asbestos body or fiber concentrations on lung tissue digestion studies.

NEOPLASTIC LESIONS OF THE PLEURA

Benign or low-grade malignant mesothelial neoplasms

Well-differentiated papillary mesotheliomas are characterized by broad papillae lined by bland cuboidal mesothelial cells (Figure 22.1). These are most common in women and are more common in the peritoneum than in the pleura.

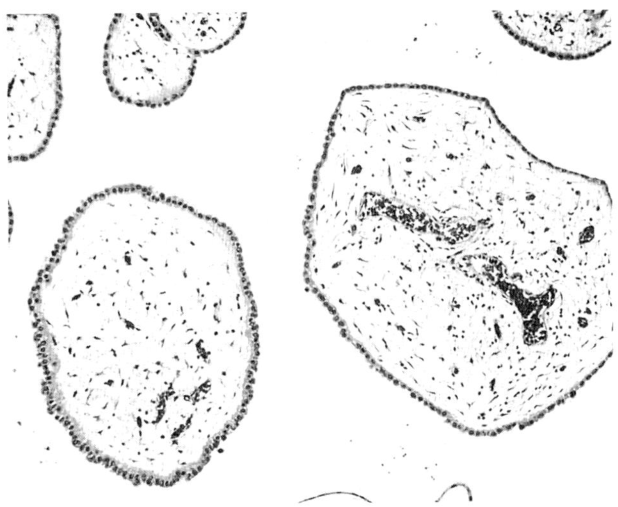

Figure 22.1 Well-differentiated papillary mesothelioma showing broad fibrous cores lined by bland cuboidal mesothelial cells. (See also Color Plate 13.)

Some are recurrent and, thus, considered of low-grade malignant potential, but even in these latter cases, patients survive for many years and do not develop metastases.[3–5]

Cystic/multicystic mesothelioma consists of a cyst or cysts lined by bland, cuboidal mesothelial cells. It has the same biological implications as well-differentiated papillary tumors.

Benign mesenchymal neoplasms of the pleura

Solitary fibrous tumor (see Chapter 38) is a well-circumscribed mass arising in the pleura and sometimes in the subpleural lung. Solitary fibrous tumor has several histopathological patterns: a cellular pattern with spindle cells to oval cells, a hemangiopericytoma pattern with staghorn blood vessels and a relatively acellular collagen pattern with slit-like spaces. Most solitary fibrous tumors are immunopositive for CD34 and this is a useful marker for confirming their diagnosis. Unlike mesotheliomas, solitary fibrous tumors are immunonegative for keratin. Other benign mesenchymal neoplasms of the pleura include lipoma and Schwannoma.[6,7]

Malignant mesothelial neoplasms

Diffuse malignant mesothelioma (see Chapter 41) is characterized grossly by a growth pattern that encases the pleura or presents as a widespread multiple studding of the pleural surface. Metastatic carcinomas and other metastatic malignancies may also grow in either of these patterns and it is necessary to obtain a tissue sample to confirm the diagnosis of diffuse malignant mesothelioma rather than other malignancies. Diffuse malignant mesothelioma has a variety of histopathological patterns and, therefore, can potentially mimic many other types of cancer on H&E staining and vice versa. Basic histopathological patterns of mesothelioma are listed in Table 22.1 (Figures 22.2 and 22.3).[4,5,8–11]

Table 22.1 Histopathology patterns of malignant mesothelioma

Histopathology patterns	
Epithelial	Tubulopapillary, epithelial/mesothelial, adenomatoid
Sarcomatous	Sarcomatous, rarely with heterologous elements (bone, cartilage)
Biphasic	Mixed epithelial and sarcomatous patterns
Desmoplastic	Predominance of connective tissue with scant cellularity in much of the tumor, usually sarcomatous, may be epithelial

Immunostains are recommended to distinguish mesotheliomas from other types of cancer. For many years there were no antibodies specific to mesotheliomas and a diagnosis of mesothelioma typically involved an attempt to exclude other types of cancer in the differential diagnosis. At present, even with a few new antibodies that are relatively specific for mesothelioma, anyone interpreting immunostains for the differential diagnosis of mesothelioma must be aware of certain caveats:

1 *Negativity for an antibody does not, by itself, confirm mesothelioma.* (i) Many of the immunostains typically used to rule out carcinoma apply primarily to lung cancers, particularly adenocarcinomas. One must remember that carcinomas from primary sites other than the lung and malignancies other than carcinoma

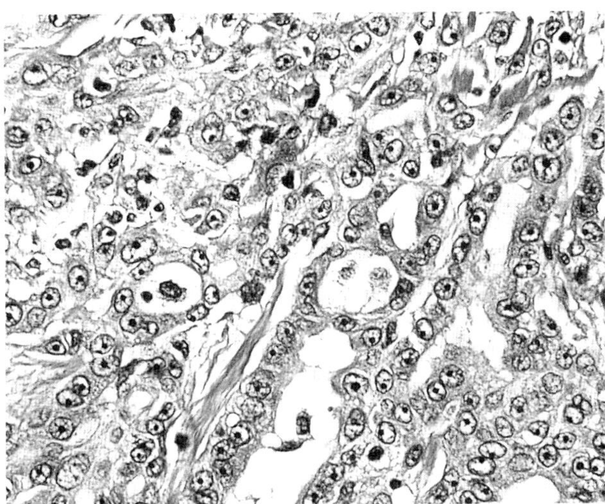

Figure 22.2 Epithelial malignant mesothelioma showing relatively bland polygonal cells with round nuclei and prominent nucleoli. (See also Color Plate 14.)

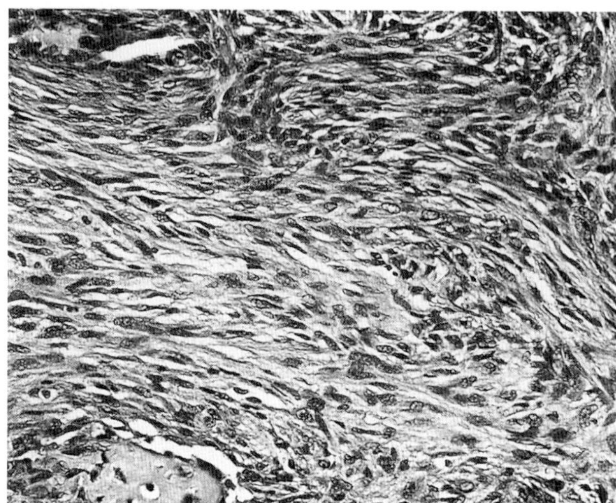

Figure 22.3 Sarcomatous malignant mesothelioma showing malignant spindle cells resembling a fibrosarcoma or malignant fibrous histiocytoma. (See also Color Plate 15.)

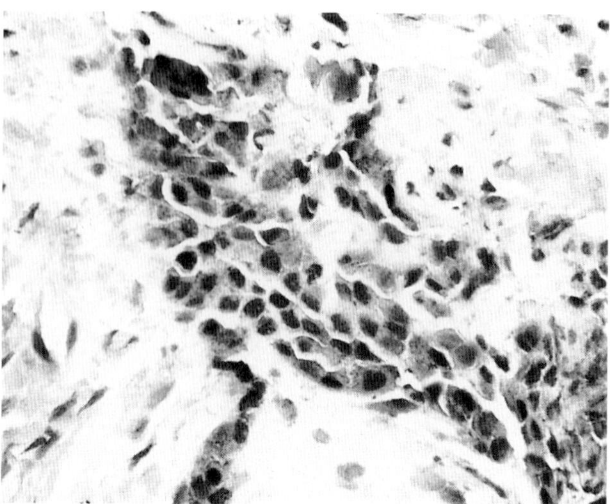

Figure 22.4 Immunostain for calretinin showing intranuclear immunopositivity in an epithelial malignant mesothelioma. (See also Color Plate 16.)

(for example, melanoma) may metastasize to the pleura. Metastatic renal cell carcinomas, for example, are typically negative for all of the traditional lung carcinoma markers such as carcinoembryonic antigen (CEA). Therefore, ruling out only adenocarcinoma of the lung by immunostains does not, by itself, confirm a diagnosis of mesothelioma. (ii) Even a well-differentiated adenocarcinoma of the lung may be immunonegative for one or more markers typically associated with lung cancer.

2. *Negativity for an antibody does not, by itself, confirm or exclude a diagnosis.* It is not unusual for poorly differentiated mesotheliomas, as well as poorly differentiated malignancies of other types, to fail to express markers seen in better-differentiated tumors of the same type. Poorly differentiated, pleomorphic and sarcomatous lung carcinomas are often negative for CEA and other lung cancer markers and only immunopositive for vimentin and keratin. Poorly differentiated and sarcomatous mesotheliomas are often negative for calretinin and other mesothelioma markers and only immunopositive for vimentin and keratin. Therefore, immunostains might not distinguish between poorly differentiated or sarcomatous mesotheliomas and poorly differentiated or sarcomatous carcinomas, or other poorly differentiated malignancies.
3. *Staining with an antibody may require interpretation according to very specific criteria before it can be considered positive.* For example, the reliability of calretinin depends on the antibody used and only nuclear immunostaining is meaningful. Cytoplasmic calretinin immunostaining may be seen in many types of carcinoma and even in mesotheliomas and should not be considered support for a diagnosis of mesothelioma in those cases. The antihuman mesothelial cell antibody HBME-1 indicates mesothelioma when staining is thick and continuous around the cell border, but indicates carcinoma when staining is thin, discontinuous or cytoplasmic. Specific criteria for interpretation also apply to other antibodies.

For the reasons given above, a panel of immunostains is recommended to distinguish diffuse malignant mesothelioma from other cancers (Figure 22.4). Characteristic immunostain results for malignant mesothelioma versus selected malignancies of other types are given in Table 22.2.[4,5,8–19]

The diagnosis of diffuse malignant mesothelioma, like the diagnosis of any other malignancy, should be based on the routine histopathology and immunostaining pattern of a tumor tissue sample when the tumor has a gross distribution potentially consistent with the diagnosis. The mere fact that an individual is reported to have a history of elevated asbestos exposure is not a basis for making the diagnosis of mesothelioma. Most individuals with a history of elevated asbestos exposure who have cancer will have cancers other than mesothelioma. Similarly, a diagnosis of mesothelioma should not be excluded simply because there is no history of asbestos exposure.

Distinguishing malignant mesothelioma from benign reactive mesothelial hyperplasias and fibrous pleuritis on biopsy can be a very difficult challenge, particularly on a small biopsy (Figure 22.5). Benign proliferations may show features that mimic those seen in malignancy and malignant mesothelioma can be very bland or biopsies may sample very early malignant lesions. Features that favor benign versus malignant mesothelial proliferations are listed in Table 22.3. Ultimately, the presence of true tissue invasion is the most reliable feature to distinguish a malignant mesothelioma but, even then, the pathologist should be aware that entrapment of benign mesothelial cells within fibrous pleuritis may mimic invasion. It should

Table 22.2 Characteristic results for selected immunostains for malignant mesothelioma versus other malignancies

	Mesothelioma	Carcinoma	Sarcoma	Melanoma
Keratin	1	1	2 (occasionally 1)	2 (rarely 1)
CK5/6	1/2	-2/1	2	2
Vimentin	1/2	2/1	1	1
Calretinin	1 (nuclear)	2 (rarely 1)	2 (rarely 1)	2
CEA, B72.3, Leu M-1, BerEP4	2	1/2	2	2
TTF-1	2	1 (lung and thyroid)	2	2
EMA	1	1	2	2 (epithelial)
HBME-1	1 (epithelial) (thick, continuous), (thin, discontinuous)	1	2	2

CK5/6, cytokeratin 5/6; TTF-1, thyroid transcription factor 1; EMA, epithelial membrane antigen; HBME-1, antihuman mesothelial cell antibody.

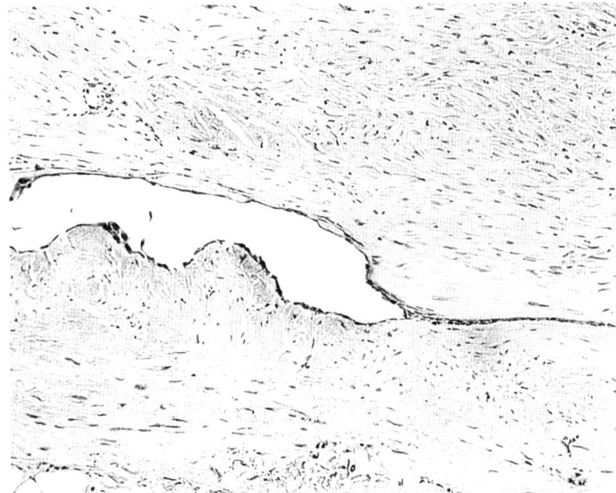

Figure 22.5 Entrapment of reactive mesothelial cells within fibrous pleuritis mimicking invasion by malignant mesothelioma. (See also Color Plate 17.)

be noted that, except for the use of keratin immunostain to assess for invasion, no current immunostains reliably distinguish between benign reactive and malignant mesothelial cells and should not be used as a basis for diagnosis. When a definitive diagnosis of benign versus malignant cannot be reached, 'atypical mesothelial hyperplasia' or similar diagnosis should be made by the pathologist and a decision about obtaining additional tissue samples, observing the patient, etc., can then be made by the clinician.[20–22]

OTHER RARE PRIMARY MALIGNANT NEOPLASMS OF THE PLEURA

Very rarely, neoplasms with all of the histopathological features of diffuse malignant mesothelioma may occur as localized, often pedunculated, masses of the pleura. These lesions have been called localized malignant mesothe-

Table 22.3 Features suggestive of benign versus malignant mesothelial proliferations

Suggestive features
Features potentially observed in benign and malignant proliferations: 1 Cellularity 2 Cytological atypia 3 Architectural atypia 4 Mitoses
Features favoring benign proliferation: 1 Active fibrin deposition with active inflammation (inflammation may also be seen in malignant mesothelioma) 2 Linear arrays of individual cells and small glands parallel to pleural surface 3 Simple, non-branching glands 4 Proliferating mesothelial cells separated by large amounts of stroma 5 Proliferating cells limited toward pleural cavity in a thickened pleura with more fibrosis toward chest 6 May show highly cellular proliferation into the pleural space but not into the underlying fibrous tissue 7 Parallel arrays of vessels/capillaries perpendicular to pleural surface
Features favoring malignant proliferation: 1 Unequivocal invasion is the most reliable criterion for the diagnosis of mesothelioma 2 Bland necrosis 3 Areas that have unequivocal malignant features: cytological malignancy, abnormal mitoses and/or frankly sarcomatoid pattern, etc. 4 Cellularity of the atypical cells throughout the full thickness of the pleura 5 Distinct tumor nodules

liomas. Although these neoplasms are amenable to surgical excision and patients generally have a good to excellent prognosis, they are most likely malignant neoplasms.[7]

Desmoplastic small round cell tumor is usually seen in children, adolescents and young adults and is usually peritoneal but can arise or extend into the pleura.[23]

Other rare primary malignancies of the pleura include the malignant variant of solitary fibrous tumor, synovial sarcoma, osteosarcoma, chondrosarcoma, angiosarcoma and malignant fibrous histiocytoma.[7,14,24]

FUTURE DIRECTIONS

The advent of experimental therapies for mesothelioma provides greater incentive for earlier diagnosis of this disease. Coincidentally, the diagnosis of mesothelioma at earlier stages of disease is increasingly possible as a result of the greater availability and popularity of techniques such as thoracoscopic biopsy. Hence, in the near future, the diagnosis of mesothelioma should entail improved patient therapy and, therefore, accurate diagnosis will be even more important than in the past. Better opportunities to provide meaningful therapy for patients will enhance interest in the development of antibodies and molecular markers for the early and accurate diagnosis of mesothelioma on biopsy.

KEY POINTS

- Carcinomas and other malignancies may grow in patterns that grossly mimic mesothelioma and it is necessary to obtain a tissue sample to confirm the diagnosis of diffuse malignant mesothelioma versus other malignancies.
- Diffuse malignant mesothelioma has a variety of histopathological patterns and, therefore, can potentially mimic many other types of cancer on H&E staining, and vice versa. Immunostains are often helpful in distinguishing diffuse malignant mesothelioma from other malignancies in these situations.
- A panel of immunostains is recommended to distinguish diffuse malignant mesothelioma from other cancers.
- Distinguishing malignant mesothelioma from benign reactive mesothelial hyperplasias and fibrous pleuritis on biopsy can be a very difficult challenge, particularly on a small biopsy.
- Unequivocal invasion is the most reliable criterion for diagnosing mesothelioma when there is a differential diagnosis of benign reactive mesothelial hyperplasia or fibrous pleuritis versus mesothelioma.

REFERENCES

● = Key primary paper
◆ = Major review article

1. Churg A. Diseases of the pleura. In: Thurlbeck WM, Churg AM (eds). *Pathology of the lung*, 2nd edn. New York: Thieme, 1995; 1067–110.
2. Yousem SA. Pulmonary apical cap: a distinctive but poorly recognized lesion in pulmonary surgical pathology. *Am J Surg Pathol* 2001; **25**: 679–83.
3. Cagle PT, Murer B. Clinicopathologic features of well-differentiated papillary mesothelioma. *Mod Pathol* 2002; **15**: 317A.
4. Roggli VL, Sanfilippo F, Shelburne JD. Mesothelioma. In: Roggli VL, Greenberg SD, Pratt PC (eds). *Pathology of asbestos-associated diseases.* Boston: Little, Brown & Company, 1992; 109–64.
5. Churg A. Neoplastic asbestos-induced disease. In: Churg A, Green FHY (eds). *Pathology of occupational lung disease*, 2nd edn. Baltimore: Williams & Wilkins, 1998; 339–91.
6. Ordonez NG. Localized (solitary) fibrous tumor of the pleura. *Adv Anat Pathol* 2000; **7**: 327–40.
7. Churg A. Localized pleural tumors. In: Cagle PT (ed.). *Diagnostic pulmonary pathology.* New York: Marcel Dekker, 2000; 719–34.
◆8. Attanoos RL, Gibbs AR. Pathology of malignant mesothelioma. *Histopathology* 1997; **30**: 403–18.
9. Hammar SP. Spindle-cell neoplasms of lung and pleura. In: Cagle PT (ed.). *Diagnostic pulmonary pathology.* New York: Marcel Dekker, 2000; 649–64.
10. Hasleton P. Biphasic pulmonary neoplasms. In: Cagle PT (ed.). *Diagnostic pulmonary pathology.* New York: Marcel Dekker, 2000; 665–83.
11. Yousem SA, Hochholzer L. Malignant mesothelioma with osseous and cartilaginous differentiation. *Arch Pathol Lab Med* 1987; **111**: 62–6.
12. Taylor DR, Page W, Hughes D, Varghese G. Metastatic renal cell carcinoma mimicking pleural mesothelioma. *Thorax* 1987; **42**: 901–2.
13. Bailey ME, Brown RW, Mody DR, Cagle PT, Ramzy I. BER-EP4 differentiates adenocarcinoma from reactive and neoplastic mesothelial cells in serous effusions: a comparison with CEA, B72.3 and Leu M-1. *Acta Cytologica* 1996; **40**: 1212–16.
14. Gaertner E, Zeren EH, Fleming MV, Colby TV, Travis WD. Biphasic synovial sarcomas arising in the pleural cavity. A clinicopathologic study of five cases. *Am J Surg Pathol* 1996; **20**: 36–45.
15. Ordonez NG. Value of cytokeratin 5/6 immunostaining in distinguishing epithelial mesothelioma of the pleura from lung adenocarcinoma. *Am J Surg Pathol* 1998; **22**: 1215–21.
16. Ordonez NG. Value of calretinin immunostaining in differentiating epithelial mesothelioma from lung adenocarcinoma. *Mod Pathol* 1998; **11**: 929–33.
●17. Khoor A, Whitsett JA, Stahlman MT, Olson SJ, Cagle PT. Utility of surfactant protein B precursor and thyroid transcription factor 1 in differentiating adenocarcinoma of the lung from malignant mesothelioma. *Hum Pathol* 1999; **30**: 695–700.
◆18. Ordonez NG. Role of immunohistochemistry in differentiating epithelial mesothelioma from adenocarcinoma. Review and update. *Am J Clin Pathol* 1999; **112**: 75–89.
19. Miettinen M, Limon J, Niezabitowski A, Lasota J. Calretinin and other mesothelioma markers in synovial sarcoma: analysis of antigenic similarities and differences with malignant mesothelioma. *Am J Surg Pathol* 2001; **25**: 610–17.
●20. Mangano WE, Cagle PT, Churg A, Vollmer RT, Roggli VL. The diagnosis of desmoplastic malignant mesothelioma and its distinction from fibrous pleurisy: a histologic and immunohistochemical analysis of 31 cases including p53 immunostaining. *Am J Clin Pathol* 1998; **110**: 191–9.

◆21. Churg A, Colby TV, Cagle PT, *et al.* The separation of benign and malignant mesothelial proliferations. *Am J Surg Pathol* 2000; **24**: 1183–200.

22. Galateau-Sallé F, Cagle PT. Non-malignant versus malignant proliferations on pleural biopsy. In: Cagle PT (ed.). *Diagnostic pulmonary pathology.* New York: Marcel Dekker, 2000; 555–67.

23. Parkash V, Gerald WL, Parma A, Miettinen M, Rosai J. Desmoplastic small round cell tumor of the pleura. *Am J Surg Pathol* 1995; **19**: 659–65.

24. Zhang PJ, Livolsi VA, Brooks JJ. Malignant epithelioid vascular tumors of the pleura: report of a series and literature review. *Hum Pathol* 2000; **31**: 29–34.

23

Pathology: cytology

MARK R WICK

Interpreting pleural fluid specimens is often a challenging task even for the experienced cytopathologists. Reactive but benign epithelial cells may closely resemble malignancies in effusion cytomorphology; conversely, carcinoma cells in pleural effusions can be deceptively bland. Mesenchymal and hematopoietic proliferations likewise may require extensive additional studies with adjunctive techniques. This chapter aims to describe current approaches for the resolution of interpretative problems in cytopathology of the pleura. Conditions such as hemothorax, chylothorax and pneumothorax relating to structural disorders of the chest are not considered herein, because their diagnosis are relatively straightforward.

GENERAL CLINICOPATHOLOGY CONSIDERATIONS IN THE DIAGNOSIS OF PLEURAL NEOPLASMS

Shortness of breath, chest pain and a flu-like illness are common presentations of patients with inflammatory or malignant pleural diseases.[1,2] Thoracentesis is typically the first diagnostic procedure employed in evaluation of fluid in the pleural cavities. In benign conditions, the cytological presentation is usually that of moderate cellularity, showing only scant mixed inflammatory cells and benign mesothelial elements, or, alternatively, a predominance of specific leukocytes. The first situation may be seen in association with cardiac, renal or hepatic insufficiency; some cases of viral pleuritis; and pneumoconioses affecting the pleura (e.g. asbestos pleuritis).[3] The second scenario accompanies empyema or parapneumonic pleural effusions, in which cases the fluid is neutrophil-rich, as well as connective tissue diseases, tuberculosis, fungal pleuritis and most viral infections.[4,5] In the last four of those disorders, many mature lymphocytes are often observed and may mimic a well-differentiated lymphoproliferative disorder.[6] Flow cytometry or immunohistology are commonly required. It is distinctly unusual to observe granulomatous histiocytic arrays in pleural cytology specimens or in pleural biopsies.

Metastatic carcinomas, melanomas and lymphomas in the pleura often shed freely into effusions, but there still remain a sizable proportion of such cases (30–40 percent) for which cytological examination is non-diagnostic. Reasons for that phenomenon are twofold: some pleural malignancies demonstrate a high degree of intercellular cohesion, with a limited tendency to seed the pleural fluid, and, second, a fibrinofibrous 'cap' often covers malignancies in the pleural soft tissue. This effectively walls off underlying tumor cells from the interserosal space. Moreover, benign mesothelial cells on the surface of the cap may shed into the pleural fluid and further obscure the true nature of the underlying pathological process. The overall efficacy of cytopathological evaluation of pleural fluid for the detection of mesothelioma approximates only 30 percent in the author's experience. The diagnostic yield is highest with epithelial mesothelioma and lowest in sarcomatoid tumors.

When processing pleural fluid samples for microscopy, it is important that a good cell-block preparation (formalin-fixed and paraffin-embedded) be obtained in order to evaluate cells by immunohistochemistry. This provision circumvents the many technical problems that can be encountered in attempting such studies with conventional cytological specimens (i.e. cytospins and filter preparations).[7] A centrifuged pellet of cells from the effusion may be suspended in nutrient solutions such as Michel's medium or RPMI medium, and submitted for flow cytometry and cytogenetic analysis. For those adjunctive techniques to be performed optimally, it is important to deliver the pleural fluid promptly (within 1 hour) to the laboratory, along with a complete clinical synopsis of the case.

If a surgical specimen is to be obtained, the author prefers video-assisted thoracoscopic (VATS) biopsies.[8] In addition to providing a more sizable and representative tissue specimen, VATS allows the surgeon to avoid sampling aforementioned fibrinofibrous 'caps' over pleural neoplasms rather than the tumors themselves.

Mesothelial hyperplasia, either in association with infection or sterile inflammation, may be so marked that it resembles mesothelioma. Benign mesothelial proliferations may yield very cellular effusion specimens (Figure 23.1), and papillary intrapleural fronds of mesothelium (Figure 23.2), simulating those of mesothelioma, may be observed in biopsy specimens.[10] Moreover, the degree of nuclear atypia that is potentially exhibited in some mesothelial hyperplasias is disturbing.[11] Inasmuch as there are currently no absolutely reliable methods to separate benign from malignant mesothelial lesions, serial sampling of pleural fluid may be necessary to establish a diagnosis. If a mesothelioma is present, it will eventually 'declare' itself. Because there is no cure for mesothelioma, little if anything is lost in waiting to assign a diagnostic label until it is certain.

Some neoplasms have such a distinctive morphology in their 'classical' forms that traditional cytopathological examination alone is capable of providing a detailed and definitive diagnosis. For example, the cells of metastatic breast carcinomas often assume a morular configuration in pleural fluid[12–14] (Figure 23.3), and may also demonstrate the presence of intracytoplasmic lumina[15] (Figure 23.4). Similarly, metastatic melanoma manifests a higher degree of nuclear and cellular pleomorphism than that seen in association with other epithelioid malignancies (Figure 23.5); intranuclear cytoplasmic invaginations and cytoplasmic pigmentation (green on Romanowsky stains) may also be noted in melanomas.[16–18] Some melanomas may assume a spindle cell pattern and even acquire myxoid or hyaline stromal changes, simulating metastatic sarcomas. The presence of numerous osteoclast-like giant cells in a background of highly pleomorphic cells may simulate malignant fibrous histiocytoma, but is a recognized feature in metastatic melanoma.[19] Another rather unusual morphological manifestation of malignant melanoma metastasized to the pleura is the presence of a heavy neutrophilic interstitial infiltrate admixed with the melanoma cells.[20] In the pleura, this appearance may suggest metastatic large-cell undifferentiated carcinoma. Other unusual patterns of malignant melanoma include a signet ring cell configuration, simulating metastatic gastric carcinoma,

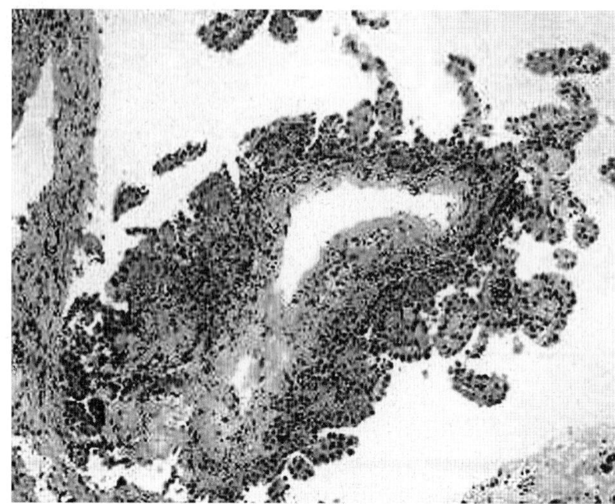

Figure 23.2 A micropapillary fragment is seen in this cell block from a pleural effusion demonstrating mesothelial hyperplasia. (See also Color Plate 19.)

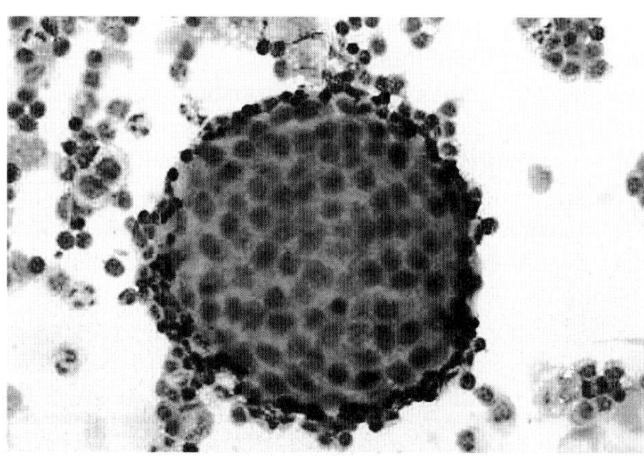

Figure 23.3 A morular, three-dimensional cellular aggregate is present in this pleural effusion specimen demonstrating metastatic ductal breast carcinoma. (See also Color Plate 20.)

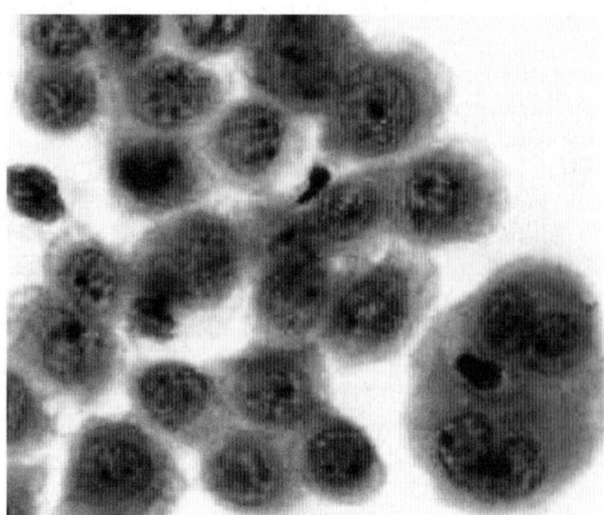

Figure 23.1 Mesothelial hyperplasia in a pleural effusion specimen. Note the dense cellularity and modest cellular pleomorphism, with intercellular spaces or 'windows.' (See also Color Plate 18.)

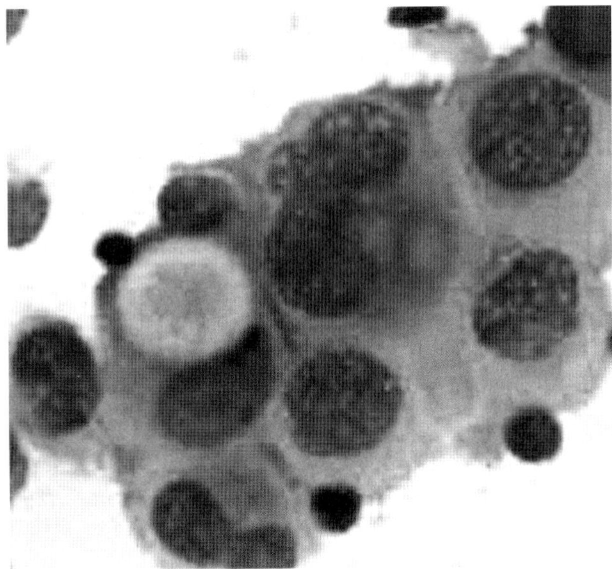

Figure 23.4 An intracytoplasmic mucus-containing inclusion is apparent in this cytological specimen of metastatic lobular mammary carcinoma in pleural fluid. (See also Color Plate 21.)

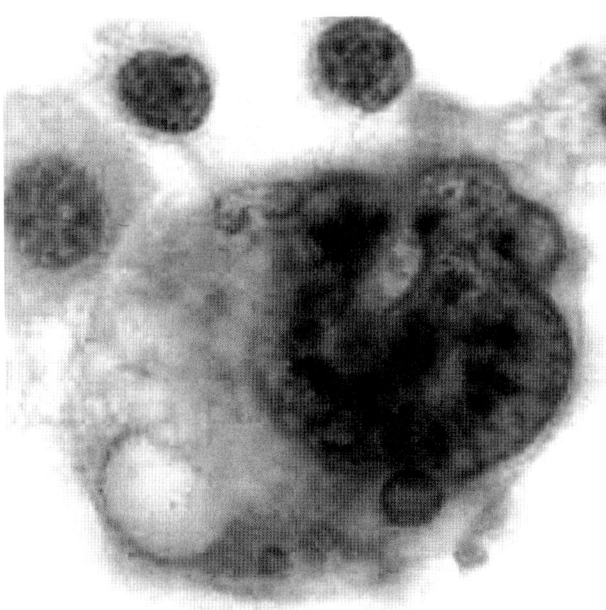

Figure 23.5 Metastatic melanoma in pleural fluid, showing marked nuclear pleomorphism. (See also Color Plate 22.)

and tumors composed of granular, uniformly epithelioid cells.[21]

There are several possible cytopathological presentations of malignant mesothelioma,[22] and these are discussed in greater detail later. The morphological appearances of this tumor type include small-cell, large-polygonal-cell and sarcomatoid lesions, or combinations thereof.

Lymphomas and leukemias uncommonly manifest themselves in the pleural spaces in the absence of known disease elsewhere in the body. This eventuality is most often seen in the context of acquired immunodeficiency syndrome and coinfection with the herpesvirus-8 agent.[24] Hematopoietic malignancies show a dispersion of dyshesive medium-sized or large polygonal cells in the pleural fluid (Figure 23.6), and Romanowsky stains often reveal irregularity of the nuclear contours and cytoplasmic vacuolization or granulation in such cellular elements[6,24–26] (Figures 23.7 and 23.8). Non-Hodgkin's lymphomas are

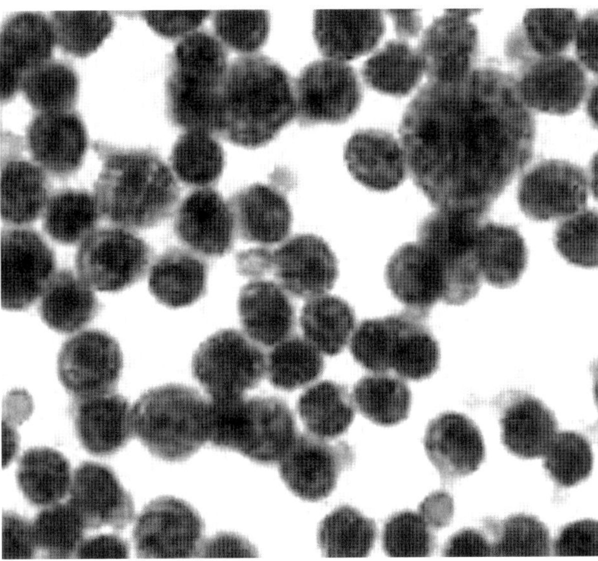

Figure 23.6 Dispersed small lymphoid cells in a lymphocyte-rich pleural effusion. The large cell in the field is a mesothelial cell. An image such as this may reflect the presence of pleural tuberculosis, collagen vascular disease or a lymphoproliferative disorder. (See also Color Plate 23.)

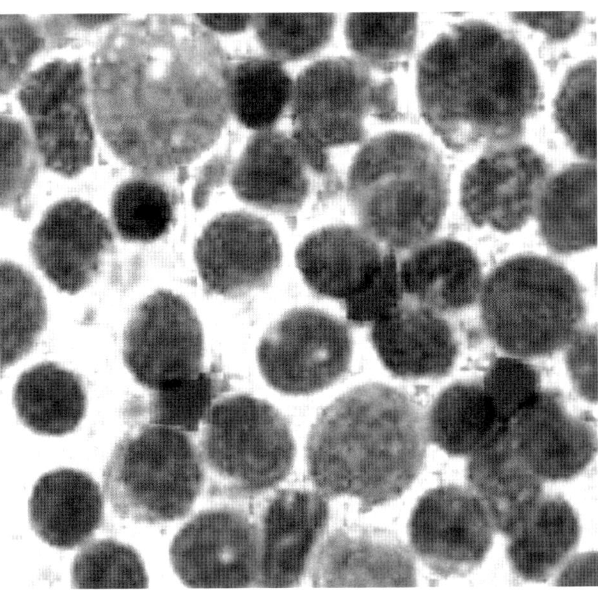

Figure 23.7 Cytoplasmic vacuoles are seen in the cells of this malignant lymphoma in pleural fluid. (See also Color Plate 24.)

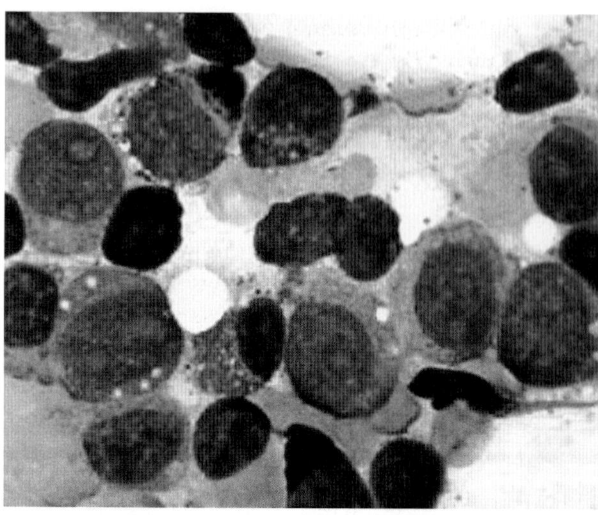

Figure 23.8 Infiltration of pleural fluid by tumor cells of acute myelogenous leukemia, with prominent cytoplasmic granulation and vacuolization. (See also Color Plate 25.)

many times more common than Hodgkin's disease as pleural lesions.

Metastatic sarcoma in the pleura is typically not problematic diagnostically for pathologists, because the patients have had a prior lesion elsewhere. Primary pleural sarcomas are extraordinarily rare, and they require immunohistochemical assessment to distinguish them from sarcomatid carcinomas and melanomas, as described below.

CYTOPATHOLOGICAL 'PARTITIONS' IN THE DIAGNOSIS OF PLEURAL NEOPLASMS

A useful method of approaching the cytopathological diagnosis of pleural neoplasms, the overwhelming majority of which are malignant, is to divide them into general groupings which share morphologic similarities.[27,28] These are presented in the following sections.

Malignant small round-cell

Small round-cell tumors (SRCT) has traditionally been used in reference to a heterogeneous group of neoplasms that occur primarily in the soft tissue in childhood and adolescence. Nonetheless, they have a propensity to involve the pleura and lungs metastatically. Moreover, some primary lesions in this general category – such as the 'Askin tumor' and synovial sarcoma – may arise in the pleura and adjacent thoracic soft tissue.[29]

These lesions share the histological image of a densely cellular proliferation with a primitive, undifferentiated appearance, and each of them may present with distant metastases to lymph nodes or viscera. SRCT is a descriptive rather than a specific diagnostic designation, and there are important therapeutic and prognostic differences attached to the different entities that comprise this group. Adjunctive techniques – especially immunohistochemical studies, cytogenetics, and flow cytometry – are critical in refining pathological interpretation and should be regarded as routine evaluation.[29,30]

Our initial focus will be on the morphological characteristics that are observed in the different tumors in this category. These principally include Ewing's sarcoma and primitive neuroectodermal tumor (both of which are considered to be part of the same neoplastic disease spectrum), juvenile-type rhabdomyosarcoma (RMS), neuroblastoma and small-cell carcinomas.

Histologically, both primitive neuroectodermal tumor (PNET) and Ewing's sarcoma (ES) are composed of relatively monomorphic cells with round to oval nuclei and scant cytoplasm.[29–33] True rosettes and pseudorosettes are potentially seen in this spectrum of neoplasms. The chromatin pattern is somewhat variable, ranging from fine and homogeneous to irregularly clumped, usually with relatively indistinct nucleoli. The presence of rosettes correlates with primitive neural differentiation (i.e. the PNET portion of the tumor spectrum), but frequently these structures are absent. Surprisingly few mitotic figures are typically visible. Cytological samples of ES/PNET typically are highly cellular and are composed of a distinctly dimorphic cell population. Large cells demonstrating 'blastic' chromatin usually predominate, and these are intermingled with smaller cells showing dense, condensed chromatin and resembling mature lymphocytes. It should be noted that a dimorphic population is not diagnostic of ES/PNET in a SRCT, because degenerative changes or pyknosis may simulate this finding. When they are present, cytoplasmic vacuoles in ES/PNET are coarse and 'punched out' in Romanowsky-stained preparations; finely vacuolated cytoplasm also may be encountered. The cytological presence of wispy cytoplasmic extensions is also possible. Histochemical positivity with the periodic acid–Schiff (PAS) reagent is more typical of the ES pole of the ES-PNET spectrum,[29] but it may indeed be seen in lesions with more neural morphological qualities as well. Yet another member of the 'Ewing family' of tumors is the desmoplastic small round-cell tumor (DSRCT). It is typically encountered in the peritoneal cavity of young patients,[34,35] but has also been described as a primary pleural lesion.[36] DSRCT differs from classical PNET in exhibiting a more fibrogenic and collagenized stroma, with compartmentalization of the tumor cells by such matrix.[32,37] It also shows divergent epithelial and myogenous differentiation, in contrast to *type ordinaire* ES and PNET.

Other tumor types may assume partial or global histological images which simulate those of ES/PNET, especially in limited pathologic samples. This includes primary or metastatic small-cell ('undifferentiated') synovial sarcoma[30,38] and lymphoblastic lymphoma. The former group demonstrates more nuclear irregularity, apoptotic cellular dropout and mitotic activity, and also may show 'lymphoglandular bodies' in cytological preparations.[25,26]

Rhabdomyosarcoma of the 'solid-alveolar' variety demonstrates a somewhat greater degree of nuclear pleomorphism than that seen in other SRCTs, occasionally with interspersed large cells possessing relatively generous amounts of eosinophilic cytoplasm[39,40] (Figure 23.9). Nuclei are not dissimilar in appearance to those of ES/PNET, and LRMS also shares potential PAS-positivity with neuroectodermal tumors. If foci suggesting an 'alveolar' (dyshesive) growth pattern are observed in a PAS-reactive SRCT, the diagnosis of rhabdomyosarcoma should be favored.

A large percentage of neuroblastoma (NB) cases present with metastases, with or without elevated urinary levels of catecholamines or their metabolites.[41,42] The primary tumors may reside in the adrenal medulla or the remainder of the sympathetic nervous system. Metastatic NB may be extremely difficult to distinguish from ES/PNET or other SRCT, particularly in small biopsies or cytological specimens. In particular, there is a rare glycogen-rich form of NB which bears a striking morphological resemblance to neuroectodermal neoplasms. Neuroblastoma is composed of primitive round to angulated cells with scant cytoplasm. Well-formed true rosettes and pseudorosettes, neuropil formation and dystrophic calcification may aid in the diagnosis of this lesion. A careful search is also worthwhile for primitive or mature ganglionic elements, represented by nucleolated cells with eccentric, relatively abundant eosinophilic cytoplasm.[43]

Small-cell neuroendocrine carcinomas (SCNCs) are, perhaps, the most important of the SRCTs that may present as a malignant pleural tumor of uncertain type, because of their relative commonality in adults.[44] The histological appearance is that of a variably-organoid proliferation of extensively apoptotic small neoplastic cells with brisk mitotic activity, often demonstrating prominent crush artifact. Cytologically, these neoplasms are composed of small cells with high nuclear-to-cytoplasmic ratios, nuclear 'smearing,' crush artifact, nuclear 'molding,' powdery chromatin, inconspicuous nucleoli, scant cytoplasm and a tendency for loose cohesion and cellular dispersion[45] (Figures 23.10 and 23.11). Staining with Romanowsky methods may reveal fine metachromatic

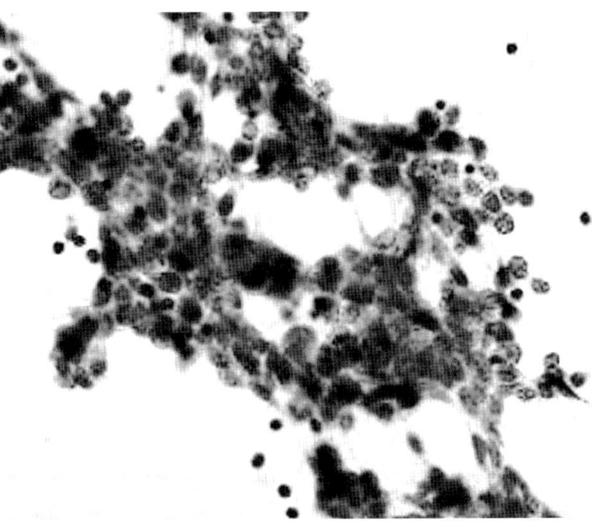

Figure 23.10 Metastatic small-cell neuroendocrine carcinoma ('oat-cell carcinoma') of the lung in pleural fluid. The tumor cells show nuclear molding and high nuclear-to-cytoplasmic ratios. (See also Color Plate 27.)

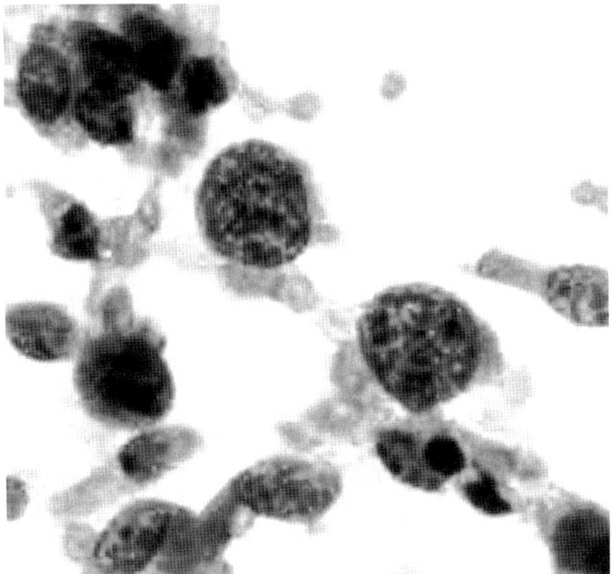

Figure 23.9 Metastatic rhabdomyosarcoma in pleural fluid, demonstrating cellular dyshesion and slight nuclear pleomorphism in small tumor cells. (See also Color Plate 26.)

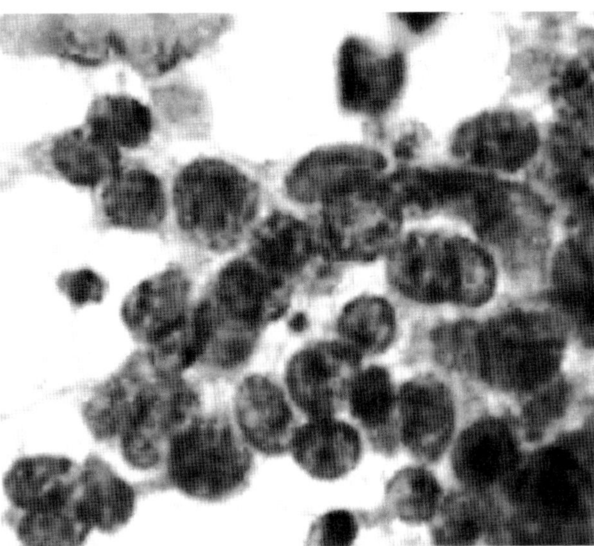

Figure 23.11 Metastatic small-cell neuroendocrine carcinoma in a pleural effusion specimen. Nuclear molding and dispersion of chromatin is evident. (See also Color Plate 28.)

cytoplasmic granules. Reactivity with argyrophilic histochemical techniques such as the Sevier–Munger, Grimelius or Churukian–Schenk procedures is helpful in recognizing that small-cell carcinomas have neuroendocrine features.

Once metastatic SCNCs are identified as such, there are few other nuances of morphology or biochemistry that can be used with certainty to predict their anatomic sources. In particular, cellular peptide and amine products are broadly shared among this group of neoplasms, regardless of their topographic origins. Hence, anatomic patterns of metastasis and the relative frequency of SCNC in various organ systems must be used as the principal data in determining the likely source. The lung is by far the most common origin for metastatic small-cell carcinomas in the pleura.

Small-cell mesotheliomas also exist, albeit rarely.[46] These tumors are rather nondescript cytologically and histologically, and they most closely simulate the appearances of small-cell carcinomas. Adjunctive pathologic studies are mandatory.

Malignant large-polygonal-cell tumors

Large-polygonal-cell tumors can be subdivided into neoplasms with amphophilic cytoplasm, cytoplasmic eosinophilia and clear-cell features.

Malignant oncocytic tumors

Cells showing intense cytoplasmic acidophilia (eosinophilia) (Figure 23.12) have been referred to using a variety of terms, including oncocyte, oxyphil, Hurthle-cell, Ashkenazy-cell and others, although one classically regards oncocytoid change to reflect to an abundance of mitochondria or other cytoplasmic organelles such as lysosomes, neuroendocrine granules, cytofilaments and smooth endoplasmic reticulum.[47]

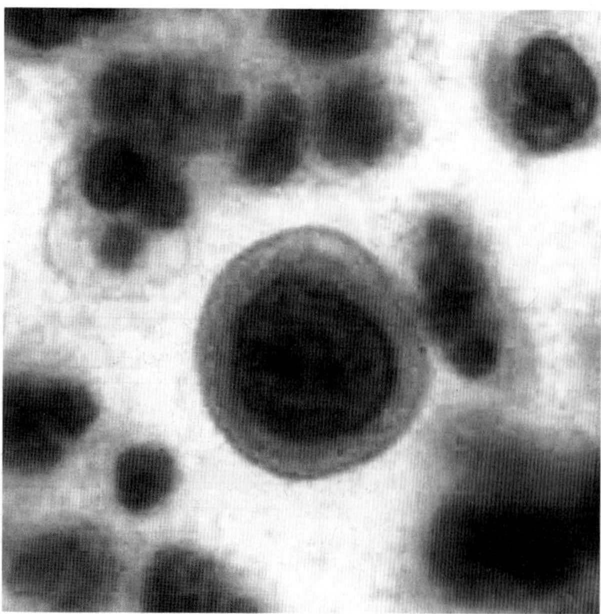

Figure 23.12 Prototypical large malignant cell with 'oncocytic' cytoplasm in metastatic large-cell carcinoma of the lung involving pleural fluid. (See also Color Plate 29.)

Oncocytic neoplasms arise most often in the salivary glands, thyroid, kidneys and parathyroid glands but can originate from virtually any organ, see Table 23.1.

Histologically, variably-organoid arrays of large cells demonstrating round nuclei, inconstant mitotic activity, dispersed chromatin and indistinct nucleoli are present. Cytologically, these tumors manifest as flat sheets, loose groups, cords and singly-dispersed polygonal cells, usually with a strikingly monotonous appearance. The polyhedral cells may be intermingled with spindled forms. The presence of neurosecretory granules, represented by fine red cytoplasmic granules, is highly suggestive of neuroendocrine differentiation and may be detected in Romanowsky stains. Amyloidaceous matrical material may be present.

Metastatic hepatocellular carcinomas (HCCs) often exhibit granular cytoplasmic eosinophilia due to lipofuscin granules and abundant endoplasmic reticulum. Up to 15 percent of HCCs show globular intracytoplasmic, PAS-negative oxyphilic inclusions, which, when present, are useful diagnostic clues. In fine-needle aspiration biopsies, the tumor cells may be seen singly, in sheets or in compact cords. Intranuclear cytoplasmic invaginations, intracellular cytoplasmic globules or bile pigment (highlighted with the Fouchet stain) may be seen.[48,49]

Malignant neoplasms with fibrillary cytoplasmic eosinophilia

Metastatic myogenic tumors, including rhabdomyosarcoma and leiomyosarcoma, may present as metastatic polygonal-cell tumors with abundant, fibrillary eosinophilic cytoplasm.[50] The presence of fusiform cells with perinuclear vacuolization may provide a clue that the tumor has smooth muscle differentiation. Cross-striations

Table 23.1 Tumors with potential clear-cell or oncocytic features which may metastasize to the pleura

Tumors
Carcinoid tumor (grade 1 neuroendocrine carcinoma) of lung
Renal cell carcinoma
Medullary carcinoma of the thyroid
Fibrolamellar hepatocellular carcinoma
Pancreatic endocrine tumors
Yolk sac tumor (endodermal sinus tumor)
Gastric carcinoma
Exocrine pancreatic adenocarcinoma

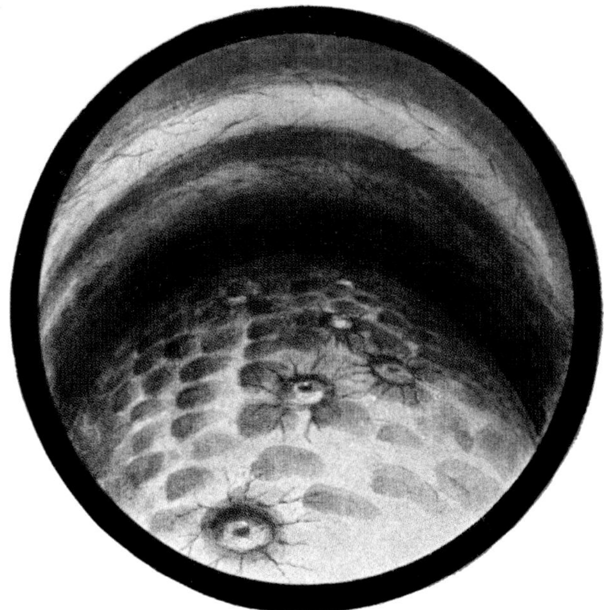

Plate 1 Illustration of neoplastic nodules on the lung surface taken from *Atlas Thoracoscopicon*. (See also Figure 1.7.)

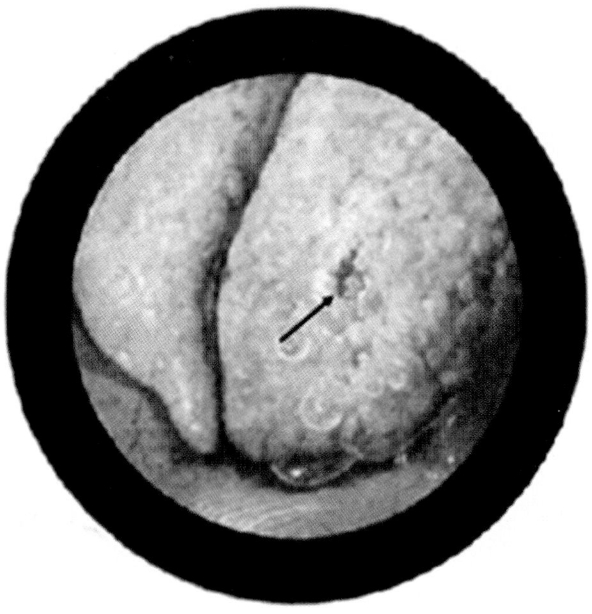

Plate 2 Sattler's illustration of the endoscopic aspect of the rupture of a lung emphysematous bulla (arrow). (See also Figure 1.9.)

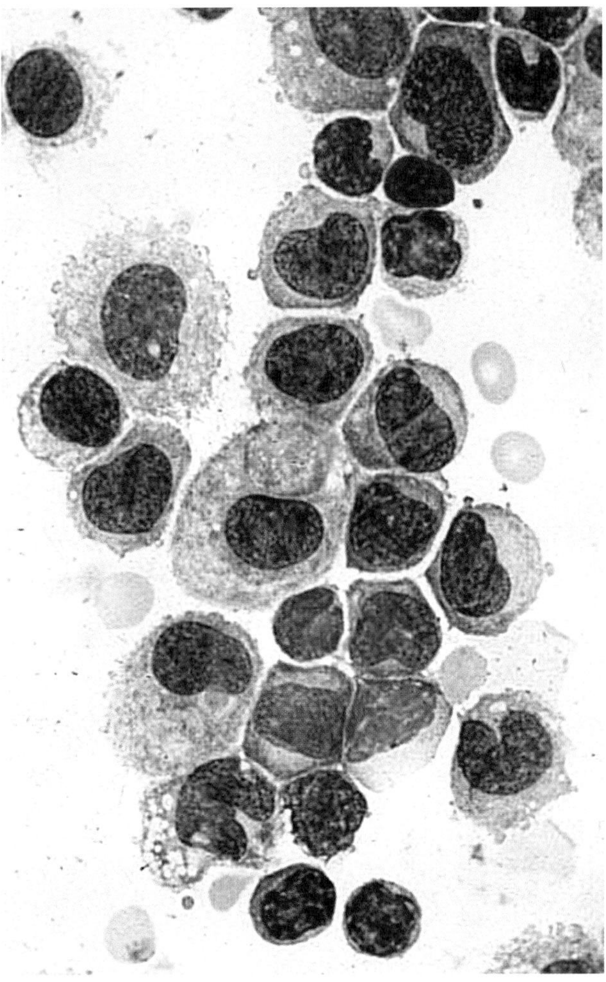

Plate 3 Typical cell smear of a pleural lavage sample from a normal, non-smoking subject; showing predominance of macrophages and lymphocytes (hematoxylin-eosin stain, ×320). (See also Figure 4.1.)

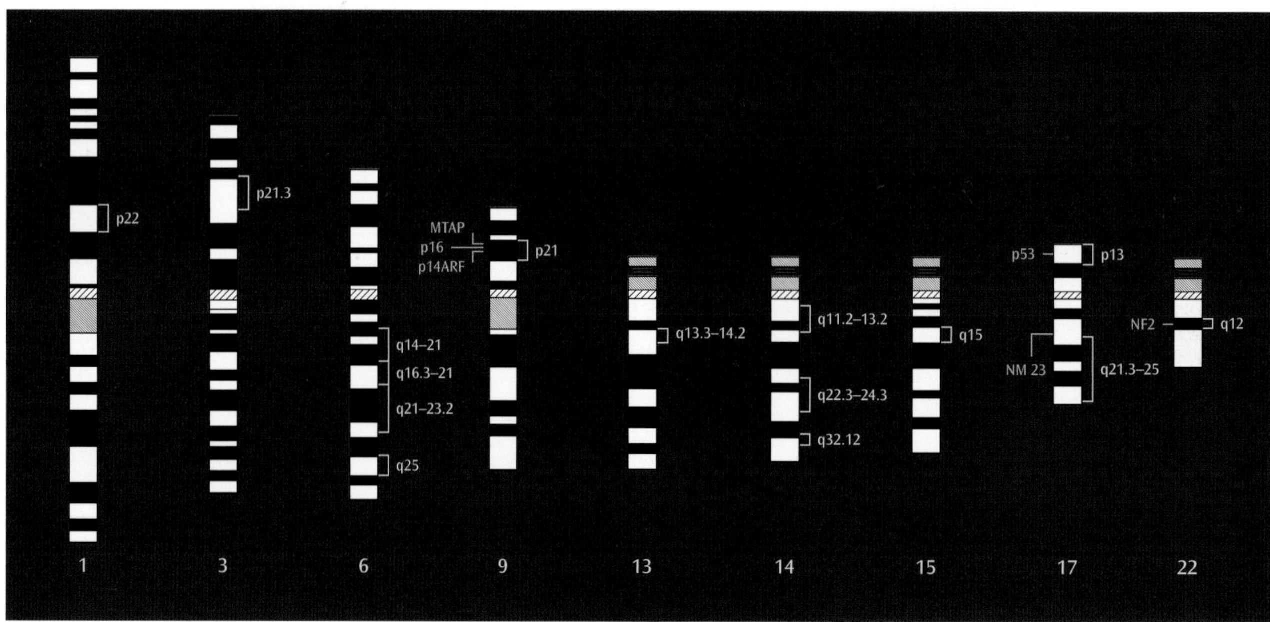

Plate 4 Idiograms of chromosomes frequently altered in malignant mesothelioma (MM), indicative of multistep tumorigenesis in this disease. Brackets demarcate minimally deleted regions (SROs) in each chromosome. Locations of TSGs (*p14*^{ARF}, *p16*^{INK4a}, *TP53* and *NF2*) known to be either mutated or homozygously deleted in MM are shown; other candidate genes (*MTAP*, *NM23*) are also indicated. (See also Figure 11.1.)

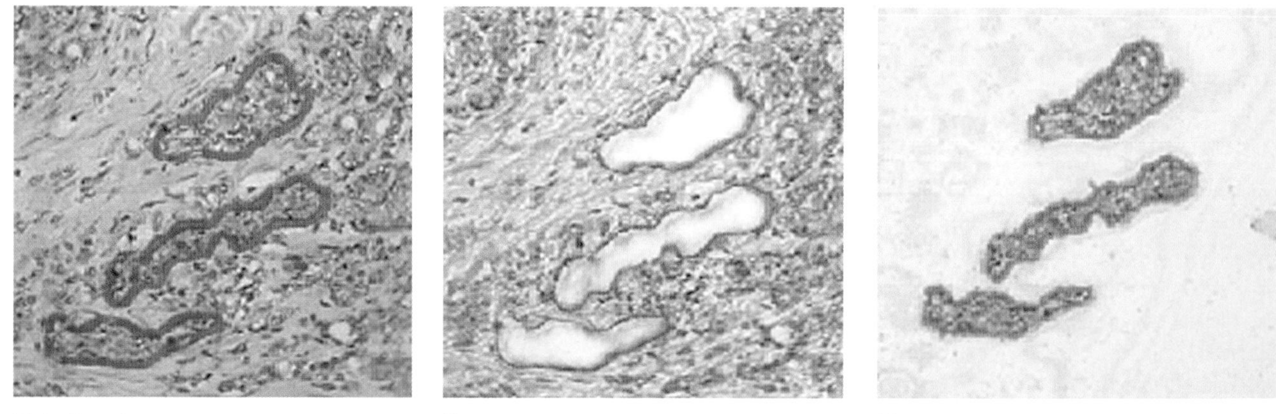

Plate 5 **Plate 6** **Plate 7**

Laser capture microdissection of cells of interest. An example shows the laser outline of the cells to be collected (Plate 5), the remaining cells after laser capture (Plate 6), and the cells collected from the outlined area (Plate 7). (See also Figure 12.2.)

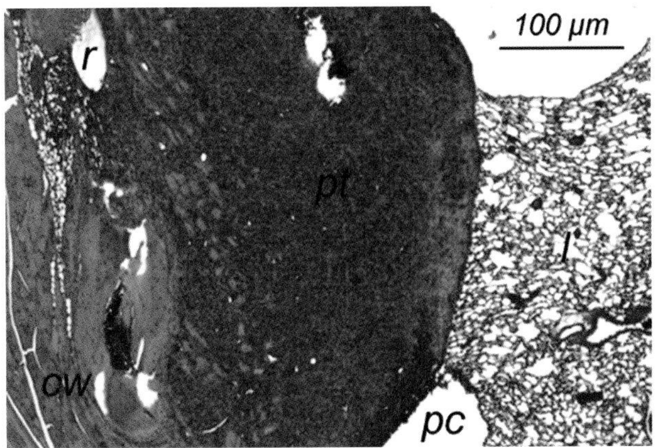

Plate 8 Histological section through a Lewis lung adenocarcinoma (LLC)-induced pleural tumor in a C57BL/6 mouse, stained with hematoxylin and eosin (× 40). Note that the tumor bridges the parietal and visceral pleurae. cw, chest wall; l, lung; r, rib; pt, pleural tumor; pc, pleural cavity. (See also Figure 14.1a.)

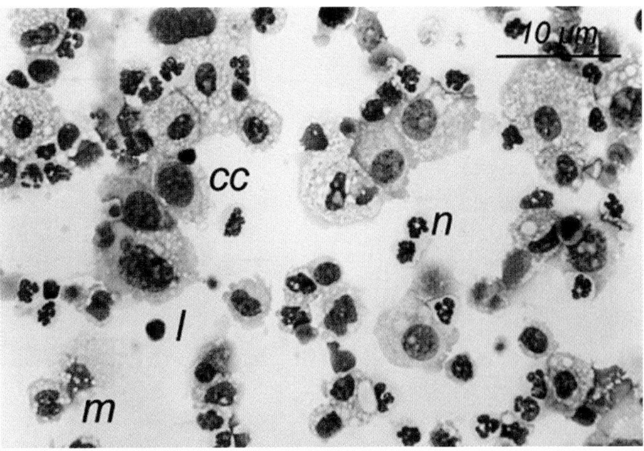

Plate 9 Cytocentrifugal preparation of malignant pleural effusion cells from the LLC-C57BL/6 model, stained with May-Grünwald-Giemsa (× 400). Alien adenocarcinoma cells are mixed with host inflammatory cells. cc, cancer cell; m, mononuclear cell; l, lymphocyte; n, neutrophil polymorphonuclear cell. (See also Figure 14.1b.)

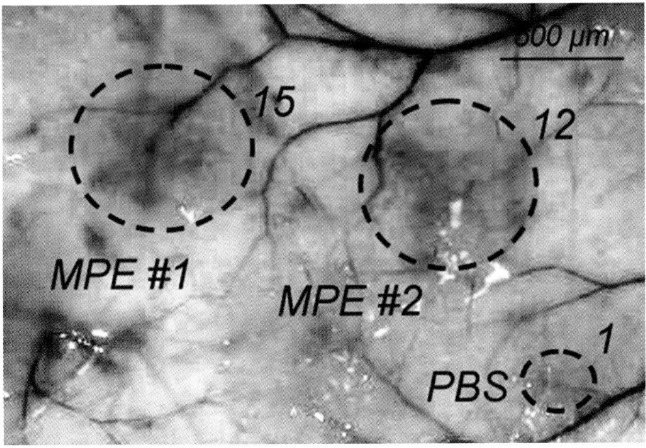

Plate 10 Vascular hyperpermeability induced in the skin of a C57BL/6 mouse by malignant pleural fluids from the LLC-C57BL/6 model, compared with PBS (negative control). After intradermal injection of 50 μL pleural fluid or PBS, the mouse received 0.8 mg Evans' blue in 200 μL normal saline. The mouse was killed and the skin inverted and photographed after 30 minutes. Circles represent areas of dye extravasation, and numbers relative surface area in respect to PBS (control). Evans' blue avidly binds to albumin; hence its extravasation indicates vascular hyperpermeability. (See also Figure 14.1c.)

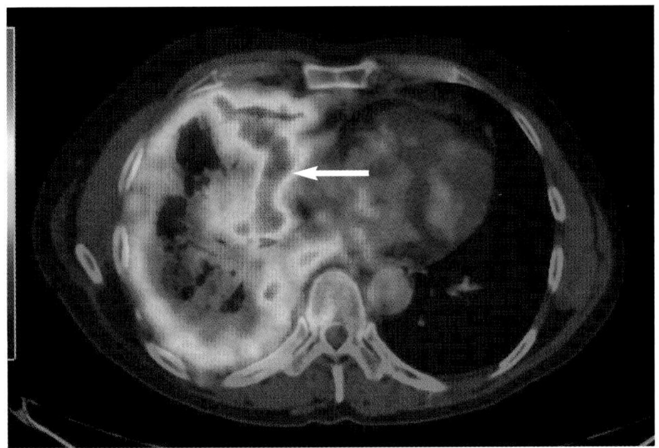

Plate 11 Positron emission tomography-computed tomography (PET-CT) scan demonstrating high grade FDG activity (arrowed) in sarcomatoid mesothelioma, with circumferential pleural thickening. (See also Figure 19.31b.)

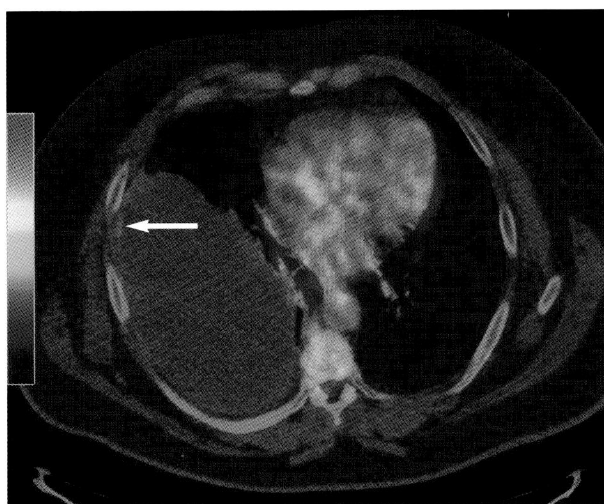

Plate 12 Integrated PET-CT scan demonstrating epithelioid mesothelioma (arrowed), with low grade fluorodeoxyglucose (FDG) activity, associated with pleural effusion. (See also Figure 19.31d.)

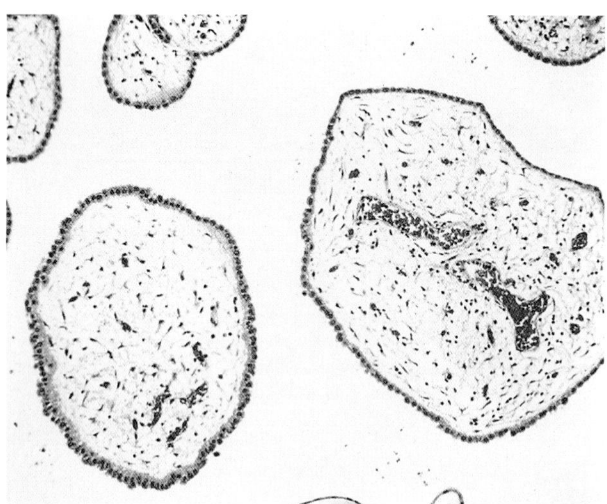

Plate 13 Well-differentiated papillary mesothelioma showing broad fibrous cores lined by bland cuboidal mesothelial cells. (See also Figure 22.1.)

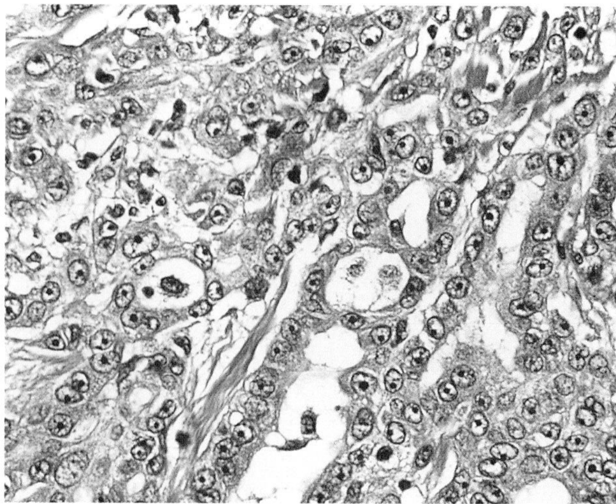

Plate 14 Epithelial malignant mesothelioma showing relatively bland polygonal cells with round nuclei and prominent nucleoli. (See also Figure 22.2.)

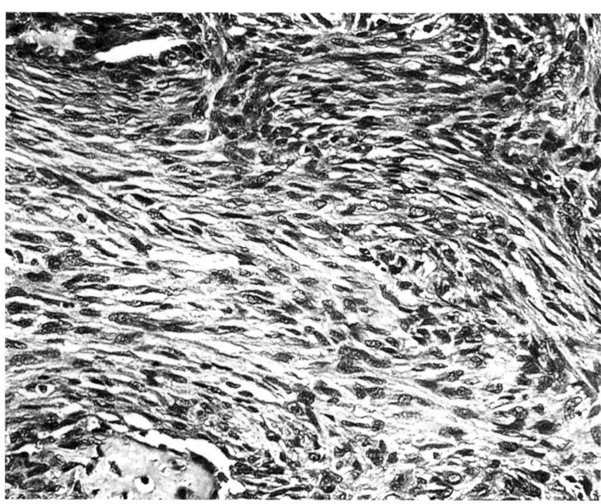

Plate 15 Sarcomatous malignant mesothelioma showing malignant spindle cells resembling a fibrosarcoma or malignant fibrous histiocytoma. (See also Figure 22.3.)

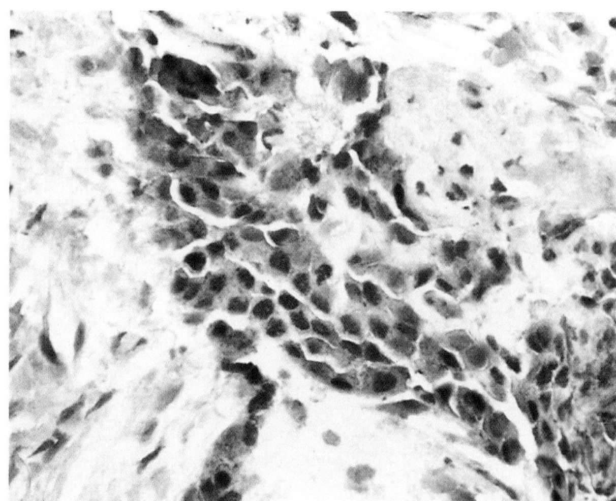

Plate 16 Immunostain for calretinin showing intra-nuclear immunopositivity in an epithelial malignant mesothelioma. (See also Figure 22.4.)

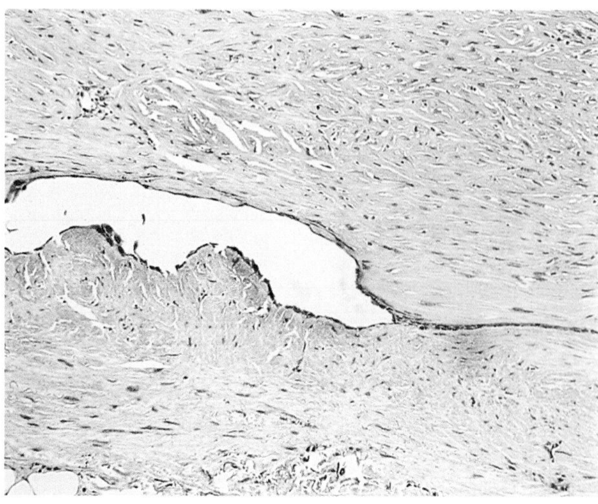

Plate 17 Entrapment of reactive mesothelial cells within fibrous pleuritis mimicking invasion by malignant mesothelioma. (See also Figure 22.5.)

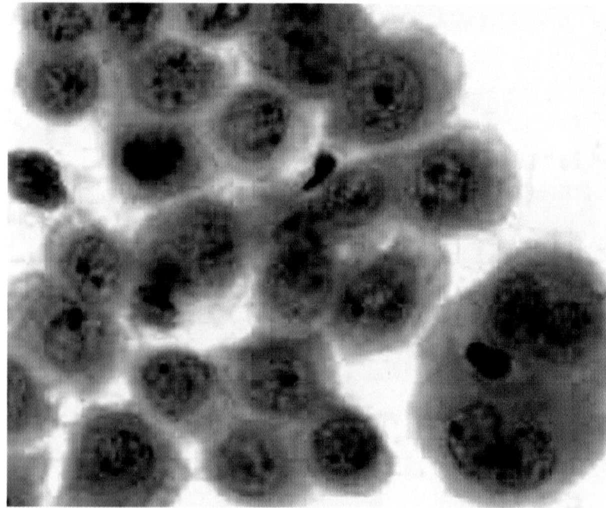

Plate 18 Mesothelial hyperplasia in a pleural effusion specimen. Note the dense cellularity and modest cellular pleomorphism, with intercellular spaces or 'windows.' (See also Figure 23.1.)

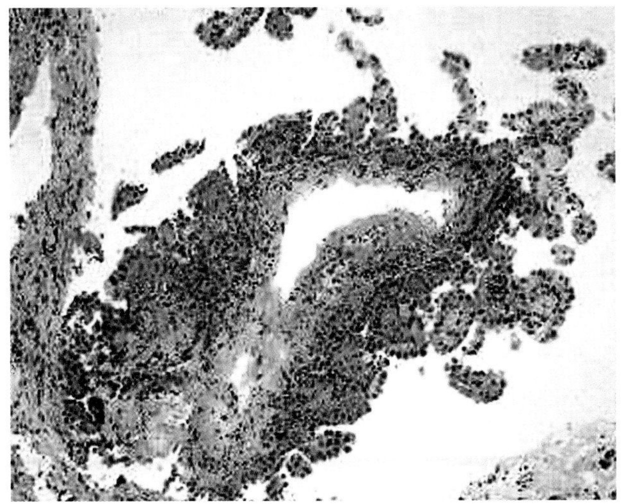

Plate 19 A micropapillary fragment is seen in this cell block from a pleural effusion demonstrating mesothelial hyperplasia. (See also Figure 23.2.)

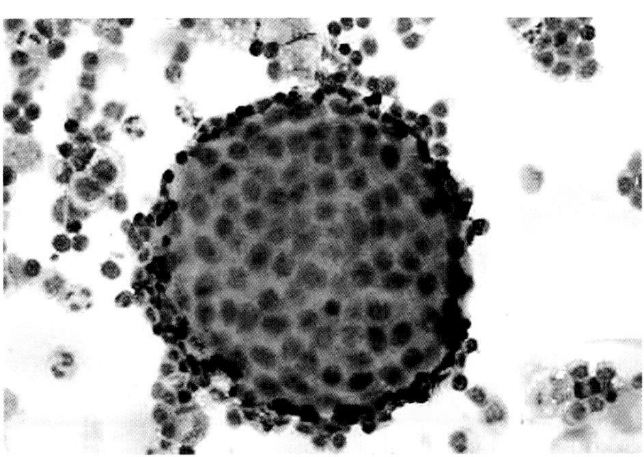

Plate 20 A morular, three-dimensional cellular aggregate is present in this pleural effusion specimen demonstrating metastatic ductal breast carcinoma. (See also Figure 23.3.)

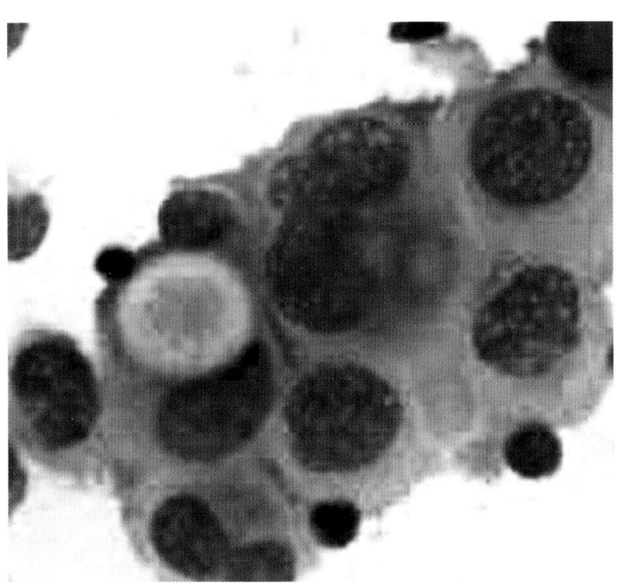

Plate 21 An intracytoplasmic mucus-containing inclusion is apparent in this cytologic specimen of metastatic lobular mammary carcinoma in pleural fluid. (See also Figure 23.4.)

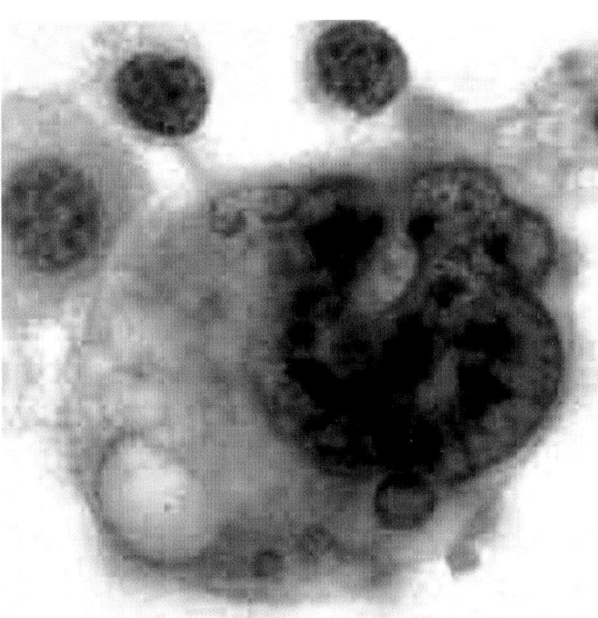

Plate 22 Metastatic melanoma in pleural fluid, showing marked nuclear pleomorphism. (See also Figure 23.5.)

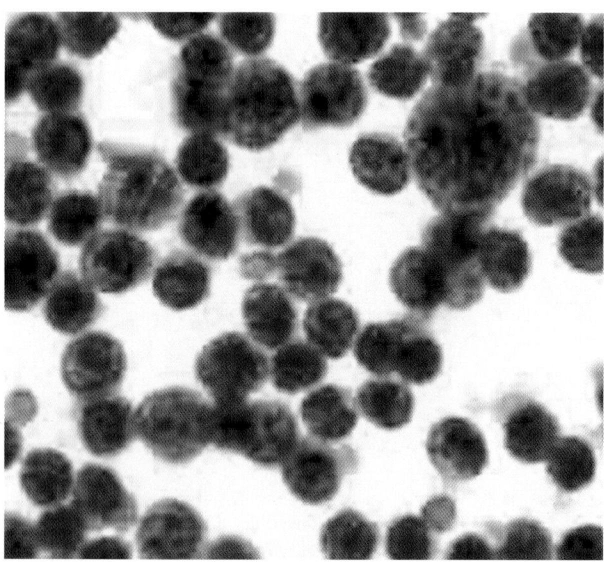

Plate 23 Dispersed small lymphoid cells in a lymphocyte-rich pleural effusion. The large cell in the field is a mesothelial cell. An image such as this may reflect the presence of pleural tuberculosis, collagen vascular disease, or a lymphoproliferative disorder. (See also Figure 23.6.)

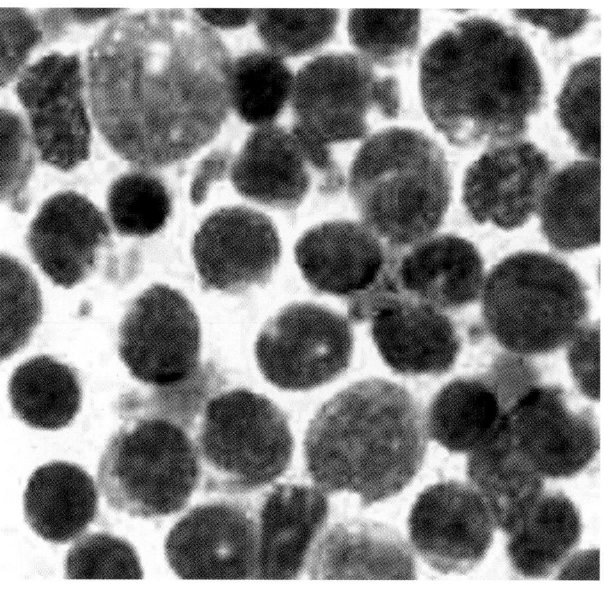

Plate 24 Cytoplasmic vacuoles are seen in the cells of this malignant lymphoma in pleural fluid. (See also Figure 23.7.)

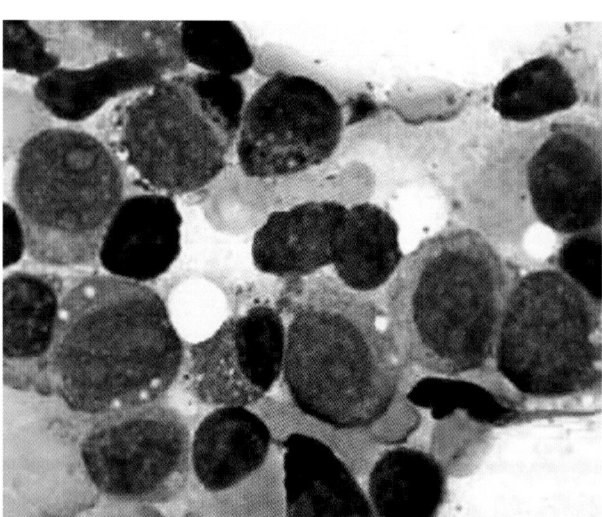

Plate 25 Infiltration of pleural fluid by tumor cells of acute myelogenous leukemia, with prominent cytoplasmic granulation and vacuolization. (See also Figure 23.8.)

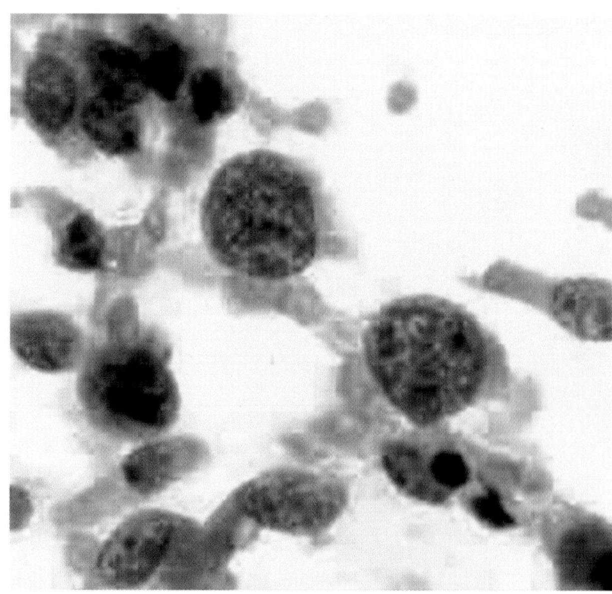

Plate 26 Metastatic rhabdomyosarcoma in pleural fluid, demonstrating cellular dyshesion and slight nuclear pleomorphism in small tumor cells. (See also Figure 23.9.)

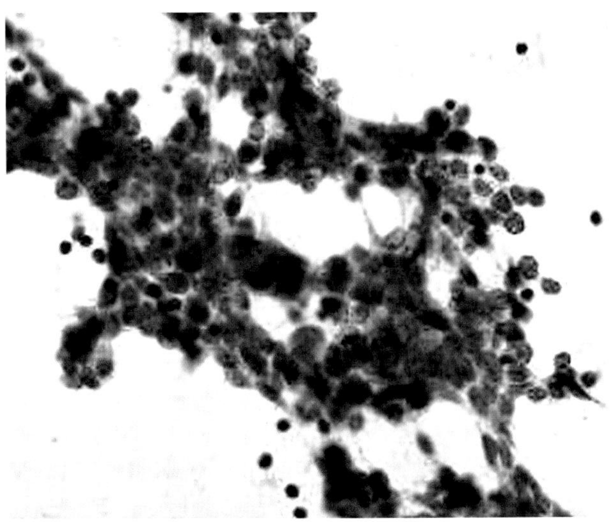

Plate 27 Metastatic small-cell neuroendocrine carcinoma ('oat-cell carcinoma') of the lung in pleural fluid. The tumor cells show nuclear molding and high nuclear-to-cytoplasmic ratios. (See also Figure 23.10.)

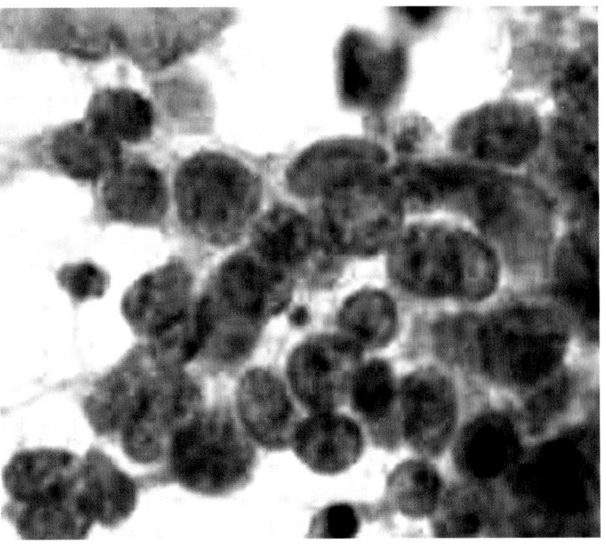

Plate 28 Metastatic small-cell neuroendocrine carcinoma in a pleural effusion specimen. Nuclear molding and dispersion of chromatin is evident. (See also Figure 23.11.)

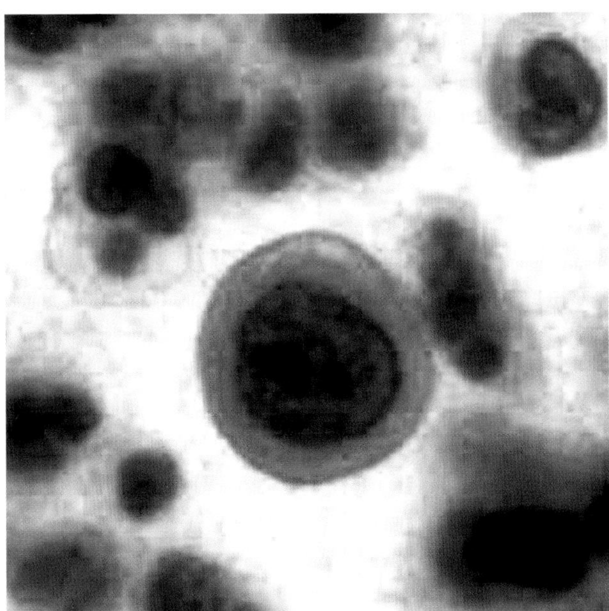

Plate 29 Prototypical large malignant cell with 'oncocytic' cytoplasm in metastatic large-cell carcinoma of the lung involving pleural fluid. (See also Figure 23.12.)

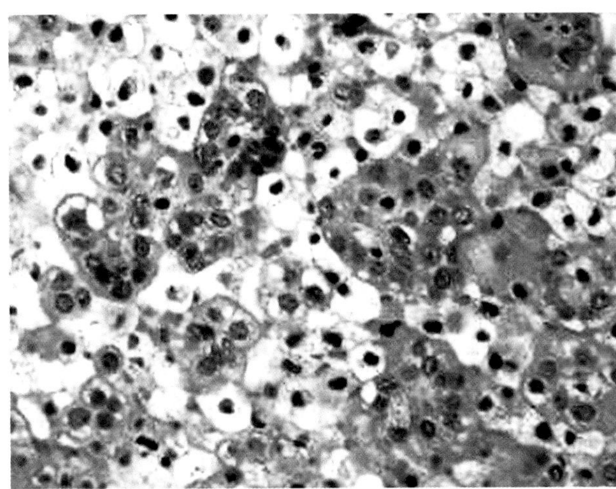

Plate 30 This mesothelioma demonstrates a combination of large 'pink' (oncocytic) cells and clear cells in this cell block preparation of pleural fluid. (See also Figure 23.13.)

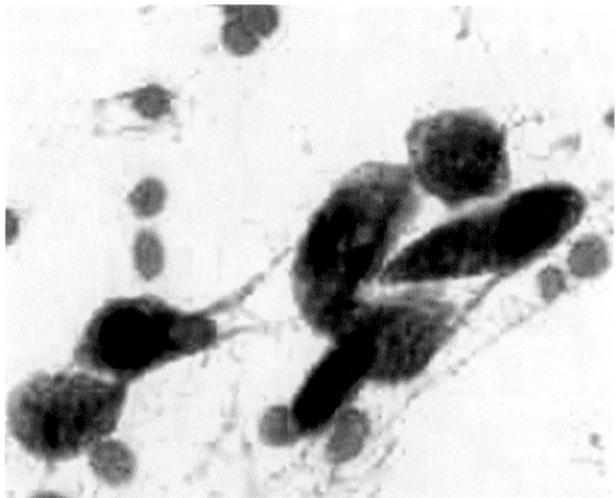

Plate 31 Dyshesive spindle cells with nuclear hyperchromasia and high nuclear cytoplasmic ratios are seen in this pleural fluid specimen. Such an image may correspond to that which is potentially seen in metastatic sarcomatoid carcinomas, mesotheliomas, or sarcomas. (See also Figure 23.14.)

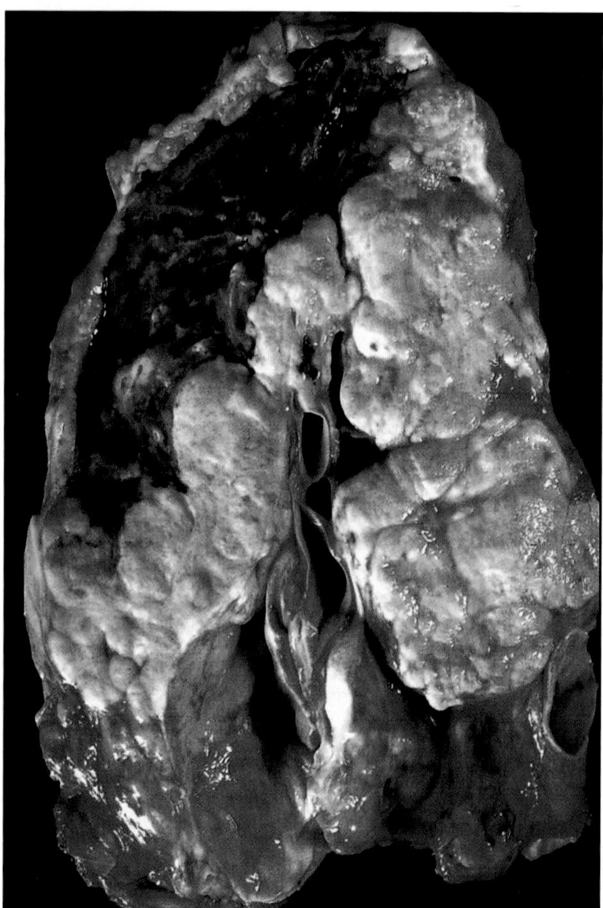

Plate 32 Autopsy photograph showing the typical configuration of end-stage pleural mesothelioma, surrounding the lungs and invading adjacent soft tissue with obliteration of the pleural space. (See also Figure 23.15.)

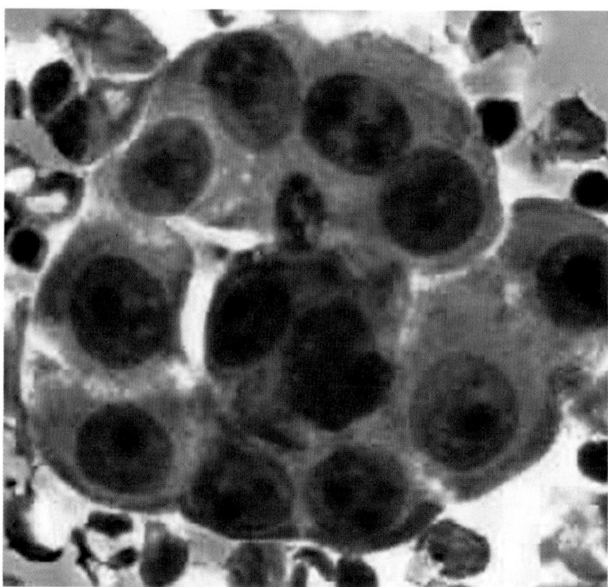

Plate 33 Pleural fluid specimen showing epithelioid malignant mesothelioma. The tumor cells exhibit increased nuclear-to-cytoplasmic ratios and nucleoli, and form a gland-like array. Intercellular windows are evident. (See also Figure 23.16.)

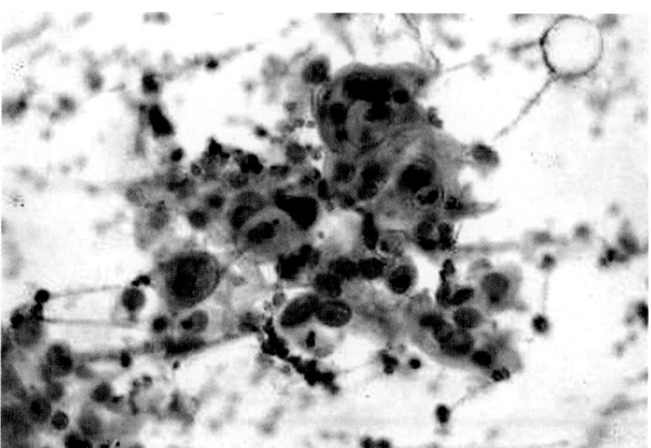

Plate 34 Sarcomatoid mesothelioma in pleural fluid. The tumor cells are irregular in size and shape and show a tendency to dyshesion, simulating the appearance of sarcoma. (See also Figure 23.17.)

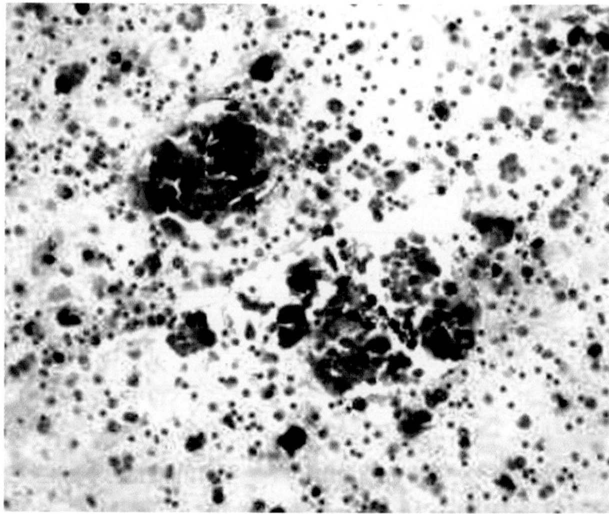

Plate 35 Immunoreactivity for cytokeratin-7 in metastatic pulmonary adenocarcinoma involving pleural fluid. (See also Figure 23.18.)

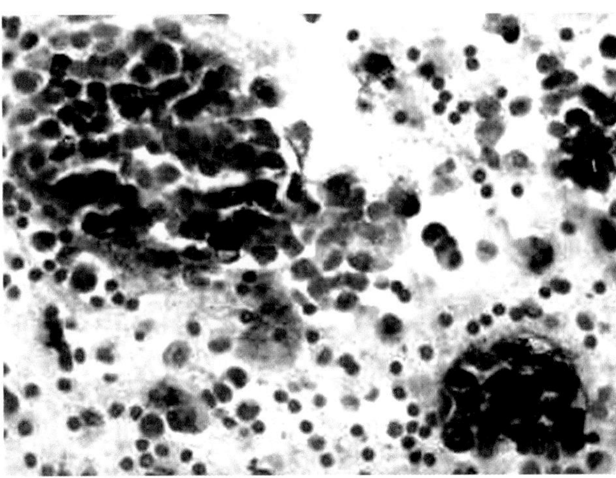

Plate 36 Labeling of tumor cells for carcinoembryonic antigen in the same case shown in figure 18. (See also Figure 23.19.)

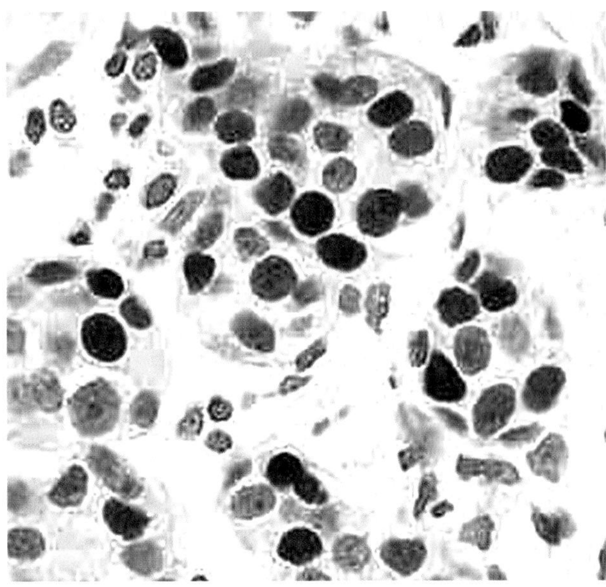

Plate 37 Nuclear positivity for thyroid transcription factor-1 in metastatic pulmonary adenocarcinoma involving pleural fluid. (See also Figure 23.20.)

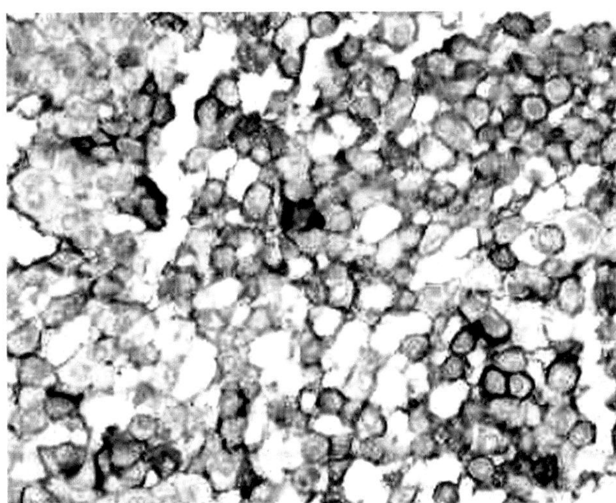

Plate 38 Diffuse immunoreactivity for thrombomodulin (CD141) is apparent in a cell block preparation of pleural fluid from a patient with epithelioid mesothelioma. (See also Figure 23.21.)

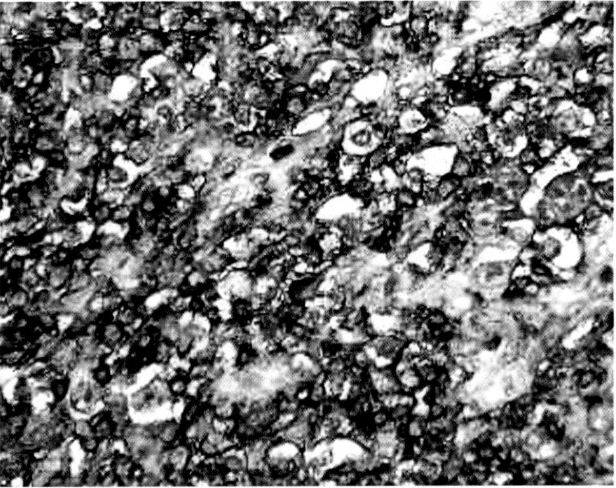

Plate 39 This cell block preparation of pleural fluid shows diffuse labeling of tumor cells for CD45 in a case of large-cell non-Hodgkin's lymphoma involving the pleural space. (See also Figure 23.22.)

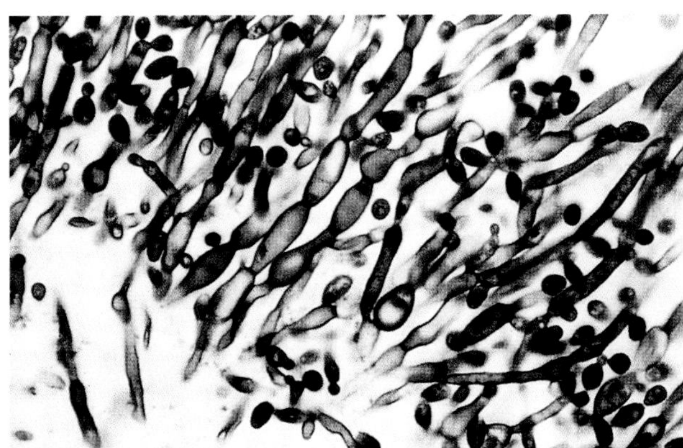

Plate 40 Candidiasis: photomicrograph (Groccot stained cytocentrifuge preparation, ×400) showing isolated or clustered pseudohyphae and spores. (See also Figure 28.1.)

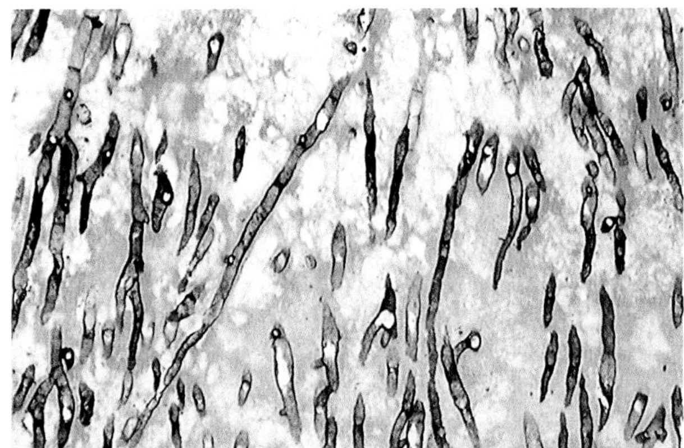

Plate 41 Aspergillosis: photomicrograph (Groccot stained cytocentrifuge preparation, ×400) showing a large number of septate hyphae. (See also Figure 28.2.)

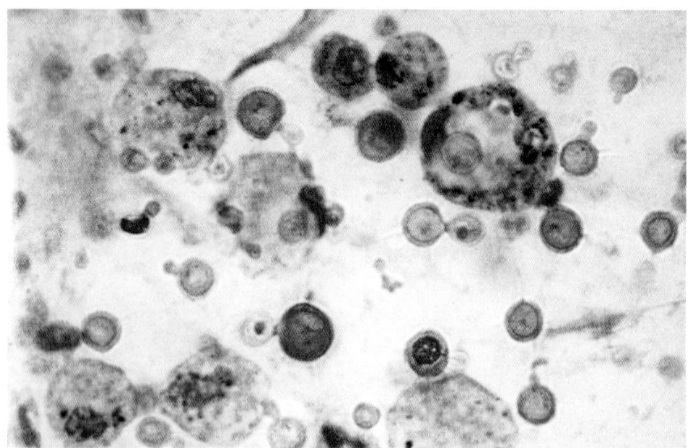

Plate 42 Cryptococcosis: photomicrograph (hematoxylin and eosin stained cytocentrifuge preparation, ×400) showing a large number of fungi inside the macrophages. (See also Figure 28.3.)

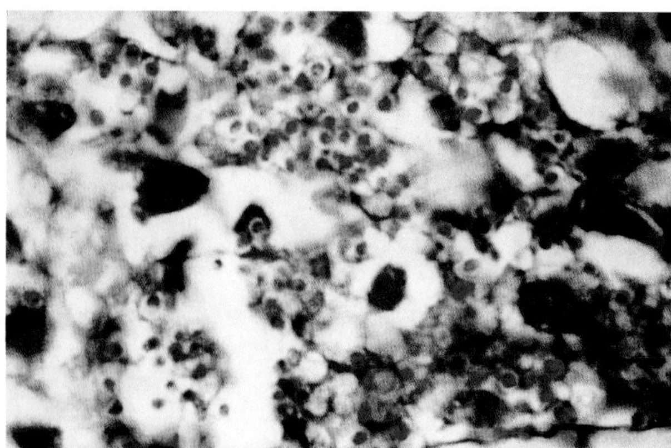

Plate 43 Histoplasmosis: photomicrograph(hematoxylin and eosin stained cytocentrifuge preparation, ×400) showing a large number of fungi inside the giant cells. (See also Figure 28.4.)

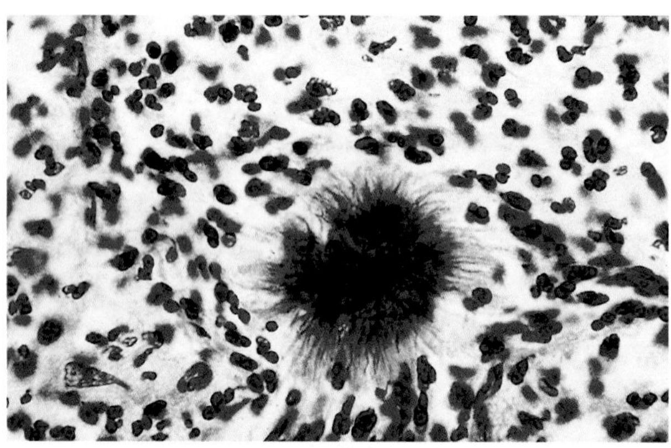

Plate 44 Actinomycosis: photomicrograph (hematoxylin and eosin stained cytocentrifuge preparation, ×400) showing sulfur granules. (See also Figure 28.5.)

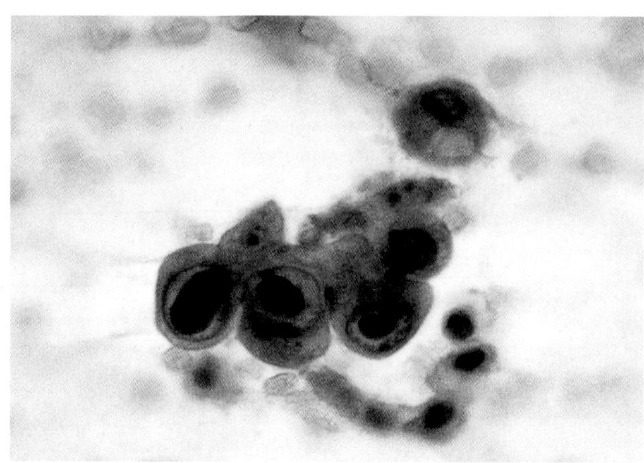

Plate 45 Cytomegalovirus: photomicrograph (Papanicolaou stained cytocentrifuge preparation, ×400) showing an intranuclear inclusion. (See also Figure 28.6.)

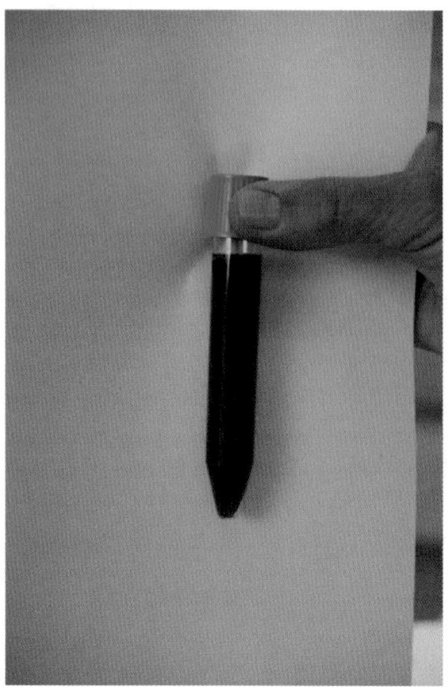

Plate 46 'Café-au-lait' color in pseudochylothorax. (See also Figure 29.1.)

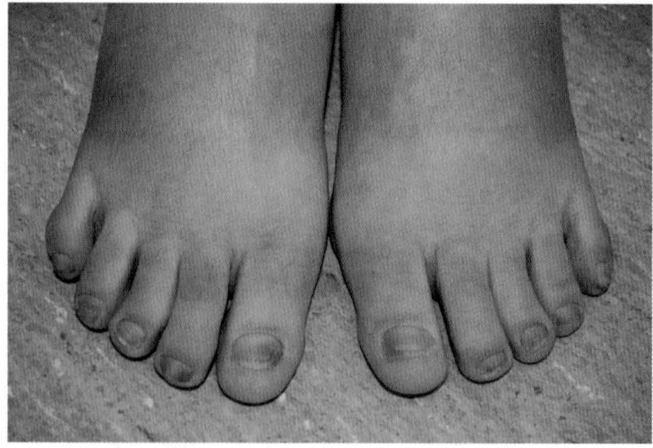

Plate 47 Typical Yellow Nails on toes and edema of the foot (and ankles). (See also Figure 29.3.)

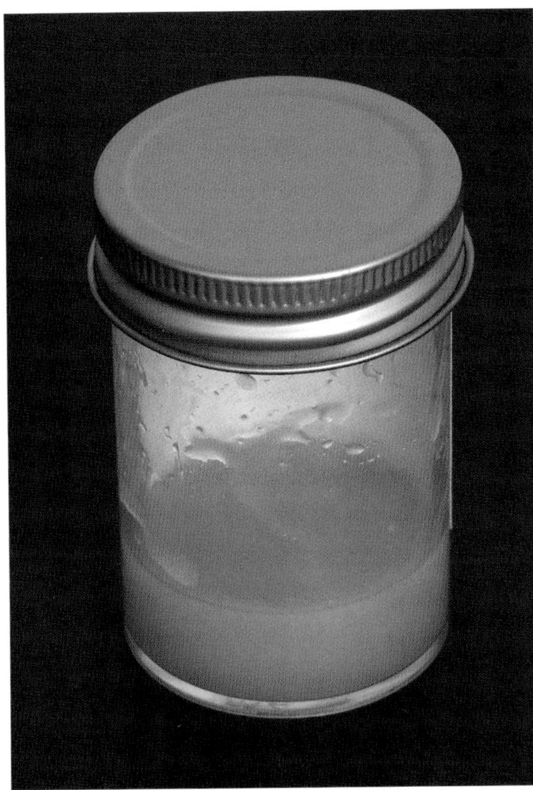

Plate 48 Pseudochylous effusion in a man with rheumatoid arthritis. (See also Figure 39.5b.)

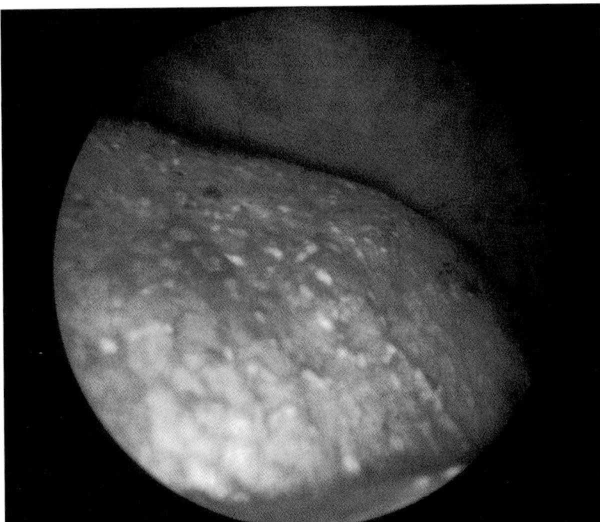

Plate 50 Lymphangiosis carcinomatosis of the lower lobe in a patient with right-sided pleural effusion. No tumor growth on the parietal pleura. (See also Figure 47.5.)

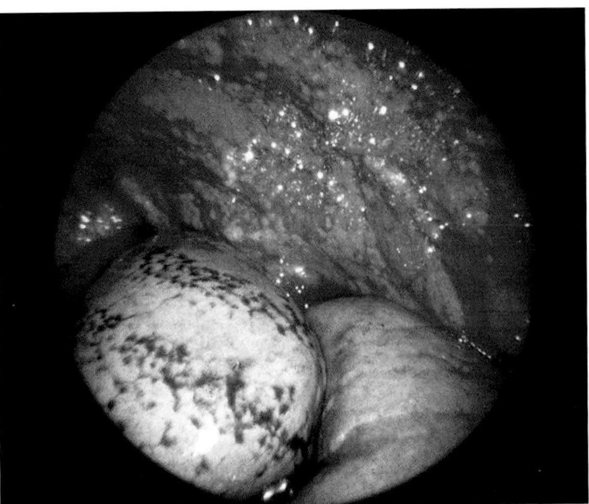

Plate 49 Thoracoscopic view into the left pleural cavity with normal upper and lower lobes of the lung. The chest wall pleura is covered by a whitish layer of small tumor nodules (diffuse malignant pleural mesothelioma). (See also Figure 47.4.)

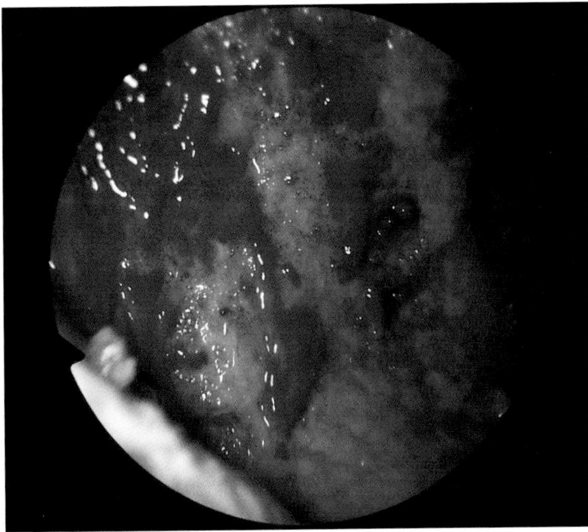

Plate 51 Larger hemorrhagic tumor nodules on the chest wall pleura (metastatic adenocarcinoma). (See also Figure 47.7.)

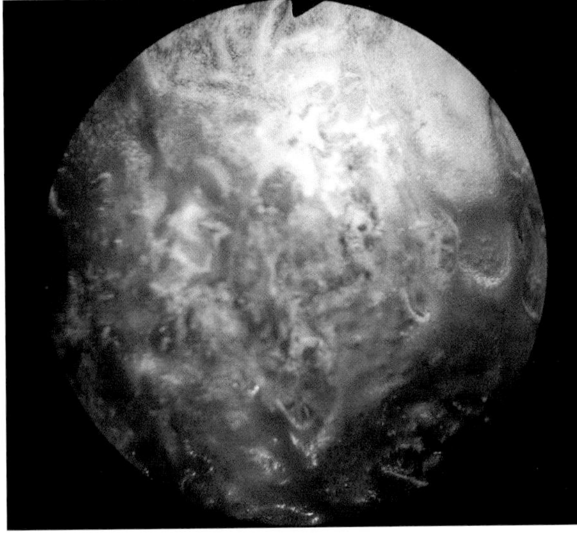

Plate 52 Same patient as in Figure 45.7 after talc poudrage. (See also Figure 47.8.)

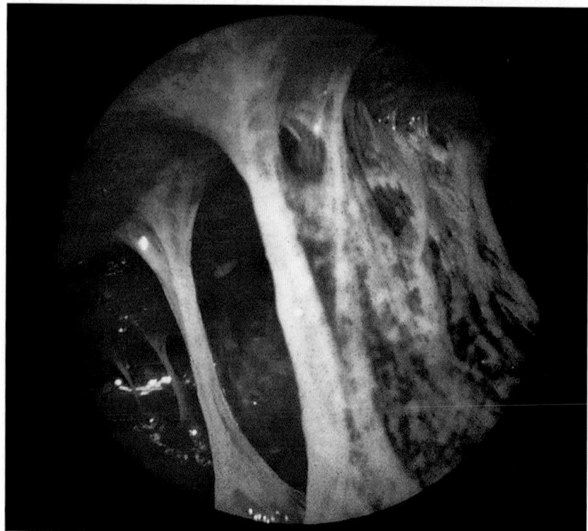

Plate 53 Tuberculous pleural effusion with fibrinous adhesions between the lung and the chest wall. (See also Figure 47.9.)

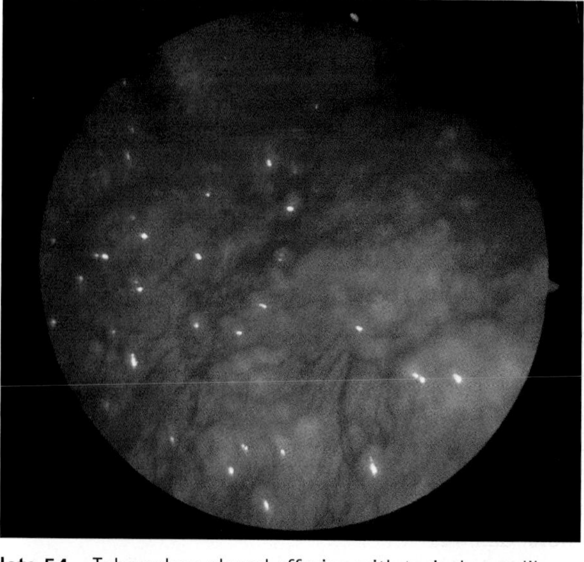

Plate 54 Tuberculous pleural effusion with typical sago-like nodules on the inflamed pleura. (See also Figure 47.10.)

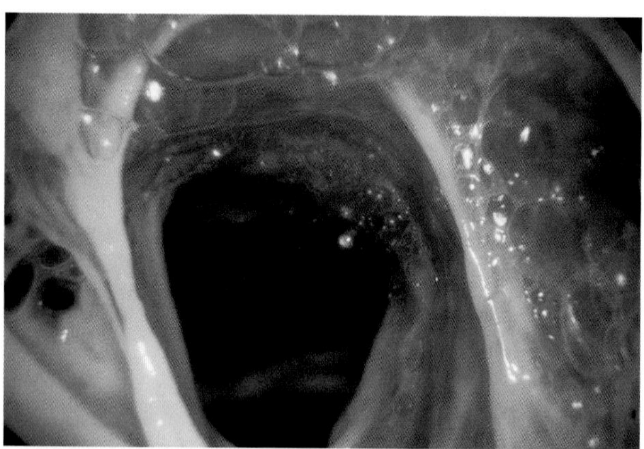

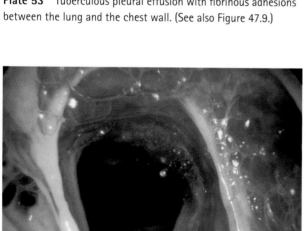

Plate 55 Thoracoscopic view of early empyema with fibrinopurulent membranes, which can be removed easily with the thoracoscopic biopsy forceps, thus restoring a single pleural space. (See also Figure 47.11.)

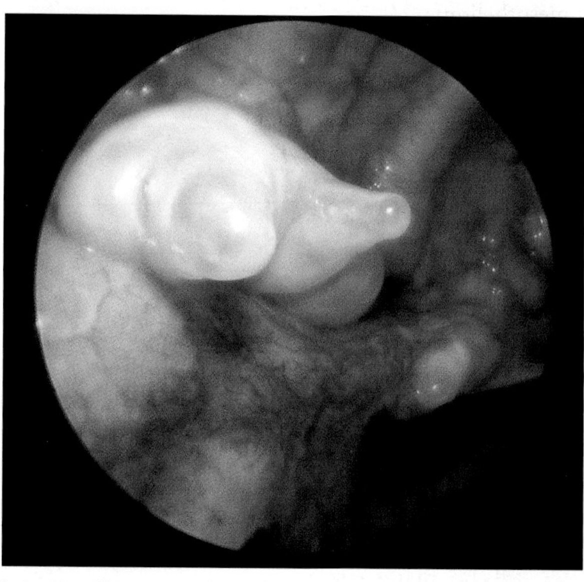

Plate 56 Thoracoscopic view of an emphysematous bulla in the apex of the right upper lobe (stage IV). (See also Figure 47.12.)

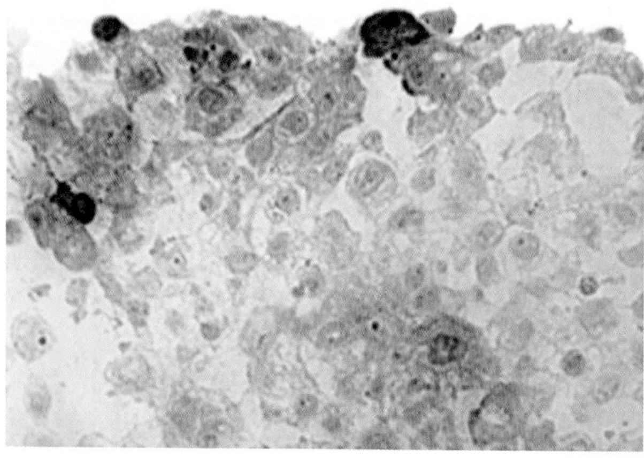

Plate 57

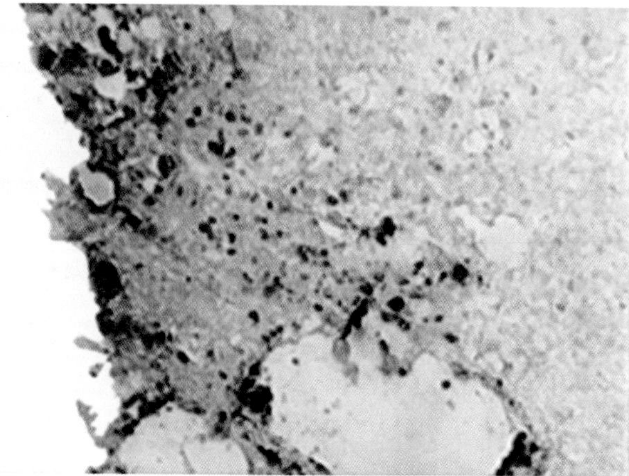

Plate 58

Gene transfer into mesothelioma. Forty-eight hours after intrapleural gene transfer, tumor biopsies were taken and stained for the transgene HSV-thymidine kinase. Immunohistochemical staining (red color) showed clear expression in the surface layers of tumor cells in both nuclear (Plate 57) and cytoplasmic (Plate 58) locations. (See also Figure 49.1.)

may be seen in occasional cells in rhabdomyosarcomas, and these can be accentuated with the phosphotungstic acid–hematoxylin method or a Mallory trichrome stain carried out on thin (2–3 μm) sections. Immunohistochemical evaluation is vital in this differential diagnosis.

Malignant neoplasms with globular cytoplasmic eosinophilia

When strictly defined by the presence of an inclusion-like mass of densely eosinophilic cytoplasm that displaces the nucleus, globular cytoplasmic eosinophilia characterizes a distinct group of heterogeneous neoplasms that are designated as 'rhabdoid'. In my opinion, malignant rhabdoid tumors demonstrate heterogeneous differentiation but have uniformly aggressive biological behavior.[51] Hence, rhabdoid cells may be part of virtually any tumors, including mesotheliomas.[52]

The presence of cross-striations and melanin would suggest rhabdomyosarcoma and malignant melanoma.[51] Only 33–66 percent of metastatic melanomas are obviously pigmented, but these figures can be maximized using Fontana–Masson stain to label for melanin.[21] Cytologically, amelanotic rhabdoid melanomas and other malignant rhabdoid tumors exhibit dispersed cells with moderate nuclear pleomorphism, anisocytosis and few other distinguishing features. Immunostains or ultrastructural studies are essential.[51]

Malignant neoplasms with diffuse cytoplasmic eosinophilia

Perhaps the most diverse and complicated diagnostic problems are attached to the group of neoplasms showing diffuse cytoplasmic eosinophilia with no other discriminating features. This constellation of tumors includes high-grade carcinomas arising in several locations, melanomas, anaplastic large-cell (AKi-1+′) non-Hodgkin's lymphomas, and sarcomas with epithelioid features.[27,47] Renal cell carcinoma, adrenocortical carcinoma and large-cell undifferentiated pulmonary carcinoma are those which most commonly assume a large-cell oncocytoid appearance with no other distinguishing features. Such epithelial malignancies are virtually superimposable on one another morphologically, and immunohistochemical or ultrastructural analyses are mandatory in discriminating between them. Likewise, amelanotic oncocytoid melanomas require similar adjunctive assessments for confident diagnostic recognition, especially if the Fontana–Masson stain is negative.

MALIGNANT CLEAR-CELL TUMORS

Malignant tumors with a potential for clear-cell change (Figure 23.13) and presentation as malignant tumors of uncertain origin and type (MTUOTs) are also diversified.

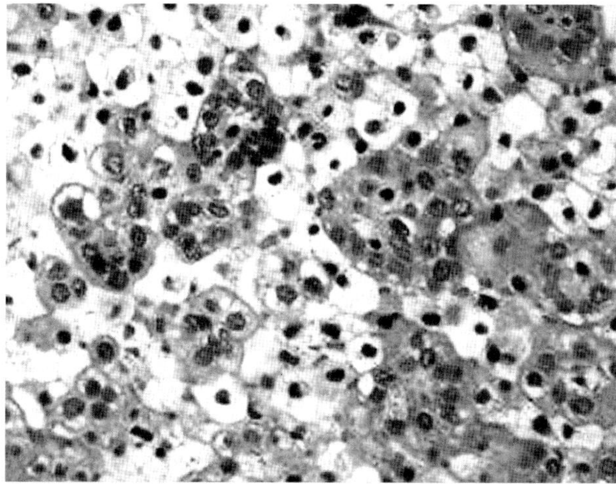

Figure 23.13 This mesothelioma demonstrates a combination of large 'pink' (oncocytic) cells and clear cells in this cell block preparation of pleural fluid. (See also Color Plate 30.)

As true of neoplasms in the preceding section, they include epithelial, mesenchymal and melanocytic lesions.[53] In addition, issues which complicate the evaluation of metastatic tumors in this category are several. They include the possibility that secondary lesions may undergo 'tumor progression' to acquire clear-cell change that reflects clonal evolution and may appear dissimilar from the primary neoplasms. Second, selected clear-cell malignancies, especially renal cell carcinoma, have the capacity to metastasize to organs in which primary clear-cell neoplasms are potentially encountered.

Malignant clear-cell tumors with a nested architecture

Among clear cell carcinomas, those arising in the kidney are best recognized and most frequently seen.[54] These tumors may secondarily involve anatomic sites that are usually spared by other metastatic lesions, and it is no exaggeration to state that renal cell carcinoma should be entertained in the differential diagnosis of virtually any clear-cell malignancy in any location. Nevertheless, the more frequent scenarios are those in which the lung and pleura, bones, liver or brain serve as the foci for metastatic renal cell carcinomas. The most reliable pathological means to address whether the kidney is indeed the source of such neoplasms is to catalogue their histological nuances. If such tumors are accompanied by significant stromal hemorrhage, a renal origin is likely.

An uncommon variant of gastric carcinoma has a tubulopapillary clear cell appearance which simulates that of renal cell carcinoma.[55] This pattern is also reminiscent of mesonephroid mullerian carcinoma of the ovaries or endometrium; all of these lesions may secondarily involve the pleural surfaces.[56] The clear-cell form of metastatic HCC is an uncommon variant that can easily be confused with other secondary tumors, especially those of renal, ovarian or adrenal origins, or with clear-cell mesothelioma.[57] Clear-cell change in all of these tumors results from accumulations of intracytoplasmic fat or glycogen, or both. Hence, immunohistochemical or cytogenetic evaluations, rather than histochemical examination, are the most helpful.

Cytologically, smears of each of the lesions in this group are generally hypercellular. They consist of loosely cohesive groups and individually scattered malignant cells with anisonucleosis, nuclear hyperchromasia, irregular prominent nucleoli and abundant finely vacuolated to clear cytoplasm.

Clear-cell thyroid carcinomas of both the papillary and follicular types have been recognized.[58] In extrathyroidal sites such as the pleura, these cancers share many microscopic features with other clear cell malignancies and immunohistology or electron microscopy must be employed to resolve such uncertainty. Cytological findings in clear-cell papillary thyroid carcinoma (CCPTC) include the presence of nuclear pseudoinclusions and grooves, similar to conventional papillary tumors. Unfortunately, these features can also be observed in metastatic renal tumors. In addition, multinucleated tumor cells may be seen in CCPTC, and these are particularly helpful because they are not a part of the cytological spectrum of other clear-cell carcinomas. Follicular formations containing colloid-like material are likewise supportive of clear-cell follicular thyroid carcinoma or CCPTC.

Clear-cell tumors lacking consistent architectural patterns

Other carcinomas that potentially assume a clear-cell image and lack a consistent growth pattern are represented by metastatic adenocarcinomas and 'hydropic' squamous carcinomas of various anatomic sources. Other than anatomic patterns of spread, there are no reliable architectural or cytological features that can be used to predict the topographic sources of these lesions. Fortunately, the immunophenotypes of clear-cell prostatic, pulmonary, renal, salivary and cutaneous tumors demonstrate many points of dissimilarity, making such profiles valuable in differential diagnosis.[53]

Metastatic melanomas composed of clear 'balloon-' or signet-ring cells are capable of imitating a multiplicity of other malignant clear-cell neoplasms, including carcinomas, sarcomas, lymphomas and germ-cell tumors.[59] The clear cells in melanomas result from cystic dilatation of premelanosomes or the cytoplasmic accumulation of lipid or acid mucin. Nuclei in these cases may be deceptively bland. In cytological preparations, the cells in clear-cell melanomas can be misinterpreted as those of an adenocarcinoma or liposarcoma. Histochemistry and immunostaining or ultrastructural studies are necessary in amelanotic tumors to define their melanocytic nature.

Metastatic classical seminoma/germinoma may be misinterpreted when it presents as a metastatic lesion. A diffuse arrangement of clear tumor cells is typical of this neoplasm, sometimes with irregular separation or compartmentalization by fibrous stroma and diffuse permeation by small mature lymphocytes.[54] Other common cytomorphological features of seminoma/germinoma include well-defined cell borders, evenly spaced nuclei and single prominent central nucleoli.[60] When present, multinucleated synctiotrophoblastic cells and epithelioid granulomas are also helpful interpretatively. Abundant intracytoplasmic glycogen is evident on PAS staining.

Malignant spindle-cell and pleomorphic tumors

Metastatic carcinomas from various organ sites may occasionally have overwhelming spindle-cell components resembling pleural sarcomas. A relatively common setting is that of a lesion composed of spindle cells for which a primary mesothelial origin cannot be excluded on radiographic and conventional pathology assessments. A proportion of these cases actually represent metastatic sarcomatoid renal cell carcinomas, and additional detailed imaging may reveal a mass in the kidney.[61,62] In such instances, the primary tumors may be entirely sarcomatoid or represent a preponderance of clear-cells with only focal spindle cell differentiation. Morphogically similar primary sarcoma-like tumors may also be encountered in the lungs, urinary tract, female genital tract, alimentary tract, pancreas, thyroid, upper airway mucosa and in pleural sarcomatoid mesothelioma.

Regardless of their specific lineages, the cytological image of sarcomatoid malignancies is much more consistent with that of a true sarcoma than with an epithelial neoplasm. Cellular dyshesion, anisocytosis, nuclear pleomorphism, unremarkable cytoplasmic details and nondescript stroma are their usual features[63] (Figure 23.14). Adjunctive studies are mandatory for diagnosis.

True spindle-cell sarcomas only exceptionally manifest as pleural metastasis in the absence of a known primary tumor; similarly, primary pleural sarcoma is extremely rare.[64]

Clinicopathological features of malignant mesothelioma

Pleural mesothelioma (Figure 23.15) is a rare tumor that may be challenging to recognize accurately. However, a firm diagnosis is crucial in the ever-growing number of legal compensation claims.[65,66]

Traditionally, three broad histopathological patterns of mesothelioma have been considered: epithelial (including oncocytoid/deciduoid, clear-cell and small-cell subtypes), sarcomatoid (including desmoplastic and 'lymphohistio-

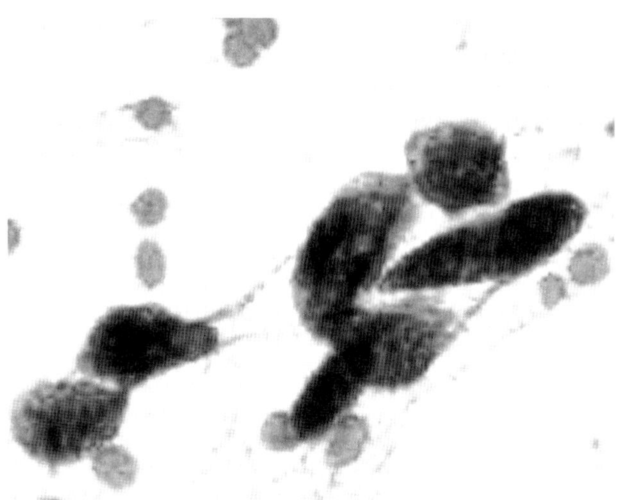

Figure 23.14 Dyshesive spindle cells with nuclear hyperchromasia and high nuclear cytoplasmic ratios are seen in this pleural fluid specimen. Such an image may correspond to that which is potentially seen in metastatic sarcomatoid carcinomas, mesotheliomas or sarcomas. (See also Color Plate 31.)

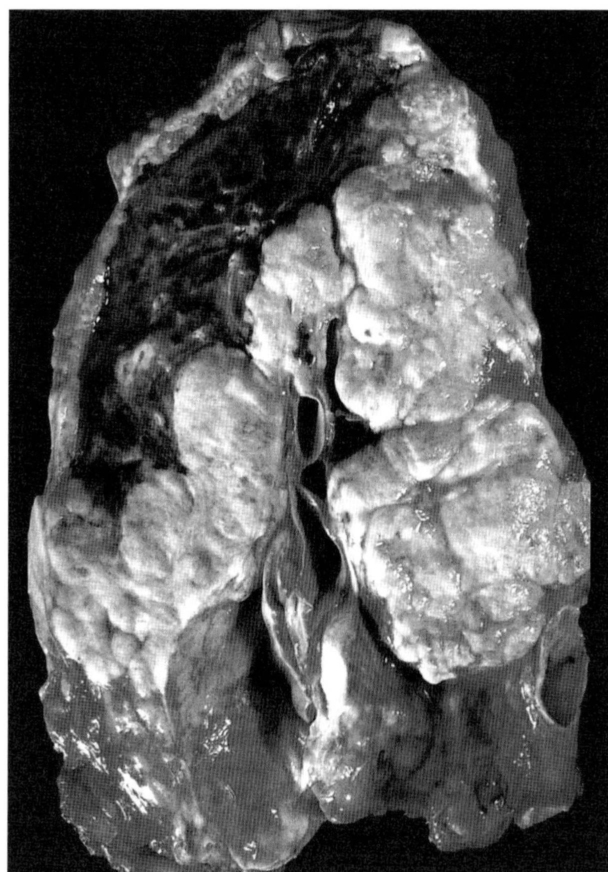

Figure 23.15 Autopsy photograph showing the typical configuration of end-stage pleural mesothelioma, surrounding the lungs and invading adjacent soft tissue with obliteration of the pleural space. (See also Color Plate 32.)

cytoid' variants), and biphasic.[67] Occasionally, unusual histopathologic features, e.g. extensive myxoid change, adenomatoid tumor-like images, 'rhabdoid features,' decidua-like configurations and bone and cartilage formation, may be present.[68] Thus, variants of mesothelioma are members of several of the cytomorphological 'partitions' presented (see above).

Epithelial mesothelioma is composed of sheets and nests of variably-atypical epithelioid cells (Figure 23.16). Mitotic figures and necrosis are uncommon, but those two features may certainly be apparent in high-grade lesions. Epithelial mesotheliomas may also show papillary or tubulopapillary growth patterns. The malignant cells may be amazingly bland cytologically and difficult to distinguish from benign reactive mesothelia. Groups of both reactive and neoplastic mesothelial cells may demonstrate intercellular spaces or 'windows,' and sufficient dispersion of such elements shows the presence of fuzzy cell membranes owing to the presence of elongated plasmalemmal microvilli. Small-cell epithelial mesothelioma demonstrates more tightly-clustered cell groups without obvious microvilli, and are exceedingly similar cytomorphologically to other small-cell malignant neoplasms.

Sarcomatoid mesothelioma comprises cytologically malignant fusiform cell proliferations that often imitate other tumors of mesenchymal origin, i.e. sarcomas.[69–71] The tumor cells have scant cytoplasm, elongated nuclei, and scattered mitotic figures (Figure 23.17). A rare subtype – the *desmoplastic* mesothelioma – is characterized by a bland appearance of the spindle cells embedded in a hypocellular, abundantly collagenized stroma,[67] resembling pleural plaques or fibrohyaline pleuritis.

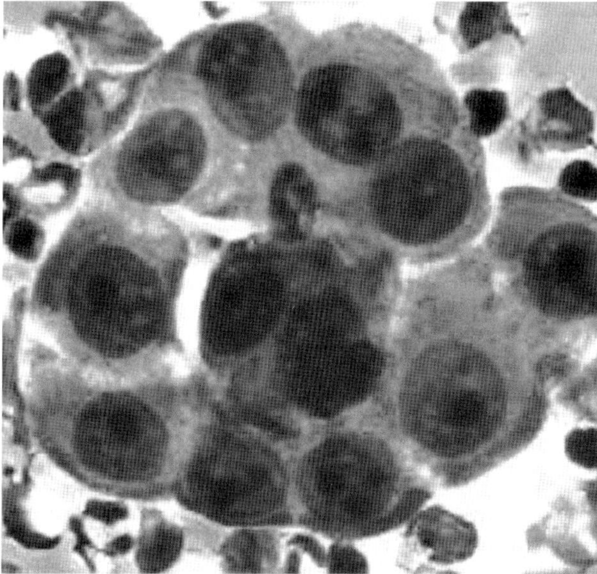

Figure 23.16 Pleural fluid specimen showing epithelioid malignant mesothelioma. The tumor cells exhibit increased nuclear-to-cytoplasmic ratios and nucleoli, and form a gland-like array. Intercellular windows are evident. (See also Color Plate 33.)

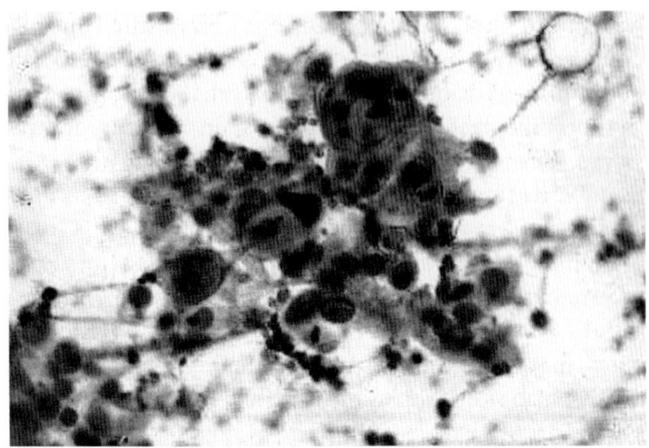

Figure 23.17 Sarcomatoid mesothelioma in pleural fluid. The tumor cells are irregular in size and shape and show a tendency to dyshesion, simulating the appearance of sarcoma. (See also Color Plate 34.)

'Lymphohistiocytoid' mesothelioma is another sarcomatoid variant, but it bears more resemblance to 'lymphoepithelioma-like' carcinomas than to sarcomas.[72] All forms of sarcomatoid mesothelioma shed poorly into pleural fluid, and manifest scarce atypical spindle cells therein in only a minority of cases.

Biphasic mesothelioma manifests a combination of the epithelial and sarcomatoid patterns.

Histochemical studies still play an important role in separating mesotheliomas from other neoplasms. The most useful histochemical procedures in this setting are the PAS stain with diastase digestion (D-PAS), the mucicarmine method and the colloidal iron procedure with hyaluronidase digestion. The presence of neutral mucin in the neoplastic cells on D-PAS or mucicarmine stains is a diagnostic feature of adenocarcinoma, though up to 5 percent of mesotheliomas may show focal labeling for mucicarmine or D-PAS.

ADJUNCTIVE STUDIES OF PLEURAL DISEASES

The pathologists are increasingly asked to determine, using cytological or biopsy specimens, the primary site for pleural malignancies – the most common ones being carcinomas, mesotheliomas and melanomas.

Biochemical tumor markers in the assessment of pleural effusion specimens

Various 'tumor markers' in pleural fluid have been examined as a means of distinguishing between benign and malignant effusions and predicting the origins of carcinomas metastasizing to the pleura. The latter goal is much less well-served than the former.

Several monoclonal antibodies directed at glycoproteins that are over-represented in malignant epithelial tumors are useful in this context, and they are best used as batteries. These include CA15.3, CA19-9, B72.3/CA72-4 and anti-carcinoembryonic antigen (CEA).[73–75] Another polypeptide which is related to keratin-19 (CYFRA-21-1) was found to have no value in this setting.[76] Most studies have shown that an elevated level of CEA (normal $\leq$5 ng/mL) is the most sensitive single indicator of pleural malignancies, and is also relatively reliable as an individual marker of metastatic carcinoma (as opposed to other neoplasms). B72.3/CA72-4 has a similar value.

In the opinion of the author, at least two of the aforementioned markers should be abnormal before a confident biochemical diagnosis of a malignant effusion can be made. None of the glycoproteins listed in this section is typically elevated in malignant mesothelioma, and false positives from benign pleural diseases can occur. Cytological examination is necessary in all cases with abnormal pleural fluid tumor marker levels, as well as situations in which the clinical suspicion for malignancy remains high.

Algorithmic immunohistochemistry of pleural malignant neoplasms of uncertain or indeterminate nature

The overwhelming number of antibodies for diagnostic immunohistology has made an algorithmic approach necessary, especially as no single reagent can provide a definitive answer in all cases. Several caveats must be heeded before immunohistochemical algorithms can be safely and effectively applied, as outlined in earlier publications.[28,77]

The statistical data used to construct the algorithms in this chapter were gathered over a period of many years using specimens (including cell blocks) fixed routinely in 10 percent neutral-buffered formalin; primary antibody incubations at 4°C for 16–18 hours; and the Elite® avidin–biotin–peroxidase complex method of immunodetection (Vector Laboratories, Burlingame, CA, USA). The antibodies that are most pertinent to differential diagnosis of tumors in the pleura are discussed below.

Immunohistological markers in the evaluation of malignant pleural tumors of uncertain nature

INTERMEDIATE FILAMENT PROTEINS

Monoclonal antibodies are now available to the complete range of keratin proteins (40–67 kDa), the intermediate filaments that are specific to epithelial tissues. Most of these probes react well with conventional, unmodified specimens; however, to maximize cytokeratin detection, proteolysis or, preferably, heat-mediated epitope retrieval, is necessary before application of primary antibodies to rehydrated paraffin sections. In most cases, the question is whether any cytokeratin is present in a given neoplasm.

Thus, mixtures of monoclonal antibodies may be prepared to cover the widest range of kilodalton sizes.[28,47,53,77–81]

One approach to the subtyping of carcinomas involves the immunohistological 'dissection' of the keratin classes which they manufacture. In fact, it has been found that monospecific antibodies to keratin 7 (a simple glandular keratin) (Figure 23.18) and keratin 20 (a 46 kDa protein that is relatively restricted to enteric-type tissues, urinary bladder and selected neuroepithelial cells) provide helpful information in this regard. In the topic under discussion here, keratin 20 is utilized as a 'secondary' reactant in the identification of MTUOTs, after application of the broadly-reactive 'screening' keratin reagent.

Vimentin is a 55 kDa protein which is expressed widely by many classes of neoplasia, but it may be used as a potentially differential indicator of certain epithelial tumor morphotypes. For example, the majority of renal cell carcinomas, thyroid carcinomas and adrenocortical carcinomas are vimentin positive.

Desmin is a 57 kDa moiety that is restricted in its distribution to cells and neoplasms that show myogenous differentiation. Thus, it is most helpful in the recognition of rhabdomyosarcomas and leiomyosarcomas. However, desmin reactivity is also present in a substantial proportion of mesotheliomas, probably as a reflection of 'divergent' differentiation in those basically epithelial tumors.

EPITHELIAL MEMBRANE ANTIGEN

Epithelial membrane antigen (EMA) is found on the surface of most epithelial cells and is actually a family of milk fat globule glycoproteins ranging in size from 40 to 425 kDa. Monoclonal antibodies to this discriminant are useful in determining the epithelial or mesenchymal nature of an undifferentiated tumor. There are some provisos to the last statement, however. First, true reactivity for EMA must be regarded as crisp labeling of the plasmalemma, with or without cytoplasmic staining as well; cytoplasmic labeling alone is a spurious finding that should be considered a negative result. Second, hepatocellular carcinomas, adrenocortical carcinomas and most malignant germ cell neoplasms are characteristically EMA negative, even though they are epithelial in nature. Also, selected malignant lymphomas may exhibit an EMA-like determinant. The use of other supplementary antibodies obviates the potential confusion that may be caused by these expressions of EMA-like moieties.

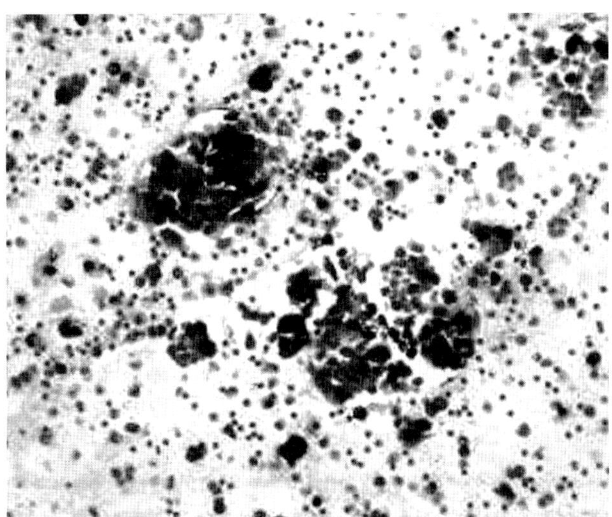

Figure 23.18 Immunoreactivity for cytokeratin-7 in metastatic pulmonary adenocarcinoma involving pleural fluid. (See also Color Plate 35.)

It has been contended that double-layered ('tram-track') EMA-labeling of the surfaces of malignant epithelioid cells is strongly suggestive of mesothelioma and that EMA positivity is restricted to malignant (and not benign) mesothelial cells. The author's experience has led to a good deal of skepticism regarding these assertions.

MOC-31

MOC-31 is a 41 kDa membrane-based glycoprotein widely-distributed in epithelial cells and tumors from many tissue sites, but not the mesothelium. This offers diagnostic distinction between serosal adenocarcinoma and mesothelioma (which typically lacks MOC-31). However, antibodies to MOC-31 fail to label several carcinomas, including hepatocellular carcinoma, germ-cell malignancies and renal cell carcinoma.

TUMOR-ASSOCIATED GLYCOPROTEIN (TAG)-72/CA72-4

The monoclonal antibodies known as B72.3 and CC49 label a plasmalemmal glycoprotein designated as tumor-associated glycoprotein-72 or CA72-4. It was isolated from a human breast carcinoma cell line and appears to be virtually 'pan-carcinomatous' in its distribution. Like MOC-31, TAG-72 is characteristically absent in mesotheliomas, adrenocortical carcinomas, hepatocellular carcinomas, renal cell carcinoma, nasopharyngeal carcinoma, thyroid carcinomas and malignant germ cell tumors.

HUMAN EPITHELIAL ANTIGEN (BER-EP4 ANTIGEN)

A monoclonal antibody designated BER-Ep4 labels two widely distributed 34 and 49 kDa glycoproteins in the cell membrane and cytoplasm of human epithelial cells. Mesotheliomas are typically non-reactive with this marker, whereas metastatic adenocarcinomas are BER-Ep4-positive. Primary pleural synovial sarcoma, which may closely mimic mesothelioma morphologically, is also commonly labeled by BER-Ep4.

CA-125

CA-125 was characterized as a glycoproteinaceous membrane constituent of ovarian carcinoma cells. A closely-similar or identical moiety was expressed by mesothelial cells and mesotheliomas. CA-125 has been detected immunohistochemically most often in neoplasms of the mullerian tract, but tumors of the biliary tree and pancreas are also reactive for this marker in roughly one-half of cases. Carcinomas in other sites are uncommonly CA-125 positive.

CA19-9

CA19-9 is a glycoprotein (sialylated lacto-N-fucopentose-119) which is related to the Le^a blood group antigen. It is labeled by the monoclonal antibody known as 1116NS19-9 which was raised against a human colonic carcinoma cell line. Carcinomas of the gastrointestinal tract, pancreas, biliary tree, urinary bladder, ovaries and endometrium manifest CA19-9 reactivity in the majority of cases, whereas tumors of other anatomic locations are only sporadically positive. Hepatocellular carcinoma and renal cell carcinoma are consistently negative for this marker.

PLACENTAL ALKALINE PHOSPHATASE

The isozyme of alkaline phosphatase that is expressed by the normal placenta is also evident as an oncofetal antigen in a relatively restricted group of somatic carcinomas. Germ-cell tumors are nearly universally positive on immunostains for placental alkaline phosphatase (PLAP). Mesotheliomas are uniformly PLAP-negative.

Seminoma and embryonal carcinoma differ from most somatic epithelial malignancies in that they do not exhibit EMA reactivity; moreover, seminomas also lack keratin in 90 percent of cases. However, anti-PLAP regularly labels examples of these germ-cell neoplasms. In addition, PLAP-positive somatic tumors uniformly express EMA, TAG-72 or the MOC-31 antigen, providing a means of distinguishing between these two broad classes of neoplasia.

CARCINOEMBRYONIC ANTIGEN

In addition to being a serological indicator for colon cancer, CEA is also expressed by many other epithelial tumors. Monoclonal antibodies to this 180 kDa family of markers represent prototypic epitope-specific probes that may be used in the selective recognition of small portions of a large antigen. Adenocarcinomas of the lung, breast and gastrointestinal tract have been uniformly reactive with a particular commercial monoclonal anti-CEA (HO62) used in the author's laboratory (Figure 23.19), and, therefore, metastatic glandular neoplasms expressing this substance are likely to have arisen in one of these anatomic sites. Mesotheliomas are consistently non-reactive for CEA.

CD15 (ANTI-LEU-M1)

CD15 is a hematopoietic cell-surface protein that is seen in myelomonocytic elements and in the Reed–Sternberg cells of Hodgkin's disease and some T-cell lymphomas. CD15 is present in adenocarcinomas from a wide spectrum of anatomic origins, but not in mesotheliomas, melanomas, sarcomas or germ-cell tumors.

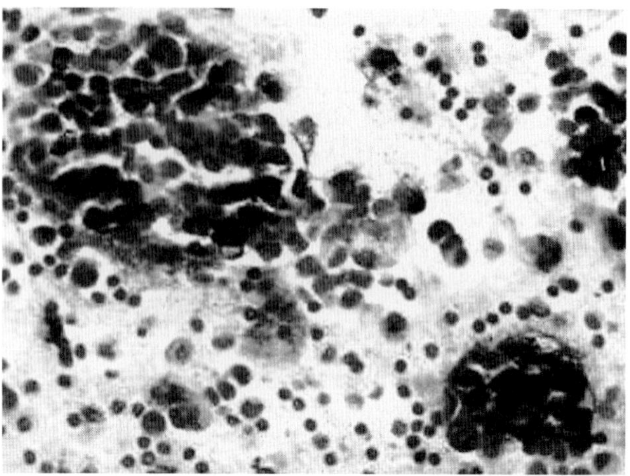

Figure 23.19 Labeling of tumor cells for carcinoembryonic antigen in the same case shown in Figure 23.18. (See also Color Plate 36.)

PROSTATE-SPECIFIC ANTIGEN AND PROSTATIC ACID PHOSPHATASE

As its name suggests, prostate-specific antigen (PSA) is restricted in its tissue distribution to epithelial cells of the prostate and prostatic adenocarcinomas. This cytoplasmic 33 kDa protein appears to be expressed at an early stage of embryonic development, inasmuch as even the most poorly differentiated prostatic malignancies display its presence. Hence, PSA represents one of few tissue-specific markers available in diagnostic immunohistochemistry and has been widely utilized in the recognition of metastatic prostate cancer. If desired, monoclonal antibodies to prostatic acid phosphatase may be utilized as corroborative reagents.

THYROGLOBULIN AND THYROID TRANSCRIPTION FACTOR-1

Thyroglobulin is a 660 kDa moiety that is restricted in its expression to the follicular thyroid epithelium and related neoplasms. The greatest utility of this marker is in the determination of origin for metastatic papillary carcinomas in the cervical lymph nodes or the lung, or for secondary deposits of more nondescript adenocarcinomas in bone. A relatively newly-described determinant, thyroid transcription factor-1 (TTF1), is a 38 kDa nuclear protein present in the majority of primary pulmonary carcinomas (Figure 23.20) but not mesotheliomas, making it valuable in that specific differential diagnosis.

GROSS CYSTIC DISEASE FLUID PROTEIN-15

Gross cystic disease fluid protein-15 (GCDFP-15) is a soluble product found in the fluid contents of fibrocystic breasts and is strongly expressed by cells with apocrine

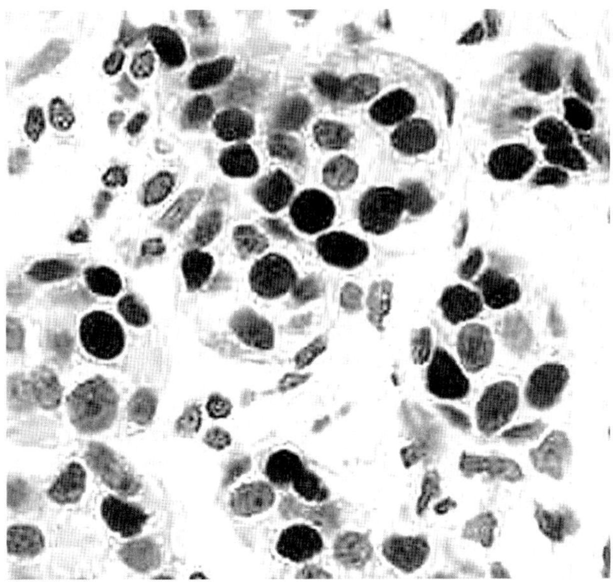

Figure 23.20 Nuclear positivity for thyroid transcription factor-1 in metastatic pulmonary adenocarcinoma involving pleural fluid. (See also Color Plate 37.)

characteristics. GCDFP-15 is present in the tumor cells of approximately 60 percent of breast carcinomas, with only minor differences among the major histological subtypes. It is much more specific for breast tumors than alpha-lactalbumin, CA15-3 or BCA225, other mammary-related proteins.

ESTROGEN RECEPTOR PROTEIN

Carcinomas of the breast and mullerian tract account for the majority of estrogen receptor protein (ERP)-positive tumors, but lesions such as thyroid carcinoma, transitional cell carcinoma of the bladder, prostatic carcinoma and even rare examples of gastric, pulmonary and hepatocellular carcinomas may express ERP. Mesothelial proliferations are uniformly ERP-negative.

S100 PROTEIN AND MELANOCYTE-RELATED MARKERS

S100 protein is expressed by normal melanocytes, Langerhans' histiocytes, cartilaginous cells, adipocytes, Schwann cells, astrocytes, oligodendroglia, ependyma, eccrine sweat glands, interdigitating reticulum cells, salivary glands and myoepithelial cells. Although S100 protein is widely employed as a screening reactant for malignant melanoma, it has become evident that certain poorly differentiated epithelial malignancies (which are keratin-reactive, unlike 99 percent of melanomas) may also express S100. Adenocarcinomas of the breasts, genitourinary tract, salivary glands and sweat glands are most notable among this group.

When melanoma appears to be the likely diagnosis (based on immunoreactivity for vimentin and S100 protein and negativity for all other determinants), several 'confirmatory' reagents can be applied, including MART-1/Melan-A, HMB-45 and anti-tyrosinase, which are best used as a panel.

CURRENT 'MESOTHELIAL' MARKERS

Calretinin is a calcium-binding protein that is virtually univerally expressed by mesothelial cells and malignant mesotheliomas. Selected adenocarcinomas (particularly poorly-differentiated colorectal tumors) may occasionally label for this marker as well. Therefore, calretinin is a useful discriminant for the broad separation of mesothelial and epithelial malignancies. Other markers with high sensitivity for mesothelial cells, but lesser specificity, are HBME-1, mesothelin, Wilms' tumor gene product (WT1 protein) and CD141 (thrombomodulin) (Figure 23.21). Calretinin and WT1 have a nuclear and cytoplasmic distribution within immunoreactive cells, whereas HBME-1 and CD141 are membrane proteins.

Another recently-studied cell membrane marker for mesothelial proliferations is podoplanin, recognized by monoclonal antibody D2-40. It labels approximately 85–90 percent of epithelial mesotheliomas and a similar proportion of sarcomatoid mesotheliomas. Podoplanin is also seen in vascular (endothelial) neoplasms, adrenocortical proliferations and germ-cell tumors;[82–84] hence, results for that protein must be interpreted in a panel-based context.

OTHER REAGENTS USED IN THE DIFFERENTIAL DIAGNOSIS OF EPITHELIAL MESOTHELIOMA

A large number of other reagents has been evaluated in the narrow differential diagnostic context of separating epithelial mesothelioma from metastatic adenocarcinomas,[81,85] see summary in Table 23.2.

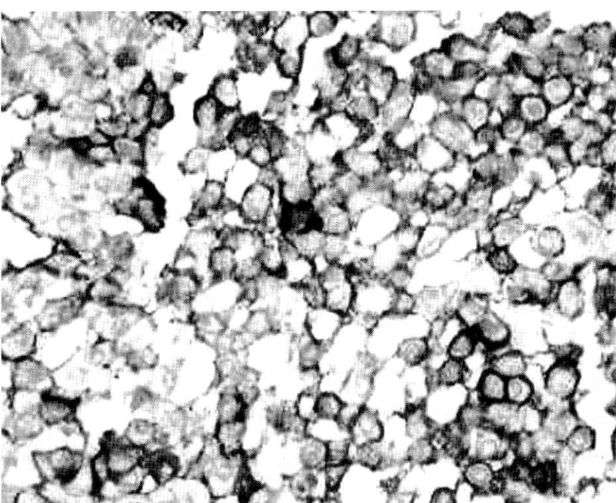

Figure 23.21 Diffuse immunoreactivity for thrombomodulin (CD141) is apparent in a cell block preparation of pleural fluid from a patient with epithelioid mesothelioma. (See also Color Plate 38.)

Table 23.2 Summary of immunohistochemical reagents used to distinguish between mesothelioma and adenocarcinoma[a]

Antibody	Mesothelioma		Adenocarcinoma	
	Result	%	Result	%
BG8	+	4	+	88
MoAb 44-3A6	+	100	+	8
Factor VIII	±	Rare	–	N.S.
Surfactant apoprotein	–	–	+	62
Anti-Lewis antigen	+	11	+	76
Tn antigen	–	–	+	62
E-cadherin	+	10	+	77
TTF-1	+	68	+	100
MoAb SM3	+	52	+	100
Secretory component (SC)	+	0–62	+	60
Pregnancy specific protein	+	0+6	+	34–59
CA 19-9	–	–	+	39
OV632	+	85–91	+	20–63
NSE	+	96	N.S.	N.S.
CD57	+	70	N.S.	N.S.
Mab 45	+	N.S.	+	N.S.
HEA-125	–	–	+	75
Anti BRG	–	–	+	83
ICAM-1	+	100	N.S.	N.S.
VCAM	+	87	N.S.	N.S.
Parathyroid hormone	+	84	+	11
CD44H	+	91	+	45
IOB 3	–	–	+	100
P63	–	0	±	10[b]

aTable modified from Reference 76.
[b]Metastatic squamous cell carcinomas are virtually 100% reactive for nuclear p63 protein
N.S., Not studied or not specified; MoAb, monoclonal antibody; NSE, neuron-specific enolase; ICAM, intercellular adhesion molecule; VCAM, vascular cell adhesion molecule; BRG, retinoblastoma-gene-related protein (other abbreviations are monoclonal antibody designations and have no expanded names).

CD45 (LEUKOCYTE COMMON ANTIGEN) AND OTHER HEMATOPOIETIC MARKERS

CD45 is a cell membrane protein that is nearly universally present in leukocytic proliferations, including leukemias and non-Hodgkin's lymphomas (Figure 23.22), but it is virtually never observed in other tumors. Thus, it is extremely valuable in the recognition of hematopoietic neoplasms in the pleura and elsewhere. There are two caveats to the latter statement; for unexplained reasons, classic Reed–Sternberg cells and Reed variant cells of Hodgkin's lymphomas do not label for CD45, and approximately 30 percent of large-cell anaplastic (Ki-1) non-Hodgkin's lymphomas also are non-reactive for this marker. Both of those tumors consistently express CD30, another highly selective determinant for lymphoid proliferations.

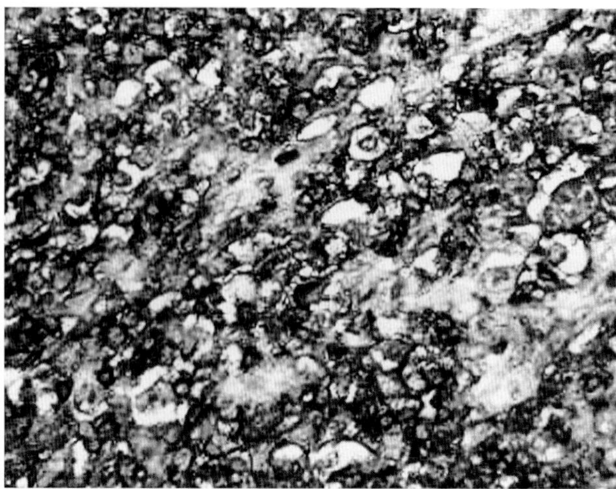

Figure 23.22 This cell block preparation of pleural fluid shows diffuse labeling of tumor cells for CD45 in a case of large-cell non-Hodgkin's lymphoma involving the pleural space. (See also Color Plate 39.)

IMMUNOHISTOLOGICAL EVALUATION OF SARCOMAS

Most sarcomas differ from metastatic sarcomatoid carcinomas and from sarcomatoid mesotheliomas in that they are keratin negative. The principal exception is synovial sarcoma,[86] which is immunoreactive for epithelial markers, including calretinin, and closely resembles mesothelioma morphologically and immunophenotypically. However, synovial sarcoma was labeled by BER-Ep4 in 90 percent of cases, compared with 13 percent for mesothelioma.[87] Conversely, mesothelial tumors were immunoreactive for Wilms' tumor protein-1 (WT1) and CD141 in the majority of cases, whereas synovial sarcoma was typically negative. Ultimately, cytogenetic studies are the most helpful in separating mesothelioma and synovial sarcoma; the latter manifests a consistent t(X;18) chromosomal translocation that is not observed in mesothelial lesions.[88]

Other immunohistochemical markers can be used to determine the lineage of a sarcoma, once it has been defined as such. These include: indicators of a generic myogenous nature, such as desmin; striated muscle differentiation (e.g. myoglobin, myogenin, myo-D1 and 'fast' myosin); proteins seen in smooth muscle cells that include calponin and caldesmon; markers of peripheral nerve sheath differentiation such as S100, CD56, CD57 and nerve growth factor receptor; proteins seen in osteogenic sarcomas, including osteopontin and osteonectin; and endothelial polypeptides such as CD31, CD34, von Willebrand factor and receptor for *Ulex europaeus* I lectin.

MUTANT P53 PROTEIN

Mutations of *p53*, an apoptosis regulation-related gene located on chromosome 17, are common events in a host of human malignancies. However, p53 is not a reliable discriminant between mesothelial hyperplasias and epithelial mesotheliomas, or between fibrous pleurisy and desmoplastic mesothelioma.[89–93] Immunostaining for 'mutant' protein is seen surprisingly often in benign reactive mesothelial lesions,[89] perhaps from amplification of the wild-type *p53* gene rather than mutation of it.

Algorithms for the immunohistological evaluation of malignant pleural tumors of unknown origin

Application of immunohistologic algorithms (Figures 23.23–28) for pleural malignancies is based on statistical data. This process yields several nodal 'branch points' in the algorithm that lead, in turn, to binary diagnostic decisions. The attentive reader will readily notice that these branch points have a certain redundancy in regard to

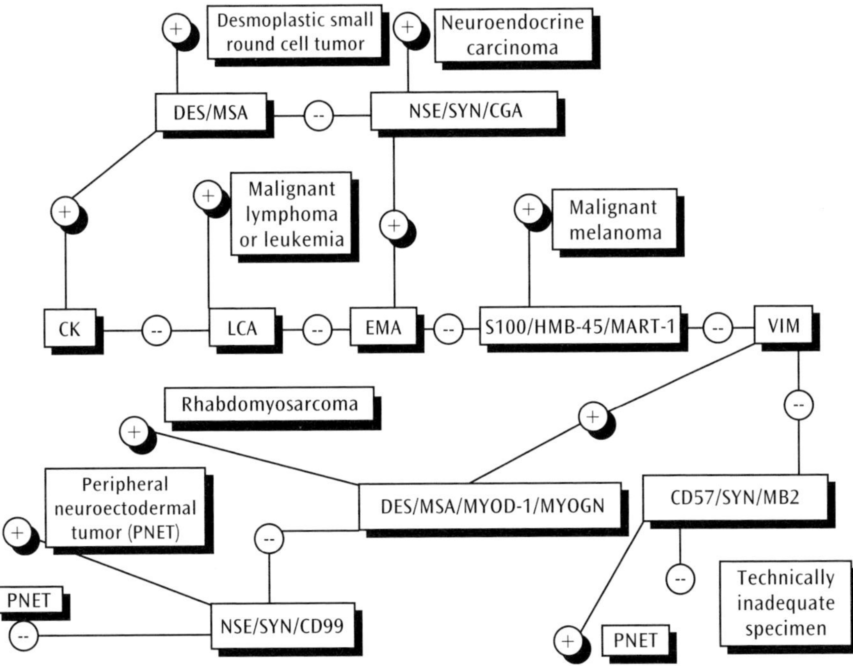

Figure 23.23 Algorithm for immunohistochemical diagnosis of small-cell malignancies.

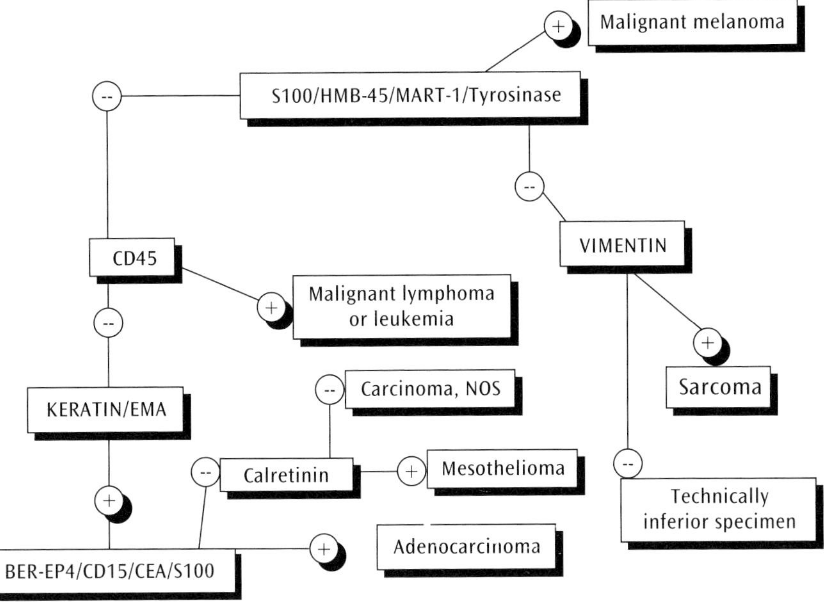

Figure 23.24 Algorithm for immunohistochemical diagnosis of generic large-cell malignancies.

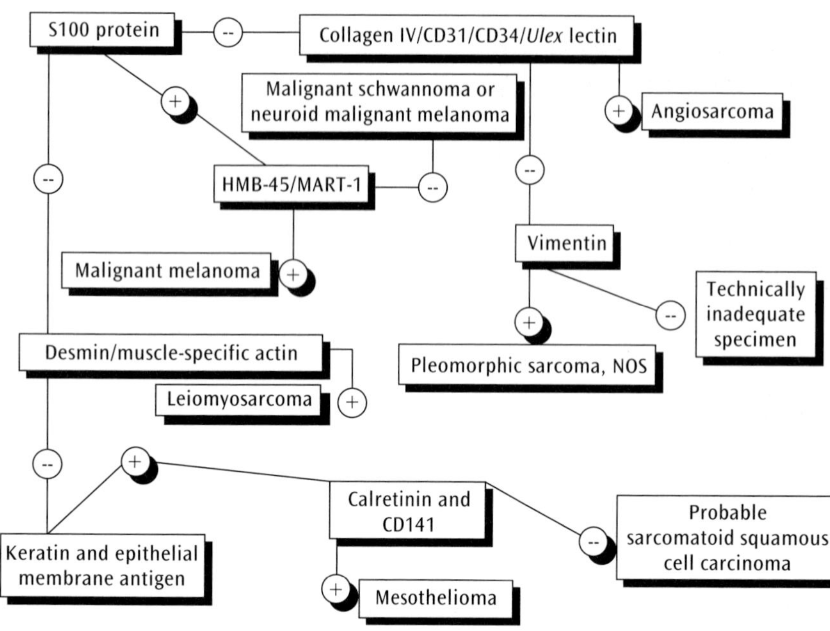

Figure 23.25 Algorithm for immunohistochemical diagnosis of pleomorphic malignancies.

PSA+ TGB–
Prostatic carcinoma
PSA– TGB+
Thyroid carcinoma
PSA/TGB
Both (–)
B72.3/MOC-31
Either or both
+
GCDFP CEA-M S100 PLAP CA-125 CA19-9 CK20 ER
+
Keratin mixture
--
Seminoma (PLAP+; VIM±) or adrenocortical carcinoma *Or* sarcoma (VIM+; PLAP–)
Both --
+
Mesothelioma
CALRET/CD141
--
VIM
--
PLAP
+
EMA
+
RCC or NPC
--
PLAP
--
ACC
+
Embryonal CA
NPC +
HCC --
-- EMA
+
Embryonal CA

GCDFP+ alone--	Breast, salivary gland
CEA+ alone--	GI tract, lung, Mullerian tract, bladder
S100+ alone--	Mullerian tract, breast, salivary gland
PLAP+ alone--	Mullerian tract, GI tract, lung, kidney, breast
CA125+ alone--	Mullerian tract, biliary tract, pancreas, lung, breast, GI tract, liver
CA19-9+ alone--	GI tract, pancreas, Mullerian tract, bladder, lung
CK20+ alone--	GI tract, Mullerian tract, pancreas, lung
ER+ alone--	Breast, Mullerian tract, bladder, liver, stomach
GCDFP+CEA+--	Breast, salivary gland
GCDFP+S100+--	Breast, salivary gland
GCDFP+PLAP+--	Breast
GCDFP+CA125+--	Breast, salivary gland
GCDFP+CA19-9+--	Salivary gland, breast
GCDFP+CK20+--	*Not described in literature*
GCDFP+ER+--	Breast
CEA+S100+--	Breast, salivary gland, Mullerian tract, stomach, biliary tract
CEA+PLAP+--	GI tract, biliary tract, lung, Mullerian tract
CEA+CA125+--	Mullerian tract, biliary tract, pancreas, lung, GI tract, breast
CEA+CA19-9+--	GI tract, pancreas, bladder, Mullerian tract, lung
CEA+CK20+--	GI or biliary tracts, pancreas, endocervix, bladder, lung
CEA+ER+--	Breast, stomach, Mullerian tract
S100+PLAP+--	Mullerian tract, breast, stomach, kidney
S100+CA125+--	Mullerian tract, breast, biliary tract
S100+CA19-9+--	Mullerian tract, biliary tree, stomach, kidney
S100+CK20+--	Mullerian tract, biliary tree, stomach
S100+ER+--	Breast, Mullerian tract
PLAP+CA125+--	Mullerian, biliary, or GI tracts
PLAP+CA19-9+--	Biliary, Mullerian, or GI tracts; lung
PLAP+CK20+--	Biliary, GI, or Mullerian tracts; pancreas
PLAP+ER+--	Breast, Mullerian tract
ALL NEGATIVE--	Renal cell carcinoma or Germ cell tumor (rare examples) or Nasopharyngeal carcinoma

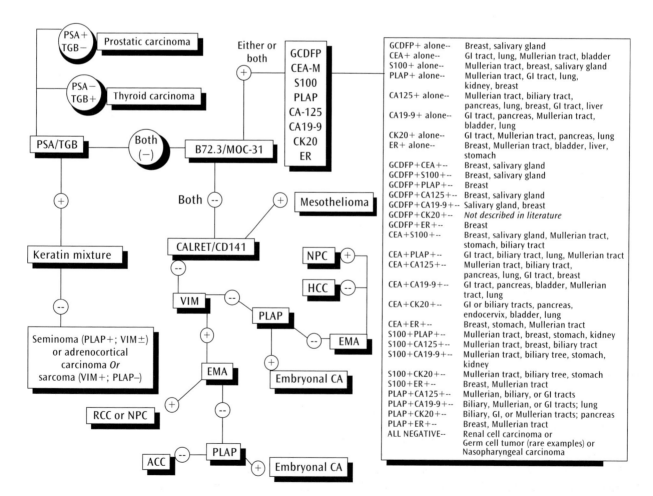

Figure 23.26 Algorithm for immunohistochemical diagnosis of epithelial malignancies of unknown origin.

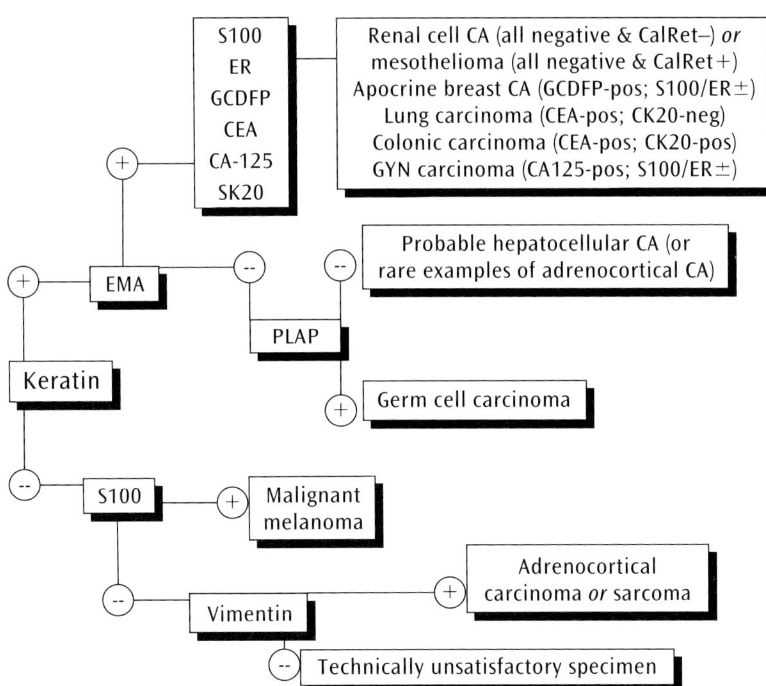

Figure 23.27 Algorithm for immunohistochemical diagnosis of oncocytic malignant neoplasms.

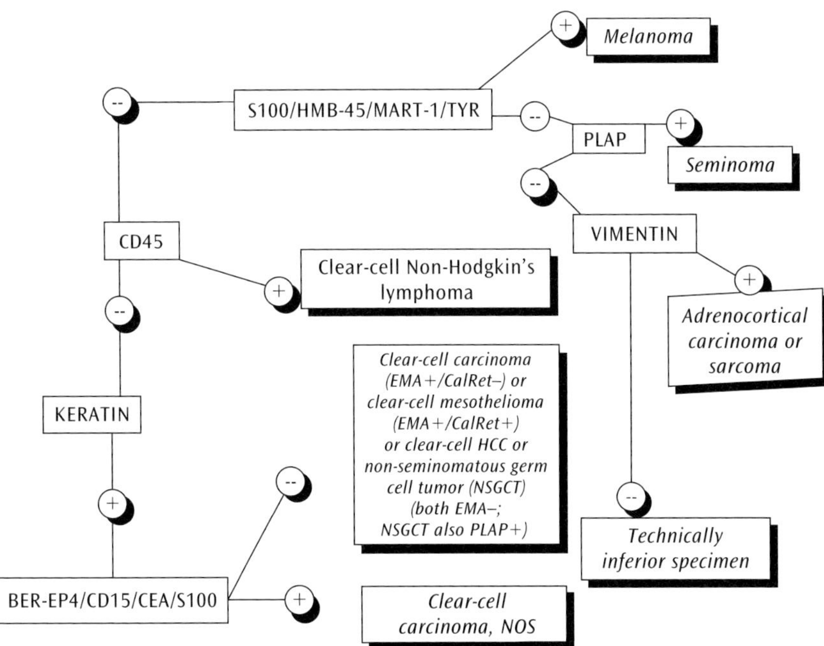

Figure 23.28 Algorithm for immunohistochemical diagnosis of clear-cell malignant neoplasms.

selected immunodeterminants; i.e. they appear at more than one place in the algorithms. This is intentional, so that the natural biological variability of certain neoplasms is adequately represented. Another critical principle of algorithmic interpretation is that one moves from data with a relatively high predictive value to those with lesser predictive values. If carried out properly, however, this 'layering' paradigm contextually enhances the specificity of antibodies that label a variety of neoplasms, because the results they produce are coupled with others that are linked to highly lineage-restrictive reagents. To state this tenet another way, algorithmic 'layering' is a way of obtaining specific information from relatively non-specific markers.

Antibody reagents in these algorithms were chosen, based on their reliability in the author's 15 years of practice. However, it should not be taken that this approach is the only workable one for the assessment of MTUOTs.

Flow cytometry in the evaluation of pleural effusions

Flow cytometry (FCM) is valuable in the assessment of lymphohematological infiltrates of the pleural space. The clonality of constituent cells can be determined quite easily by such means if >5 mL of properly-prepared fresh specimen is submitted, and a B-lymphocytic, T-lymphocytic or myeloid lineage can be assigned based on cell-surface marker characteristics.[25] If necessary, lymphoid gene rearrangement analyses can be performed.

Flow cytometry has a limited role in the assessment of pleural diseases. Cytometric evaluations has inadequate accuracy in distinguishing benign from malignant effusions,[94–97] or adenocarcinoma from mesothelioma.[98,99] FCM studies with rather small cohorts suggested that DNA-aneuploidy and an S (proliferative) phase of the cell cycle (SPF) number <5 or 6 may correlate with shortened survival in mesothelioma.[100–103] In that vein, it should be noted that a measurement equivalent to that of the SPF can be obtained immunohistochemically with the antibody known as MIB-1/Ki-67.[104]

Cytogenetic evaluation of pleural diseases

Cytogenetic analyses, by classical karyotypic methods, fluorescence *in-situ* hybridization, comparative genomic hybridization, or other molecular methods, have contributed to our understanding of the subcellular alterations in various human malignancies. Many well-characterized chromosomal markers of lymphoid neoplasms are recognized, e.g. t(8;14) translocation of Burkitt's lymphoma, t(14;18) translocation of follicular lymphomas, t(2;5) translocation seen in a proportion of anaplastic large-cell lymphomas, 11q23 deletion seen in small-lymphocytic lymphoma/chronic lymphocytic leukemia, translocations affecting 3q27 in some diffuse large-cell non-Hodgkin's lymphomas and t(15;17) translocation in acute promyelocytic leukemia.[105–111] Such cytogenetic tests may aid the diagnosis of lymphoma in the pleural fluid.

Similarly, cytogenetic studies have potential application to 'solid' tumor pathology in the pleura. For example, Ewing's sarcoma/PNET demonstrates a reproducible t(11;22) translocation that distinguishes it from other small-cell neoplasms.[29,30]

The cytogenetics of mesothelioma are detailed separately in this text (see Chapter 11).

KEY POINTS

- Special processing is recommended if flow cytometry or cytogenetic studies of pleural effusions are desired. The specimen should be centrifuged and a cellular pellet should be suspended in nutrient medium for such evaluations.
- Pleural biopsies are much better acquired with video-assisted thoracoscopic technique than by 'closed' needle sampling.
- Benign-reactive and malignant pleural lesions can be remarkably similar cytologically, regardless of their cellular lineages. Hence, this area is a difficult one in cytopathological diagnosis.
- Malignant tumors can be generically divided on cytological grounds into small round-cell, large polygonal-cell and spindle-cell-pleomorphic lesions. This system facilitates differential diagnosis.
- Immunohistochemical algorithms can be linked with cytological categories to yield logical schemes for diagnostic interpretation. Flow cytometry is best applied to pleural effusions in the evaluation of clonality (malignancy) of hematolymphoid proliferations. It has much less utility in the differential diagnosis and prognostication of 'solid' tumors.
- Cytogenetic evaluation is a helpful adjunct in the characterization of hematolymphoid and mesenchymal malignancies in pleural fluid.

REFERENCES

● = Key primary paper
◆ = Major review article

1. Antman KH. Clinical presentation and natural history of benign and malignant mesothelioma. *Semin Oncol* 1981; **8**: 313–20.
2. Belani CP, Ziskind AA, Dhawan M, Lemmon CC. Management of malignant pleural and pericardial effusions. In: Aisner J, Arriagada R, Green MR, Martini N, Perry MC (eds). *Comprehensive textbook of thoracic oncology.* Baltimore: Williams & Wilkins, 1996; 880–905.
3. Gaensler EA, Kaplan AI. Asbestos pleural effusion. *Ann Intern Med* 1971; **74**: 178–91.
4. Luse SA, Reagan JW. A histologic study of effusions. I. Effusions not associated with malignant tumors. *Cancer* 1954; **7**: 1155–66.
5. Reda MG, Raigelman W. Pleural effusion in systemic lupus erythematosus. *Acta Cytol* 1980; **24**: 553–56.
●6. Das DK, Gupta SK, Ayyagari S, *et al.* Pleural effusions in non-Hodgkin's lymphomas: a cytomorphologic, cytochemical, and immunologic study. *Acta Cytol* 1987; **31**: 119–24.
7. Leong ASY, Suthipinatwong C, Vinyuvat S. Immunostaining of cytologic preparations: a review of technical problems. *Appl Immunohistochem Mol Morphol* 1999; **7**: 214–20.
8. Galan GG, Tarrazona-Hervas V, Morcillo-Aixela A, *et al.* The indications for and results of videothoracoscopic surgery:

reflections on 152 procedures. *Arch Bronchopneumonol* 1999; **35**: 477–482.
9. Sakuraba M, Masuda K, Hebisawa A, Sagara Y, Komatsu H. Diagnostic value of thoracoscopic pleural biopsy for pleurisy under local anesthesia. *ANZ J Surg* 2006; **76**: 722–4.
10. Matsubara O, Mark EJ, Ritter JH: Pseudoneoplastic lesions of the lungs, pleural surfaces, and mediastinum. In: Wick MR, Humphrey PA, Ritter JH (eds). *Pathology of pseudoneoplastic lesions*. Philadelphia: Lippincott-Raven, 1997; 97–129.
11. Kutty CPK, Remeniuk E, Varkey B. Malignant-appearing cells in pleural effusion due to pancreatitis. *Acta Cytol* 1981; **25**: 412–16.
●12. Ashton PR, Hollingsworth AS, Johnston WW: The cytopathology of metastatic breast cancer. *Acta Cytol* 1975; **19**: 1–6.
13. Danner DE, Gmelich JT. A comparative study of tumor cells from metastatic carcinoma of the breast in effusions. *Acta Cytol* 1975; **19**: 509–18.
14. Mallonee MM, Lin F, Hassanein K. A morphologic analysis of the cells of ductal carcinoma of the breast and of adenocarcinoma of the ovary in pleural and abdominal effusions. *Acta Cytol* 1987; **31**: 441–7.
15. Spriggs AI, Jerrome DW. Intracellular mucus inclusions: a feature of malignant cells in effusions in the serous cavities, particularly due to carcinoma of the breast. *J Clin Pathol* 1975; **28**: 929–36.
16. Yamada T, Itou V, Watanabe Y, *et al.* Cytologic diagnosis of malignant melanoma. *Acta Cytol* 1972; **16**: 70–6.
17. Hajdu SI, Savino A. Cytologic diagnosis of malignant melanoma. *Acta Cytol* 1973; **11**: 320–7.
●18. Longatto-Filho A, deCarvalho LV, Santos GD, *et al.* Cytologic diagnosis of melanoma in serous effusions: a morphologic and immunocytochemical study. *Acta Cytol* 1995; **39**: 481–4.
19. Denton KJ, Stretch J, Athanasou N. Osteoclast-like giant cells in malignant melanoma. *Histopathology* 1992; **20**: 179–181.
20. Suster S, Moran CA. Unusual manifestations of metastatic tumors to the lungs. *Semin Diagn Pathol* 1995; **12**: 193–206.
21. Nakhleh RE, Wick MR, Rocamora A, Swanson PE, Dehner LP. Morphologic diversity in malignant melanomas. *Am J Clin Pathol* 1990; **93**: 731–40.
22. Roberts GH, Campbell GH. Exfoliative cytology of diffuse mesothelioma. *J Clin Pathol* 1972; **25**: 557–82.
●23. Ansari MQ, Dawson DB, Nador R, *et al.* Primary body cavity-based AIDS-related lymphomas. *Am J Clin Pathol* 1996; **105**: 221–9.
24. Melamed MR. The cytological presentation of malignant lymphomas and related diseases in effusions. *Cancer* 1963; **16**: 413–31.
●25. O'Hara MF, Cousar JB, Glick AD, *et al.* Multiparametric approach to the diagnosis of hematopoietic-lymphoid neoplasms in body fluids. *Diagn Cytopathol* 1985; **1**: 33–8.
●26. Spriggs AE, Vanhegan RI. Cytological diagnosis of lymphoma in serous effusions. *J Clin Pathol* 1981; **34**: 1311–25.
♦27. Cerilli LA, Wick MR. Metastatic malignancies of unknown origin: a histological and cytological approach to diagnosis. *Pathol Case Rev* 2001; **6**: 137–45.
28. Wick MR, Cerilli LA. Applications of immunohistochemistry in the diagnosis of undifferentiated tumors. In: Lloyd RV (ed.). *Morphology methods*. Totowa: Humana Press, 2001; 323–60.
29. Askin FB, Perlman EJ. Neuroblastoma and peripheral neuroectodermal tumors. *Am J Clin Pathol* 1998; **109** (Suppl): S23–30.
●30. Winters JL, Geil JD, O'Connor WN. Immunohistology, cytogenetics, and molecular studies of small round cell tumors of childhood: a review. *Ann Clin Lab Sci* 1995; **25**: 66–78.
31. DeAlava E, Pardo J. Ewing tumor: tumor biology and clinical applications. *Int J Surg Pathol* 2001; **9**: 7–17.
32. Sahu K, Pai RR, Khadilkar UN. Fine needle aspiration cytology of the Ewing's sarcoma family of tumors. *Acta Cytol* 2000; **44**: 332–36.
33. Kumar PV. Fine needle aspiration cytologic findings in malignant small cell tumor of the thoracopulmonary region (Askin tumor). *Acta Cytol* 1994; **38**: 702–6.
34. Ordonez NG. Desmoplastic small round cell tumor. I. A histopathologic study of 39 cases with emphasis on unusual histological patterns. *Am J Surg Pathol* 1998; **22**: 1303–13.
35. Wolf AN, Ladanyi M, Paull G, Balugrund JE, Westra WH. The expanding clinical spectrum of desmoplastic small round-cell tumor: a report of two cases with molecular confirmation. *Hum Pathol* 1999; **30**: 430–435.
36. Parkash V, Gerald WL, Parma, Miettinen M, Rosai J. Desmoplastic small round cell tumor of the pleura. *Am J Surg Pathol* 1995; **19**: 659–65.
37. Bian Y, Jordan AG, Rupp M, *et al.* Effusion cytology of desmoplastic small round cell tumor of the pleura. *Acta Cytol* 1993; **37**: 77–82.
38. Argani P, Askin FB, Colombani P, Perlman EJ. Occult pulmonary synovial sarcoma confirmed by molecular techniques. *Pediatr Dev Pathol* 2000; **3**: 87–90.
♦39. Hajdu SI, Hajdu EO. Exfoliative cytology of malignant lymphoreticular, soft tissue, and bone neoplasms. *Pathol Annu* 1976; **11**: 317–34.
40. Nishikawa A, Tanaka T, Kanai N, *et al.* Exfoliative cytopathology of alveolar rhabdomyosarcoma. *Acta Pathol Jpn* 1987; **37**: 1003–1007.
41. Wong JW, Pitlik D, Abdul-Karim FW. Cytology of pleural, peritoneal, and pericardial fluids in children. A 40-year summary. *Acta Cytol* 1997; **41**: 467–73.
42. Helson L, Krochmal P, Hajdu SI. Diagnostic value of cytologic specimens obtained from children with cancer. *Ann Clin Lab Sci* 1975; **5**: 294–7.
43. Farr GH, Hajdu SI. Exfoliative cytology of metastatic neuroblastoma. *Acta Cytol* 1972; **16**: 203–6.
44. Sahn SA. Pleural effusion in lung cancer. *Clin Chest Med* 1993; **14**: 189–200.
45. Banner BF, Warren WH, Gould VE. Cytomorphology and marker expression of malignant neuroendocrine cells in pleural effusions. *Acta Cytol* 1986; **30**: 99–104.
●46. Mayall FG, Gibbs AR. The histology and immunohistochemistry of small-cell mesothelioma. *Histopathology* 1992; **20**: 47–51.
●47. Nappi O, Ferrara G, Wick MR. Neoplasms composed of eosinophilic polygonal cells: an overview with consideration of different cytomorphologic patterns. *Semin Diagn Pathol* 1999; **16**: 82–90.
48. Rosendale BE, Dusenberry D. Cytology of hepatocellular carcinoma in serous fluids: a report of three cases. *Diagn Cytopathol* 1996; **15**: 127–31.
49. Falconieri G, Zanconati F, Colautti I, *et al.* Effusion cytology of hepatocellular carcinoma. *Acta Cytol* 1995; **39**: 893–7.
50. Hajdu SI, Koss LG. Cytologic diagnosis of metastatic myosarcomas. *Acta Cytol* 1969; **13**: 545–51.
51. Wick MR, Ritter JH, Dehner LP. Malignant rhabdoid tumors: a clinicopathologic review and conceptual discussion. *Semin Diagn Pathol* 1995; **12**: 233–48.
52. Puttagunta L, Vriend RA, Nguyen GK. Deciduoid epithelioid mesothelioma of the pleura with focal rhabdoid change. *Am J Surg Pathol* 2000; **24**: 1440–3.
♦53. Nappi O, Mills SE, Swanson PE, Wick MR. Clear cell tumors of unknown nature and origin: a systematic approach to diagnosis. *Semin Diagn Pathol* 1997; **14**: 164–74.
54. Humphrey PA. Clear cell neoplasms of the urinary tract and male reproductive system. *Semin Diagn Pathol* 1997; **14**: 240–52.
55. Ritter JH, Mills SE, Gaffey MJ, Nappi O, Wick MR. Clear cell tumors of the alimentary tract and abdominal cavity. *Semin Diagn Pathol* 1997; **14**: 213–19.
56. Matias-Guiu X, Lerma E, Prat J. Clear cell tumors of the female genital tract. *Semin Diagn Pathol* 1997; **14**: 233–9.
57. Murakata LA, Ishak KG, Nzeako UC. Clear cell carcinoma of the liver: a comparative immunohistochemical study with renal clear-cell carcinoma. *Mod Pathol* 2000; **13**: 874–81.

58. Ropp BG, Solomides C, Palazzo J, Bibbo M. Follicular carcinoma of the thyroid with extensive clear-cell differentiation: a potential diagnostic pitfall. *Diagn Cytopathol* 2000; **23**: 222–3.
59. Perniciaro C. Dermatopathologic variants of malignant melanoma. *Mayo Clin Proc* 1997; 72: 273–79.
●60. Hajdu SI, Nolan MA. Exfoliative cytology of malignant germ cell tumors. *Acta Cytol* 1975; **19**: 255–60.
61. Azuma T, Nishimatsu H, Nakagawa T, *et al.* Metastatic renal cell carcinoma mimicking pleural mesothelioma. *Scan J Urol Nephrol* 1999; **33**: 140–1.
62. Kutty K, Varkey B. Incidence and distribution of intrathoracic metastases from renal cell carcinoma. *Arch Intern Med* 1984; **144**: 273–6.
63. Silverman JF, Dabbs DJ, Finley JL, Geisinger KR. Fine needle aspiration biopsy of pleomorphic (giant cell) carcinoma of the pancreas: cytologic, immunocytochemical, and ultrastructural findings. *Am J Clin Pathol* 1988; **89**: 714–20.
64. Bonomo L, Feragalli B, Sacco R, Merlino B, Storto ML. Malignant pleural disease. *Eur J Radiol* 2000; **34**: 98–118.
●65. Newhouse M. Epidemiology of asbestos-related tumors. *Semin Oncol* 1981; **8**: 250–7.
●66. Peterson JT, Greenberg SD, Buffler P. Non-asbestos-related malignant mesothelioma: a review. *Cancer* 1984; **54**: 951–60.
67. Attanoos RL, Gibbs AR. Pathology of malignant mesothelioma. *Histopathology* 1997; **30**: 403–18.
68. Wick MR, Mills SE. Mesothelial proliferations: an increasing morphological spectrum. *Am J Clin Pathol* 2000; **113**: 619– 22.
69. Carter D, Otis CN. Three types of spindle cell tumors of the pleura: fibroma, sarcoma, and sarcomatoid mesothelioma. *Am J Surg Pathol* 1988; **12**: 747–53.
70. Cagle PT, Truong LD, Roggli VL, Greenberg SD: Immunohistochemical differentiation of sarcomatoid mesotheliomas from other spindle cell neoplasms. *Am J Clin Pathol* 1989; **92**: 566–71.
♦71. Rdzanek M, Fresco R, Pass HI, Carbone M. Spindle cell tumors of the pleura: differential diagnosis. *Semin Diagn Pathol* 2006; **23**: 44–55.
72. Khalidi HS, Medeiros LJ, Battifora H. Lymphohistiocytoid mesothelioma: an often-misdiagnosed variant of sarcomatoid malignant mesothelioma. *Am J Clin Pathol* 2000; **113**: 649–54.
●73. Villena V, Lopez-Encuentra A, Echave-Sustaeta J, *et al.* Diagnostic value of CA72-4, carcinoembryonic antigen, CA15-3, and CA19-9 assay in pleural fluid: a study of 207 patients. *Cancer* 1996; **78**: 736–40.
●74. Mezger J, Stotzer O, Schilli G, Bauer S, Wilmanns W. Identification of carcinoma cells in ascitic and pleural fluid: comparison of four panepithelial antigens and carcinoembryonic antigen. *Acta Cytol* 1992; **36**: 75–81.
75. Shimokata K, Totani Y, Nakanishi K, *et al.* Diagnostic value of cancer antigen 15-3 (CA15-3) detected by monoclonal antibodies (115D8 and DF3) in exudative pleural effusions. *Eur Respir J* 1988; **1**: 341–4.
●76. Romero S, Fernandez C, Arriero JM, *et al.* CEA, CA15-3, and CYFRA 21-1 in serum and pleural fluid of patients with pleural effusions. *Eur Respir J* 1996; **9**: 17–23.
●77. DeYoung BR, Wick MR. Immunohistologic analysis of metastatic carcinomas of unknown origin: an algorithmic approach. *Semin Diagn Pathol* 2000; **17**: 184–93.
♦78. Ordonez NG. What are the current best immunohistochemical markers for the diagnosis of epithelioid mesothelioma? A review and update. *Hum Pathol* 2007; **38**: 1–16.
79. Kachali C, Eltoum I, Horton D, Chhieng DC. Use of mesothelin as a marker for mesothelial cells in cytologic specimens. *Semin Diagn Pathol* 2006; **23**: 20–4.
80. Li Q, Bavikatty N, Michael CW. The role of immunohistochemistry in distinguishing squamous cell carcinoma from mesothelioma and adenocarcinoma in pleural effusions. *Semin Diagn Pathol* 2006; **23**: 15–19.
●81. Saad RS, Lindner JL, Lin X, Liu YL, Silverman JE. The diagnostic utility of D2-40 for malignant mesothelioma versus pulmonary carcinoma with pleural involvement. *Diagn Cytopathol* 2006; **34**: 801–6.
82. Kahn HJ, Bailey D, Marks A. Monoclonal antibody D2-40, a new marker of lymphatic endothelium, reacts with Kaposi's sarcoma and a subset of angiosarcomas. *Mod Pathol* 2002; **15**: 434–40.
83. Lau SK, Weiss LM, Chu PG. D2-40 immunohistochemistry in the differential diagnosis of seminoma and embryonal carcinoma: a comparative immunohistochemical study with KIT (CD117) and CD30. *Mod Pathol* 2007; **20**: 320–5.
84. Browning L, Parker A, Bailey D. D2-40 is a sensitive and specific marker in differentiating primary adrenal cortical tumors from both metastatic clear cell renal cell carcinoma and pheochromocytoma. *J Clin Pathol* 2008; **61**: 293–6.
●85. Wick MR, Moran CA, Mills SE, Suster S. Immunohistochemical differential diagnosis of pleural effusions, with emphasis on malignant mesothelioma. *Curr Opin Pulm Med* 2001; **7**: 187–92.
86. Gaertner E, Zeren EH, Fleming MV, Colby TV, Travis WD. Biphasic synovial sarcomas arising in the pleural cavity: a clinicopathologic study of five cases. *Am J Surg Pathol* 1996; **20**: 36–45.
87. Miettinen M, Limon J, Niezabitowski A, Lasota J. Calretinin and other mesothelioma markers in synovial sarcoma: analysis of antigenic similarities and differences with malignant mesothelioma. *Am J Surg Pathol* 2001; **25**: 610–17.
88. Argani P, Zakowski MF, Klimstra DS, Rosai J, Ladanyi M. Detection of the *SYT-SSX* chimeric RNA of synovial sarcoma in paraffin-embedded tissue and its application in problematic cases. *Mod Pathol* 1998; **11**: 65–71.
89. Cury PM, Butcher DN, Corrin D, Nicholson AG. The use of histological and immunohistochemical markers to distinguish pleural malignant mesothelioma and *in-situ* mesothelioma from reactive mesothelial hyperplasia and reactive pleural fibrosis. *J Pathol* 1999; **189**: 251–7.
90. Mayall FG, Jacobson G, Wilkins R. Mutations of p53 gene and SV40 sequences in asbestos-associated and non-asbestos-associated mesotheliomas. *J Clin Pathol* 1999; **52**: 291–3.
●91. Stoetzer OJ, Munker R, Darsow M, Wilmanns W. p53-immunoreactive cells in benign and malignant effusions: diagnostic value using a panel of monoclonal antibodies and comparison with CEA staining. *Oncol Rep* 1999; **6**: 455–8.
●92. Mangano WE, Cagle PT, Churg A, Vollmer RT, Roggli VL. The diagnosis of desmoplastic malignant mesothelioma and its distinction from fibrous pleurisy: a histologic and immunohistochemical analysis of 31 cases including p53 immunostaining. *Am J Clin Pathol* 1998; **110**: 191–9.
♦93. Churg A, Colby TV, Cagle PT, *et al.* The separation of benign and malignant mesothelial proliferations. *Am J Surg Pathol* 2000; **24**: 1183–1200.
●94. Ceyhan BB, Demiralp E, Celikel T. Analysis of pleural effusions using flow cytometry. *Respiration* 1996; **63**: 17–24.
●95. Joseph MG, Banerjee D, Harris P, Gibson S, McFadden RG. Multiparameter flow cytometric DNA analysis of effusions: a prospective study of 36 cases compared with routine cytology and immunohistochemistry. *Mod Pathol* 1995; **8**: 686–93.
96. Pinto MM. DNA analysis of malignant effusions: comparison with cytologic diagnosis and carcinoembryonic antigen content. *Anal Quant Cytol Histol* 1992; **14**: 222–6.
97. Nance KV, Silverman JF. The utility of ancillary techniques in effusion cytology. *Diagn Cytopathol* 1992; **8**: 185–9.
98. Esteban JM, Sheibani K. DNA ploidy analysis of pleural mesotheliomas: its usefulness for their distinction from lung adenocarcinomas. *Mod Pathol* 1992; **5**: 626–30.
99. El-Naggar AK, Ordonez NG, Garnsey L, Batsakis JG. Epithelioid pleural mesotheliomas and pulmonary adenocarcinomas: a comparative DNA flow-cytometric study. *Hum Pathol* 1991; **22**: 972–8.

●100. Emri S, Akbulut H, Zorlu F, *et al.* Prognostic significance of flow cytometric DNA analysis in patients with malignant pleural mesothelioma. *Lung Cancer* 2001; **33**: 109–14.

101. Isobe H, Sridhar KS, Doria R, *et al.* Prognostic significance of DNA aneuploidy in diffuse malignant mesothelioma. *Cytometry* 1995; **19**: 86–91.

102. Pyrhonen S, Laasonen A, Tammilehto L, *et al.* Diploid predominance and prognostic significance of S-phase cells in malignant mesothelioma. *Eur J Cancer* 1991; **27**: 197–200.

103. Dazzi H, Thatcher N, Hasleton PS, Chatterjee AK, Lawson RA. DNA analysis by flow cytometry in malignant pleural mesothelioma: relationship to histology and survival. *J Pathol* 1990; **162**: 51–5.

104. Comin CE, Anichini C, Boddi V, Novelli L, Dini S. MIB-1 proliferation index correlates with survival in pleural malignant mesotheliomas. *Histopathology* 2000; **36**: 26–31.

105. Macintyre E, Willerford D, Morris SW. Non-Hodgkin's lymphoma: molecular features of B-cell lymphoma. *Hematology* 2000; **1**: 180–204.

106. Kuppers R, Dalla-Favera R. Mechanisms of chromosomal translocation in B-cell lymphomas. *Oncogene* 2001; **20**: 5580–94.

107. Karnolsky IN. Cytogenetic abnormalities in chronic lymphocytic leukemia. *Folia Med* 2000; **42**: 5–10.

●108. Hegde U, Wilson WH. Gene expression profiling of lymphomas. *Curr Oncol Rep* 2001; **3**: 243–249.

109. Appelbaum FR, Rowe JM, Radich J, Dick JE. Acute myeloid leukemia. *Hematology* 2001; **2**: 62–86.

110. Lin RJ, Sternsdorf T, Tini M, Evans RM. Transcriptional regulation in acute promyelocytic leukemia. *Oncogene* 2001; **20**: 7204–15.

111. Padua RA, McGlynn A, McGlynn H. Molecular, cytogenetic, and genetic abnormalities in MDS and secondary AML. *Cancer Treat Res* 2001; **108**: 111–57.

24

Effusions from cardiac diseases

GARY T KINASEWITZ, KELLIE R JONES

INCIDENCE/EPIDEMIOLOGY

Pleural effusions are a common manifestation of heart disease. The incidence and characteristics of the effusion will vary depending upon the nature of the underlying cardiac disorder. When the underlying cardiac disorder is severe enough to result in congestive heart failure, transudative pleural effusions will develop in a majority of patients. Given the prevalence of heart disease in Western society, it is not surprising that congestive heart failure is the most common cause of transudative pleural effusions.[1] Pericardial disease is less common, but both acute and chronic pericardial disease can also give rise to pleural effusions, even in the absence of heart failure. Depending on the etiology of the pericardial disease, the pleural fluid may be either a transudate or an exudate.

The frequency with which pleural effusions are detected varies with the population studied and the methods employed. The routine chest radiograph will reveal effusions in 58 to 73 percent of unselected patients admitted to the hospital with congestive heart failure.[2,3] Weiner-Kronish and colleagues[4] found pleural effusions by ultrasound examination in half of a group of patients admitted to a coronary care unit with congestive heart failure. However, the incidence of pleural effusion in heart failure patients increases when more sensitive techniques such as computed tomography (CT) or autopsy are employed. Kataoka[5] prospectively evaluated 60 patients with decompensated congestive heart failure of varying etiologies admitted to a special Heart Failure Unit in the hospital. He found 87 percent of the patients had pleural effusions using CT examination. Less than half of these effusions were visible on the routine postero-anterior (PA) chest radiograph. Race and colleagues[6] found pleural fluid in over 90 percent of autopsied patients who died of heart failure. In 72 percent the effusions exceeded 250 mL, large enough to be detected on a radiograph. The effusions were bilateral in 88 percent of patients with unilateral right and left-sided effusions accounting for 8 and 4 percent of cases, respectively.

The incidence of pleural effusions in patients with pericardial disease depends on the underlying etiology. Weiss and Spodick[7] found pleural effusions by routine radiographic examination in 35 of 133 consecutive patients with pericardial disease of varying etiologies. Only 37 percent had bilateral effusions; the majority (60 percent) were left sided and only one isolated right-sided sided effusion was observed. Some diseases, such as malignancy and rheumatoid arthritis, can cause effusions because of pericardial involvement and by affecting the pleura. It is not surprising that the incidence of pleural effusion in association with such disorders is even higher than when the disorder also involves the pericardium. [8–11]

PATHOGENESIS

The normal mechanisms responsible for the filtration of pleural fluid from the pleural capillaries and its reabsorption are reviewed in detail in Chapter 5, Physiology: fluid and solute exchange in normal physiological states. The interstitium of the lung ordinarily plays no role in the reabsorption of pleural fluid under normal conditions.[12] However, experimental studies have suggested that it may be the major source of pleural fluid in patients with congestive heart failure.

Allen and colleagues[13] produced left atrial hypertension and pulmonary edema in sheep by means of a left atrial balloon catheter and found that the volume of pleural fluid formed correlated with the amount of pulmonary edema. Pleural effusions did not develop unless pulmonary edema was present. Broaddus *et al.*[14] produced pulmonary edema in sheep by infusing them with large volumes of saline and found that as much as 25 percent of the infused volume escaped into the pleural cavity. The resolution of alveolar edema requires the reabsorption of the alveolar fluid into the interstitium of the lung for subsequent removal by the pulmonary lymphatics.[15] This reabsorption of alveolar fluid into the interstitium of the lung raises lung interstitial pressure and promotes the leak of fluid from the subpleural lung through the visceral mesothelium into the pleural space. The mesothelium *per se* is a very porous membrane that offers little resistance to the flow of fluid.[16]

Acute elevations in systemic venous pressure produced by volume loading and vena caval obstruction can also induce pleural effusions in experimental animals.[17,18] The effusions which develop are a consequence of increased filtration from the pleural capillaries and decreased reabsorption due to the combined effects of increased pleural capillary hydrostatic pressure and lymphatic outflow obstruction of the pleural lymphatics which ultimately empty into the superior vena cava. Lowering of the plasma oncotic pressure due to saline infusion undoubtedly is yet another factor contributing to the formation of pleural fluid in these animals. However, hypoalbuminemia in the absence of venous hypertension is unlikely to cause pleural effusions in humans.[19] When the obstruction to lymphatic outflow is chronic, the lymphatic pumping mechanism can compensate for the venous obstruction.[20] Once lymphatic flow is restored, both the edema fluid in the lung and the associated pleural effusions resolve.[21]

The clinical correlate of these experimental studies is that pleural effusions are common in patients with left heart failure but rare in those with right heart failure. Weiner-Kronish and colleagues[4] prospectively studied 37 patients admitted to a coronary care unit with congestive heart failure and found that 19 (51 percent) had pleural effusions. The pulmonary capillary wedge pressure was significantly greater and alveolar edema was more common in the patients with pleural effusions (Table 24.1). Sixteen of 19 patients with pleural effusions (but only 3 of 18 without effusions) had a pulmonary capillary wedge pressure ≥20 mmHg. In contrast, no significant difference in right atrial pressure was noted between those with and without pleural effusions. Subsequently, these investigators studied a group of 18 patients with right atrial hypertension due to pulmonary vascular disease and normal pulmonary capillary wedge pressures.[22] Pleural effusions were not found in any of these patients with isolated right heart failure. Thus, while right ventricular failure may facilitate the formation of pleural effusions, left ventricular failure appears to be essential for their development.

The pathogenesis of pleural effusions in patients with pericardial disease is less clear. In some patients, it is likely that the pericardium and pleura are affected by the same process. For example, the incidence of pleural effusions is high in patients with tuberculous pericarditis, and infection of the mesothelium lining of both the pericardial and pleural cavities is usually present.[9] Simultaneous involvement of the pericardium and pleura probably accounts for the finding of malignant effusions in over one-third of patients with malignant pericardial disease.[8] Malignant invasion of the mediastinal lymph nodes, through which the pleural and pericardial lymphatics drain, contributes to the simultaneous development of pericardial and pleural effusions. However, the frequent occurrence of unilateral left-sided pleural effusions in those with idiopathic and acute inflammatory pericardial disease is more difficult to explain.[7] The left sided effusion may represent a sympathetic response to contiguous inflammation or be due to an impairment in lymphatic drainage. The former mechanism probably accounts for the simultaneous presence of both pericardial and pleural effusions in patients with acute pancreatitis.[23]

CLINICAL PRESENTATION

The clinical presentation is generally typical of patients with congestive heart failure. Increasing dyspnea, orthopnea and edema are the most common presenting symptoms. Patients with heart failure rarely complain of pleuritic pain. Frequently, the effusions may be asymptomatic radiographic findings in a patient with known congestive heart failure. Physical examination commonly reveals evidence of biventricular failure with distended

Table 24.1 Hemodynamic and radiographic findings in heart failure patients

	Effusion present (n = 19)	Effusion absent (n = 18)
Pulmonary arterial pressure (mmHg)	38.0 ± 1.5	30.7 ± 2.1*
Pulmonary wedge pressure (mmHg)	24.1 ± 1.3	17.2 ± 1.5*
Right atrial pressure (mmHg)	12.6 ± 1.5	9.8 ± 1.0
Alveolar edema on chest radiography (n)	8	4

Values are mean ±SEM; *$p < 0.05$ effusion present versus effusion absent. Data from reference 4.

neck veins, rales, an S_3 gallop and peripheral edema. Dullness to percussion at the lung base, decreased fremitus and egophony indicate the presence of a pleural effusion.

In contrast to the painless dyspnea of the patient with heart failure, patients with pericarditis typically complain of chest pain that may be pleuritic in nature as well as dyspnea.[24] A pericardial friction rub is frequently audible and the electrocardiogram (ECG) may display the typical diffuse ST-segment elevations. Low voltage on the ECG and distant heart sounds in a patient with cardiomegaly are highly suggestive but uncommon clinical findings.[24] Hypotension, tachycardia and pulsus paradoxus may signal impending tamponade. When the pericarditis is one manifestation of a systemic disease such as lupus erythematosus or rheumatoid arthritis, other stigmata of the underlying disorder may be readily appreciated.

RADIOLOGY

Most patients have bilateral effusions and cardiomegaly apparent on the PA chest radiograph. Additional radiographic signs of heart failure including pulmonary vascular engorgement, increased septal markings and alveolar edema may be present.[2] Generally, the effusions are of moderate size, 300–1000 mL, and occupy less than half a hemithorax.[25] Minor differences in the size of the effusions in each hemithorax are not uncommon. Several investigators have found that predominantly right-sided and predominantly left-sided effusions occurred with equal frequency.[26,27]

Unless heart failure develops in the setting of an acute myocardial infarction, the absence of cardiomegaly in a patient with bilateral effusions should raise the suspicion of some other disease. Rabin and Blackman[28] found effusions due to heart failure in only 3 of 78 patients who presented with this clinical picture. Malignancy and serositis accounted for over half the bilateral effusions in this study. Unilateral effusions do occur in patients with heart failure but they are less common (Table 24.2). Unilateral right-sided effusions have been observed in 16 percent of patients while unilateral left-sided effusions were detected in 7 percent of patients with heart failure, a difference that probably is not clinically significant.[5,6] A superimposed process such as thromboembolism should be suspected whenever a unilateral effusion is found in a patient with heart failure. The presence of a large left-sided effusion in a patient with cardiomegaly should raise the suspicion of pericarditis.[3,7]

When pleural effusions develop in a patient with heart failure, the fluid is usually free flowing and will layer on a decubitus radiograph. However, unusual loculations may occur, particularly in the presence of previous pleural disease. The presence of a pseudotumor which might be mistaken for a lung mass may be suspected by its characteristic convex radiographic appearance within a fissure and confirmed if the 'mass' disappears with diuretic therapy (Figure 24.1).[29]

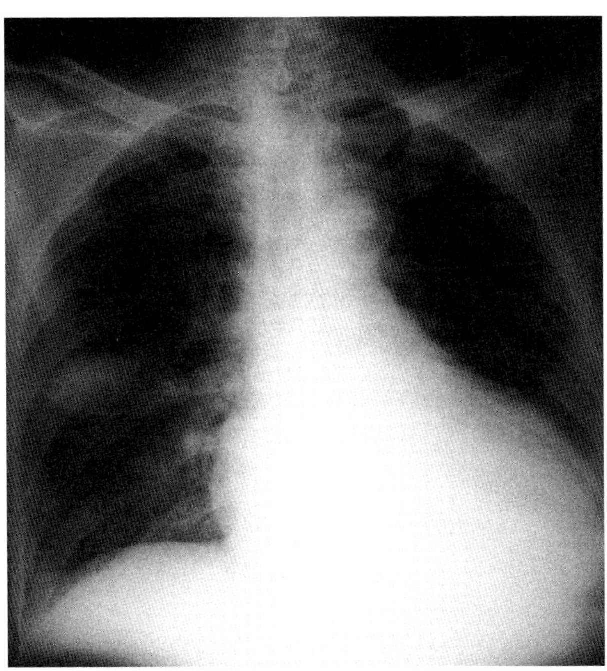

Figure 24.1 Loculated pleural effusion or 'pseudotumor' in the minor fissure of the right lung. The mass disappeared after diuretic therapy. Courtesy of Thomas Johnson M.D.

Table 24.2 Intrathoracic distribution of pleural effusions in heart failure patients

Author	Ref no.	Method of detection	*n*	Bilateral effusions	%	Right only	%	Left only	%
Weiss and Spodick	3	Chest radiograph	70	51	73	13	19	6	9
Peterman and Brothers	26	Chest radiograph	54	49	91	2	4	3	6
Woodring	27	Chest radiograph	120	87	73	18	15	15	13
Porcel *et al.*	43	Chest radiograph	197	117	59	62	31	18	9
Katoaka and Takada	25	Computed tomography	52	44	85	6	12	2	4
Race *et al.*	6	Autopsy	290	255	88	24	8	11	4
Total of all series			783	603	77	125	16	55	7

Ultrasound may occasionally be helpful in localizing a small or loculated effusion for thoracentesis.[30,31] The effusion will appear as an echo-free area beneath the chest wall that changes shape with respiration.[32] Pericardial effusions may be recognized as an echo-free space between the epicardium and pericardium associated with flattening of the pericardial echo relative to the epicardial echo.[33] Diastolic collapse of the right atrium and right ventricular free wall indicates the presence of tamponade.[34] CT may be helpful to identify or exclude an additional pulmonary process (Figure 24.2).

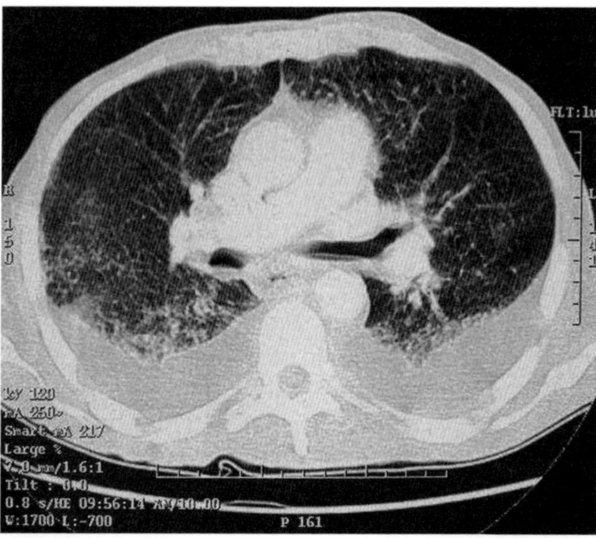

(a)

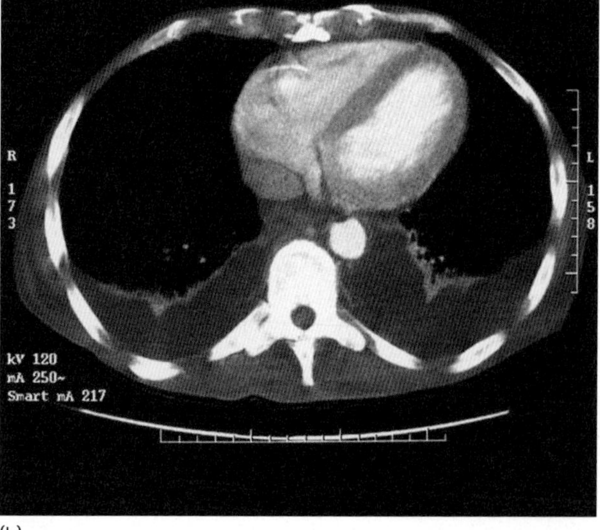

(b)

Figure 24.2 (a) Chest computed tomography scan of a patient with congestive heart failure reveals increased septal markings and bilateral effusions of equal size. (b) Mediastinal windows in the same patient clearly demonstrate the bilateral effusions and cardiomegaly.

PLEURAL FLUID CHARACTERISTICS

Patients who present with the typical findings of cardiomegaly and bilateral pleural effusions probably do not require diagnostic thoracentesis.[35,36] If the effusions resolve with diuretic therapy, the diagnosis can be considered clinically confirmed. However, patients with atypical presentations, including those with marked asymmetry in the size of their effusions, those without cardiomegaly and those with clinical findings such as pleuritic pain or fever that raise suspicion of an additional process, should undergo thoracentesis.

The effusions which develop in patients due to congestive heart failure are transudates with a low protein concentration (pleural fluid to serum ratio less than 0.5) and a low absolute lactate dehydrogenase (LDH) value (less than two-thirds the upper limit of normal) and a pleural fluid to serum LDH ratio of less than 0.6.[37] The fluid typically contains less then 1000 cells/mm^3, the majority of which are lymphocytes and mesothelial cells.[38]

When thoracentesis is delayed to observe the effect of diuretic therapy, there is the possibility that a transudate may be converted into an exudate. Pleural fluid is primarily removed via lymphatic reabsorption but additional water may be directly reabsorbed into the pleural capillaries if the venous hypertension is corrected. This increases the concentrations of protein and LDH within the pleural space and, in some patients, it may be sufficient to convert a transudative effusion into one with exudative characteristics. Shinto and Light[39] performed a repeat thoracentesis on 12 patients who presented with heart failure and an initial thoracentesis demonstrating transudative fluid. Repeat thoracentesis 12–48 hours later demonstrated only small increases of less than 20 percent in the protein and LDH concentrations and in only one patient had the fluid acquired the characteristics of an exudate. Chako *et al.*[40] studied eight patients with transudative effusions due to heart failure but waited 6 (±2) days before performing a second thoracentesis.[40] The mean weight loss was greater in this study and the protein and LDH concentrations increased by 45 and 70 percent, respectively. These increases were sufficient to convert the transudates to exudates in three of the eight patients.

Romero-Candeira and colleagues[41] expanded on these observations by performing multiple thoracenteses at 48-hour intervals in 21 patients with congestive heart failure of varying etiologies who had transudative effusions on initial presentation. The final thoracentesis was performed 5 (±2) days after the initial one. The protein concentration increased by 43 percent and the LDH activity increased by 63 percent with diuretic therapy and 67 percent of the effusions met one or more of Light's criteria and would have been misclassified as exudates by the results of the final thoracentesis.[41] Because of hemoconcentration during diuretic therapy, the plasma protein concentration also increased so that normal plasma to pleural fluid albumin and total protein gradients were preserved in 80 percent of these patients. Nonetheless, these more specific indicators still would have misclassified 20 percent of the effusions as exudates. It is clear that when thoracentesis is delayed for several days while the patient is being treated for congestive heart failure, the results of pleural fluid chemistries must be interpreted with caution. The presence of a plasma to pleural fluid albumin gradient greater than 1.2 g/dL indicates that the effusion was formed as a transudate irrespective of whether or not it meets traditional protein and LDH criteria at the time of thoracentesis.[42]

B-type natriuretic peptide (BNP) is secreted by the cardiac ventricles in response to acute distention. Porcel and colleagues[43] found that BNP levels greater than 1500 pg/mL in the pleural fluid distinguished 44 patients with effusions due to heart failure from 73 controls with hepatic hydrothorax or exudates of varying etiology. Gegenhuber *et al.*[44] found that plasma BNP levels were elevated in patients with effusions due to heart failure and that the elevated plasma levels persisted at 24 hours despite removing most of the effusion by thoracentesis. Since pleural fluid originates as an ultrafiltrate of plasma, it is not surprising that the plasma and pleural fluid BNP levels are highly correlated.[45] An elevated BNP level may help identify the cardiac origin of an effusion in a patient with heart failure, even if the effusion meets one or more of Light's criteria for an exudate after diuresis.

Because congestive heart failure is such a common condition, it is not uncommon to encounter a patient who has an exudative effusion caused by a coexistent condition such as pneumonia. Generally, the etiology of the effusion is obvious in such cases. Gotsman *et al.*[46] reported on 47 patients with exudative effusions in the setting of congestive heart failure. Infection, cardiac surgery and malignancy accounted for most of the identified etiologies. However, 20 of the 47 patients had no other obvious cause for their exudative effusions. Patients with no obvious cause were more likely to have received acute diuretic therapy compared with those with transudates.

We recently reviewed our experience with 770 patients seen at our medical center with congestive heart failure and radiographic evidence of pleural effusions.[47] The majority had typical clinical presentation and were treated medically without thoracentesis. Only 175 had a thoracentesis and in this select group, 89 patients had exudates. Exudates were significantly more common in those who had a remote history of coronary artery bypass grafting (CABG). A non-cardiac cause was ultimately identified in 77 of these patients including 11 who had undergone CABG one or more years prior to the development of the effusion. The effusions in four of the remaining patients could be explained by red blood cell (RBC) contamination during a traumatic tap, leaving only eight patients of the original 770 patients with unexplained exudates. All of these patients had received diuretic therapy prior to thoracentesis. Thus, unexplained exudates are rare in patients with congestive heart failure. The presence of an exudate in a patient who has not had previous chest surgery should prompt a search for an etiology other than congestive heart failure.

Exudates are much more likely when patients with pericardial disease develop an effusion. In general, the pleural and pericardial fluid will have the same characteristics. Indeed, examination of the pleural fluid can often establish the nature of the underlying problem. The finding of malignant cells or positive acid-fast smears of the pleural fluid will indicate the probable cause of the pericardial disease.[8,9] High anti-nuclear antibody (ANA) titers may be found in both the pericardial and the pleural fluid from patients with lupus erythematosis.[48] Pericardial effusions due to heart failure do occur; Kataoka *et al.*[5] found pericardial effusions in 20 percent of patients with decompensated congestive heart failure, whereas 87 percent of these patients had pleural effusions. None of the pericardial effusions were large. Both the pericardial and pleural fluid have the characteristics of a transudate.

TREATMENT

The pleural membranes *per se* are intact in the patient with congestive heart failure so that restoration of a normal balance of Starling forces should permit the reabsorption of the pleural fluid. Diuretics, afterload reduction and digitalis are the mainstays of therapy. Howard and Dunn demonstrated that aggressive diuretic therapy with continuous IV furosemide will reduce the length (and associated cost) of hospital stay without any increase in morbidity.[49] If treatment of the underlying heart failure is successful, the effusion will resolve.

Since they often have the same etiology, the pleural effusions in patients with pericardial disease will respond to treatment of the underlying process. Anti-inflammatory therapy for serositis and anti-tuberculous therapy for the patient with tuberculosis will effectively treat both the pleural effusion and the pericardial disease. However, if there is clinical evidence of tamponade, immediate pericardial drainage is necessary and can be lifesaving. Malignant pericardial disease usually signals far advanced disease and often requires definitive local therapy for its control. Pericardial sclerosis with doxycycline or bleomycin may prevent the reaccumulation of fluid in about three-quarters of treated patients.[50–52] Alternatively, a pericardial window can be created to allow the fluid to drain into the pleural or peritoneal cavities or the preperitoneal subcutaneous space.[53–56] Pericardiectomy may be required for the patient with symptomatic constrictive pericardial disease.[11]

When a patient with large pleural effusion remains dyspneic despite intensive medical therapy, therapeutic thoracentesis is indicated. Often the removal of 500–1000 mL of fluid may produce immediate and dramatic symptomatic relief, even before there is an increase in vital capacity or the partial pressure of arterial O_2 (PaO_2). The beneficial effects of therapeutic thoracentesis include a reduction in the resting volume of the chest wall which enables the inspiratory muscles to operate on a more advantageous portion of their length–tension relationship.[57]

Occasionally, one encounters a patient with severe heart failure whose pleural effusion remains refractory to conventional therapy. In this unusual patient, if therapeutic thoracentesis improves the patient's symptoms, pleurodesis may be considered. Either doxycycline or talc may be used as sclerosing agents.[58,59] Unilateral pleurodesis runs the risk of worsening fluid accumulation in the opposite hemithorax.[60] Bilateral pleurodesis may increase the risk of alveolar edema, though clinical experience has not supported this theoretical possibility.[59]

An alternative for the management of the refractory effusion is pleural peritoneal shunting. A subcutaneous catheter is implanted to connect the pleural and peritoneal cavities. The Le Veen shunt has a one-way valve that directs flow from the pleural to the peritoneal cavity during expiration when the pleural pressure exceeds that in the peritoneal cavity.[61] The Denver shunt has a compressible pumping chamber that transports fluid from the pleural to the peritoneal cavity where it is reabsorbed.[62,63] It has been successfully employed to provide symptomatic relief of dyspnea in patients with refractory effusions caused by congestive heart failure.[63,64]

FUTURE DIRECTIONS

The pathogenesis of pleural fluid accumulation in cardiac disease is clear, but the explanation for its presence in atypical locations such as a pseudotumor, or the predominance of left-sided effusions with pericardial disease, remains to be elucidated. BNP is a promising marker indicating a cardiac contribution to a pleural effusion. Cardiac disease is so common in our society that physicians can expect to encounter patients with an effusion caused by cardiac failure and a concomitant second problem contributing to the effusion. While additional testing such as cytological examination may identify the second problem, one still must rely on clinical intuition and the recognition of an atypical presentation to prompt additional testing. A marker for the 'complicated' cardiac effusion is needed.

KEY POINTS

- Congestive heart failure is the most common cause of transudative pleural effusions.
- Pleural effusions caused by heart failure are bilateral in over 80 percent of patients.
- A large left-sided effusion in a patient with cardiomegaly should raise suspicion of pericardial disease.
- Right heart failure facilitates the development of pleural effusions, but left heart failure is essential.
- Bilateral effusions in a patients with a normal sized heart are usually not caused by congestive heart failure.
- A transudative effusion from congestive heart failure can be transformed into an exudate by several days of diuretic therapy.
- Pleural and pericardial effusions in patients with pericardial disease generally have the same etiology.
- Effective treatment of the underlying cardiac disorder usually results in resolution of the pleural effusions.

REFERENCES

● = Key primary paper
◆ = Major review article
* = Paper that represents the first formal publication of a management guideline

1. Marel M, Zrustova M, Stastny B, *et al.* The incidence of pleural effusion in a well-defined region: Epidemiologic study in central Bohemia. *Chest* 1993; **104**: 1486–9.
2. Logue RB, Rogers JV Jr, Gay BB Jr. Subtle roentgenographic signs of left heart failure. *Am Heart J* 1963; **65**: 464–73.
3. Weiss JM, Spodick DH. Laterality of pleural effusions in congestive heart failure. *Am J Cardiol* 1984; **53**: 951–3.
●4. Wiener-Kronish JP, Matthay MA, Callen PW, *et al.* Relationship of pleural effusions to pulmonary hemodynamics in patients with congestive heart failure. *Am Rev Respir Dis* 1985; **132**: 1253–6.
5. Kataoka H. Pericardial and pleural effusions in decompensated chronic heart failure. *Am Heart J* 2000; **139**: 918–23.
6. Race GA, Scheifly CH, Edwards JE. Hydrothorax in congestive heart failure. *Am J Med* 1957; **22**: 83–9.
●7. Weiss JM, Spodick DH. Association of left pleural effusion with pericardial disease. *N Engl J Med* 1983; **308**: 696–7.
8. DeCamp MM, Mentzer SJ, Swanson SJ, *et al.* Malignant effusive disease of the pleura and pericardium. *Chest* 1997; **112**: 291S–5.
9. Casas E, Blanco JR, Ibarra V, *et al.* Incidence of pericardial infusion in pulmonary tuberculosis. *Int J Tuberc Lung Dis* 2000; **4**: 1173–5.
10. Hara KS, Ballard DJ, Ilstrup DM, *et al.* Rheumatoid pericarditis: Clinical features and survival. *Medicine* 1990; **69**: 81–91.
11. Kelly CA, Bourke JP, Malcolm A, *et al.* Chronic pericardial disease in patients with rheumatoid arthritis: a longitudinal study. *Q J Med* 1990; **75**: 461–70.
12. Kinasewitz GT, Groome LJ, Marshall RP, *et al.* Role of pulmonary lymphatics and interstitium in visceral pleural fluid exchange. *J Appl Physiol* 1984; **56**: 355–63.
13. Allen S, Gabel J, Drake R. Left atrial hypertension causes pleural effusion formation in unanesthetized sheep. *Am J Physiol* 1989; **257**: H690–2.
14. Broaddus VC, Wiener-Kronish JP, Staub NC. Clearance of lung edema into the pleural space of volume-loaded anesthetized sheep. *J Appl Physiol* 1990; **68**: 2623–30.
15. Staub NC. Pulmonary edema. *Physiol Rev* 1974; **54**: 678–809.
16. Payne DK, Kinasewitz GT, Gonzalez E. Comparative permeability of canine visceral and parietal pleura. *J Appl Physiol* 1988; **65**: 2558–64.

17. Mellins RB, Levine OR, Fishman AP. Effect of systemic and pulmonary venous hypertension on pleural and pericardial fluid accumulation. *J Appl Physiol* 1970; **29**: 564–9.
18. Pang LM, Mellins RB, Rodriguez-Martinez F. Effect of acute lymphatic obstruction on fluid accumulation in the chest in dogs. *J Appl Physiol* 1975; **39**: 985–9.
19. Eid A, Keddissi JI, Kinasewitz GT. Hypoalbuminemia as a cause of pleural effusions. *Chest* 1999; **115**: 1066–9.
20. Szabó G, Magyar Z. Effect of increased systemic venous pressure on lymph pressure and flow. *Am J Physiol* 1967; **212**: 1469–74.
21. Allen SJ, Drake RE, Laine GA, *et al.* Effect of thoracic duct drainage on hydrostatic pulmonary edema and pleural effusion in sheep. *J Appl Physiol* 1991; **71**: 314–16.
22. Wiener-Kronish JP, Goldstein R, Matthay RA, *et al.* Lack of association of pleural effusion with chronic pulmonary arterial and right atrial hypertension. *Chest* 1987; **92**: 967–70.
23. Maringhini A, Ciambra M, Patti R, *et al.* Ascites, pleural, and pericardial effusions in acute pancreatitis: A prospective study of incidence, natural history, and prognostic role. *Dig Dis Sci* 1996; **41**: 848–52.
24. Agner RC, Gallis HA. Pericarditis: Differential diagnostic considerations. *Arch Intern Med* 1979; **139**: 407–12.
25. Kataoka H, Takada S. The role of thoracic ultrasonography for evaluation of patients with decompensated chronic heart failure. *J Am Coll Cardiol* 2000; **35**: 1638–46.
26. Peterman TA, Brothers SK. Pleural effusions in congestive heart failure and in pericardial disease. *N Engl J Med* 1983; **309**: 313.
27. Woodring JH. Distribution of pleural effusion in congestive heart failure: what is atypical? *South Med J* 2005; **98**: 518–23.
28. Rabin CB, Blackman NS. Bilateral pleural effusion: its significance in association with a heart of normal size. *J Mt Sinai Hosp* 1957; **24**: 45–63.
29. Van Gelderen WFC. Vanishing pleural fluid collections in cardiac failure simulating lung tumours. *Australas Radiol* 1994; **38**: 93–6.
30. Weingardt JP, Guico RR, Nemcek AA Jr, *et al.* Ultrasound findings following failed clinically directed thoracenteses. *J Clin Ultrasound* 1994; **22**: 419–26.
31. Wu RG, Yuan A, Liaw YS, *et al.* Image comparison of real-time gray-scale ultrasound and color doppler ultrasound for use in diagnosis of minimal pleural effusion. *Am J Respir Crit Care Med* 1994; **150**: 510–14.
32. Matalon TA, Neiman HL, Mintzer RA. Noncardiac chest sonography. *Chest* 1983; **83**: 675–8.

∗33. Horowitz MS, Schultz CS, Stinson EB. Sensitivity and specificity of echocardiographic diagnosis of pericardial effusion. *Circulation* 1974; **50**: 239–47.

∗34. Singh S, Wann SL, Schuchard GH, *et al.* Right ventricular and right atrial collapse in patients with cardiac tamponade – a combined echocardiographic and hemodynamic study. *Circulation* 1984; **70**: 966.

●35. Hall WJ, Mayewski RJ. Diagnostic thoracentesis and pleural biopsy in pleural effusions. *Ann Intern Med* 1985; **103**: 799–802.

36. Sokolowski JW, Burgher LW, Jones FL Jr, *et al.* Guidelines for thoracentesis and needle biopsy of the pleura. *Am Rev Respir Dis* 1989; **140**: 257–8.
37. Light RW, MacGregor IM, Luchsinger PC, *et al.* Pleural effusions: The diagnostic separation of transudates and exudates. *Ann Intern Med* 1972; **77**: 507–13.
38. Light RW, Erozan YS, Ball WC Jr. Cells in pleural fluid. *Arch Intern Med* 1973; **132**: 854–60.
39. Shinto RA, Light RW. Effects of diuresis on the characteristics of pleural fluid in patients with congestive heart failure. *Am J Med* 1990; **88**: 230–4.
40. Chakko SC, Caldwell SH, Sforza PP. Treatment of congestive heart failure: Its effect on pleural fluid chemistry. *Chest* 1989; **95**: 798–802.
41. Romero-Candeira S, Fernandez C, Martin C, *et al.* Influence of diuretics on the concentration of proteins and other components of pleural transudates in patients with heart failure. *Am J Med* 2001; **110**: 681–6.
42. Broaddus VC. Diuresis and transudative effusions – Changing the rules of the game. *Am J Med* 2001; **110**: 732–5.

●43. Porcel JM, Vives M, Cao G, *et al.* Measurement of pro-brain natriuretic peptide in pleural fluid for the diagnosis of pleural effusions due to heart failure. *Am J Med* 2004; **116**: 417–20.

44. Gegenhuber A, Mueller T, Dieplinger B, *et al.* Plasma B-type natriuretic peptide in patients with pleural effusions: preliminary observations. *Chest* 2005; **128**: 1003–9.
45. Kolditz M, Halank M, Schiemanck CS, *et al.* High diagnostic accuracy of NT-proBNP for cardiac origin of pleural effusions. *Eur Respir J* 2006; **28**: 144–50.
46. Gotsman I, Fridlender Z, Meirovitz A, *et al.* The evaluation of pleural effusions in patients with heart failure. *Am J Med* 2001; **111**: 375–8.
47. Eid A, Keddissi JI, Samaha M, *et al.* Exudative effusions in congestive heart failure. *Chest* 2002; **122**: 1518–23.
48. Wang D-Y, Yang P-C, Yu W-L, *et al.* Serial antinuclear antibodies titre in pleural and pericardial fluid. *Eur Respir J* 2000; **15**: 1106–10.
49. PA Howard, MI Dunn. Aggressive diuresis for severe heart failure in the elderly. *Chest* 2001; **119**: 807–10.
50. Maher EA, Shepherd FA, Todd TJR. Pericardial sclerosis as the primary management of malignant pericardial effusion and cardiac tamponade. *J Thorac Cardiovasc Surg* 1996; **112**: 637–43.
51. Vaitkus PT, Hermann HC, LeWinter MM. Treatment of malignant pericardial effusion. *J Am Med Assoc* 1994; **272**: 59–64.
52. Yano T, Yokoyama H, Inoue T, *et al.* A simple technique to manage malignant pericardial effusion with a local instillation of bleomycin in non-small cell carcinoma of the lung. *Oncology* 1994; **51**: 507–9.
53. Hazelrigg SR, Mack MJ, Landreneau RJ, *et al.* Thoracoscopic pericardiectomy for effusive pericardial disease. *Ann Thorac Surg* 1993; **56**: 792–5.

◆54. Piehler JM, Pluth JR, Schaff HV, *et al.* Surgical management of effusive pericardial disease: Influence of extent of pericardial resection on clinical course. *J Thorac Cardiovasc Surg* 1985; **90**: 506–16.

55. Olson JE, Ryan MB, Blumenstock DA. Eleven years experience with pericardial–peritoneal window in the management of malignant and benign pericardial effusions. *Ann Surg Oncol* 1995; **2**: 165–9.
56. Van Trigt P, Douglas J, Smith PK, *et al.* A prospective trial of subxiphoid pericardiotomy in the diagnosis and treatment of large pericardial effusion. *Ann Surg* 1993; **218**: 777–82.
57. Estenne M, Yernault JC, De Troyer A. Mechanism of relief of dyspnea after thoracocentesis in patients with large pleural effusions. *Am J Med* 1983; **74**: 813–19.
58. Sudduth CD, Sahn SA. Pleurodesis for nonmalignant pleural effusions. *Chest* 1992; **102**: 1855–60.
59. Glazer M, Berkman N, Lafair JS, *et al.* Successful talc slurry pleurodesis in patients with nonmalignant pleural effusion: Report of 16 cases and review of the literature. *Chest* 2000; 117: 1404–9.
60. Davidoff D, Naparstek Y, Eliakim M. The use of pleurodesis for intractable pleural effusion due to congestive heart failure. *Postgrad Med J* 1983; **59**: 330–1.
61. Dorsey JS, Cogordan JA. Pleuroperitoneal shunt for intractable pleural effusion. *Can J Surg* 1984; **27**: 598–9.
62. Ponn RB, Blancaflor J, D'Agostino RS, *et al.* Pleuroperitoneal shunting for intractable pleural effusions. *Ann Thorac Surg* 1991; **51**: 605–9.
63. Cimochowski GE, Joyner LR. Pleural peritoneal shunting for benign and malignant pleural effusions. *Surg Annu* 1989; **21**: 49–71.
64. Little AG, Kadowaki MH, Ferguson MK, *et al.* Pleuro-peritoneal shunting: Alternative therapy for pleural effusions. *Ann Surg* 1988; **208**: 443–50.

25

Effusions from malignancy

FRANCISCO RODRIGUEZ-PANADERO

INTRODUCTION

Malignant pleural effusion is one of the most common problems faced by clinicians in their everyday practice. However, it is less commonly recognized that a pleural malignancy can occur without the presence of effusion. This is not unusual in cases of mesothelioma, where the effusion can be very small or even absent from the beginning of the disease. However, metastatic neoplasms can also be present without any effusion in the pleural space. In one autopsy series from our group we found metastatic pleural involvement in 29 percent of 191 cases with a malignant tumor elsewhere, but pleural effusion was present in little more than half of these cases.[1] Therefore, the incidence of malignant pleural effusion in this particular autopsy series was 15 percent. This fact would be particularly relevant when 'dry' diffuse pleural involvement is suspected in cases of lung cancer that might otherwise be subjected to resection surgery. Therefore, exploratory thoracoscopy is often advocated in those circumstances, just before proceeding to thoracotomy.

In a prospective study including 1000 consecutive patients who were submitted to thoracentesis, Villena and coworkers[2] found that the etiology of the effusion was malignant in 364 patients (36 percent), and it is widely recognized that the incidence of malignant pleural effusion has increased in recent years. Approximately one-third of the malignant pleural effusions are related to lung cancer, and metastatic carcinoma of the breast is the second most frequent cause. While mesothelioma incidence began to decline a few years ago in some countries that banned asbestos use early, it is still rising in many countries, and is not expected to decline before year 2020.[3]

PATHOGENESIS

The pleura can be invaded directly from neighboring structures (lung, chest wall – including breast in some cases – diaphragm and mediastinum), but most of the pleural malignancies arise, according to two necropsy studies, from tumor emboli to the visceral pleura, with secondary seeding to the parietal pleura (Figures 25.1 and 25.2).[1,4] The effusion can develop as a direct consequence of neoplastic pleural involvement, but it can also occur in cases with lymphatic blockade at the mediastinal level (Figure 25.3). This last mechanism was invoked by Meyer in 1966,[4] and confirmed by us in another necropsy study many years later.[5] However, the exact mechanisms involved in the development of effusion in the presence of tumor implants in the pleural space are not fully understood. It is likely that increased pleural permeability caused directly by the tumor and the accompanying inflammation are responsible for the development of the effusion.[6] In some circumstances, a malignant tumor can coexist with an effusion without direct pleural involvement, and those effusions were defined by Sahn as 'paramalignant'.[7] We found this phenomenon in up to 17 percent of patients having a malignant tumor elsewhere. Pulmonary embolism, pneumonia and lymphatic mediastinal blockade were found to be the most frequent causes in a necropsy study from our group.[8]

CLINICAL PRESENTATION

Most of the malignant effusions present with dyspnea on exertion, which is progressive as the effusion is becoming

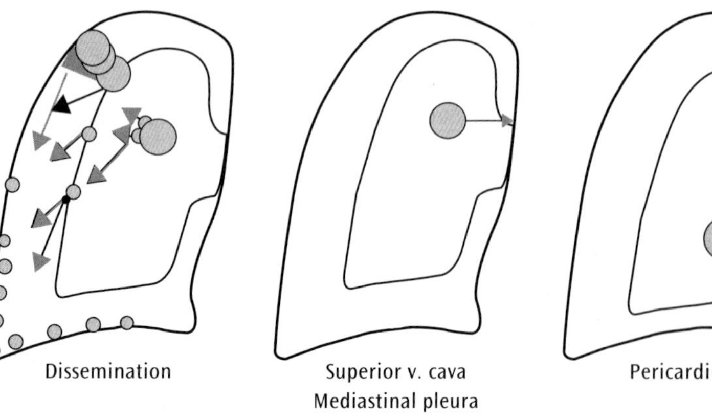

Figure 25.1 Possible mechanisms of pleural involvement by lung cancer. The tumor can embolize to the visceral pleura, and then reach the parietal pleura directly or through secondary seeding of cells. Also, the mediastinal surface of the pleura can be involved by direct tumor invasion, followed by widespread cell seeding within the pleural cavity.

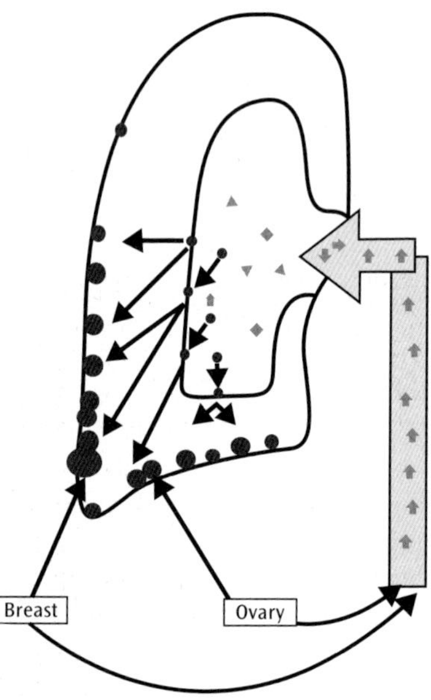

Figure 25.2 Metastatic pleural involvement in extrathoracic tumors, according to autopsy studies (see references 1 and 4). In most cases, microscopic tumor embolization to the lungs and then to the visceral pleura occurs. The parietal pleura is involved through secondary seeding from tumors on the visceral pleura. Breast cancer can invade the pleura both directly or through blood-borne metastasis. Ovarian cancers can metastasize by hematogenous routes and through tumor implantations on the diaphragm.

larger. Typically, it is more marked when the patient is lying on one side (the one contralateral to the effusion), and it is rapidly relieved after thoracentesis. If not, severe carcinomatous involvement of the underlying lung should be suspected. Cough is another typical symptom, especially in patients with large effusions. It can improve after thoracentesis. It is my experience that these coughing patients tend to have less tolerance to therapeutic thoracentesis and are more prone to develop pneumothorax as a complication of the procedure. Thoracentesis should therefore be carried out very carefully on these patients and be stopped as soon as they begin to cough. Monitoring of the pleural pressure during therapeutic thoracentesis would be advisable in such cases[9] (see also Chapter 18, Pleural manometry).

Chest pain is not frequent at the time of presentation of the effusion, with the marked exception of mesothelioma, which usually presents with early pain even before the effusion develops clinically. Pain in mesothelioma is usually diffuse on the affected hemithorax, has no clear pleuritic characteristics (i.e. it varies little with respiratory movements) and progresses over time.

When pain is present in patients with carcinomatous effusions it is usually less diffuse than in mesothelioma and chest wall involvement by the tumor should be suspected.

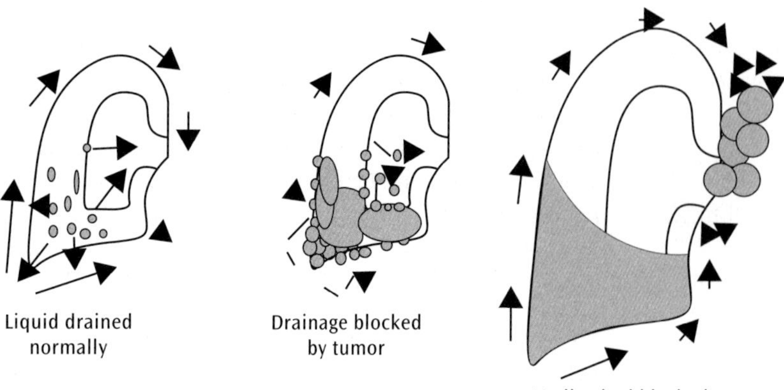

Figure 25.3 Pathophysiological mechanisms of malignant pleural effusions. Most of the liquid is removed from the pleural space through the lymphatics in the parietal pleura. This mechanism can be impaired by direct pleural involvement of the tumor, or by distant lymphatic blockade at the mediastinal level.

RADIOGRAPHIC APPEARANCE OF MALIGNANT EFFUSIONS

Pleural effusions associated with metastatic carcinomas are usually moderate to large at the time of clinical presentation, and rarely have a multiloculated appearance initially. This is related to the fact that most of the metastatic tumor lesions show a very high fibrinolytic activity.[10] However, the effusion can be small and loculated at presentation in many cases of mesothelioma.

It is essential to evaluate the position of the mediastinum in the presence of an effusion suspicious of being malignant, since it provides very useful information for the management of patients. Thus, a large effusion with contralateral mediastinal shift is very likely to be malignant, usually requires an immediate therapeutic thoracentesis and is a good candidate for pleurodesis (Figure 25.4). If a patient has a large effusion where the mediastinum is midline or shifted ipsilaterally, a more careful approach is indicated. In this setting, the following four conditions should be considered, according to Sahn:[11]

- carcinoma of the ipsilateral mainstem bronchus resulting in atelectasis (see Figure 25.5). This can also occur in cases of endobronchial metastasis from a distant tumor;
- a fixed mediastinum caused by malignant tumor and/or lymph nodes;
- malignant mesothelioma (the radiodensity represents predominantly tumor with a small to moderate effusion);
- extensive tumor infiltration of the ipsilateral lung radiographically mimicking a large effusion.

Ultrasound examination can be very useful in evaluating an effusion suspected of being malignant, both for diagnostic[12,13] or interventional purposes[14] or to detect complications, such as cardiac tamponade.[15]

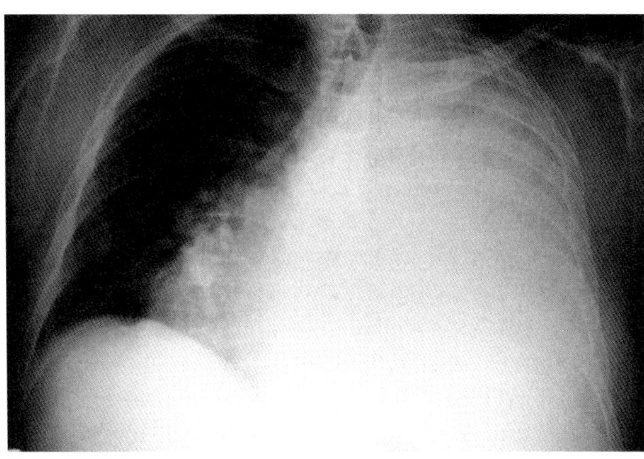
(a)

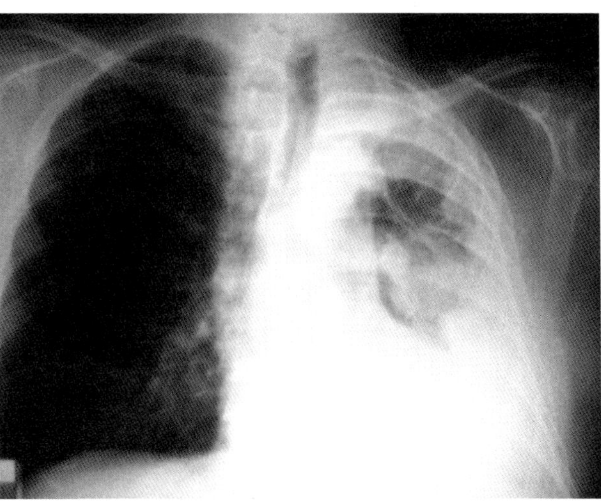
(b)

Figure 25.4 (a) Lung cancer with massive pleural effusion and contralateral mediastinal shift. Many therapeutic thoracenteses were required, and large amounts of fluid removed. (b) Same patient, 11 months after talc poudrage.

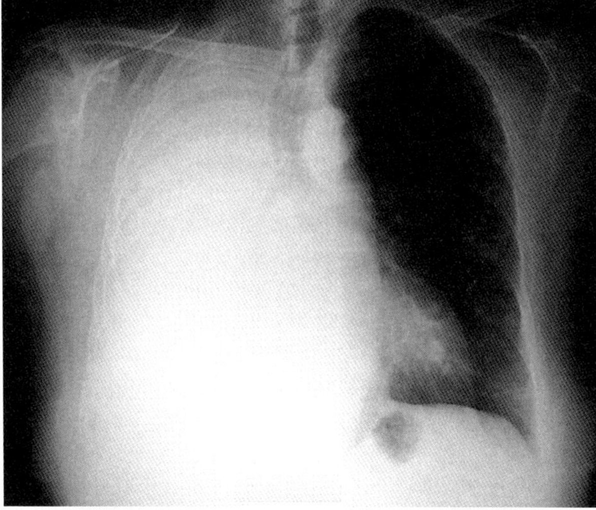

Figure 25.5 Lung cancer with central bronchial obstruction. Pleurodesis should not be attempted in this type of case unless diagnostic/therapeutic bronchoscopy has been performed.

DIAGNOSIS OF MALIGNANT PLEURAL EFFUSIONS

According to the European Respiratory Society/American Thoracic Society (ERS/ATS) Consensus Statement on Management of Malignant Pleural Effusions,[16] malignancy should be considered and a diagnostic thoracentesis performed in any individual with a unilateral effusion or bilateral effusion and a normal heart size on the chest radiograph. The following routine tests are recommended for pleural fluid (see Chapter 17): nucleated cell count and differential count, total proteins, lactate dehydrogenase (LDH), glucose, pH, amylase (in case of effusions with suspected pancreatic origin) and cytology. The pleural fluid differential white cell count typically shows a predominance of either lymphocytes or other mononuclear cells. The presence of neutrophils or eosinophils is much less common but does not exclude a malignant effusion. Adenosine deaminase (ADA) determination is routinely recommended in countries with medium to high prevalence of tuberculosis. It can yield false positive results in some cases of mesothelioma and lymphoma.

Almost all malignant effusions are exudates, but a few can be transudates (approximately 1 percent in our thoracoscopy series). Malignant transudative effusions can occur in lung cancer with obstruction of the mainstem bronchus, but also in lymphoma and other malignancies.[17] Blockade of lymphatic drainage may be invoked as one of the possible pathogenetic mechanisms,[18] but an underlying cardiac failure or other conditions that are usually associated with transudative effusions should also be taken into account.[19]

Approximately one-third of malignant effusions will demonstrate a pleural fluid pH of less than 7.30 at presentation (118 out of 359 with pH measured at the time of diagnostic thoracoscopy in our series); this low pH correlates with glucose values of less than 60 mg/dL. The cause of these low glucose, low pH malignant effusions appears to be an increased tumor burden,[20] resulting in decreased glucose transfer into the pleural space and decreased efflux of acidic byproducts of glucose metabolism.[21] For that reason, malignant effusions with these properties have been shown to have a higher diagnostic yield on cytology and poorer response to pleurodesis (Figure 25.6), and they are associated with a decreased overall survival.[22,23] When considering pleural pH as a predicting factor for survival, one has to take into account that patients with mesothelioma tend to survive longer than those with metastatic pleural carcinoma;[24] they also have a tendency to show a lower pH because of the marked pleural thickening caused by mesothelioma.

Heffner and coworkers[25] found in a metanalysis study that although pH was by itself an independent predictor of survival, it had insufficient predictive accuracy for selecting patients for pleurodesis, and this lack of predictive power was probably associated to the influence of mesothelioma cases in their study.

In conclusion, pH can be helpful in clinical practice when used in conjunction with the patient's performance status, primary tumor type and response to therapeutic thoracentesis.

Pleural fluid cytology is the simplest definitive method available for obtaining a diagnosis of malignant pleural effusion. The diagnostic yield is dependent on such factors as extent of disease and the nature of the primary malignancy. Thus, in our thoracoscopy series including 545 patients with malignant pleural effusion, the yield of cytology ranged from 80 percent in metastatic breast cancer to 70 percent in lung cancer, 56 percent in mesothelioma, 40 percent in lymphoma and 20 percent in sarcoma (unpublished data) (Figure 25.7). The cytological diagnosis of malignancy can therefore be very difficult in some cases of mesothelioma and lymphoma, and the diagnosis with these tumors frequently requires a more invasive procedure, such as thoracoscopy.

In our experience, low pH/glucose malignant effusions have a significantly higher yield of cytology than those with normal pH levels (Figure 25.8).

Most of the current guidelines recommend the addition of a biopsy procedure when a first cytology is negative in effusions of unknown origin.[26] Percutaneous needle pleural biopsy is frequently advised in those circumstances.[2,27] However, closed pleural biopsy adds little to the cytological diagnosis in most cases and this is related to the scarce and irregular distribution of the tumor lesions in the pleural cavity when cytology is negative.[28] With recent advances of image techniques some authors prefer computed tomography (CT)-guided needle biopsy, which could replace

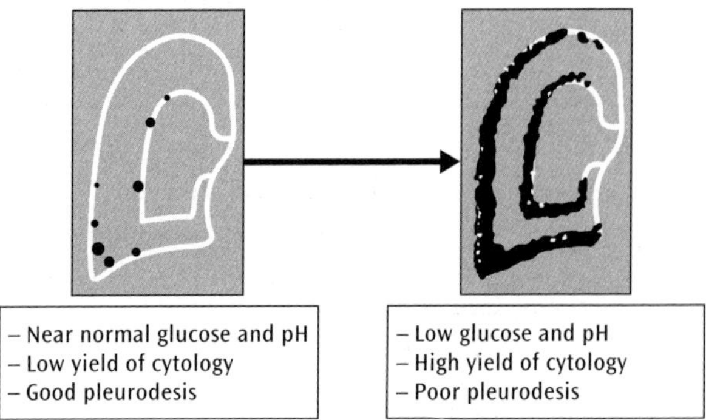

Figure 25.6 Cytology, pleurodesis and glucose–pH relationships. Because neoplastic disease progresses in most of the cases, it would be advisable to perform pleurodesis as soon as possible.

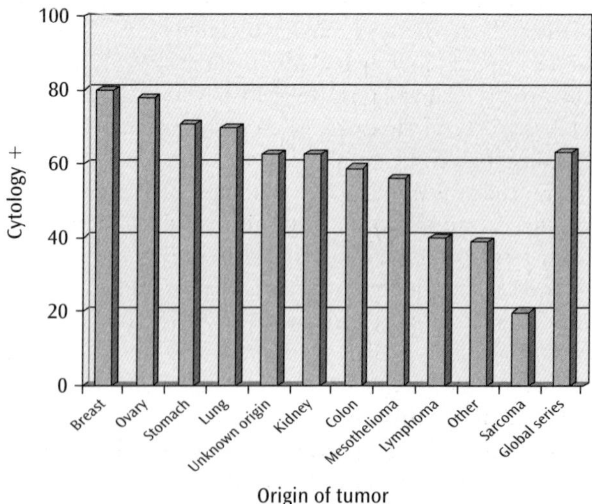

Figure 25.7 Sensitivity of cytology in our thoracoscopy series, including 545 consecutive patients with malignant pleural effusion. The yield varies widely between tumors of different origins.

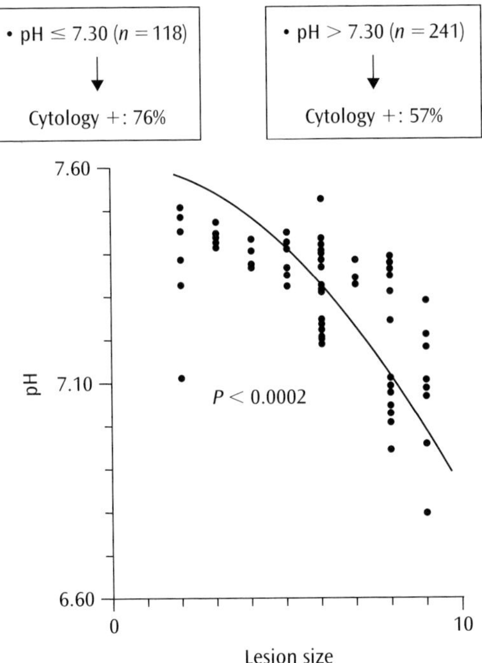

Figure 25.8 Relation between positive cytology and pH in 359 patients with malignant pleural effusion in our thoracoscopy series. Pleural pH shows a strong correlation with tumor burden found at thoracoscopy.

blind needle biopsy in more than two-thirds of the cases.[29] This applies especially to patients with a significant pleural thickening that is suspicious for malignancy.

The yield of blind needle biopsy is higher when the pleural lesions are diffuse, as in tuberculosis and advanced neoplastic disease. In contrast, thoracoscopy has a very high yield in malignant effusions. It can be performed with local anesthesia and a single port of entry, and it has little more complications than needle biopsy (the technique of medical thoracoscopy is further discussed in Chapter 47).[30] In a prospective study including 150 patients, Boutin and coworkers[31] found a positive yield of Abrams needle biopsy in 36 percent of the cases, whereas thoracoscopy obtained the diagnosis in up to 87 percent. In another prospective study, Loddenkemper *et al.*[32] obtained similar results comparing simultaneous Tru-cut needle biopsy and thoracoscopy. However, pleural needle biopsy can be performed on an outpatient basis,[33] whereas thoracoscopy is much more complex and always requires hospitalization.

Our current policy is therefore to perform needle biopsy of the pleura only in young patients (in whom tuberculous pleurisy is more likely, at least in countries with relatively high prevalence of tuberculosis) and in those patients that reject thoracoscopy or are too sick to tolerate it.

Although tumor markers in pleural fluid cannot be considered as a definitive diagnosis, they can be of help in selecting patients for further investigation with more invasive techniques when they are clearly positive. In a study involving 416 patients, Porcel *et al.*[34] found that a panel of several tumour markers in pleural fluid (CEA, CA 125, CA 15-3, and CYFRA 21-1) reached 54 percent sensitivity, whereas combined use of cytology and the tumour marker panel performed best in diagnosing malignant effusions (sensitivity 69 percent). More than one-third of cytology-negative malignant pleural effusions could be identified by at least one marker.

Flow cytometry may play an interesting role in the study of pleural effusions suspected of being malignant. It can complement cytology in many cases,[35] particularly in lymphocytic effusions where lymphoma is suspected.[36]

MANAGEMENT OF MALIGNANT PLEURAL EFFUSIONS

The approach to an effusion suspicious of being malignant (i.e. lasting for more than 2 weeks and not clearly related to other conditions) should take into account the size of the effusion in the chest radiograph as a first step (see algorithms in Figures 25.9–25.12). If the effusion is small (less than one-third of the hemithorax) and cytology is positive, the best choice would be to apply chemotherapy if the primary is known to be sensitive to that treatment (breast, ovary, small-cell lung cancer, lymphoma, etc.) and to observe the evolution of the pleural effusion. When cytology is negative and/or the primary is unknown, thoracoscopy would be recommended, since the diagnosis yield is high, large specimens can be taken under visual control for special studies (immunohistochemistry and others), and talc poudrage for pleurodesis can be performed at the same time.

For management of large effusions, the approach depends mainly upon the position of the mediastinum. If there is a contralateral mediastinal shift, diagnostic and therapeutic thoracentesis should be carried out without delay. If a positive cytology is obtained and the primary is

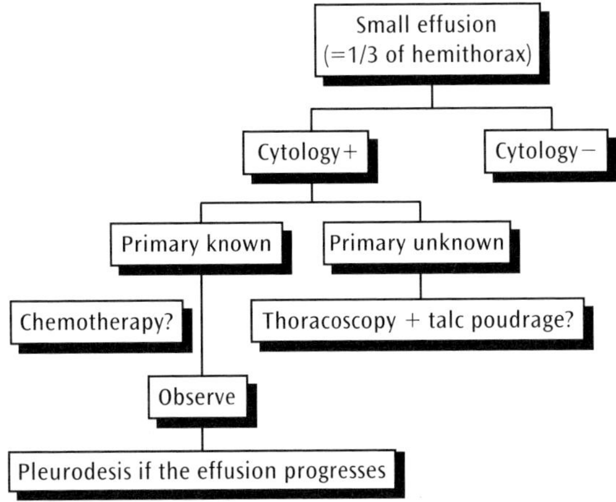

Figure 25.9 Management of small effusions with positive cytology.

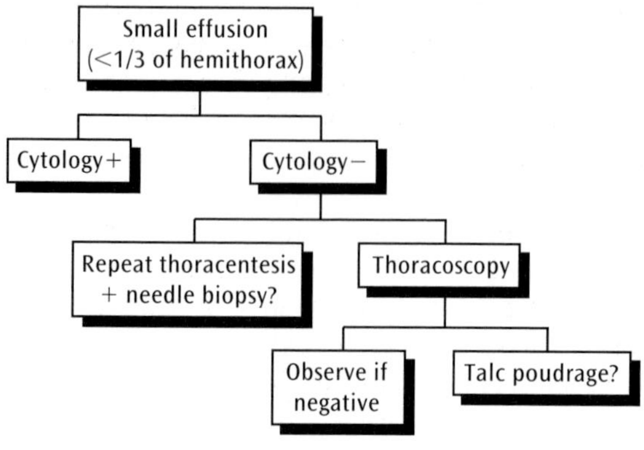

Figure 25.10 Management of small effusions when the first cytological examination is negative. The next investigation recommended is a pleural biopsy, preferably via thoracoscopy (which also allows talc pleurodesis in the same setting if malignant lesions are confirmed).

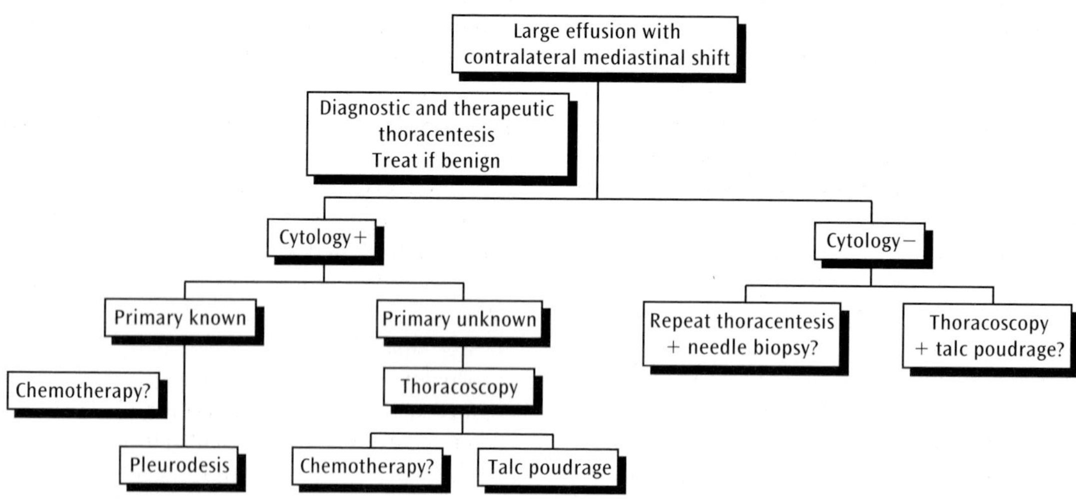

Figure 25.11 Management of large effusions with contralateral mediastinal shift.

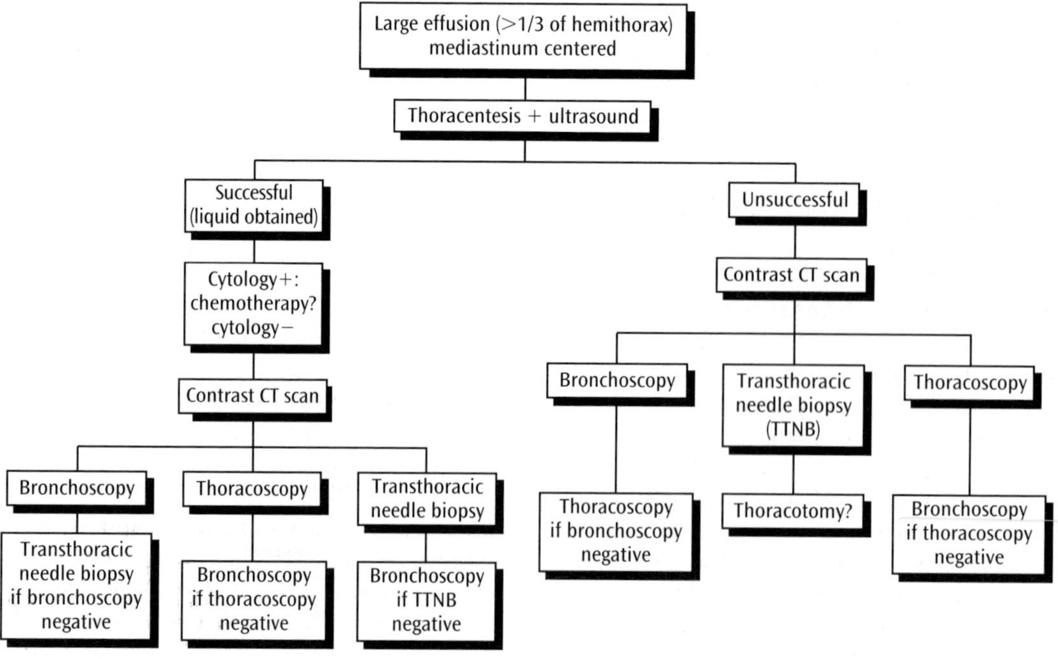

Figure 25.12 Management of apparently large effusions with the mediastinum is not displaced or ipsilaterally shifted.

known, chemotherapy could be tried in selected patients, but a pleurodesis procedure would be needed in most. If the first cytology is negative, thoracoscopy and talc pleurodesis would be strongly recommended as the second step following the initial thoracentesis.

Approximately two-thirds of patients with malignant effusions require pleurodesis sooner or later.[37] In the presence of a large and recurrent effusion the choice is clearly pleurodesis, preferably using talc (see below). This should be carried out as early as possible in order to prevent the development of a trapped lung, which could prevent lung re-expansion and make a successful pleurodesis problematic.

When there appears to be a large effusion and the mediastinum is midline or ipsilaterally shifted, a contrast CT scan would be recommended as the first approach. The CT scan can be helpful in choosing bronchoscopy, thoracoscopy or transthoracic needle biopsy (TTNB) to obtain the diagnosis. Exploratory thoracotomy should be the choice if all those procedures fail, but according to my experience it is seldom needed for diagnosis in effusions suspicious of being malignant.

Diagnostic and therapeutic bronchoscopy is mandatory if a central bronchial obstruction is suspected (see Figure 25.5). Management of trapped lung can be much more complex: it can be detected on contrast CT scans, and pleural pressure measurement during thoracentesis might be useful. In patients with mediastinum centered or with ipsilateral shift, the likelihood of a precipitous drop in pleural pressure is increased, and either pleural pressure should be monitored during thoracentesis or only a small volume of fluid removed.

When the effusion is relatively small (less than one-third of the hemithorax), the question is whether pleurodesis is necessary. The answer is obvious if the effusion remains stable and well tolerated. However, in an undefined proportion of cases the effusion would enlarge and, as the disease advances, be accompanied by a trapped lung at which time successful pleurodesis will become unlikely.

MANAGEMENT OF PLEURAL EFFUSION IN SPECIAL CONDITIONS

Pleural effusion and ipsilateral lung cancer

The finding of pleural effusion coexisting with lung cancer is usually associated with a poor prognosis,[9,38] and the tumor, node, metastasis (TNM) staging is problematic in this circumstance, because the true nature of the effusion needs to be established. The incidence of this problem has been estimated in 7–15 percent of all lung cancers,[16] but it is probably higher if we include pleural effusions only detectable on CT scan or at thoracotomy. In one series including 971 consecutive patients with lung cancer, Martín Díaz and coworkers[39] found pleural effusion in 188 cases (19 percent), and only 72 (7 percent) were visible on chest X-ray films. The remaining 116 effusions were detected on CT or ultrasound examination, or were found only at thoracotomy. Although cytology was positive in 40 percent of the effusions that were visible on chest radiographs, pleural metastases were actually found in up to 75 percent of cases.

If the mediastinum is midline or shows an ipsilateral shift, obstruction of the mainstem bronchus should be suspected (see Figure 25.5), and bronchoscopy performed. In the remaining cases, we strongly recommend performing exploratory thoracoscopy before attempting tumor resection, in order to detect unsuspected pleural metastases.[40–42]

When the effusion is found at thoracotomy only, one could think about the possibility of a paramalignant pleural effusion (associated with obstructive pneumonitis, atelectasis or lymphatic blockade), and resection of the tumor has to be considered. However, the prognosis is poorer in those patients than in those without pleural effusion.[43]

Pleural cytology can be eventually positive without macroscopically visible lesions on the pleural surface, and this appears to be associated with a better prognosis.[44] In some cases with tight adhesions between the lung and chest wall, tumor resection could be achieved despite positive cytology.[41,45]

The finding of a positive cytology in pleural lavage performed at thoracotomy has been associated with a worse prognosis in cases submitted to resection.[46–48]

The success rate of pleurodesis in pleural effusion secondary to lung cancer appears to be lower than in other malignancies (65 percent complete success in our thoracoscopy series, compared with an average 76 percent in the remaining cases of metastatic carcinomas). Although the presence of trapped lung might play a role, we found no clear differences in this respect in our thoracoscopy series. Another likely explanation would be that complete lung re-expansion is hard to achieve in the presence of lung cancer, compared with other metastatic malignancies.

Pleural effusion in mesothelioma

Pleural effusion may be absent or scarce in a number of cases of malignant mesothelioma (Figure 25.13) and, as pointed out above, pleural fluid pH can be significantly lower than in other malignancies at presentation. Although this does not relate to a shorter survival when compared with pleural metastatic carcinomas, it is associated with a lower rate of successful pleurodesis in our experience (59 percent in mesothelioma versus 76 percent average in metastatic carcinomas, excluding lung cancer). Both low pH and failure of pleurodesis are probably associated with the marked diffuse pleural thickening that is observed in mesothelioma cases, which prevent a good apposition between the visceral and parietal pleural layers.

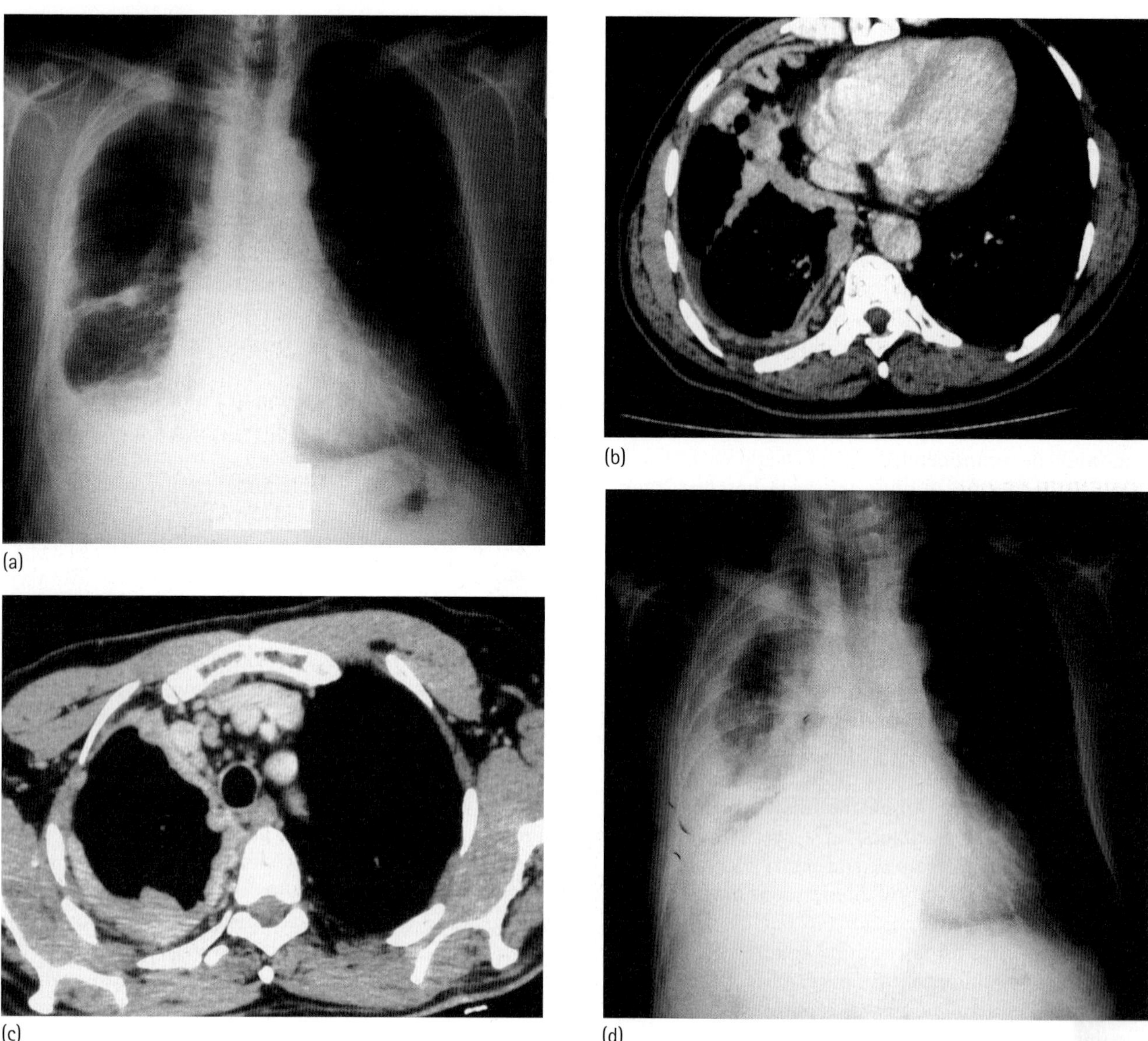

(a) (b) (c) (d)

Figure 25.13 Malignant mesothelioma in a 75-year-old man with a past history of asbestos exposure. No pleural fluid obtained. (a) Chest radiograph at presentation (with chest pain). (b and c) Appearance on computed tomography scan. (d) Chest radiograph 17 months later. Only palliative treatment for chest pain was applied.

Cytological diagnosis is rather difficult with mesothelioma because it is sometimes hard to establish a clear distinction between mesothelioma and metastatic adenocarcinoma. Also, differentiating between reactive and malignant mesothelial cells can be difficult. Cytology was positive for malignancy in 56 percent in our cases of mesothelioma, but the cytological diagnoses was correct only in two-thirds of cases.

Pleural effusion in lymphoma

Pleural involvement by lymphoma can show no significant differences with other types of effusions at presentation, but there are a few details that should be taken into account:

- The aspect of the pleural fluid can be chylous more frequently than in other malignancies because the thoracic duct can be disrupted by lymphoma involvement: among 51 cases of lymphoma in our thoracoscopy series, we found a chyliform appearance in 15.6 percent of the cases, while it was present in only 2 percent in our series overall. A right-sided chylous pleural effusion in lymphoma is mostly associated with involvement of the thoracic duct at the lower part of the paravertebral zone in the hemithorax (see also Chapter 29, Effusions from lymphatic disruptions).

- Cytological diagnosis can be difficult in lymphoma, because a lymphocytic pleural effusion is frequently found and the lymphocytes show a normal appearance in many cases. Cytology was positive in only 40 percent of our cases, compared with 63.5 percent in the total series. Flow cytometry analysis can be helpful in suspected cases of lymphoma.[35,36]
- When there is a chylothorax coexisting with lymphoma, pleurodesis can be very effective if oral feeding is stopped for a few days before, during and after the pleurodesis attempt (we had a 72 percent successful talc pleurodesis in our lymphoma series, including those with chyliform effusion).

CONSIDERATIONS ON PLEURODESIS FOR MALIGNANT PLEURAL EFFUSIONS

Pleurodesis is addressed separately in Chapter 46. Here, I emphasize the key points regarding its role in the management of malignant pleural effusions (MPE).

Indications and contraindications for pleurodesis

The main indication for pleurodesis in MPE is a symptomatic, recurrent effusion, especially if contralateral mediastinal shift is present. The main indication for treatment in those cases is relief of dyspnea, which is dependent on both the volume of the effusion and the underlying condition of the lungs and pleura. In this circumstance, therapeutic thoracentesis and pleurodesis attempt (simultaneous or sequential) is mandatory. If dyspnea is not relieved by thoracentesis, other causes should be investigated, such as lymphangitic carcinomatosis, atelectasis, thromboembolism and tumor embolism. When pleurodesis is indicated, it should be performed as early as possible in order to prevent development of a trapped lung, which could provoke a failure in lung re-expansion and failed pleurodesis. Although a drainage of less than 150 mL per day is considered a requisite for pleurodesis by some authors, we believe that a successful pleurodesis can be achieved in many patients with large amounts of fluid removed before the procedure.

In patients with ipsilateral mediastinal shift, it is unlikely that removal of pleural fluid will provide significant relief of dyspnea. Hence, pleurodesis is rarely indicated and other therapeutic measures should be considered (see below).

According to a prospective study from our group, serial determinations of pH and D-dimer in pleural fluid are of help in predicting which patients are more likely to need a pleurodesis procedure.[49] Patients who eventually required pleurodesis often showed a preceding decline in pleural fluid pH over serial determinations. In addition, the median pleural fluid D-dimer levels were higher in the group requiring pleurodesis.

CONTRAINDICATIONS TO PLEURODESIS IN MPE

If thoracoscopic pleurodesis is considered, patients with severe chronic obstructive pulmonary disease (COPD) and consequent respiratory insufficiency, with hypoxemia (partial pressure of O_2 [PO_2] <50 mmHg) and hypercapnia, will not tolerate induction of a pneumothorax without further deterioration of the gas exchange, and are therefore not suitable candidates for thoracoscopy. Patients with unstable cardiovascular status should not undergo thoracoscopy. Moreover, thoracoscopic pleurodesis should not be attempted in patients with a significant contralateral involvement of the lung, since they are likely to develop an acute respiratory insufficiency (Figure 25.14). The presence of a bilateral pleural effusion might also be problematic, unless all the effusion is removed from the contralateral side before attempting pleurodesis on one side. Simultaneous pleurodesis should not be attempted since the likelihood of developing complications is high.

When talc poudrage is not feasible, other alternatives should be considered, including talc slurry or doxycycline application through the chest tube after removing the pleural fluid.

Choice of sclerosing agent

According to the ERS/ATS consensus statement on Management of Malignant Pleural Effusions,[16] which included a comprehensive review of the success with the most relevant agents, talc was found to be the best sclerosant regarding rate of success. In a recent multicenter study, Dresler *et al.*[50] obtained similar overall efficacy for talc poudrage and 'slurry' forms of administration; however, they found that poudrage was better in metastatic lung and breast carcinomas. In a randomized series including 57 patients in total, Yim *et al.*[51] found no significant difference in results when comparing talc poudrage and slurry. However, in another randomized study comparing talc poudrage and slurry in 55 patients with malignant pleural effusion, Mañes and coworkers[52] in our group found a significantly higher rate of recurrences with talc slurry than with poudrage. Therefore, this issue is not definitely solved, and our group is currently working in broadening our randomized series. Potential disadvantages of slurry include lack of uniform distribution and accumulation in dependent areas of the pleural cavity, with subsequent incomplete pleurodesis and multiple loculations. Also, we have found that most of the talc administered in the slurry form might be eventually eliminated through the chest tube with the saline solution after the drain is unclamped.[53] The addition of some iodide compound (thymol or povidone) has not been demonstrated to improve the pleurodesis outcome experimentally.[54]

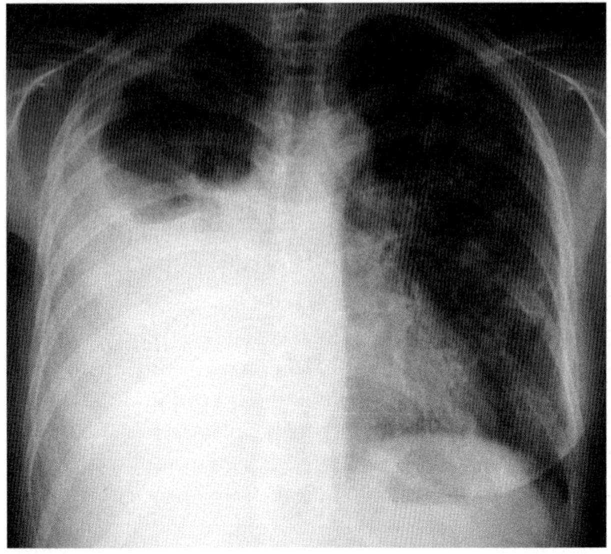

(a)

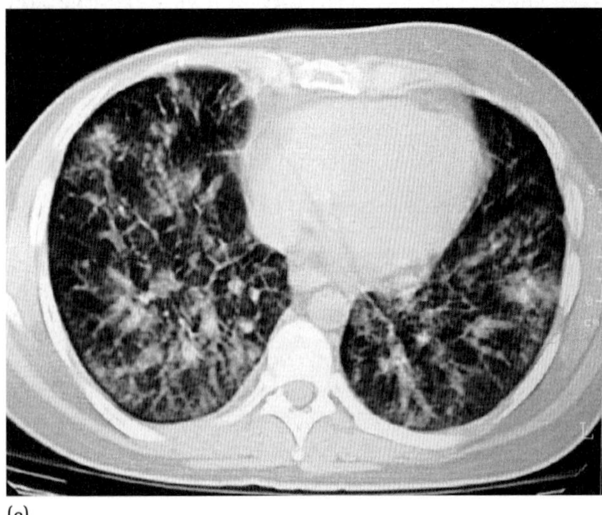

(c)

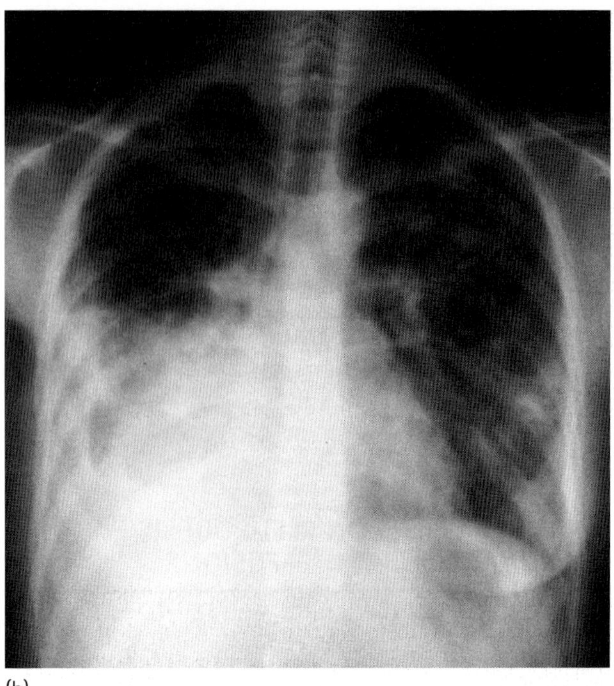

(b)

Figure 25.14 A 32-year-old woman with advanced breast cancer and *Pneumocystics carinii* infection acquired after intensive chemotherapy. Thoracoscopic talc pleurodesis should not be attempted in the presence of diffuse bilateral lung involvement. Doxycycline pleurodesis was attempted without success, and a small-bore catheter was inserted to relieve dyspnea. (a) Chest radiograph, prior to thoracentesis. (b) Immediately after therapeutic thoracentesis. (c) Appearance of computed tomography scan a few days before development of the pleural effusion.

Moreover, iodide might provoke severe adverse effects when instilled into the pleural space.[55]

Side effects and complications of pleurodesis

Pain and transient fever, due to release of pro-inflammatory mediators, are common side effects associated with pleurodesis performed with practically any sclerosant. However, there are other worrying complications that have been reported with the procedure, as discussed below.

RE-EXPANSION EDEMA

In order to prevent re-expansion lung edema, careful and graded suction should be applied. We usually leave the drain connected to water-seal without suction for at least 3 hours following the pleurodesis procedure, and then apply increasing suction gradually.

PERSISTENT AIR LEAK

Air leak can occur during lung re-expansion,[56] especially in patients with necrotic tumor nodules in the visceral pleura. In our experience, this especially occurs in patients that have been submitted to previous chemotherapy, even if no biopsies of the visceral pleural were taken (Figure 25.15).

ACUTE RESPIRATORY DISTRESS OR PNEUMONITIS

Acute respiratory distress or pneumonitis has been described in some cases of talc pleurodesis.[50,57–59] The precise pathophysiological mechanism responsible for this severe complication is still unclear, but it appears that a high dose of talc used might have played a significant role in some cases. Also, the size of talc particles used for pleurodesis appears to be critical.[60] In a study on experimental talc slurry pleurodesis, Kennedy and coworkers[61] found prominent perivascular infiltrates with mononuclear

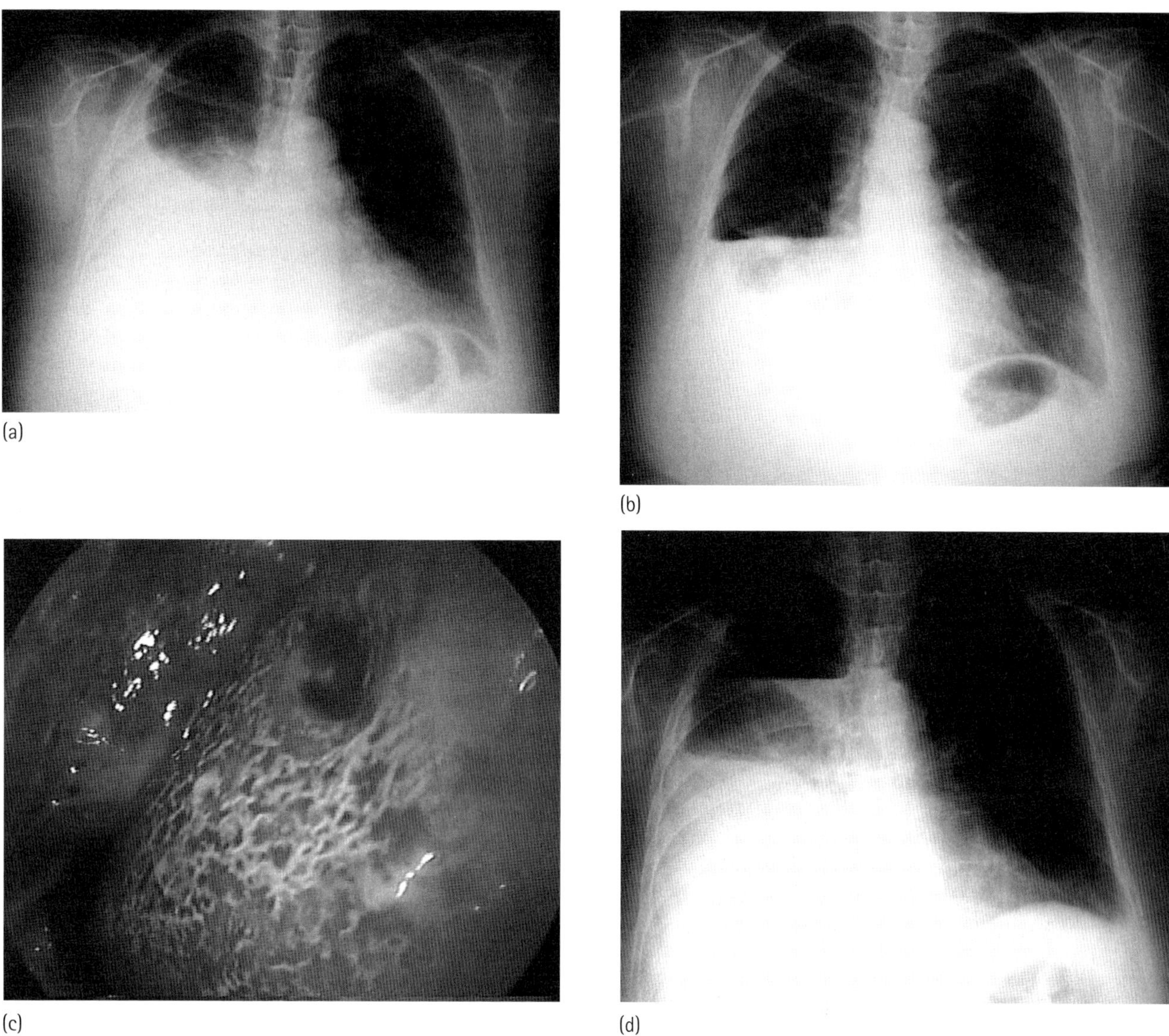

Figure 25.15 Metastatic cancer of the colon. Chemotherapy was given, but the effusion could not be controlled. (a) Chest radiograph before thoracentesis. (b) Iatrogenic pneumothorax occurred after therapeutic thoracentesis. (c) Necrotic tumor nodules and diffuse lymphangitis were observed on the visceral pleura at thoracoscopy. One of them (top of the figure, dark umbilicated lesion) was spontaneously ruptured, with no biopsy performed. (d) Air leak and persistence of pneumothorax was observed after unsuccessful talc pleurodesis.

inflammation in the underlying lung, and they speculated that some mediators might spread through the pulmonary circulation.

There is some concern about the systemic absorption of the sclerosing agents, and this is suspected to be the rule for almost all of the soluble agents that are instilled into the pleural space. In contrast, talc is thought to persist in the pleura for a long time, thus accounting, at least in part, for its better results in pleurodesis. However, there are some disturbing reports on the finding of talc particles in distant organs after talc pleurodesis, both in animals[62] and humans.[63] Our experience with four autopsies in patients that had undergone thoracoscopic talc poudrage is, however, completely different, since no talc was found beyond the pleura in any case. It seems that the size of particles may play an important role in the whole process,[64] and a recent European multicenter study on safety of talc poudrage using large-size particle talc (with 25.6 μm median diameter) found no cases of acute respiratory distress in a series including 558 patients.[65]

POSSIBLE ACTIVATION OF THE SYSTEMIC COAGULATION

One special aspect to be considered is the possible activation of the systemic coagulation following pleurodesis. Agrenius and coworkers[66,67] reported an increase in coagulation and inhibition of fibrinolytic activity in the pleural space after instillation of quinacrine as a sclerosing agent. Since it is assumed that a fibrin mesh formation is a necessary step for the fibrotic process, these findings make sense in the context of the mechanisms which lead to pleural symphysis. We also demonstrated similar effects after talc pleurodesis in our patients,[10] and were subsequently concerned about the possible systemic implications of the pleural coagulation/fibrinolysis imbalance that is involved in the pleurodesis process itself. Prompted by this concern and by our finding of two cases of massive pulmonary embolism after talc pleurodesis, we performed a preliminary study on simultaneous pleural/plasma determination of markers for coagulation and fibrinolysis. We found that an activation of the systemic coagulation is frequently observed after talc poudrage[68] and that this side effect can be partially controlled with prophylactic heparin.[69] The relevance of this finding in clinical practice is still unclear, but some early deaths (less than 30 days) following pleurodesis procedures (up to 43 percent in the series of Seaton and coworkers[70]) may in part be related to an undetected pulmonary embolism, and not to advanced neoplastic disease, as is commonly believed.

OTHER ALTERNATIVES TO PLEURODESIS IN MALIGNANT EFFUSIONS

When pleurodesis fails or is contraindicated, several options are available as discussed below.

Repeat pleurodesis

Repeat pleurodesis is especially appropriate in patients that have a good performance status and with a high recurrence rate. According to our experience, a second talc poudrage procedure, with increased dosage of talc, can be helpful.

Pleuroperitoneal shunt

A pleuroperitoneal shunt can be useful in patients that have a trapped lung and that are in a generally good condition, provided that they have no significant ascites.[71]

Parietal pleurectomy

Parietal pleurectomy by thoracotomy is very effective in controlling the effusion, but it is associated with significant morbidity. Instead, thoracoscopic parietal pleural abrasion or partial pleurectomy can be effectively performed through video-assisted thoracoscopic surgery (VATS).

Indwelling pleural catheter

In patients with an expected short survival (poor performance status and usually presenting with very low pleural pH), placement of an indwelling pleural catheter connected to a vacuum bottle or a disposable bag can be an acceptable choice. Tremblay and Michaud[72] have reported very good results in a series of 250 cases treated with a tunneled pleural catheter for MPEs.

Repeated thoracentesis

In cases with very poor general condition, repeated thoracenteses may be the only choice available. However, this option should be kept as a last choice since discomfort, risks of infection and protein depletion can significantly adversely affect the already poor quality of life of those patients.

PROSPECTS FOR CLINICAL STUDIES

Although I can foresee a wide spectrum of improvements in diagnosis and management of malignant pleural effusion in a near future, I believe that several points deserve special attention, as detailed below.

Advanced techniques for diagnosis in malignant pleural effusions

The increasing application of genetic and molecular biology techniques to pleural pathology is expected to bring a spectacular improvement in diagnosis of pleural involvement by malignancy, and this would not always need pleural biopsy, since many studies can be performed on pleural fluid samples.[73]

Course of small, asymptomatic malignant pleural effusions

Since late pleurodesis attempts are more likely to fail than earlier interventions, it might be suggested that pleurodesis be performed at an early stage, once the malignant nature of the effusion is known. Many of these patients, however, have few symptoms attributable to the effusion and are not likely to seek relief or treatment for it. Prospective studies are therefore needed in order to provide reliable management guidelines. As referred to earlier in this chapter, our group has undertaken one of these prospective studies, and found that about one-third of the malignant effusions that occupy less than 30 percent of the hemithorax would never require a pleurodesis procedure. This is obviously a preliminary conclusion, and we need more prospective studies, searching especially for markers that reliably predict the evolution of the effusion in a given patient. To date, we found that determination of pH and D-dimer in pleural fluid serial samples can reasonably give a clue on the future evolution (see section on 'Management of malignant pleural effusions' in this chapter).

Systemic complications and side effects of pleurodesis

This is clinically relevant, especially regarding dissemination of talc particles, which have provoked a growing concern about the use of talc for pleurodesis. Correct calibration of the talc to be used and determination of the optimal size of particles is of utmost importance. Another problem to be addressed is the potential triggering of coagulation in the systemic circulation. Since it is likely that this untoward event occurs with other sclerosing agents as well, such information would be useful in developing preventive measures.

Prevention of pleural fluid formation

Development of MPEs appears to be associated with several angiogenic factors, especially vascular endothelial growth factor (VEGF); hence, anti-angiogenic therapies would be a promising approach. I believe this is an area research effort should focus on, with the aim of eventually abolishing the need for pleurodesis.

KEY POINTS

- Malignant pleural effusion accounts for more than one-third of the effusions that require thoracentesis. Approximately one-third of the malignant effusions are related to lung cancer, while metastatic breast carcinoma is the second most frequent cause.
- The pleura can be involved by direct tumor invasion but most pleural metastases arise from tumor emboli to the visceral pleura, with secondary seeding to the parietal pleura.
- Most patients with MPEs present with progressive dyspnea on exertion. Chest pain is more commonly associated with malignant mesothelioma.
- The position of the mediastinum is critical in radiographic evaluation for management of MPE. A massive effusion with contralateral mediastinal shift requires therapeutic thoracentesis followed by chemical pleurodesis if the lung re-expands. When the mediastinum is centered or ipsilaterally shifted, contrast CT and/or ultrasound will help guide the best next step of investigation.
- Pleural fluid cytology is the simplest diagnostic test for MPEs. Thoracoscopy is the investigation of choice if the first cytological examination is negative and malignancy is suspected.
- Talc pleurodesis, particularly via thoracoscopic poudrage, is the most cost-effective procedure for pleurodesis in MPE.
- Placement of an indwelling pleural catheter connected to a vacuum bottle or a disposable bag can be considered as a valid alternative in patients for whom chemical pleurodesis is not suitable.

REFERENCES

● = Key primary paper
◆ = Major review article
∗ = Paper that represents the first formal publication of a management guideline

●1. Rodriguez-Panadero F, Borderas Naranjo F, Lopez-Mejias J. Pleural metastatic tumours and effusions. Frequency and pathogenic mechanisms in a post-mortem series. *Eur Resp J* 1989; **2**: 366–9.
2. Villena V, López Encuentra A, Echave-Sustaeta J, Álvarez Martínez C, Martín Escribano P. [Prospective study of 1000 consecutive patients with pleural effusion]. *Arch Bronconeumol* 2002; **38**: 21–6.
3. Peto J, Decarli A, La Vecchia C, Levi F, Negri E. The European mesothelioma epidemic. *Br J Cancer* 1999; **79**: 666–72.
●4. Meyer PC. Metastatic carcinoma of the pleura. *Thorax* 1966; **21**: 437–43.
5. Rodríguez Panadero F, Borderas Naranjo F, López Mejías J. [Lymphatic mediastinal blockade as cause of pleural effusion.] *Med Clin (Barc)* 1987; **89**: 725–7.
6. Light RW, Hamm H. Malignant pleural effusion: would the real cause please stand up? *Eur Respir J* 1997; **10**: 1701–2.
7. Sahn SA. Pleural diseases related to metastatic malignancies. *Eur Respir J* 1997; **10**: 1907–13.
8. Rodríguez Panadero F, Borderas Naranjo F, López Mejías J. [Benign pleural effusions in cancer patients. Frequency and etiopathogenic mechanism in a series of autopsy cases]. *Rev Clin Esp* 1988; **183**: 311–12.
9. Villena V, López-Encuentra A, Pozo F, De Pablo A, Martín-Escribano P. Measurement of pleural pressure during therapeutic thoracentesis. *Am J Respir Crit Care Med* 2000; **162**: 1534–8.
10. Rodríguez-Panadero F, Segado A, Martín Juan J, *et al.* Failure of talc pleurodesis is associated with increased pleural fibrinolysis. *Am J Respir Crit Care Med* 1995; **151**: 785–90.
◆11. Sahn SA. Malignancy metastatic to the pleura. In: Antony VB (ed.). *Clinics in chest medicine. Diseases of the pleura.* Philadelphia: W.B. Saunders Company, 1998: 351–61.
12. Wernecke K. Sonographic features of pleural disease. *Am J Roentgenol* 1997; **168**: 1061–6.
13. Gorg C, Restrepo I, Schwerk WB. Sonography of malignant pleural effusion. *Eur Radiol* 1997; **7**: 1195–8.

14. Macha HN, Reichle G, von Zwehl D, *et al.* The role of ultrasound assisted thoracoscopy in the diagnosis of pleural disease. Clinical experience in 687 cases. *Eur J Cardiothorac Surg* 1993; **7**: 19–22.
15. Kaplan LM, Epstein SK, Schwartz SL, Cao QL, Pandian NG. Clinical, echocardiographic, and hemodynamic evidence of cardiac tamponade caused by large pleural effusions. *Am J Respir Crit Care Med* 1995; **151**: 904–8.
*16. Antony VB, Loddenkemper R, Astoul P, *et al.* Management of malignant pleural effusions. *Eur Respir J* 2001; **18**: 402–19.
17. Moltyaner Y, Miletin MS, Grossman RF. Transudative pleural effusions. False reassurance against malignancy. *Chest* 2000; **118**: 885.
18. Fernandez C, Martin C, Aranda I, Romero S. Malignant transient pleural transudate: a sign of early lymphatic tumoral obstruction. *Respiration* 2000; **67**: 333–6.
19. Assi Z, Caruso JL, Herndon J, Patz Jr EF. Cytologically proved malignant pleural effusions. Distribution of transudates and exudates. *Chest* 1998; **113**: 1302–4.
20. Rodriguez-Panadero F, Lopez-Mejias J. Low glucose and pH levels in malignant effusions; Diagnostic significance and prognostic value in respect to pleurodesis. *Am Rev Respir Dis* 1989; **139**: 663–7.
21. Good JT, Taryle DA, Sahn SA. The pathogenesis of low glucose, low pH malignant effusions. *Am Rev Respir Dis* 1985; **131**: 737–41.
22. Sahn SA., Good JT Jr. Pleural fluid pH in malignant effusions: Diagnostic, Prognostic, and therapeutic implications. *Ann Int Med* 1988; **108**: 345–9.
23. Sanchez-Armengol A, Rodriguez-Panadero F. Survival and talc pleurodesis in metastatic pleural carcinoma, revisited. Report on 125 cases. *Chest* 1993; **104**: 1482–5.
24. Rodríguez-Panadero F, Del Rey Pérez JJ. Survival of malignant pleural mesotheliomas as compared to metastatic carcinomas. *Eur Respir Rev* 1993; **3**: 208–10.
25. Heffner JE, Nietert PJ, Barbieri C. Pleural fluid pH as a predictor of survival for patients with malignant pleural effusions. *Chest* 2000; **117**: 79–86.
26. Antunes G, Neville E, Duffy J, Ali N. BTS guidelines for the management of malignant pleural effusions. *Thorax* 2003; **58** (Suppl 2): ii29–38.
27. Escudero Bueno C, García Clemente M, Cuesta Castro B, *et al.* Cytologic and bacteriologic analysis of fluid and pleural biopsy specimens with Cope's needle. Study of 414 patients. *Arch Intern Med* 1990; **150**: 1190–4.
●28. Canto A, Rivas J, Saumench J, Morera R, Moya J. Points to consider when choosing a biopsy method in cases of pleurisy of unknown origin. *Chest* 1983; **84**: 176–9.
29. Maskell NA, Gleeson FV, Davies RJ. Standard pleural biopsy versus CT-guided cutting-needle biopsy for diagnosis of malignant disease in pleural effusions: a randomised controlled trial. *Lancet* 2003; **361**: 1326–30.
◆30. Loddenkemper R. Thoracoscopy: State of the art. *Eur Respir J* 1998; **11**: 213–21.
31. Boutin C, Viallat JR, Cargnino P, Farisse P. Thoracoscopy in malignant pleural effusions. *Am Rev Respir Dis* 1981; **124**: 588–92.
32. Loddenkemper R, Grosser H, Gabler A, *et al.* Prospective evaluation of biopsy methods in the diagnosis of malignant pleural effusions: intrapatient comparison between pleural fluid cytology, blind needle biopsy and thoracoscopy. *Am Rev Respir Dis* 1983; **127** (Suppl 4): 114.
33. Villena V, Lopez Encuentra A, De Pablo A, *et al.* Diagnóstico ambulatorio de los pacientes que precisan biopsia pleural. Estudio de 100 casos consecutivos. [Ambulatory diagnosis of the patients requiring a pleural biopsy. Study of 100 consecutive cases]. *Arch Bronconeumol* 1997; **33**: 395–8.
34. Porcel JM, Vives M, Esquerda A, *et al.* Use of a panel of tumor markers (carcinoembryonic antigen, cancer antigen 125, carbohydrate antigen 15-3, and cytokeratin 19 fragments) in pleural fluid for the differential diagnosis of benign and malignant effusions. *Chest* 2004; **126**: 1757–63.
35. Ceyhan BB, Demiralp E, Celikel T. Analysis of pleural effusions using flow cytometry. *Respiration* 1996; **63**: 17–24.
36. Kayser K, Blum S, Beyer M, *et al.* Routine DNA cytometry of benign and malignant pleural effusions by means of the remote quantitation server Euroquant: a prospective study. *J Clin Pathol* 2000; **53**: 760–4.
◆37. Rodríguez-Panadero F, Anthony VB. Pleurodesis: State of the art. *Eur Respir J* 1997; **10**: 1648–54.
38. Naito T, Satoh H, Ishikawa H, *et al.* Pleural effusion as a significant prognostic factor in non-small cell lung cancer. *Anticancer Res* 1997; **17**: 4743–6.
39. Martín Díaz E, Arnau Obrer A, Martorell Cebollada M, Cantó Armengod A. La toracocentesis en la evaluación del cáncer de pulmón con derrame pleural. [Thoracocentesis for the assessment of lung cancer with pleural effusion]. *Arch Bronconeumol* 2002; **38**: 479–84.
40. Rodríguez-Panadero F. Lung cancer and ipsilateral pleural effusion. *Ann Oncol* 1995; **6** (Suppl 3): S25–7.
41. Cantó A, Arnau A, Guijarro R, Centeno A, Marorell M. Actitud quirúrgica en el carcinoma broncopulmonar que se acompaña de un derrame pleural homolateral. *Arch Bronconeumol* 1992; **28**: 332–6.
42. Roberts JR, Blum MG, Arildsen R, *et al.* Prospective comparison of radiologic, thoracoscopic, and pathologic staging in patients with early non-small cell lung cancer. *Ann Thorac Surg* 1999; **68**: 1154–8.
43. Sawabata N, Matsumura A, Motohiro A, *et al.* Malignant minor pleural effusion detected on thoracotomy for patients with non-small cell lung cancer: Is tumor resection beneficial for prognosis? *Ann Thorac Surg* 2002; **73**: 412–15.
44. Cantó A, Arnau A, Galbis J, *et al.* [The so-called malignant pleural effusion: A new review of direct data obtained with diagnostic pleuroscopy]. *Arch Bronconeumol* 1996; **32**: 453–8.
45. Usuda K, Saito Y, Endo C, *et al.* Cytologic assessment of peroperative pleural effusion and prognosis in lung cancer patients who underwent resection. *Tohoku J Exp Med* 1992; **167**: 219–30.
46. Kondo H, Asamura H, Suemasu K, *et al.* Prognostic significance of pleural lavage cytology immediately after thoracotomy in patients with lung cancer. *J Thorac Cardiovasc Surg* 1993; **106**: 1092–7.
47. Higashiyama M, Doi O, Kodama K, *et al.* Pleural lavage cytology immediately after thoracotomy and before closure of the thoracic cavity for lung cancer without pleural effusion and dissemination: clinicopathologic and prognostic analysis. *Ann Surg Oncol* 1997; **4**: 409–15.
48. Dresler CM, Fratelli C, Babb J. Prognostic value of positive pleural lavage in patients with lung cancer resection. *Ann Thorac Surg* 1999; **67**: 1435–9.
49. Romero Romero B, Diaz-Cañaveral L, Laserna E, *et al.* The need for chemical pleurodesis in patients with malignant pleural effusion is associated to decline of pH and high levels of D-dimer in serial pleural fluid samples. *Am J Respir Crit Care Med* 2001; **163**: A903.
50. Dresler CM, Olak J, Herndon JE, *et al.* Phase III intergroup study of talc poudrage vs talc slurry sclerosis for malignant pleural effusion. *Chest* 2005; **127**: 909–15.
51. Yim AP, Chan AT, Lee TW, Wan IY, Ho JK. Thoracoscopic talc insufflation versus talc slurry for symptomatic malignant pleural effusion. Ann Thorac Surg 1996; **62**: 1655–8.
52. Mañes N, Rodriguez-Panadero F, Bravo JL, Hernandez H, Alix A. Talc pleurodesis: Prospective and randomized study. Clinical follow-up. *Chest* 2000; **118** (Suppl): 131S.
◆53. Rodriguez-Panadero F, Jannsen JP, Astoul P. Thoracoscopy: general overview and place in the diagnosis and management of pleural effusion. *Eur Respir J* 2006; **28**: 409–21.

54. Xie C, McGovern JP, Wu W, Wang NS, Light RW. Comparisons of pleurodesis induced by talc with or without thymol iodide in rabbits. *Chest* 1998; **113**: 795–9.
55. Olivares-Torres CA, Laniado-Laborin R, Chaves-Garcia C, *et al.* Iodopovidone pleurodesis for recurrent pleural effusions. *Chest* 2002; **122**: 581–3.
56. Chang YC, Patz EF Jr, Goodman PC. Pneumothorax after small-bore catheter placement for malignant pleural effusions. *AJR Am J Roentgenol* 1996; **166**: 1049–51.
57. Rinaldo JE, Owens GR, Rogers RM. Adult respiratory distress syndrome following intrapleural instillation of talc. *J Thorac Cardiovasc Surg* 1983; **85**: 523–6.
58. Bouchama A, Chastre J, Gaudichet A, Soler P, Gibert C. Acute pneumonitis with bilateral pleural effusion after talc pleurodesis. *Chest* 1984; **86**: 795–7.
59. Rehse DH, Aye RW, Florence MG. Respiratory failure following talc pleurodesis. *Am J Surg* 1999; **177**: 437–40.
●60. Maskell NA, Lee YC, Gleeson FV, *et al.* Randomized trials describing lung inflammation after pleurodesis with talc of varying particle size. *Am J Respir Crit Care Med* 2004; **170**: 377–82.
61. Kennedy L, Harley RA, Sahn SA, Strange C. Talc slurry pleurodesis: Pleural fluid and histologic analysis. *Chest* 1995; **107**: 1707–12.
62. Campos Werebe E, Pazetti R, Milanez de Campos JR, *et al.* Systemic distribution of talc after intrapleural administration in rats. *Chest* 1999; **115**: 190–3.
63. Milanez de Campos JR, Campos Werebe E, Vargas FS, *et al.* Respiratory failure due to insuflated talc. *Lancet* 1997; **349**: 251–2.
●64. Ferrer J, Villarino MA, Tura JM, Traveria J, Light RW. Talc preparations used for pleurodesis vary markedly from one preparation to another. *Chest* 2001; **119**: 1901–5.
●65. Jannscn JP, Collier G, Astoul P, *et al.* Safety of talc poudrage in malignant pleural effusion. *Lancet* 2007; **369**: 1535–9.
●66. Agrenius V, Chmielewska J, Widström O., Blombäck M. Increased coagulation activity of the pleura after tube drainage and quinacrine instillation in malignant pleural effusion. *Eur Respir J* 1991; **4**: 1135–9.
●67. Agrenius V, Chmielewska J, Widström O, Blombäck M. Pleural fibrinolytic activity is decreased in inflammation as demonstrated in quinacrine pleurodesis treatment of malignant pleural effusion. *Am Rev Resp Dis* 1989; **140**: 1381–5.
68. Rodriguez-Panadero F, Segado A, Torres I, *et al.* Thoracoscopy and talc poudrage induce an activation of the systemic coagulation system. *Am J Respir Crit Care Med* 1995; **151**: A357.
69. Rodriguez Panadero F, Segado A, Martin Juan J, *et al.* Activation of systemic coagulation in talc poudrage can be (partially) controlled with prophylactic heparin. *Am J Respir Crit Care Med* 1996; **153**: A458.
70. Seaton KG, Patz EF Jr, Goodman PC. Palliative treatment of malignant pleural effusions: Value of small-bore catheters, thoracostomy and doxycycline sclerotherapy. *Am J Roentgenol* 1995; **164**: 589–91.
71. Petrou M, Kaplan D, Goldstraw P. The management of recurrent malignant pleural effusions: The complementary role of talc pleurodesis and pleuro-peritoneal shunting. *Cancer* 1995; **75**: 801–5.
72. Tremblay A, Michaud G. Single-center experience with 250 tunnelled pleural catheter insertions for malignant pleural effusion. *Chest* 2006; **129**: 362–8.
●73. Mohanty SK, Dey P. Serous effusions: Diagnosis of malignancy beyond cytomorphology. An analytic review. *Postgrad Med J* 2003; **79**: 569–74.

26

Effusions from infections: parapneumonic effusion and empyema

NAJIB M RAHMAN, ROBERT JO DAVIES

THE CLINICAL IMPORTANCE OF INFECTION IN THE PLEURAL SPACE

Pleural infection remains an important disease with a significant clinical impact on respiratory specialists, physicians in general internal medicine and thoracic surgeons. Diagnosis is often challenging and a sophisticated multidisciplinary management strategy is required, including physicians, surgeons, radiologists and microbiologists. This disease is associated with a considerable morbidity and mortality. Despite this background, there is great variation in the management of these patients[1–18] with an evidence-based optimal pattern of care still to be established. Recently published studies confirm previous findings of an overall mortality for pleural infection of up to 20 percent[19–21] which rises further to about 35 percent in the immunocompromised host. [22] This mortality appears to be 'disease associated' in that it occurs over the 6 months after initial presentation[20,21] and by implication is probably amenable to reduction with improved care. Patients who survive 6 months after their episode of pleural infection have a survival similar to normal subjects over the next 4 years (Figure 26.1). The actual mortality risk from empyema is substantially influenced by the presence of comorbid disease. In our unit, over a 4-year period, all of the patients who died from their pleural infection had comorbid disease.[21] In addition to this mortality, up to 30 percent of patients will fail treatment with chest tube drainage and antibiotics alone and will require surgical drainage of their pleural collection.[20]

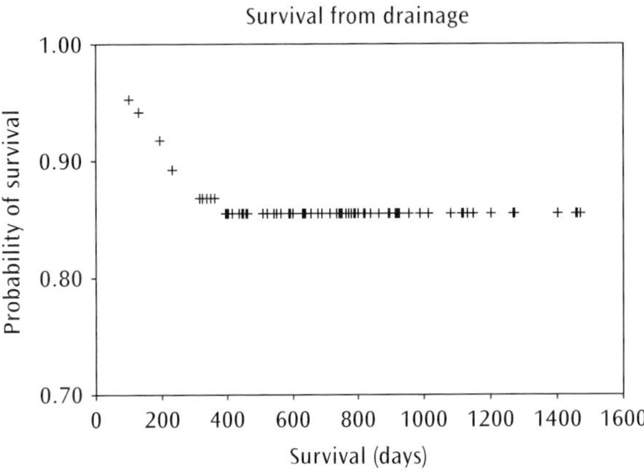

Figure 26.1 Kaplan–Meier plot showing patient survival from the time of presentation with pleural infection.[21]

Simple parapneumonic effusions arise in up to 57 percent of cases of cases of pneumonia[23] and approximately 65 000 patients develop frank pleural infection in the USA and the UK each year.[23,24] Of these 65 000 about 23 000 either require surgery or die. This chapter describes the current knowledge of this disorder and highlights optimal methods for diagnosis and treatment where possible.

HISTORICAL PERSPECTIVE

The first recorded description of empyema is attributed to the Egyptian physician Imhotep in around 3000BC,[25] in which he described '*An abscess with prominent head from the breast*', perhaps suggestive of empyema complicated by chest wall invasion (empyema necessitans). However, the first reliable description of pleural empyema and its treatment is attributed to Hippocrates in about 500BC, who treated cases of pleural infection with open thoracic drainage.[26] This remained the primary treatment for this disorder until the First World War, though Hewitt and Bulau[27,28] described methods for closed pleural drainage using a chest tube and an underwater seal decades before (1876–1891). Napoleon's surgeon, Guillaume Dupuytren (1777–1835), after whom digital contractures associated with liver disease are named, succumbed to empyema after announcing that we would 'rather die at the hands of God than of surgeons'.[29,30] The famous Italian tenor Enrico Caruso (1873–1921) is likely to have died from empyema. One of the most graphic historical accounts of pleural empyema was written by the Oxford physician, Sir William Osler, (after whom our Unit is named) who described his own, ultimately terminal, illness in 1919, after refusing thoracic surgery for his condition.[31]

The influenza pandemic of 1919, during the First World War, led to clusters of empyema cases among the fit young army recruits living in army camps. The treatment of choice was open surgical drainage resulting in a mortality as high as 70 percent in some outbreaks,[32,33] probably attributable to respiratory failure induced by the large open pneumothorax produced by the thoracotomy.[32] Since *Streptococcus haemolyticus* infection was responsible for many of these cases, it is interesting to consider that the streptokinase produced by this organism may have prevented fibrinous adhesions forming in the pleural cavity, exacerbating the problem by facilitating complete lung collapse.[34,35] The US Army Empyema Commission was formed to address this problem and this proved to be a landmark event in the care of this disorder.[34] The Commission noted that dogs with empyema died more often if treated with early open drainage rather than delayed intervention, and it advocated the closed tube drainage techniques described by Hewitt and Bulau.[27,28] Their summary recommendations were:

1. Adequate pus drainage with a closed chest tube.
2. Avoidance of early open drainage.
3. Obliteration of the pleural space.
4. Proper nutritional support.

The implementation of these changes reduced the mortality to 4.3 percent[35] and they remain the core aims of physical and supportive therapy to this day.

The next major advance was the discovery of penicillin that further decreased empyema mortality in the 1940s and was also associated in a change in the microbiology of the disease to produce the modern bacterial spectrum described below.

Intrapleural fibrinolytic therapy was tried by Tillett and Sherry[36] in the 1940s but did not become standard practice because of frequent antigenic side effects from this impure product.

Surgical techniques improved beyond open drainage in the late nineteenth century, when thoracoplasty was described by Estlander (1897) and Schede (1890).[37,38] This eliminated the empyema cavity but required major surgery and was disfiguring. Decortication of the pleura was first described by Fowler and Beck at the end of the nineteenth century[39,40] and most recently video-assisted thoracoscopic surgery (VATS) has been introduced to allow pleural debridement without formal thoracotomy in some patients.[41]

THE EPIDEMIOLOGY OF PLEURAL INFECTION

Pleural infection affects patients of all ages but is more common in the elderly[21] and in childhood.[42] Men are affected twice as often as women.[43,44] Its incidence is higher in those with diabetes, alcoholism and substance abuse, rheumatoid arthritis and coincidental chronic lung disease.[4,20,43,45] Diabetes is present in 10 to 23 percent of patients, five times the background prevalence of this disease[4,19,20,43] and excess alcohol intake is present in 6 to 10 percent of patients.[19,20,43,46] Poor dentition and risk factors for aspiration (seizures, gastro-esophageal reflux, mental retardation, alcohol use and sedative drug use) are believed to be associated with an increased prevalence of anaerobic infection.[19]

The markedly different bacteriological patterns observed in pneumonia and empyema (see below) suggests that they are microbiologically distinct diseases. Other causes include surgery, trauma and iatrogenic insults,[20,43,47–49] including thoracentesis for pneumothorax or pleural effusion (Table 26.1). Up to one-third of cases occur without any as yet identified risk factors.[19] Where the pleural infection is acquired in hospital, the prognosis is worse, and recent evidence suggests that the microbiological pattern of infection influences mortality independent of this (see below).[50] The duration of recovery is also prolonged in these patients with the median hospital stay being 58 days for hospital-acquired empyema in one representative series,[51] compared with 12–13 days for the entire group in randomised trials.[20] Hospital-acquired infections also exhibit a microbiology that is strikingly different from that of community-acquired empyema (Figure 26.2).[43,50] The clinical picture of hospital-acquired

Table 26.1 Frequency and cause of 701 patients with pleural infection[19,42,46–48]

Causes of pleural space infection	Frequency (%)
Parapneumonic effusion	70
Post-bacterial pneumonia	
Hospital-acquired pneumonia	
Primary empyema	4
Postoperative	12
Traumatic	3
Blunt trauma	
Penetrating trauma	
Iatrogenic	4
e.g. post chest tube insertion	
Abdominal infection	2
e.g. subphrenic abscess	
Miscellaneous	5
Esophageal perforation	
Bacteremia	
Rupture of lung abscess into pleural space	
intravenous drug abuse (contaminated needles)	

empyema is sufficiently different from that of community-acquired disease that it should probably be considered a different entity from both the epidemiological and therapeutic standpoints.

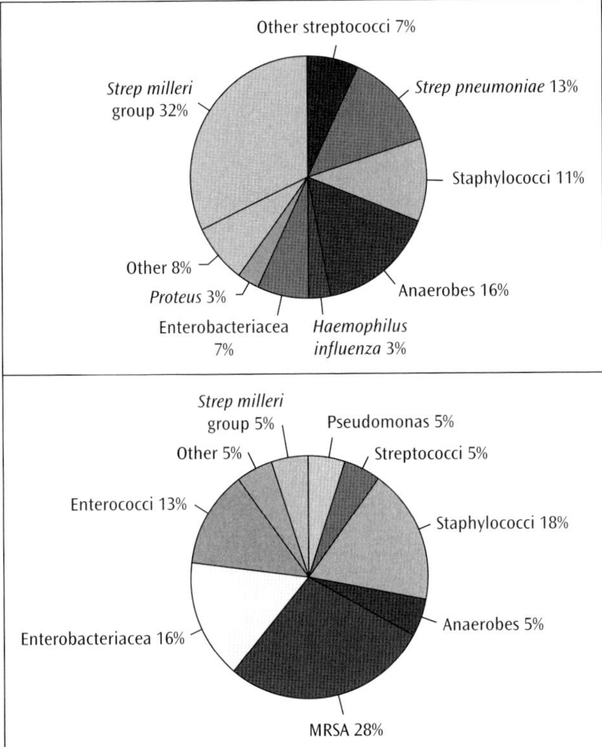

Figure 26.2 Bacteriology in positive isolates from the MIST1 cohort.[43,50]

THE PATHOPHYSIOLOGY OF PLEURAL INFECTION

This can be divided into three stages as discussed below.

Development of the initial pleural effusion: 'the exudative phase'

Animal work suggests that a pleural effusion may be a necessary substrate for sustained pleural infection. In animal models of empyema, direct inoculation of bacteria into the pleural cavity in the absence of pleural effusion results either in overwhelming sepsis or spontaneous recovery – and not sustained bacterial growth as characterizes clinical empyema.[52,53] However, experiments in rabbits suggest that empyema (in rabbits) may be induced by direct inoculation of bacteria without an initial pleural effusion if the bacteria are in a thicker broth.[54,55] The development of the initial effusion is due to increased permeability of the pleural membranes, in response to inflammation in the underlying lung parenchyma, which is thought to result in transfer of interstitial fluid across the visceral pleura. Indirect clinical evidence suggests that pleural inflammation alone is insufficient to result in significant pleural fluid, as many patients complain of pleuritic chest pain during a pneumonic illness, and yet only a minority develop radiologically detectable pleural fluid.

Given the correct circumstances, fluid moves into the pleural space due to locally increased capillary vascular permeability and the activation of immune processes such as neutrophil migration. Pro-inflammatory cytokines including interleukin (IL)-6, IL-8 and tumor necrosis factor alpha (TNF-α) produce changes in the anatomical shape of pleural mesothelial cells creating intercellular 'gaps' which further enhance permeability and additional fluid accumulates.[56–58] The accumulating pleural fluid has a normal glucose level (>40 mg/dL) and pH (>7.20), with no detectable bacteria, and hence no microbiological or biochemical evidence of bacterial invasion. The effusion will usually resolve spontaneously with antibiotic therapy for the underlying pneumonia.

The evolution of infection: 'the fibropurulent phase'

If inflammation persists within the lung parenchyma, secondary bacterial invasion of the pleural space occurs at some stage, with profound pathological effects on the normal pleural physiology. The high levels of fibrinolytic activity which characterize the normal pleural space are rapidly depressed[59] and titres of specific inhibitors of fibrinolytic activity such as tissue plasminogen activator inhibitor (PAI) 1 and 2 rise.[59] Levels of PAI 1 and 2 and mediators such as TNF-α are directly released from mesothelial cells[59] and are increased in infected pleural fluid compared with fluid from malignancy and other causes.[59,60] This leads to fibrin deposition over the visceral and parietal pleura, with the division of the pleural space by fibrinous septae, producing fluid loculation and pleural adhesions. While effusions of any cause may become loculated, the depression of the fibrinolytic system (elevated PAI level, depressed tissue plasminogen activator [tPA]) has only been observed in pleural infection, and not in effusions secondary to malignancy or transudates.[59,60] This division of the pleural cavity provides the skeleton for the later invasion of fibrous tissue and the 'natural' process of scarring and healing. However, it also creates multiple separate pockets of infected pleural fluid, and hence impairs the drainage of pus and is a major factor in reducing chest tube efficacy. Bacterial metabolism and neutrophil phagocytic activity induced by bacterial cell wall-derived fragments and proteases lead to increased lactic acid production[61] and thus a fall in pleural fluid pH and glucose – the biochemical hallmarks of early transition to the infected state.[62] As the numbers of neutrophils in the pleural space rise, lactate dehydrogenase is released producing the high levels typically seen in infected pleural fluids,[24,63] and ultimately the pleural fluid becomes frankly purulent, secondary to bacterial and inflammatory cell death and lysis.

Natural healing: 'the organizing stage'

Finally, there is the proliferation of fibroblasts and the evolution of pleural scarring, with animal model data suggesting this process is driven by mediators such as platelet-derived growth factor-like growth factor (PDGF)[64] and transforming growth factor beta (TGF-β).[54,56,59,65] This forms an inelastic peel on both pleural surfaces with dense fibrous septations across the pleural cavity. As this solid fibrous peel replaces the soft fibrin, lung re-expansion is prevented, impairing lung function. Interesting recent evidence points to a potential therapeutic target in the mediators thought to drive this process; the administration of anti-TGF-β antibodies during pleural infection results in significantly less pleural thickening, in a well established animal model of empyema.[55] The establishment of the phase of scar tissue formation is another important clinical landmark. It marks the point where pus drainage with a chest tube, even if supplemented by fibrinolytics that may lyse fibrin but not collagenous fibrous tissue, is likely to fail. Interestingly there is marked inter-individual variation and sometimes a prolonged delay in the rapidity with which this happens. Approximately 50 percent of patients do not have collagenous fibrous pleural scarring even 3 weeks after the onset of pleural infection,[66] implying that tube drainage and thoracoscopic surgery may still be effective in patients with a long history at presentation. The subsequent clinical course after the organizing stage is entered is also variable, with some patients undergoing spontaneous resolution of pleural thickening at 12 weeks[67] while others develop chronic sepsis and lung function deficits.[65]

In summary, pleural infection is a progressive process in which a self-resolving parapneumonic pleural effusion can progress to a complicated, multi-septated fibrotic collection that is only amenable to surgery. This evolution does not occur in a linear fashion but is summarized in Table 26.2 using the classification of Light and colleagues.[68]

Table 26.2 Light's classification of parapneumonic effusions and empyema[68]

Parapneumonic effusion	
Class 1 – Non-significant	Small <10 mm thick on decubitus No thoracentesis needed
Class 2 – Typical parapneumonic	>10 mm thick Glucose >40 mg/dL, pH > 7.2, Gram stain and culture negative
Class 3 – Borderline complicated	pH 7.0–7.2 or LDH > 1000 Gram-stain negative and culture negative
Class 4 – Simple complicated	pH < 7.0 Gram-stain or culture positive Not loculated or frank pus
Class 5 – Complex complicated	pH < 7.0 Gram-stain or culture positive Multiple loculation
Class 6 – Simple empyema	Frank pus Single locule or free flowing
Class 7 – Complex empyema	Frank pus, multiple loculations Often requires decortication

LDH, lactate dehydrogenase.

CLINICO-PATHOLOGICAL STAGE CORRELATIONS IN PLEURAL INFECTION

Several terms to describe the stages of evolution of pleural infection are used when applied to the clinical situation. While these terms are closely related to the pathological stages as defined above, they are primarily used as a tool to predict clinical course and guide clinical decision making, and are hence different. Knowledge of the hierarchy of clinical terms is important to avoid unnecessary investigations and prevent diagnoses from being missed. Each stage is associated with a change in pleural fluid characteristics, which reflect the pathological progression described above (Table 26.3).

Simple parapneumonic effusion

Simple parapneumonic effusion correlates to the exudative phase. The effusion is free flowing without evidence of bacterial infection in the pleural space, the term 'simple' being used to describe the clinical course of effusion without any evidence of bacterial or white cell activity. Previous series[24] suggest that these effusions are most likely to resolve without recourse to chest drainage or surgery.

Complicated parapneumonic effusion

Complicated parapneumonic effusion correlates with the early fibrinopurulent stage. There is biochemical evidence of early bacterial invasion, and fibrinous septations begin to form. 'Complicated' refers to the likely requirement for intercostal drain or surgery to resolve the pleural effusion. Biochemical parameters are used both to define this stage and as an indication that intercostal drain insertion should be instituted (see below).

Empyema

Empyema correlates to the late fibrinopurulent stage, and is defined as frank pus in the pleural space (i.e. macroscopic evidence of bacterial and inflammatory cell death) regardless of biochemical and microbiological parameters. The presence of frank pus in the pleural space is treated with immediate drainage.

Microbiology-positive pleural fluid – 'pleural infection'

The presence of any organism (other than likely contaminants from non-sterile sampling) in pleural fluid is diagnostic of pleural infection. Regardless of biochemical parameters or macroscopic appearance, this condition is treated with intercostal drainage (Figure 26.3).

The term 'parapneumonic effusion' assumes that underlying lung parenchymal bacterial infection is a necessary prerequisite to empyema formation. While many cases evolve in this manner, the different microbiological pattern seen in pleural infection is strongly suggestive of a different aetiology in at least a substantial minority of cases, and in the absence of direct risk factors (e.g. oesophageal perforation, thoracic trauma). Preliminary data suggests that underlying lung consolidation is not seen in 30 percent of pleural infection on thoracic CT scanning, and this may be associated with specific bacterial subtypes.[69] It is therefore probably more accurate to use the term 'pleural infection' either requiring drainage or not, rather than the terms simple and complicated parapneumonic effusion.

BACTERIOLOGY

There is substantial variation in the reported microbiology of pleural infection according to clinical context and series.

Table 26.3 Pleural fluid characteristics according to stage of pleural infection

	Simple parapneumonic effusion	Complicated parapneumonic effusion	Empyema
Appearance	May be turbid	May be cloudy	Pus
Biochemical markers	pH > 7.30	pH < 7.20	n/a
	LDH may be elevated	LDH > 1000 IU/L	
	Glucose > 60 mg/dL	Glucose < 35 mg/dL	
	or		
	Glucose pleural/serum ratio > 0.5		
Nucleated cell count	Neutrophils usually < 10 000/μL	Neutrophils abundant (usually > 10 000/μL)	n/a
Gram's stain	Negative	May be positive	May be positive
Culture	Negative	May be positive	May be positive

LDH, lactate dehydrogenase.

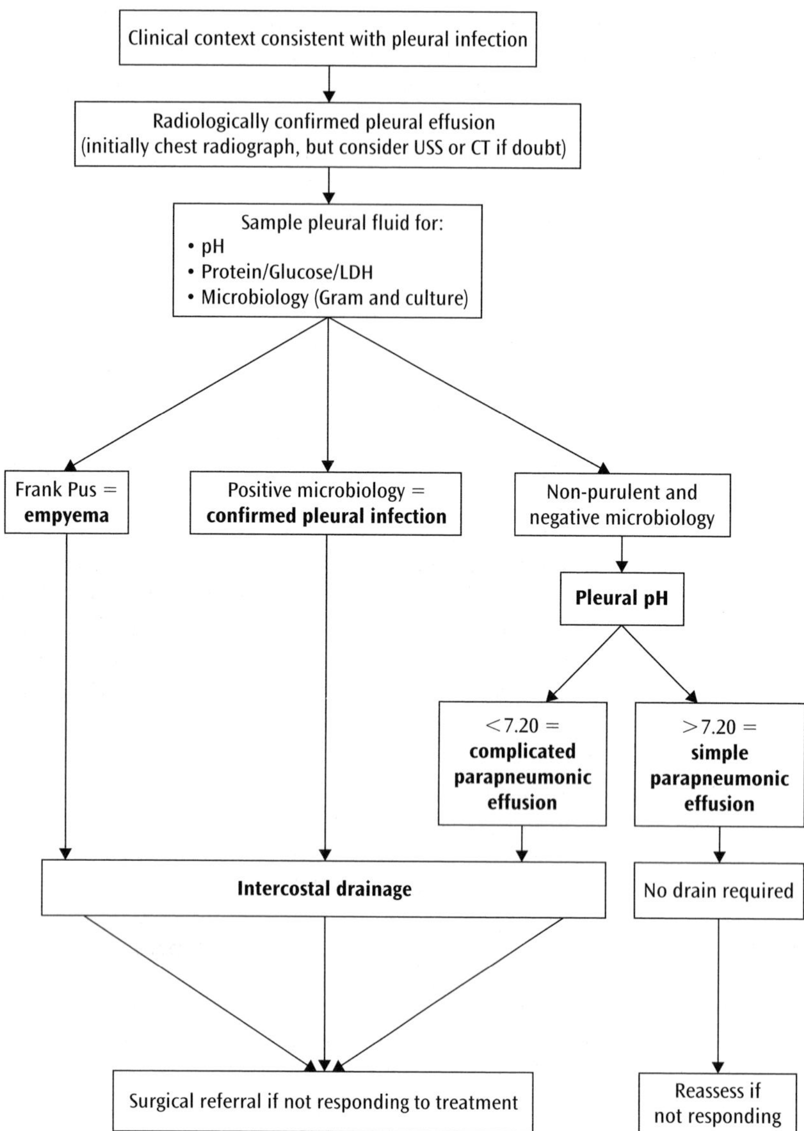

Figure 26.3 Algorithm for the diagnosis of pleural infection. CT, computed tomography; LDH, lactate dehydrogenase; USS, ultrasound scan.

Despite this variation, there emerges a consistent microbiological pattern which is distinct between community- and hospital-acquired empyema, and is furthermore distinct from the microbiology of pneumonia.

Detailed microbiological data were recently reported[50] from the largest randomized trial in pleural infection (the MIST1 study[20]). This represents the largest single cohort of well-defined microbiology in pleural infection. In this study, a microbiological diagnosis was achieved using standard methods in 58 percent (mirroring previous data), with a further 16 percent achieving diagnosis using nucleic acid amplification techniques (bacterial DNA polymerase chain reaction).[50] The use of DNA amplification reduced the number of cases remaining microbiologically undiagnosed from 42 percent with standard techniques to 26 percent.[50] While blood cultures were positive in only 12 percent of cases, they were often the only positive microbiological test in these patients.[50] The majority of culture positive cases (35 percent of entire group, = 62 percent of microbiology-positive samples) were due to a single aerobic organism, 9 percent due to a single anaerobic organism and 13 percent due to polymicrobial infection. A distinct microbiological pattern was seen in community- and hospital-acquired disease.[50]

Combining all previous data over the past 10 years[4,50,70–116] (Table 26.4), a microbiological diagnosis was reached in 1253 out of 2501 cases (50.1 percent) with aerobic organisms the most frequent organisms identified from infected pleural fluid. These are most commonly Gram-positive organisms from streptococcal species followed by *Staphylococcus aureus*. In the modern era, around 25 percent of culture positive cases are caused by *Streptococcus pneumoniae* whereas it accounted for 60 percent of cases prior to the advent of antibiotics.[50,117] However, many currently culture negative cases may be due to this bacterium in patients who may have been administered antibiotics prior to sampling.

Table 26.4 A summary of the bacteriology of all positive cultures from clinical studies between 1996 and 2006 published in the English language where details of bacteriology were presented[4,50,70–73,75–78,80–86,89,91,92,94–96,100,103–107,112,114–116]

Organism	Number	% of total
Aerobes – Gram positive	948	63
Streptococci	680	45
Streptococcus milleri group	169	11.2
Streptococcus pneumoniae	346	22.9
Streptococcus pyogenes	36	2.4
Other streptococcus species	117	7.8
Staphylococci	248	16
Staphylococcus aureus	197	13.1
Methicillin resistant *S. aureus*	40	2.7
Staphylococcus epidermidis	11	0.7
Enterococcus spp.	20	1
Aerobes – Gram negatives	228	15
Escherichia coli	52	3.4
Klebsiella	64	4.2
Other coliforms	37	2.4
Proteus	15	1
Enterobacter spp.	18	1.2
Pseudomonas aeruginosa	42	2.8
Anaerobes	206	14
Fusobacterium	51	3.4
Bacteroides	51	3.4
Peptostreptococcus	50	3.3
Mixed anaerobes/unclassified	21	1.4
Prevotella	31	2.1
Clostridium	2	0.1
Mycobacterium tuberculosis	22	1.4
Actinomyces spp.	7	0.5
Other	96	6
Total	1508	100

Gram-negative aerobic organisms are also common causes of pleural infection. The most frequent of these are *Haemophilus influenzae*, *Escherichia coli*, *Pseudomonas* spp. and *Klebsiella pneumoniae* (Table 26.4).

Anaerobic pleural infection is more likely to have an insidious clinical onset, with less fever and greater weight loss. The delayed clinical diagnosis of anaerobic empyema is therefore frequent, and a high clinical index of suspicion should be maintained if life-threatening and entirely treatable disease is not to be overlooked. Anaerobic infection is commonly associated with poor dental hygiene and aspiration pneumonia and often has a mixed bacterial flora. The frequency of anaerobic organisms isolated from published series of pleural infection ranges from 14 to 32 percent of positive cultures,[4,50,70–78,80–82,84–86,89,91,92,94–96,101,103–107,112,114–118] with an overall combined rate of 14 percent (Table 26.4). The anaerobic pathogens most commonly identified are *Peptostreptococcus*, *Fusobacterium*, *Bacteroides* and *Prevotella* species. The positive diagnostic rate from pleural fluid culture may be significantly increased if aerobic and anaerobic 'blood culture' bottles are inoculated with the fresh pleural fluid sample and are sent to complement the standard 'sterile vial' sample.[119,120]

Microbiology from the MIST1 trial cohort showed very substantial differences between community-acquired empyema and hospital-acquired infection, and probably represents the best base for empirical antibiotic choices. Within this cohort, community-acquired disease (whether arising following an evident community-acquired pneumonia or as a 'primary empyema' without obvious underlying parenchymal lung infection) was caused by streptococcal disease in over 50 percent of microbiology positive cases (largely *Streptococcus pneumoniae* and *Streptococcus intermedius*[50]). Staphylococci, anaerobes and Gram-negative organisms accounted for the majority of the remainder of cases. This translates to around 50 percent of microbiologically positive cases associated with penicillin-resistant organisms,[50] and 30 percent associated with anaerobic infection (often as co-infection with aerobes), which has clear implications for empirical antibiotic choices (see later).

In contrast, hospital-acquired empyema, which occurs after hospital acquired pneumonia, surgery or iatrogenic causes, was dominated by *Staphylococcus*, Gram-negative organisms (e.g. Enterobactericae, coliforms), *Enterococcus* species and a high proportion of methicillin-resistant *Staphylococcus aureus* (MRSA = 28 percent) (Figure 26.2).[50] This observation fits with previous surgical series where 14 percent of the culture positive cases were attributable to MRSA.[47] Streptococcal disease was almost absent as a cause of hospital-acquired empyema, resulting in bacteria resistant to standard antibiotic therapies for pneumonia in the majority of cases of hospital-acquired disease.[50] The so called 'atypical' organisms (e.g. *Mycoplasma*, *Legionella*) were not detected as a cause of pleural infection.[50]

Previous data from lung abscess treatment has suggested that 'mixed' infections are associated with a poorer prognosis,[121,122] although this does not appear to be true for pleural infection.[50] Mortality is higher in hospital- than in community-acquired disease.[50] Streptococcal disease has a 1-year mortality of 17 percent.[50] The survival with culture-negative disease intriguingly mirrors that of streptococcal disease,[50] perhaps lending weight to the theory that culture-negative disease is frequently a result of antibiotic-treated streptococcal disease. In contrast to this, mortality in patients with Gram-negative disease, staphylococcal and mixed aerobic disease is much higher at 45 percent at 1 year.[50] This difference in prognosis seen between bacterial subgroups may be a potential area for targeting more aggressive therapy in the future (Figure 26.4).

Gram-negative empyema is more frequent in patients with underlying diseases, especially those with diabetes or alcoholism.[4] Some bacterial pneumonias more commonly

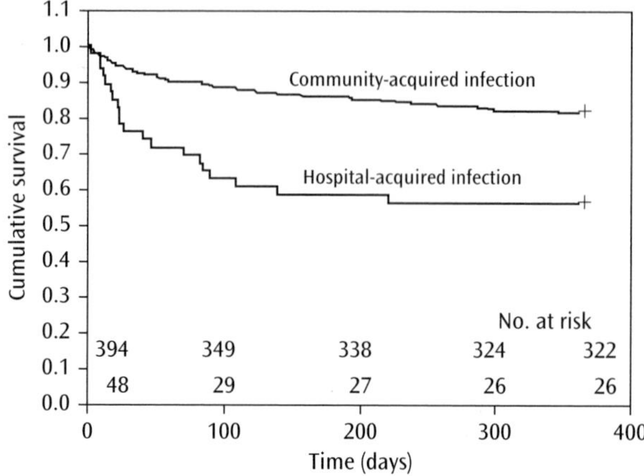

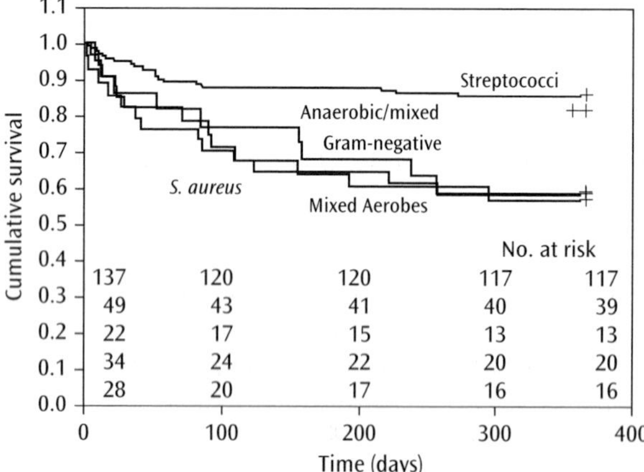

Figure 26.4 Survival curves in patients with different sources of infection (upper) and with different bacteriological subtypes (lower). Reproduced from Maskell *et al.*[50]

progress to pleural infection than others, with *S. aureus* and Gram-negative enteric bacteria such as *K. pneumoniae* having a particular proclivity to cause pleural infection.[123]

Fungal pleural empyema may be becoming more frequent. A study from a tertiary care hospital over a 7-year period reported 67 such cases. *Candida* species accounted for 64 percent and *Aspergillus* spp. 12 percent of the fungal empyemas.[124]

Combining all the literature reporting the bacteriology of empyema represents 2501 cases and strongly suggests that the microbiology of pleural infection and pneumonia are quite distinct, and should be treated as separate syndromes. Indeed, treatment of empyema with standard antibiotics for community- and hospital-acquired pneumonia is likely to result in resistant organisms being treated with ineffective antibiotics. It is postulated that the microenvironment of the infected pleural space (low partial pressure of O_2 [PO_2], acidic environment) may be the driving factor for different microbiology seen in pleural infection.

THE DIAGNOSIS AND CLINICAL ASSESSMENT OF PLEURAL INFECTION

The diagnosis of pleural infection is first dependent on the diagnosing physician having a high suspicion for the disorder. The usual clinical presentation is either a patient with pneumonia whose chest radiograph suggests pleural fluid or whose clinical progress is unsatisfactory, or a patient in whom radiographic pleural opacity and clinical indices suggest infection (fever, raised inflammatory markers, etc.).

In the context of pneumonia, the clinical dilemma is when to drain a pleural fluid collection. Up to 57 percent of pneumonia patients develop pleural fluid at some point in their clinical course.[23] However, only 4 percent of these develop frank pleural infection[48] and require pleural space drainage. There are no clinical features that predict patients who will eventually need drainage and pleural effusion sampling is always required to assess whether the effusion is infected.[5,6,24]

Diagnostic thoracocentesis in the context of pleural infection may be difficult. The fibrinous loculation of the pleural space can result in a multiloculated collection that is not easy to access as the diaphragm may be elevated and distorted by the pleural inflammatory tissue. As even small collections of infected pleural fluid probably warrant drainage, this risks major organ trauma during aspiration. In this situation, image-guided aspiration (usually thoracic ultrasound) is mandatory, permitting fluid sampling in 97 percent of cases, and preventing organ trauma and complications[125–128] (Figure 26.5).

Pleural fluid analysis is then the appropriate tool for the definitive identification of infection. The presence of overt pus is diagnostic of empyema, and no further biochemical tests are required for diagnosis. Performing Gram's stain and culture will identify bacteria in a proportion of non-purulent fluids and aids antibiotic choice. Approximately 40 percent of infected pleural effusions are culture negative[21,50] and in this situation biomarkers of intrapleural white cell and bacterial metabolism – pleural fluid pH, lactate dehydrogenase and glucose concentrations – are of the greatest diagnostic value. There are a number of large case series[62,129] and a detailed metanalysis[130] of the clinical strength of these indices (Figure 26.6). These show that pleural fluid pH alone is the optimal index for diagnosis and should be performed as routine in any potentially infected pleural fluid, which is not obviously purulent or Gram's stain-/culture-positive. Figure 26.3 gives a suggested flow diagram for the diagnosis of pleural infection that is based on this approach. If access to rapid pH measurement is unavailable, the measurement of pleural fluid glucose concentration is nearly as useful.

The exact level of pleural fluid acidity that should warrant treatment (i.e. intercostal drainage insertion) as a presumed infection is a matter of some debate. A range of suggested thresholds around pH 7.2 have been advocated, perhaps individually influenced by the patient's exact clinical circumstances. Pleural fluid pH should be measured

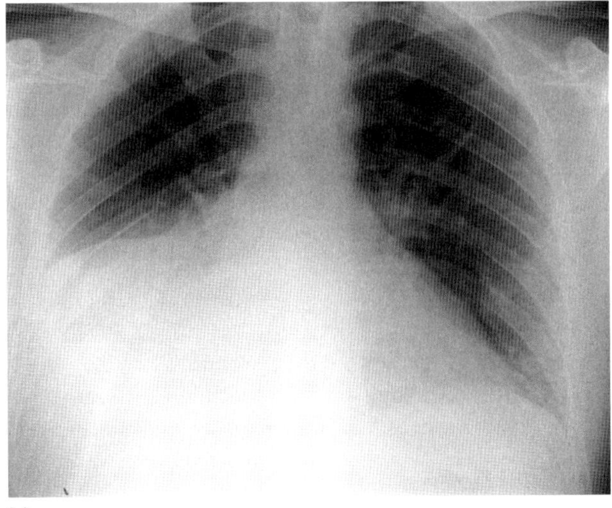

(a)

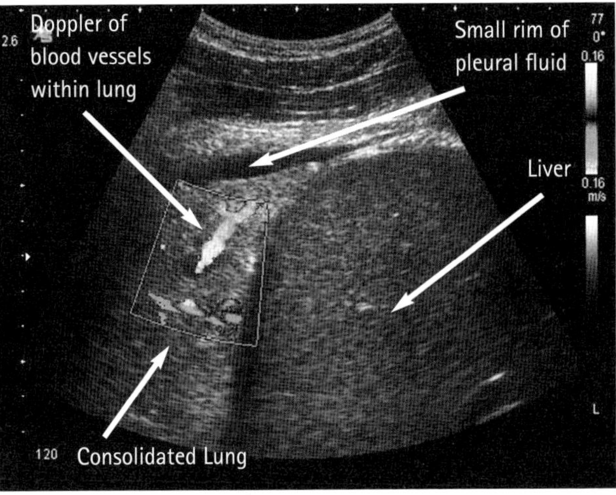

(b)

Figure 26.5 (a) Chest radiography of a 30-year-old man admitted with infective symptoms and thought to have a pleural effusion on chest X-ray, which prompted an attempt at 'bind' pleural aspiration (failed). (b) Subsequent ultrasound image revealing heavily consolidated lung and a tiny amount of pleural fluid as the cause for the chest radiograph appearance. Normal blood flow through consolidated lung is shown.

using a blood gas analyzer, as methods such as litmus paper or a pH meter have been shown to produce inaccurate results.[131] In the absence of reliable pH measurement, pleural fluid glucose may be used.[130] Since pleural pH is not 100 percent sensitive for the diagnosis of pleural infection (with scattered cases without an acidic effusion appearing in most case series), a single easy to remember threshold of 7.2 is probably as useful as a more complex algorithm. The physician must then always interpret this result in the clinical context and with common sense. Furthermore, diagnostically significant variations in pleural fluid appearance and pH have been shown in different locules in patients with pleural infection.[132] Although biochemical parameters are the most sensitive

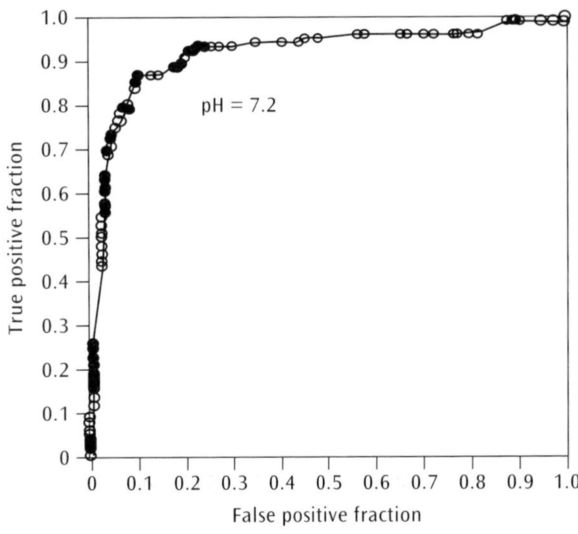

Figure 26.6 Receiver operating characteristic (ROC) curve for the diagnostic accuracy of pleural fluid pH for pleural infection.[130]

guide of need for intercostal drainage, they must be interpreted in the context of the clinical scenario, and resampling of pleural fluid is advocated if clinical parameters are not improving. Furthermore, a minority of patients with an initial pleural fluid pH of >7.2 will progress to require thoracic surgery, reinforcing the need for clinical evaluation above any single test. The occasional scenario where the biology of the disease renders pH unhelpful should also be remembered. In particular, *Proteus mirabilus* infection tends to be associated with a high pleural pH due to the urea splitting activity of this bacterium, which generates an alkaline medium.[75,76]

DIFFERENTIAL DIAGNOSIS

The most common problem with differential diagnosis is the failure to make the correct positive diagnosis. The potentially indolent presentation of pleural infection can produce a patient with anorexia, weight loss, little fever, raised blood inflammatory markers and sometimes no respiratory symptoms. In this situation, respiratory disease may not be considered in the differential diagnosis at all. Alternatively, this presentation associated with a smooth round subpleural chest radiograph opacity leads to an incorrect diagnosis of bronchial malignancy. The best protection against these errors is to have a low threshold for considering the diagnosis – which is particularly important as this is an eminently treatable disorder.

At the other end of the spectrum, not all patients with a fever and an acidic/turbid/apparently 'purulent' pleural effusion have a pleural infection. Pleural involvement occurs in up to 5 percent of patients with rheumatoid arthritis with the majority of these patients being male.[133] Patients often have markedly acidic pleural fluid with a low glucose level and present with pleuritis. The differentiation between this and a complicated parapneumonic effusion is challenging. This differential diagnosis is generally easily established by the recognition of the coincident joint disease and measurement of the serum rheumatoid factor. However, the not-uncommon scenario of the patient with rheumatoid arthritis who also has a pleural infection must also be remembered. Interestingly, the prevalence of pleural effusion in patients with rheumatoid effusion seems to be declining and there is a clinical suspicion that this may relate to the use of modern disease modifying therapy such as methotrexate.

Pleural malignancy may also present with fever and an acidic pleural effusion. Here, the systemic inflammatory response is probably related to tumor-induced cytokine production. Such patients may have a particularly short survival,[134–136] and low pleural fluid pH has been related to poor pleurodesis success and poorer prognosis.[137–140] It can be impossible to resolve this differential diagnosis with certainty at presentation, with the patient requiring treatment for presumed infection until the correct diagnosis is established by later biopsies or clinical follow up. The demonstration of predominantly neutrophils on the pleural fluid smear supports the diagnosis of pleural infection while the demonstration of mononuclear cells supports the diagnosis of malignancy.

In a patient with thick opaque pleural fluid that is not malodorous, then chylothorax and pseudochylous effusion enter the differential diagnosis. This differential can usually be established by bench centrifugation of the pleural fluid (10 minutes at 3000 r.p.m.). This leaves a clear supernatant in empyema as the cell debris is separated whereas chylous and pseudochylous effusions remain milky.[141] The diagnosis is then confirmed by the measurement of pleural fluid triglyceride and cholesterol levels and by microscopy for cholesterol crystals.

Occasionally, pleural sepsis secondary to esophageal rupture can be confused with primary empyema, especially in the elderly where the rupture may not be associated with a clear history of vomiting or chest pain. In these circumstances the diagnostic clues include: the presence of food particles in the pleural fluid, a raised pleural fluid amylase of salivary origin and possibly the presence of a hydropneumothorax on chest radiograph. Once suspected, imaging of the esophagus (e.g. oral contrast enhanced computed tomography (CT) scan – Figure 26.7) is required and a prompt thoracic surgical consultation is indicated.

Patients with pulmonary embolism can occasionally present a diagnostic challenge as the patient may present with fever, pleuritic pain and a pleural effusion. The pleural fluid biochemistry is not usually suggestive of pleural infection, but is non-specific and CT pulmonary angiography may sometimes be needed to evaluate this possibility.[142]

Finally, if pancreatitis is suspected then a pleural fluid amylase can be ordered and this diagnosis rejected if the level is normal.[143]

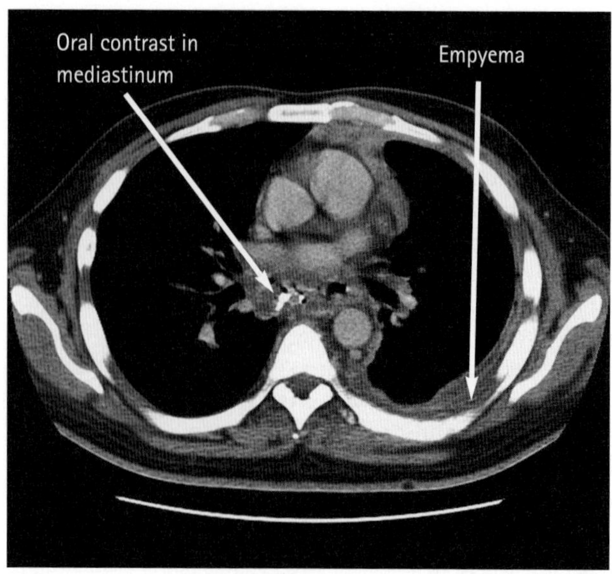

Figure 26.7 Oral contrast enhanced computed tomography scan demonstrating esophageal leak as the cause of empyema. The patient was discovered to have necrotic nodes eroding into the esophagus from tuberculosis.

PREDICTORS OF CLINICAL OUTCOME IN PLEURAL INFECTION

Pleural infection has a high mortality and morbidity and presents a clinical challenge in the timing of surgical intervention. Surgery is associated with a significant morbidity,[144–146] but is a necessary step in the recovery of a major subset of these patients. Accordingly, repeated efforts have been made to identify robust predictors of outcome that can be identified early in a patient's clinical course, allowing the early selection of those who will require surgery. Unfortunately, most studies of this question have been confounded by marked variations in patient management that are themselves likely to influence patient outcome (though whether for good or ill is often not known). These reports suggest that frankly purulent pleural fluid,[21] co-morbid diabetes,[4] delayed referral and pleural drainage,[84,147,148] the presence of pleural fluid loculation[149] and (counter-intuitively) in one study a low pleural fluid white count[149] may predict a poor outcome. However, in the largest randomized trial of pleural infection to date,[20] which included patients with pleural infection on established guidelines, purulence and loculation were not associated with a poor outcome.

There is only one prospective cohort study where the clinical management was delivered to all patients according to a consistent protocol (removing the confounding effects of varied management).[21] In this study, 85 subjects were managed with a consistent antibiotic regimen, chest tube drainage and intrapleural streptokinase. Only one subject was lost to follow up, with detailed outcome being available for up to 4 years or death in many subjects. In this study, the only statistical predictor of outcome was the presence of frankly purulent pleural fluid at presentation, and this was not sufficiently discriminatory to be clinically helpful.[21] Thus, it seems that there are no clinically reliable predictors of which patients will fail a brief trial of chest drainage and antibiotics at presentation. This is illustrated by the case of a previously fit 19-year-old female patient who presented with a 2-day history and a pleural effusion which was acidic, pH = 6.8, but remarkably innocent looking. The fluid was Gram-smear- and culture-positive for *S. pneumoniae*. She had no pleural thickening on thoracic CT scan and was promptly treated with tube drainage and intravenous antibiotics. Despite this she rapidly deteriorated and required surgical drainage only 36 hours later. In contrast, in one series of 26 patients who underwent thoracoscopy for chronic empyema of at least 3 weeks duration, over 50 percent had no evidence of intrapleural scar tissue – being still at the fibrinopurulent stage of their infection.[66] The clinical implication of the absence of any robust predictors of outcome is that all patients, regardless of individual clinical features at presentation, warrant management in a consistent manner.

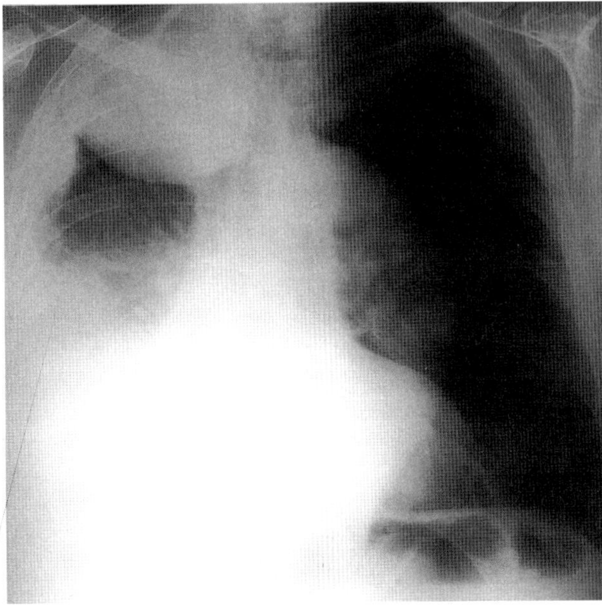

Figure 26.8 The characteristic D-shaped chest radiograph opacity of a pleural empyema.

RADIOLOGY

Pleural effusions are often obvious on the chest radiograph though infected effusions are often loculated and atypical in appearance. The presence of fever, pulmonary infiltrates and fluid should always alert the clinician to the possibility of a parapneumonic collection (Figure 26.8). The lateral chest radiograph may confirm pleural fluid not suspected on the postero-anterior image.[24] Pleural fluid loculation often results in a 'D' shaped subpleural opacity, which can easily be misinterpreted as a lung mass by an inexperienced observer. In the ventilated patient who is often imaged supine, free fluid may layer out posteriorly and then be represented as a hazy opacity of one hemithorax with preserved vascular shadows.[150]

Thoracic ultrasound enables the exact localization of any pleural fluid collection and so facilitates image-guided diagnostic aspiration if required.[128,151] It can detect the presence of as little as 5 mL of pleural fluid and is also highly effective in detecting loculations not seen on CT images (Figure 26.9). However, the technique is limited by the fact that it may not identify some separate fluid loculations in inaccessible areas of the thorax.

In patients with complex pleural fluid collections, contrast enhanced thoracic CT with contrast in the tissue phase (about 90 seconds after injection) is the imaging method of choice. It provides detailed information about fluid loculation (though it does not show septations within loculations), pinpoints the position of existing chest tubes and can identify any airway obstruction caused by tumour or foreign body. In addition, CT with intravenous contrast can usually differentiate between pleural empyema and

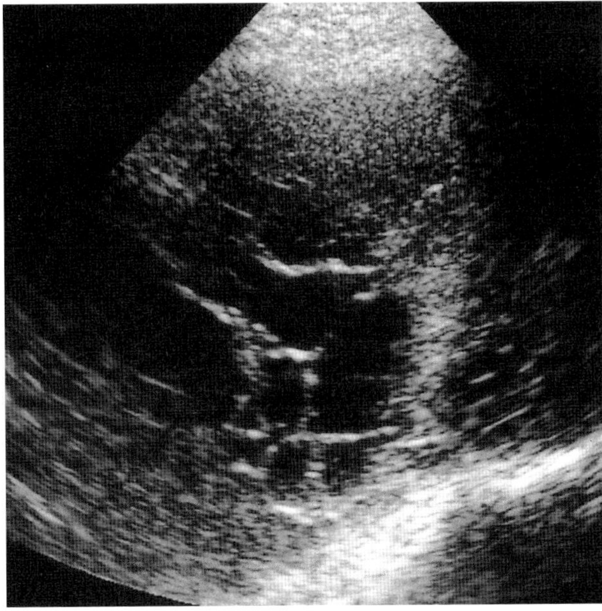

Figure 26.9 The typical pleural ultrasound appearance of pleural infection. The pleural space is divided into a multiseptated collection with varying echogenic appearances within the divided fluid, indicating varying degrees of fluid purulence.

lung abscess. Empyemas are usually lenticular in shape with compression of the surrounding lung parenchyma and the 'split pleura' sign is often noted (Figure 26.10), caused by enhancement of both parietal and visceral pleural surfaces which are separated by the pleural fluid collection. Lung abscesses, however, are usually round

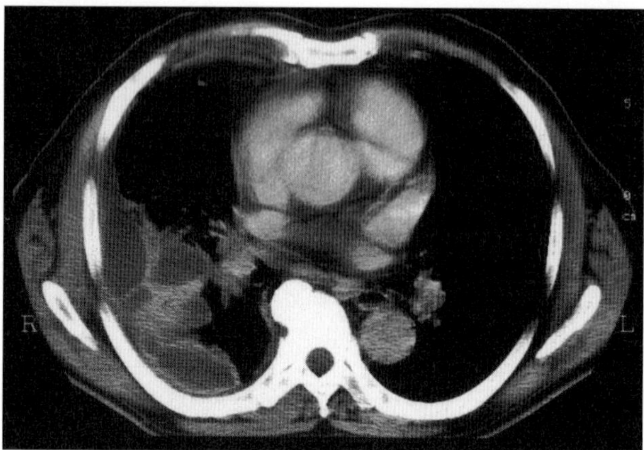

Figure 26.10 A contrast-enhanced computed tomography appearance of pleural empyema showing a multiloculated pleural collection. The 'split pleura' sign with enhancing pleural tissue visible on both the visceral and parietal pleural surfaces is shown.

with thick and irregular walls with indistinct boundaries between lung parenchyma and collection.[152,153] Other discriminatory signs are shown in Table 26.5.

Magnetic resonance imaging (MRI) is usually reserved for patients who cannot undergo CT because of hypersensitivity to intravenous contrast or who are at particular risk for irradiation, such as young women (where the breasts are radiosensitive).[154,155] In complex loculated effusions the multiplanar capability of MRI can also be used to advantage,[156] reliably identifying loculations and chest wall infiltration[157] (Figure 26.11). However, differentiation of infective effusion from malignant disease is not possible. Whereas thoracic CT is unable to differentiate pleural thickening from pleural infection or malignancy,[158] fluorodeoxyglucose (FDG) positron emission tomography (PET) scanning may permit identification of pleural thick-

Table 26.5 Differentiating between a lung abscess and empyema on contrast enhanced thoracic computed tomography[150,152,153]

Lung abscess	Empyema
Often round in shape	Lenticular in shape
Vessels passing through or near	No vessels closely associated
Indistinct boundary between lung parenchyma and collection	Compression of surrounding lung parenchyma
Thick and irregular wall, making contact with chest wall at acute angle	Smooth margins creating obtuse angles, following contours of chest

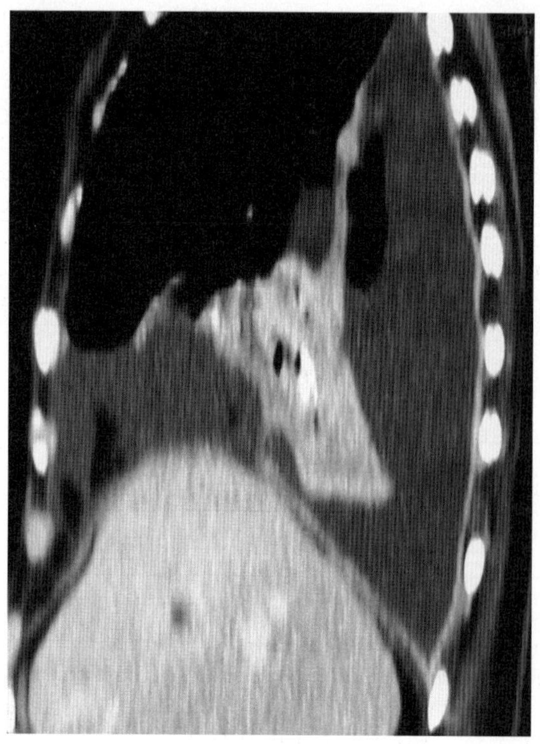

(a)

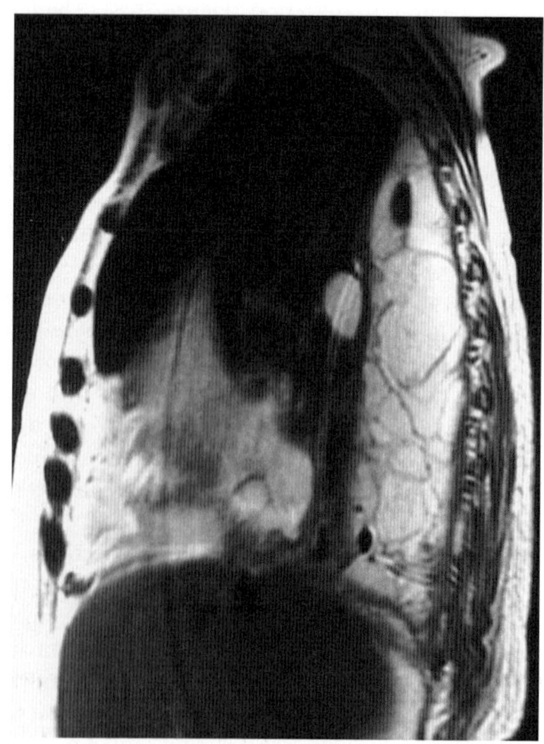

(b)

Figure 26.11 Computed tomography scan (a) and magnetic resonance imaging (MRI) scan (b), T2 weighted images of septated pleural effusion. The septations are clearly demonstrated on the MRI image. Image courtesy of Dr Fergus Gleeson, Oxford.

ening (cold on PET scanning[159,160]), but is unable to reliably separate infection and malignancy in the context of pleural effusion.

ANTIBIOTICS

All patients with parapneumonic effusions or empyema should receive antibiotics from the time of diagnosis. Where possible, the antibiotics prescribed should be guided by bacterial culture results. However, these results are usually not immediately available and approximately 40 percent of cases will be persistently culture-negative.[4,50,70–116] The patient's clinical setting and the underlying cause of the empyema should therefore dictate the initial choice of empirical antibiotic therapy, which will be required for the duration of therapy in 40 percent of cases.

Community-acquired pleural infection

In order to provide cover for penicillin-resistant organisms and anaerobes described above, a combination of a second generation cephalosporin or aminopenicillin plus a β-lactamase inhibitor plus anaerobic cover will provide adequate empirical cover for the duration of therapy. Given the low prevalence of *Legionella* and *Mycoplasma* in pleural infection,[50] in contrast to community-acquired pneumonia, addition of a macrolide is unnecessary.

Hospital-acquired pleural infection

A combination of a broad-spectrum antibiotic (such as a carbapenems or the anti-pseudomonal penicillins) and an agent active against MRSA is required for the hospital-acquired subgroup, to provide cover for multiresistant organisms and anaerobes.[50] Postoperative, trauma and iatrogenic related empyema will also require anti-staphylococcal coverage as the incidence of MRSA empyema is substantial in the hospital-acquired group.[50] Although the majority of hospital-acquired infections are treated intravenously for the duration of treatment, oral regimens exist which cover the majority of likely pathogens. Exact regimens will be influenced by local practice and bacterial resistance patterns, but suitable illustrative regimes are shown in Table 26.6. Oral regimens are not recommended for the treatment of hospital-acquired infection, but may be required for the long-term treatment of patients with hospital-acquired disease who are unfit for invasive procedures.

Penicillins, cephalosporins, clindamycin, carbapenems and metronidazole all show good and similar penetration of the pleural space.[161–163] However, aminoglycosides appear to penetrate poorly into the pleural space and may be inactive in purulent, acidic pleural fluid. They should therefore be avoided in treating pleural infection.[161,162] In all cases, positive pleural fluid or blood cultures should be used to narrow antibiotic therapy tailored to the organism(s) found. However, mixed infections occur in up to 13 percent of cases, especially relevant to anaerobic bacteria, and these organisms may be difficult to isolate. Consideration should therefore be given to continuing concurrent anaerobic antibiotics, even when a positive microbiological diagnosis has been made.

The duration of antibiotic treatment depends on the bacteriology, the efficacy of pleural drainage and the speed of resolution of the patient's symptoms. There are no studies directly addressing the length of treatment required in pleural infection, although at least 2 weeks therapy is not uncommon (following paradigms for the treatment of pulmonary abscess). It is our practise to give at least the first week of antibiotic therapy intravenously, with a subsequent change to oral regimens dictated by the patient's response. A combination of an oral aminopenicillin with a beta lactamase inhibitor (or clindamycin and ciprofloxacin in penicillin-allergic patients) is often adequate as oral sustained therapy. Decisions on the length of treatment can be guided by repeated measurements of serum markers of the acute-phase reaction, such as the C-reactive protein. The monitoring of fever lysis is also

Table 26.6 Possible empirical antibiotic regimens for pleural infection

	Suggested antibiotic regimen	
	Oral	**Intravenous**
Hospital-acquired[a]	Clindamycin 300 mg qds + ciprofloxacin 500 mg bd (+ rifampicin 300 mg bd if MRSA is suspected)	Meropenem 500 mg tds + vancomycin 1 g bd
Community-acquired	Co-Amoxiclav 625 mg tds + metronidazole 400 mg tds OR clindamycin 300 mg qds + ciprofloxacin 500 mg bd	Cefuroxime 1.5 g tds (or co-amoxiclav 1.2 g tds) + metronidazole 500 mg tds (meropenem 500 mg in penicillin-allergic patients)

[a]Oral regimens are not recommended for hospital-acquired infection, but may be required for long-term treatment (see text).
MRSA, methicillin-resistant *Staphylococcus aureus*.

valuable, though elderly patients and those with indolent, often anaerobic empyema, frequently fail to mount a fever and here indices such as the C-reactive protein seem particularly helpful.

CHEST CATHETER DRAINAGE

The optimal size of catheter for the drainage of an infected pleural space remains a cause of vigorous debate. Previous management guidelines have suggested that larger bore catheters are required to allow drainage of high viscosity empyema fluid, citing evidence that inadequate tube bore is a predictor of need for surgery.[21,23,164,165] However, flexible smaller bore catheters are less traumatic to insert and more comfortable for the patient after insertion, extrapolating data from catheter treatment of malignant pleural effusion.[166] Numerous observational series, including hundreds of patients, show that good outcomes can be achieved with smaller catheters (<12 F).[127,128,167–173]

Given the extent and importance of the 'chest tube size' debate, consideration of the background to this argument is appropriate. There are three reasons why infected pleural fluid may resist drainage through a catheter: drainage may fail if the fluid is of high viscosity and directly blocks the tube; it may fail because the balance of forces drawing it down the tube is inadequate; and it may fail if the fluid is partitioned by fibrinous septae. Although a large-bore tube may improve the first problem, smaller bore catheters can be kept clear by flushing and a large-bore tube is unlikely to decrease the other difficulties. During the chest tube drainage of non-septated pleural contents, provided that the sucker does not block, the negative tube tip pressure is transmitted through the pleural fluid to the lung surface. Therefore, whether fluid flow occurs at all is related to the balance between the negative suction pressure and the compliance of the underlying lung and not to catheter bore. In contrast, the rate at which fluid drains is clearly dependent on tube calibre, as well as fluid viscosity. Therefore, provided that the tube does not block, the rapidity of chest tube drainage might be improved by increasing the drain size, but the likelihood of eventual successful drainage is unchanged. In the presence of a multi-septated effusion the advantages of a large drain seem even smaller. Here, as some fluid drainage occurs, the fibrinous septae distort, distributing the drainage forces across the many locules as well as the lung surface. It is the pressure gradients developed across the walls of these locules that predict whether they will rupture and drain, not the rapidity of flow down the drainage catheter. Here again, provided that the catheter is patent, its bore would seem to be irrelevant.

There is some indirect evidence in support of the above arguments. *In vitro* studies suggest that increased tube bore is associated with increased fluid flow, but the increase in flow is small with catheters above 7 F.[174] Two small studies have directly compared small- and large-bore catheters for the drainage of intra-abdominal pus, both of which reported no advantage of drains larger than 8 F.[175,176] Assessing clinical studies over the last 18 years of treatment of pleural infection in which different catheter sizes were used, no difference between outcomes with different catheter size are reported.[75,77,78,86,171,177] The use of regular saline flushes and suction may prevent small catheter blockage and aid the drainage of pus.

INTRAPLEURAL FIBRINOLYTICS

Background

The use of intrapleural fibrinolytic agents to chemically disrupt the fibrinous pleural septations of empyema (Figure 26.12) has been used to aid the drainage of infected pleural fluids for over 50 years. It was first described in 1949 by Tillet and Sherry,[36] who used partially purified streptococcal fibrinolysin that contained both streptokinase and strepdornase (a DNAse) to drain infected post-operative haemothoraces. This was associated with immunological side effects and the use of this agent failed to become routine practice. Subsequently, the availability of highly purified streptokinase and non-antigenic urokinase was, in part, responsible for renewed interest in this therapy.

Streptokinase is a proteolytic enzyme derived from a bacterial protein of group C beta-haemolytic streptococci. It forms a complex with plasminogen that then converts

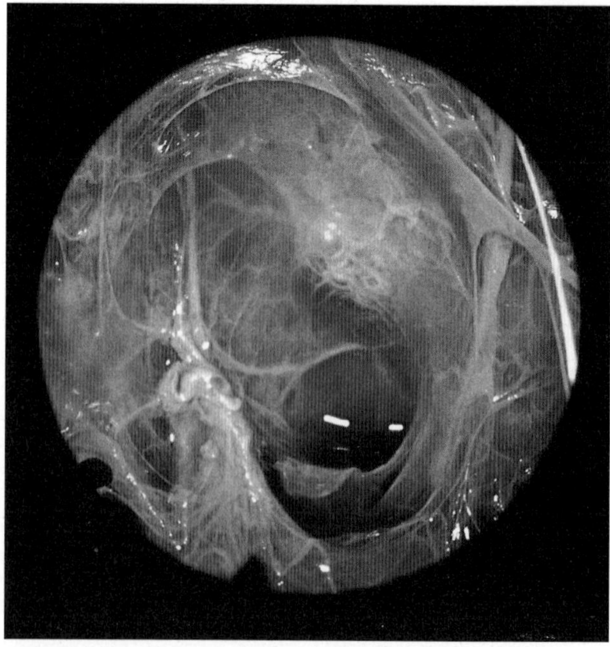

Figure 26.12 The macroscopic appearance of pleural fibrinous septation at thoracoscopy in an infected malignant pleural effusion.

additional circulating plasminogen to plasmin. Plasmin lyses fresh fibrin clots and digests prothrombin and fibrinogen.[178] Because it is derived from a bacterial source it is antigenic,[179] unlike urokinase.

Streptokinase is usually administered as a solution of 250 000 IU in 30 mL of sterile saline via the chest tube and the tube clamped for 2–4 hours before returning to normal drainage. This has been given daily[71,77,83,85,95] or repeated twice daily for several days.[20] Urokinase can be used in a similar fashion with 100 000 IU as the standard daily dose.[78]

These agents theoretically improve pleural pus drainage through the disruption of fibrinous septae and the dissolution of the visceral fibrinous pleural rind. Lysis of this rind may then aid lung expansion and so help to obliterate the infected pleural space. Uncontrolled observational case series[2,10,16,17,51,89,180,181] report good outcomes for patients treated with these drugs.

The safety of intrapleural fibrinolytic agents

Potential side effects of fibrinolytic therapy include hemorrhage, pleuritic pain after drug administration and fever.[77,89,181] There have been a few case reports of both systemic and local hemorrhage after intrapleural fibrinolytic administration,[182–184] but the majority of the published studies report no bleeding complications.[2,3,10,16,17,83,86,92,101,107,108,111,116,181] Within the MIST1 cohort, there was a serious adverse event rate of 3 percent in the placebo arm and 7 percent of the streptokinase arm, largely due to immunological reactions to the streptokinase and with no excess of bleeding complications.[20]

Studies of whether fibrinolytic drugs given into the pleural space induce systemic activation of fibrinolytic mechanisms are also reassuring. Systemic fibrinolytic activation is best quantified from the thrombin time, fibrinogen levels and the presence of fibrinogen degradation products. Two studies have assessed whether these change after the administration of intrapleural streptokinase. They studied a total of 26 patients with thrombin time, fibrinogen levels and fibrinogen degradation products being quantified before and after the administration of up to 1.5 million units of intrapleural streptokinase given in repeated doses. Neither of these studies revealed any detectable changes in the coagulation indices when compared with baseline.[185,186]

A further important safety issue relates to the systemic antigenic effects of intrapleural streptokinase and hence the necessity for the use of a different fibrinolytic drug for later clinical indications such as myocardial infarction. Anti-streptokinase immunoglobulin (Ig)G detectable in blood after prior exposure to streptokinase or streptococcal infection is associated with reduced fibrinolytic efficacy and hence reduced efficacy in achieving coronary reperfusion.[187] Within the MIST1 study, at 3 months there was a highly significant rise in anti-streptococcal antibodies in the streptokinase arm compared with placebo.[20] Assessing whether it does induce a systemic antibody response is complicated by the fact that many pleural infections are themselves streptococcal and hence are likely to induce an antibody response as a direct consequence of the bacterial infection. Currently, cautious best practice would seem to indicate that subjects who have had intrapleural streptokinase should be managed as if they had received intravenous streptokinase. These patients should be given a streptokinase exposure card and an alternative fibrinolytic agent used if needed.

Randomized trials using fibrinolytics

To date, 14 randomized trials have been published using intrapleural fibrinolytics: 10 in adults[20,71,76–78,85,86,101,111,177] and four in children[92,107,108,116] (Table 26.7). Eight of these studies are 'efficacy' studies assessing fibrinolytic versus placebo[20,78,85,86,107,111,116,177] (two pediatric[107,116]), one assesses chest drainage plus fibrinolytic versus chest drainage only[101] (i.e. no placebo) and one is a comparison of two different fibrinolytic agents.[77]. The remaining three studies assess the early use of VATs versus a drainage plus fibrinolytic strategy[76,92,108] (two pediatric[92,108]).

The randomized trials of fibrinolytic therapy until 2004 all assessed clinical surrogates for treatment success, usually using volume of fluid drained, radiographic outcome or length of hospital stay as outcome measures (Table 26.7). A selected few assessed the need for surgical drainage as a primary outcome measure, but the criteria for surgical drainage were not clear and may simply be a further surrogate for poor radiographic outcomes. The majority of these studies found significant benefit for the use of intrapleural fibrinolytic therapy. These studies were all small, the largest number of cases in a single study being 60, and the total number of patients in these studies amounting to 272 (100 of these being children). A meta-analysis conducted in 2004 assessing the publishes studies at the time concluded that while there seemed to be evidence of benefit from intrapleural thrombolytic therapy (decreased hospital stay, improved radiographic appearance, lower surgical rate), there was insufficient evidence to recommend its use routinely.[188]

The first randomised trial to demonstrate improvement in clinically meaningful outcomes with intrapleural fibrinolytic, such as clinical success rate and need for surgery, was conducted by Diacon *et al.*[86] in 2004. A total of 44 patients were randomized to intrapleural streptokinase or intrapleural saline in addition to pleural rinses through the chest drain, and decisions about further management, including surgery, were made in a blinded and consistent manner. After 3 days of intrapleural therapy, there was no difference between the active and placebo groups, whereas after 7 days, there was a significantly increased clinical success rate and a significantly lower surgical rate in the streptokinase group.[86] However, this study was not

Table 26.7 Randomized controlled trials of fibrinolytic therapy in adult empyema

Author	Interventions	Number of patients	Doses	Trial methodology	Results
Bouros *et al.*[77]	SK versus UK	50 25 SK versus 25 UK	250 000 IU SK 100 000 IU UK repeated daily if required	Randomized Double blind	Similar fluid drainage both groups Two patients in each group required surgery Transient fever 7/25 SK, versus 0/25 UK
Davies *et al.*[85]	SK versus saline	24 12 SK versus 12 saline	250 000 IU SK daily for 3 days	Randomized Double blind	Significantly greater volume of pleural fluid drainage in SK group ($p < 0.001$) and radiographic improvement ($p < 0.05$) Higher surgical referral rate in control group (0/13 versus 3/12, non-significant)
Bouros *et al.*[78]	UK versus saline	31 15 UK versus 16 saline	100 000 IU SK daily for 3 days	Randomized Double blind	Faster mean time to defervescence and shorter hospital stay in UK group ($p < 0.01$) Significantly greater radiographic improvement in UK group
Tuncozgur *et al.*[177]	UK versus saline	49 24 UK versus 25 saline	100 000 IU UK for 5 days	Randomized Blinding unclear	Shorter time to defervesence ($p < 0.01$), shorter hospital stay ($p < 0.001$) in UK group, volume drained greater with UK ($p < 0.001$). Lower decortication rate (60% versus 29%, $p < 0.001$) Decision to surgery included radiological assessment High rate of failure in saline group
Talib *et al.*[111]	SK versus saline	24	250 000 IU SK for 6 days 12 SK versus 12 saline	Randomized Non-blinded	Increased drainage, shorter duration of drainage in SK group. Significant difference in radiographic improvement ($p < 0.001$)
Diacon *et al.*[86]	SK versus saline	44	250 000 IU SK daily and continued as needed 22 SK versus 22 saline	Randomized Placebo controlled High rate of withdrawal Wide inclusion criteria Surgical referral based on radiology	One mortality in each group. Longer duration of SK treatment (4.5 versus 3 days). No difference in outcome after 3 days, but after 7 days, higher clinical success rate ($p < 0.01$) and fewer surgical referrals ($p < 0.02$)
Maskell *et al.*[20]	SK versus saline	430	250 000 IU SK bd for 3 days 208 SK versus 222 saline	Randomized Double blind	No difference in mortality, need for surgery or combined endpoint. No difference in hospital stay, radiographic outcome or lung function at 3 months. No difference between groups in subgroups (purulent, short clinical history) Surgical referral based on clinical opinion (not radiographic alone)
Misthos *et al.*[101]	Intercostal drain versus intercostal drain + SK	127 70 intercostal drain versus 57 intercostal drain + SK	250 000 IU SK od for 3 days (tube clamped for 4 hours)	Randomized Non-controlled, non-blinded	Higher treatment success in SK group (67% versus 87%, $p < 0.05$) Shorter hospital stay and lower mortality in SK group ($p < 0.001$)

SK, streptokinase; UK, urokinase.

powered to address surgical outcomes and there was a high rate of subject withdrawal (Table 26.7).

Against this background, the MIST1 trial[20] reported its findings in 2005. The study recruited 454 patients across 52 UK hospitals, and was powered to address whether streptokinase altered combined death and surgical rate. Patients were recruited on the basis of established criteria for pleural infection (appropriate clinical scenario and one or more of: pleural fluid pH <7.2, purulent pleural fluid, microbiologically positive fluid) and randomized to intrapleural streptokinase (250 000 IU bd for 3 days) or intrapleural saline (bd for 3 days) in addition to standard local care (chest drain, antibiotics).[20] Intrapleural agents were given to 430 patients and primary outcome data was available in 99 percent. No difference was found in the combined rate of death and surgery at 3 months (primary outcome measure) in the placebo and streptokinase (SK) groups, the outcome occurring in around 30 percent of patients (Figure 26.13). There was no difference between SK and placebo groups in death or surgery analyzed separately, length of hospital stay, radiographic change or lung function at 3 months. Subgroup analyses demonstrated no difference between streptokinase and placebo regardless of characteristic studied (pleural fluid purulence, complicated parapneumonic effusion, short clinical history, initial amount of radiographic effusion). There was a small excess of adverse effects in the SK group, mainly associated with allergic or immunological reactions, but no excess of systemic thrombolysis or bleeding.[20]

A study in 127 patients was published later in 2005, assessing intrapleural streptokinase ($n = 47$) versus normal chest drainage ($n = 70$), with no placebo used.[101] Once again, treatment success, length of hospital stay and surgical referral were lower in the streptokinase group, and this study found a significant mortality benefit in the SK group (4.2 percent versus 1.7 percent, $p < 0.001$). However, the study was not placebo controlled, and therefore by definition unblinded, which made the differences in the surgical and hospital stay outcomes questionable.

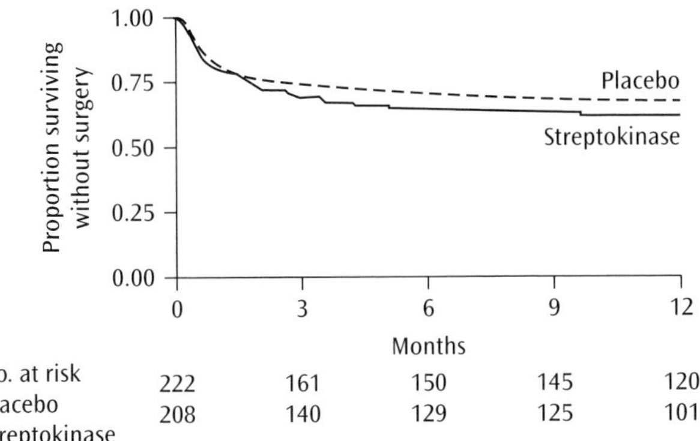

Figure 26.13 Primary result of the MIST1 study, showing no difference between placebo and streptokinase in outcome (death + surgical rate) at 12 months.[20]

A meta-analysis performed in 2006[189] and including the five methodologically sound trials (575 patients in total) concluded that the routine use of fibrinolytic therapy for all patients was not supported by the current evidence, although it suggested that some patients may benefit from treatment given the trial heterogeneity.[189]

Does the MIST1 trial therefore end 50 years of clinical investigation into intrapleural thrombolytics? There is direct evidence that fibrinous septations are divided by intrapleural streptokinase in malignant pleural effusion.[190] There are reasons to believe that fibrinolytic agents other than streptokinase may be more efficacious in breaking down adhesions and loculations intrapleurally. The mode of action of streptokinase relies upon a minimum level of plasminogen in order to produce fibrinolytic plasmin, and there is evidence that the intrapleural concentration of plasminogen is low. Agents such as direct plasminogen activators are not limited by the endogenous plasminogen level and therefore may be more successful in dividing septations within an infected pleural space. There are several case reports and series in both adults[191,192] and children[193–198] reporting success using intrapleural tPA, with an apparently good safety profile. Clearly, further randomized studies are needed to elucidate the role of this agent in pleural infection, and a UK based randomized trial using tPA in the treatment of pleural infection is currently under way.

OTHER FIBRINOLYTICS STUDIES

Whether one fibrinolytic agent is better than another was addressed by Bouros *et al.*[77] who compared streptokinase and urokinase. This study was effectively a pilot of only 50 patients and allows a power calculation of the size of study that would be needed to establish whether there is a difference between the two drugs. In this study both agents failed in 8 percent of subjects. If it is assumed that the failure rates do differ and are 8 percent versus 12 percent, a randomized study of 3000 subjects would be needed to assess whether there is a difference at the 5 percent level with 95 percent power.

Intrapleural DNAse

Another potentially therapeutic intrapleural agent in pleural infection is DNAse. The capacity of DNAse to reduce pus viscosity is well recognized. This is central to its nebulized use in cystic fibrosis to reduce sputum viscosity.[199] This effect has been studied on pus samples gathered from pleural empyemas. In the first of these studies, 20 samples of purulent pleural exudate were collected from experimental empyemas in rabbits.[200] These samples were then incubated *in vitro* with streptokinase, urokinase, combination streptokinase and streptodornase (streptodornase is streptococcal DNAse) or saline. Liquefaction of the exudates was only achieved with the combination streptokinase and streptodornase.[200] The second study involved nine specimens of pus collected from patients with either pleural empyema or abscess elsewhere.[201] These specimens were also incubated with saline, combination streptokinase and streptodornase, human recombinant DNAse or combination human recombinant DNAse and streptokinase. Each of the DNAse-containing incubations again effectively reduced the pus viscosity by over 95 percent with little change seen in the other groups.[201]

Nutrition

Adequate nutrition was identified as a key aim of therapy, and an important determinant of outcome in pleural infection during the First World War. Unfortunately, it is still sometimes overlooked, while complex modern therapies with adjunctive intrapleural agents and/or early minimally invasive surgery receive much attention. Empyema patients characteristically suffer the protracted catabolic consequences of chronic infection, including immunodeficiency and slow recovery. In one series of 80 patients with infected pleural fluid, a low blood albumin level was the most important determinant of a fatal outcome.[202] It is therefore essential to provide adequate nutritional support from the time of diagnosis. This may require nasogastric or occasionally intravenous feeding.

Bronchoscopy

A small number of empyema patients have a proximal obstructing lesion as the cause of their empyema. In a UK series of 119 cases, 40 percent underwent bronchoscopy and bronchial disease was identified in only five (<4 percent of the total sample).[19] Bronchoscopy is therefore not routinely appropriate in these patients.[6] However, failure of the empyema to resolve or clinical or radiographic features of bronchial obstruction should indicate either thoracic computed tomography or bronchoscopy to identify any bronchial pathology.

Surgery for pleural infection

Medical therapy will fail in up to 30 percent of patients with empyema,[20,118] and these patients are referred for surgical options. There is currently no definitive data that helps define the point at which a patient with empyema should proceed to surgical intervention. Previous observational studies have suggested that the presence of purulent fluid or loculations increase the chances of surgical intervention,[21] whereas other studies have not found these parameters to be predictive.[20,152] Many such patients will recover fully without surgical interventions and surgical options are associated with significant morbidity. It is likely that patients with late fibropurulent or organizing empyema will require a surgical procedure to establish complete drainage and adequate lung re-expansion, and a proportion of these patients may require additional surgery.[203]

Management guidelines suggest that surgical referral should be made after 7 days of failed medical therapy.[6] There are currently a number of surgical options available to achieve these goals and include;

1. VATS;
2. mini-thoracotomy;
3. open thoracotomy with decortications;
4. rib resection with open drainage.

Formal thoracotomy with decortication is a major procedure, and the techniques involved have changed little over the past 50 years.[204] This procedure involves removal of all fibrous tissue and blood clot from the visceral pleura and evacuation of all the pus and fibrous tissue from the pleural cavity. This eliminates sepsis and allows the lung to re-expand. The outcome from thoracotomy and decortication is excellent, with reported success rates of 95 percent[118] in these highly selected patients, although its morbidity is substantial. Thoracotomy in general is associated with significant morbidity;[99] one study reported that over 80 percent will have post-thoracotomy pain at 3 months, decreasing only slightly to 61 percent at 1 year, and between 3 and 5 percent of patients experience severe pain.[146] Around two-thirds of patients require treatment for pain up to 6 months after thoracotomy.[145] A longer follow-up study reported 55 percent of patients experiencing chronic pain over 1 year after surgery, with 45 percent experiencing pain at 2 years, 38 percent at 3 years and 30 percent over 4 years after surgery.[144] While the reported pain intensity was low, 23 percent of patients felt it interfered with their lives, and 9 percent required daily analgesia or intervention (anaesthetic block or referral to pain clinic).[144]

The increasingly popular mini-thoracotomy is similar to a formal thoracotomy and decortication but involves a much smaller incision. This is possible as the operation is assisted by the use of a camera that allows the surgeon to work with open instruments through the small incision.

The introduction of VATS in the late 1980s offered a less traumatic alternative to thoracotomy and its use in the treatment of pleural infection has become widespread.[66,205–210] Its exact niche is still under evaluation, but recent studies suggest that VATS is effective and is a less invasive strategy than thoracotomy and decortication in certain patient cohorts. Published retrospective series on VATS management of empyema are generally favorable, with reduced hospital inpatient time, postoperative complications and length of operating time.[18,76,99,113,207–214] Conversion rates to formal thoracotomy are highly variable in previous studies, ranging from 8 to 59 percent.[18,99,113,211–215] Most VATS failures are with empyema in the organizing stage of the disease, and non-blinded studies have cited certain bacteriological patterns and delayed referral (more than around 25 days), as predictive of VATS failure.[18,214]

There are now two randomized prospective trials comparing VATS treatment to intercostal drainage in association with fibrinolytics in adults[71,76] (Table 26.8). Wait *et al.*[71] randomized 20 patients to chest tube drainage with intrapleural streptokinase or VATS. Twenty patients were randomized, nine to chest tube with fibrinolytics and 11 to VATS surgery. Five of the nine controls failed to resolve with medical therapy compared with only one of the patients randomized to VATS.[71] However, the positive result in this trial is actually attributable to the very high control failure rate of 53 percent[71] (compared with approximately 20 percent in most other studies), and the primary outcome (clinical response at 3 days post randomization) was assessed in an unblinded manner, which renders the result liable to substantial observer bias. A Cochrane review conducted in 2005 evaluating surgical versus non-surgical treatment of empyema[71] was only able to include this study (as the only randomized study at the time) and concluded that the study was both underpowered and methodologically flawed, suggesting that further evidence was required.[71]

There has since been a larger randomized prospective trial comparing VATS to tube drainage in 70 adult subjects.[76] A significantly lower proportion of patients undergoing VATS as primary therapy required subsequent thoracotomy and decortication (17 percent versus 37 percent, $p < 0.05$),[76] and VATS was associated with a shorter hospital stay. However, the decision to proceed to thoracotomy was not made blind to initial treatment allocation, and details of the tube only group (size of tube, use of flushes, suction and thrombolytics) are not described.

A VATS procedure is well tolerated with a low complication rate in studies assessing complications for all indications including pleural infection.[216] The postsurgical morbidity rate is very much lower than for thoracotomy in a retrospective case series[217] (96 percent of patients symptom free at 2 years), although there are no direct comparative studies. Therefore, the early indications are that VATs may be a valuable tool in the management of empyema, but larger and more robust studies are needed to demonstrate this.

There are a number of retrospective, non-randomized studies suggesting benefit from early VATS in pediatric empyema, in terms of length of hospital stay, tube dwell time and analgesic use.[74,110,198,218,219] A study aggregating the previous retrospective evidence on VATS in children suggested an overall lower in hospital mortality rate from primary operative management compared with primary tube drainage,[220] but the pooled papers reviewed were highly likely to suffer from selection bias being non-randomized. There are two randomized studies assessing the use of VATS in pediatric empyema,[92,108] with conflicting results (Table 26.8). Kurt *et al.*[92] compared primary VATS with primary tube drainage in 18 patients, with thrombolytic therapy permitted in both limbs after initial intervention. They found a decreased length of hospital stay, decreased tube dwell time and decreased analgesic use in the VATS group.[92] However, in a larger study, Sonnappa *et al.*[108] randomized 60 children to VATS or chest tube + urokinase. No difference in terms of hospital stay, failure rate or radiological outcome at 6 months was seen between the groups, with VATS being substantially more expensive ($11 000 versus $9000).[108] Therefore, further investigation is required to fully elucidate the role of VATS in paediatric empyema, although the largest randomized study to date has shown no benefit (and a cost harm) for VATs.

Medical thoracoscopy (thoracoscopy performed under local anesthetic and sedation usually by a physician) is very commonly used in the investigation and management of patients with malignant pleural disease, and there is now increased interest in its use for infected pleural effusion. A retrospective series of 127 patients was recently published,[79] in which medical thoracoscopy was used as primary therapy for cases of multiloculated pleural infection identified at thoracic ultrasound. This included cases of failed chest tube drainage. 'Successful' treatment was achieved using medical thoracoscopy as primary therapy in 91 percent of cases, with a 6 percent thoracotomy conversion rate.[79] Further studies are needed to elucidate the role of medical thoracoscopy in the treatment of pleural infection.

Unfortunately, there are no radiological techniques that reliably predict which group of empyema patients requiring surgical intervention may be amenable to VATS, although authors have suggested that delayed referral and certain bacteriological patterns are associated with worse outcomes from VATs.

Open drainage by rib resection has the advantage that it can be performed under local or general anesthesia. It is not as major a procedure as decortication and therefore often more appropriate for patients at high operative risk.[204] In this procedure, segments of one to three ribs overlying the lower part of the empyema are resected and a large-bore tube inserted. This can be connected to a colostomy bag to enable the patient to leave hospital. One disadvantage of this technique is the length of time needed to achieve complete healing (median time 6 months).[204] A modified version of the rib resection 'open window thoracostomy' can also be used. This was devised by Eloesser[221] and involves the formation of a skin-lined track connecting the empyema cavity.

Treatment options in patients with persisting sepsis who are not fit enough for a general anesthesia

The frail patient who is a poor risk for general anesthesia or who declines surgical intervention despite failure of their empyema to resolve with standard drainage and antibiotics, presents a particular clinical challenge. There

Table 26.8 Randomized trials of surgery for pleural infection

Author	Interventions	Number of patients	Doses	Trial methodology	Results
Wait *et al.*[71]	SK versus VATS	20 9 SK versus 11 VATS	250 000 IU SK daily for 3 days	Randomized Assessor unblinded High rate of medical therapy failure	Reduced hospital stay in VATS group 5/9 required VATS in SK group All surgery in SK group managed with VATS
Bilgin *et al.*[76]	VATS versus intercostal drain	70	n/a 35 VATS versus 35 intercostal drain	Randomized Assessor unblinded	Lower need for decortication in VATS group (17% versus 37%, $p < 0.05$). Shorter hospital stay with VATS ($p < 0.05$). One death in drain group only.
Sonnappa *et al.*[108]	(Pediatric) VATS versus drain + UK	60 children (30 drain + UK) versus (24 VATS, 4 VATS + mini-thoracotomy, 1 repeat VATS)	40 000u or 10 000 IU UK bd for 3 days (according to child age)	Randomized Assessor unblinded	No difference in length of hospital stay, failure rate or radiological outcome at 6 months. Lower cost in UK group ($p < 0.001$)
Kurt *et al.*[92]	(Paediatric) VATS versus intercostal drain (fibrinolytic permissible after in both groups)	18 children 10 VATS versus 8 intercostal drain	Reteplase 0.02 IU/kg up to 4 times/day for up to 5 days	Randomized Assessor unblinded	Shorter length of stay, less analgesic use, fewer radiographs and fewer subsequent intervenions required in VATS group None of VATS group required fibrinolytic

SK, streptokinase; VATS, video-assisted thoracoscopic surgery.

are several options available in this situation. It is advisable to re-image the thorax (often with CT) to evaluate the position and size of any residual pleural collections. Placement of additional image-guided drains is then possible. This is particularly useful if individual loculations are present which do not appear to be communicating with the previously drained main cavity. Changing the bore of catheter from small to large (or vice versa) is reasonable, given that it is not clear if one or the other is clinically superior in this situation, where other options are not available. In addition to these measures, careful review of the microbiology is required with a consideration of a change of antimicrobials in culture-negative cases. The pleural collection can often be drained by rib resection under local anaesthesia. This procedure allows the surgeon to ensure that all intrapleural loculations are broken down by mechanical means, and that a drain is inserted under direct vision aiding dependent drainage.[11] More recently, long-term indwelling pleural catheters have been used for the treatment of recurrent malignant pleural effusion,[222] and may have a role in the treatment of pleural infection where surgical options are not possible, although there are no current data.

Empyema in patients with human immunodeficiency virus (HIV) infection

As in all other respiratory infections, the clinical features of empyema in subjects with HIV infection differ from those in the immunocompetent host. Patients with HIV infection are at risk of empyema caused both by the usual pathogens and a range of opportunistic organisms. The clinical presentation is similar to that in HIV-negative subjects, with fever, cough, chest pain, shortness of breath and weight loss occurring frequently.[223] In a USA study of 599 HIV-positive individuals requiring at least one period of inpatient care over a 3-year period, three-quarters of infectious effusions were due to common pneumonia pathogens, 15 percent were due to tuberculosis and 7 percent to *Pneumocyctis carinii*.[224] In areas with a high prevalence of tuberculosis (such as Africa), tuberculosis can account for about half of all empyemas. In this setting, the mortality can be as high as 33 percent.[22] Other opportunistic infections reported to cause pleural infection in HIV-positive subjects empyema include *Salmonella paratyphi, Listeria* spp, *Cryptococcus neoformans, Corynebacterium parvum* and *Rhodococcus equi*.[223,225–229] A recent study assessed patients with HIV treated surgically for pleural infection.[230] Twenty-five percent of patients in this study presented with empyema as the first manifestation of HIV/acquired immune deficiency syndrome (AIDS). The microbiology associated was broadly similar to that in immunocompetent individuals, with a predominance of Gram positives, but organisms such as fungi (*Candida*), tuberculosis and *P. carinii* were more commonly seen.[230]

FUTURE DIRECTIONS

There is increasing interest in molecular techniques for the diagnosis of pleural infection (e.g. bacterial DNA amplification), and further work is needed to assess this technique.

Although the current evidence suggests that intrapleural fibrinolytic therapy is not associated with a change in long-term outcome, there is interest in newer fibrinolytic agents (for example, direct plasminogen activators) either alone or in conjunction with DNase. A multi-centre randomized trial is currently under way in the UK assessing these two agents.

The provision of VATs has transformed thoracic surgery, but its exact role in empyema therapy has not been the subject of a adequately powered randomized trial, compared with more traditional methods of surgery or medical management. There are early indications that medical thoracoscopy may be useful as an early treatment, but further evaluation is required.

KEY POINTS

- All patients with a pleural effusion in association with sepsis or rate pneumonic illness require a diagnostic pleural fluid aspiration.
- Pleural fluid pH should be assessed in all non-purulent possibly infected effusions and a pH of less than 7.2 indicates that formal drainage is required.
- A high index of suspicion for pleural infection is needed in patients with known risk factors (e.g. diabetes, alcohol abuse)
- The bacteriology of empyema is substantially different from that of pneumonia, and different antibiotic regimens are required
- The bacteriology of hospital-acquired empyema is substantially different from community-acquired empyema and these conditions require quite different empirical antibiotic regimens from presentation
- Adequate nutrition is an important determinant of outcome and therefore needs to be addressed at the time of diagnosis.
- There remains no definitive predictors of outcome in patients with pleural infection. All cases should therefore require rapid diagnosis and prompt treatment.
- Routine use of intrapleural fibrinolytics therapy to alter clinically meaningful outcomes is not supported by the current randomized evidence.
- Patients not fit for general anaesthesia with persistent pleural sepsis require further imaging and possible additional tube placement. Medical and surgical options not requiring general anaesthesia should be considered.

REFERENCES

● = Key primary paper
◆ = Major review article

1. Berger HA, Morganroth ML. Immediate drainage is not required for all patients with complicated parapneumonic effusions. *Chest* 1990; **97**: 731–5.
2. Bergh NP, Ekroth R, Larsson S, Nagy P. Intrapleural streptokinase in the treatment of haemothorax and empyema. *Scand J Thorac Cardiovasc Surg* 1977; **11**: 265–68.
●3. Bouros D, Schiza S, Tzanakis N, Drositis J, Siafakas N. Intrapleural urokinase in the treatment of complicated parapneumonic pleural effusions and empyema. *Eur Respir J* 1996; **9**: 1656–9.
4. Chen KY, Hsueh PR, Liaw YS, Yang PC, Luh KT. A 10-year experience with bacteriology of acute thoracic empyema: emphasis on *Klebsiella pneumoniae* in patients with diabetes mellitus. *Chest* 2000; **117**: 1685–9.
◆5. Colice GL, Curtis A, Deslauriers J, *et al.* Medical and surgical treatment of parapneumonic effusions: an evidence-based guideline. *Chest* 2000; **118**: 1158–71.
◆6. Davies CW, Gleeson FV, Davies RJ. BTS guidelines for the management of pleural infection. *Thorax* 2003; **58** (Suppl 2): ii18–28.
7. Davies RJ, Gleeson FV. The diagnosis and management of pleural empyema. *Curr Opin Infect Dis* 1998; **11**: 163–8.
8. de Souza A, Offner PJ, Moore EE, *et al.* Optimal management of complicated empyema. *Am J Surg* 2000; **180**: 507–11.
9. Heffner JE. Infection of the pleural space. *Clin Chest Med* 1999; **20**: 607–22.
10. Henke CA, Leatherman JW. Intrapleurally administered streptokinase in the treatment of acute loculated nonpurulent parapneumonic effusions. *Am Rev Respir Dis* 1992; **145**: 680–4.
11. Kaplan DK. Treatment of empyema thoracis. *Thorax* 1994; **49**: 845–6.
12. Mattison LE, Coppage L, Alderman DF, Herlong JO, Sahn SA. Pleural effusions in the medical ICU: prevalence, causes, and clinical implications. *Chest* 1997; **111**: 1018–23.
13. Moulton JS, Benkert RE, Weisiger KH, Chambers JA. Treatment of complicated pleural fluid collections with image-guided drainage and intracavitary urokinase. *Chest* 1995; **108**: 1252–9.
14. Ogirala RG, Williams MH Jr. Streptokinase in a loculated pleural effusion. Effectiveness determined by site of instillation. *Chest* 1988; **94**: 884–6.
15. Ryan JM, Boland GW, Lee MJ, Mueller PR. Intracavitary urokinase therapy as an adjunct to percutaneous drainage in a patient with a multiloculated empyema. *AJR Am J Roentgenol* 1996; **167**: 643–7.
16. Taylor RF, Rubens MB, Pearson MC, Barnes NC. Intrapleural streptokinase in the management of empyema. *Thorax* 1994; **49**: 856–9.
17. Willsie-Ediger SK, Salzman G, Reisz G, Foreman MG. Use of intrapleural streptokinase in the treatment of thoracic empyema. *Am J Med Sci* 1990; **300**: 296–300.
18. Waller DA, Rengarajan A, Nicholson FH, Rajesh PB. Delayed referral reduces the success of video-assisted thoracoscopic debridement for post-pneumonic empyema. *Respir Med* 2001; **95**: 836–40.
●19. Ferguson AD, Prescott RJ, Selkon JB, Watson D, Swinburn CR. The clinical course and management of thoracic empyema. *QJM* 1996; **89**: 285–9.
●20. Maskell NA, Davies CW, Nunn AJ, *et al.* UK Controlled trial of intrapleural streptokinase for pleural infection. *N Engl J Med* 2005; **352**: 865–74.
●21. Davies CW, Kearney SE, Gleeson FV, Davies RJ. Predictors of outcome and long-term survival in patients with pleural infection. *Am J Respir Crit Care Med* 1999; **160**: 1682–7.
22. Desai G, Amadi W. Three years' experience of empyema thoracis in association with HIV infection. *Trop Doct* 2001; **31**: 106–7.
◆23. Sahn SA. Management of complicated parapneumonic effusions. *Am Rev Respir Dis* 1993; **148**: 813–17.
◆24. Light RW, Girard WM, Jenkinson SG, George RB. Parapneumonic effusions. *Am J Med* 1980; **69**: 507–12.
25. Breasted JH. *The Edwin Smith surgical papyrus.* Chicago: University of Chicago Press, 1980.
26. Birmingham A.L. Hippocrates, Aphorisms 44. In: Adams LB (ed.). *The genuine works of Hippocrates: the classics of surgery.* Delran: Gryphon Editions, 1985: 768–71.
27. Meyer JA. Gotthard Bulau and closed water-seal drainage for empyema, 1875–1891. *Ann Thorac Surg* 1989; **48**: 597–9.
28. Hewitt C. Drainage for empyema. *Br Med J* 1876; **1**: 317.
29. Warren P. *The surgical treatment of cardiac and pulmonary disease.* University of Manitoba Website http://www.umanitoba.ca/faculties/medicine/units/medical_humanities/history/notes/surgery. 2004, accessed 11-6-2007.
30. Tubiana R. History. In: Tubiana R, Leclercq C, Hurst LC, Badalamente M, Mackin E (eds). *Dupuytren's disease.* London: Martin Dunitz, 2000: 1–11.
31. Bryan CS. *Osler: Inspirations from a great physician.* New York: Oxford University Press, 2002.
32. Graham E.A. Open pnuemothorax: its relations to the treatment of empyema. *Am J Med Sci* 1918; **156**: 839–71.
33. Graham EA. Principles involved in the treatment of acute and chronic empyema. 1924. *J Am Coll Surg* 2005; **201**: 157.
34. Empyema commission. Cases of empyema at Camp Lee. *J Am Med Assoc* 1918; **71**: 366–73.
35. Stone WJ. The management of postpneumonic empyema based on 310 cases. *Am J Med Sci* 1919; **158**.
●36. Tillett WS, Sherry S. The effect in patients of streptococcal fibrinolysin (streptokinase) and streptococcal deoxyribonuclease on fibrinous, purulent and sanguinous pleural exudations. *J Clin Invest* 1949; **28**: 173–90.
37. Estlander JA. Sur le resection des cotes dans l'empyeme chronique. *Rev Mens* 1897; **8**: 885.
38. Schede M. Die Behandlung der Empyeme. *Verh Innere Med Weisbaden* 1890; **9**: 41.
39. Fowler GR. A case of thoracoplasty for the removal of a large cicatricial fibrous growth from the chest interior. *Med Rec* 1893; **44**: 938.
40. Beck C. Thoracoplasty in America and visceral pleurectomy with a report of a case. *J Am Med Assoc* 1897; **28**: 58.
41. Hornick P, Townsend ER, Clark D, Fountain SW. Videothoracoscopy in the treatment of early empyema: an initial experience. *Ann R Coll Surg Engl* 1996; **78**: 45–8.
42. Givan DC, Eigen H. Common pleural effusions in children. *Clin Chest Med* 1998; **19**: 363–71.
43. Maskell NA, Davies CW, Jones E, Davies RJ. The characteristics of 300 patients partcipating in the MRC/BTS multicentre intrapleural streptokinase vs. placebo trial (ISRCTN-39138989). *Am J Resp Crit Care Med* 2002; **165**: B11. American Thoracic Society Meeting, Atlanta.
◆44. Strange C, Sahn SA. The definitions and epidemiology of pleural space infection. *Semin Respir Infect* 1999; **14**: 3–8.
45. Lemmer JH, Botham MJ, Orringer MB. Modern management of adult thoracic empyema. *J Thorac Cardiovasc Surg* 1985; **90**: 849–55.
46. Jerng JS, Hsueh PR, Teng LJ, *et al.* Empyema thoracis and lung abscess caused by *viridans* streptococci. *Am J Respir Crit Care Med* 1997; **156**: 1508–14.
47. Smith JA, Mullerworth MH, Westlake GW, Tatoulis J. Empyema thoracis: 14-year experience in a teaching center. *Ann Thorac Surg* 1991; **51**: 39–42.
48. Snider GL, Saleh SS. Empyema of the thorax in adults: review of 105 cases. *Dis Chest* 1968; **54**: 410–15.

49. Yeh TJ, Hall DP, Ellison RG. Empyema thoracis: A review of 110 cases. *Am Rev Respir Dis* 1963; **88**: 785–90.

●50. Maskell NA, Batt S, Hedley EL, *et al.* The bacteriology of pleural infection by genetic and standard methods and its mortality significance. *Am J Respir Crit Care Med* 2006; **174**: 817–23.

◆51. Alfageme I, Munoz F, Pena N, Umbria S. Empyema of the thorax in adults. Etiology, microbiologic findings, and management. *Chest* 1993; **103**: 839–43.

●52. Sahn SA, Taryle DA, Good JT Jr. Experimental empyema. Time course and pathogenesis of pleural fluid acidosis and low pleural fluid glucose. *Am Rev Respir Dis* 1979; **120**: 355–61.

53. Mavroudis C, Ganzel BL, Katzmark S, Polk HC Jr. Effect of hemothorax on experimental empyema thoracis in the guinea pig. *J Thorac Cardiovasc Surg* 1985; **89**: 42–9.

●54. Sasse SA, Jadus MR, Kukes GD. Pleural fluid transforming growth factor-beta1 correlates with pleural fibrosis in experimental empyema. *Am J Respir Crit Care Med* 2003; **168**: 700–5.

●55. Kunz CR, Jadus MR, Kukes GD, *et al.* Intrapleural injection of transforming growth factor-beta antibody inhibits pleural fibrosis in empyema. *Chest* 2004; **126**: 1636–44.

◆56. Kroegel C, Antony VB. Immunobiology of pleural inflammation: potential implications for pathogenesis, diagnosis and therapy. *Eur Respir J* 1997; **10**: 2411–18.

●57. Broaddus VC, Boylan AM, Hoeffel JM, *et al.* Neutralization of IL-8 inhibits neutrophil influx in a rabbit model of endotoxin-induced pleurisy. *J Immunol* 1994; **152**: 2960–7.

●58. Broaddus VC, Hebert CA, Vitangcol RV, *et al.* Interleukin-8 is a major neutrophil chemotactic factor in pleural liquid of patients with empyema. *Am Rev Respir Dis* 1992; **146**: 825–30.

59. Idell S, Girard W, Koenig KB, McLarty J, Fair DS. Abnormalities of pathways of fibrin turnover in the human pleural space. *Am Rev Respir Dis* 1991; **144**: 187–94.

60. Aleman C, Alegre J, Monasterio J, *et al.* Association between inflammatory mediators and the fibrinolysis system in infectious pleural effusions. *Clin Sci (Lond)* 2003; **105**: 601–7.

●61. Sahn SA, Reller LB, Taryle DA, Antony VB, Good JT Jr. The contribution of leukocytes and bacteria to the low pH of empyema fluid. *Am Rev Respir Dis* 1983; **128**: 811–15.

●62. Light RW, MacGregor MI, Ball WC Jr, Luchsinger PC. Diagnostic significance of pleural fluid pH and PCO_2. *Chest* 1973; **64**: 591–6.

◆63. Miserocchi G. Physiology and pathophysiology of pleural fluid turnover. *Eur Respir J* 1997; **10**: 219–25.

64. Mutsaers SE, Kalomenidis I, Wilson NA, Lee YC. Growth factors in pleural fibrosis. *Curr Opin Pulm Med* 2006; **12**: 251–8.

◆65. Hamm H, Light RW. Parapneumonic effusion and empyema. *Eur Respir J* 1997; **10**: 1150–6.

66. Landreneau RJ, Keenan RJ, Hazelrigg SR, Mack MJ, Naunheim KS. Thoracoscopy for empyema and hemothorax. *Chest* 1996; **109**: 18–24.

67. Neff CC, vanSonnenberg E, Lawson DW, Patton AS. CT follow-up of empyemas: pleural peels resolve after percutaneous catheter drainage. *Radiology* 1990; **176**: 195–7.

68. Light RW. *Pleural diseases*, 3rd edn. Baltimore: Williams and Wilkins, 1995.

69. Rahman NM, Batt S, Gleeson FV, *et al.* The relationship between lung parenchymal CT appearances and pleural bacteriology in pleural infection [abstract]. *Am J Respir Crit Care Med* 2006; **173**: A11.

70. Ahmed RA, Marrie TJ, Huang JQ. Thoracic empyema in patients with community-acquired pneumonia. *Am J Med* 2006; **119**: 877–83.

●71. Wait MA, Sharma S, Hohn J, Dal Nogare A. A randomized trial of empyema therapy. *Chest* 1997; **111**: 1548–51.

72. Alfaro C, Fergie J, Purcell K. Emergence of community-acquired methicillin-resistant *Staphylococcus aureus* in complicated parapneumonic effusions. *Pediatr Infect Dis J* 2005; **24**: 274–6.

73. Azoulay E, Fartoukh M, Galliot R, *et al.* Rapid diagnosis of infectious pleural effusions by use of reagent strips. *Clin Infect Dis* 2000; **31**: 914–19.

74. Bailey KA, Bass J, Rubin S, Barrowman N. Empyema management: twelve years' experience since the introduction of video-assisted thoracoscopic surgery. *J Laparoendosc Adv Surg Tech A* 2005; **15**: 338–41.

◆75. Barnes NP, Hull J, Thomson AH. Medical management of parapneumonic pleural disease. *Pediatr Pulmonol* 2005; **39**: 127–34.

●76. Bilgin M, Akcali Y, Oguzkaya F. Benefits of early aggressive management of empyema thoracis. *ANZ J Surg* 2006; **76**: 120–2.

●77. Bouros D, Schiza S, Patsourakis G, *et al.* Intrapleural streptokinase versus urokinase in the treatment of complicated parapneumonic effusions: a prospective, double-blind study. *Am J Respir Crit Care Med* 1997; **155**: 291–5.

●78. Bouros D, Schiza S, Tzanakis N, *et al.* Intrapleural urokinase versus normal saline in the treatment of complicated parapneumonic effusions and empyema. A randomized, double-blind study. *Am J Respir Crit Care Med* 1999; **159**: 37–42.

79. Brutsche MH, Tassi GF, Gyorik S, *et al.* Treatment of sonographically stratified multiloculated thoracic empyema by medical thoracoscopy. *Chest* 2005; **128**: 3303–9.

80. Buckingham SC, King MD, Miller ML. Incidence and etiologies of complicated parapneumonic effusions in children, 1996 to 2001. *Pediatr Infect Dis J* 2003; **22**: 499–504.

81. Castellote J, Lopez C, Gornals J, Domingo A, Xiol X. Use of reagent strips for the rapid diagnosis of spontaneous bacterial empyema. *J Clin Gastroenterol* 2005; **39**: 278–81.

82. Chen LE, Langer JC, Dillon PA, *et al.* Management of late-stage parapneumonic empyema. *J Pediatr Surg* 2002; **37**: 371–4.

●83. Chin NK, Lim TK. Controlled trial of intrapleural streptokinase in the treatment of pleural empyema and complicated parapneumonic effusions. *Chest* 1997; **111**: 275–9.

84. Chu MW, Dewar LR, Burgess JJ, Busse EG. Empyema thoracis: lack of awareness results in a prolonged clinical course. *Can J Surg* 2001; **44**: 284–8.

●85. Davies RJ, Traill ZC, Gleeson FV. Randomised controlled trial of intrapleural streptokinase in community acquired pleural infection. *Thorax* 1997; **52**: 416–21.

●86. Diacon AH, Theron J, Schuurmans MM, Van de Wal BW, Bolliger CT. Intrapleural streptokinase for empyema and complicated parapneumonic effusions. *Am J Respir Crit Care Med* 2004; **170**: 49–53.

87. Dzielicki J, Korlacki W. The role of thoracoscopy in the treatment of pleural empyema in children. *Surg Endosc* 2006; **20**: 1402–5.

88. Freitas M, Castelo A, Petty G, Gomes CE, Carvalho E. *Viridans* streptococci causing community acquired pneumonia. *Arch Dis Child* 2006; **91**: 779–80.

89. Jerjes-Sanchez C, Ramirez-Rivera A, Elizalde JJ, *et al.* Intrapleural fibrinolysis with streptokinase as an adjunctive treatment in hemothorax and empyema: a multicenter trial. *Chest* 1996; **109**: 1514–19.

90. Kalfa N, Allal H, Lopez M, *et al.* Thoracoscopy in pediatric pleural empyema: a prospective study of prognostic factors. *J Pediatr Surg* 2006; **41**: 1732–7.

91. Kuboi S, Nomura H. Clinical background of cases showing a positive culture of pleural effusion at Shin-Kokura Hospital over a period of 5 years. *J Infect Chemother* 2006; **12**: 264–8.

●92. Kurt BA, Winterhalter KM, Connors RH, Betz BW, Winters JW. Therapy of parapneumonic effusions in children: video-assisted thoracoscopic surgery versus conventional thoracostomy drainage. *Pediatrics* 2006; **118**: e547–53.

93. Lahti E, Mertsola J, Kontiokari T, *et al.* Pneumolysin polymerase chain reaction for diagnosis of pneumococcal pneumonia and empyema in children. *Eur J Clin Microbiol Infect Dis* 2006; **25**: 783–9.

94. Le Monnier A, Carbonnelle E, Zahar JR, *et al.* Microbiological diagnosis of empyema in children: comparative evaluations by

culture, polymerase chain reaction, and pneumococcal antigen detection in pleural fluids. *Clin Infect Dis* 2006; **42**: 1135–40.
95. Lim TK, Chin NK. Empirical treatment with fibrinolysis and early surgery reduces the duration of hospitalization in pleural sepsis. *Eur Respir J* 1999; **13**: 514–18.
96. Lindstrom ST, Kolbe J. Community acquired parapneumonic thoracic empyema: predictors of outcome. *Respirology* 1999; **4**: 173–9.
97. Manuel PJ, Vives M, Esquerda A, Ruiz A. Usefulness of the British Thoracic Society and the American College of Chest Physicians guidelines in predicting pleural drainage of non-purulent parapneumonic effusions. *Respir Med* 2006; **100**: 933–7.
98. Margenthaler JA, Weber TR, Keller MS. Predictors of surgical outcome for complicated pneumonia in children: impact of bacterial virulence. *World J Surg* 2004; **28**: 87–91.
99. Melloni G, Carretta A, Ciriaco P, *et al.* Decortication for chronic parapneumonic empyema: results of a prospective study. *World J Surg* 2004; **28**: 488–93.
100. Menezes-Martins LF, Menezes-Martins JJ, Michaelsen VS, *et al.* Diagnosis of parapneumonic pleural effusion by polymerase chain reaction in children. *J Pediatr Surg* 2005; **40**: 1106–10.
●101. Misthos P, Sepsas E, Konstantinou M, *et al.* Early use of intrapleural fibrinolytics in the management of postpneumonic empyema. A prospective study. *Eur J Cardiothorac Surg* 2005; **28**: 599–603.
102. Mitri RK, Brown SD, Zurakowski D, *et al.* Outcomes of primary image-guided drainage of parapneumonic effusions in children. *Pediatrics* 2002; **110**: e37.
103. Ozel SK, Kazez A, Kilic M, *et al.* Conservative treatment of postpneumonic thoracic empyema in children. *Surg Today* 2004; **34**: 1002–5.
104. Paganini H, Guinazu JR, Hernandez C, *et al.* Comparative analysis of outcome and clinical features in children with pleural empyema caused by penicillin-nonsusceptible and penicillin-susceptible *Streptococcus pneumoniae*. *Int J Infect Dis* 2001; **5**: 86–8.
105. Saglani S, Harris KA, Wallis C, Hartley JC. Empyema: the use of broad range 16S rDNA PCR for pathogen detection. *Arch Dis Child* 2005; **90**: 70–3.
106. Satish B, Bunker M, Seddon P. Management of thoracic empyema in childhood: does the pleural thickening matter? *Arch Dis Child* 2003; **88**: 918–21.
●107. Singh M, Mathew JL, Chandra S, Katariya S, Kumar L. Randomized controlled trial of intrapleural streptokinase in empyema thoracis in children. *Acta Paediatr* 2004; **93**: 1443–5.
●108. Sonnappa S, Cohen G, Owens CM, *et al.* Comparison of urokinase and video-assisted thoracoscopic surgery for treatment of childhood empyema. *Am J Respir Crit Care Med* 2006; **174**: 221–7.
109. Soriano T, Alegre J, Aleman C, *et al.* Factors influencing length of hospital stay in patients with bacterial pleural effusion. *Respiration* 2005; **72**: 587–93.
110. Subramaniam R, Joseph VT, Tan GM, Goh A, Chay OM. Experience with video-assisted thoracoscopic surgery in the management of complicated pneumonia in children. *J Pediatr Surg* 2001; **36**: 316–19.
●111. Talib SH, Verma GR, Arshad M, Tayade BO, Rafeeque A. Utility of intrapleural streptokinase in management of chronic empyemas. *J Assoc Physicians India* 2003; **51**: 464–8.
112. Tsai TH, Jerng JS, Chen KY, Yu CJ, Yang PC. Community-acquired thoracic empyema in older people. *J Am Geriatr Soc* 2005; **53**: 1203–9.
113. Wurnig PN, Wittmer V, Pridun NS, Hollaus PH. Video-assisted thoracic surgery for pleural empyema. *Ann Thorac Surg* 2006; **81**: 309–13.
114. Yao CT, Wu JM, Liu CC, *et al.* Treatment of complicated parapneumonic pleural effusion with intrapleural streptokinase in children. *Chest* 2004; **125**: 566–71.
115. Ozol D, Oktem S, Erdinc E. Complicated parapneumonic effusion and empyema thoracis: microbiologic and therapeutic aspects. *Respir Med* 2006; **100**: 286–91.
●116. Thomson AH, Hull J, Kumar MR, Wallis C, Balfour LI. Randomised trial of intrapleural urokinase in the treatment of childhood empyema. *Thorax* 2002; **57**: 343–7.
117. Estrera AS, Platt MR, Mills LJ, Shaw RR. Primary lung abscess. *J Thorac Cardiovasc Surg* 1980; **79**: 275–82.
118. LeMense GP, Strange C, Sahn SA. Empyema thoracis. Therapeutic management and outcome. *Chest* 1995; **107**: 1532–7.
119. Runyon BA, Antillon MR, Akriviadis EA, McHutchison JG. Bedside inoculation of blood culture bottles with ascitic fluid is superior to delayed inoculation in the detection of spontaneous bacterial peritonitis. *J Clin Microbiol* 1990; **28**: 2811–12.
120. Ferrer A, Osset J, Alegre J, *et al.* Prospective clinical and microbiological study of pleural effusions. *Eur J Clin Microbiol Infect Dis* 1999; **18**: 237–41.
121. Andersen MN, McDonald KE. Prognostic factors and results of treatment in pyogenic pulmonary abscess. *J Thorac Cardiovasc Surg* 1960; **39**: 573– 8.
122. Hagan JL, Hardy JD. Lung abscess revisited. A survey of 184 cases. *Ann Surg* 1983; **197**: 755–62.
123. Torres A, Serra-Batlles J, Ferrer A, *et al.* Severe community-acquired pneumonia. Epidemiology and prognostic factors. *Am Rev Respir Dis* 1991; **144**: 312–18.
124. Ko SC, Chen KY, Hsueh PR, Luh KT, Yang PC. Fungal empyema thoracis: an emerging clinical entity. *Chest* 2000; **117**: 1672–8.
125. Eibenberger KL, Dock WI, Ammann ME, *et al.* Quantification of pleural effusions: sonography versus radiography. *Radiology* 1994; **191**: 681–4.
126. Jones PW, Moyers JP, Rogers JT, *et al.* Ultrasound-guided thoracentesis: is it a safer method? *Chest* 2003; **123**: 418–23.
127. O'Moore PV, Mueller PR, Simeone JF, *et al.* Sonographic guidance in diagnostic and therapeutic interventions in the pleural space. *AJR Am J Roentgenol* 1987; **149**: 1–5.
128. Stavas J, vanSonnenberg E, Casola G, Wittich GR. Percutaneous drainage of infected and noninfected thoracic fluid collections. *J Thorac Imaging* 1987; **2**: 80–7.
129. Potts DE, Taryle DA, Sahn SA. The glucose-pH relationship in parapneumonic effusions. *Arch Intern Med* 1978; **138**: 1378–80.
●130. Heffner JE, Brown LK, Barbieri C, DeLeo JM. Pleural fluid chemical analysis in parapneumonic effusions. A meta-analysis. *Am J Respir Crit Care Med* 1995; **151**: 1700–8.
131. Lesho EP, Roth BJ. Is pH paper an acceptable, low-cost alternative to the blood gas analyzer for determining pleural fluid pH? *Chest* 1997; **112**: 1291– 2.
132. Maskell NA, Gleeson FV, Darby M, Davies RJ. Diagnostically significant variations in pleural fluid pH in loculated parapneumonic effusions. *Chest* 2004; **126**: 2022–4.
133. Joseph J, Sahn SA. Connective tissue diseases and the pleura. *Chest* 1993; **104**: 262–70.
134. Romano M, Catalano A, Nutini M, *et al.* 5-lipoxygenase regulates malignant mesothelial cell survival: involvement of vascular endothelial growth factor. *FASEB J* 2001; **15**: 2326–36.
135. Strizzi L, Vianale G, Catalano A, Muraro R, Mutti L, Procopio A. Basic fibroblast growth factor in mesothelioma pleural effusions: correlation with patient survival and angiogenesis. *Int J Oncol* 2001; **18**: 1093– 8.
136. Edwards JG, Cox G, Andi A, *et al.* Angiogenesis is an independent prognostic factor in malignant mesothelioma. *Br J Cancer* 2001; **85**: 863–8.
137. Aelony Y, Yao JF, King RR. Prognostic value of pleural fluid pH in malignant epithelial mesothelioma after talc poudrage. *Respiration* 2006; **73**: 334–9.
138. Heffner JE, Heffner JN, Brown LK. Multilevel and continuous pleural fluid pH likelihood ratios for evaluating malignant pleural effusions. *Chest* 2003; **123**: 1887–94.
139. Heffner JE, Nietert PJ, Barbieri C. Pleural fluid pH as a predictor of

survival for patients with malignant pleural effusions. *Chest* 2000; **117**: 79–86.

140. Martinez-Moragon E, Aparicio J, Sanchis J, *et al.* Malignant pleural effusion: prognostic factors for survival and response to chemical pleurodesis in a series of 120 cases. *Respiration* 1998; **65**: 108–13.

◆141. Light RW, Erozan YS, Ball WC Jr. Cells in pleural fluid. Their value in differential diagnosis. *Arch Intern Med* 1973; **132**: 854–60.

◆142. Light RW. Pleural effusion due to pulmonary emboli. *Curr Opin Pulm Med* 2001; **7**: 198–201.

143. Light RW. Pleural effusions. *Med Clin North Am* 1977; **61**: 1339–52.

144. Dajczman E, Gordon A, Kreisman H, Wolkove N. Long-term postthoracotomy pain. *Chest* 1991; **99**: 270–4.

145. Kalso E, Perttunen K, Kaasinen S. Pain after thoracic surgery. *Acta Anaesthesiol Scand* 1992; **36**: 96–100.

146. Perttunen K, Tasmuth T, Kalso E. Chronic pain after thoracic surgery: a follow-up study. *Acta Anaesthesiol Scand* 1999; **43**: 563–7.

147. Cham CW, Haq SM, Rahamim J. Empyema thoracis: a problem with late referral? *Thorax* 1993; **48**: 925–7.

148. Ashbaugh DG. Empyema thoracis. Factors influencing morbidity and mortality. *Chest* 1991; **99**: 1162–5.

149. Huang HC, Chang HY, Chen CW, Lee CH, Hsiue TR. Predicting factors for outcome of tube thoracostomy in complicated parapneumonic effusion for empyema. *Chest* 1999; **115**: 751–6.

150. Armstrong P. *Imaging of diseases of the chest*, 3rd edn. London: Mosby; 2001.

151. Wu RG, Yuan A, Liaw YS, *et al.* Image comparison of real-time gray-scale ultrasound and color Doppler ultrasound for use in diagnosis of minimal pleural effusion. *Am J Respir Crit Care Med* 1994; **150**: 510–14.

◆152. Kearney SE, Davies CW, Davies RJ, Gleeson FV. Computed tomography and ultrasound in parapneumonic effusions and empyema. *Clin Radiol* 2000; **55**: 542–7.

153. Stark DD, Federle MP, Goodman PC, Podrasky AE, Webb WR. Differentiating lung abscess and empyema: radiography and computed tomography. *AJR Am J Roentgenol* 1983; **141**: 163–7.

154. Brenner DJ. Radiation risks potentially associated with low-dose CT screening of adult smokers for lung cancer. *Radiology* 2004; **231**: 440–5.

155. Beir V. National Reserach Council. Committee on the Biological Effects of Ionising Radiations. *Health effects of exposure to low levels of ionizing radiation.* Washington, DC: National Academy Press, 1990.

156. Davis SD, Henschke CI, Yankelevitz DF, Cahill PT, Yi Y. MR imaging of pleural effusions. *J Comput Assist Tomogr* 1990; **14**: 192–8.

◆157. Evans AL, Gleeson FV. Radiology in pleural disease: state of the art. *Respirology* 2004; **9**: 300–12.

158. Waite RJ, Carbonneau RJ, Balikian JP, *et al.* Parietal pleural changes in empyema: appearances at CT. *Radiology* 1990; **175**: 145–50.

159. Duysinx B, Nguyen D, Louis R, *et al.* Evaluation of pleural disease with 18-fluorodeoxyglucose positron emission tomography imaging. *Chest* 2004; **125**: 489–93.

160. Duysinx BC, Larock MP, Nguyen D, *et al.* 18F-FDG PET imaging in assessing exudative pleural effusions. *Nucl Med Commun* 2006; **27**: 971–6.

161. Taryle DA, Good JT Jr, Morgan EJ III, Reller LB, Sahn SA. Antibiotic concentrations in human parapneumonic effusions. *J Antimicrob Chemother* 1981; **7**: 171–7.

162. Hughes CE, Van Scoy RE. Antibiotic therapy of pleural empyema. *Semin Respir Infect* 1991; **6**: 94–102.

163. Niwa T, Nakamura A, Kato T, *et al.* Pharmacokinetic study of pleural fluid penetration of carbapenem antibiotic agents in chemical pleurisy. *Respir Med* 2006; **100**: 324–31.

164. Light RW. Management of parapneumonic effusions. *Arch Intern Med* 1981; **141**: 1339–41.

165. Miller KS, Sahn SA. Chest tubes. Indications, technique, management and complications. *Chest* 1987; **91**: 258–64.

166. Patz EF Jr, Goodman PC, Erasmus JJ. Percutaneous drainage of pleural collections. *J Thorac Imaging* 1998; **13**: 83–92.

167. Merriam MA, Cronan JJ, Dorfman GS, Lambiase RE, Haas RA. Radiographically guided percutaneous catheter drainage of pleural fluid collections. *AJR Am J Roentgenol* 1988; **151**: 1113–16.

168. Silverman SG, Mueller PR, Saini S, *et al.* Thoracic empyema: management with image-guided catheter drainage. *Radiology* 1988; **169**: 5–9.

169. Ulmer JL, Choplin RH, Reed JC. Image-guided catheter drainage of the infected pleural space. *J Thorac Imaging* 1991; **6**: 65–73.

170. vanSonnenberg E, Nakamoto SK, Mueller PR, *et al.* CT- and ultrasound-guided catheter drainage of empyemas after chest-tube failure. *Radiology* 1984; **151**: 349–53.

171. Crouch JD, Keagy BA, Delany DJ. 'Pigtail' catheter drainage in thoracic surgery. *Am Rev Respir Dis* 1987; **136**: 174–5.

172. Hunnam GR, Flower CD. Radiologically guided percutaneous catheter drainage of empyemas. *Clin Radiol* 1988; **39**: 121–6.

173. Klein JS, Schultz S, Heffner JE. Interventional radiology of the chest: image-guided percutaneous drainage of pleural effusions, lung abscess, and pneumothorax. *AJR Am J Roentgenol* 1995; **164**: 581–8.

174. Park JK, Kraus FC, Haaga JR. Fluid flow during percutaneous drainage procedures: an in vitro study of the effects of fluid viscosity, catheter size, and adjunctive urokinase. *AJR Am J Roentgenol* 1993; **160**: 165–9.

175. Gobien RP, Stanley JH, Schabel SI, *et al.* The effect of drainage tube size on adequacy of percutaneous abscess drainage. *Cardiovasc Intervent Radiol* 1985; **8**: 100–2.

176. Rothlin MA, Schob O, Klotz H, Candinas D, Largiader F. Percutaneous drainage of abdominal abscesses: are large-bore catheters necessary? *Eur J Surg* 1998; **164**: 419–24.

●177. Tuncozgur B, Ustunsoy H, Sivrikoz MC, *et al.* Intrapleural urokinase in the management of parapneumonic empyema: a randomised controlled trial. *Int J Clin Pract* 2001; **55**: 658–60.

178. Barletta JF. Streptokinase and urokinase for the treatment of pleural effusions and empyemas. *Ann Pharmacother* 1999; **33**: 495–8.

179. Bruserud O, Elsayed S, Pawelec G. At least five antigenic epitopes on the streptokinase molecule are recognized by human CD4+ TCR alpha beta+ T cells. *Mol Immunol* 1992; **29**: 1097–104.

180. Bouros D, Schiza S, Panagou P, Drositis J, Siafakas N. Role of streptokinase in the treatment of acute loculated parapneumonic pleural effusions and empyema. *Thorax* 1994; **49**: 852–5.

181. Aye RW, Froese DP, Hill LD. Use of purified streptokinase in empyema and hemothorax. *Am J Surg* 1991; **161**: 560–2.

182. Srivastava P, Godden DJ, Kerr KM, Legge JS. Fatal haemorrhage from aortic dissection following instillation of intrapleural streptokinase. *Scott Med J* 2000; **45**: 86–7.

183. Temes RT, Follis F, Kessler RM, Pett SB Jr, Wernly JA. Intrapleural fibrinolytics in management of empyema thoracis. *Chest* 1996; **110**: 102–6.

184. Godley PJ, Bell RC. Major hemorrhage following administration of intrapleural streptokinase. *Chest* 1984; **86**: 486–7.

185. Davies CW, Lok S, Davies RJ. The systemic fibrinolytic activity of intrapleural streptokinase. *Am J Respir Crit Care Med* 1998; **157**: 328–30.

186. Berglin E, Ekroth R, Teger-Nilsson AC, William-Olsson G. Intrapleural instillation of streptokinase. Effects on systemic fibrinolysis. *Thorac Cardiovasc Surg* 1981; **29**: 124–6.

187. Juhlin P, Bostrom PA, Torp A, Bredberg A. Streptokinase antibodies inhibit reperfusion during thrombolytic therapy with streptokinase in acute myocardial infarction. *J Intern Med* 1999; **245**: 483–8.

●188. Cameron R, Davies HR. Intrapleural fibrinolytic therapy versus conservative management in the treatment of parapneumonic effusions and empyema. *Cochrane Database Syst Rev* 2004; **2**: CD002312.

●189. Tokuda Y, Matsushima D, Stein GH, Miyagi S. Intrapleural fibrinolytic agents for empyema and complicated parapneumonic effusions: a meta-analysis. *Chest* 2006; **129**: 783–90.

190. Maskell NA, Gleeson FV. Images in clinical medicine. Effect of intrapleural streptokinase on a loculated malignant pleural effusion. *N Engl J Med* 2003; **348**: e4.
191. Walker CA, Shirk MB, Tschampel MM, Visconti JA. Intrapleural alteplase in a patient with complicated pleural effusion. *Ann Pharmacother* 2003; **37**: 376–9.
192. Skeete DA, Rutherford EJ, Schlidt SA, *et al.* Intrapleural tissue plasminogen activator for complicated pleural effusions. *J Trauma* 2004; **57**: 1178–83.
193. Feola GP, Shaw LC, Coburn L. Management of complicated parapneumonic effusions in children. *Tech Vasc Interv Radiol* 2003; **6**: 197–204.
194. Bishop NB, Pon S, Ushay HM, Greenwald BM. Alteplase in the treatment of complicated parapneumonic effusion: a case report. *Pediatrics* 2003; **111**: E188–90.
195. Wells RG, Havens PL. Intrapleural fibrinolysis for parapneumonic effusion and empyema in children. *Radiology* 2003; **228**: 370–8.
196. Weinstein M, Restrepo R, Chait PG, *et al.* Effectiveness and safety of tissue plasminogen activator in the management of complicated parapneumonic effusions. *Pediatrics* 2004; **113**: e182–5.
197. Ray TL, Berkenbosch JW, Russo P, Tobias JD. Tissue plasminogen activator as an adjuvant therapy for pleural empyema in pediatric patients. *J Intensive Care Med* 2004; **19**: 44–50.
198. Gates RL, Hogan M, Weinstein S, Arca MJ. Drainage, fibrinolytics, or surgery: a comparison of treatment options in pediatric empyema. *J Pediatr Surg* 2004; **39**: 1638–42.
199. Jaffe A, Bush A. Cystic fibrosis: review of the decade. *Monaldi Arch Chest Dis* 2001; **56**: 240–7.
●200. Light RW, Nguyen T, Mulligan ME, Sasse SA. The *in vitro* efficacy of varidase versus streptokinase or urokinase for liquefying thick purulent exudative material from loculated empyema. *Lung* 2000; **178**: 13–18.
●201. Simpson G, Roomes D, Heron M. Effects of streptokinase and deoxyribonuclease on viscosity of human surgical and empyema pus. *Chest* 2000; **117**: 1728–33.
202. Nwiloh J, Freeman H, McCord C. Malnutrition: an important determinant of fatal outcome in surgically treated pulmonary suppurative disease. *J Natl Med Assoc* 1989; **81**: 525–9.
203. Martella AT, Santos GH. Decortication for chronic postpneumonic empyema. *J Am Coll Surg* 1995; **180**: 573–6.
204. Katariya K, Thurer RJ. Surgical management of empyema. *Clin Chest Med* 1998; **19**: 395–406.
205. Lackner RP, Hughes R, Anderson LA, Sammut PH, Thompson AB. Video-assisted evacuation of empyema is the preferred procedure for management of pleural space infections. *Am J Surg* 2000; **179**: 27–30.
206. Waller DA, Rengarajan A. Thoracoscopic decortication: a role for video-assisted surgery in chronic postpneumonic pleural empyema. *Ann Thorac Surg* 2001; **71**: 1813–16.
207. Angelillo Mackinlay TA, Lyons GA, Chimondeguy DJ, *et al.* VATS debridement versus thoracotomy in the treatment of loculated postpneumonia empyema. *Ann Thorac Surg* 1996; **61**: 1626–30.
208. Cunniffe MG, Maguire D, McAnena OJ, Johnston S, Gilmartin JJ. Video-assisted thoracoscopic surgery in the management of loculated empyema. *Surg Endosc* 2000; **14**: 175–8.
209. Powell LL, Allen R, Brenner M, Aryan HE, Chen JC. Improved patient outcome after surgical treatment for loculated empyema. *Am J Surg* 2000; **179**: 1–6.
210. Podbielski FJ, Maniar HS, Rodriguez HE, Hernan MJ, Vigneswaran WT. Surgical strategy of complex empyema thoracis. *JSLS* 2000; **4**: 287–90.
211. Solaini L, Prusciano F, Bagioni P. Video-assisted thoracic surgery in the treatment of pleural empyema. *Surg Endosc* 2007; **21**: 280–4.
212. Petrakis IE, Kogerakis NE, Drositis IE, *et al.* Video-assisted thoracoscopic surgery for thoracic empyema: primarily, or after fibrinolytic therapy failure? *Am J Surg* 2004; **187**: 471–4.
213. Luh SP, Chou MC, Wang LS, Chen JY, Tsai TP. Video-assisted thoracoscopic surgery in the treatment of complicated parapneumonic effusions or empyemas: outcome of 234 patients. *Chest* 2005; **127**: 1427–32.
214. Lardinois D, Gock M, Pezzetta E, *et al.* Delayed referral and Gram-negative organisms increase the conversion thoracotomy rate in patients undergoing video-assisted thoracoscopic surgery for empyema. *Ann Thorac Surg* 2005; **79**: 1851– 6.
215. Hope WW, Bolton WD, Stephenson JE. The utility and timing of surgical intervention for parapneumonic empyema in the era of video-assisted thoracoscopy. *Am Surg* 2005; **71**: 512–14.
216. Katlic MR. Video-assisted thoracic surgery utilizing local anesthesia and sedation. *Eur J Cardiothorac Surg* 2006; **30**: 529–32.
217. Stammberger U, Steinacher C, Hillinger S, *et al.* Early and long-term complaints following video-assisted thoracoscopic surgery: evaluation in 173 patients. *Eur J Cardiothorac Surg* 2000; **18**: 7–11.
218. Goldschlager T, Frawley G, Crameri J, *et al.* Comparison of thoracoscopic drainage with open thoracotomy for treatment of paediatric parapneumonic empyema. *Pediatr Surg Int* 2005; **21**: 599–603.
219. Suchar AM, Zureikat AH, Glynn L, *et al.* Ready for the frontline: is early thoracoscopic decortication the new standard of care for advanced pneumonia with empyema? *Am Surg* 2006; **72**: 688–92.
220. Avansino JR, Goldman B, Sawin RS, Flum DR. Primary operative versus nonoperative therapy for pediatric empyema: a meta-analysis. *Pediatrics* 2005; **115**: 1652–9.
221. Eloesser L. Of an operation for tuberculous empyema. *Ann Thorac Surg* 1969; **8**: 355–7.
222. Tremblay A, Michaud G. Single-center experience with 250 tunnelled pleural catheter insertions for malignant pleural effusion. *Chest* 2006; **129**: 362–8.
223. Furman AC, Jacobs J, Sepkowitz KA. Lung abscess in patients with AIDS. *Clin Infect Dis* 1996; **22**: 81–5.
224. Afessa B. Pleural effusion and pneumothorax in hospitalized patients with HIV infection: the Pulmonary Complications, ICU support, and Prognostic Factors of Hospitalized Patients with HIV (PIP) Study. *Chest* 2000; **117**: 1031–7.
225. Minkin R, Shapiro JM. *Corynebacterium afermentans* lung abscess and empyema in a patient with human immunodeficiency virus infection. *South Med J* 2004; **97**: 395–7.
226. Shapiro JM, Romney BM, Weiden MD, White CS, O'Toole KM. *Rhodococcus equi* endobronchial mass with lung abscess in a patient with AIDS. *Thorax* 1992; **47**: 62–3.
227. Marron A, Roson B, Mascaro J, Carratala J. *Listeria monocytogenes* empyema in an HIV infected patient. *Thorax* 1997; **52**: 745–6.
228. Mulanovich VE, Dismukes WE, Markowitz N. Cryptococcal empyema: case report and review. *Clin Infect Dis* 1995; **20**: 1396–8.
229. Wolday D, Seyoum B. Pleural empyema due to *Salmonella paratyphi* in a patient with AIDS. *Trop Med Int Health* 1997; **2**: 1140–2.
230. Khwaja S, Rosenbaum DH, Paul MC, *et al.* Surgical treatment of thoracic empyema in HIV-infected patients: severity and treatment modality is associated with CD4 count status. *Chest* 2005; **128**: 246–9.

27

Effusions from infections: tuberculosis

ESTEBAN PÉREZ-RODRIGUEZ, RICHARD W LIGHT

INTRODUCTION

Tuberculous pleurisy results from *Mycobacterium tuberculosis* infection of the pleura. It manifests as a pleural effusion with exudative characteristics and can be found either isolated or in association with pulmonary tuberculosis (TB).

Pleural TB is one of the most frequent extrapulmonary manifestations of tuberculosis.[1] In a summary of five studies carried out in Africa on human immunodeficiency virus (HIV)-positive patients, pleural tuberculosis represented approximately 60 percent of all cases of extrapulmonary TB.[2–6] The incidence of coexisting pulmonary TB is estimated to be between 34 and 50 percent.[7]

Since the introduction of anti-tuberculous agents and measures for its control, the incidence of TB has decreased significantly in the developed world. With new infections being controlled, pleural disease now is seen more as a reactivation than a primary infection.

INCIDENCE AND EPIDEMIOLOGY

Today, TB is one of the most frequent causes of death from an identifiable pathogen in the world. According to data from the World Health Organization (WHO), eight million new cases of TB and 1.9 million deaths occur each year. This represents 7 percent of all causes of deaths and 26 percent of preventable deaths in developing countries.[8,9] Ninety-five percent of all TB cases and 98 percent of all deaths caused by TB occur in underdeveloped countries, especially in sub-Saharan areas and parts of Asia such as Indonesia, Bangladesh and Pakistan.[10]

Poverty, lack of TB control policies, war, prison settings and HIV co-infection have all contributed to the continual spread of TB in many parts of the world.[11] Nine percent of all new TB cases in adults were attributable to HIV infection, especially in the African region (31 percent) and in some industrialized countries, notably the USA (26 percent). In South Africa alone there were two million co-infected adults. The HIV pandemic presents a massive challenge to global TB control.[12] Also, correctional facilities have often been cited as reservoirs for tuberculosis. In Europeans prisons, the incidence of TB is up to 83 times higher in prisoners than in civilians.[13]

Pleural effusion is one of the most frequent extrapulmonary manifestations of tuberculosis. Its frequency as a percentage of the total number of cases of tuberculosis differs among countries. In Spain, the pleura is affected in 23 percent of all patients with TB[14] while in the USA, only 4 percent are affected, with an annual incidence of 1000 cases. Pleural and pulmonary TB coexist in 34–50 percent of patients.[7,15]

The incidence of pleural TB was reported to be increased (29–60 percent) in HIV patients in some studies.[16,17] However, Mlika-Cabane *et al.*[18] prospectively studied the radiographic characteristics of 146 cases of thoracic TB in Tanzania of which 80 cases were HIV-positive (55 percent). There were no significant differences in the incidence of pleural effusions between HIV-positive (41 percent) and negative (35 percent) patients. These same authors also studied 158 patients with thoracic TB in Burundi and found that the incidence of pleural TB was similar in positive subjects (24 percent) as in negative subjects (28 percent). When these authors combined the data from Tanzania and Burundi and calculated the probability of a TB patient being HIV positive, the presence of pleural effusion did not predict HIV seropositivity. Pleural effusion was present in 58 of 185 (31 percent) of the HIV-positive and 38 of 119 (32 percent) of the negative subjects. Similar results were obtained in Zimbabwe,[19] where no association was found between the presence of pleural effusion and HIV status in a study of 422 patients (202 HIV-positive and 220 negative).

This disparity in the results could be explained by the immunological status of the HIV positive subjects. Jones *et al.*[20] observed that pleural TB in HIV-positive patients was more frequent in patients with high CD4 counts.

Tuberculous pleural effusion is one of the most frequent causes of exudates in large series of pleural effusions in immunocompetent patients. If we exclude patients with underlying pulmonary disease, TB is the most common cause of pleural exudates in many areas of the world.[21,22]

ETIOLOGY AND PATHOGENESIS

Pleural TB reflects a compartmentalized activation of immunity mediated by cells in the pleural space. Mycobacterial proteins access this space through rupture of a subpleural focus 6–12 weeks after a primary infection,[23] and rarely from a vertebral focus by direct extension.[24] With fewer new infections, pleural disease now more commonly represents reactivation than primary infection and is present in approximately 7 percent of cases of active pulmonary TB. In a study from Maryland, USA, organisms isolated from patients with pleural TB were significantly less likely to be genotypically clustered than patients presenting with pulmonary TB, suggesting that pleural TB is more frequently reactivation TB than is pulmonary TB.[25] In a study in Edinburgh, UK, from 1980–91, Moudgil *et al.*[26] attributed 64 percent of the new cases of pleural TB to reactivation TB.

In an animal model with pleural effusion induced by the intrapleural injection of purified protein derivative (PPD) in sensitized animals, neutrophils were the predominant cells in the initial phase, and after the third day lymphocytes predominated.[27] (See also Chapter 14, Experimental models: pleural disease other than mesothelioma.) The pleural fluid in TB is predominantly lymphocytic. Many of the lymphocytes are T-helper type 1 (Th1) cells,[28] and the CD4/CD8 ratio observed was 4.3 in pleural fluid, while it was 1.6 in peripheral blood.[29–31]

This cellular component reflects the immunological reaction of tuberculous pleurisy in which mesothelial cells, neutrophils, lymphocytes, monocytes and their cytokines are involved. The most probable hypothesis for the pathogenesis of pleural TB suggests that the endothelial and mesothelial cells are incipient protagonists of the process.[32]

These cells, exposed to inflammatory stimuli derived from mycobacteria (glycolipids and lipoproteins) mediated chemokine expression in pleural mesothelial cells, release interleukin (IL)-1 to IL-6, tumor necrosis factor alpha (TNF-α) as well as alpha and beta chemokines. Alpha chemokines (IL-8, neutrophil activating protein [NAP-2]) are chemotactic for neutrophils, lymphocytes or both, while beta chemokines (macrophage inflammatory protein [MIP-1] and monocyte chemoattractant protein [MCP-1]) are chemotactic for monocytes and macrophages.[33–35]

Mohammed *et al.*[33–34] reported that pleural fluid from patients with tuberculosis pleuritis contained significantly ($p < 0.001$) more biologically active MIP-1 and MCP-1 than did fluids from patients with congestive heart failure. Unfortunately, they did not measure these cytokines in other types of exudative pleural fluids. Antigenic MIP-1 and MCP-1 were detected by immunocytochemistry in pleural biopsy sections from patients with tuberculous pleurisy. *In vitro*, pleural mesothelial cell stimulated with Bacillus Calmette-Guérin (BCG) produced MIP-1 and MCP-1. Reverse transcription-polymerase chain reaction studies confirmed that BCG and interferon (IFN)-γ induced MIP-1 and MCP-1 expression in mesothelial cells, demonstrating that Th1 and Th2 cytokines may regulate the C-C chemokines expression in mesothelial cells and thus play a biologically important role in the recruitment of mononuclear cells to the pleural space. Also, large concentrations of IL-8 have been found by Pace *et al.*[36] in cancer and tuberculosis pleural effusions. The concentration of IL-8 correlated best with lymphocyte recruitment and not with neutrophil recruitment. This chemotactic activity was partly blocked by anti-IL-8 antibody and was stimulated by the induction of messenger RNA for IL-8 and IL8 protein production in pleural macrophages. These findings demonstrate that pleural macrophages and mesothelial cells produce IL-8 in tuberculous pleurisy and this is an important factor for the recruitment of lymphocytes into pleural space.[37]

This explains why the pleural fluid from the patient with TB is predominantly lymphocytic. In fact, values higher than 85 percent are reported to be very suggestive of this diagnosis,[38–40] and a predominance of neutrophils are only found in the early phase of TB.[41]

In HIV-positive patients, it seems reasonable to hypothesize that pleural TB would be manifested with a less intense immunological response. The findings of Kitinya *et al.*[42] support this. In their series of 57 patients with pleural TB, 69 percent of the 36 HIV-positive patients had mycobacteria in the pleural fluid, whereas only 38 percent of the 21 HIV-negative patients had mycobacteria in the pleural fluid. Also, the presence of granulomas on biopsy was *less* frequent in the HIV-positives (61 percent) than in the HIV-negatives (90 percent).

Some authors[43,44] report that HIV-positive patients respond to tuberculous infection with local recruitment of T lymphocytes, despite their decrease in the serum. Jones *et al.*[20] found that patients with HIV and pleural TB with CD4 counts >200/μL were more likely to develop a pleural effusion (8 of 29, 28 percent) than those with CD4 counts

<200/μL (6 of 58, 10 percent). This suggests that the immune state must be relatively well preserved in order for pleural TB to develop.

Although the immune mechanisms linked to the activation of the Th1 cells are important in the development of tuberculous pleural effusion, pleuritis after the primary infection does not confer protection from subsequent TB, as 65 percent of untreated patients develop active pulmonary disease[45,46] after the tuberculous pleuritis resolves.

SYMPTOMS AND LABORATORY FINDINGS

Pleural tuberculosis affects men more frequently than women, with an approximate ratio of 3:1 and affects mainly young adults with a mean age around 35 years.[47] However, more recent studies report an older mean age with 10–15 percent of the patients being over the age of 70 years.

The clinical presentation is usually acute or subacute and the interval from the beginning of symptoms to the diagnosis is less than 1 month in most patients. The most common symptoms are: cough 71–94 percent; fever 71–100 percent; chest pain 78–82 percent; and dyspnea 12–15 percent.[48,49] Rarely are patients asymptomatic, but this is more common among the aged. Physical examination reveals a decrease in the breath sounds over the affected area and dullness to percussion. A pleural friction rub is seldom present. The Mantoux skin test is negative in 30 percent of the cases with the standard five-unit test, more than half are negative with one unit test. However, the skin test usually becomes become positive with repetition after 2–6 weeks.[48,49]

In patients with HIV, the clinical presentation of TB is different.[50] In Tanzania, Richter *et al.*[51] found that HIV-positive patients with pleural TB present with a more prolonged interval between the beginning of symptoms and diagnosis than do the HIV-negative patients. The HIV-positive patients are also more symptomatic, with fever, dyspnea, night sweats and asthenia, while the physical examination often reveals hepatomegaly, splenomegaly and lymphadenopathy. The Mantoux skin test is more frequently negative in HIV-positive (47 percent) than in HIV-negative patients (12 percent).

The rate of identification of mycobacteria in sputum from patients with isolated pleural TB is low (4–7 percent) but is much higher (28–50 percent) if there are associated pulmonary infiltrates.[49,52] Routine laboratory studies are nonspecific. A frequent finding is a high sedimentation rate with normal leukocyte count.[49]

Thoracentesis shows a clear yellow or a serosanguineous liquid. The pleural fluid is an exudate and usually contains predominantly lymphocytes – a finding very suggestive of TB pleuritis if the patient is young.[53] The pleural fluid may contain predominantly neutrophils in the very early phase.[41] Eosinophilia >10 percent is exceptional and practically excludes the diagnosis, as long as this finding is obtained in the first thoracentesis.[54] A finding of >5 percent of mesothelial cells is exceptional in pleural TB and serves to exclude the diagnosis.[55]

RADIOLOGY

Approximately 30 percent of patients with pleural TB present with ipsilateral radiological disease in the lung parenchyma as assessed with the chest radiograph. This percentage may be as high as 86 percent with chest computed tomography (CT).[56]

The pleural effusion is generally unilateral and small to moderate in size. Massive effusions are observed in 12–29 percent of cases, and tuberculosis is one of the three most frequent causes of massive pleural exudates: malignancy and empyema being the other two.[57,58] Joseph *et al.*[59] reported that massive effusions were more frequent in HIV-positive patients. Less than 10 percent of tuberculous effusions are bilateral and bilateral effusions are generally in HIV-positive patients.

Identifying whether pleural TB is a primary infection or a reinfection can be quite difficult.[60] Some authors have reported that patients with pleural tuberculosis were significantly less likely to be genotypically clustered than patients presenting with pulmonary tuberculosis.[25] Normally, radiological criteria are used to differentiate primary and reinfection tuberculosis. Primary TB manifests as lymphadenopathy or lower lobe infiltrates. In cases reported as pleural TB reactivation, the following characteristics are described: advanced age, tobacco habit, alcohol abuse, significant weight loss, presence of *Mycobacterium* in sputum and pleural effusions of smaller volume. However, 8–20 percent of patients with pulmonary TB have atypical radiological appearances,[60] and diagnosis often requires the use of immunological criteria.[61]

DIAGNOSIS

The clinical likelihood of the diagnosis of pleural TB varies depending on the prevalence of TB and HIV co-infection. In a significant percentage of cases, pleural TB is found in adults and elderly people. Elderly individuals tend to have additional comorbidities, making the diagnosis more difficult. We have reported a diagnosis sensitivity of 58 percent using age, clinical data and thorax X-ray.[62]

Pleural fluid with TB pleuritis is usually an exudate containing predominantly lymphocytes, with few eosinophils (<10 percent), or mesothelial cells (<5 percent).[63]

A definitive diagnosis of tuberculous pleurisy requires demonstration of *M. tuberculosis* in sputum or pleural specimens or the presence of caseating granulomas in the pleura. Sputum culture is positive in 30–50 percent of patients with pleural and pulmonary tuberculosis, but in only 4 percent in patients with isolated pleural effusion.[64] However, this increased to 55 percent with sputum induction.[65] The sensitivity of pleural fluid culture for the diagnosis of tuberculous pleuritis is 23–86 percent and that of needle pleural biopsy is 39–71 percent.

The finding of necrotizing caseating granulomas in biopsy specimens is most likely to provide a diagnosis (in 51–88 percent of cases) (Table 27.1).[1,21,26,50,66,67,68,69] The use of all the above-mentioned tests provides a diagnosis in 82–98 percent. Increasing numbers of specimens obtained by blind pleural biopsy in pleural TB does not significantly increase the diagnostic performance. This is probably because tuberculous pleuritis is a diffuse process affecting the entire pleural surface, unlike malignant disease in which involvement of the parietal pleural is patchy or non-existent.[70]

Diagnostic performance of the various tests differs depending on HIV status. Anergy is more frequent in HIV-positive patients (47–59 percent) than HIV-negative patients (12–24 percent). The likelihood of isolation of mycobacteria from sputum is higher in HIV-positive patients (53 versus 23 percent).[42,52] Direct smear of pleural fluid (15 versus 8 percent) and culture of pleural biopsy tissue (91 versus 78 percent) are more likely to yield mycobacteria in HIV-positive patients. Findings of granulomas are less frequent (77 versus 88 percent) in HIV positive patients. Kitinya *et al.*[42] described three morphological types of TB related to HIV status – reactive, hyporeactive and non-reactive – according to whether well formed, poorly formed or no granulomas were present on biopsy. In 36 HIV-positive patients, 14 were non-reactive or hyporeactive, while this occurred in only 2 out of 21 HIV-negative patients. In the 14 non-reactive/hyporeactive HIV-positive patients, the culture was positive in 11, compared with 14 out of 22 of the reactive patients. These data contrast with those of other authors and can probably be explained by the different CD4 status in the series studied, as reported by Jones *et al.*[20]

The low sensitivity of finding mycobacteria in the pleural fluid explains why blind pleural biopsy has been the conventional diagnostic procedure for tuberculous pleurisy for the last 40 years. Pleural biopsy is an invasive technique, is difficult to perform on infants, takes a long time for culture results and requires experience. Alternative methods have been developed that attempt to diagnose TB pleuritis from tests on the pleural fluid.

New alternatives for diagnosis have been aimed at the actual detection of mycobacteria (BACTEC [see below] and polymerase chain reaction [PCR]) and at identifying biomarkers based on understanding of the immunological mechanisms of TB pleuritis (adenosine deaminase [ADA], ADA isoenzymes, IFN-γ, lysozyme, tuberculostearic acid, SC5b-9, IL-2, IL-6, IL-12).

The radiometric mycobacterial culture system (BACTEC; Becton Dickinson, Franklin Lakes, NJ, USA) accelerates diagnosis by 2–3 weeks compared with conventional culture. Bedside inoculation of pleural fluid provides more positive results (11 of 24) than laboratory inoculation (4 of 24).[71,72]

For the detection of *M. tuberculosis* deoxyribonucleic acid (DNA) in sputum samples, PCR (Amplicor kit; Roche Molecular Systems, Branchburg, NJ, USA) has a false positive rate of less than 1 percent.[73,74] In pleural fluid, various investigators have reported disparate results with PCR (sensitivity 61–94 percent and specificity 78–100 percent);[75–77] hence, its clinical use is not recommended. Querol *et al.*[76] found that the sensitivity of PCR was 100 percent in pleural tuberculosis with positive cultures and 60 percent in cases with negative cultures, in both cases superior to both pleural fluid acid-fast bacilli (AFB) smear (14 percent) and culture (52 percent). However, other authors have reported much poorer results.

The most promising new test in the diagnosis of pleural tuberculosis is ADA. In 1973, Piras *et al.*[78] first reported that the ADA levels were elevated in the cerebrospinal fluid of patients with tuberculous meningitis, and in 1978 the

Table 27.1 Diagnosis of tuberculous pleuritis

Authors	No. of cases	Fluid culture positive %	Biopsy histology positive %	Biopsy culture positive %
Seibert *et al.*[1]	70	58	84	67 (12/18)
Valdes *et al.*[21]	81	38	76.5	56.8
Moudgil *et al.*[26]	62	54	60	NR
Chan *et al.*[50]	83	23	51	40 (2/5)
Antoniskis *et al.*[66]	59	77	58	52
Maartens *et al.*[67]	62	47	84	71
Kirsch *et al.*[68]	30	NR	80	60
Valdes *et al.*[69]	254	37	80	56

NR, not reported.

same authors reported that the pleural fluid ADA levels were elevated in tuberculous pleuritis.

There is much evidence supporting the usefulness of an increased level of pleural fluid ADA in establishing the diagnosis of tuberculous pleurisy (Table 127.2).[79–88] Nevertheless, high levels of ADA can also be found in other diseases such as empyemas, malignant lymphomas and collagen–vascular diseases. Its use in the diagnosis of pleural TB shows a sensitivity of 77–100 percent and a specificity of 81–97 percent.

Bañales *et al.*[82] performed a metanalysis of 2251 cases in which ADA was carried out by the Blake–Berman method.[87] They reported a sensitivity of 99 percent and a specificity of 89 percent. There were 116 false positives (5.7 percent) and these included 20 carcinomas, 18 lymphomas, 52 empyemas and 6 mesotheliomas. The cut-off level varied between 40 and 71 IU/L, which identified the need for individual cut-off levels of reference in respective centers.

In a study of 405 cases of pleural effusion including 91 due to TB, Valdes *et al.*[80] found a sensitivity of 100 percent and specificity of 95 percent using a cut-off value equal to or greater than 47 IU/L. The number of false positives was 16 (3.5 percent) (malignant 10, parapneumonic 1 and empyema 5). In a series of 129 patients under the age of 35 of whom 39 had TB, these same authors found a sensitivity of 100 percent and specificity of 87.5 percent using a cut-off value of 47 IU. All the false positives were empyemas. The study suggested that biopsy may be unnecessary in regions where the prevalence of TB is high in individuals under the age of 35 with ADA higher than 47 IU, given that false-positive empyemas are easily identifiable.

Burgess *et al.*[79] analyzed the diagnostic performance of individual ADA and of that associated with the value of lymphocytes in pleural fluid. In a series of 303 cases of which 143 were TB, they found a sensitivity of 91 percent and a specificity of 81 percent using an ADA cut-off value of 50 IU. When the patients were also required to have a lymphocyte/neutrophil ratio equal or greater than 0.75, the sensitivity fell to 88 percent while the specificity increased to 95 percent.

Pérez-Rodriguez *et al.*,[85] in their initial series of 304 consecutive patients with pleural effusion undergoing thoracentesis, including 48 with pleural TB, found the sensitivity and specificity of using ADA test (with a cut-off level of 40 IU) to be 87.5 and 96.8 percent, respectively. Six were false negatives (1.9 percent) and eight were false positives (2.6 percent), including four empyemas, three lymphomas and a melanoma.

In view of the above, one can conclude that the ADA level is a good parameter for identifying pleural TB. Adding the criteria of pleural fluid lymphocyte/neutrophil ratio above 0.75 and an age limit of <35 years both improve diagnostic specificity.

In HIV-positive patients, the immunological response is diminished (as observed by Kitinya *et al.*[42]) and one might expect the ADA to be less useful diagnostically. However, Riantawan *et al.*[44] found that the diagnostic utility of ADA was as good in HIV patients ($n = 37$) as in HIV-negative ($n = 52$) ones. The average levels of ADA were 110 and 114 IU, respectively, and when a cut-off value of 60 IU was applied, the sensitivity in both groups was 95 percent. The percentage of lymphocytes in serum was less in the HIV positive subjects than in the HIV-negative subjects, while in pleural fluid the lymphocyte percentage was similar in both groups.

Some authors believe that ADA is a better negative predictive parameter than the combination of symptoms plus

Table 27.2 Utility of adenosine deaminase (ADA) in the diagnosis of tuberculous pleurisy

Authors	No.	No. of cases of tuberculous pleurisy	Cut-off level U/L	Sensitivity %	Specificity %
Maertens *et al.*[67]	109	82	45	77	83
Burgess *et al.*[79,a]	303	143	50	91	81
Valdes *et al.*[80,a]	405	91	47	100	95
Valdes *et al.*[81,a]	350	76	47	100	91
Bañales J *et al.*[82,b]	218	82	70	98	96
Segura *et al.*[83,b]	600	170	71	100	92
Ocañ *et al.*[84,b]	182	46	45	100	97
Pérez-Rodriguez *et al.*[85,b]	304	48	40	88	97
De Oliveira *et al.*[86]	276	54	40	91	96
Blake Berman[87]	202	82	–	95	96
Maritz *et al.*[88]	368	107	–	93	81
Total	3317	981	40–71	93.9%	91.3%

[a]Galanti and Giusti method; [b]Blake–Berman method.

lymphocytes in pleural fluid plus PPD. In a series of 19 pleural effusions of unidentified etiologies with positive PPD and ADA less than 47 IU, none developed tuberculosis during a 69-month follow-up.[89]

ADA in pleural fluid represents the sum of two isoenzymes ADA1 + ADA2.[34] ADA1 is ubiquitous and is necessary for the breakdown of the substrate adenosine to 2′deoxyadenosine. This enzyme is important because a low level of 2′deoxyadenosine is essential for the proper functioning of immune cells. In contrast, ADA2 is not ubiquitous, and coexists with ADA1 only in monocytes and macrophages.

Gakis[90] demonstrated that the level of ADA in monocytes and macrophages is always low, except on certain occasions in which ADA2 is dramatically increased due to infections by intracellular organisms. From this it can be deduced that ADA1 is produced by lymphocytes and monocytes, while ADA2 is only produced by monocytes. This explains why some studies find a correlation between ADA and monocytes but not lymphocytes in pleural TB, and why ADA in false-positive cases is primarily ADA1.[91]

For a better discriminating capability in the diagnosis of pleural TB, some authors have used the levels of ADA2 and found a high sensitivity and specificity of 100 and 91 percent, respectively.[92] Another measure that has been used is the ADA1/ADA total. With this measure a cut-off level of 0.42 (values <0.42 representing TB) yielded an improved sensitivity of 100 percent and specificity of 97–98.6 percent (Table 27.3).

The levels of ADA in the pleural fluid decline with time, at ambient temperatures. However, the addition of stabilizing agents (glycerol and ethylene glycol each at 5 percent concentration) to pleural fluid specimens allows the transport of the specimens to distant laboratories at ambient temperatures without a decline in the ADA levels.[93]

Pleural fluid levels of IFN-γ are increased in pleural TB compared with other exudative effusions. When a cut-off value of 140 pg/mL or 3.9 U/mL is used, a sensitivity of 74–100 percent and a specificity of 91–100 percent have been reported.[80,94] False positives have been described in parapneumonic effusions, lymphoproliferative disorders and other malignancies. The cost and speed of results have limited its routine use.

Pleural fluid levels of lysozyme are also frequently higher in pleural TB than in pleural fluids of other etiologies. It is an enzyme present in the epithelioid cells of granulomas, activated macrophages and certain tumor cells. Its diagnostic effectiveness in pleural TB has been described with varying sensitivities (66–100 percent) and a low specificity (66 percent).[80,95] False positives have been reported in parapneumonic effusions, empyemas, malignancies, post-thoracic surgery, collagen–vascular disease, heart failure and, on rare occasions, pleural sarcoidosis. Its routine use is not recommended.

Other less relevant parameters studied are: tuberculostearic acid, monoclonal antibodies, SC5b-9 and other cytokines (IL-2, -3, -4, -5, -6, -10 and -12).

Tuberculostearic acid is a structural component of mycobacteria and actinomycetes. Measured in pleural fluid, its sensitivity for diagnosing tuberculous pleuritis is reported as 68–90 percent and its specificity 52 percent.[96,97]

Anti-mycobacterial antibodies have seldom been studied in pleural TB.[98] The only one to have been developed to date is anti-P32 (antigen specific to mycobacteria). P32 antigen is restricted to *Mycobacterium tuberculosis, bovis, kansasi* and *avium*. Pleural fluid and the corresponding sera were obtained from five patients with pleural TB and 14 patients from pleural effusions of other origins. The pleural fluids and sera from patients with pleural TB contained a significantly higher proportion of antiP32 IgG and IgA antibodies than samples obtained from non-tuberculous pleural effusions.

A monoclonal antibody against soluble phase-terminal complement complex (SC5b-9) has been analyzed in pleural fluid to differentiate tuberculous effusions from malignant effusions and effusions of other causes. In one study, 26 patients with TB pleural effusions had a significantly higher SC5b-9 level than did the 38 cases of pleural effusions of other etiologies. With a cut-off level of 2.0 mg/L, the specificity and sensitivity of SC5b-9 for pleural TB was 74 and 100 percent, respectively.[99]

In tuberculous pleuritis, high pleural fluid levels of IL-2, IL-6 and IL-12 and TNF-α have been described (see also Chapter 8, Immunology). The levels of IL-2 and IL-6 have been found up to 15 times higher in pleural fluid than in serum.[100] IL-12 has also been reported to be elevated in pleural TB and its low levels have been related to poor

Table 27.3 Adenosine deaminase (ADA) and ADA1/ADA$_{pleural}$ activity in the diagnosis of tuberculous pleuritis

Authors	ADA				$ADA_1/ADA_{pleural}$			
	Total (TB)	S %	Sp %	Ef %	Total (TB)	S %	Sp %	Ef %
Valdés *et al.*[80]	350 (76)	100	93	–	101 (76)	100	97	98
Pérez-Rodriguez *et al.*[91]	103 (27)	89	92	91	103 (27)	100	99	99

ADA, adenosine deaminase; TB, no. with tuberculous pleuritis; S, sensitivity; Sp, specificity; Ef, efficiency.

prognoses.[101] However, these cytokines have never been shown to have significant diagnostic utility, because their levels overlap with those in exudates of other causes.

In summary, non-invasive diagnosis using a ADA cut-off level of 40 IU with lymphocyte/neutrophil ratio above 0.75 can be used to diagnose pleural tuberculosis in patients <35 years old from countries with a high prevalence of tuberculosis and a low level of mycobacterial resistance[102,103] (Figure 27.1, diagnostic algorithm). In other situations, closed pleural biopsy is required, though more invasive procedures such as thoracoscopy are usually not necessary.[104]

TREATMENT AND MANAGEMENT

In most cases, pleural TB without treatment resolves spontaneously in 2–4 months. However, if no treatment is received, 65 percent (92 out of 114) of patients end up developing pulmonary tuberculosis in the following 5 years.[45] This is the rationale of treatment for tuberculous pleuritis.

Treatment of patients with tuberculosis should generally be monitored by official public health centers to ensure: administration of correct therapy, which helps prevent the emergence of resistant mycobacteria; coordination of contact tracing; monitoring of the pattern of resistances to drugs in the community; adequate education of patients; and identification of possible outbreaks.[105] Therapy of pleural TB, as for pulmonary TB, is based on the use of therapeutic regimens with combination of drugs directed at reducing the population of mycobacteria without creating resistance and at sterilizing the lesions during the prolonged treatment phase. Duration of treatment, number of drugs, use of steroids, therapeutic drainage and intrapleural urokinase are aspects of possible controversy.

One of the most widely recommended therapeutic regimens is a 6-month treatment course. An initial phase with isoniazid (5–10 mg/kg.day up to 300 mg/day), rifampin (600 mg/day) and pyrazinamide (1.5–2 g/day) administered daily for 2 months is followed by isoniazid and rifampin daily during the following 4 months.[106] If the patient lives in a region with more than 4 percent primary resistance to isoniazid, comes from an area where high

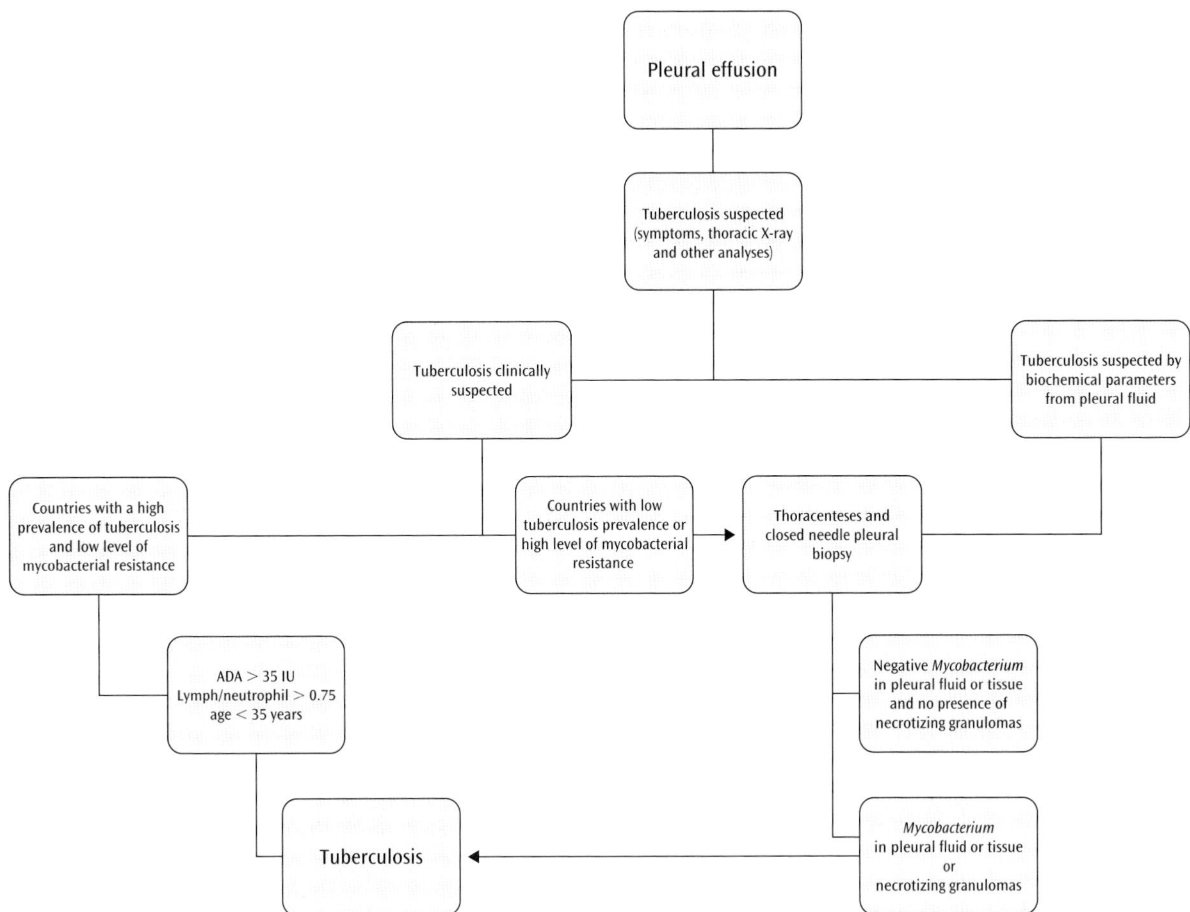

Figure 27.1 Diagnostic algorithm. ADA, adenosine deaminase.

levels of resistant microorganisms are reported, has received anti-TB drugs previously or has been exposed to patients with known multi-resistant TB, ethambutol (15 mg/kg.day) should be added until the results of the sensitivity studies become known.[107] The scarce bacillary presence in pleural fluid and biopsy suggests that a less intense regimen may be adequate. The use of only two drugs, isoniazid and rifampin, daily for 6 months has been shown to be effective in immunocompetent patients as well as HIV-positive patients, without any evidence of relapse (0 percent) during a follow-up for more than 3 years.[108,109] There is complete resolution after 6 months in 75 percent of cases and in practically all cases 14 months after the initiation of treatment.[110] During the initial phase of treatment, some patients may show an increase of pleural effusion, and this does not necessarily indicate a therapeutic failure.[111]

Generally, the same treatment regime is recommended for HIV-positive patients. However, treatment should be prolonged if the clinical or bacteriological response is slow or less than optimal.[112,113]

Systemic corticosteroids have been proposed in the treatment of pleural tuberculosis because pleural tuberculosis is associated with inflammation and fibrosis, and steroids can reduce the degree of pleural inflammation.[31] A recent review by Matchaba *et al.*[114] found that only 3 out of 10 studies met randomization, double blind, placebo-controlled criteria.[7,115,116] They analyzed the effects of corticoids in terms of symptoms, residual pleural fluid and residual pachypleuritis and concluded that there is insufficient evidence to define whether steroids are useful in pleural TB.

Reasonable management of pleural TB could include performing a therapeutic thoracentesis at the same time as the diagnostic thoracentesis is carried out, especially in large-volume effusions, with the intention of draining all the fluid possible and initiating the antituberculous treatment. Routine drainage with a pigtail catheter does not reduce the level of residual pleural thickening.[117] Some authors have used intrapleural urokinase in loculated TB pleural effusions,[118] but there are no randomized studies evaluating this treatment and it is not recommended.

COMPLICATIONS

Residual pleural thickening, empyema and thoracic wall infection are the most frequently described complications. Others, such as non-Hodgkin's lymphomas, sarcomas and other malignancies can present themselves after chronic inflammatory processes[119,120] but these complications are very unusual.

Residual pleural thickening is the most frequent complication. Its incidence varies according to the time of evaluation and the degree of thickness. At the conclusion of treatment, 43–50 percent of patients have pleural thickening of more than 2 mm[121,122] and 20 percent have more than 10 mm. The relationship between residual pleural thickening and different variables (low concentration of glucose in fluid and low pH level, high lysozyme level and TNF-α level, presence of mycobacteria in pleural fluid or biopsy, high effusion level, duration of symptoms, low hemoglobin level and loss of weight)[121,123] have been weak. Residual pleural thickening has been reported to be less in HIV-positive than in HIV-negative patients.[124] However, functional sequelae related to the pleural thickening are infrequent.[125]

Tuberculous empyema (pus in pleural fluid) is an unusual complication, normally related to the presence of bronchopleural fistulae.[126] The response to medical treatment is limited by loculated pleural effusion and pleural thickening[127] and in these cases drainage and decortication are should be considered.[128,129] However, good results have been reported with repeated thoracentesis and medical treatment for 24 months.[130]

Isolated cases of empyema necessitatis and costal involvement by proximity due to *M. tuberculosis* have been described.[131,132] On rare occasions, fistulas and abscesses of the thoracic wall in the path of the pleural biopsy have been reported.[133] In our experience this happened once in 106 biopsy cases.

FUTURE DIRECTIONS OF DEVELOPMENT

1. Reinforce mechanisms for prevention: education, vaccinations, chemoprophylaxis and adequate treatments, available in any geographical area of the world.
2. Facilitate diagnosis:
   (i) Obviate the necessity for pleural biopsy for diagnosis through the search for parameters in the pleural fluid (ADA, ADA isoenzymes, IFN-γ, PCR). This would allow for easier diagnoses in regions with limited health care resources. Improving the diagnostic rate may result in provision of treatment to populations that are currently not diagnosed, including children who are may not be able to cooperate with pleural biopsy, and those who live in areas where there are no trained personel to perform pleural biopsy.
   (ii) Improve, standardize and make reproducible the diagnostic methods that are offering better performances in various geographic areas with different prevalences of the disease.
3. Develop therapeutic aspects:
   (i) Given that pleural tuberculosis has a low mycobacterial population, are three anti-TB drugs needed? Can the treatment be shortened?
   (ii) In the adjuvant treatment, are corticoids useful (when, how, why, for what)? Is pleural drainage necessary? Could intrapleural fibrinolytic drugs be useful if there is an increase in procoagulant activity? Could treatments with IFN-γ or IL-12 be useful?

4. Predict complications: identify parameters in pleural fluid with predictive capabilities for pachypleuritis that have not been studied to date (TNF-β, procoagulants/fibrinolitics, others).

KEY POINTS

- Pleural tuberculosis is one of the most frequent types of extrapulmonary tuberculosis. It coexists with pulmonary tuberculosis in 34–50 percent of cases and is the most frequent cause of a pleural exudate in the absence of underlying lung disease in patients under the age of 35.
- A clinical picture suggestive of tuberculosis has a high prediction rate (60–70 percent) but the diagnosis requires confirmation in order to justify treatment. Without treatment, pleural tuberculosis is self-limited after 2–4 months in healthy individuals, but 65 percent will develop active extrapleural tuberculosis in the following 5 years.
- Pleural effusion due to tuberculosis is frequently caused by an immunological response to antigenic components of the mycobacteria more than the presence of a high bacillary population in the pleural space, as demonstrated by the infrequency of isolation of mycobacteria by culture.
- Diagnostic confirmation is obtained through the identification of mycobacteria in pleural fluid and/or biopsy with the presence of necrotizing granulomas. The sensitivity of demonstration of mycobacteria in pleural fluid by direct studies (Ziehl stain, Auramina) is very low (<10 percent) compared with that of 23–77 percent by pleural fluid cultures and 52–71 percent by culturing pleural tissue. The presence of granulomas (51–84 percent) on pleural tissues is the most frequent finding that establishes the diagnosis. The combination of these tests allows for diagnosis in more than 90 percent of cases.
- Alternative diagnostic methods have been developed. Among these are ADA determination, IFN-γ and the identification of mycobacteria by means of PCR. Pleural fluid ADA measurement is currently the most effective method (sensitivity 77–100 percent, specificity 81–97 percent). In patients below 35 years of age, a pleural fluid ADA >35 IU/L with a lymphocyte/neutrophil ratio >0.75 is sufficient for the diagnosis of tuberculous pleuritis in countries with a high prevalence of tuberculosis and low incidence of drug-resistant mycobacteria.
- A widely recommended therapeutic regimen includes rifampin, isoniazid and pyrazinamide. Therapeutic drainage of the effusion can significantly improve the symptoms. There is insufficient evidence to justify the routine use of corticoids as adjuvant therapy.
- Pleural thickening (>2–10 mm) complicates up to 43 percent of cases. Neither pleural fluid biochemistry nor type of treatment predicts the development of pleural thickening. Empyema is an unusual complication that requires pleural drainage and prolonged anti-tuberculous treatment.

REFERENCES

● = Key primary paper
◆ = Major review article

1. Seibert AF, Haynes JR, Middleton R, Bass JB. Tuberculous pleural effusion. Twenty-year experience. *Chest* 1991; **99**: 883–6.
2. Mehta J, Dutt A, Harvill L, *et al.* Epidemiology of extrapulmonary tuberculosis. *Chest* 1991; **99**: 1134–8.
◆3. Mlika-Cabanne N, Brauner M, Kamanfu G, *et al.* Radiographic abnormalities in tuberculosis and risk of coexisting human immunodeficiency virus infection. Methods and preliminary results from Bujumbura, Burundi. *Am J Respir Crit Care Med* 1995; **152**: 794–9.
4. Elliott A. Luo N, Tembo G, *et al.* Impact of HIV on tuberculosis in Zambia: a cross sectional study. *BMJ* 1990; **301**: 412–15.
5. Batungwanayo J, Taelman H, Allen S, *et al.* Pleural effusion, tuberculosis and HIV-1 infection in Kigali, Rwanda. *AIDS* 1993; **7**: 73–9.
6. Aktogu S, Yorgancioglu A, Cirak K, *et al.* Clinical spectrum of pulmonary and pleural tuberculosis; a report of 5480 cases. *Eur Respir J* 1996; **9**: 2031–5.
7. Wyser C, Walzl G, Smedema J, *et al.* Corticosteroids in the treatment of tuberculous pleurisy. A double-blind, placebo-controled, randomised study. *Chest* 1996; **110**: 333–8.
8. Dye C, Scheele S, Dolin P, Pathania V, Raviblione MC. Global burden of tuberculosis: estimated incidence, prevalence and mortality by country. *J Am Med Assoc* 1999; **282**: 677–86.
9. Raviglione MC, Snider DE, Kochi A. Global epidemiology of tuberculosis: morbidity and mortality of a worldwide epidemic. *J Am Med Assoc* 1995; **273**: 220–6.
10. Murray CJ, Styblo K, Rouillon A. Tuberculosis in developing countries: burden, intervention and cost. *Bull Int Union Tuberc Lung Dis* 1990; **65**: 6–24.
11. Rose AMC, Watson JM, Graham C, *et al.* Public Health Laboratory Service/British Thoracic Society/Department of Health Collaborative Group. Tuberculosis at the end of the 20th century in England and Wales: results of a national survey in 1998. *Thorax* 2001; **56**: 173–9.
12. Corbett EL, Watt CJ, Walker N, *et al.* The growing burden of tuberculosis: Global trends and interactions with the HIV epidemic. *Arch Intern Med* 2003; **163**: 1009–21.
13. Aerts A, Hauer B, Wanlin M, Veen J. Tuberculosis and tuberculosis control in European prisons. *Int J Tuberc Lung Dis* 2006; **10**: 1215–23.
14. Vidal R, de Gracia J, Fite E, Monso E, Martin N. Estudio controlado de 637 pacientes con tuberculosis: diagnostico y resultados terapeuticos con esquemas terapeuticos de 9 y 6 meses. *Med Clin* 1986; **87**: 368–70.

15. Liam CK, Lim KH, Wong CM. Tuberculosis pleurisy as a manifestation of primary and reactivation disease in a region with a high prevalence of tuberculosis. *Int J Tuberc Lung Dis* 1999; **3**: 816–22.
16. Kramer F, Modilevsky T, Waliany AR, Leedom JM, Barnes PF. Delayed diagnosis of tuberculosis in patients with human immunodeficiency virus infection. *Am J Med* 1990; **89**: 451–6.
17. Davies PDO. The association between HIV and tuberculosis in the developing world. In: Davies PDO (ed.). *Clinical tuberculosis.* London: Arnold, 1995: 253.
◆18. Mlika-Cabanne N, Brauner M, Mugusi F, *et al.* Radiographic abnormalities in tuberculosis and risk of coexisting human deficiency virus infection. Results from Dar-es-Salaam, Tanzania, and scoring system. *Am Rev Respir Crit Care Med* 1995; **152**: 786–93.
◆19. Pozniak AL, MacLeod GA, Ndlovu D, *et al.* Clinical and radiographic features of tuberculosis associated with human immunodeficiency virus in Zimbabwe. *Am J Respir Crit Care Med* 1995; **152**: 1558–61.
20. Jones BE, Young SM, Antoniskis D, *et al.* Relationship of the manifestations of tuberculosis to CD4 cell counts in patients with human immunodeficiency virus infection. *Am J Respir Crit Care Med* 1993; **148**: 1292–7.
◆21. Valdes L, Alvarez D, San José E, *et al.* Value of adenosine deaminase in the diagnosis of tuberculous pleural effusions in young patients in a region of high prevalence of tuberculosis. *Thorax* 1995; **50**: 600–603.
22. Pérez-Rodriguez E, Ortiz de Saracho J, Sanchez JJ, *et al.* Is adenosine deaminase in pleural effusion an expression of lymphocytic or monocytic activity? *Eur Respir J* 1995; **8**: 309s.
23. Stead W, Eichenholz A, Stauss HK. Operative and pathologic findings in twenty-four patients with syndrome of idiopathic pleurisy with effusion, presumably tuberculous. *Am Rev Tuberc* 1955; **71**: 473–502.
24. Stevenson F. The natural history of pleural effusion and orthopaedic tuberculosis. *J Bone Joint Surg Br* 1955; **37**: 80–91.
25. Torgersen J, Dorman SE, Baruch N, Hooper N, Cronin W. Molecular epidemiology of pleural and other extrapulmonary tuberculosis: a Maryland state review. *Clin Infect Dis* 2006; **42**: 1375–82.
26. Moudgil H, Sridhar G, Leitch AG. Reactivation disease: the commonest form of tuberculosis pleural effusion in Edinburgh,1980–1991. *Respir Med* 1994; **88**: 301–4.
27. Widstrom O, Nilsson BS. Pleurisy induced by intrapleural BCG in immunized guinea pigs. *Eur J Respir Dis* 1982; **63**: 425–34.
28. Okamoto M, Hasegawa Y, Hara T, *et al.* T-helper type 1/T-helper type 2 balance in malignant pleural effusions compared to tuberculosis pleural effusions. *Chest* 2005; **128**: 4030-5.
29. Rossi GA, Balbi B, Manca F. Tuberculous pleural effusions: evidence for a selective presence of PPD-specific T-lymphocytes at site of inflammation in the early phase of the infection. *Am Rev Respir Dis* 1987; **136**: 575–9.
30. Fujiwara H, Okuda Y, Fukakawa T, Tsuyuguchi I. *In vitro* tuberculin reactivity of lymphocytes from patients with tuberculous pleurisy. *Infect Immun* 1982; **35**: 402–9.
31. Baganha FM, Pego A, Lima AA, Gaspar EV, Cordeiro RA. Serum and pleural adenosine deaminase: correlation with lymphocytic populations. *Chest* 1990; **97**: 605–10.
◆32. Pérez-Rodriguez E, Jimenez Castro D. The use of adenosine deaminase isoenzymes in the diagnosis of tuberculous pleuritis. *Curr Opin Pulm Med* 2000; **6**: 259–66.
33. Mohamed KA, Nasreen N, Ward MJ, *et al. Mycobacterium* mediated chemokine expression in pleural mesothelial: role of C–C chemokines in tuberculosis. *J Infect Dis* 1998; **178**: 1450–8.
●34 Mohamed KA, Nasreen N, Ward MJ, *et al.* Helper T cell type 1 and 2 cytokines regulate C–C chemokine expression in mouse pleural mesothelial cells. *Am J Respir Crit Care Med* 1999; **159**: 1653–9.
●35. Nasreen N, Mohammed KA, Ward MJ, Antony VB. *Mycobacterium*-induced transmesothelial migration of monocytes into pleural space: role of intercellular adhesion molecule-1 in tuberculous pleurisy. *J Infect Dis* 1999; **180**: 1616–23.
●36. Pace E, Gjomarkaj M, Melis M, *et al.* Interleukin-8 induces lymphocyte chemotaxis into the pleural space: role of pleural macrophages. *Am J Respir Crit Care Med* 1999; **159**: 1592–9.
37. Park JS, Kim YS, Jee YK, *et al.* Interleukin-8 production in tuberculosis pleurisy: role of mesothelial cells stimulated by cytokine network involving tumor necrosis factor-alpha and interleukine-1beta. *Scand J Immunol* 2003; **57**: 463–9.
38. Light RW. Tuberculous pleural effusions. In: Light RW (ed.). *Pleural diseases*, 3rd edn. Baltimore: Williams and Wilkins, 1995: 154–66.
39. Sahn SA. State of the art: The pleura. *Am Rev Respir Med* 1988; **138**: 184–234.
40. Perez-Rodriguez E, Jimenez Castro D, Gaudo Navarro J. Valoracion diagnostica del derrame pleural. *Rev Clin Esp* 2000; **200**: 74–7.
41. Antony VB, Sahn SA, Antony AC, Repine JE. Bacillus Calmette–Guerin-stimulated neutrophils release chemotaxins for monocytes in rabbit pleural spaces and *in vitro. J Clin Invest* 1985; **76**: 1514–21.
◆42. Kitinya JN, Richter C, Perenboom R, *et al.* Influence of HIV status on pathological changes in tuberculous pleuritis. *Tuberc Lung Dis* 1994; **75**: 195–8.
43. Law KF, Jagirdar J, Weiden MD, *et al.* Tuberculosis in HIV-positive patients: cellular response and immune activation in the lung. *Am J Respir Crit Care Med* 1996; **153**: 1377–84.
◆44. Riantawan P, Chaowalit P, Wongsangiem M, Rojanaraweewong P. Diagnostic value of pleural fluid adenosine deaminase in tuberculous pleuritis with reference to HIV coinfection and a Bayesian analysis. *Chest* 1999; **116**: 97–103.
45. Sibley JC. A study of 200 cases of tuberculous pleurisy with effusion. *Am Rev Tuberc* 1950; **62**: 314–23.
46. Roper W, Waring JJ. Primary serofbrinous pleural effusion in military personnel. *Am Rev Tuberc* 1955; **71**: 616–34.
◆47. Aktogu S, Yorgancioglu A, Cirak K, Kose T, Dereli SM. Clinical spectrum of pulmonary and pleural tuberculosis: a report of 5480 cases. *Eur Respir J* 1996; **9**: 2031–5.
48. Berger HW, Mejia E. Tuberculous pleurisy. *Chest* 1973; **63**: 88–92.
49. Chan C, Arnold M, Chan CY, Mak T, *et al.* Clinical and pathological features of tuberculous pleural effusion and its long-term consequences. *Respiration* 1991; **58**: 171–5.
50. Barnes PF, Bloch AB, Davidson PT, Snider DE. Tuberculosis in patients with human immunodeficiency virus infection. *N Engl J Med* 1991; **324**: 1644–50.
◆51. Richter C, Perenboom R, Mtoni I, *et al.* Clinical features of HIV-seropositive and HIV-seronegative patients with tuberculous pleural effusion in Dar es Salaam. Tanzania. *Chest* 1994; **106**: 1471–5.
◆52. Arriero JM, Romero S, Hernandez L, *et al.* Tuberculous pleurisy with or without radiographic evidence of pulmonary disease. Is there any difference? *Int J Tuberc Lung Dis* 1998; **2**: 513–17.
53. Light RW, Erozan YS, Ball WC. Cells in pleural fluid. Their value in differential diagnosis. *Arch Intern Med* 1973; **132**: 854–60.
◆54. Diaz Nuevo G, Jimenez Castro D, Perez-Rodriguez E, Prieto Yaya E, Sueiro Bendito A. Pleural eosinophilia: its diagnostic and prognostic significance. *Rev Clin Esp* 1999; **199**: 573–5.
55. Spriggs AI, Boddington MM. Absence of mesothelial cells from tuberculous pleural effusions. *Thorax* 1960; **15**: 169–71.
56. Kim HJ, Lee HJ, Kwon SY, *et al.* The prevalence of pulmonary parenchymal tuberculosis in patients with tuberculous pleuritis.*Chest* 2006; **129**: 1253–8.
57. Porcel JM, Vives M. Etiology and pleural fluid characteristics of large and massive effusions. *Chest* 2003; **124**: 978–83.
58. Gil Montoro D, Perez-Rodriguez E, de Francisco G, *et al.* Derrames pleurales masivos: incidencia y significado en 1098 casos. *Rev Patol Respir* 2001; **4**: 67–70.
59. Joseph J, Strange C, Sahn SA. Pleural effusions in hospitalized patients with AIDS. *Ann Intern Med* 1993; 118: 856–9.
60. Navio P, Jimenez D, Pérez-Rodriguez E, *et al.* Atypical locations of

pulmonary tuberculosis and the influence of the roentgenographic patterns and sample type in its diagnosis: *Respiration* 1997; **64**: 296–9.
61. Farman DP, Speir WA Jr. Initial roentgenographic manifestations of bacteriologically proven *Mycobacterium tuberculosis*. Typical or atypical? *Chest* 1986; **89**: 75–7.
62. Jimenez Castro D, Díaz Nuevo G, Izquierdo Alonso JL, Pérez-Rodriguez E. Valor diagnóstico de presunción en los derrames pleurales. *Rev Patol Respir* 2001; **4**: 5–8.
◆63. Ferrer J. Pleural tuberculosis. *Eur Respir J* 1997; **10**: 942–7.
◆64. Morehead RS. Tuberculosis of the pleura. *South Med J* 1998; **91**: 630–6.
65. Conde MB, Loivos AC, Rezende VM, *et al.* Yield of sputum induction in the diagnosis of pleural tuberculosis. *Am J Respir Crit Care Med* 2003; **167**: 723–5.
66. Antoniskis D, Amin K, Barnes P. Pleuritis as a manifestation of reactivation tuberculosis. *Am J Med* 1990; **89**: 447–50.
67. Maertens G, Bateman ED. Tuberculous pleural effusions: Increased culture yield with beside inoculation of pleural fluid and poor diagnostic value of adenosine deaminase. *Thorax* 1991; **46**: 96–9.
68. Kirsch CM, Kroe DM, Azzi RL, *et al.* The optimal number of pleural biopsy specimens for a diagnosis of tuberculous pleurisy. *Chest* 1997; **112**: 702–6.
◆69. Valdes L, Alvarez D, San José E, *et al.* Tuberculous pleurisy: a study of 254 patients. *Arch Intern Med* 1998; **158**: 2017–21.
70. Jimenez D, Perez-Rodriguez E, Diaz G, Fogue L, Light RW. Determining the optimal number of specimens to obtain with needle biopsy of the pleura. *Respir Med* 2002; **96**: 14–17.
71. Maartens G, Bateman ED. Tuberculous pleural effusions: Increased culture yield with beside inoculation of pleural fluid and poor diagnostic value of adenosine deaminase. *Thorax* 1991; **46**: 96–9.
72. Schluger NW, Rom WN. Current approaches to the diagnosis of active pulmonary tuberculosis. *Am J Respir Crit Care Med* 1994; **149**: 264–7.
73. Schirm J, Oostendorp LA, Mulder JG. Comparison of Amplicor, in-house PCR, and conventional culture for detection of *Mycobacterium tuberculosis* in clinical samples. *J Clin Microbiol* 1995; **33**: 3221–4.
74. Bennedsen J, Thomsen VO, Pfyffer GE, *et al.* Utility of PCR in diagnosing pulmonary tuberculosis. *J Clin Microbiol* 1996; **34**: 1407–11.
75. Nagesh BS, Sehgal S, Jindal SK, Arora SK. Evaluation of polymerase chain reaction for detection of *Mycobacterium tuberculosis* in pleural fluid. *Chest* 2001; **119**: 1737–41.
◆76. Querol JM, Minguez J, Garcia Sanchez E, *et al.* Rapid diagnosis of pleural tuberculosis by polymerase chain reaction. *Am J Respir Crit Care Med* 1995; **152**: 1977–81.
77. Villena V, Rebollo MJ, Aguado JM, *et al.* Polymerase chain reaction for the diagnosis of pleural tuberculosis in immunocompromised and immunocompetent patients. *Clin Infect Dis* 1998; **26**: 212–14.
●78. Piras MA, Gakis G, Budroni M, Andreoni G. Adenosine deaminase activity in pleural effusions: an aid to differential diagnosis. *Br Med J* 1978; **2**: 1751–2.
◆79. Burgess LJ, Maritz FJ, Le Roux I, Talijaard JJ. Combined use of pleural adenosine deaminase with lymphocyte/neutrophil ratio. Increased specificity for the diagnosis of tuberculous pleuritis. *Chest* 1995; **109**: 414–19.
◆80. Valdes L, San José E, Alvarez D, *et al.* Diagnosis of tuberculous pleurisy using the biologic parameters adenosine deaminase, lysozyme and interferon gamma. *Chest* 1993; **103**: 458–65.
◆81. Valdes L, San José E, Alvarez D, Valle JM. Adenosine deaminase (ADA) isoenzyme analysis in pleural effusion: diagnostic role, relevance to the origin of increased ADA in tuberculous pleurisy. *Eur Respir J* 1996; **9**: 747–75.
82. Bañales JL, Pineda PR, Fitzgerald JM, *et al.* Adenosine deaminase in the diagnosis of tuberculosis pleural effusions. A report of 218 patients and review of the literature. *Chest* 1991; **99**: 355–7.
83. Segura RM, Pascual C, Ocaña I, *et al.* Adenosine deaminase in body fluids: a useful diagnostic tool in tuberculosis. *Clin Biochem* 1989; **22**: 141–8.
84. Ocaña I, Martinez Vazquez JM, Segura RM, Fernandez de Sevilla T, Capdevila JA. Adenosine deaminase in pleural fluid: test for diagnosis of tuberculous pleural effusion. *Chest* 1983; **84**: 51–3.
85. Perez-Rodriguez E, Ortiz de Caracho J, Sanchez JJ, *et al.* Pleural adenosine deaminase (ADAp) and its iso-enzymes in tuberculous effusions. *Eur Respir J* 1995; **8**: 554s.
86. De Oliveira HG, Rossatto ER, Prolla JC. Pleural fluid adenosine deaminase and lymphocyte proportion: clinical usefulness in the diagnosis of tuberculosis. *Cytopathology* 1994; **5**: 27–32.
●87. Blake J. Berman P. The use of adenosine deaminase assays in the diagnosis of tuberculosis. *S Afr Med J* 1982; **62**: 19–21.
88. Maritz FJ, Malan C, Le Roux I. Adenosine deaminase estimations in the differentiation of pleural effusions. *S Afr Med J* 1982; **62**: 556–8.
89. Ferrer JS, Muñoz XG, Orriols RM, Light RW, Morell FB. Evolution of idiopathic pleural effusion: a long-term follow-up study. *Chest* 1996; **109**: 1508–13.
●90. Gakis C. Adenosine deaminase (ADA) isoenzymes ADA1 and ADA2: diagnostic and biological role. *Eur Respir J* 1996; **9**: 632–3.
◆91. Perez-Rodriguez E, Perez-Walton IJ, Sanchez Hernandez JJ, *et al.* ADA1/ADAp ratio in pleural tuberculosis: an excellent diagnostic parameter in pleural fluid. *Respir Med* 1999; **93**: 816–21.
92. Inase N, Tominaga S, Yasui M, *et al.* Adenosine deaminase 2 in the diagnosis of tuberculous pleuritis. *Kekkaku* 2005; **80**: 731–4.
93. Miller KD, Barnette R, Light RW. Stability of adenosine deaminase during transport. *Chest* 2004; **126**: 1933–7.
94. Villena V, Lopez-Encuentra A, Echave-Sustaeta J, *et al.* Interferon-gamma in 388 immunocompromised and immunocompetent patients for diagnosing pleural tuberculosis. *Eur Respir J* 1996; **9**: 2635–9.
95. Moriwaki Y, Kohjiro N, Itoh M, *et al.* Discrimination of tuberculous from carcinomatous pleural effusion by biochemical markers: adenosine deaminase, lysozyme, fibronectin and carcinoembryobnic antigen. *Jpn J Med* 1989; **28**: 478–84.
96. Yew WW, Chan CY, Kwan S, Cheung SW, French GL. Diagnosis of tuberculosis pleural effusions by the detection of tubercolostearic acid in pleural aspirates. *Chest* 1991; **100**: 1261–3.
97. Muranishi H, Nakashima M, Hirano H, *et al.* Simultaneous measurements of adenosine deaminase activity and tuberculostearic acid in pleural effusions for the diagnosis of tuberculous pleuritis. *Intern Med* 1992; **31**: 752–5.
98. Van Vooren JP, Farber CM, De Bruyn J, Yernault JC. Antimycobacterial antibodies in pleural effusion. *Chest* 1990; **97**: 88–90.
99. Hara N, Abe M, Inuzuka S, Kawarada Y, Shigematsu N. Pleural SC5b-9 in differential diagnosis of tuberculous, malignant and other effusions. *Chest* 1992; **102**: 1060–64.
100. Barnes PF, Lu S, Abrams JS, *et al.* Cytokine production at the site of disease in human tuberculosis. *Infect Immun* 1993; **61**: 3482–9.
101. Zhang M, Gately MK, Wang E, *et al.* Interleukin 12 at the site of disease in tuberculosis. *J Clin Invest* 1994; **93**: 1733–9.
102. Laniado-Laborin R. Adenosine deaminase in the diagnosis of tuberculosis pleural effusion: is it really an ideal test? A word of caution. *Chest* 2005; **127**: 417–18.
103. Diacon AH, Van de Wal BW, Wyser C, *et al.* Diagnostic tools in tuberculosis pleurisy: a direct comparative study. *Eur Respir J* 2003; **22**: 589–91.
104. Sakuraba M, Masuda K, Hebisawa A, Sagara Y, Komatsu H. Thoracoscopic pleural biopsy for tuberculosis pleurisy under local anesthesia. *Ann Thorac Cardiovasc Surg* 2006; **12**: 245–8
105. Small PM, Fujiwara PI. Medical progress: Management of tuberculosis in the United States. *New Engl J Med* 2001; **345**: 189–200.
106. Bass JB, Farer LS, Hopewell PC, *et al.* Treatment of tuberculosis and tuberculosis infection in adults and children. *Am J Respir Crit Care Med* 1994; **149**: 1359–74.

107. Joint Tuberculosis Committee of the British Thoracic Society. Chemotherapy and management of tuberculosis in the United Kingdom: recommendations 1998. *Thorax* 1998; **53**: 536–48.

◆108. Dutt AK, Moers D, Stead WW. Tuberculous pleural effusion: 6-month therapy with isoniazid and rifampin. *Am Rev Respir Dis* 1992; **145**: 1429–32.

◆109. Cañete C, Galarza I, Granados A, *et al.* Tuberculous pleural effusion: experience with six months of treatment with isoniazide and rifampicin. *Thorax* 1994; **49**: 1160–61.

110. Ormerod LP, McCarthy OR, Rudd RM, Horsfield N. Short-course chemotherapy for tuberculous pleural effusion and culture-negative pulmonary tuberculosis. *Tuberc Lung Dis* 1995; **76**: 25–7.

111. Al-Majed SA. Study of paradoxical response to chemotherapy in tuberculous pleural effusion. *Respir Med* 1996; **90**: 211–14.

112. Prevention and treatment of tuberculosis among patients infected with human immunodeficiency virus: principles of therapy and revised recommendations. *MMWR Morb Mortal Wkly Rep* 1998; **47**: 1–58.

113. Zumla A, Malon P, Henderson J, Grange JM. Impact of HIV infection on tuberculosis. *Postgrad Med J* 2000; **76**: 259–68.

◆114. Matchaba PT, Volmink J. Steroids for treating tuberculous pleurisy. *Cochrane Database Syst Rev* 2000; **2**: CD001876.

115. Lee CH, Wang WJ, Lan RS, *et al.* Corticosteroids in the treatment of tuberculous pleurisy: a double-blind, placebo-controlled, randomized study. *Chest* 1988; **94**: 1256–9.

116. Galarza I, Cañete C, Granados A, Estopa R, Manresa F. Randomised trial of corticosteroids in the treatment of tuberculous pleurisy. *Thorax* 1995; **50**: 1305–307.

117. Lai YF, Chao TY, Wang YH, Lin AS. Pigtail drainage in the treatment of tuberculous pleural effusions: a randomized study. *Thorax* 2003; **58**: 149–51.

118. Cases Viedma E, Lorenzo Dus MJ, Gonzalez-Molina A, Sanchis Aldas JL. A study of loculated tuberculous pleural effusions treated with intrapleural urokinase. *Respir Med* 2005; **100**: 2037–42.

119. Fujiwara T, Kasahara H, Tanohata K, Nagase M. Fast spin-echo MR imaging of non-Hodgkin lymphoma arising from chronic tuberculous empyema. *J Thorac Imaging* 1995; **10**: 82–4.

120. Takanami I, Imamura T, Morota N, Kodaira S. Malignant fibrous histiocytoma of the chest wall developing after pleuropneumonectomy performed for tuberculous pyothorax: report of an unusual case. *J Thorac Cardiovasc Surg* 1994: **108**: 395–6.

◆121. de Pablo A, Villena V, Echave Sustaeta J, Encuentra A. Are pleural fluid parameters related to the development of residual pleural thickening in tuberculosis? *Chest* 1997; **112**: 1293–7.

122. Barbas CS, Cukier A, de Varvalho CR, Barbas-Filho JV, Light RW. The relationship between pleural fluid findings and the development of pleural thickening in patients with pleural tuberculosis. *Chest* 1991; **100**: 1264–7.

123. Flores J, Pérez-Rodriguez E, Ferrando C, *et al.* Parámetros no terapéuticos que definen el pronóstico de la tuberculosis pleural. *Arch Bronconeumol* 1993; **29**: 104–105.

124. Lawn SD, Evans AJ, Sedgwick PM, Acheampong JW. Pulmonary tuberculosis: radiological features in west Africans coinfected with HIV. *Br J Radiol* 1999; **72**: 339–44.

125. Candela A, Andujar J, Hernandez L, *et al.* Functional sequelae of tuberculous pleurisy in patients correctly treated. *Chest* 2003; **123**: 1996–2000.

126. Jenssen AO. Chronic calcified pleural empyema. *Scand J Respir Dis* 1969; **50**: 19–27.

127. Elliot AM, Berning SE, Iseman M, Peloquin CA. Failure of drug penetration and acquisition of drug resistance in chronic tuberculous empyema. *Tuberc Lung Dis* 1995; **76**: 463–7.

128. Ali S, Siddiqui A, McLaughlin J. Open drainage of massive tuberculous empyema with progressive reexpansion of the lung: an old concept revisited. *Ann Thorac Surg* 1996; **62**: 218–24.

◆129. Mushegera CK, Mbuyi Muamba JM, Kabemba MJ. Indications and results of pleuropulmonary decortications in the university hospital of Kinshasa. *Acta Chir Belg* 1996; **96**: 217–22.

130. Neihart RE, Hof DG. Successful nonsurgical treatment of tuberculous empyema in an irreducible pleural space. *Chest* 1985; **88**: 792–4.

131. Peterson MW, Austin JH, Yip CK, McManus RP, Jaretzki A. CT findings in transdiaphragmatic empyema necessitatis due to tuberculosis. *J Comput Assist Tomogr* 1987; **11**: 704–6.

132. Ip M, Chen NK, So SY, Chiu SW, Lam WK. Unusual rib destruction in pleuropulmonary tuberculosis. *Chest* 1989; **95**: 242–4.

133. Guest JL Jr, Anderson JN, Simmons EM Jr. Dumbbell granulomatous abscess of the chest wall following needle biopsy of the pleura. *South Med J* 1976; **69**: 1513–15.

28

Effusions from infections: atypical infections

LISETE R TEIXEIRA, FRANCISCO S VARGAS

FUNGI

Pleural disease associated with fungal infection represents less than 1 percent of all pleural effusions.[1]

Candidiasis

Candida sp. is the most common pathogen in fungal pleural empyema (Figure 28.1); the species known as *albicans* is found in more than 50 percent of cases.[2] Empyema has been reported as a complication of gastropleural fistula, spontaneous esophageal rupture and after chest or abdominal surgeries.[3] Since *Candida* sp. commonly colonize the skin, chest tube drainage or repeated thoracentesis after inadequate aseptic procedures predisposes to fungal infection.[2,3]

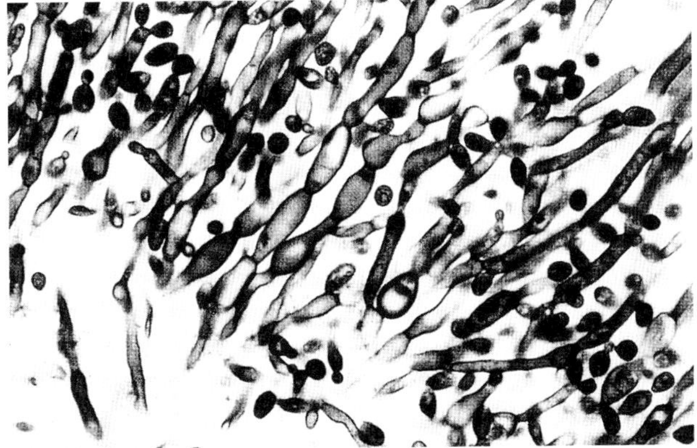

Figure 28.1 Candidiasis: photomicrograph (Groccot stained cytocentrifuge preparation, ×400) showing isolated or clustered pseudohyphae and spores. (See also Color Plate 40.)

The pleural effusion is a yellowish exudate and turbid or frankly purulent with high levels of lactate dehydrogenase (LDH) and low levels of glucose.[1]

Among the several therapeutic options, caspofungin has been suggested to be more effective and less toxic than amphotericin B. The intrapleural instillation of antifungal agents is considered a complementary treatment. In patients with poor control of the infection, decortication can be tried.[4]

Aspergillosis

Tuberculosis, malignant diseases, granulocytopenia and the use of corticosteroids, cytotoxic agents and multiple antibiotics have been implicated in the development of aspergillosis.[5]

The route of the pleural infection is through a bronchopleural or a pleurocutaneous communication. *Aspergillus* can reach the structures adjacent to the pleura, resulting in osseous involvement or the appearance of cutaneous empyema necessitatis.[6]

The pleural effusion is an exudate or an empyema with symptoms of fever, dyspnea, productive cough or haemoptysis.[1] When colonies of hyphae (Figure 28.2) are seen in the pleural fluid or in histological sections (pleural biopsy), a presumptive diagnosis can be made, but it should be confirmed by culture. Immunological tests serve as important aids in the diagnosis, particularly in patients with negative cultures. The detection of circulating antibodies or *Aspergillus* antigens is useful in establishing the etiology.[7] The appearance of pleural empyema with an air–fluid level upon radiological study is indicative of a bronchopleural fistula requiring immediate treatment.[6]

Antifungal drugs and surgery (drainage and resection) should be considered in the treatment of the pleural

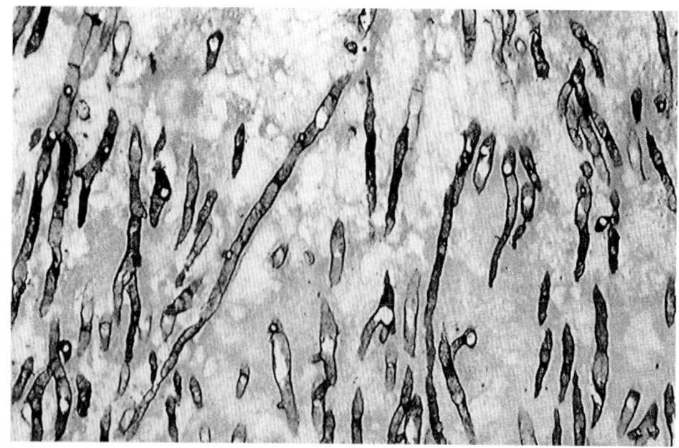

Figure 28.2 Aspergillosis: photomicrograph (Groccot stained cytocentrifuge preparation, ×400) showing a large number of septate hyphae. (See also Color Plate 41.)

effusion. Systemic antifungal agents, such as itraconazole or amphotericin B, produce poor results, because the access to the pleural cavity is difficult. New agents, including oxiconazole, may have therapeutic benefits. Positive results have been achieved with the intrapleural instillation of antifungal agents and the local administration of aerosolized amphotericin B.[6,8]

Surgical decortication or pleuropneumonectomy is associated with a high rate of postoperative complications. Another option involves thoracostomy followed by placement of gauze impregnated with amphotericin B.[6,8]

Cryptococcosis

The genus *Cryptococcus* (Figure 28.3) which is found throughout the world, contains many species, but only *Cryptococcus neoformans* is considered a human pathogen, and rarely produces pleural effusions.[9] Some predisposing conditions are: malignant lymphoma, diabetes mellitus, renal failure, treatment with immunosuppressive drugs and acquired immune deficiency syndrome (AIDS).[10]

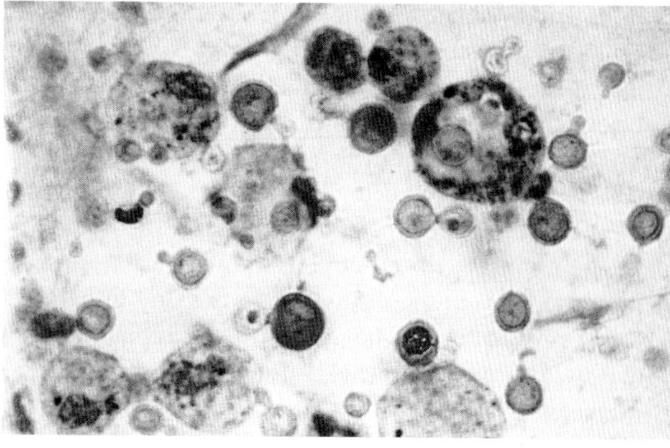

Figure 28.3 Cryptococcosis: photomicrograph (hematoxylin and eosin stained cytocentrifuge preparation, ×400) showing a large number of fungi inside the macrophages. (See also Color Plate 42.)

The organism is usually found in bird excreta that have accumulated over long periods. At least four serotypes (A, B, C and D) with epidemiological differences have been identified. Serotypes A and D are the most common with the highest prevalence of serotype A in Japan, South Asia, Brazil, Australia and Southern California.[7]

The respiratory tract is thought to be the major portal of entry for *C. neoformans*, but most cases of pulmonary infection go unrecognized because they are mild or asymptomatic. The rare pleural involvement appears to occur from extension of a subpleural pulmonary cryptoccocal nodule into the pleural space.[7,11]

The effusion, usually unilateral, may vary in size and is associated with underlying lung parenchymal lesions, interstitial infiltrates, masses, alveolar consolidation and lymphadenopthy. The pleural fluid is an exudate, frankly bloody or serosanguinous. In approximately 50 percent of cases, the lymphocytes are the predominant cells. Culture of the fluid is positive in about half of the patients; in the remaining cases, the diagnosis is made by histological study, culture of lung tissue or identification of cryptococcal antigen in the blood, pleural fluid or cerebrospinal fluid.[11]

Serious underlying illness is frequently present. Cryptococcal pleural effusion most commonly occurs in patients with associated diseases such as AIDS, leukemia or lymphoma. It is also observed in patients who have received a transplant or who are being treated with corticosteroids and/or immunosuppressant drugs, which depress the immune response.[11] Patients with pleural cryptococcosis are candidates for therapy with amphotericin B and/or fluconazole.[7,11]

Coccidioidomycosis

Coccidioidomycosis is caused by the fungus *Coccidioides immitis*, endemic in certain areas of the Americas. However, the number of cases has been increasing due to tourism and turnover of military personnel.[12,13]

Coccidioidomycosis is acquired by inhalation of spores, the incubation period is usually 10–16 days and approximately 60 percent of infections are asymptomatic.[12–14]

The symptoms are self-limited (flu-like illness) with recovery after 3–6 weeks. Hematogenous dissemination tends to occur in patients with underlying diseases.[12,14]

Pleural effusion has been reported in 7–20 percent of symptomatic cases. Effusions are usually left-sided and rarely on the right or bilateral. Generally, they are small and clear completely in a few days. In approximately 2 percent of cases the effusion is large, clearing in several weeks or persisting for more than 1 year. In approximately 50 percent of patients, a pulmonary infiltrate is observed;

adenopathy is seen in 20 percent of cases. The cause of the pleural effusion may be the contiguous spread of infection from pneumonia, the rupture of a subpleural granuloma, or an immune complex pleuritis in response to coccidioidal antigen.[12,15]

The pleural fluid is exudative with no other relevant biochemical findings. The fluid nucleated cell count is usually less than 10 000/mL with a predominance of mononuclear cells; eosinophilia is rare (<7 percent). The diagnosis is made by culture, serology and/or skin testing. The pleural biopsy may reveal the presence of granulomas, sometimes with caseation; however, culture of the biopsy is the most sensitive test, with yields approaching 100 percent. Pleural fluid cultures are positive in only about 20 percent patients and sputum culture in fewer than 15 percent of cases.[12,15]

Chronic or residual pleural effusion is seen in about 3 percent of cases. The pleural effusion ranges from slight to massive occupying the entire hemithorax; it may clear after many months. Empyema may follow the pleural effusion or may result from rupture of a chronic pulmonary lesion.[12]

Specific local management of patients that have pleural effusions is not required, empyema should be submitted to a chest tube drainage. Medical treatment consists of the administration of amphotericin B or the azoles (euconazole or itraconazole). Fluconazole is effective in 55 percent of the patients. Exceptionally, surgical lung resection should be considered to prevent the rupture of a cavity into the pleural space.[13]

Histoplasmosis

The etiological agent *Histoplasma capsulatum* is a dimorphic fungus, whose growth is favored in warm humid soils containing high concentrations of chicken, pigeon or bat feces. It is an endemic mycosis in certain areas of America, East Asia, Oceania, Africa and in the Middle-East. In Europe, the sporadic cases reported in Italy, German, France, Greece and Switzerland were imported from the endemic areas.[16]

Histoplasmosis is acquired through inhalation of airborne spores and is almost never transmitted from person to person. The granulomatous inflammatory response to *H. capsulatum* in immunocompetent hosts generally resolves the infection over several weeks.[17]

The clinical pulmonary forms are: (1) acute; (2) chronic and (3) progressive. Approximately 90 percent of the acute pulmonary infections are asymptomatic. Most clinically apparent acute pulmonary infections are mild-to-moderate in severity, with non-specific symptoms. Chronic pulmonary disease, which often mimics tuberculosis, occurs almost exclusively in patients with underlying severe chronic obstructive pulmonary disease. Progressive disseminated pulmonary histoplasmosis occurs commonly among infants and immunocompromised adults.[16]

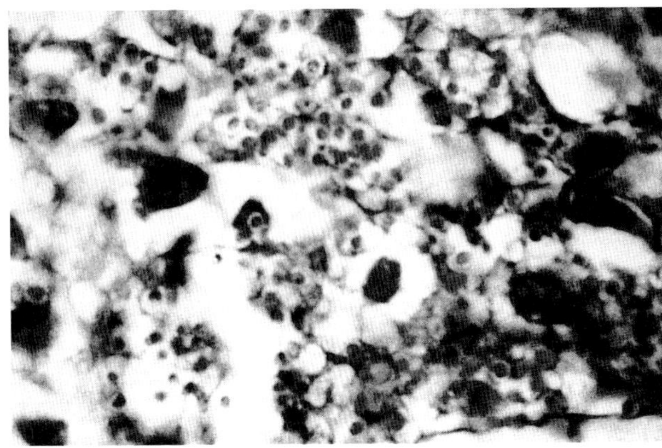

Figure 28.4 Histoplasmosis: photomicrograph(hematoxylin and eosin stained cytocentrifuge preparation,×400) showing a large number of fungi inside the giant cells. (See also Color Plate 43.)

The *H. capsulatum* organism (Figure 28.4) rarely (1–5.7 percent of patients) produces a pleural effusion, but when it does it is generally unilateral and small. The effusion is caused by contiguous spread from the lung parenchyma, by hematogenous spread or by simultaneous pericardial infection. Pleural involvement is associated with an inflammatory response as a result of hypersensitivity to a *H. capsulatum* antigen. The final result is the development of a pleural effusion.[16,18,19]

Associated symptoms of pleuritis include chest pain, fever, anorexia and malaise. The pleural fluid is exudative, characterized by a high protein concentration with a predominance of lymphocytes.[18,19]

Definitive diagnosis requires growth of the fungus: cultures, serological tests and antigen detection. Serological tests are important because of the difficulty in detecting the organism. Antigen detection in serum and urine with radioimmunoassay is useful in immunocompromised patients.[17]

In the normal host, the pleural effusion is self-limited and generally resolves without specific therapy. However, slow resolution, fungal empyema, bronchopleural fistula and extensive pleural fibrosis requiring pleurectomy have also been observed. Medical treatment includes antifungal drugs and corticosteroids.[18,19]

Blastomycosis

Human blastomycosis, caused by *Blastomyces dermatitidis*, occurs principally in the Ohio and Mississipi River valleys, USA. Although the disease is commonly known as North American blastomycosis, it has been reported from other continents.[7]

The respiratory tract is the portal of entry in pulmonary blastomycosis, clinically characterized by fever, chills, cough and pleuritic chest pain. Although pleural thickening is common (88 percent), pleural effusion is rare (2–15 percent).[7,17,20] The pleural fluid is an exudate with a high level of protein with a mix of lymphocytes and neutrophils. A cytological examination showing the characteristic yeast forms is considered diagnostic. However, the usual method for diagnosis is culture, which takes 2–6 weeks. The accuracy of the pleural biopsy is around 59 percent.[1,20]

The South American blastomycosis, caused by *Paracoccidioides brasiliensis* rarely causes pleural effusion. Anecdotal cases have been reported, the pleural effusions may be unilateral or bilateral with a small amount of fluid.[21]

The treatment includes antifungal drugs and trimethoprim–sulfamethoxazole.[20,21]

Sporotrichosis

Sporotrichosis is caused by the fungus *Sporothrix schenckii,* which is found in decaying vegetation, sphagnum moss and soil. The usual mode of infection is by cutaneous inoculation of the organism. Infection can be related to zoonotic spread from infected cats or scratches from digging animals.[22]

Extracutaneous manifestations are unusual. Pulmonary sporotrichosis has rarely been reported; when present, it simulates tuberculosis.[22] Morissey and Caso[23] described a case of a pleural exudate with fungus stains positive for *S. schenkii.* Examination of the pleura revealed noncaseating granulomas. Cultures of fluid and pleural tissue were negative for mycobacteria.

Treatment includes local measures (hyperthermia), solution of potassium iodide, azoles, polyenes and allylamines.[22]

BACTERIA

Actinomyces or *Nocardia*

Pleural disease caused by *Actinomyces* (anaerobic) or *Nocardia* (aerobic) often resembles the disease caused by mycobacteria or fungi.

Actinomycosis

Human actinomycosis is caused mainly by *Actinomyces israelii,* a normal commensal of the oropharynx. The thoracic infection is caused by aspiration associated with periodontitis or following dental procedures. Alcohol abuse may increase the risk because it increases the likelihood of aspiration.[24]

Thoracic actinomycosis is more common among males, mainly during the fifth and sixth decades of life. The lung lesion is suppurative with necrosis and abscess formation. The prevalence of pleural effusion is between 50 and 80 percent.[24,25]

The clinical picture is similar to that observed in tuberculosis or fungal infections. The chest radiograph shows an infiltrative consolidation with multiple cavities associated to pleural thickening or effusion. Nowadays destruction of ribs or vertebrae is uncommon and sinus tracts of the chest wall are rarely seen.[24,25]

The pleural fluid is exudative with a predominance of lymphocytes or an empyema with a predominance of polymorphonuclear leukocytes. Sulfur granules in the pleural fluid are strongly suggestive of actinomycosis (Figure 28.5). The granules are yellow-white on inspection and appear as irregular masses of branched, Gram-positive filaments.[1,25] The fluid is an important source for isolation of the organisms; it should be Gram-stained and cultured anaerobically. Video-assisted thoracic surgery (VATS) seems to be the most effective diagnostic method.[24]

The local management of the pleural effusion includes tube thoracostomy if the fluid is an empyema; decortication is sometimes necessary. The specific treatment consists of prolonged administration of high doses of antibiotics.[1,24]

Nocardiosis

Nocardiosis is usually caused by *Nocardia asteroides,* a Gram-positive aerobic bacteria. Other pathogenic human species include *Nocardia brasiliensis* and *Nocardia caviae.*[9]

Nocardia species are not human commensals; their presence in the upper respiratory tract should be considered as evidence of infection. They produce an acute, subacute or chronic pneumonia.[9,26]

The signs and symptoms of nocardiosis include anorexia, weight loss, dyspnea, cough with purulent sputum and occasionally hemoptysis. The presence of pleuritic pain suggests pleural involvement. Patients with pleural disease (25–50 percent of cases) usually have parenchymal infiltrates and cavitation.[9,27]

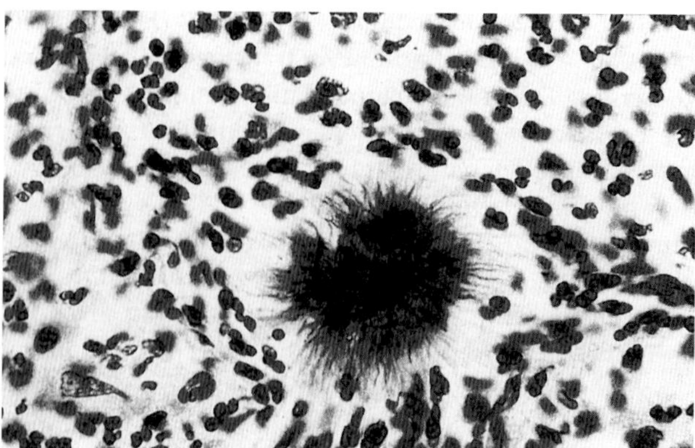

Figure 28.5 Actinomycosis: photomicrograph (hematoxylin and eosin stained cytocentrifuge preparation, ×400) showing sulfur granules. (See also Color Plate 44.)

The pleural fluid ranges from a serous exudate to frank pus. When *Nocardia* are not identified in pleural effusion, bronchoscopy provides material for identification.[28] The organism is aerobic and easily cultured on blood agar. The presence of *N. asteroides* in the sputum does not mean the presence of pulmonary disease; 45 percent of patients with positive culture did not have radiographic abnormalities. If nocardiosis is suspected clinically, transbronchial biopsy, percutaneous lung aspiration, needle biopsy or open lung biopsy must be performed.[27]

Sulfonamides or trimethoprim–sulfamethoxazole are the drugs of choice. The antibiotics are used in conjunction with appropriate surgical management of the pleural effusion.[9,26]

Chlamydiae and Rickettsiae

These organisms are grouped together because of their small size, the association with eukaryotic cells and the similarity of identification techniques.

The Chlamydiae are among the more common pathogens. Although recently the Chlamydiae have been related to multiple diseases, including respiratory infections, an extensive search in Medline did not reveal any report of pleural effusion.

The order Rickettsiales includes a very diverse group of microorganisms. Recent characterizations at the molecular level demonstrate a relationship between the genera *Coxiella* and *Rickettsia*, excluded from this classification is the genus *Ehrlichlia*.[7]

Q FEVER

Q fever is caused by the rickettsial agent *Coxiella burnetti*. It is acquired by the inhalation of contaminated dust particles or by drinking infected and unpasteurized milk.[7] Half of patients do not exhibit any respiratory symptoms and one-third have pleuritic chest pain.[29]

Pleural effusion is usually small and found in 10–35 percent of patients. The fluid is a mononuclear exudate, although on occasion there has been an eosinophilic effusion. The related increase of adenosine deaminase (ADA) activity is probably due to the lymphocytic activation. The diagnosis is established by demonstrating a positive *C. burnetti* complement fixation reaction. The treatment of choice is tetracycline or its derivatives (minocycline and doxycicline).[1,29]

ROCKY MOUNTAIN SPOTTED FEVER

The causative agent is *Rickettsia rickettsii*, which is acquired by humans through a tick bite. The reports of pleural effusions are restricted to the south-eastern and coastal Atlantic states of North America. The clinical picture manifests 5–7 days after the contact and is characterized by the triad of fever, rash and a history of tick exposition. Pleural effusion and pulmonary infiltrate are present in 10–36 percent of patients. The pleural and lung lesions are probably due to vasculitis with increased permeability of the capillaries. The characteristics of the pleural fluid have not been well-defined. The treatment of choice is doxycycline.[1,30]

Ehrlichiosis

There are two human ehrlichial diseases: a monocytic disease caused by *Ehrlichia chaffeensis* and a granulocytic disease caused by *Anaplasma phagocytophilum*. The disease is not uncommon.The symptoms begin 7 days after a tick bite and are characterized by high fever, headache, myalgias, nausea, vomiting and anorexia. Monoclonal antibodies have been used to detect the organism.[31]

Pulmonary infiltrates and a pleural effusion develop in approximately 50 percent of patients. The infiltrates probably represent non-cardiogenic pulmonary edema with a pathogenesis similar to the hantavirus syndrome. The treatment of choice is tetracycline or doxycycline.[1,31]

Mycoplasma pneumoniae

The organism is a small bacterium derived from ancestral anaerobic bacteria (clostridia). Bronchopneumonia involving one or more lobes develops in 3–10 percent of infected patients.[32] Pleural effusion, generally small, occurs in 5–20 percent of patients; empyema is a rare complication.[1,33] The pathogenesis of pleural effusion is unclear, but it is speculated that the presence of *M. pneumoniae* DNA may elicit stronger immunological reaction causing lung damage, with interleukin (IL)-8 and IL-18 playing a role in the reaction.[1,33] The diagnosis is established by increasing specific antibody titers or by isolating *M. pneumoniae* from the pleural fluid. The detection of *M. pneumoniae* DNA in throat swab specimens through the application of polymerase chain reaction (PCR) has been found to be a sensitive and specific diagnostic technique and the positive PCR results using pleural fluid samples have been found to be strongly associated with the abnormalities observed on the radiograms.[34]

Macrolides are the drugs of choice. No specific treatment is necessary for pleural effusion; however, a diagnostic thoracentesis should exclude a complicated parapneumonic effusion.[1,33]

PARASITES

Amebiasis

Amebiasis, a parasitic disease caused by *Entamoeba histolytica*, is common in third-world countries. Humans acquire the disease by ingesting the cyst. After the ingestion, the trophozoites develop, colonize the intestine, migrate to the liver and give rise to liver abscess.[1] A solitary rupture into the pleural cavity producing a pleural effusion is much less common than directly into the lungs. The pleural fluid is described as 'chocolate sauce' or 'anchovy paste'.[1,35]

The patients complain of shortness of breath, cough and pleuritic chest pain with an abrupt worsening when a transdiaphragmatic rupture occurs. The chest radiograph shows a small to massive pleural effusion, occasionally with a contralateral mediastinum shift, and elevation of the hemidiaphragm and atelectasis at the base.[1,35]

The diagnosis is confirmed by the pleural fluid appearance and by serological test for amebiasis. Amoebas are seen in the exudative fluid in less than 10 percent of patients.[1,35]

The treatment of choice is metronidazole associated with a therapeutic thoracocentesis or a tube thoracostomy. One-third of patients have a bacterial infection of the pleural space, and should be treated with antibiotics.[1]

Echinococcosis–hydatidosis

Human echinococcosis is caused by three species of *Echinococcus*: *E. granulosus* (producing cystic hydatic in 90 percent of cases), *E. multilocularis* and *E. vogeli*.[7] When feces containing the parasite's eggs are ingested by humans, larvae emerge in the duodenum, enter the blood and lodge in the liver or in the lung. *Echinococcus* has a worldwide distribution; however, it is seen more often in most sheep- and cattle-raising areas.[1]

The organs most commonly affected are the liver and the lungs. Pleural involvement is rare, it may be secondary to hematogenous dissemination of the larvae, however, it usually follows the rupture of a pulmonary or hepatic cyst releasing its contents into the pleural cavity. Since the cyst is not fertile after rupture in about 90 percent of cases, pleural hydatidosis is rare, occurring in less than 10 percent of the episodes. When the cyst ruptures into the pleural space, the patient becomes acutely ill, with chest pain, dyspnea and occasionally goes into shock. In about 50 percent of patients, the rupture occurs simultaneously into the pleural space and into the tracheobronchial tree.[36]

In geographic areas where echinococcosis occurs frequently, the diagnosis is usually apparent from the clinical picture, radiological findings and results of serological and skin tests. In non-endemic areas, where physicians are unfamiliar with echinococcosis, the diagnosis is suspected only after the cytological examination of the pleural fluid with demonstration of echinococcal scoleces. Eosinophils are frequently present in the pleural fluid, unless it becomes secondarily infected.[1,37] The biochemical characteristics of the pleural fluid have not been reported.

In patients with a rupture of a hydatid cyst, a thoracotomy to remove the parasite is recommended. Medical treatment with benzimidazole compounds such as mebendazole or albendazole should be considered as a supplement.[1,36,37]

Paragonimiasis

Paragonimiasis is caused by numerous species of lung flukes, (genus *Paragonimus*). The pulmonary form is the most common presentation of *Paragonimus westermani* and *Paragonimus miyazakii*. It is a food-borne parasitic disease common in southeast Asia.[38]

Humans acquire paragonimiasis by eating undercooked crustaceans contaminated with metacercariae of the worm. After ingestion, the metacercariae hatch in the duodenum and the larval fluke bore through the intestinal wall, enter the peritoneal cavity and travel through the diaphragm to reach the visceral pleura and lung. In the lung, the adult remains for years producing eggs which are expectorated or swallowed and excreted in the stools. Once in water, the eggs turn into ciliated miracidia that infect freshwater snails. Another larval form develops and is liberated as cercariae that penetrate crayfish and crabs. Adult lung flukes can live in the human host for as long as 20 years, highlighting the need for clinicians to be aware of the disease in areas where the disease is not endemic.[1]

In pulmonary paragonimiasis, pleural disease occurs in approximately 60 percent of patients. The pleural involvement is represented in 60 percent by pleural effusion (80 percent unilateral), in 30 percent by hydropneumothorax (half are bilateral) and in 10 percent by pleural thickening. Pleural paragonimiasis should be suspected in oriental patients or in patients who have traveled to the Orient.[1,39]

The diagnosis is made by detecting eggs in sputum, stool, bronchoscopic lavage or biopsy specimens, or by the presence of a positive anti-*Paragonimus* antibody test. The pleural fluid is an eosinophilic exudate with low pH (<7.10), low glucose (<10 mg/dL) and high LDH (>1000 IU/L). The pleural fluid white-cell count is usually less than 2000/mm^3 with marked eosinophilia. The blood and sputum commonly show an elevated number of eosinophils.[1,39,40]

It has been demonstrated that the levels of immunoglobulin (Ig)E and *P. westermani*-specific IgE and IgG immunoglobulins are elevated and higher in the pleural fluid than in the serum, suggesting that these antibodies are produced in the pleural space. Recently, it was demonstrated that interleukin (IL)-5 concentrations in pleural effusions are higher in paragonimiasis than in transudates, empyema, lung cancer or tuberculosis and that these levels are correlated with the percentage of eosinophils in peripheal blood and pleural fluid.[1,39,40]

The drug of choice to treat is praziquantel or bithionol. Pulmonary disease is rarely fatal. Thoracotomy with decortication may be necessary when pleural surfaces are abnormally thickened and penetration of the drugs into the pleural space insufficient to eradicate the infection.[1,39,40]

Trichomoniasis

Three species of *Trichomonas* sp. can parasitize humans: *T. vaginalis* (cause of vaginitis), *T. hominis* (a non-pathogenic protozoan) and *T. tenax (*a rare cause of pulmonary disease, including pleural effusion).[7]

In the few cases of pleural effusion caused by *T. tenax*, the characteristics of the patients are similar: alcohol abusers with poor oral hygiene. Despite its rarity, pleural infection with *Trichomonas* should be considered in high-risk patients such as those with cancer, chronic lung disease and immunosuppression.[41]

The *Trichomonas* species present in the lung or in the pleural fluid are generally part of a mixed microbial flora. Antibiotic therapy should include metronidazole (1.5 g/day) for 10 to 20 days.[7,41]

Loiasis

Human infection by the filarial parasite *Loa loa* is characterized by migratory angioedema and subconjunctival migration of adult parasites. Pulmonary involvement and pleural effusion are rare. The fluid is an eosinophilic exudate with microfilariae. Diethylcarbamazine is used in the loiasis treatment.[42]

VIRUSES

Pleural effusions caused by viral infections tend to be small and self-limiting. For these reasons, in the majority of cases, the fluid is not collected. Moreover, most hospitals are not equipped to perform virus cultures. These facts explain why the effusions are usually not recognized.

Adenovirus

A pleural effusion is observed in approximately 40 percent of patients principally in infections with adenovirus types 3 and 7. The illness is endemic throughout the year and occurs in all age groups although it is more common among school-age children.[43]

The pleural fluid is a paucicellular exudate with a predominance of mononuclear cells. In the acute phase, thoracocentesis may reveal an increased number of polymorphonuclear leukocytes. The diagnosis is established by documenting increasing complement fixation titers or culturing viruses from the fluid. At times, cytological evaluation can be diagnostic of viral infection.[1,43]

Hantavirus

Hantaviruses are members of the genus *Hantavirus*, carried by infected rodents and transmitted to humans who inhale excreta. The person-to-person transmission of *Hantavirus* has been presumed in a few cases. *Hantavirus* causes two different syndromes: the hantavirus pulmonary syndrome (southwestern USA) and the hemorrhagic fever renal syndrome (Asia and Europe).[44]

The largest number of cases of hantavirus pulmonary syndrome has been reported from the 'Four Corners' (New Mexico, Arizona, Utah and Colorado) but there are confirmed cases from all regions of the USA and Canada. The entity results from infection with the named *Muerto Canyon virus* or *Sin Nombre virus* (without name), transmitted to humans via contact with infected deer mice (*Peromyscus maniculatus*). Edema and pleural effusion are common. The effusion may be due to either primary cardiac dysfunction or profound vascular leak.[44]

The pleural fluid can be either a transudate during the initial phase (maximal cardiopulmonary dysfunction), or an exudate (recovery of cardiac function) due to capillary leaks. The chest radiograph shows a normal-sized heart with bilateral infiltrates and the laboratory tests show the triad: thrombocytopenia, a left shift in the myeloid series and large immunoblastoid lymphocytes.[44,45]

Nephropathia epidemica is a similar syndrome caused by a *Hantavirus* called *Puumala hantavirus* which is genetically related to the *Sin Nombre virus.* It is a mild and benign form of hemorrhagic fever with acute renal dysfunction. In contrast to the hantavirus pulmonary syndrome, in nephropathia epidemica the fluid volume overload is related to the renal failure and seems to contribute to the pleural effusion. However, the presence of hypoproteinemia and leukocytosis suggest that capillary leakage and inflammation are also important features.[45]

The specific diagnosis is based on the determination of antibodies for IgM and IgG. The treatment remains supportive; however, it appears that intravenous ribavirin or amantidine are effective. The use of methylprednisolone has been related to a better prognosis.[45]

Cytomegalovirus

Although *Cytomegalovirus* (CMV) and *Pneumocystis carinii* are the most common opportunistic infections in AIDS patients, the presence of a pleural effusion is uncommon. Moreover, CMV-infected cells are rarely identified in the pleural fluid (Figure 28.6). These inclusions have been observed in the mesothelial cells, but they are not specific.[46]

It is not well understood how the CMV infection produces a pleural effusion. It is likely that the infected cells enter into the pleural space through small leaks caused by recurrent pneumothorax, a frequent complication of *P. carinii* pneumonia. It has been suggested that the obstruction of peripheral bronchioles leads to local air trapping with overextension and rupture of the alveoli. This sequence enables cells infected with virus to spread into the pleural space, causing a pleural effusion.[46,47]

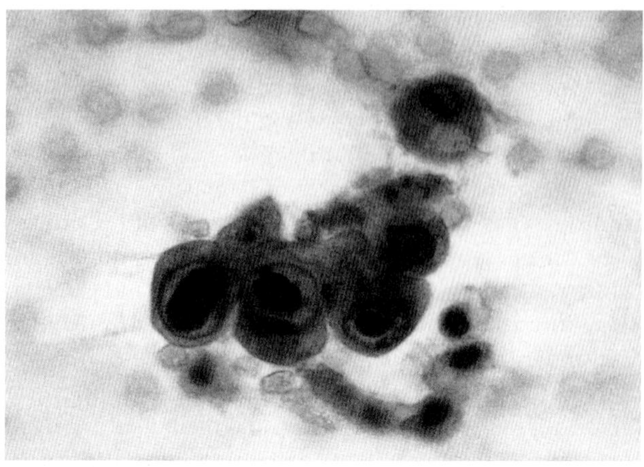

Figure 28.6 *Cytomegalovirus*: photomicrograph (Papanicolaou stained cytocentrifuge preparation, ×400) showing an intranuclear inclusion. (See also Color Plate 45.)

Herpes virus

Pulmonary infection with *Herpes simplex virus* manifests as a pneumonitis, especially in the immunocompromised host. The presence of pleural effusion is uncommon and the isolation of the viruses from the pleural fluid is rarely achieved. The disease has been described predominantly in men with advanced *Human immunodeficiency virus* (HIV) infection. The exudative and lymphocitic pleural effusion shows a characteristic cytomorphological appearance, resembling an immunoblastic not Burkitt or Burkitt-like lymphoma and a clear immunophenotypic indetermination (non-B, non-T-cell).[48]

Hepatitis

Pleural effusion in patients with acute viral hepatitis, is apparently uncommon (1–70 percent).[1] Because most of the patients have right-sided pleural effusion, it could be speculated that it is a local reaction. However, reported cases with bilateral effusion without hypoproteinemia argue against this hypothesis.[49]

The effusion is an exudate with predominance of mononuclear cells, with hepatitis soluble antigens. It is small and predominantly right-sided and does not produce respiratory symptoms.[1]

Mononucleosis

Infectious mononucleosis occurs in older children and adolescents. Pulmonary infiltrates are well recognized but pleural effusion is uncommon.[50] Diagnosis is usually made clinically in conjunction with a positive Monospot; *Epstein–Barr virus* (EBV) serology can be used to confirm the diagnosis.[51]

The pleural effusion is a small or large exudate with a predominance of lymphocytes; empyema has been described. Unilateral or bilateral effusions are seen with approximately equal frequency. Most of the cases resolve spontaneously.[50,51]

Dengue fever

Dengue fever is transmitted to human beings by mosquitoes. The chief characteristic is the increase of the capillary permeability with leakage of plasma. Pleural effusion is common (50–95 percent) and generally is a bilateral small exudate.[1,52]

KEY POINTS

- Pleural diseases caused by atypical infections are uncommon.
- The early diagnosis and treatment are important for infection control.
- The majority of these infections are considered opportunistic infections and are most commonly seen in immunosuppressed patients with AIDS, malignancies or chronic diseases.
- Although pleural fungal infections represent less than 1 percent of all pleural effusions, the identification of these patients is essential for effective treatment.
- A search for the etiological agent is important since mycobacteria, fungi and the higher bacteria (*Actinomyces* and *Nocardia*) produce similar clinical, radiographic and pleural fluid findings.
- The use of appropriate diagnostic tests, including pleural biopsy and serologic techniques, are current approaches to the management of atypical pleural effusions.
- The microbiological study should be carried out in the pleural fluid. The microbiological evaluation of sputum, blood or lung tissue might contribute to the final diagnosis.
- The specific fungi treatment is carried out with the azoles derivatives, specially euconazole or itraconazole or with amphotericin B.
- Pleural effusion secondary to parasitic infections are uncommon in the USA, but not in developing countries.
- A significant fraction of undiagnosed pleural effusions is caused by viral infections.

REFERENCES

● = Key primary paper
◆ = Major review article

1. Light RW. *Pleural diseases*, 5th edn. Baltimore: Lippincott Williams & Wilkins, 2007.
●2. Chen KY, Ko SC, Hsueh PR, *et al.* Pulmonary fungal infection. Emphasis on microbiological spectra, patient outcome, and prognostic factors. *Chest* 2001; **120**: 177–84.
3. Schacherer D, Mayer S, Borisch I, *et al.* Esophagobronchial and esophagomediastinal fistula, pleural and pericardial effusion due to severe pseudodiverticulosis of the esophagus. *Z Gastroenterol* 2006; **44**: 491–5.
4. Mora Duarte J, Betts R, Rotstein C, *et al.* Comparison of caspofungin and amphotericin B for invasive candidiasis. *N Engl J Med* 2002; **347**: 2020–29.
5. Wex P, Utta E, Drozdz W. Surgical treatment of pulmonary and pleuro-pulmonary *Aspergillus* disease. *Thorac Cardiovasc Surg* 1993; **41**: 64–70.
6. Soto-Hurtado EJ, Marín-Gámez E, Segura-Dominguez N, *et al.* Pleural aspergillosis with bronchopleurocutaneous fistula and costal bone destruction: a case report. *Lung* 2005; **183**: 417–23.
7. Murray PR. *Manual of clinical microbiology*, 6th edn. Washington, DC: ASM Press, 1995.
8. Regnard JF, Icard P, Nicolosi M, *et al.* Aspergilloma: A series of 89 surgical cases. *Ann Thorac Surg* 2000; **69**: 898–903.
◆9. George RB, Penn RL, Kinasewitz GT. Mycobacterial, fungal, actinomycotic, and nocardial infections of the pleura. *Clin Chest Med* 1985; **6**: 63–75.
10. Kawabata T, Matsuyama W, Higashimoto I, *et al.* Pleural cryptococcosis with idiopathic CD4 positive T-lymphocytopenia. *Intern Med* 2004; **43**: 977–81.
◆11. Young EJ, Hirsh DD, Fainstein V, *et al.* Pleural effusions due to *Cryptococcus neoformans:* a review of the literature and report of two cases with Cryptococcal antigen determinations. *Am Rev Respir Dis* 1980; **121**: 743–7.
◆12. Batra P. Pulmonary coccidioidomycosis. *J Thorac Imaging* 1992; **7**: 29–38.
13. Osaki T, Morishita H, Maeda H, *et al.* Pulmonary coccidioidomycosis that formed a fungus ball with 8-years duration. *Intern Med* 2005; **44**: 141–4.
14. Chiller TM, Galgiani JN, Stevens DA. Coccidioidomycosis. *Infect Dis Clin North Am* 2003; **17**: 41–57.
15. Mortara L, Bayer AS. Fever, cough, pleuritic chest pain and pleural fluid eosinophilia in a 30-year-old-man. *Chest* 1994; **105**: 918–9.
16. Kapotsis GE, Daniil Z, Malagan K, *et al.* A young male with chest pain, cough and fever. *Eur Respir J* 2004; **24**: 506–9.
17. Fraser RS, Muller NL, Colman N, Pare PD. *Histoplasmosis.* In: *Diagnosis of diseases of the chest*, 4th edn. Philadelphia: W Saunders, 1999: 876–90.
18. Kilburn CD, McKinsey S. Recurrent massive pleural effusion due to pleural, pericardial and epicardial fibrosis in histoplasmosis. *Chest* 1991; **100**: 1715–17.
19. Carter AB, Hunninghake GW. Massive pleural effusion in diffuse granulomatous disease. *Chest* 1997; **112**: 284–8.
20. Alvarez GG, Burns BF, Desjardins M, *et al.* Blastomycosis in a young African man presenting with a pleural effusion. *Can Respir J* 2006; **13**: 441–4.
21. Pellegrino A, De Capriles CH, Magaldi S, *et al.* Case report: Severe juvenile type paracoccidioiidomycosis with hepatitis C. *Am J Trop Med* 2003; **68**: 301–3.
●22. Kauffman CA, Hajjeh R, Chapman R. Practice guidelines for the management of patients with sporotrichosis. *Clin Infect Dis* 2000; **30**: 684–7.
23. Morissey R, Caso R. Pleural sporotrichosis. *Chest* 1983; **84**: 507.
●24. Kobashi Y, Yoshida K, Miyashita N, *et al.* Thoracic actinomycosis with mainly pleural involvement. *J Infect Chemother* 2004; **10**: 172–7.
◆25. Fife TD, Finegold SM, Grennan T. Pericardial actinomycosis: case report and review. *Rev Infect Dis* 1991; **13**: 120–26.
26. Yoshida K, Bandoh S, Fujita J, *et al.* Pyothorax caused by *Nocardia otitidiscaviarum* in a patient with rheumatoid vasculitis. *Intern Med* 2004; **43**: 615–19.
27. Uttamchandani RB, Daikos GL, Reyes RR, *et al.* Nocardiosis in 30 patients with advanced human immunodeficiency virus infection: clinical features and outcome. *Clin Infect Dis* 1994; **18**: 348–53.
28. Toukap NA, Hainaut P, Moreau M, *et al.* Nocardiosis: a rare cause of pleuropulmonary disease in the immunocompromised host. *Acta Clin Belg* 1996; **51**:161–5.
29. Okikamoto N, Asaoka N, Osaki K, *et al.* Clinical features of Q fever pneumonia. *Respirology* 2004; **9**: 278–82.
30. Byrd RP Jr, Vasquez J, Roy TM. Respiratory manifestations of tick-borne diseases in the southeastern United States. *South Med J* 1997; **90**: 1–4.
31. Scully RE, Mark Ej, Neely WF. Human granulocytic ehrlichiosis. Case records of the Massachusetts General Hospital. *N Engl J Med* 2001; **345**: 1627–34.
◆32. Waites KB, Talkington DF. *Mycoplasma pneumonie* and its role as a human pathogen. *Clin Microbiol Rev* 2004; **17**: 697–728.
33. Shuvy M, Rav-Acha M, Izhar U, *et al.* Massive empyema caused by *Mycoplasma pneumoniae* in an adult: a case report. *BMC Infect Dis* 2006; **6**: 18.
34. Narita M, Matsuzono Y, Itakura O, *et al.* Analysis of mycoplasmal pleural effusion by the polymerase chain reaction. *Arch Dis Child* 1998; **78**: 67–9.
35. Kumar R, Dasan B, Choudhury S, *et al.* Hemoptysis demonstrated on Tc99m-sulfur colloid scanning. A rare complication of amoebic liver abscess. *Clin Imaging* 2002; **26**: 296–8.
◆36. Skerrett SJ, Plorde JJ. Parasitic infections of the pleura space. *Semin Respir Med* 1992; **13**: 242–58.
37. Pfefferkorn U, Viehl CT, Barras JP. Rupture hydatid cyst in the right thorax: differential diagnosis to pleural empyema. *Thorac Cardiovasc Surg* 2005; **53**: 250–51.
38. Singh TN, Kananbala S, Devi KS. Pleuropulmonary paragonimiasis mimicking pulmonary tuberculosis – a report of three cases. *Indian J Med Microbiol* 2005; **23**: 131–4.
●39. Mukae H, Taniguchi H, Matsumoto N, *et al.* Clinicoradiologic features of pleuropulmonary paragonimus westermani on Kyusyu Island, Japan. *Chest* 2001; **120**: 514–20.
40. Robertson KB, Janssen WJ, Saint S, *et al.* Clinical problem-solving – the missing piece. *N Engl J Med* 2006; **355**: 1913–18.
41. Lewis KL, Doherty DE, Ribes J, *et al.* Empyema caused by trichomonas. *Chest* 2003; **123**: 291–2.
42. Klion AD, Eisenstein EM, Smirniotopoulos TT, *et al.* Pulmonary involvement in Loiasis. *Am Rev Respir Dis* 1992; **145**: 961–3.
●43. Hong JY, Lee HJ, Piedra PA, *et al.* Lower respiratory tract infections due to adenovirus in hospitalized Korean children: epidemiology, clinical features, and prognosis. *Clin Infect Dis* 2001; **32**: 1423–9.
44. Bustamante EA, Levy H, Simpson SQ. Pleural fluid characteristics in Hantavirus pulmonary syndrome. *Chest* 1997; **112**: 1133–6.
●45. Fabbri M, Maslow MJ. Hantavirus pulmonary syndrome in the United States. *Curr Infect Dis Rep* 2001; **3**: 258–65.
46. Delfs-Jegge S, Dalquen P, Hurwitz N. Cytomegalovirus-infected cells in a pleural effusion from an acquired immunodeficiency syndrome patient. *Acta Cytol* 1994; **38**: 70–72.
47. Beers MF, Sohn M, Swartz M. Recurrent pneumothorax in AIDS patients with pneumocystis pneumonia: A clinicopathological report of three cases and review of the literature. *Chest* 1990; **98**: 266–70.
●48. Nador RG, Cesarman E, Chadburn A, *et al.* Primary effusion lymphoma: a distinct clinicopathologic entity associated with the Kaposi's sarcoma-associated herpes virus. *Blood* 1996; **88**: 645–56.

49. Selimoglu MA, Ziraatci O, Tan H, *et al.* A rare complication of hepatitis A: pleural effusion. *J Emerg Med* 2005; **28**: 229–30.
50. Cloney DL, Kugler JÁ, Donowitz LG, *et al.* Infectious mononucleosis with pleural effusion. *South Med J* 1988; **81**: 1441–2.
51. Chen J, Konstantinopoulos PA, Satyal S, *et al.* Just another simple case of infectious mononucleosis? *Lancet* 2003; **361**: 1182.
52. Avirutnan P, Malasit P, Seliger B. Dengue virus infection of human endothelial cells leads to chemokine production, complement activation and apoptosis. *J Immunol* 1998; **161**: 6338–46.

29

Effusions from lymphatic disruptions

GUNNAR HILLERDAL

DEFINITIONS

Chylus or chyle is lymph coming mainly from the gastrointestinal tract. Except for medium-chained triglycerides, most types of fat will be resorbed into the lymphatics of the intestines and delivered to the general circulation via the thoracic duct. This explains the peculiar composition of chylus with high levels of triglycerides, cholesterol and chylomicrons. The content varies with whether the person is fasting or has just enjoyed a meal rich in calories, i.e. fat. Eating will considerably increase the flow of chylus and its content of fat components.

Chylothorax is the occurrence of chylus in the pleural space and results from leakage of the thoracic duct due to damage of the wall, either by trauma or blockage of the duct with subsequent rupture. The diagnosis is made by analysis of the pleural fluid.

Pseudochylothorax or cholesterol pleurisy is a pleural fluid with a very high content of cholesterol and occurs when a fluid has been present for a long time in the pleural space surrounded by a fibrotic pleura with poor vascularization. There are no chylomicrons in the fluid and usually the level of triglycerides is also low. The cholesterol has been formed in the encapsulated fluid and has no connection with lymphatic vessels or chylus.

Both conditions have a common characteristic: the pleural fluid is usually thick, opalescent, whitish or the colour of café-au-lait or chocolate milk, due to the very high fat content. Apart from that, and the high level of cholesterol, the two conditions have nothing in common.

INCIDENCE AND EPIDEMIOLOGY

Chylothorax is a rare disease, which has become more common with increasing activities of thoracic surgeons. The incidence after chest surgery, mainly coronary artery surgery, is around 0.5 percent[1–3] and is by far the most common cause. The other causes of chylothorax, i.e. after lymphomas, traffic accidents, etc., are of a sporadic occurrence.

Pseudochylothorax is an even rarer occurrence. The most common causes, large fibrotic pleural peels after tuberculosis pleurisy or pneumothorax treatment, are now very rare because there are few such patients alive.

Etiology of chylothorax

Chylothorax is caused by leakage of chyle from the thoracic duct. This leakage is secondary to trauma, weakening of the wall, or blockage of the duct (Table 29.1). The thoracic duct is fairly weak and even an intense sudden stretching of it can cause rupture, for example a forceful cough or emesis. It has also been described after the strains of childbirth both in mother and child, more usually in the infant.[19] It must be remembered that when a fairly trivial damage such as a cough causes a chylothorax, some underlying cause must always be suspected and appropriate investigations started. Similarly, when chylothorax develops in a child, a malformation must be the first suspicion.

Table 29.1 Causes of chylothorax

Causes of chylothorax
A. Traumatic:
Non-iatrogenic:
Any accident with damage or stretching of the chest wall or thoracic spine
Forceful cough or emesis
Childbirth
Iatrogenic:
Surgery of chest
Head and neck surgery
Radiation (often late sequale)
Sclerotherapy of the esophagus[4]
B. Diseases:
Malignant:
Lymphomas[5]
Other malignancies[6]
Benign tumors:
Retrosternal goiter[7]
Diseases affecting the lymph vessels:
Sarcoidosis[8,9]
Lymphangioleiomyomatosis
Hemangiomatosis (Gorham's syndrome)[10]
Congenital
Filiariasis[11]
Tuberculosis[12]
Amyloidosis
Yellow nail syndrome
Diseases affecting venous pressure:
Thrombosis of the superior vena cava or other central veins
Heart failure with increased venous pressure[13–15]
Transdiaphragmal movement of chylous ascites[15–17]
C. Congenital[18]
D. Idiopathic[18]

Traumatic rupture of the duct can be an early or late complication of traffic accidents but the vast majority of cases are now seen after various types of surgery involving heart, lung, or the head and neck region. It can occur even after thoracoscopic surgery. The incidence of chylothorax after chest surgery of various kinds is, as mentioned, around 0.5 percent.[1–3] The most common cause in childhood is a postoperative complication to surgery of cardiac malformations.[18]

Of the non-traumatic causes, the most common is a malignant lymphoma. Whenever a chylothorax of unknown etiology occurs, the first suspicion should be of an underlying malignant lymphoma. The lymphoma is most often of the non-Hodgkin's type. Malignant cells are not seen in the pleural fluid and, if the chylothorax is the first symptom of the disease, the diagnosis can cause great difficulties.[5] Other malignancies can cause blockage of the ductus by metastatic spread, but this is a fairly rare occurrence.[6]

Apart from those diseases which directly affect the lymph vessels and where chylothorax is common, it is usually an extremely rare complication of most of the different diseases listed in Table 29.1. For example, case reports in the world literature of chylothorax as a complication of sarcoidosis, goiter or tuberculosis are easily counted on one hand.

Congenital chylothorax is caused by malformation of the thoracic duct more often than by the trauma of birth.[20]

One differential diagnosis could be parenteral nutrition via a subclavian vein with penetration of the vessel and leakage into the pleura of the parenteral fluid. Analysis of the pleural content and comparison with the intravenous solution can give the diagnosis.[21]

Anatomy of the thoracic duct and pathogenesis of chylothorax

The lymph vessels from the lower parts of the body combine with those from the peritoneal cavity and come together behind the aorta below the diaphragm and form the thoracic duct. Usually, there is a widening of the duct where it starts, which has been termed the cisterna chyli. The duct passes through the diaphragm behind the aorta and continues upwards on the right side of the vertebral column between the azygos vein and the aorta. At the height of the third or fourth vertebra it turns to the left, crosses the midline and continues upwards behind the esophagus, medially of and behind the subclavian artery. It then turns laterally again, often after making a small loop up into the neck region, and finally empties into the left vena subclavia between the jugular and the vertebral veins.

This anatomy explains why chylothoraces most often occur on the right side. The largest part of the duct is within the right hemithorax and this is also where it is most easily damaged due to stretching. When the leakage from the duct occurs where it passes over the mid-line, a bilateral chylothorax can occur.[22,23] If the duct is damaged at the level of the aorta, the chylothorax tends to appear on the left side.[7,24,25] What has been described here is, however, only the most common anatomy. There can be very large variations. Two or more branches of the duct can be seen. The most common variation of this is one main duct and a number of small collaterals. Where the duct crosses the midline can also vary and it can even empty into the right subclavian artery.

When the duct starts to leak, a collection of chyle below the pleura is formed. This is called a 'chyloma' and usually is very short-lived because the pleura soon ruptures and the chylus empties into the pleural space. Thus, chylomas are only rarely seen clinically, for instance as a swelling of the supraclavicular fossa.[13] The rupture of a 'chyloma' can be a very dramatic clinical event with acute chest pain causing dyspnoea and tachycardia, suggesting myocardial infarction or pulmonary embolism. Such episodes seem to occur particularly after traumatic rupture of the thoracic duct. Depending on where the rupture occurs, some very rare entities can be found: chylomediastinum, where the chylus collects in the mediastinum without breaking through the pleura[26] and chylopericardium, where it empties into the pericardial sac.[27–29] Very rarely, when an abnormal communication between the ductus and the bronchi is formed or when there is a broncopleural fistula in chylothorax, chyloptysis can occur.[30]

The thoracic duct contains many valves forcing the chylus in one direction only. Movement of the thorax propels the chyle forwards. There are numerous small connections with veins, making it possible to ligate the ductus without any resulting problems.

Apart from its protein and fat content, the chyle also contains a large number of lymphocytes and is bacteriostatic. The normal daily flow in an adult is around 2 L.[31,32] The flow of chylus increases substantially with intake of food and drink, and decreases to a small trickle with starvation. With repeated thoracenteses or continuous drainage of a chylothorax, large amounts of fat, proteins and lymphocytes are lost, quickly resulting in negative effects on the patient's nutritional and immunological status.

CLINICAL PRESENTATION

The clinical presentation of chylothorax is as for any other pleural effusion, the main symptom being dyspnea. The chest X-ray shows the effusion, which should lead to a diagnostic thoracentesis. The typical whitish fluid should alert the clinician to the possibility of the diagnosis.

Diagnosis of chylothorax

The diagnosis is by analysis of the fats within the pleural fluid. Triglyceride levels greater than 1.2 mmol/L are highly suggestive of a chylous effusion. In equivocal cases with lower triglycerides, a lipid electrophoresis can clarify the diagnosis.[33] Very low triglycerides virtually exclude the diagnosis of chylothorax, but it should be remembered that after prolonged fasting the levels can be quite low. In these cases, one can measure the pleural levels of triglycerides after a meal containing a lipid composition, when the levels should increase, thereby proving that the pleural effusion is in fact a chylothorax.

Cholesterol values should also be measured simultaneously. High triglyceride levels can occur in pseudochylothorax,[34] but in this disease the cholesterol level is always very high (more than 200 mg/dL) and at microscopy cholesterol crystals can be seen, which are thought to be diagnostic.

Cells are also increased, usually more than 1000/μL. There is a dominance of monocytes and, in particular, of lymphocytes.

The gross appearance of the fluid can be misleading, and in any pleural effusion of undetermined cause, a lipoprotein analysis can be helpful.[34] Another differential diagnosis of a turbid or milky fluid is an empyema; centrifugation of the fluid will in the case of an empyema show a clear supernatant. The clinical picture is also different in most cases, the patient with empyema being obviously ill, with high fever, etc. The cell picture in empyemas is also different with almost 100 percent granulocytes. In rare cases, a chylothorax can become secondarily infected.

Investigations

Once the diagnosis of chylothorax has been established, investigations as to the cause should be carried out. If there is no history of trauma or surgery, or if the trauma seems to be fairly trivial (such as a violent cough), a malignant lymphoma should be excluded. A computed tomography (CT) scan of the thorax and upper abdomen should be performed to visualize any enlarged lymph nodes or other signs of tumor, and to enable scrutiny of the lungs. Lymphography can be made to show where the leakage or blockage is situated.[34] This can be of importance for the clinical decisions of where to take biopsies.

If no cause has been found, thoracic surgery might be necessary. Biopsies of any suspect area should be taken, and before the operation it should also be decided whether ligation of the ductus should be performed at the same setting. Biopsy of the lung, especially any suspicious part seen at CT, should be performed, since this is the best way to diagnose a lymphangioleiomyomatosis. It should be remembered, however, that even thoracic surgery might not give a definitive diagnosis. A malignant lymphoma can be very difficult to diagnose. In all unclear cases, treatment of the chylothorax should be performed and the patient then followed up.

Treatment

A large effusion causes respiratory distress, which can be relieved by thoracentesis. However, the chylus usually soon reaccumulates, and repeated thoracenteses can be necessary. Apart from the diminished quality of life, the patient will lose protein and other nutrients, so some alternative therapy will become necessary in these cases. A number of different treatments have been tried (Table 29.2).

Treatment of the underlying disease is important and will in some cases cause the chylothorax to disappear. Examples are corticosteroids in sarcoidosis[8] or treatment of heart failure. In many instances, for example malignant lymphomas, specific treatment will have a good effect on the underlying disease,[5] but the damage to the ductus can remain and consequently so can the chylothorax; therefore, further measures will be necessary.

A low-fat diet, with medium-chain triglycerides, which to the large extent are absorbed directly into the blood, will cause the chyle to decrease in amount, but there will still be

Table 29.2 Treatment of chylothorax

Treatment of chylothorax
A. Treatment of the underlying disease (lymphoma, other malignancy)
B. Conservative measures:
Repeated thoracocenteses
Continuous drainage
Pharmacologic: Octreotide
Diminishing food intake
Low-fat diet, medium-chain triglyceride diet
Total parenteral nutrition
C. Medical pleurodesis (instillation of talc or other sclerosing agent)
D. Surgical measures:
Pleuro-peritoneal pump
Fibrin glue to close the leak in the duct[35]
Ligation of the thoracic duct
By thoracoscopy
By thoracotomy
Pleurectomy

a flow.[36] This can be tried for up to 2 weeks. The next step is total parenteral nutrition, which will diminish the chylous flow through the ductus even further. In around 50 percent of patients with traumatic chylothorax, spontaneous healing will occur with conservative treatment[3,37] and occurs even more in children.[18,20] Thus, a trial of such treatment is usually recommended.[1,38,39] The longer the time of conservative therapy, the more patients will be cured spontaneously. Conservative measures are often effective, especially in children.[20] For example, in 39 children with mainly postoperative chylothorax, the effusion had disappeared after 14 days in 15 and after 45 days in 30.[18] Thus, especially in children, it seems advisable to wait a longer time, but this will necessitate long hospitalization and a risk of complications such as empyema.

In recent years, a new pharmacological treatment has been of great value: subcutaneously injected octreotide. This is a peptide which regulates the release of growth hormone and thyrotropin, and also has effects on the gastro-intestinal tract, where it inhibits glandular secretion, neurotransmission, smooth-muscle contraction and absorption of nutrients. Adverse effects are nausea, abdominal cramps, diarrhea, malabsorption of fat and flatulence. Long-term treatment can cause an increase in the number of cholesterol gallstones. Because of the inhibition of absorption of fats and other nutrients, octreotide has been shown to be useful in chylothorax from many different causes.[40–42]

If conservative measures fail, further therapy becomes necessary. One can try with medical pleurodesis, but in the end surgery might become necessary. Thoracoscopic intervention, a minimally invasive procedure, is now recommended by many, especially if the patient's nutritional status is already poor.[2]

Chemical pleurodesis for pleural effusions has been used with varying success for decades. Many different drugs have been used, the choice of which depended less on scientific investigations than on local customs. All of these different drugs have also been used for chylothorax. Examples are tetracycline, bleomycin[43] and talc.[44] Talc is now the most popular substance and good results have been reported. The general impression is that it is more difficult to achieve a chemical pleurodesis in chylothorax than in malignant pleurisy, probably due to the normal pleura and perhaps a neutralizing effect of the chyle.

An alternative to pleurodesis where for some reasons this is not feasible, is the pleuro-peritoneal shunt, which in principle is a one-way subcutaneous connection between the pleura and the peritoneum with a pump that can be activated by light pressure. It requires daily pumping and thus a cooperative patient. It has been used in some cases of chylothorax[11,37] With time, the rupture in the duct often heals, making it possible to remove the shunt, and it is therefore recommended especially for infants and children.[45]

When conservative measurements and pleurodesis have failed, ligation of the thoracic duct is an alternative. It is successful in up to 90 percent of patients.[46] However, as mentioned, there can be large variations in the anatomy of the duct and there can also be smaller tributaries which can leak, and therefore sometimes a full thoracotomy is necessary.[47] If the patient has drunk full cream before the operation, the leakage is often visible at surgery,[48] but whether this procedure is worthwhile is controversial. The ductus is ligated shortly above the diaphragm, and where the leakage occurs is thus unimportant if it occurs in the main duct. The surgical procedure can also be performed by thoracoscopy with good results.[49,50] Due to the rich network of collaterals there are never any problems with lymph stasis afterwards.

SOME DISEASES WITH SPECIAL ASPECTS OF CHYLOTHORAX

Lymphomas

Most commonly, a non-Hodgkin's lymphoma causes the chylothorax. In most instances the lymphoma is diagnosed before the complication of chylothorax occurs, but it can also be the first manifestation of the disease. As already mentioned, even if the malignant disease can be treated, it is often necessary to treat the chylothorax separately.[5, 38, 43] Chemical pleurodesis is one option and the best alternative seems to be talc,[40] ligation of the thoracic duct is another, and sometimes these two measures can be combined.

The etiology behind the chylothorax is probably invasion of the thoracic duct wall by lymphoma cells, causing it to become more brittle. Lymphoma cells are, however, usually not seen in biopsies of the pleura or the duct.[5] Chylothorax can be the first symptom of the lymphoma, and definitive diagnosis is sometimes not made until months or years later. Thus, treatment of the chylothorax even without knowledge of the underlying diagnosis is mandatory in these cases.

Lymphangioleiomyomatosis

This disease of unknown etiology is rare and occurs only in women and in their reproductive years. Cells which resemble smooth muscle cells proliferate in the lymphatic vessels and in the lung, causing reticulonodular infiltrates which are slowly progressive and in the end result in pulmonary insufficiency.[50–52] Chylothorax occurs in a large proportion – in 28 percent in one series[50] but in only 13 percent in another review.[51] Pneumothorax and hemoptysis are other symptoms. The prognosis is poor. Pleurodesis or thoracic duct ligation can control the chylothorax, as can octreotide in some reports, but the lung disease is progressive. Some beneficial effects are probably seen with oophorectomy and/or progesterone treatment.

ETIOLOGY AND PATHOGENESIS OF PSEUDOCHYLOTHORAX

If an exudate remains for a long time – months or years – in a fibrotic area of a grossly thickened pleura, it has a tendency to become enriched with cholesterol. Thus, this 'cholesterol pleurisy' is seen in fluid which is encapsulated. The fibrotic scar tissue which forms the walls of the chamber is poorly vascularized and so there is little absorption of any substances in the fluid. Earlier theories suggested that blood cells, both red and white, which reached the fluid became necrotic and disintegrated. Cholesterol from the cell walls is poorly absorbed in these circumstances, and thus with time its levels would increase. However, analysis has shown that there is a predominant binding of the cholesterol to high-density lipoprotein (HDL), which implies that it is derived from serum lipoproteins rather than from cellular debris.[34]

Probably due to osmotic effects, the cholesterol effusion can slowly enlarge. Over some years, an original small space can increase to a liter or more. Since the pleural fibrosis is often associated with changes in the lungs, often causing a lowered lung function, this thickened pleura can cause considerable dyspnea and a poor quality of life.[53] The fluid is opaque, sometimes whitish but more commonly brown (Figure 29.1).

The kind of thick peel which leads to cholesterol pleurisy can be seen after tuberculous pleurisy, therapeutic pneumothorax or in chronic rheumatoid pleurisy, which are the three most common causes.[53–55] However, the first two causes are becoming increasingly rare in a modern industrialized society. Other causes are traumatic (i.e. large bleeding in the pleura which gets organized), remnants of poorly treated empyemas and other diseases which can cause extensive fibrosis of the pleura. Coronary artery bypass surgery can cause a long-standing postoperative pleural effusion with development of pleural fibrosis, and the pleural fluid can show the typical composition of a pseudochylothorax.[56] A long-standing, thick pleural fibrosis due to some of the mentioned causes more often than not contains a central fluid collection, and this is where the cholesterol will start to build up. In most cases, it will never be diagnosed.

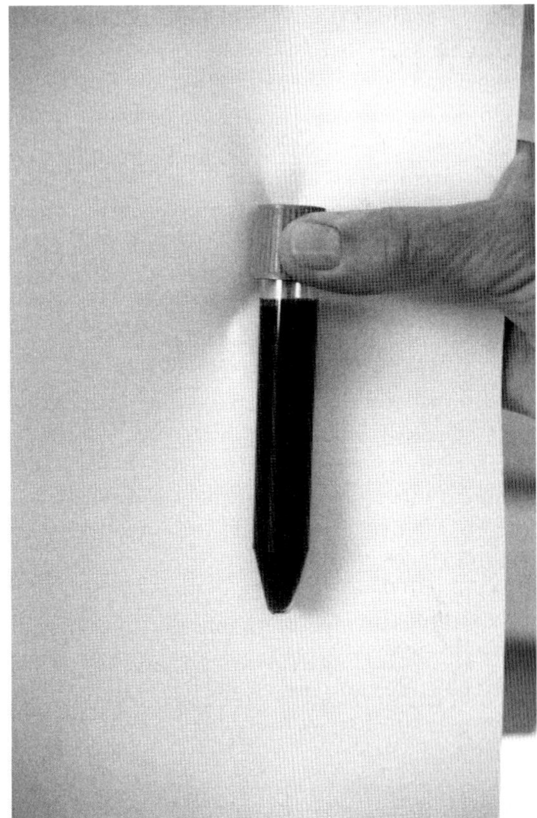

Figure 29.1 'Café-au-lait' color in pseudochylothorax. (See also Color Plate 46.)

I have not seen any report on cholesterol pleurisy in persons with asbestos-related diffuse pleural thickening. Possibly, this type of pleural fibrosis contains too dense fibrotic tissue, and there is no central pool of fluid, and thus the conditions for cholesterol pleurisy do not exist.

Pseudochylothorax of small or moderate size is fairly common in patients with large pleural peels. In most cases there is a benign course, and it is only if the patient has symptoms or if there has been a substantial increase in the size that any intervention is needed. However, any thick peel around part of or the whole of a lung should be carefully noted by the radiologist. Such peels practically always contain an area with fluid, and thus there is a risk of complications. Earlier chest X-rays should always be searched for, and it is not sufficient to look at one that is only 1 or 2 years older but rather one taken 10 or more years ago.

If the thickening has increased considerably in size, or if no earlier films can be recovered and there is a large pleural thickening and the patient has some symptoms, thoracentesis should be performed. This is important not only to relieve dyspnoea but also to prevent complications which can occur in untreated cholesterol pleurisy. A CT scan is very helpful to illustrate the anatomy. Great care should be taken before a pleural peel is declared to be 'inactive'.

Apart from respiratory insufficiency, the pseudochylothorax fluid can cause a number of complications. Infections can occur, the most common of which is a reactivation of tuberculosis. Cultures for tuberculosis (TB) should always be made on the fluid at puncture. Even if the cultures are negative, a patient with some complications from a pseudochylothorax due to old TB who has never had modern tuberculosis treatment (which applies to the majority of these patients) should be treated with a course of chemotherapy.

Non-specific infection also occurs and can be difficult to treat. Another complicating infection can be a fungal one, and particularly the *Aspergillus* species can cause very troublesome infections which are hard to treat.[57] Any infection can also lead to bronchopleural or pleurocutaneous fistulas.

Two points should be stressed regarding thoracocentesis in these patients: first, the peel is often of considerable thickness and in addition calcified, which can make puncture difficult. Second, the walls around the fluid are stiff and thus cannot adapt easily when the fluid is withdrawn, and therefore a negative pressure can develop if forceful suction is applied. This is immediately felt by the patient and further fluid removal is painful and meaningless, unless air is allowed to enter to equalize the pressures. This can be helpful in delineating the cavity later (Figure 29.2).

YELLOW NAIL SYNDROME

In 1966, Emerson described a triad of yellow nails, lymphedema, and pleural effusion[58] (Figure 29.3). The etiology is thought to be a dysfunction of the lymphatics. In the nails, this causes disfiguration, thickening and a yellow color. In the pleural space, there is a large daily flow of fluid, and almost all of this fluid is resorbed via the lymphatic vessels in the parietal pleura. It is thought that in yellow nail syndrome these vessels are also affected, which causes collection of fluid in the pleura.

The syndrome is defined as at least two of the three cardinal findings. Often, the patient also has a long-standing cough and/or repeated infections which turn out to be due to small bronchiectasies. Yellow nails without pleural effusion is more common than the full-blown syndrome but still rare. Pleural effusions can develop after many years of yellow nails.

The amount of fluid is highly variable and in many cases small, while in others there can be considerable amounts which need to be treated. The fluid is an exudate and not chylus since the mechanism is different from what occurs in chylothorax. In rare cases, however, the fluid is a frank chylothorax.

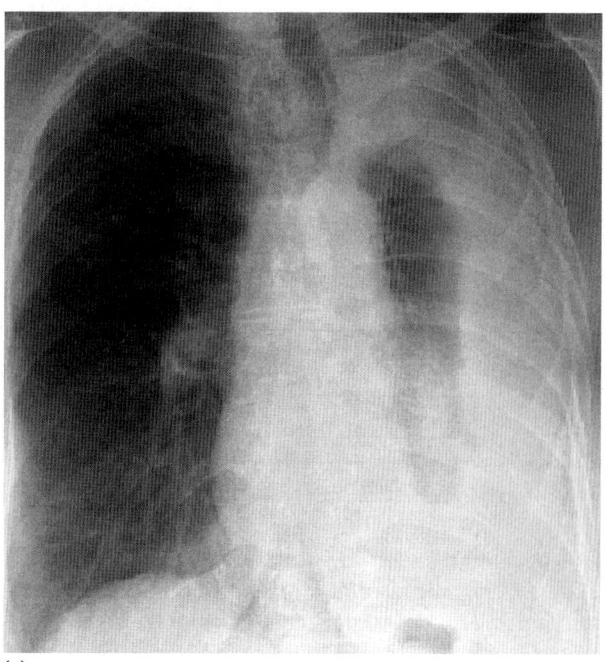
(a)

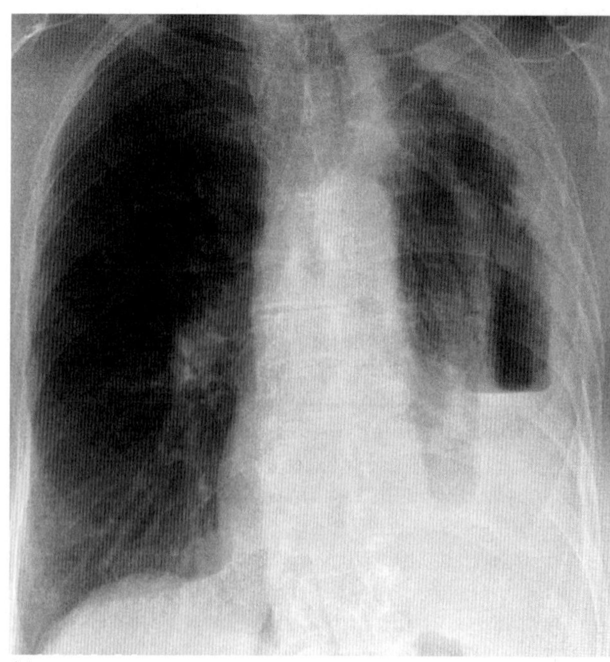
(b)

Figure 29.2 Pseudochylothorax, before and after thoracocentesis with letting in of air.

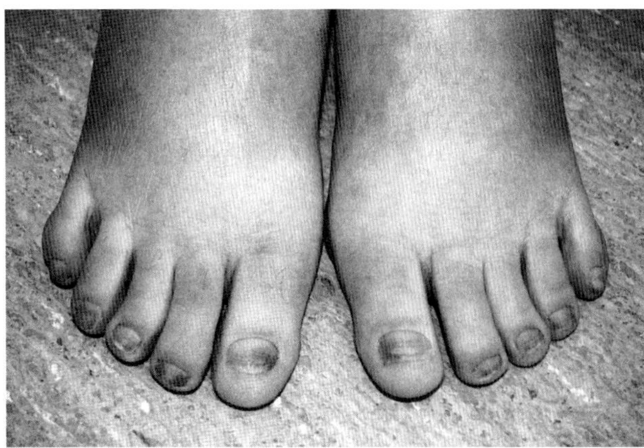

Figure 29.3 Typical yellow nails on toes and edema of the foot (and ankles). (See also Color Plate 47.)

The yellow nail syndrome can be secondary to a number of diseases: congenital hypoplastic lymphatics, autoimmune diseases, various malignant tumors and in some chronic infections. In many instances, no etiology can be established.

Treatment is difficult. In some cases cure has been described if the causative disease has been treated, for example surgery of a carcinoma.[59] For the pleural effusion, pleurodesis or pleuroperitoneal shunting can solve the problem.[60] In the rare cases where a chylothorax is found, octreotide treatment can have an effect.[61]

FUTURE DIRECTIONS

Chylothorax is still a problem, but progress in its treatment has been made. The introduction of octreotide has considerably improved outcome in many cases of chylothorax, but randomized studies are missing so far and might be indicated in some diseases. In the yellow nail syndrome, too little is still known about the pathogenesis; it remains a fascinating but difficult to treat disease. Hopefully, further studies will give us an effective treatment.

KEY POINTS

- Chylothorax is a rare complication of damage to the thoracic duct: analysis of the pleural fluid shows high levels of triglycerides and cholesterol; the cells are mainly lymphocytes. Trauma or lymphoma are the most common causes. Conservative treatment with subcutaneously injected octreotide and/or low-fat diet or total parenteral nutrition should be tried first, especially in children and in traumatic causes; the next step is pleurodesis and/or ligation of the thoracic duct
- Pseudochylothorax is a long-standing collection of fluid in a thick pleural fibrosis with very high levels of cholesterol: treatment is rarely necessary; complications are respiratory insufficiency, infections and fistulas.
- Yellow nail syndrome is a rare disease with disfigured and yellow nails, often accompanied by lymphedema and pleural effusions. It is usually secondary to autoimmune disease or malignancy; congenital cases occur. Treatment of the underlying cause, if possible, is recommended, otherwise pleurodesis or possibly pleuropulmonary shunting are recommended.

REFERENCES

• = Key primary paper
◆ = Major review article

1. Shimizu J, Hayashi Y, Oda M, *et al.* Treatment of postoperative chylothorax by pleurodesis with the streptococcal preparation OK-432. *Thorac Cardiovasc Surgeon* 1994; **42**: 233– 6.
2. Wakim R, Bellamy J, Irani M. La réintervention précoce dans le chylothorax après chirurgie thoracique. *Ann Chir* 1995; **49**: 863–8.
3. Terzi A, Furlan G, Magnanelli G, Terrini A, Ivic N. Chylothorax after pleuro-pulmonary surgery: a rare but unavoidable complication. *Thorac Cardiovasc Surgeon* 1994; **42**: 81–4.
4. Nygaard SD, Berger HA, Fick RB. Chylothorax as a complication of oesophagal sclerotherapy. *Thorax* 1992; **47**: 134–5.
5. O'Callaghan AM, Mead GM. Chylothorax in lymphoma: mechanism and management. *Ann Oncol* 1995; **6**: 603–7.
6. Mogulkoc H, Önal B, Oykay N, Gunel O, Bayindir U. Chylothorax, chyloperitoneum and lymphoedema – the presenting features of signet-cell carcinoma. *Eur Respir J* 1999; **13**: 1489–91.
7. Delgado C, Martin M, de la Portilla F. Retrosternal goiter associated with chylothorax. *Chest* 1994; **106**: 1924–5.
8. Jarman PR, Whyte MKB, Sabroe I, Hughes JMB. Sarcoidosis presenting with chylothorax. *Thorax* 1995; **50**: 1324–5.
9. Parker MJM, Torrington KG, Philips YY. Sarcoidosis complicated by chylothorax. *South Med J* 1994; **87**: 860–2.
10. Tie MLH, Poland GA, Rosenow EC. Chylothorax in Gorham's syndrome. *Chest* 1994; **105**: 208–13.
11. Kitchen ND, Hocken DB, Greenalgh RM, Kaplan DK. Use of the Denver pleuroperitoneal shunt in the treatment of chylothorax secondary to filiariasis. *Thorax* 1991; **46**: 144–5.
12. Antón PA, Rubio J, Casán P, Franquet T. Chylothorax due to *Mycobacterium tuberculosis*. *Thorax* 1995; **50**: 1019.
13. Boix MM, Gonzalez GO, Martinez JJM, *et al.* Quilotorax secundario a insuficiencia cardiaca. *Rev Clin Esp* 1987; **181**: 507–9.
14. Brenner WI, Boal BH, Reed GE. Chylothorax as a manifestation of rheumatic mitral stenosis. *Chest* 1978; **73**: 672–3.
15. Moss R, Hinds S, Fedullo AJ. Chylothorax: a complication of the nephrotic syndrome. *Am Rev Respir Dis* 1989; **140**: 1436–7.
16. Villena V, de Pablo A, Martin-Escribano P. Chylothorax and chylous ascites due to heart failure. *Eur Respir J* 1995; **8**: 1235–9.
17. Muns G, Rennard SI, Floreani AA. Combined recurrence of chyloperitoneum and chylothorax after retroperitoneal surgery. *Eur Respir J* 1995; **8**: 185–7.
18. ◆ Buttiker V, Fanconi S, Burger R. Chylothorax in children. Guidelines for diagnosis and management. *Chest* 1999; **116**: 682–7.

19. Cammarata SK, Brush RE, Hyzy RC. Chylothorax after childbirth. *Chest* 1991; **99**: 1539–40.
20. van Straaten HLM, Gerards LJ, Krediet TG. Chylothorax in the neonatal period. *Eur J Pediatr* 1993; **52**: 2–5.
21. Wolthuis A, Lamdewé RBM, Theunissen PHMH, Westerhuis LWJJM. Chylothorax or leakage of total parenteral nutrition? *Eur Respir J* 1998; **12**: 1233–5.
22. Restoy EG, Cueto FB, Arenas EE, Duch AA. Spontaneous bilateral chylothorax: uniform features of a rare condition. *Eur Respir J* 1988; **1**: 872–3.
23. Flaherty S, Ellison R. Bilateral chylothorax following thymectomy: resolution following unilateral drainage. *Mil Med* 1994; **159**: 627–8.
24. Janssen JP, Joosten HJM, Postmus PE. Thoracoscopic treatment of postoperative chylothorax after coronary bypass surgery. *Thorax* 1994; **49**: 1273.
25. Cheng WC, Chang CN, Lin TK. Chylothorax after endoscopic sympathectomy; case report. *Neurosurgery* 1994; **35**: 330–2.
26. Riquet M, Darse-Derippe J, Saab M, *et al.* Chylome médiastin après médiastinoscopie. A propos d'une observation. *Rev Mal Respir* 1993; **10**: 473–6.
27. de Winter RJ, Bresser P, Remer JWP, Kromhout JG, Reekers J. Idiopathic chylopericardium with bilateral reflux of chyle. *Am Heart J* 1994; **127**: 936–9.
28. Rose DM, Colvin SB, Danilowicz D, Isom OW. Cardiac tamponade secondary to chylopericardium following cardiac surgery: case report and review of the literature. *Ann Thorac Surg* 1982; **34**: 333–6.
29. Dunn RP. Primary chylopericardium: a review of the literature and an illustrated case. *Am Heart J* 1975; **89**: 369–77.
30. Chyloptysis in adults. Presentation, recognition, and differential diagnosis. *Chest* 2004; **125**: 336–40.
31. MacFarlane JR, Holman CW. Chylothorax. *Am Rev Respir Dis* 1972; **105**: 287–91.
◆32. Valentine VG, Raffn TA. The management of chylothorax. *Chest* 1992; **102**: 586–91.
●33. Staats BA, Ellefson RD, Budahn LL, *et al.* The lipoprotein profile of chylous and nonchylous pleural effusions. *Mayo Clin Proc* 1980; **55**: 700–4.
34. Hamm H, Pfalzer B, Fabel H. Lipoprotein analysis in a chyliform pleural effusion: implications for pathogenesis and diagnosis. *Respiration* 1991; **58**: 294–300.
35. Ngan H, Fok M, Wong J. The role of lymphography in chylothorax following thoracic surgery. *Br J Radiol* 1988; **61**: 1032–6.
36. Akaogi E, Mitsui K, Sohara Y, *et al.* Treatment of postoperative chylothorax with intrapleural fibrin glue. *Ann Thorac Surg* 1989; **48**: 116–18.
37. Jensen GL, Mascioloi EA, Meyer LP, *et al.* Dietary modification of chyle composition in chylothorax. *Gastroenetrology* 1989; **87**: 761–5.
◆38. Paes ML, Powell H. Chylothorax: an update. *Br J Hosp Med* 1994; **51**: 482–90.
39. Marts BC, Naunheim KS, Fiore AC, Pennington DG. Conservative versus surgical management of chylothorax. *Am J Surg* 1992; **164**: 532–5.
◆40. Lamberts SWJ, van der Lely AJ, de Herder WW, Hofland LJ. Octreotide. *New Engl J Med* 1996; **334**: 246–54.
●41. Kalomenidis I. Octerotide and chylothorax. *Curr Opin Pulm Med* 2006; **12**: 264–7.
42. Mares DC, Mather PN. Medical thoracoscopic talc pleurodesis for chylothorax due to lymphoma. *Chest* 1998; **114**: 731–5.
43. Fogli L, Gorini P, Belcastro S. Conservative management of traumatic chylothorax: a case report. *Intensive Care Med* 1993; **19**; 176–7.
44. Norum J, Aasebo U. Intrapleural bleomycin in the treatment of chylothorax. *J Chemother* 1994; **6**: 427–30.
45. Graham DD, McGahren ED, Tribble CG, Daniel TM, Rodgers BM. Use of video-assisted thoracic surgery in the treatment of chylothorax. *Ann Thorac Surg* 1994; **57**: 1507–12.
46. Murphy MC, Newman BM, Rodgers BM. Pleuroperitoneal shunts in the management of persistent chylothorax. *Ann Thorac Surg* 1989; **48**: 195–200.
47. Noel AA, Gloviczki P, Bender CE, *et al.* Treatment of symptomatic primary chylous disorders. *J Vasc Surg* 2001; **34**: 785–91.
48. Zoetmulder F, Rutgers E, Baas P. Thoracoscopic ligation of a thoracic duct leakage. *Chest* 1994; **106**: 1233–4.
49. Kent RB, Pinson TW. Thoracoscopic ligation of the thoracic duct. *Surg Endosc* 1993; **7**: 52–3.
●50. Taylor JR, Ryu J, Colby TV, Raffin TA. Lymphangioleiomyomatosis: clinical course in 32 patients. *N Engl J Med* 1990; **323**: 1254–60.
51. Johnson S. Lymphangioleiomyomatosis. *Eur Respir J* 2006; **27**: 1056–65.
52. Almoosa KF, McCormack FX, Sahn SA. Pleural disease in lymphangioleiomyomatosis. *Clin Chest Med* 2006; **27**: 355–68.
●53. Hillerdal G. Chyliform (cholesterol) pleural effusion. *Chest* 1985; **88**: 426–8.
54. Ferguson GC. Cholesterol pleural effusion in rheumatoid lung disease. *Thorax* 1966; **21**: 577–82.
55. Debieuvre D, Gury JP, Ory P, Jobard JM. Association pseudochylothorax et tuberculose pleurale. *Rev Pneumol Clin* 1994; **50**: 175–7.
56. Garcia-Pachon E, Fernandez LC, Lopez-Azorin F, Padilla-Navas I. Pseudo-chylothorax in pleural effusion due to coronary artery bypass surgery. *Eur Respir J* 1999; **13**: 1487–8.
57. Hillerdal G. Pulmonary aspergillus infection invading the pleura. *Thorax* 1981; **36**: 745–51.
●58. Emerson PA. Yellow nails, lymphedema, and pleural effusions. *Thorax* 1966; **21**: 247–53.
59. Iqbal M, Rossoff LJ, Marzouk KA, Steinberg HN. Yellow nail syndrome. Resolution of yellow nails after successful treatment of breast cancer. *Chest* 2000; **117**: 1516–18.
60. Brofman JD, Hall JB, Scott W, Little AG. Yellow nails, lymphedema and pleural effusion. *Chest* 1990; **97**: 743–5.
61. Makrilakis K, Pavlatos S, Giannikoupolos G, Toubanakis C, Katsilambros N. Successful Octreotide treatment of chylous pleural effusion and lymphedema in the Yellow Nail Syndrome. *Ann Int Med* 2004; **141**: 246–7.

30

Effusions from vascular causes

JOSÉ M PORCEL, RICHARD W LIGHT

PLEURAL EFFUSIONS CAUSED BY PULMONARY EMBOLI

Incidence and epidemiology

Pulmonary embolism is a common disease, with an incidence of approximately 200 per 100 000 person-years.[1] It is the fourth leading cause of pleural effusion in the USA following congestive heart failure, parapneumonic effusions and malignant pleural effusions;[2] it has been estimated that 180 000 cases of pleural effusion from pulmonary emboli occur each year. This estimate is based on the fact that at least 600 000 persons have a pulmonary embolic event each year[3] and at least 30 percent of those with pulmonary emboli have a pleural effusion.[2] In an epidemiological study from the Czech Republic in the early 1990s, pulmonary embolism was the fourth leading cause of pleural effusion.[4] However, in most series of patients who undergo thoracentesis, pulmonary embolism accounts for less than 5 percent of pleural effusions. Two reasons may explain this apparent paradox. First, the majority of pleural effusions associated with pulmonary embolism cause only blunting of the costrophrenic angles, which preclude a safe thoracentesis. Second, most patients with moderate or high clinical probability of pulmonary embolism are immediately anticoagulated while awaiting confirmatory tests, and this increases the risk of a diagnostic thoracentesis which is not necessary once the diagnosis of pulmonary embolus is established.

Pulmonary embolus is probably responsible for a significant percentage of undiagnosed pleural effusions. For example, Storey and coworkers[5] reported the etiology of a series of 133 patients with pleural effusions and noted that only three were caused by pulmonary emboli, but causes of the pleural effusions were not determined in 25 patients. One wonders how many of these 25 patients with pleural effusions of undetermined etiology had pulmonary emboli, since these authors did not do any routine evaluation for pulmonary embolism. Gunnels[6] reported on a series of 27 patients with exudative pleural effusion who did not have any diagnosis after the initial work-up, which included a needle biopsy of the pleura but no evaluation for pulmonary embolus. She reported that during the follow-up period, two of the 19 patients without malignant disease died and both had pulmonary emboli at autopsy.[6] Pulmonary emboli might have been discovered in more patients if the diagnosis was considered.

Pathogenesis

Although the precise pathogenesis of the pleural effusions associated with pulmonary emboli is not known, the fact that the associated pleural fluid can either be an exudate or (rarely) a transudate suggests that there may be two separate mechanisms.

The mechanism for the exudative pleural effusion is probably related to increased permeability of the pulmonary capillaries to fluid and protein. As a result of the increased permeability, excess fluid enters the interstitial spaces of the lung and some of this interstitial fluid traverses the visceral pleural. In the experimental situation, more than 20 percent of interstitial fluid exits the lung by passing through the visceral pleura.[7] Leckie and Tothill[8] have shown that patients with exudative pleural effusion secondary to pulmonary emboli have a large amount of protein entering and leaving the pleural space.

The factor(s) responsible for the increased permeability of the pulmonary capillaries is not definitely known; it is probable that the increased permeability results from the release of cytokines or inflammatory mediators from the platelet-rich thrombi. Ischemia of the capillaries in the visceral pleura probably does not play a significant role since these capillaries are supplied by the bronchial circulation,[9] and probably do not develop ischemia with pulmonary emboli. However, ischemia of the capillaries distal to the embolus may play a contributory role in increasing the vascular permeability. One cytokine that may be at least partly responsible for the increased vascular permeability is vascular endothelial growth factor (VEGF). This is one of the most potent agents known for increasing vascular permeability. Platelets contain large quantities of VEGF.[10] The pleural fluid levels of VEGF were very high in one patient with a pleural effusion secondary to pulmonary emboli.[11]

The mechanism for the rare transudative pleural effusions associated with pulmonary embolism is probably related to increased pressures in either the pulmonary or systemic circulation. Pulmonary embolism is associated with both increased pulmonary arterial pressures and increased systemic vascular pressures from the associated right heart failure. Increased pressures in either of these locations can lead to increased pleural fluid formation, although it is more likely that increased pressure in the systemic capillaries[12] rather than increased pulmonary artery pressure[13] is directly related to the accumulation of pleural fluid.

Clinical presentation

RISK FACTORS

There are many factors that predispose patients to pulmonary embolism. The most common are major surgery, previous venous thromboembolism, trauma, immobility (e.g. infection, acute rheumatism, falls without fractures, prolonged air travel), malignancy and its treatment, estrogen therapy, hereditable and acquired thrombophilia (e.g. activated protein C resistance, prothrombin G20210A mutation, antiphospholipid antibody syndrome), pregnancy and the postpartum state, and hospitalization for medical conditions including heart failure, stroke and chronic lung disease. Less common risk factors are advanced age, obesity, central venous catheters, acute infections, or certain medical disorders such as myeloproliferative diseases, nephrotic syndrome, inflammatory bowel disease or paroxysmal nocturnal hemoglobinuria.[14,15] Importantly, approximately 20 percent of patients with pulmonary embolism have no predisposing factors.[16,17] Pulmonary embolism is thought to be a disease of old people, yet 12 percent of 400 patients with pulmonary embolism in one series were under 40 years old.[18]

SYMPTOMS AND SIGNS

Patients with pulmonary emboli present with three different symptom complexes: (1) pleuritic chest pain or hemoptysis (pulmonary infarction); (2) isolated dyspnea; and (3) syncope with circulatory collapse. In the Registro Informatizado de la Enfermedad TromboEmbólica (RIETE) registry, of 3391 patients with pulmonary embolism who had no chronic lung disease or heart failure, 1709 patients presented with pleuritic chest pain or hemoptysis and 27 percent had pleural effusion, 1083 presented with isolated dyspnea and 12 percent had pleural effusion while 599 presented with circulatory collapse and 16 percent had pleural effusion.[19]

Multiple symptoms can occur with pulmonary embolism. In the RIETE study, the proportion of 4444 patients with the following symptoms was: dyspnea, 83 percent; chest pain, 52 percent; leg pain or swelling, 37 percent; cough, 20 percent; syncope, 14.5 percent; fever >38°C, 12 percent; and hemoptysis, 7 percent.[20]

Physical findings also vary in patients with pulmonary emboli. When two reports are combined,[16,17] the proportion of 357 patients with the following physical findings was: tachypnea ≥20/minute, 68 percent; rales, 31 percent; tachycardia >100/minute, 26 percent; accentuated pulmonic component of second heart sound, 27 percent; and wheezes, pleural friction rub and Homans' sign, less than 5 percent each.

ARTERIAL BLOOD GASES AND ELECTROCARDIOGRAPHY

Approximately one of every four patients with pulmonary embolism has a normal pulse oximetry or partial pressure of alveolar O_2 (PaO_2).[21] Electrocardiographic abnormalities historically considered to be suggestive of pulmonary embolism, such as the S1Q3T3 pattern or the right bundle branch block, are actually present in approximately 15 percent of patients.[20]

CHEST RADIOGRAPHS

Pleural effusions occur in 20–50 percent of patients with pulmonary embolism. Worsley and associates[22] reviewed the chest radiographs of 383 patients in the Prospective Investigation of Pulmonary Embolism Diagnosis (PIOPED) study with angiographically proven pulmonary emboli and reported that 36 percent had a pleural effusion. Two large multicenter studies comprising 2319[23] and 4033[20] patients with pulmonary embolism reported that the incidence of pleural effusion was 23 and 21 percent, respectively, when assessed by chest radiograph.

Recently, Porcel and colleagues[24] reviewed the radiological characteristics of pleural effusions in 230 patients with pulmonary embolism. Pleural effusions were observed in 32 and 47 percent of patients by chest radiograph and computed tomography (CT), respectively. Several concepts arose from this investigation. First, pleural effusions secondary to pulmonary embolism are usually unilateral and small. Among the 73 patients with a pleural effusion visible on the chest radiograph, 34 (47 percent) had unilateral left-sided effusions, 28 (38 percent) had unilateral right-sided effusions and 11 (15 percent) had bilateral effusions. In 66

(90 percent) of the 73 patients, effusions occupied a third or less of the hemithorax, while in the remaining 7 (10 percent) patients the effusions were large or massive.[24] Second, pulmonary embolism should be considered in the differential diagnosis of a loculated pleural effusion, in addition to complicated parapneumonic effusion, tuberculosis, hemothorax and long-standing malignant effusion. CT demonstrated fluid loculations in 21 percent of patients with pleural effusion for whom the diagnosis of pulmonary embolism was deferred for a mean of 12 days after symptoms developed.[24] Third, contrary to some previous findings,[25] the size of the effusions tended to be smaller if pulmonary infarction was present. Peripheral wedge-shaped opacities, likely to represent pulmonary infarction, were observed in 50 (38 percent) of 133 patients with pulmonary embolism on CT scan. The frequency of pleural effusion was not significantly different in patients with or without pulmonary infarction (50 percent versus 46 percent), but effusion median volumes were smaller in the former (200 mL) than in the latter (600 mL).[24] There are two possible explanations for this finding: (1) large amounts of pleural fluid with the resulting passive atelectasis may conceal the identification of some parenchymal opacities; and (2) ischemia may induce mesothelial cells to secrete various coagulation cascade proteins, such as the tissue factor. The resulting procoagulant activity and fibrin deposition in the pleural space may lead to a spontaneous pleurodesis, thereby precluding pleural fluid accumulation. Finally, an absolute correlation between the sidedness of the pleural effusion and that of the pulmonary embolism is lacking. Of the 93 patients with pleural effusion detected by chest radiograph or CT, the pulmonary embolism was unilateral in 61 and the pleural effusion was on the ipsilateral side in 38 and on the contralateral side in 7, whereas it was bilateral in 16. The pulmonary embolism was bilateral in 31 patients and the pleural effusion was also bilateral in 6, but unilateral in 25 patients.[24] The presence of an effusion on the opposite side of an intraluminal filling defect may simply reflect the poor sensitivity of conventional computed tomographic pulmonary angiography (CTA) for emboli in subsegmental pulmonary arteries.

PLEURAL FLUID FINDINGS

The pleural fluid findings associated with pulmonary embolism vary widely and do not help in establishing a diagnosis. Nonetheless, in patients with more than a minimal pleural effusion, thoracentesis should be attempted, at least to exclude other potential etiologies. In our experience, even in fully-anticoagulated patients pending confirmatory tests for pulmonary embolism, thoracentesis can be safe if performed with a 25-gauge needle, preferably under ultrasound guidance. If the diagnosis of pulmonary embolism is already established, a thoracentesis is indicated if the patient is febrile to rule out a pleural infection or if the effusion is increasing in size to rule out a hemothorax.

Classically, it has been taught that the pleural effusion secondary to pulmonary embolism may be a transudate or an exudate, but two recent series cast doubt on this dogma. In these two studies, pleural effusions from 60 and 26 patients with pulmonary embolism, respectively, all fell into the exudative category when Light's criteria were applied.[24,26] In fact, the potential transudative nature of the effusions associated with pulmonary embolism is reported in a single publication that had significant methodological limitations.[27]

The pleural fluid is yellow and not blood-tinged or bloody in approximately 40 percent of patients.[24,26] The pleural fluid white blood cell (WBC) count ranges from under 100 to more than 50 000 cells/mm^3.[24,26,27] The differential WBC may reveal predominantly neutrophils, lymphocytes, mononuclear cells, mesothelial cells or eosinophils.

Investigations

CLINICAL PROBABILITY OF PULMONARY EMBOLISM

An important component for the strategy for the optimal diagnosis of pulmonary embolism using noninvasive tests is the classification of the clinical probability of pulmonary embolism as high, intermediate or low according to well-validated prediction rules (e.g. modified Wells and Geneva scores).[28,29] Table 30.1 presents two approaches to estimate the pretest clinical probability of pulmonary embolism. Although widely used, the Wells score[28] contains a highly subjective variable, the physician's opinion as to whether pulmonary embolism is the most likely diagnosis. On the other hand, the revised Geneva score[29] is standardized and relies exclusively on clinical variables, but it should be tested in a formal outcome study. Prospective studies using these algorithms have shown that the prevalence of pulmonary embolism with low, intermediate and high clinical probability scores is approximately 10, 30 and 70 percent, respectively.[30]

The diagnosis of pulmonary embolism should be considered in every patient with an undiagnosed pleural effusion. If the patient has a predisposing factor for pulmonary emboli and has pleuritic chest pain or dyspnea that is out of proportion to the size of the effusion, the patient should be started on heparin treatment and a test for pulmonary embolism should be performed before a thoracentesis is attempted.[31]

D-DIMER

The best screening test for pulmonary embolus is measurement of the D-dimers in the peripheral blood. D-dimers are degradation products that result from the breakdown of cross-linked fibrin by plasmin. Fibrin is cross-linked by factor XIII and is the primary component of thrombus material. Increased levels of D-dimer are found in condi-

Table 30.1 Estimation of pretest clinical probability of pulmonary embolism

Prediction rules	
Wells criteria	
Clinical signs and symptoms of deep venous thrombosis	3
Alternative diagnosis less likely than pulmonary embolism	3
Heart rate >100 beats/minute	1.5
Surgery or bedridden for ≥3 days in the previous 4 weeks	1.5
Previous deep venous thrombosis or pulmonary embolism	1.5
Hemoptysis	1
Active cancer (treatment within 6 months, or palliative)	1
Clinical probability	
Low	<2
Intermediate	2–6
High	>6
Pulmonary embolism likely	>4
Pulmonary embolism unlikely	≤4
Revised Geneva score	
Heart rate	
75–94 beats/minute	3
≥95 beats/minute	5
Pain on lower-limb deep venous palpation and unilateral edema	4
Unilateral lower limb pain	3
Previous deep venous thrombosis or pulmonary embolism	3
Surgery or fracture of the lower limbs within 1 month	2
Active malignant condition (or considered cured <1 year)	2
Hemoptysis	2
Age >65 years	1
Clinical probability	
Low	<4
Intermediate	4–10
High	≥11

tions that result in the activation of the fibrinolytic system. Thus, D-dimer tests lack specificity for thromboembolism, although it appears that normal levels should be useful in excluding it.[32] Elevated levels of D-dimer are also found in patients with recent surgery, infection, malignancy and liver disease. More than 50 percent of hospitalized patients have elevated levels of D-dimer. Nevertheless, if the levels are normal and an appropriate test is used, the diagnosis of pulmonary embolus can be excluded. However, if the D-dimer test is positive, an additional test is necessary to definitely diagnose pulmonary embolism.[32]

It is important for physicians to understand the characteristics and limitations of the test that is performed at their hospital. Rapid enzyme-linked immunosorbent assay (ELISA) tests (e.g. VIDAS, Instant IA, Nycocard), and latex immunoturbidimetric assays (e.g. Tinaquant, HemosIL D-dimer HS, Liatest, Plus) have a high sensitivity in screening for venous thromboembolism (approximately 95 percent), while the red cell (e.g. SimpliRED) or the first-generation latex agglutination tests are, in general, much less sensitive.[33]

The utility of using a D-dimer test as a screening test has been demonstrated in a recent prospective cohort study that included 3306 patients with suspected pulmonary embolism.[34] Patients were categorized as having pulmonary embolism 'likely' ($n = 1100$), or 'unlikely' ($n = 2206$) using the dichotomized version of the Wells clinical decision rule. If the D-dimer test was negative (VIDAS D-dimer assay or the Tinaquant assay) in patients with an unlikely clinical probability score, pulmonary embolism was considered excluded and no additional tests were performed. When the D-dimer test was performed on 2206 patients with pulmonary embolism unlikely, it was normal in 1057 (48 percent). These patients did not undergo further evaluation or receive treatment and only four (0.4 percent) developed a pulmonary embolus during the subsequent 3 months.[34]

PERFUSION LUNG SCANS

For the past several decades, the perfusion lung scan has been the primary test by which the possibility of pulmonary embolus has been evaluated. If the lung scan is negative, a pulmonary embolus is virtually ruled out. If the perfusion lung scan is a high-probability lung scan, 87 percent of the patients will have a pulmonary embolism and when a high-probability lung scan is coupled with a high clinical probability of embolism, the positive predicted value increases to 96 percent.[2] Nevertheless, the utility of the lung scan is limited by the fact that many patients with a high suspicion of pulmonary embolism will have an intermediate- or low-probability lung scan and therefore will require additional diagnostic tests. For example, in the PIOPED study, 931 patients underwent both scintigraphy and pulmonary angiography. Of the 116 patients with high-probability scans and definitive angiograms, 102 (88 percent) had pulmonary embolism. Of the 322 patients with intermediate-probability scans, 105 (33 percent) had pulmonary embolism, while of the 493 patients with low-probability scans, 59 (12 percent) had pulmonary embolism.[35] In the PIOPED study, 164 patients from 266 (62 percent) with positive arteriograms did not have high probability lung scans.

If a pleural effusion is present, the perfusion lung scan is more difficult to interpret.[36] A large effusion severely restricts the ability of the lung to expand and causes a shift of perfusion to the contralateral lung. The presence of the pleural fluid itself makes interpretation of the lung scans more difficult. An apparent perfusion defect can be caused by the presence of fluid anywhere in the chest. If perfusion and ventilation scans are obtained with the patient in different positions, then the lung scan may be misinterpreted as a ventilation/perfusion mismatch.[2] If a patient has more than a small pleural effusion, it is preferable to perform a therapeutic thoracentesis before the lung scan is obtained.[2]

PULMONARY ARTERIOGRAMS

The pulmonary arteriogram remains the gold standard for diagnosing pulmonary emboli. However, pulmonary arteriography still has some limitations. First, the arteriography must be performed in a special facility to which the patient must be transported. Second, there are limitations in the interpretation of pulmonary arteriograms. The interpretation of the pulmonary angiogram is influenced heavily by three factors: (1) the location of the thromboembolic obstruction; (2) the quality of the images; and (3) the experience of the interpreters.[2] Angiography with digital subtraction is less time-consuming and has a diagnostic accuracy similar to pulmonary arteriograms and greater than film-screen angiography.[37]

COMPUTED TOMOGRAPHIC ANGIOGRAPHY

In recent years, spiral CTA has largely surpassed perfusion lung scanning,[38] although the latter is still used, particularly when CTA is contraindicated because of renal failure, allergy to radiographic contrast material or concerns for radiation exposure (e.g. pregnancy, women of reproductive age).

In general, the sensitivity of single-detector CTA in diagnosing pulmonary embolism has ranged from 75 to 100 percent, with a specificity that averages 95 percent.[39,40] In the past several years, CT technology has evolved from single-detector CT to multidetector CT and from 4-slice to 64-slice scanners, which has significantly improved resolution and thus sensitivity for the detection of subsegmental pulmonary embolism.

If CTA scans are used for the diagnosis of pulmonary emboli, it is important that the pulmonary arteries be examined on the video monitor and not just on the hard copies of the scans. False-positive and false-negative results are common when the length of the pulmonary artery is not scrutinized on the monitor. In a meta-analysis that included 4657 patients with suspected pulmonary embolism who did not receive anticoagulation after negative results on CTA, the 3-month risks for a subsequent venous thromboembolic event and fatal pulmonary embolism were 1.4 and 0.51 percent, respectively.[41] This, and other studies,[42] suggest that CTA is at least as accurate as invasive pulmonary angiography to rule out pulmonary embolism.

Stein and colleagues[43] investigated the use of multidetector CTA alone and combined with imaging of the pelvic and thigh veins (CTA/CTV) in 824 patients with suspected pulmonary embolism. They reported that the sensitivity of CTA/CTV (90 percent) in the diagnosis of pulmonary embolism exceeds that of CTA alone (83 percent), with similar specificity (95 percent). However, an accompanying editorial questions if the small increase in the negative predictive value from 95 to 97 percent is enough to justify the additional irradiation by CTV.[44] To reduce radiation, the PIOPED II investigators recommend CTV of only the femoral and popliteal veins.[45]

We believe that CTA is the best way to evaluate the possibility of pulmonary emboli in patients with a pleural effusion. Patients with a pleural effusion are likely to have an embolus in the central, lobar, segmental or subsegmental pulmonary arteries and these are the areas in which CTA can detect an embolus. The additional advantage of obtaining a CTA in a patient with a pleural effusion who is being evaluated for pulmonary embolism is that the CTA can also demonstrate pulmonary infiltrates or masses, pleural nodules or thickening, or mediastinal abnormalities, which may provide clues to the etiology of the pleural effusion if a pulmonary embolus is not present.

DUPLEX ULTRASONOGRAPHY OF LEG VEINS

An alternative approach to the diagnosis of pulmonary emboli is to study the legs to see if there is any evidence of deep venous thrombosis. The basis for this approach is that approximately 90 percent of pulmonary emboli originate in the legs. The best method by which to evaluate the proximal veins of the legs is probably duplex ultrasonography with venous compression. This test has a sensitivity that exceeds 90 percent and a specificity that exceeds 95 percent.[35,40] If deep venous thrombosis is demonstrated with ultrasonography, the diagnosis of pulmonary embolus is likely. The patient needs to be anticoagulated and usually no further diagnostic tests directed toward the pleural effusions are indicated. Unfortunately, deep venous thrombosis is not demonstrated in about 40 percent of patients with pulmonary embolism,[20,46] and in these patients additional studies are necessary to delineate the etiology of the pleural effusion. Among patients with negative multidetector CTA scans, leg ultrasonography yielded an incremental rate of detection of venous thrombosis of only 0.9 percent in one study.[47] Thus, it seems that patients undergoing multidetector CT scanning do not require ultrasonography as a complementary diagnostic test.

THORACIC ULTRASONOGRAPHY

Recently, a prospective multicenter study reported the accuracy of thoracic ultrasound in the diagnosis of 352 patients suspected of having pulmonary embolism.[48] Pulmonary embolism was considered definite when two or more typical triangular or rounded pleural-based lesions were demonstrated, and probable when one typical lesion with pleural effusion was present. Pulmonary embolism was diagnosed in 194 patients, mostly by CTA. In 49 percent of these patients, investigators found small pleural effusions by thoracic ultrasound. Ultrasonography had a sensitivity of 74 percent, and a specificity of 95 percent for diagnosing peripheral pulmonary embolism.[48]

For unstable patients with suspected massive pulmonary embolism, echocardiography searching for right ventricular enlargement or poor ventricular function, in combination with leg ultrasonography, are recommended as rapidly obtainable bedside tests.[45]

SUMMARY

The following procedure is recommended when patients with pleural effusion are evaluated for pulmonary emboli. If the clinical probability of pulmonary embolus is not high, then a D-dimer test (one with a high sensitivity for pulmonary emboli) should be obtained. If this is negative, it is unlikely that the patient has a pulmonary embolus and no further evaluation for pulmonary emboli is usually indicated.[49,50] If the clinical probability of pulmonary embolus is high or if the D-dimer test is positive, additional tests are indicated. One can proceed with the combination of CTA and CT venography of the femoral and popliteal veins.[45] If no venous thrombosis or pulmonary embolism is demonstrated, a pulmonary digital subtraction angiography or serial leg ultrasonography should be obtained if the clinical probability of pulmonary embolus is high (Figure 30.1).

Treatment and management

In the treatment of patients with pulmonary embolus, the presence of a pleural effusion does not alter the therapy. The primary treatment is anticoagulation (normally heparin followed by vitamin-K antagonists). The presence of bloody pleural fluid should not serve as a contraindication to anticoagulation, since the vast majority of such patients will not have significant bleeding into their pleural space if they are anticoagulated.

Either unfractionated heparin or low molecular weight heparin (LMWH) is appropriate for the initial treatment of pulmonary embolism.[51] The advantages of LMWH compared with conventional heparin include the following: (1) it is not necessary to monitor coagulation parameters; (2) outpatient treatment is possible; (3) heparin-induced thrombocytopenia is less frequent; and (4) heparin-associated osteopenia is less frequent. The duration of anticoagulation with vitamin-K antagonists varies according to the risk of recurrent pulmonary embolism. Patients with a first episode of pulmonary embolism and a transient risk factor can be treated for 3–6 months. An extended-duration therapy (>12 months or indefinite) should be considered for idiopathic or recurrent pulmonary embolism.[51]

Therapeutic thoracentesis is usually not necessary in the treatment of the pleural effusion secondary to pulmonary embolus because the effusions tend to be small.

Complications

The two primary complications related to the pleural effusion in patients with pulmonary embolus are hemothorax and pleural infection. If a pleural effusion enlarges in size or if a contralateral pleural effusion develops after the initiation of anticoagulant therapy in a patient with a pleural effusion caused by pulmonary embolism, the patient probably has one of these two complications or recurrent pulmonary emboli.

Patients who develop hemothorax as a complication of therapy for pulmonary embolus usually develop an increase in the size of their pleural effusion 4–7 days after anticoagulant therapy is initiated.[52,53] The coagulation studies in patients who develop this complication are usually within an acceptable therapeutic range. The pathogenesis of the hemothoraces in these instances is not clear. Although they have been attributed to rupture of the pulmonary infarction,[54] the evidence for this is somewhat lacking. The treatment for spontaneous hemothorax complicating anticoagulant therapy is transfusion, as needed, plus the immediate discontinuation of the anticoagulant therapy and insertion of chest tubes.[2] If brisk bleeding persists, a thoracotomy with resection of the infarcted lobe may be necessary.[54]

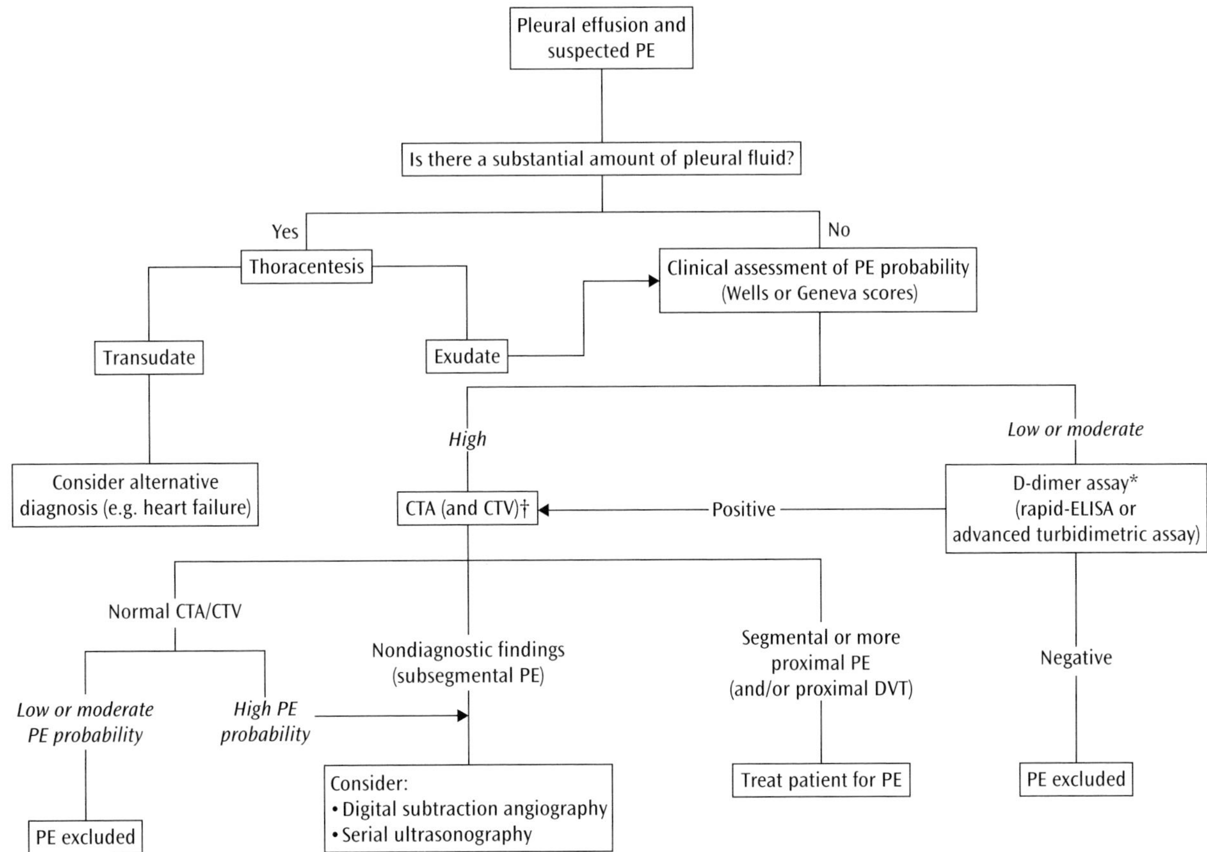

Figure 30.1 Suggested workup for patient with pleural effusion and suspected pulmonary embolus. PE, pulmonary embolism; CTA, computed tomographic pulmonary angiography; CTV, computed tomographic venography; ELISA, enzyme-linked immunosorbent assay; DVT, deep venous thrombosis.
*If measured by latex agglutination a normal D-dimer is only sufficient to exclude PE if the clinical probability of PE is low
†If multidetector CTA is used, evaluation for deep venous thrombosis may not be necessary

PLEURAL EFFUSIONS CAUSED BY OTHER PULMONARY VASCULAR DISEASES

There are other pulmonary vascular diseases that cause pleural effusions in addition to non-septic pulmonary emboli. These include the superior vena cava (SVC) syndrome, thoracic aortic dissection, septic pulmonary emboli, sickle cell anemia and pulmonary veno-occlusive disease.

Superior vena cava syndrome

The SVC syndrome results from the obstruction of SVC, with severe reduction in venous return from the head, neck, and upper extremities. A recent study focuses on the pleural findings in patients with SVC syndrome caused by malignant (e.g. lung cancer) or benign (e.g. intravascular device) conditions.[55] Pleural effusions were demonstrated in 44 of the 67 patients (66 percent) with radiological studies, either chest radiographs or CT scans, regardless of the etiology. Ten effusions were unilateral left-sided, 17 were unilateral right-sided and the remaining 17 were bilateral. The majority of pleural effusions were small; 61 percent occupied less than 25 percent of the affected hemithorax, and only three patients with malignancy had large effusions. Pleural fluid was analyzed in 22 patients; none had transudates and four met the standard criteria of chylothorax.[55] The reason for the exudative nature of these effusions is elusive, while the chylous effusions probably result from the increased hydrostatic pressure in the SVC and thoracic duct and its subsequent non-traumatic rupture. Pleural fluid cytology was positive in 9 of the 17 effusions sampled from patients with malignancy, which suggests that at least in some cases the effusions were secondary to pleural metastases rather than to the SVC occlusion.

Thoracic aortic dissection

Thoracic aortic dissection is a catastrophic life-threatening condition that typically presents with severe, sharp, tearing chest pain. In one series, CT scan detected pleural effusion in 42 of 48 (87.5 percent) patients with thoracic aortic dissection.[56] Pleural effusions appeared at a mean of 4.5 days (range 1–15 days) after the onset of dissection, but they were seen on the first day of hospitalization in 18 patients. Effusions were bilateral in 31 patients (74 percent) and left sided in the remainder 11 patients (26 percent). Thoracentesis was performed in six patients because of dyspnea secondary to a massive pleural effusion, and the pleural fluid was bloody in half of these cases. Most of the effusions resolved before discharge from the hospital. Others authors have reported effusions to be less common. For example, Sato *et al*,[57] found pleural effusions in 16 of 66 (24 percent) patients with thoracic aortic dissection, mostly (13 patients) of the Standford type B (i.e. no involvement of the ascending aorta). However, it was unclear what reference standard, either chest radiograph or CT, was used to identify the effusions. In rare cases, pleural effusion or hemothorax, rather than chest or back pain, is the first sign of thoracic aortic dissection.[58] The presence of pleural effusion is neither an indication nor a contraindication for surgery.

Septic pulmonary emboli

Septic emboli occur when fragments of the thrombus contain organisms, usually bacteria but occasionally fungi or parasites. Most septic emboli originate from the heart in association with endocarditis of the tricuspid valve (e.g. intravenous drug users), a ventricular septal defect, from an infected venous catheter (including pacemaker leads) or septic thrombophlebitis. The organism most commonly associated with septic emboli is *Staphylococcus aureus*.

Patients with septic emboli present with a picture of the systemic inflammatory response syndrome. The chest radiograph usually reveals multiple, ill-defined, round or wedge-shaped opacities in the periphery of the lung. The opacities may be uniform or may vary widely in size, reflecting recurrent showers of emboli. Cavitation is frequent and many occur rapidly; the cavities are usually thin-walled and many have no fluid level.[59]

The reported incidences of pleural effusion with right-sided endocarditis have varied from 25 to 69 percent. In one study, unilateral or bilateral effusions were present by chest radiograph in 7 of 13 patients (54 percent) with septic pulmonary embolism, and by CT in two additional effusions (sensitivity 69 percent).[60] Two patients required drainage of the pleural space by tube thoracostomy or thoracoscopy. However, a review article concluded that the incidence of pleural effusion with right-sided endocarditis is approximately 25 percent.[61] The pleural fluid is an exudate, but the cultures are negative in the majority of cases. The differential count can reveal neutrophils, lymphocytes or monomesothelial cells. One interesting characteristic of the pleural fluid is that the lactate dehydrogenase level is usually relatively high and may be elevated to 10 times or more the upper limit for serum.

Lemierre's syndrome is a special case of septic emboli in which an oropharyngeal infection is followed by internal jugular vein septic thrombophlebitis and metastatic emboli, most frequently to the lungs and joints.[62] Patients frequently present with symptoms and signs of septic emboli to the lungs including dyspnea, pleuritic chest pain, fever and hemoptysis. The syndrome is most commonly associated with the anaerobic Gram-negative rod *Fusobacterium necrophorum*. The diagnosis is established with evidence of metastatic infection and internal jugular vein thrombophlebitis. The diagnostic procedure of choice is a contrast-enhanced CT of the neck and chest, which typically reveals distended veins with enhancing walls, low-attenuation intraluminal filling defects and localized soft tissue edema.[63] The treatment should include an extended course of a β-lactamase-resistant antibiotic and surgical drainage of any purulent fluid collections. The role of anticoagulant therapy remains controversial.

Pleural effusions occur with Lemierre's syndrome as with any septic emboli. In one review of 109 patients reported in the literature during a 20-year period, 43 percent had pleural effusion.[64] Empyema and pneumothorax have also been reported.[65] If the fluid is infected, tube thoracostomy or thoracoscopy with the breakdown of adhesions may be necessary.[66]

Sickle cell anemia

There is a high incidence of pleural effusions in patients with sickle cell anemia who develop acute chest syndrome. This syndrome is characterized by fever, cough, pleuritic chest pain, dyspnea, leukocytosis and new lung opacities on radiographs. The acute chest syndrome is the leading cause of death in sickle cell disease. This syndrome occurs in up to 50 percent of patients who have sickle cell disease and is second only to pain as a cause for hospitalization.[67] The pathogenesis of the syndrome is probably multifactorial. Possible etiological factors include infection (e.g. *Chlamydia pneumoniae*, *Mycoplasma pneumoniae* and respiratory viruses), *in situ* microvascular thrombosis and fat embolism from infarcted bone marrow.

When patients are seen with acute chest syndrome, the chest radiograph frequently shows bilateral patchy areas of consolidation. The incidence of pleural effusion with the acute chest syndrome is 35–55 percent.[68,69] In a report of 107 episodes of the acute chest syndrome in 77 adults, unilateral pleural effusions were present in 35 percent while bilateral pleural effusions were present in an additional 14 percent.[68] In another study, a pleural effusion was present in 55 percent of 537 patients with acute chest syndrome.[69]

The seriousness of the syndrome is attested to by a mortality of approximately 5 percent.[68] Treatment is supportive and consists of antibiotics, oxygen, analgesics and transfusion or mechanical ventilation in the more severe cases.

Pulmonary veno-occlusive disease

Pulmonary veno-occlusive disease is a rare abnormality characterized pathologically by evidence of repeated pulmonary venous thrombosis and clinically by pulmonary arterial hypertension, pulmonary edema, or both. The characteristic histological feature of pulmonary veno-occlusive disease is obstruction of pulmonary venules and veins by intimal fibrosis; intravascular fibrous septa are nearly always present. The etiology and pathogenesis of this disease are unknown and may be related to more than one source or mechanism.[70]

Clinically, the patients typically have slowly progressive dyspnea and orthopnea punctuated by attacks of acute pulmonary edema. Physical examination reveals signs of pulmonary hypertension. Small pleural effusions are present in the majority of patients.[71] In one series, chest CT scans were obtained on eight patients with veno-occlusive disease and five of these patients had bilateral pleural effusions.[71] The pleural effusion occupied less than 5 percent of the hemithorax in four patients, but in the fifth patient the effusions occupied one-third of the volume of the thoracic cavity.[71] In another series, CT showed a pleural effusion in 4 (27 percent) of 15 patients with pulmonary veno-occlusive disease compared with 2 (13 percent) of 15 patients with primary pulmonary hypertension.[72] The chest radiographs may also show Kerley B lines, which result from chronic pulmonary capillary hypertension, with consequent transudation of fluid into the interstitial spaces of the lung.

The characteristics of the pleural fluid have not been delineated, but it is likely that the pleural fluid is a transudate. The pleural effusions probably are related to the increased interstitial fluid that results from the obstruction of the pulmonary veins, since 20 percent of the fluid that enters the interstitial spaces of the lung exits the lung by traversing the visceral pleura.[7] The key factor in pleural effusion with pulmonary veno-occlusive disease is that the presence of pleural effusions in a patient with pulmonary hypertension is uncommon unless the patient has veno-occlusion disease. Accordingly, the presence of pleural effusions in a patient with pulmonary hypertension may suggest the diagnosis of pulmonary veno-occlusive disease.

Pulmonary veno-occlusive disease can be diagnosed definitively only by surgical lung biopsy.[70] The prognosis of pulmonary veno-occlusive disease is grim, with most patients dying within 2 years of diagnosis. The only treatment that significantly improves the prognosis of patients with pulmonary veno-occlusive disease is lung transplantation.[70]

HEMOTHORAX

Etiology

Hemothorax is the presence of a significant amount of blood in the pleural space. To establish the diagnosis of hemothorax, the hematocrit on the pleural fluid should be at least 50 percent that of the peripheral blood. Blood entering the pleural space coagulates rapidly. Presumably as a result of physical agitation produced by movement of the heart and the lungs, the clot may be defibrinated. Loculations occurs early in the course of hemothorax, as with empyema.

Most hemothoraces result from penetrating or blunt chest trauma. Approximately 40 percent of patients with blunt chest trauma develop hemothorax, often in association with pneumothorax.[2] An occasional hemothorax results from iatrogenic manipulation, such as placement of a subclavian venous catheter or following open-heart surgery. On rare occasions, a hemothorax results from a medical condition such as metastatic malignant pleural disease, anticoagulant therapy, or thoracic endometriosis (Table 30.2).

Spontaneous hemopneumothorax, defined as the accumulation of more than 400 mL of blood in the pleural space in association with spontaneous pneumothorax, is a rare condition occurring in young patients (less than 35 years) that may be life threatening.[73] It complicates approximately 3 percent of spontaneous pneumothoraces and one-third of patients may experience hemodynamic instability with hypovolemic shock.[73] The bleeding into the pleural space can result from a torn apical vascular adhesion.

Table 30.2 Causes of hemothorax

Causes
Traumatic (penetrating or blunt chest trauma)
Iatrogenic
Heart or lung surgery
Placement of a subclavian vein-catheter
Pleural procedures (thoracentesis, chest tube insertion, pleural biopsy)
Lung biopsy
Non-traumatic
Malignant pleural disease
Anticoagulant therapy
Intrapleural fibrinolytics
Pulmonary embolism
Catamenial
Bleeding disorders
Aortic dissection or rupture
Spontaneous hemopneumothorax

Diagnosis

In patients with penetrating or blunt chest trauma, the diagnosis of hemothorax is usually established by the demonstration of a pleural effusion with a chest radiograph or with ultrasound. In spontaneous hemopneumothorax, the finding of pneumothorax with an ipsilateral air–fluid level is characteristic. The use of chest CT scans for the evaluation of patients with severe chest injury has led to the identification of hemothoraces not seen on supine chest radiographs (occult hemothoraces). For example, Stafford *et al.*[74] obtained chest radiographs and chest CT scans in 410 patients with blunt or penetrating chest trauma and reported that the chest radiograph missed hemothoraces in 88 patients (21 percent), and pneumothorax in 75 patients (18 percent).

When a diagnostic thoracentesis reveals pleural fluid that appears to be pure blood, a hematocrit should always be obtained on the pleural fluid. Frequently, even though the pleural fluid appears to be blood, the hematocrit on the pleural fluid is less than 5 percent. A hemothorax should be considered to be present only when the pleural fluid hematocrit is equal to or greater than 50 percent of the peripheral blood hematocrit.[75]

Treatment

The treatment of choice for patients with hemothorax is the immediate insertion of a chest tube, which has the following advantages: (1) it allows more complete evacuation of the blood from the pleural space; (2) it stops the bleeding if the bleeding is from pleural lacerations; (3) it allows one to quantify easily the amount of continued bleeding; (4) it may decrease the incidence of subsequent empyema because blood is a good culture medium; (5) the blood drained from the pleural space may be autotransfused; and (6) the rapid evacuation of pleural blood decreases the incidence of subsequent fibrothorax.[2]

Large-bore chest tubes (size 28 F to 32 F) should be inserted in patients with hemothorax because the blood frequently clots. Chest tubes should be removed as soon as they stop draining or cease to function (e.g. <50 mL over 6 hours) because they can serve as conduits for pleural infection. It is recommended that patients who are treated with tube thoracostomy for traumatic hemothorax be given antibiotics (e.g. cefazolin) empirically in order to reduce the incidence of empyema and pneumonia.[76] One exception to prompt-chest tube insertion is suspicion of a dissection or transection of the aorta, since intercostal drainage in this situation can lead to rapid exsanguination. Video-assisted thoracoscopic surgery (VATS) is feasible and safe for stable patients with continued and uncontrollable bleeding, clotted hemothorax early after the injury or complex empyema.[77]

In traumatic hemothorax, immediate thoracotomy is indicated for massive bleeding (i.e. initial chest tube output greater than 1500 mL), continued pleural hemorrhage (i.e. >200 mL/hour for several hours), suspected aortic injury or cardiac tamponade, sucking chest wounds or major bronchial air leaks.[2]

The four main pleural complications of traumatic hemothorax are the retention of clotted blood in the pleural space, empyema, delayed pleural effusion and fibrothorax.[2] Some hemothoraces remain only partially drained by tube thoracostomy. In a recent study, 11 percent of 596 patients treated with tube thoracostomy for traumatic hemothorax were found to have retention of clotted blood.[78] The residual clot, a source for significant complications such as empyema or fibrothorax, should probably be removed if occupies at least a third of the involved hemithorax between 2 and 4 days after the initial injury.[2] A chest CT scan is useful for distinguishing between a retained clotted collection and a parenchymal process, such as pneumonia or contusion. The optimal method for removal of the clotted blood is VATS.[79] When thoracoscopy is not readily available, consideration can be given to intrapleural fibrinolytics (if applied within ten days of injury)[80] or thoracotomy.

The treatment of empyema complicating hemothorax is similar to that of any bacterial infection of the pleural space. The development of pleural thickening weeks or months after the hemothorax appears to be more common when there is an associated pneumothorax or empyema. Decortication for fibrothorax should be postponed for several months following the injury in most cases because the pleural thickening frequently diminishes with time.[2]

Video-assisted thoracoscopic surgery should be considered an initial treatment option in all patients with spontaneous hemopneumothorax who are hemodynamically stable.[81] Treatment of hemothorax secondary to anticoagulant therapy and catamenial hemothorax is reviewed elsewhere in this book.

FUTURE DIRECTIONS

The combination of a highly sensitive D-dimer assay and multidetector CTA will become the standard for diagnosing pulmonary embolism as the cause of a pleural effusion. Additional studies in either animals or humans will be carried out, which will delineate the exact pathogenesis of the pleural effusion that occurs with pulmonary embolus. Additional studies will also be carried out to characterize the pleural fluid that occurs with the acute chest syndrome secondary to sickle cell anemia and with veno-occlusive disease. The role of fibrinolytics in retained clotted hemothorax warrants further investigation.

KEY POINTS

- Pulmonary embolism should be considered in the differential diagnosis of all patients with an undiagnosed exudative pleural effusion.

- The possibility of pulmonary embolus is best assessed with the combination of a high-sensitivity D-dimer assay and CTA in patients with a pleural effusion.
- Pleural effusions secondary to pulmonary embolism are usually small and unilateral, but may become loculated if diagnosis is delayed.
- Pleural effusions can result from SVC syndrome, acute aortic dissection, septic pulmonary emboli, sickle cell anemia and pulmonary veno-occlusive disease.
- Diagnosis of spontaneous hemopneumothorax must be considered in young adolescents presenting with spontaneous onset of chest pain and dyspnea along with radiographic findings of hydropneumothorax and/or signs of significant hypovolemia.
- The majority of traumatic hemothoraces are managed nonoperatively by tube thoracostomy.

REFERENCES

● = Key primary paper
◆ = Major review article

1. Hyers TM. Pulmonary embolism. In: Wachter RM, Goldman L, Hollander H (eds.). *Hospital medicine*, 2nd edn. Philadelphia: Lippincott Williams & Wilkins, 2005; 505–14.
◆2. Light RW. *Pleural diseases*, 5th edn. Philadelphia: Lippincott Williams & Wilkins, 2007.
3. Tapson VF, Humbert M. Incidence and prevalence of chronic thromboembolic pulmonary hypertension: from acute to chronic pulmonary embolism. *Proc Am Thorac Soc* 2006; **3**: 564–7.
4. Marel M, Arustova M, Stasny B, Light RW. Incidence of pleural effusion in a well-defined region: Epidemiologic study in Central Bohemia. *Chest* 1993; **104**:1486–9.
5. Storey DD, Dines DE, Coles DT. Pleural effusion: a diagnostic dilemma. *J Am Med Assoc* 1976; **236**: 2183–6.
6. Gunnels JJ. Perplexing pleural effusion. *Chest* 1978; **74**: 390–3.
7. Wiener-Kronish JP, Broaddus VC, Albertine KH, *et al.* Relationship of pleural effusions to increased permeability pulmonary edema in anesthetized sheep. *J Clin Invest* 1988; **82**: 1422–9.
8. Leckie WJH, Tothill P. Albumin turnover in pleural effusions. *Clin Sci* 1965; **29**: 339–52.
9. Albertine KH, Wiener-Kronish JP, Roos PJ, Staub NC. Structure, blood supply, and lymphatic vessels of the sheep's visceral pleura. *Am J Anat* 1982; **165**: 277–94.
10. Jelkmann W. Pitfalls in the measurement of circulating vascular endothelial growth factor. *Clin Chem* 2001; **47**: 617–23.
11. Cheng C-S, Rodriguez RM, Perkett EA, *et al.* Vascular endothelial growth factor in pleural fluid. *Chest* 1999; **115**: 760–5.
12. Mellins RB, Levine OR, Fishman AP. Effect of systemic and pulmonary venous hypertension on pleural and pericardial fluid accumulation. *J Appl Physiol* 1970; **29**: 564–9.
13. Wiener-Kronish JP, Matthay MA, Callen PW, *et al.* Relationship of pleural effusions to pulmonary hemodynamics in patients with congestive heart failure. *Am Rev Respir Dis* 1985; **132**: 1253–6.
14. Anderson FA Jr, Spencer FA. Risk factors for venous thromboembolism. *Circulation* 2003; **107**(23 Suppl 1): 19–116.
15. Edelsberg J, Hagiwara M, Taneja C, Oster G. Risk of venous thromboembolism among hospitalized medically ill patients. *Am J Health Syst Pharm* 2006; **63**(20 Suppl 6): S16–22.
16. Stein PD, Henry JW. Clinical characteristics of patients with acute pulmonary embolism stratified according to their presenting syndromes. *Chest* 1997; **112**: 974–9.
17. Miniati M, Prediletto R, Formichi B, *et al.* Accuracy of clinical assessment in the diagnosis of pulmonary embolism. *Am J Respir Crit Care Med* 1999; **159**: 864–71.
18. Stein PD, Huang HL, Afzal A, Noor HA. Incidence of acute pulmonary embolism in a general hospital. Relation to age, sex, and race. *Chest* 1999; **116**: 909–13.
19. Lobo JL, Zorrilla V, Aizpuru F, *et al.* Clinical syndromes and clinical outcome in patients with pulmonary embolism: findings from the RIETE registry. *Chest* 2006; **130**: 1817–22.
●20. Monreal M, Muñoz-Torrero JF, Naraine VS, *et al.* Pulmonary embolism in patients with chronic obstructive pulmonary disease or congestive heart failure. *Am J Med* 2006; **119**: 851–8.
21. Maloba M, Hogg K. Best evidence topic report. Diagnostic utility of arterial blood gases for investigation of pulmonary embolus. *Emerg Med J* 2005; **22**: 435–6.
22. Worsley DF, Alavi A, Aronchick JM, *et al.* Chest radiographic findings in patients with acute pulmonary embolism: observations from the PIOPED study. *Radiology* 1993; **189**: 133–6.
23. Elliott CG, Goldhaber SZ, Visani L, DeRosa M. Chest radiographs in acute pulmonary embolism: results from the international cooperative pulmonary embolism registry. *Chest* 2000; **118**: 33–8.
●24. Porcel JM, Madroñero AB, Pardina M, *et al.* Analysis of pleural effusions in acute pulmonary embolism: radiological and pleural fluid data from 230 patients. *Respirology* 2007; **12**: 234–9.
25. Bynum LJ, Wilson JE III. Radiographic features of pleural effusions in pulmonary embolism. *Am Rev Respir Dis* 1978; **117**: 829–34.
●26. Romero-Candeira S, Hernandez-Blasco L, Soler MJ, Munoz A, Aranda I. Biochemical and cytologic characteristics of pleural effusions secondary to pulmonary embolism. *Chest* 2002; **121**: 465–9.
27. Bynum LJ, Wilson JE III. Characteristics of pleural effusions associated with pulmonary embolism. *Arch Intern Med* 1976; **136**: 159–62.
28. Wells PS, Anderson DR, Rodger M, *et al.* Excluding pulmonary embolism at the bedside without diagnostic imaging: management of patients with suspected pulmonary embolism presenting to the emergency department by using a simple clinical model and D-dimer. *Ann Intern Med* 2001; **135**: 98–107.
29. Le Gal G, Righini M, Roy PM, *et al.* Prediction of pulmonary embolism in the emergency department: the revised Geneva score. *Ann Intern Med* 2006; **144**: 165–71.
30. Dalen JE. New PIOPED recommendations for the diagnosis of pulmonary embolism. *Am J Med* 2006; **119**: 1001–2.
31. Light RW. Pleural effusion due to pulmonary emboli. *Curr Opin Pulm Med* 2001; **7**: 198–201.
32. Nijkeuter M, Huisman MV. Diagnostic methods in pulmonary embolism. *Eur J Intern Med* 2005; **16**: 247–56.
33. Stein PD, Hull RD, Patel KC, *et al.* D-dimer for the exclusion of acute venous thrombosis and pulmonary embolism: a systematic review. *Ann Intern Med* 2004; **140**: 589–602.
●34. van Belle A, Buller HR, Huisman MV, *et al.* Effectiveness of managing suspected pulmonary embolism using an algorithm combining clinical probability, D-dimer testing, and computed tomography. *J Am Med Assoc* 2006; **295**: 172–9.
35. The PIOPED Investigators. Value of the ventilation/perfusion scan in acute pulmonary embolism: results of the Prospective Investigation of Pulmonary Embolism Diagnosis (PIOPED). *J Am Med Assoc* 1990; **263**: 2753–9.
36. Mele FM, Caride VJ. Pleural effusions: patterns on ventilation-perfusion lung scans. *Clin Nucl Med* 1998; **23**: 571–5.

37. Smith TP, Ryan JM, Brodwater BK. Acute pulmonary thromboembolism: comparison of the diagnostic capabilities of conventional film-screen and digital angiography. *Chest* 2002; **122**: 968–72.
38. Weiss CR, Scatarige JC, Diette GB, *et al.* CT pulmonary angiography is the first-line imaging test for acute pulmonary embolism: a survey of US clinicians. *Acad Radiol* 2006; **13**: 434–46.
39. Hogg K, Brown G, Dunning J, *et al.* Diagnosis of pulmonary embolism with CT pulmonary angiography: a systematic review. *Emerg Med J* 2006; **23**: 172–8.
◆40. Segal JB, Eng J, Tamariz LJ, Bass EB. Review of the evidence on diagnosis of deep venous thrombosis and pulmonary embolism. *Ann Fam Med* 2007; **5**: 63–73.
41. Moores LK, Jackson WL Jr, Shorr AF, Jackson JL. Meta-analysis: outcomes in patients with suspected pulmonary embolism managed with computed tomographic pulmonary angiography. *Ann Intern Med* 2004; **141**: 866–74.
●42. Quiroz R, Kucher N, Zou KH, *et al.* Clinical validity of a negative computed tomography scan in patients with suspected pulmonary embolism: a systematic review. *J Am Med Assoc* 2005; **293**: 2012–7.
●43. Stein PD, Fowler SE, Goodman LR, *et al.* Multidetector computed tomography for acute pulmonary embolism. *N Engl J Med* 2006; **354**: 2317–27.
44. Perrier A, Bounameaux H. Accuracy or outcome in suspected pulmonary embolism. *N Engl J Med* 2006; **354**: 2383–5.
◆45. Stein PD, Woodard PK, Weg JG, *et al.* Diagnostic pathways in acute pulmonary embolism: recommendations of the PIOPED II investigators. *Am J Med* 2006; **119**: 1048–55.
●46. Girard P, Sanchez O, Leroyer C, *et al.* Deep venous thrombosis in patients with acute pulmonary embolism. Prevalence, risk factors, and clinical significance. *Chest* 2005; **128**: 1593–1600.
47. Perrier A, Roy PM, Sanchez O, *et al.* Multidetector-row computed tomography in suspected pulmonary embolism. *N Engl J Med* 2005; **352**: 1760–8.
●48. Mathis G, Blank W, Reissig A, *et al.* Thoracic ultrasound for diagnosing pulmonary embolism: a prospective multicenter study of 352 patients. *Chest* 2005; **128**: 1531–8.
●49. Kearon C, Ginsberg JS, Douketis J, *et al.* An evaluation of D-dimer in the diagnosis of pulmonary embolism: a randomized trial. *Ann Intern Med* 2006; **144**: 812–21.
◆50. Qaseem A, Snow V, Barry P, *et al.* Current diagnosis of venous thromboembolism in primary care: a clinical practice guideline from the American College of Physicians and the American College of Family Physicians. *Ann Intern Med* 2007; **146**: 454–8.
◆51. Snow V, Qaseem A, Barry P, *et al.* Management of venous thromboembolism: a clinical practice guideline from the American College of Physicians and the American College of Family Physicians. *Ann Intern Med* 2007; **146**: 204–10.
52. Rostand RA, Feldman RL, Block ER. Massive hemothorax complicating heparin anticoagulation for pulmonary embolus. *South Med J* 1977; **70**:1128–30.
53. Mrug M, Mishra PV, Lusane HC, Cunningham JM, Alpert MA. Hemothorax and retroperitoneal hematoma after anticoagulation with enoxaparin. *South Med J* 2002; **95**: 936–8.
54. Wick MR, Ritter JH, Schuller D. Ruptured pulmonary infarction: a rare, fatal complication of thromboembolic disease. *Mayo Clin Proc* 2000; **75**: 639–42.
●55. Rice TW, Rodriguez RM, Barnette R, Light RW. Prevalence and characteristics of pleural effusions in superior vena cava syndrome. *Respirology* 2006; **11**: 299–305.
●56. Hata N, Tanaka K, Imaizumi T, *et al.* Clinical significance of pleural effusion in acute aortic dissection. *Chest* 2002; **121**: 825–30.
57. Sato F, Kitamura T, Kongo M, *et al.* Newly diagnosed acute aortic dissection. Characteristics, treatment modifications, and outcomes. *Int Heart J* 2005; **46**: 1083–98.
58. Little S, Johnson J, Moon BY, Mehta S. Painless left hemorrhagic pleural effusion. An unusual presentation of dissecting ascending aortic aneurysm. *Chest* 1999; **116**: 1478–80.
59. Han D, Lee KS, Franquet T, *et al.* Thrombotic and nonthrombotic pulmonary arterial embolism: spectrum of imaging findings. *Radiographics* 2003; **23**: 1521–39.
●60. Cook RJ, Ashton RW, Aughenbaugh GL, Ryu JH. Septic pulmonary embolism. Presenting features and clinical course of 14 patients. *Chest* 2005; **128**: 162–6.
61. Sexauer WP, Quezado Z, Lippmann ML, Goldberg SK. Pleural effusions in right-sided endocarditis: characteristics and pathophysiology. *South Med J* 1992; **85**: 1176–80.
62. Riordan T, Wilson M. Lemierre's syndrome: more than a historical curiosa. *Postgrad Med J* 2004; **80**: 328–34.
◆63. Armstrong AW, Spooner K, Sanders JW. Lemierre's Syndrome. *Curr Infect Dis Rep* 2000; **2**: 168–73.
64. Chirinos JA, Lichtstein DM, Garcia J, Tamariz LJ. The evolution of Lemierre syndrome: report of 2 cases and review of the literature. *Medicine (Baltimore)* 2002; **81**: 458–65.
65. Gowan RT, Mehran RJ, Cardinal P, Jones G. Thoracic complications of Lemierre syndrome. *Can Respir J* 2000; **7**: 481–5.
66. Alifano M, Venissac N, Guillot F, Mouroux J. Lemierre's syndrome with bilateral empyema thoracis. *Ann Thorac Surg* 2000; **69**: 930–1.
◆67. Siddiqui AK, Ahmed S. Pulmonary manifestations of sickle cell disease. *Postgrad Med J* 2003; **79**: 384–90.
68. Maitre B, Habibi A, Raided-Thoraval F, *et al.* Acute chest syndrome in adults with sickle cell disease. *Chest* 2000; **117**: 1386–92.
●69. Vichinsky EP, Neumayr LD, Earles AN, *et al.* Causes and outcomes of the acute chest syndrome in sickle cell disease. National Acute Chest Syndrome Study Group. *N Engl J Med* 2000; **342**: 1855–65.
70. Mandel J, Mark EJ, Hales CA. Pulmonary veno-occlusive disease. *Am J Respir Crit Care Med* 2000; **162**: 1964–73.
71. Swensen SJ, Tashjian JH, Myers JL, *et al.* Pulmonary venoocclusive disease: CT findings in eight patients. *AJR Am J Roentgenol* 1996; **167**: 937–40.
72. Resten A, Maitre S, Humbert M, *et al.* Pulmonary hypertension: CT of the chest in pulmonary venooclusive disease. *AJR Am J Roentgenol* 2004; **183**: 65–70.
●73. Hsu NY, Shih CS, Hsu CP, Chen PR. Spontaneous hemopneumothorax revisited: clinical approach and systemic review of the literature. *Ann Thorac Surg* 2005; **80**: 1859–63.
74. Stafford RE, Linn J, Washington L. Incidence and management of occult hemothoraces. *Am J Surg* 2006; **192**: 722–6.
◆75. Porcel JM, Light RW. Thoracentesis. http://pier.acponline.org/physicians/procedures/physpro899/physpro899. [Data accessed: 2006 Nov 6]. In: PIER [online database]. Philadelphia: American College of Physicians; 2007.
76. Sanabria A, Valdivieso E, Gomez G, Echeverry G. Prophylactic antibiotics in chest trauma: a meta-analysis of high-quality studies. *World J Surg* 2006; **30**: 1843–7.
77. Ambrogi MC, Lucchi M, Dini P, Mussi A, Angeletti CA. Videothoracoscopy for evaluation and treatment of hemothorax. *J Cardiovasc Surg (Torino)* 2002; **43**: 109–12.
78. Oguzkaya F, Akcali Y, Bilgin M. Videothoracoscopy versus intrapleural streptokinase for management of post traumatic retained haemothorax: a retrospective study of 65 cases. *Injury* 2005; **36**: 526–9.
79. Navsaria PH, Vogel RJ, Nicol AJ. Thoracoscopic evacuation of retained posttraumatic hemothorax. *Ann Thorac Surg* 2004; **78**: 282–6.
80. Inci I, Ozcelik C, Ulku R, Tuna A, Eren N. Intrapleural fibrinolytic treatment of traumatic clotted hemothorax. *Chest* 1998; **114**: 160–5.
◆81. Ng CSh, Yim AP. Spontaneous hemopneumothorax. *Curr Opin Pulm Med* 2006; **12**: 273–7.

31

Effusions in immunocompromised hosts

BEKELE AFESSA, JOHN J MULLON

INTRODUCTION

The immune system is composed of two components: non-specific and specific. The non-specific immune system does not require prior exposure to infectious agents or other antigens and consists of mucous membrane and skin barriers, complements and leukocytes. The specific immune system requires prior contact with infectious agents or other antigens and consists of macrophages, humoral immunity and cell-mediated immunity. Immunocompromised hosts have primary or secondary defects in their immune system (Tables 31.1 and 31.2). Serious immune deficiency is uncommon in solid tumors unless treated with immunosuppressants. Neutropenic patients are prone to infections with pyogenic or enteric bacteria. With prolonged neutropenia, fungal infections also occur. Humoral immune deficiency and defects in the complement system are associated with infection by pyogenic bacteria. Patients with cellular immune deficiency are predisposed to fungal and viral infections. Overall, the diagnostic importance of pleural fluid analysis in the immunocompromised host is similar to that of the immunocompetent patient. However, because of the wider differential diagnoses and the adverse impact of delayed diagnosis, a more aggressive diagnostic evaluation and management are recommended. This chapter will focus on pleural diseases that develop in the main immunocompromised conditions.

Table 31.1 The main primary immune deficiencies

Primary immune deficiences	
Humoral	Phagocytic
X-linked agammaglobulinemia	Neutropenia
Autosomal recessive agammaglobulinemia	Congenital
Common variable immunodeficiency	Cyclic
Hyperimmunoglobulin M syndromes	Chronic granulomatous disease
Immunoglobulin A deficiency	Leukocyte adhesion deficiency
Immunoglobulin G subclass deficiency	Hyperimmunoglobulin E syndrome
Combined humoral and cellular deficiency	Myeloperoxidase deficiency
Severe combined immune deficiency (SCID)	Chediak–Higashi syndrome
Inherited complement deficiencies	

Table 31.2 Underlying conditions in patients with secondary immune deficiency

Underlying conditions	
Immunosuppressive therapy	Malignancy
For malignancy	Hodgkin's disease
For autoimmune disease	Chronic lymphocytic leukemia
Conditioning for BMT	Multiple myeloma
Treatment or prevention of GVHD in HSCT recipients	Solid tumors
Treatment or prevention of rejection in solid organ transplant recipients	Others
HIV infection	Diabetes mellitus
Splenectomy	Renal insufficiency
Autoimmune diseases	Hepatic cirrhosis
Systemic lupus erythematosus	Malnutrition
Rheumatoid arthritis	Alcoholism
Radiation	Aging
Allogeneic blood transfusion	Burn

GVHD, graft-versus-host disease; HIV, human immunodeficiency virus; HSCT, hematopoietic stem cell transplant.

PLEURAL DISEASES IN PATIENTS WITH HUMAN IMMUNODEFICIENCY VIRUS INFECTION

Epidemiology

An estimated 39.5 million people are living with human immunodeficiency virus (HIV) worldwide.[1] Pleural effusions are seen in approximately 7–27 percent of hospitalized patients with HIV.[2] Bacterial infections, tuberculosis and Kaposi sarcoma (KS) are the three leading causes of pleural effusion in patients with HIV.[2–4] In nine publications of 623 HIV infected patients with pleural effusion, 64.7 percent were associated with infections, 26.6 percent with non-infectious etiology and no cause was identified in 8.7 percent (Table 31.3).[2,5]

Infectious causes

BACTERIAL

Although the incidence of bacterial pneumonia in patients with HIV has decreased since the introduction of highly active anti-retroviral therapy (HAART), it still occurs in approximately 9 percent of hospitalized patients. Its incidence is higher in injection drug users and those with advanced immunosuppression. Pleural effusion is present in 12–47 percent of HIV infected patients with bacterial pneumonia.[2] Empyema occurs in approximately 1.1 percent of patients with pleural effusion (Table 31.3).[2] In a recent study from West Africa, empyema was found in 8 of the 35 HIV infected patients with pleural effusion (23 percent).[5] Bacterial pneumonia in HIV infected patients is

Table 31.3 Causes of pleural effusion in patients with human immunodeficiency virus (HIV) infection

Causes	Number	Causes	Number
Non-infectious	166	Infectious	403
Renal failure	17	Bacterial pneumonia	185
Hypoalbuminemia	23	Empyema	7
Kaposi's sarcoma	62	*Mycobacterium tuberculosis*	165
Lymphoma	19	*Mycobacterium avium* complex	4
Bronchogenic carcinoma	8	*Pneumocystis jiroveci*	25
Pancreatitis	7	*Cytomegalovirus*	1
Hepatic cirrhosis	7	*Aspergillus* spp	2
Congestive heart failure	10	*Cryptococcus neoformans*	7
Pericarditis	1	*Nocardia* spp	3
Atelectasis	4	*Leishmanai donovani*	2
Acute respiratory distress syndrome	1	Septic emboli	2
Pulmonary embolism	5	Unknown	54
Trauma	1		
Surgery	1		

commonly caused by *Streptococcus pneumoniae*, *Staphylococcus aureus*, *Haemophilus influenzae* and *Pseudomonas aeruginosa*.[2] However, parapneumonic effusions and empyema can be caused by other pathogens such as *Rhodococcus equi*, *Legionella pneumophila*, *Salmonella* spp. and *Bordetella bronchiseptica*.

In the absence of pulmonary nodules, unilateral effusion with focal air space consolidation suggests parapneumonic effusion.[6] In addition to antibiotics, the management of complicated pleural effusions and empyemas requires serial thoracentesis, urgent drainage and close clinical surveillance to discern the need for decortication or rib resection, and open drainage.[2] Video-assisted thoracoscopic surgery (VATS) has been shown to be efficacious and safe for the treatment of empyema in HIV-infected patients.[7]

TUBERCULOSIS

Approximately two billion people are infected with *Mycobacterium tuberculosis*.[8] Although tuberculosis is a worldwide pandemic, over 75 percent of it occurs in Africa and Asia. Of the two million annual deaths due to tuberculosis, 250 000 of them are associated with HIV infection. Pleural effusion is seen in 8–21 percent of HIV infected patients with pulmonary tuberculosis.[2,5] In certain regions of the world, tuberculosis is the most common cause of pleural effusion.[5] Among HIV infected patients with tuberculosis, the frequency of pleural effusion is higher in patients with CD4+ lymphocyte counts above 200 cells/μL.[9]

Chest radiograph findings of unilateral effusion with miliary nodules and/or mediastinal lymphadenopathy suggest tuberculosis.[6] The diagnostic approach to tuberculous pleuritis in patients with HIV is similar to that in other patients.[10] The tuberculin skin test is positive in 12–63 percent of HIV infected patients with tuberculous pleurisy, with positivity higher in those with higher CD4 counts.[9] Sputum should be obtained for acid-fast bacilli (AFB) smear and mycobacterial culture, even in the absence of parenchymal involvement. The pleural fluid AFB smear is positive in 6–15 percent.[2] Positive pleural fluid AFB smear is more likely when the blood CD4+ lymphocyte count is <200 cells/μL. Pleural biopsy AFB has been reported to have positive rates of 44 and 69 percent.[2] Pleural fluid and biopsy cultures are each positive in 30–50 percent of pleural tuberculosis. In the appropriate clinical setting, the diagnosis of tuberculous pleurisy can be established by demonstrating granulomas in pleural biopsy. Despite the depressed T-lymphocyte function, granulomas have been reported in 44–88 percent of HIV infected patients.[2]

Although tuberculous pleural effusions are usually characterized by lymphocytosis and paucity of mesothelial cells and eosniophils in non-HIV infected patients, cases of tuberculous pleurisy with numerous mesothelial cells have been reported in patients with HIV.[11] The roles of polymerase chain reaction (PCR), lysozyme, interferon gamma (IFN-γ) and adenosine deaminase (ADA) measurements in pleural fluid for the diagnosis of tuberculous pleuritis have not been clearly defined because of their inability to provide culture and drug sensitivity information. In one study from Thailand, pleural fluid ADA level at a cutoff value of 60 U/L had sensitivity, specificity and positive and negative predictive values of 95 percent or higher for the diagnosis of pleural tuberculosis, independent of patients' HIV status.[12] The diagnostic use of ADA in areas with low incidence of tuberculosis may lead to high false-positive rates, although the finding of a low ADA level has high negative predictive value and may be useful in excluding tuberculous pleurisy.

Most HIV infected patients with tuberculous pleurisy should be started on four-drug therapy, consisting of isoniazid, rifampin, pyrazinamide and ethambutol. The majority of HIV infected patients with tuberculous pleuritis respond favorably to treatment. In one study from South Carolina, the mortality of HIV infected patients with pleural tuberculosis was 9 percent after an average follow-up period of 31 months.[13] In contrast, higher mortality rates have been reported from Africa.[2] There is insufficient evidence for the efficacy of corticosteroids in the treatment of tuberculosis pleurisy.[14]

PNEUMOCYSTIS JIROVECII

Pleural effusions have been reported in 6–15 percent of HIV infected patients with *Pneumocystis jirovecii* pneumonia (PCP).[2] Approximately 4 percent of pleural effusions in HIV infected patients are associated with PCP (Table 31.3). However, confirmed *Pneumocystis jirovecii* involvement of the pleura is limited to few case reports. *Pneumocystis* pleural disease appears to be an anatomic extension of smoldering subpleural PCP and it can be diagnosed by staining pleural fluid for the organism.[2] Treatment requires antibiotics for the underlying PCP and tube thoracostomy if a bronchopleural fistula is present.

MISCELLANEOUS INFECTIOUS CAUSES

Pleural effusion has been reported in 5 percent of HIV infected patients with pulmonary cryptococcosis and may precede meningitis.[15] There are case reports of pleural effusions associated with various infections including histoplasmosis, candidiasis, amebiasis, microfilariasis and *Mycobacterium avium* complex.

Malignant causes

Ninety percent of the malignancies reported in acquired immune deficiency syndrome (AIDS) are either KS or non-Hodgkin's lymphoma (NHL).[2] Most of the AIDS-defining malignancies are associated with secondary viral infections by *Human herpes virus* (HHV)-8, *Epstein–Barr virus* (EBV) or *Human papilloma virus*.[16] Since the wide-spread use of HAART, the incidence rates of KS and NHL have declined. However, KS remains the most common AIDS-associated malignancy in the developed world and is one of the most common cancers in developing nations. Compared with empyema, KS and lymphoma are more likely to be associated with bilateral pleural effusions.[6] Current treatment options for HHV-8 associated disease are ineffective, unavailable or toxic.[17]

KAPOSI SARCOMA

Kaposi sarcoma affects mainly homosexual and bisexual men. Pulmonary KS occurs in 47–75 percent of HIV infected patients with cutaneous KS and may present without mucocutaneous involvement.[2] Pleural effusions occur in 15–89 percent of pulmonary KS.[2] Most KS-associated pleural effusions are visibly bloody or blood-tinged.[2] Although uncommon, chylous effusion associated with KS has been reported.[18]

A chest radiograph finding of bilateral effusions with intrapulmonary nodules, and/or hilar lymphadenopathy suggests KS.[6] However, it is difficult to make a definitive diagnosis of pleural KS. Since there are no characteristic KS cells and most KS lesions are found in the visceral pleura, pleural fluid and closed needle biopsies are usually non-diagnostic. Thoracoscopic surgical finding of the characteristic KS lesions in the pleura establishes the diagnosis. In most cases, the presumptive diagnosis of pleural KS can be made in the appropriate clinical setting by visualization of the characteristic endobronchial lesions bronchoscopically and excluding other causes.

Although radiation therapy, chemotherapy and biological modifiers have been used to treat KS, the major goal of treatment of pleural KS is palliation. HAART is associated with regression of KS and improved survival. Thoracentesis and tube thoracostomy are used to drain large, symptomatic, pleural effusions associated with KS. However, the effusions recur and sclerotherapy is usually ineffective. Thoracoscopic talc pleurodesis, pleuroperitoneal shunt or indwelling pleural catheter are other alternatives. The median survival of patients with pulmonary KS is 2–10 months, and this is shorter with pleural involvement.[2]

NON-HODGKIN'S LYMPHOMA

The incidence of NHL has declined and it occurs mainly in patients who are refusing or failing HAART. Among a cohort of 304 439 adults with AIDS in the USA, 14 lymphomas, 4 of which involved the pleura, were identified.[19] Pulmonary involvement, with pleural effusion in 68 percent, is reported in 1–14 percent of AIDS-related NHL.[2] Pleural effusions are absent in AIDS related primary pulmonary lymphoma. The diagnostic yield of pleural fluid and closed needle pleural biopsy are 75 and 100 percent, respectively. Despite chemotherapy, prognosis is poor.

PRIMARY EFFUSION LYMPHOMA

Primary effusion lymphoma (PEL), or body-cavity-based lymphoma, is a form of NHL characterized by pleural, pericardial or peritoneal lymphomatous effusions in the absence of a solid tumor mass.[20] It is associated with HHV-8 and accounts for 1–3 percent of all AIDS-related lymphomas.[2] Although PEL affects mainly homosexuals with advanced AIDS, it has also been reported in injection drug users. The median CD4+ lymphocyte counts range between 34 and 84 cells/μL at the time of PEL diagnosis.

The PEL cells are immunophenotypically indeterminate, lacking B- and T-cell-associated antigens, but expressing markers associated with the late stages of B-cell differentiation. Infection of the tumor clone with HHV-8 constitutes the genetic hallmark of PEL.[2] Although EBV infects PEL cells, it is absent in some, in contrast to HHV-8, which is present in all.

Radiographic studies in PEL show pleural effusion without detectable mass, parenchymal opacities or lymphadenopathy.[2] In addition to pleural effusion, plain chest radiographs and computed tomography show pleural thickening, pericardial thickening and pericardial and peritoneal effusions. Pleural fluid analysis shows elevated lactate dehydrogenase and protein. PCR of the fluid shows HHV-8. Although lymphoma spread outside of the body cavity is unusual in PEL, minor involvement of the lymph nodes and bone marrow have been reported.[2]

Although some patients with PEL have been treated with chemotherapy, the impact of treatment on outcome is either unknown or poor. Tube thoracostomy drainage of the pleural effusion can be used for palliation. The reported median survival of patients with PEL is less than 7 months.[2,21]

OTHER MALIGNANCIES

Bronchogenic carcinoma is an uncommon cause of pleural effusion in HIV infected patients. There are reports of malignant mesothelioma in HIV infected patients without history of asbestos exposure.[22]

Multicentric Castleman's disease is a lymphoproliferative disorder of the plasma cell type, which has been reported in patients with HIV infection. Tissues involved by the disease frequently contain HHV-8.[20] Reports of HIV infected patients with Castleman's disease show pleural effusion in 24 percent. Other manifestations include dyspnea, cough, malaise, fever, hepatosplenomegaly and lymphadenopathy. Patients with Castleman's disease respond to treatment with steroids and chemotherapy. However, relapse of the disease and deterioration to lymphoma are frequent.

Miscellaneous causes

Renal failure, cardiac dysfunction, hypoalbuminemia, pancreatitis, liver failure and other conditions listed in Table 31.3 should be included in the differential diagnosis of pleural effusions in AIDS.

IMMUNE RECONSTITUTION INFLAMMATORY SYNDROME

The use of HAART may lead to the immune reconstitution inflammatory syndrome (IRIS), associated with transient deterioration following initial improvement.[23] In HIV infected patients with tuberculous infection, IRIS may lead to unmasking of previously undiagnosed or worsening of mycobacterial disease.[23] In a study of five patients with IRIS and tuberculosis infection, chest radiograph showed pleural effusion in one.[24] The other radiographic abnormalities of the syndrome included marked mediastinal lymphadenopathy and new pulmonary infiltrates. The discontinuation of HAART is usually effective in improving symptoms of IRIS but may lead to progression of the HIV disease.[23]

PNEUMOTHORAX

The incidence of pneumothorax in AIDS is between two and seven per 1000 person-years.[2] In hospitalized patients with HIV, the pneumothorax rate is 1–2 percent and increases to 4–12 percent in those with PCP. Risk factors for pneumothorax include cigarette smoking, injection drug use, aerosolized pentamidine, PCP, pulmonary tuberculosis and radiographic presence of cysts, pneumatoceles or bullae.[2] PCP is the most common cause of pneumothorax in patients with HIV, followed by pulmonary tuberculosis. Nodules, which may stain positive for *Pneumocystis jirovecii*, can be found on the lung surface and pleura in patients with pneumothorax and PCP. There are case reports of pneumothorax associated with pulmonary cryptococcosis and lymphoid interstitial pneumonitis.[25]

Conservative management of pneumothorax in patients with HIV is associated with high failure rate and prolonged hospitalization. Needle drainage, tube thoracostomy, Heimlich valve, pleurodesis, pleurectomy, VATS and thoracotomy may be used in the treatment of pneumothorax.[2,4] The reported success rates of tube thoracostomy in the drainage of pneumothorax range between 20 and 82 percent.[2] The recurrence rates range between 11 and 65 percent.[2]

Pneumothorax in PCP is an independent risk factor for increased mortality. The overall mortality rate of pneumothorax in AIDS is approximately 34 percent, ranging between 10 and 81 percent. In patients with recurrent pneumothorax or in those with PCP and on positive-pressure mechanical ventilation, the mortality approaches 100 percent.

PLEURAL DISEASES IN TRANSPLANT RECIPIENTS

Thousands of patients undergo solid organ and hematopoietic stem cell transplantation (HSCT) annually worldwide.[26,27] Immunosuppressed transplant recipients are at high risk for the development of infections and malignancies. The incidence of pleural diseases in transplant recipients varies according to the transplant type. Causes of pleural effusion in transplant recipients include immunosuppressant medications, infections and malignancies (Table 31.4). Some of the pleural complications, such as post-transplant infection and post-transplant lymphoproliferative disorder (PTLD) relate to the level and duration of immunosuppression and are not organ-specific.[28] Infectious pleural complications are likely to occur more frequently in HSCT recipients during the immediate post-transplant period as the result of the pre-transplant conditioning regimen and leukopenia.

Pleural effusions develop in almost all lung and heart, as well as the majority of liver, transplant recipients in the immediate post-transplant period because of the proximity of the surgical sites to the pleura. Pleural effusion is less common in kidney transplantation. However, approximately 21 percent of kidney transplant recipients admitted to the intensive care unit (ICU) have pleural effusion.[29] The majority of intestinal transplant recipients also receive

Table 31.4 Causes of pleural effusion in transplant recipients

Causes of pleural effusion in transplant recipients
Infections
Bacterial
Viral
Mycobacterial
Fungal
Protozoan
Neoplasm
PTLD
Lymphoma
Lung cancer
Mesothelioma
Miscellaneous
Surgery
Rejection
Reperfusion lung injury
Obstruction of pulmonary venous anastomosis
GVHD
Urinothorax
Budd–Chiari syndrome
Medications (including imatinib and GCSF)
Capillary leak syndrome

GCSF, granulocyte colony-stimulating factor; GVHD, graft-versus-host disease; PTLD, post-transplant lymphoproliferative disorder.

other solid organ transplant. There is paucity of data about pulmonary and pleural complications in intestinal transplant recipients. Pleural effusion develops in 10–39 percent of HSCT recipients.[30]

Infectious causes

Viruses, bacteria, mycobacteria, fungi and protozoa cause parapneumonic effusions and empyema in transplant recipients. Parapneumonic effusions and empyemas develop in 3–5 percent of lung transplant recipients and they are more frequent in double than single lung transplant recipients.[31,32] In a study of 68 living lobar lung transplant recipients, empyema developed in two and both requiring decortication.[33] Approximately 30 percent of liver transplant recipients may develop bacterial pneumonia, some with parapneumonic effusion, in the postoperative period.[34]

The diagnostic evaluation and treatment of transplant recipients with parapneumonic effusion and empyema are similar to those of other patients with these diseases.

BACTERIA

The common pathogens causing parapneumonic effusions and empyema in transplant recipients include *P. aeruginosa, Klebsiella pneumoniae, Acinetobacter baumannii* and *S. aureus. Listeria monocytogenes* is rarely isolated from the pleural fluid of transplant recipients.[35] *Burkholderia cepacia* is often isolated from empyema of lung transplant recipients with cystic fibrosis.[32] Parapneumonic pleural effusions and empyema may accompany *Legionella* pneumonia in transplant recipients.[36]

Because chyle is bacteriostatic, infected chylothorax is uncommon. However, infected chylothorax has been reported in a kidney transplant recipient.[37]

MYCOBACTERIA

In endemic areas and in patients at high risk for *M. tuberculosis* infection, tuberculous pleural effusion should be included in the differential diagnoses. The measurement of ADA activity in pleural fluid provides a good tool for the diagnosis of tuberculous pleural effusion in transplant recipients.[38]

FUNGI

Candidiasis and Aspergillosis infections are common in transplant recipients, especially those with prolonged neutropenia. However, pleural involvement is uncommon. *Candida albicans* has been associated with empyema requiring decortication and chest tube drainage in a cardiac transplant recipient.[39] Hemothorax may be seen in transplant recipients with *Aspergillus* pneumonia.[40] There are case reports of pleural involvement by cryptococcal, histoplasma, *Pneumocystis*, *Mucor*, *Rhizopus* and *Chaetomium* fungal infections.

OTHER INFECTIONS

Although an infrequent cause of pneumonia in transplant recipients, *Toxoplasma gondii* may be associated with pleural effusion.[41] Small pleural effusions associated with cytomegalovirus pneumonia are seen in approximately 26 percent of heart transplant and 22 percent of HSCT recipients.[42,43]

Malignant causes

POST-TRANSPLANT LYMPHOPROLIFERATIVE DISORDER

This disorder includes a heterogeneous group of diseases ranging from a benign reactive lymphoid hyperplasia to a high-grade malignant lymphoma.[44] In a review of 4747 solid organ transplant and HSCT recipients, thoracic involvement by PTLD was reported in 11 (0.2 percent): 1 of 343 heart (0.3 percent), 3 of 83 lung (0.4 percent), 3 of 1573 kidney (0.2 percent), 2 of 371 kidney–pancreas (0.5 percent), 0 of 715 liver and 2 of 1662 (0.1 percent) hematopoietic stem cell transplant recipients.[45]

An EBV-associated PTLD may manifest as pleural effusion, usually with involvement of solid organs. Although approximately 90 percent of PTLDs are of B-cell origin, T-cell phenotype involving the pleura have been reported. PTLD may manifest as primary effusion without solid organ involvement.[46,47] Chylothorax has been reported in a heart transplant recipient with PTLD.[40] Flow cytometric studies of the pleural fluid can be diagnostic for PTLD. The treatment of PTLD involves reduction of immunosuppression.

OTHER HEMATOLOGICAL MALIGNANCIES

Transplant recipients are at risk for the development of NHL with pleural effusion. There are reports of pleural effusions caused by Burkitt-like lymphoma, HHV-8 associated KS and PEL in solid organ transplant recipients.[48,49] Relapse of the underlying hematological malignancy may involve the pleura in HSCT recipients.[50]

NON-HEMATOLOGICAL MALIGNANCIES

Transplant recipients with smoking and asbestos exposure history are at high risk for bronchogenic carcinoma and malignant mesothelioma. Several reports have shown an increased risk of secondary malignancy following HSCT, some of them associated with malignant pleural effusion.[51,52]

Miscellaneous causes

LUNG TRANSPLANT RECIPIENTS

The pleural effusion that occurs in lung transplant recipients in the early postoperative period is bloody, exudative and neutrophil predominant.[31,53,54] In single lung transplant recipients, the effusion develops on the same side as the graft.[31] Pleural fluid output as well as its cellularity, lactate dehydrogenase, and total protein content decrease rapidly over the first week following lung transplant.[53] Less than 1 percent of cells in the pleural fluid are of donor origin by the eighth day of transplant.[55] Late postoperative pleural effusions, usually exudative with lymphocyte predominance, occur in approximately 20 percent of lung transplant recipients. In the absence of infection or rejection, the effusions resolve without recurrence and no pleural fluid analysis is needed.

Pleural complications are more common in double than in single lung transplantation. Stenosis or thrombosis of pulmonary venous anastomosis may cause venous outflow impairment leading to unilateral edema and pleural effusion.[56] The pulmonary reimplantation response, a form of non-cardiogenic pulmonary edema that begins soon after lung transplant and resolves in days to weeks, may be associated with pleural effusion.[57] Reperfusion injury, rejection and infection may lead to graft failure after lung transplant resulting in capillary leak syndrome with pleural effusion.[55] The pleural effusion in acute lung rejection is exudative with lymphocyte predominance. Acute rejection occurs in most recipients and is characterized by a dramatic response to steroid therapy.

Pleural complications, commonly air leak and loculated pleural effusion, occur in approximately 35 percent of living lobar lung recipients.[33] Pleural effusions in lung transplant recipients may result from subpleural hematoma, chylothorax and hemothorax.[32] Persistent chylothorax and hemothorax may necessitate thoracic duct and bronchial artery ligation.[32]

HEART TRANSPLANT RECIPIENTS

Although pleural effusion develops in almost all patients postoperatively, it usually has no clinical significance. Pericardial tamponade and massive pleural effusion requiring pericardial window and chemical pleurodesis has been reported following cardiac transplantation.[58]

LIVER TRANSPLANT RECIPIENTS

The majority of liver transplant recipients develop pleural effusion, most in the first post-transplant week.[59] The effusions are predominantly on the right side. The postoperative effusions are usually asymptomatic and transudative and resolve spontaneously. If indicated, they can be drained percutaneously. If postoperative pleural effusions in liver transplant recipients get larger, subdiaphragmatic processes, such as hematoma, biloma and abscess, should be suspected.[60]

Although stenosis of the suprahepatic inferior vena caval anastomosis is rare after liver transplantation, it may cause significant obstruction to venous drainage from the allograft liver resulting in Budd–Chiari syndrome with massive ascites and pleural effusion.[61] Pleural effusion has been reported in 16.5 percent of liver transplant recipients treated with sirolimus.[62]

KIDNEY TRANSPLANT RECIPIENTS

During the early post-transplant period, urinary obstruction due to a failed ureteroneocystotomy or ureteral injury may lead to retroperitoneal urinoma with subsequent urinothorax.[63] Urinothorax can result from a perirenal lymphocele during the later period after transplantation.[55,64] Lymphocytic, exudative pleural effusion secondary to sarcoidosis, that resolved following corticosteroid therapy, has been described in a kidney transplant recipient.[65]

HEMATOPOIETIC STEM CELL TRANSPLANT RECIPIENTS

Hepatic veno-occlusive disease is a common complication of allogeneic HSCT. Up to half of allogeneic HSCT recipients with hepatic veno-occlusive disease may develop pleural effusion.[66,67] HSCT recipients with severe acute or chronic graft-versus-host disease (GVHD) may develop pleural effusions associated with pericardial effusion and ascites.[68–70] Capillary leak syndrome with pleural effusion may be precipitated by the administration of granulocyte colony-stimulating factor (GCSF) in HSCT recipients.[71] Pleural effusion has also been reported in HSCT recipients following imatinib administration.[72]

Pneumothorax

Pneumothorax develops in approximately 10 percent of lung transplant recipients, the most common cause being transbronchial lung biopsy.[31,32] The pneumothoraces usually resolve spontaneously or with tube thoracostomy. Pneumothoraces have been reported in 7.0 percent of liver transplant[73] and 4.5 percent of heart transplant recipients.[40] In HSCT recipients, pneumothorax may complicate bronchoiolitis obliterans associated with chronic GVHD.[74]

PLEURAL DISEASES IN HEMATOLOGICAL MALIGNANCIES

Nearly all hematological malignancies can present with, or develop, pleural effusions during their clinical course. Approximately 20–30 percent of lymphomas are associated with pleural effusion, especially if they involve the mediastinum.[30] Acute and chronic leukemias and myelodysplastic syndromes are rarely accompanied by pleural involvement.

Pleural involvement by the primary lymphoma is the most common cause of effusion in patients with lymphoma. Other causes include drug toxicity, underlying infections, radiation therapy, secondary malignancy or, rarely, autoimmune diseases.[30] The size of the effusions may vary from very small to massive. Depending on the size and the cause of the effusion, patients may be asymptomatic or present with life-threatening respiratory failure or hemodynamic compromise. Although the first diagnostic evaluation is usually thoracentesis, it may not give a specific diagnosis because of the sparse malignant cells in the pleural fluid. Closed or thoracoscopic pleural biopsy is required for diagnosis if pleural fluid cytology fails to determine the cause of the effusion. Although pleural effusions in lymphomas are usually exudates, they may also be transudates caused by venous compression or as reaction to lymphomatous involvement of lung parenchyma. Obstruction of the thoracic duct by lymphoma or radiation induced fibrosis may lead to chylothorax.[30] In most patients with lymphoma, the pleural fluid responds to treatment of the primary disease, whereas resistant or relapsing cases may necessitate pleurodesis.

Pyothorax-associated lymphoma, mostly reported from Japan, is a non-Hodgkin's lymphoma that develops in the pleural cavity after a long-standing history of pyothorax, usually in patients who have undergone therapeutic pneumothorax for the treatment of pulmonary tuberculosis.[75] It develops in approximately 2 percent of patients with chronic pyothorax, 19–64 years after the therapeutic pneumothorax. In the majority of these patients, the lymphoma cells are large atypical B cells, and express latent gene products of EBV. Most of the patients are elderly with multiple co-morbidities. Treatment includes chemotherapy, radiation therapy and surgery, alone or in combination.[75] The 5-year survival rate is approximately 35 percent.

Although rare during life, pleural infiltration with malignant cells is a common finding at autopsy of patients with acute leukemia.[30] Pleural effusions are uncommon in chronic lymphocytic and myelocytic leukemias. The effusions may be hemorrhagic if they are due to leukemic pleural infiltration. Bacterial, viral and fungal infections cause pleural effusion in patients with leukemia.[76–78] Extramedullary hematopoiesis may cause pleural effusion in chronic myelocytic leukemia.

Pleural effusion occurs in approximately 6 percent of patients with multiple myeloma and may be caused by nephrotic syndrome, pulmonary embolism and congestive heart failure. Myelomatous pleural involvement is rare, occurring in <1 percent of cases and mostly in IgA type multiple myeloma.

PLEURAL EFFUSION IN PRIMARY IMMUNE DEFICIENCIES

Approximately 50 000 new cases of primary immune deficiencies are diagnosed annually in the USA.[79] The diagnoses are delayed until adolescence or early adulthood in approximately 40 percent. Humoral deficiencies are the most common.[80] Infectious complications are frequent manifestations of primary immune deficiencies (Table 31.5). Although pulmonary infections are common, the incidence of parapneumonic effusions and empyema has not been well described.[81]

PLEURAL DISEASES IN OTHER IMMUNOCOMPROMISED PATIENTS

The spleen acts as a mechanical filter for particulate antigens and microorganisms in the circulation and plays roles in both the non-specific and specific immune responses.[82] In addition to congenital asplenia and splenectomy, functional hyposplenism is associated with sickle cell disease, celiac disease, sarcoidosis, systemic lupus erythematosus, ulcerative colitis and amyloidosis. Polysaccharide capsular organisms, including *S. pneumoniae, H. influenzae* and *Neisseria meningitidis*, are the most common pathogens causing sepsis in patients with hyposplenism. Although patients with hyposplenism are at high risk for complicated parapneumonic effusions and empyema, there is paucity of data in the published literature.

Table 31.5 Complications associated with primary immune defects

Immune defect	Presentation
Complement	Rheumatoid disorders Recurrent infection (pyogenic)
Neutrophil	Pneumonia (*Staphylococcus aureus, Pseudomonas, Candida, Aspergillus*)
Humoral	Pneumonia (encapsulated bacteria and viruses)
Cellular or combined	Opportunistic infections (viral, *Pneumocystis*, mycobacterial)

Immunosuppressant medications that are utilized to treat malignancies and connective tissue diseases may be associated with pleural effusions and are discussed in Chapters 32 and 33.

FUTURE DIRECTIONS

The global spread of HIV infection and the utilization of immunosuppressant medications and transplant to treat various diseases have led to an increased number of immunocompromised hosts. Infectious and non-infectious pleural complications occur as the result of immunodeficiency. Despite the heterogeneity of the conditions causing immunodeficiency, future prevention should focus on minimizing the level of immunosuppression and finding prophylactic measures to reduce the risk of pleural complications. Currently, the diagnostic approach to pleural effusion does not differ significantly between the immunocompromised host and immunocompetent patients. Studies are needed to define the best diagnostic approach to pleural effusion in the various groups of immunocompromised patients. Newer and better antibiotics and anti-neoplastic medications are likely to improve the outcome of pleural complications in the immunocompromised host. However, research aimed at restoration of immunocompetence should be given high priority.

KEY POINTS

- Immunocompromised patients are at risk for the development of infectious and non-infectious pleural complications.
- The causes of pleural effusion vary depending on the type and severity of the immunodeficiency. Parapneumonic effusion and empyema associated with bacterial pneumonias are the most common causes. Depending on the underlying conditions and patients' geographic location, immunocompromised patients may develop uncommon infectious pleural complications including mycobacterial, fungal, viral and parasitic.
- Pleural effusions associated with non-Hodgkin's lymphoma (including primary effusion lymphoma), Kaposi sarcoma and immune reconstitution inflammatory syndrome may develop in patients with AIDS.
- Causes of pleural effusion in transplant recipients include immunosuppressant medications, infections and malignancies. Pleural effusion in the immediate post-transplant period is common in lung, heart and liver transplant recipients. PTLD is associated with severe and prolonged immunosuppression. Other causes of pleural effusions in transplant recipients include hepatic veno-occlusive disease, GCSF, GVHD and capillary leak syndrome
- Pyothorax-associated lymphoma is reported mostly from Japan. It develops in the pleural cavity after a long-standing history of pyothorax, usually in patients who have undergone therapeutic pneumothorax for the treatment of pulmonary tuberculosis.
- The diagnostic importance of pleural fluid analysis in the immunocompromised host is similar to that of the immunocompetent patient. However, because of the wider differential diagnoses and the adverse impact of delayed diagnosis, more aggressive diagnostic evaluation and timely management are recommended.

REFERENCES

● = Key primary paper
◆ = Major review article

1. UNAIDS. AIDS Epidemic Update: December 2006. Available from: http://www.who.int/hiv/mediacentre/news62/en/index.html
◆2. Afessa B. Pleural effusions and pneumothoraces in AIDS. *Curr Opin Pulm Med* 2001; **7**: 202–9.
3. Beck JM. Pleural disease in patients with acquired immune deficiency syndrome. *Clin Chest Med* 1998; **19**: 341–9.
◆4. Light RW, Hamm H. Pleural disease and acquired immune deficiency syndrome. *Eur Respir J* 1997; **10**: 2638–43.
5. Domoua K, Daix T, Coulibaly G, *et al.* [Aetiologies of pleural effusions in HIV-infected patients in Abidjan, Cote-d'Ivoire]. *Bull Soc Pathol Exot* 2006; **99**: 15–16.
6. Miller RF, Howling SJ, Reid AJ, *et al.* Pleural effusions in patients with AIDS. *Sex Transm Infect* 2000; **76**: 122–5.
7. DiMaio JM, Wait MA. The thoracic surgeon's role in the management of patients with HIV infection and AIDS. *Chest Surg Clin N Am* 1999; **9**: 97–111.
8. World Health Organization. 2006. Tuberculosis facts. Available from: http://www.who.int/tb/en
9. Jones BE, Young SM, Antoniskis D, *et al.* Relationship of the manifestations of tuberculosis to CD4 cell counts in patients with human immunodeficiency virus infection. *Am Rev Respir Dis* 1993; **148**: 1292–7.
10. American Thoracic Society/Centers for Disease Control and Prevention/Infectious Diseases Society of America: controlling tuberculosis in the United States. *Am J Respir Crit Care Med* 2005; **172**: 1169–227.
11. Jones D, Lieb T, Narita M, *et al.* Mesothelial cells in tuberculous pleural effusions of HIV-infected patients. *Chest* 2000; **117**: 289–91.
12. Riantawan P, Chaowalit P, Wongsangiem M, *et al.* Diagnostic value of pleural fluid adenosine deaminase in tuberculous pleuritis with reference to HIV coinfection and a Bayesian analysis. *Chest* 1999; **116**: 97–103.
13. Frye MD, Pozsik CJ, Sahn SA. Tuberculous pleurisy is more common in AIDS than in non-AIDS patients with tuberculosis. *Chest* 1997; **112**: 393–7.

14. Elliott AM, Luzze H, Quigley MA, *et al.* A randomized, double-blind, placebo-controlled trial of the use of prednisolone as an adjunct to treatment in HIV-1-associated pleural tuberculosis. *J Infect Dis* 2004; **190**: 869–78.
15. Batungwanayo J, Taelman H, Bogaerts J, *et al.* Pulmonary cryptococcosis associated with HIV-1 infection in Rwanda: a retrospective study of 37 cases. *AIDS* 1994; **8**: 1271–6.
16. Bernstein WB, Little RF, Wilson WH, *et al.* Acquired immunodeficiency syndrome-related malignancies in the era of highly active antiretroviral therapy. *Int J Hematol* 2006; **84**: 3–11.
17. Casper C, Wald A. The use of antiviral drugs in the prevention and treatment of Kaposi sarcoma, multicentric Castleman disease and primary effusion lymphoma. *Curr Top Microbiol Immunol* 2007; **312**: 289–307.
18. Maradona JA, Carton JA, Asensi V, *et al.* AIDS-related Kaposi's sarcoma with chylothorax and pericardial involvement satisfactorily treated with liposomal doxorubicin. *AIDS* 2002; **16**: 806.
19. Mbulaiteye SM, Biggar RJ, Goedert JJ, *et al.* Pleural and peritoneal lymphoma among people with AIDS in the United States. *J Acquir Immune Defic Syndr* 2002; **29**: 418–21.
20. Hengge UR, Ruzicka T, Tyring SK, *et al.* Update on Kaposi's sarcoma and other HHV8 associated diseases. Part 2: pathogenesis, Castleman's disease, and pleural effusion lymphoma. *Lancet Infect Dis* 2002; **2**: 344–52.
21. Boulanger E, Gerard L, Gabarre J, *et al.* Prognostic factors and outcome of human herpesvirus 8-associated primary effusion lymphoma in patients with AIDS. *J Clin Oncol* 2005; **23**: 4372–80.
22. Behling CA, Wolf PL, Haghighi P. AIDS and malignant mesothelioma – is there a connection? *Chest* 1993; **103**: 1268–9.
23. Lipman M, Breen R. Immune reconstitution inflammatory syndrome in HIV. *Curr Opin Infect Dis* 2006; **19**: 20–5.
24. Buckingham SJ, Haddow LJ, Shaw PJ, *et al.* Immune reconstitution inflammatory syndrome in HIV-infected patients with mycobacterial infections starting highly active anti-retroviral therapy. *Clin Radiol* 2004; **59**: 505–13.
25. Schroeder SA, Beneck D, Dozor AJ. Spontaneous pneumothorax in children with AIDS. *Chest* 1995; **108**: 1173–6.
26. Transplants in the US by state. The Organ Procurement and Transplantation Network. Available from: http://www.optn.org/latestData/rptData.asp
27. Report on state of the art in blood and marrow transplantation. Center for International Blood & Marrow Transplant Research. *CIBMTR Newsletter.* Available from: http://www.optn.org/latestData/rptData.asp
◆28. Judson MA, Sahn SA. The pleural space and organ transplantation. *Am J Respir Crit Care Med* 1996; **153**: 1153–65.
29. Candan S, Pirat A, Varol G, *et al.* Respiratory problems in renal transplant recipients admitted to intensive care during long-term follow-up. *Transplant Proc* 2006; **38**: 1354–6.
◆30. Alexandrakis MG, Passam FH, Kyriakou DS, *et al.* Pleural effusions in hematologic malignancies. *Chest* 2004; **125**: 1546–55.
●31. Ferrer J, Roldan J, Roman A, *et al.* Acute and chronic pleural complications in lung transplantation. *J Heart Lung Transplant* 2003; **22**: 1217–25.
32. Herridge MS, de Hoyos AL, Chaparro C, *et al.* Pleural complications in lung transplant recipients. *J Thorac Cardiovasc Surg* 1995; **110**: 22–6.
33. Backhus LM, Sievers EM, Schenkel FA, *et al.* Pleural space problems after living lobar transplantation. *J Heart Lung Transplant* 2005; **24**: 2086–90.
34. Ma YK, Yan LN, Li B, *et al.* Diagnosis and treatment of bacterial pneumonia in liver transplantation recipients: report of 33 cases. *Chin Med J (Engl)* 2005; **118**: 1879–85.
35. Janssens W, Van Raemdonck D, Dupont L, *et al.* *Listeria* pleuritis 1 week after lung transplantation. *J Heart Lung Transplant* 2006; **25**: 734–7.
36. Thacker WL, Benson RF, Schifman RB, *et al.* *Legionella tucsonensis* sp. nov. isolated from a renal transplant recipient. *J Clin Microbiol* 1989; **27**: 1831–4.
37. Natrajan S, Hadeli O, Quan SF. Infected spontaneous chylothorax. *Diagn Microbiol Infect Dis* 1998; **30**: 31–2.
38. Chung JH, Kim YS, Kim SI, *et al.* The diagnostic value of the adenosine deaminase activity in the pleural fluid of renal transplant patients with tuberculous pleural effusion. *Yonsei Med J* 2004; **45**: 661–4.
39. Canver CC, Patel AK, Kosolcharoen P, *et al.* Fungal purulent constrictive pericarditis in a heart transplant patient. *Ann Thorac Surg* 1998; **65**: 1792–4.
●40. Lenner R, Padilla ML, Teirstein AS, *et al.* Pulmonary complications in cardiac transplant recipients. *Chest* 2001; **120**: 508–13.
41. Collet G, Marty P, Le Fichoux Y, *et al.* Pleural effusion as the first manifestation of pulmonary toxoplasmosis in a bone marrow transplant recipient. *Acta Cytol* 2004; **48**: 114–16.
42. Schulman LL, Reison DS, Austin JH, *et al.* Cytomegalovirus pneumonitis after cardiac transplantation. *Arch Intern Med* 1991; **151**: 1118–24.
43. Abe K, Suzuki K, Kamata N, *et al.* [High-resolution CT findings in cytomegalovirus pneumonitis after bone marrow transplantation]. *Nippon Igaku Hoshasen Gakkai Zasshi* 1998; **58**: 7–11.
44. Harris NL, Ferry JA, Swerdlow SH. Posttransplant lymphoproliferative disorders: summary of Society for Hematopathology Workshop. *Semin Diagn Pathol* 1997; **14**: 8–14.
●45. Halkos ME, Miller JI, Mann KP, *et al.* Thoracic presentations of posttransplant lymphoproliferative disorders. *Chest* 2004; **126**: 2013–20.
46. Ohori NP, Whisnant RE, Nalesnik MA, *et al.* Primary pleural effusion posttransplant lymphoproliferative disorder: Distinction from secondary involvement and effusion lymphoma. *Diagn Cytopathol* 2001; **25**: 50–3.
47. Lamba M, Jabi M, Padmore R, *et al.* Isolated pleural PTLD after cardiac transplantation. *Cardiovasc Pathol* 2002; **11**: 346–50.
48. Wolford JF, Krause JR. Posttransplant mediastinal Burkitt-like lymphoma. Diagnosis by cytologic and flow cytometric analysis of pleural fluid. *Acta Cytol* 1990; **34**: 261–4.
49. Jones D, Ballestas ME, Kaye KM, *et al.* Primary-effusion lymphoma and Kaposi's sarcoma in a cardiac-transplant recipient. *N Engl J Med* 1998; **339**: 444–9.
50. Park J, Park SY, Cho HI, *et al.* Isolated extramedullary relapse in the pleural fluid of a patient with acute myeloid leukemia following allogeneic BMT. *Bone Marrow Transplant* 2002; **30**: 57–9.
51. Germing U, Kobbe G, Sohngen D, *et al.* Early occurrence of an adenocarcinoma after allogeneic bone marrow transplantation in a patient with AML. *Oncol Rep* 1999; **6**: 855–7.
52. Motherby H, Ross B, Kube M, *et al.* Pleural carcinosis confirmed by adjuvant cytological methods: a case report. *Diagn Cytopathol* 1998; **19**: 370–4.
53. Judson MA, Handy JR, Sahn SA. Pleural effusions following lung transplantation. Time course, characteristics, and clinical implications. *Chest* 1996; **109**: 1190–4.
54. Shitrit D, Izbicki G, Fink G, *et al.* Late postoperative pleural effusion following lung transplantation: characteristics and clinical implications. *Eur J Cardiothorac Surg* 2003; **23**: 494–6.
●55. Judson MA, Sahn SA, Hahn AB. Origin of pleural cells after lung transplantation: from donor or recipient? *Chest* 1997; **112**: 426–9.
56. Liguori C, Schulman LL, Weslow RG, *et al.* Late pulmonary venous complications after lung transplantation. *J Am Soc Echocardiogr* 1997; **10**: 763–7.
57. Khan SU, Salloum J, O'Donovan PB, *et al.* Acute pulmonary edema after lung transplantation: the pulmonary reimplantation response. *Chest* 1999; **116**: 187–94.
58. Lee JT, Durzinsky DS, Wilson WR, *et al.* Pericardial tamponade and massive pleural effusion complicating orthotopic heart transplantation. *J Cardiovasc Surg (Torino)* 1999; **40**: 377–9.

●59. Hong SK, Hwang S, Lee SG, *et al.* Pulmonary complications following adult liver transplantation. *Transplant Proc* 2006; **38**: 2979–81.

60. Spizarny DL, Gross BH, McLoud T. Enlarging pleural effusion after liver transplantation. *J Thorac Imaging* 1993; **8**: 85–7.

61. Zajko AB, Claus D, Clapuyt P, *et al.* Obstruction to hepatic venous drainage after liver transplantation: treatment with balloon angioplasty. *Radiology* 1989; **170**: 763–5.

62. Montalbano M, Neff GW, Yamashiki N, *et al.* A retrospective review of liver transplant patients treated with sirolimus from a single center: an analysis of sirolimus-related complications. *Transplantation* 2004; **78**: 264–8.

63. Carcillo J Jr, Salcedo JR. Urinothorax as a manifestation of nondilated obstructive uropathy following renal transplantation. *Am J Kidney Dis* 1985; **5**: 211–13.

64. DeCamp MM, Tilney NL. Late development of intractable lymphocele after renal transplantation. *Transplant Proc* 1988; **20**: 105–9.

65. Schmidt RJ, Bender FH, Chang WW, *et al.* Sarcoidosis after renal transplantation. *Transplantation* 1999; **68**: 1420–3.

66. Ozkaynak MF, Weinberg K, Kohn D, *et al.* Hepatic veno-occlusive disease post-bone marrow transplantation in children conditioned with busulfan and cyclophosphamide: incidence, risk factors, and clinical outcome. *Bone Marrow Transplant* 1991; **7**: 467–74.

67. van den Bosch MA, van Hoe L. MR imaging findings in two patients with hepatic veno-occlusive disease following bone marrow transplantation. *Eur Radiol* 2000; **10**: 1290–3.

68. Seber A, Khan SP, Kersey JH. Unexplained effusions: association with allogeneic bone marrow transplantation and acute or chronic graft-versus-host disease. *Bone Marrow Transplant* 1996; **17**: 207–11.

69. Toren A, Nagler A. Massive pericardial effusion complicating the course of chronic graft-versus-host disease (cGVHD) in a child with acute lymphoblastic leukemia following allogeneic bone marrow transplantation. *Bone Marrow Transplant* 1997; **20**: 805–7.

70. Ueda T, Manabe A, Kikuchi A, *et al.* Massive pericardial and pleural effusion with anasarca following allogeneic bone marrow transplantation. *Int J Hematol* 2000; **71**: 394–7.

71. Oeda E, Shinohara K, Kamei S, *et al.* Capillary leak syndrome likely the result of granulocyte colony-stimulating factor after high-dose chemotherapy. *Intern Med* 1994; **33**: 115–19.

72. Goldsby R, Pulsipher M, Adams R, *et al.* Unexpected pleural effusions in 3 pediatric patients treated with STI-571. *J Pediatr Hematol Oncol* 2002; **24**: 694–5.

73. Duran FG, Piqueras B, Romero M, *et al.* Pulmonary complications following orthotopic liver transplant. *Transpl Int* 1998; **11**(Suppl 1): S255–9.

74. Afessa B, Litzow MR, Tefferi A. Bronchiolitis obliterans and other late onset non-infectious pulmonary complications in hematopoietic stem cell transplantation. *Bone Marrow Transplant* 2001; **28**: 425–34.

75. Narimatsu H, Ota Y, Kami M, *et al.* Clinicopathological features of pyothorax-associated lymphoma; a retrospective survey involving 98 patients. *Ann Oncol* 2007; **18**: 122–8.

76. Desselle BC, Bozeman PM, Patrick CC. Diagnostic utility of thoracentesis for neutropenic children with cancer. *Clin Infect Dis* 1995; **21**: 887–90.

77. Mori M, Imamura Y, Maegawa H, *et al.* Cytology of pleural effusion associated with disseminated infection caused by varicella-zoster virus in an immunocompromised patient. A case report. *Acta Cytol* 2003; **47**: 480–4.

78. Trudo FJ, Gopez EV, Gupta PK, *et al.* Pleural effusion due to herpes simplex type II infection in an immunocompromised host. *Am J Respir Crit Care Med* 1997; **155**: 371–3.

79. Verbsky JW, Grossman WJ. Cellular and genetic basis of primary immune deficiencies. *Pediatr Clin North Am* 2006; **53**: 649–84.

80. Ballow M. Primary immunodeficiency disorders: antibody deficiency. *J Allergy Clin Immunol* 2002; **109**: 581–91.

81. Hollingsworth CL. Thoracic disorders in the immunocompromised child. *Radiol Clin North Am* 2005; **43**: 435–47.

82. Sumaraju V, Smith LG, Smith SM. Infectious complications in asplenic hosts. *Infect Dis Clin North Am* 2001; **15**: 551–65.

32

Effusions from connective tissue diseases

DEMOSTHENES BOUROS, DIMITRIS A VASSILAKIS†

INTRODUCTION

Rheumatoid arthritis and systemic lupus erythematosus (SLE) are the most common connective tissue diseases (CTD), where pleural disease is observed, however, the reported prevalence, natural history and course of the pleural involvement varies considerably. Limited reliable data are available for the other CTD, which are rare themselves.

It is important to recognize that the prevalence and severity of pleural involvement critically depends upon the nature of the population studied. Given the high rate of progress in medicine, patients with milder disease are increasingly recognized, which changes our view on the clinical spectrum of these diseases. Additionally, the use of newer imaging techniques allows the detection of previously unsuspected effusions of doubtful clinical significance. The prevalence of pleural disease depends upon whether patients are investigated for symptomatic pleural disease, screened radiographically or undergo computed tomography (CT) by protocol.

In CTD, additionally, pleural involvement may result from renal or cardiac disease, pulmonary emboli and pneumonia or empyema. In these cases the effusion is not an active autoimmune pleuritis. A further problem is the existence of overlap autoimmune syndromes. Finally, there are no controlled data on treatment.

This review was mainly based on a MedLine (PubMed) search of (primarily) English literature using as keywords 'pleural effusion', 'pleura', 'pleural' and the individual names of the diseases presented below.

†Deceased.

SYSTEMIC LUPUS ERYTHEMATOSUS

Incidence

Pleural effusions are common in SLE and are included in the American Rheumatism Association diagnostic criteria for SLE.[1] Approximately 30–50 percent of patients develop a pleural effusion during the course of their illness.[2–7] Pleural abnormalities are found at autopsy in 40–93 percent,[8–11] but represent in some cases, secondary cardiopulmonary complications of SLE.[10] There is no clear gender association. Pleural effusions are variably reported to be more prevalent in females[2] or males.[12,13] Pleuritic pain was reported in almost half of the patients in one series, with 14 experiencing repeated episodes,[14] and a chest radiographic study disclosed a prevalence of pleural effusion of approximately 35 percent.[15] However, since many patients with transient pleural disease are asymptomatic, the exact prevalence is difficult to determine. The clinical features of SLE, including the frequency of pleural disease, also vary significantly between ethnic groups.[16–21]

Clinical manifestations

Pleuritic pain occurs in most patients with lupus pleuritis.[5] It is often distressing and may be prolonged,[14] occasionally necessitating pleurectomy.[22] Although many patients present with painless pleural effusions,[23] frequent findings include fever, pleural rub and tachycardia.[5] Lupus pleuritis is the first manifestation of SLE in only 5–10 percent,[24] but is an early feature in 25–30 percent, usually preceded by arthralgia, and is sometimes associated with pneumonitis and pericarditis.[15] The presence of pleural disease is usually accompanied with multisystem involvement.[25] The prevalence of pleural disease at presentation increases in the elderly,[26] but is also frequent in children.[27–29] Pleuritis is also a frequent feature of drug-induced lupus syndromes (not covered here, see Chapter 33, Effusions caused by drugs). Finally, pleural effusions may result from complications of SLE.

Radiographic imaging

On chest radiography, pleural effusions are generally small, but occasionally massive.[30–36] They are bilateral in approximately 50 percent, with no predilection for the right or left side[4] and may, in serial chest radiographs, often change sides.[14]

Diagnosis

In patients with known SLE, the diagnosis is often obvious, but in patients with pleuritis associated with non-specific arthritis, the major differential diagnosis is rheumatoid pleural disease (distinction between the two is covered in the section on rheumatoid arthritis). SLE pleuritis should be considered in any patient with an exudative pleural effusion of unknown etiology.[15] Measurement of lactic acid has been proposed a rapid tool to distinguish between bacterial pleural inflammation and other causes of exudative effusions.[37] However, a new pleural effusion in patients with SLE remains a diagnostic challenge.[38]

Pleural fluid analysis

The pleural fluid is usually exudative, yellow or serosanguineous.[5,15] Hemothorax has also been reported.[36,39] Neutrophils or monocytes predominate, but lymphocytes are common in chronic effusions.[3,5] Pleural fluid eosinophilia is generally considered to rule out underlying SLE.[40] The pleural fluid pH is usually higher than 7.20, the glucose concentrations are slightly decreased,[5,41] but usually higher than 60 mg/dL, and lactate dehydrogenase (LDH) levels are less than the upper normal limits of serum LDH.[3]

Reductions in pleural fluid complement levels have been observed,[1–3,15,42–44] possibly reflecting complement conversion by immune complexes.[3,5,42–44] Immune complex deposition may engender pleural effusions by increasing capillary permeability.[45] Elevated CA-125 levels have been reported in the pleural fluid of a number of connective tissue diseases, including SLE.[46,47]

Fluid lupus cells

Lupus erythematosus (LE) cells are found occasionally in serous effusions in SLE[5,48–54] and may appear at the onset or later in the disease course.[55] Some have regarded the presence of LE cells in serous effusions as virtually diagnostic of SLE,[48–51] an approach which is no longer favored since they are subject to observer variation,[50] are not easy to detect and have also been reported in effusions from rheumatoid joints,[56] malignant pleural effusions[57] and in pleural fluid, without clinical evidence of SLE.[55] Additionally, LE cells are not found in the pleural fluid of all patients with lupus pleuritis[58] and are usually associated with the presence of serum LE cells; thus, the added diagnostic value of pleural fluid LE cells is questionable.[58]

Pleural fluid antinuclear antibodies

Pleural fluid antinuclear antibodies (ANA) titers >1:60 and pleural fluid to serum ANA ratios >1 are suggestive but not diagnostic of SLE pleuritis; high pleural fluid titers (up to 1:640) are seen occasionally in patients with non-SLE exudative effusions.[59,60] Sometimes, demonstrable pleural fluid ANA may be absent.[61] Patients with SLE pleuritis sometimes have higher pleural fluid ANA, ssDNA, dsDNA, smooth muscle and ribonucleoprotein titers than in the serum.[59,62] Pleural fluid ANA titer levels may be useful in distinguishing between lupus pleuritis and other causes of pleural disease in SLE patients, in which pleural fluid ANA titers tend to be low or absent.[58] The authors in a recent study regarding the diagnostic value of ANA in SLE pleural effusion reached the same conclusion.[63]

Treatment

Due to the small number of reported patients, the best type of intervention remains uncertain.[64] Pleuritic pain in SLE may respond to non-steroidal anti-inflammatory agents, and almost always responds to corticosteroid therapy. Sometimes, high doses may be needed for large effusions and severe pleuritis.[65] Immunosuppressants (azathioprine and hydroxychloroquine) may be efficacious[32,66,67] and monthly cyclosporine courses have been used with a good outcome.[67] Recurrent pleural effusions usually respond to pleurodesis.[32,68,69]

Prognosis

Small effusions do not require any treatment, usually resolve spontaneously and have no known prognostic significance.[15] Conversely, pleuritic pain appears to be an adverse prognostic marker,[15,70,71] with a mean survival of less than 4 years in affected cases.[15]

RHEUMATOID ARTHRITIS

Incidence

Pleural involvement in rheumatoid arthritis (RA) was first observed in the mid-nineteenth century.[72] It has been found at autopsy in half of the patients.[4] On the other hand, clinical evidence of pleural disease is found in less than 5 percent of RA patients, while 20 percent experience pleuritic pain at some stage.[73–75] Pleuritic pain seems to be more prevalent in male patients.[73,76] In one study with RA, only 17 (3.3 percent) had pleural effusions, with higher prevalence in males (7.9 percent) than females (1.6 percent).[73] In another radiological/clinical study of 309 RA patients, chest radiographic evidence of pre-existing pleural disease was detected in 24 percent of males and 16 percent of females (compared with 16 and 8 percent of control subjects).[76]

Clinical manifestations

Most of the patients are asymptomatic, the effusions are small and resolve spontaneously.[77] The pleural effusion may present in the absent of arthritis.[78] In large effusions, breathlessness may result from pulmonary compression due to the size of the effusion. Occasional complaints are fever, cough and pleuritic pain.[79] The presence of pleural disease has not been linked to more severe systemic disease, but is associated with a higher prevalence of cardiac and ocular lesions.[73] In a study of 1968 subjects, 81 percent of patients who were found to have rheumatoid pleural effusions were male, and the average age of onset was 51 years (range 35–69 years).[73] In over half of the cases, rheumatoid effusions are associated with subcutaneous nodules[73,70,80] and usually follow the onset of joint manifestations. Only very rarely (6 percent) do effusions precede arthritis and, in 11 percent, pleural and systemic disease present concurrently.

Radiographic imaging

Effusions are bilateral in 25 percent in chest radiographs,[73] with no predilection for either side.[80] Effusions are usually small or moderate, but are occasionally massive,[81,82] and may be transient, chronic or recurrent.[83] Up to one-third of patients have simultaneous parenchymal lesions (interstitial lung disease or necrobiotic nodules).[73,83]

Diagnosis

The typical pleural effusion in RA is exudative with high titers of rheumatoid factor, low pH, low glucose and high LDH levels. The diagnostic likelihood is increased with male gender, age >50, long-standing arthritis and the presence of subcutaneous nodules. However, the diagnosis is usually made by the exclusion of other causes.

Differential diagnosis

Differential diagnosis from SLE is challenging in patients with coexisting arthritis and pleural effusions. Effusions in SLE are distinguished from these of RA by low (1:40) titers of rheumatoid factor, glucose concentrations in excess of 80 mg/dL, LDH levels lower than the upper normal limits of serum LDH and pH > 7.35.

It uncommon for pleural effusions in RA to stay undiagnosed for long. In a study of 40 patients with exudative pleural effusions undiagnosed after exhaustive evaluation and followed for 5 years, rheumatoid pleural disease was eventually diagnosed in only one instant and no cause was ever identified in 32.[84]

Fluid analysis

The fluid is exudative and non-odorous and may be cloudy, greenish yellow or opalescent.[85] Glucose levels exceed 30 mg/100 mL in 20–30 percent, but it has been argued that normal glucose concentrations may indicate causes other than RA.[80] Other biochemical findings include pH >7.20, LDH levels more than twice the upper limit of the normal serum value, low complement and immune complex levels and rheumatoid factor titers (>1:320) that exceed serum titers.[79] Whole complement activity and C3, C4 levels are less in RA pleural fluid than in non-rheumatoid effusions.[44] The complement cascade is activated through both classic and the alternative pathways in rheumatic pleurisy; in one study, determinations of SC5b-9 and C4d/C4 content in pleural fluid most accurately distinguished between rheumatic, tuberculous and malignant effusions.[86]

As in empyema and tuberculous effusions, the activity of adenosine deaminase in rheumatoid effusions is higher in pleural fluid than in serum, indicating local synthesis of ADA by cells within the pleural cavity in RA.[87]

Fluid cytology

In a study of 24 patients with RA pleuritis,[88] on the cytological examination of the pleural fluid, a characteristic triad of giant multinucleated macrophages, elongated macrophages and a background of granular debris was found. The above features have also been observed in other studies,[83,89] but in none of 10 000 non-rheumatoid effusions.[88]

'Rheumatoid arthritis cells' or 'RA cells' ('ragocytes' with characteristic inclusion bodies, representing phagocytic vacuoles or phagosomes, larger than lysosomes seen in granular leukocytes) may be present,[90] but they have no diagnostic value[88,91] since they may also be seen in tuberculous effusions and empyema.[83]

Glucose

In a pleural effusion – with confirmed absence of bacteria and acid-fast bacilli – with a fluid glucose concentration of 25 mg/100 mL or less, despite normal serum glucose concentrations, the diagnosis of RA is the most prominent.[92] In 76 rheumatoid effusions, pleural glucose levels were less than 20 mg/dL in 63 percent, and less than 50 mg/dL in 83 percent.[80]

The mechanism for low pleural glucose levels in RA is unknown. Administering glucose increases serum but not pleural glucose concentrations.[75,92] However, glucose in the pleura is not utilized rapidly; the addition of glucose to pleural fluid *in vitro* is not associated with significant cellular glucose utilization.[75] It has been suggested that the rheumatoid inflammatory process may influence the activity of enzymes contributing to cellular membrane carbohydrate transport[92] or produces substances interfering with glucose entry into pleural fluid.[75]

Cholesterol

High concentrations of total lipids and cholesterol have been observed in some rheumatoid effusions.[75,80,93] The presence of cholesterol crystals in an occasional patient may give rise to an 'opalescent sheen'.[80] Chronicity or high cellularity are probably necessary for the development of a high pleural fluid lipid or cholesterol content.[75,80]

Infection

Although it has a highly variable prevalence, empyema is not uncommon in RE. In one study, 16 percent of all adult cases with empyema were RA patients. These patients were half of the 10 patients observed during a 5-year period with RA effusion.[94] In another study, only one of 19 patients with RA and a pleural effusion had an empyema.[73] Among 67 patients with non-tuberculous empyema, three were associated with RA in another study.[95] Middle-aged males seem to be particularly susceptible.[95] Causative factors may be corticosteroid therapy, a rheumatoid susceptibility to infection, pre-existing chronic bronchopulmonary infection, pre-existing rheumatoid effusions, altered biochemical characteristics of pleural fluid and the formation of broncho-pleural fistulas through necrotic rheumatoid nodules.[94]

Biopsy

Most cases of needle biopsy of the pleura have shown nonspecific granulomatous or fibrotic changes.[73,96] Only rarely are pleural rheumatoid nodules demonstrated which are diagnostic.[96,97] At thoracoscopy the parietal pleura has a granular appearance and the histopathological changes in tissue gained from thoracoscopic biopsies are often diagnostic.[85]

Treatment

Most effusions are asymptomatic and do not require specific treatment. Initial treatment with non-steroidal anti-inflammatory agents may suffice. Some patients respond to corticosteroids,[73,83,93,98] but others do not,[4,99,100] and effusions may recur despite continuing steroid therapy. Repeated aspirations have been used to control effusions. At times, persistent symptomatic effusions or pleural thickening necessitate decortication.[101–103] In cases of empyema, drainage and antibiotics are used.[77,104]

Intrapleural installation of corticosteroids has been attempted with varying results.[99,105] Decortication should be considered in patients with symptomatic pleural thickening, although it can be technically difficult.[103] The significance of pleural thickening can be estimated by serial pleural pressure measurements during therapeutic thoracentesis; a rapid drop in pleural pressure denotes trapping of the lung by thickened pleura.[106]

Long-term outcome

Rheumatoid effusions resolve within 4 weeks in 50 percent and within 4 months in two-thirds of patients,[73] but may also persist for years in approximately 20 percent.[4]

SYSTEMIC SCLEROSIS

Pleural effusions have been observed with both diffuse[46,107,108] and limited[109] scleroderma, but are uncommon. In a study evaluating the prevalence of serositis in systemic sclerosis (SSc), none of 37 patients (including 19 with limited SSc) had a pleural effusion. In the same study, reviewing medical records, pleural effusions were identified in only four of 58 other SSc patients (7 percent),[110] while pericardial effusions were present in 17 percent.

Since a percentage of SSc patients develop SLE overlap, the above-mentioned low prevalence of pleural effusions in these patients makes the association uncertain.[111]

In two cases, pleural effusions in SSc have been associated with elevated serum and pleural fluid CA125 levels,[46,107] which were seen to decrease with resolution of the effusion in one case.[46]

POLYMYOSITIS/DERMATOMYOSITIS

Pleuritic pain is occasionally reported in these conditions,[112–114] but obvious clinical or radiographic evidence of pleural disease is rare. In a clinicopathological analysis of 65 autopsy cases, none of the patients with polymyositis or dermatomyositis had pleural effusions clinically or at autopsy.[112] Two patients with massive pleural effusions have been described, both presenting with marked pyrexia and a good response to corticosteroid therapy.[115] Although cardiomyopathy and hypothyroidism might have contributed to pleural fluid accumulation in one case, no confounding features were present in the second patient, a 34-year-old man with dermatomyositis and coexisting interstitial lung disease.

SJÖGREN'S SYNDROME

There are limited data regarding the epidemiology of pleural disease in Sjögren's syndrome (SS). There were no patients with pleural effusion in various series regarding the prevalence of pleural effusion in patients with primary SS.[116–119] In contrast, 5 of 343 secondary SS patients exhibited pleural involvement.[120] Pleuritic pain was confined to patients with secondary SS.[119]

In the few reports of pleural effusions associated with primary SS, they were usually bilateral,[116,121,122] but may be unilateral.[123] The fluid is lymphocytic and exudative, with normal glucose levels and pH and low adenosine deaminase levels.[122–124] Studies of serum and pleural fluid in one patient disclosed rheumatoid factor and anti-SS-A antibody, immune complexes and activation of complement, all localized to the pleural fluid.[116] Analysis of pleural fluid T-cell receptor beta-chain variable (V beta) regions revealed overexpression of V beta gene products, including V beta 2 and V beta 13, previously shown to be over-represented in salivary glands of SS patients.[116]

ANKYLOSING SPONDYLITIS

Infection of cavities within the apical fibrotic tissue in patients with ankylosing spondylitis (AS) may lead to underlying pleural thickening or even empyema. Only a few cases of other forms of pleural disease in AS have been reported,[125–127] since pleural involvement is rare.[128] Pleural disease has been identified in 2 of 53 patients (one tuberculous, one non-tuberculous effusion),[129] 2 of 255 patients (idiopathic bilateral pleural calcification)[130] and 1 of 200 patients (unexplained pleural thickening).[131] In all the above cases the finding may represent the pleural sequelae of tuberculous or non-tuberculous infection, rather than a direct complication of AS. Finally, in a radiographic study of 2080 patients with AS, 10 patients were discovered with non-apical pleural disease, which did not differ significantly form the prevalence in controls. Three patients had transient pleural exudates with normal pleural fluid glucose concentrations, and one had an empyema.[132]

MIXED CONNECTIVE TISSUE DISEASE

Pleural effusions have been noted in half of the patients during the course of the illness.[133–136] Pleuritic chest pain is reported in approximately 40 percent.[137] Unlike SLE, however – despite the high prevalence of inflammatory pleural disease, often associated with pericarditis – pleural involvement is seldom an initial manifestation of disease.[138] In the few reported cases, in which pleural involvement is the cardinal presenting feature of mixed connective tissue disease (MCTD), pleural effusions were sometimes associated with pericarditis[138,139] and were bilateral[140] or unilateral.[141] In general, pleural effusions are small and resolve spontaneously.[133]

EOSINOPHILIA–MYALGIA SYNDROME

Pleural effusions do occur in patients with eosinophilia–myalgia syndrome (EMS). In one large series of 1531 patients, pleural effusions were found in 12 percent of the 178 who had chest radiographs.[142] The prevalence was 33 percent in another study.[143] Effusions are usually bilateral and the fluid is a sterile eosinophilic exudative.[143,144] Pleural involvement is not necessarily clinically significant and has no documented therapeutic or prognostic implication.

ANGIO-IMMUNOBLASTIC LYMPHADENOPATHY

Pleural effusions occur in angio-immunoblastic lymphadenopathy (AIL). Half of the patients in one study were found to have a pleural effusion which was usually associated with ascites and pedal edema.[145] The characteristics of the pleural fluid are not well described. In a Japanese series, with a review of the Japanese literature, pleural effusions were found in 50 percent, including all five index cases plus 8 of 21 patients previously reported in the local literature.[146]

CHURG–STRAUSS SYNDROME

Pleural involvement in the Churg–Strauss syndrome (CSS) was generally regarded as rare, based upon a single long-term follow-up study of 96 patients.[147] In a review of the English literature before 1984, however,[148] pleural disease was found to be more common. Eighteen of 61 patients (30 percent) with chest radiographs had an effusion. In a more recent study, two of nine patients with CSS had a pleural effusion.[149] Thoracentesis yielded an acidotic exudative effusion with low glucose, low C3, eosinophilia and a markedly increased rheumatoid factor[150] in a case report. Pleural biopsy was characteristic in a second case CSS.[151]

WEGENER'S GRANULOMATOSIS

In the reported studies on patients with Wegener's granulomatosis (WG), presenting mainly small groups of patients, minor pleural involvement is not infrequent. Effusions were present on thorax radiography in up to half of the cases,[152–155] or less often on CT.[156] There is even a report of a patient with a pleural effusion which was the presenting symptom of the disease.[157] Pleural thickening has occasionally been evident on chest radiography[155] or CT.[158] Pleural aspiration has shown an exudative neutrophil predominant effusion with protein levels ranging from 3.8 to 5.7 mg/dL.[154]

Pleural effusions in WG are seldom clinically important and generally resolve spontaneously, or regress with the introduction of corticosteroid and/or immunosuppressive treatment.

MISCELLANEOUS DISEASES

Pleural effusions occasionally accompany other connective tissue diseases, including polyarteritis nodosa,[159] temporal arteritis,[160–162] giant cell arteritis,[163,164] Kawasaki disease,[165] Adamantiadis–Behçet's syndrome,[166] human adjuvant disease[167] and adult-onset Still's disease.[168–170] The major difficulty in characterizing pleural involvement in these disorders is the fact that these disorders are rare.

FUTURE DIRECTIONS

Multicenter studies are necessary in order to obtain a better picture of the pleural involvement, which seems to be a rare manifestation of diseases that are often uncommon themselves. These studies would aid diagnosis, natural history and best treatment options for pleural disease in connective tissue diseases.

Thoracoscopy, a procedure which is becoming widely available, could be of significant help in this investigation.

KEY POINTS

- Pleural effusion is the most common thoracic manifestation of SLE, with an incidence of approximately 50 percent, and may be accompanied by multisystem involvement. The SLE effusion is a non-specific exudate, which may have low glucose and low pH. The added diagnostic value of pleural fluid LE cells is questionable. The best type of intervention remains uncertain, but most of the patients respond to corticosteroid therapy.
- The typical pleural effusion in RA is exudative, with high titers of rheumatoid factor, low pH, low glucose and high lactate dehydrogenase levels. The diagnostic likelihood is increased with male gender, age >50, long-standing arthritis and the presence of subcutaneous nodules. However, the diagnosis is usually made by exclusion of other causes.
- Pleural effusions have been observed with both diffuse and limited scleroderma, but are uncommon. The same applies to polymyositis/dermatomyositis.
- Pleural disease sometimes occurs in secondary SS due to RA or SLE, with the prevalence observed in the last two disorders, but it is rare in primary SS.
- Pleural involvement in CSS was regarded as rare, however, recently pleural disease was found to be more common.
- Pleural effusion in patients with WG, in studies presenting mainly small groups of patients, is not infrequent.

REFERENCES

● = Key primary paper
◆ = Major review article

1. Cohen AS, Reynolds WE, Franklin EC. Preliminary criteria for the classification of systemic lupus erythematosus. *Bull Rheum Dis* 1971; **21**: 643–8.
◆2. Pines A, Kaplinsky N, Olchovsky D, Rozenman J, Frankl O. Pleuro-pulmonary manifestations of systemic lupus erythematosus: clinical features of its subgroups. Prognostic and therapeutic implications. *Chest* 1985; **88**: 129–35.
●3. Halla JT, Schrohenloher RE, Volanakis JE. Immune complexes and other laboratory features of pleural effusions: a comparison of rheumatoid arthritis, systemic lupus erythematosus, and other diseases. *Ann Intern Med* 1980; **92**: 748–52.
◆4. Hunninghake GW, Fauci AS. Pulmonary involvement in the collagen vascular diseases. *Am Rev Respir Dis* 1979; **119**: 471–503.
●5. Good JT Jr, King TE, Antony VB, Sahn SA. Lupus pleuritis. Clinical features and pleural fluid characteristics with special reference to pleural fluid antinuclear antibodies. *Chest* 1983; **84**: 714–18.

◆6. Alarcon-Segovia D, Alarcon DG. Pleuro-pulmonary manifestations of systemic lupus erythematosus. *Dis Chest* 1961; **39**: 7–17.

●7. Man BL, Mok CC. Serositis related to systemic lupus erythematosus: prevalence and outcome. *Lupus* 2005; **14**: 822–6.

8. Ropes MW. *Systemic lupus erythematosus.* Cambridge: Harvard University Press; 1976.

◆9. Miller LR, Greenberg SD, McLarty JW. Lupus lung. *Chest* 1985; **88**: 265–9.

●10. Haupt HM, Moore GW, Hutchins GM. The lung in systemic lupus erythematosus. Analysis of the pathologic changes in 120 patients. *Am J Med* 1981; **71**: 791–8.

11. Gross M, Esterly J R, Earle R H. Pulmonary alterations in systemic lupus erythematosus. *Am Rev Respir Dis* 1972; **105**: 572–7.

●12. Miller MH, Urowitz MB, Gladman DD, Killinger DW. Systemic lupus erythematosus in males. *Medicine (Baltimore)* 1983; **62**: 327–34.

13. Mayor AM, Vila LM. Gender differences in a cohort of Puerto Ricans with systemic lupus erythematosus. *Cell Mol Biol* (*Noisy-le-grand*) 2003; **49**: 1339–44.

◆14. Harvey AM, Shulman LE, Tumulty PA, *et al.* Systemic lupus erythematosus: a review of the literature and clinical analysis of 138 cases. *Medicine (Baltimore)* 1954; **33**: 291–437.

15. Winslow WA, Ploss LN, Loitman B. Pleuritis in systemic lupus erythematosus: it's importance as an early manifestation in diagnosis. *Ann Intern Med* 1958; **49**: 70–88.

●16. Segasothy M, Phillips PA. Systemic lupus erythematosus in Aborigines and Caucasians in central Australia: a comparative study. *Lupus* 2001; **10**: 439–44.

17. Camilleri F, Mallia C. Male SLE patients in Malta. *Adv Exp Med Biol* 1999; **455**: 173–9.

●18. Molina JF, Molina J, Garcia C, *et al.* Ethnic differences in the clinical expression of systemic lupus erythematosus: a comparative study between African-Americans and Latin Americans. *Lupus* 1997; **6**: 63–7.

19. Chang CC, Shih TY, Chu SJ, *et al.* Lupus in Chinese male: a retrospective study of 61 patients. *Chung Hua I Hsueh Tsa Chih (Taipei)* 1995; **55**: 143–50.

20. Costallat LT, Coimbra AM. Systemic lupus erythematosus in 18 Brazilian males: clinical and laboratory analysis. *Clin Rheumatol* 1993; **12**: 522–5.

21. Al Rawi Z, Al Shaarbaf H, Al Raheem E, Khalifa SJ. Clinical features of early cases of systemic lupus erythematosus in Iraqui patients. *Br J Rheumatol* 1983; **22**: 165–71.

22. Bell R, Lawrence DS. Chronic pleurisy in systemic lupus erythematosus treated with pleurectomy. *Br J Dis Chest* 1979; **73**: 314–16.

23. Wang DY, Chang DB, Kuo SH, *et al.* Systemic lupus erythematosus presenting as pleural effusion: report of a case. *J Formos Med Assoc* 1995; **94**: 746–9.

24. Mitra B, Sengupta P, Saha K, Sarkar N, Pal J. Systemic lupus erythematosus presenting with recurrent pleural effusion without any systemic manifestation. *J Assoc Physicians India* 2005; **53**: 1073–6.

25. Paran D, Fireman E, Elkayam O. Pulmonary disease in systemic lupus erythematosus and the antiphospholipid syndrome. *Autoimmun Rev* 2004; **3**: 70–5.

26. Baker SB, Rovira JR, Campion EW, Mills JA. Late onset systemic lupus erythematosus. *Am J Med* 1979; **66**: 727–32.

27. Chantarojanasiri T, Sittirath A, Preutthipan A, Tapaneya-Olarn W, Suwanjutha S. Pulmonary involvement in childhood systemic lupus erythematosus. *J Med Assoc Thai* 1999; **82**(Suppl 1): S144–8.

28. Gedalia A, Molina JF, Molina J, *et al.* Childhood-onset systemic lupus erythematosus: a comparative study of African Americans and Latin Americans. *J Natl Med Assoc* 1999; **91**: 497–501.

●29. Nadorra RL, Landing BH. Pulmonary lesions in childhood onset systemic lupus erythematosus: analysis of 26 cases, and summary of literature. *Pediatr Pathol* 1987; **7**: 1–18.

30. Bouros D, Panagou P, Papandreou L, Kottakis I, Tegos C. Massive bilateral pleural effusion as the only first presentation of systemic lupus erythematosus. *Respiration* 1992; **59**: 173–5.

31. Elborn JS, Conn P, Roberts SD. Refractory massive pleural effusion in systemic lupus erythematosus treated by pleurectomy. *Ann Rheum Dis* 1987; **46**: 77–80.

32. Kaine JL. Refractory massive pleural effusion in systemic lupus erythematosus treated with talc poudrage. *Ann Rheum Dis* 1985; **44**: 61–4.

33. Bulgrin JG, Dubois EL, Jacobson G. Chest roentgenographic changes in systemic lupus erythematosus. *Radiology* 1960; **74**: 42.

34. Taylor TL, Ostrum H. The roentgen evaluation of systemic lupus erythematosus. *Am J Roentgenol* 1959; **82**: 95.

35. Mathlouthi A, Ben M'rad S, Merai S, *et al.* Massive pleural effusion in systemic lupus erythematosus: thoracoscopic and immunohistological findings. *Monaldi Arch Chest Dis* 1998; **53**: 34–6.

36. Mulkey D, Hudson L. Massive spontaneous unilateral hemothorax in systemic lupus erythematosus. *Am J Med* 1974; **56**: 570.

37. Brook I. Measurement of lactic acid in pleural fluid. *Respiration* 1980; **40**: 344–8.

38. Wang DY. Diagnosis and management of lupus pleuritis. *Curr Opin Pulm Med* 2002; **8**: 312–16.

39. Passero FC, Myers AR. Hemopneumothorax in systemic lupus erythematosus. *J Rheumatol* 1980; **7**: 183–6.

40. Lakhotia M, Mehta SR, Mathur D, Baid CS, Varma AR. Diagnostic significance of pleural fluid eosinophilia during initial thoracocentesis. *Indian J Chest Dis Allied Sci* 1989; **31**: 259–64.

41. Carr DT, Lillington GA, Mayne JG. Pleural-fluid glucose in systemic lupus erythematosus. *Mayo Clin Proc* 1970; **45**: 409–12.

42. Hunder GG, McDuffie FC, Huston KA, Elveback LR, Hepper NG. Pleural fluid complement, complement conversion, and immune complexes in immunologic and nonimmunologic diseases. *J Lab Clin Med* 1977; **90**: 971–80.

43. Glovsky MM, Louie JS, Pitts WH Jr, Alenty A. Reduction of pleural fluid complement activity in patients with systemic lupus erythematosus and rheumatoid arthritis. *Clin Immunol Immunopathol* 1976; **6**: 31–41.

44. Hunder GG, McDuffie FC, Hepper NG. Pleural fluid complement in systemic lupus erythematosus and rheumatoid arthritis. *Ann Intern Med* 1972; **76**: 357–63.

45. Andrews BS, Arora NS, Shadforth MF, Goldberg SK, Davis JS. The role of immune complexes in the pathogenesis of pleural effusions. *Am Rev Respir Dis* 1981; **124**: 115–20.

●46. Kimura K, Ezoe K, Yokozeki H, Katayama I, Nishioka K. Elevated serum CA125 in progressive systemic sclerosis with pleural effusion. *J Dermatol* 1995; **22**: 28–31.

●47. Yucel AE, Calguneri M, Ruacan S. False positive pleural biopsy and high CA125 levels in serum and pleural effusion in systemic lupus erythematosus. *Clin Rheumatol* 1996; **15**: 295–7.

48. Carel RS, Shapiro MS, Cordoba O, Taragan R, Gutman A. LE cells in pleural fluid. *Arthritis Rheum* 1979; **22**: 936–7.

49. Keshgegian AA. Lupus erythematosus cells in pleural fluid. *Am J Clin Pathol* 1978; **69**: 570–1.

50. Naylor B. Cytological aspects of pleural, peritoneal and pericardial fluids from patients with systemic lupus erythematosus. *Cytopathology* 1992; **3**: 1–8.

51. Yoshiyuki OR, Shioya S, Handa K, Shimizu K. Lupus erythematosus cells in pleural fluid cytologic diagnosis in two patients. *Acta Cytol* 1977; **21**: 215–17.

52. Reda MG, Baigelman W. Pleural effusion in systemic lupus erythematosus. *Acta Cytol* 1980; **24**: 553–7.

53. Makashir R, Jayaram G. Lupus erythematosus cells in pleural fluid. *Diagn Cytopathol* 1988; **4**: 273–4.

54. Sethi S, Pooley RJ, Yu GH. Lupus erythematosus (LE) cells in pleural fluid: initial diagnosis of systemic lupus erythematosus by cytologic examination. *Cytopathology* 1996; **7**: 292–4.

55. Chao TY, Huang SH, Chu CC. Lupus erythematosus cells in pleural effusions: diagnostic of systemic lupus erythematosus? *Acta Cytol* 1997; **41**: 1231–3.
56. Hunder GG, Pierre RV. In vivo LE cell phenomenon. *Arthritis Rheum* 1970; **13**: 570–1.
57. Greis M, Atay Z. Zytomorphologische Begleitreaction bei malignen Pleuraerguessen. *Pneumonologie* (suppl) 1990; **44**: 262–4.
●58. Wang DY, Yang PC, Yu WL, *et al.* Comparison of different diagnostic methods for lupus pleuritis and pericarditis: a prospective three-year study. *J Formos Med Assoc* 2000; **99**: 375–80.
●59. Khare V, Baethge B, Lang S, Wolf RE, Campbell GD Jr. Antinuclear antibodies in pleural fluid. *Chest* 1994; **106**: 866–71.
●60. Win T, Groves AM, Phillips GD. Antinuclear antibody positive pleural effusion in a patient with tuberculosis. *Respirology* 2003; **8**: 396–7.
●61. Ferreiro JE, Reiter WM, Saldana MJ. Systemic lupus erythematosus presenting as chronic serositis with no demonstrable antinuclear antibodies. *Am J Med* 1984; **76**: 1100–5.
●62. Riska H, Fyhrquist F, Selander RK, Hellstrom PE. Systemic lupus erythematosus and DNA antibodies in pleural effusions. *Scand J Rheumatol* 1978; **7**: 159–60.
63. Porcel JM, Ordi-Ros J, Esquerda A, *et al.* Antinuclear antibody testing in pleural fluid for the diagnosis of lupus pleuritis. *Lupus* 2007; **16**: 25–7.
64. Breuer GS, Deeb M, Fisher D, Nesher G. Therapeutic options for refractory massive pleural effusion in systemic lupus erythematosus: a case study and review of the literature. *Semin Arthritis Rheum* 2005; **34**: 744–9.
65. Brasington RD, Furst DE. Pulmonary disease in systemic lupus erythematosus. *Clin Exp Rheumatol* 1985; **3**: 269–76.
66. Ben Chetrit E, Putterman C, Naparstek Y. Lupus refractory pleural effusion: transient response to intravenous immunoglobulins. *J Rheumatol* 1991; **18**: 1635–7.
67. Sherer Y, Langevitz P, Levy Y, Fabrizzi F, Shoenfeld Y. Treatment of chronic bilateral pleural effusions with intravenous immunoglobulin and cyclosporin. *Lupus* 1999; **8**: 324–7.
●68. McKnight KM, Adair NE, Agudelo CA. Successful use of tetracycline pleurodesis to treat massive pleural effusion secondary to systemic lupus erythematosus. *Arthritis Rheum* 1991; **34**: 1483–4.
●69. Gilleece MH, Evans CC, Bucknall RC. Steroid resistant pleural effusion in systemic lupus erythematosus treated with tetracycline pleurodesis. *Ann Rheum Dis* 1988; **47**: 1031–2.
70. Cook RJ, Gladman DD, Pericak D, Urowitz MB. Prediction of short term mortality in systemic lupus erythematosus with time dependent measures of disease activity. *J Rheumatol* 2000; **27**: 1892–5.
●71. Cervera R, Khamashta MA, Font J, *et al.* Morbidity and mortality in systemic lupus erythematosus during a 5-year period. A multicenter prospective study of 1,000 patients. European Working Party on Systemic Lupus Erythematosus. *Medicine (Baltimore)* 1999; **78**: 167–75.
72. Fuller HM. *On rheumatism, rheumatic gout and sciatica: Their pathology, symptoms and treatment.* New York: S. S. & W. Wood, 1854.
73. Walker WC, Wright V. Pulmonary lesions and rheumatoid arthritis. *Medicine (Baltimore)* 1968; **47**: 501–20.
●74. Hyland RH, Gordon DA, Broder I, *et al.* A systematic controlled study of pulmonary abnormalities in rheumatoid arthritis. *J Rheumatol* 1983; **10**: 395–405.
75. Dodson WH, Hollingsworth JW. Pleural effusion in rheumatoid arthritis. Impaired transport of glucose. *N Engl J Med* 1966; **275**: 1337–42.
●76. Jurik AG, Davidsen D, Graudal H. Prevalence of pulmonary involvement in rheumatoid arthritis and its relationship to some characteristics of the patients. A radiological and clinical study. *Scand J Rheumatol* 1982; **11**: 217–24.
◆77. Balbir-Gurman A, Yigla M, Nahir AM, Braun-Moscovici Y. Rheumatoid pleural effusion. *Semin Arthritis Rheum* 2006; **35**: 368–78.
78. Allan JS, Donahue DM, Garrity JM. Rheumatoid pleural effusion in the absence of arthritic disease. *Ann Thorac Surg* 2005; **80**: 1519–21.
79. Halla JT, Schronhenloher RE, Volanakis JE. Immune complexes and other laboratory features of pleural effusions. *Ann Intern Med* 1980; **92**: 748–52.
80. Lillington GA, Carr DT, Mayne GJ. Rheumatoid pleurisy with pleural effusion. *Arch Intern Med* 1971; **128**: 764–8.
81. Brennan SR, Daly JJ. Large pleural effusions in rheumatoid arthritis. *Br J Dis Chest* 1979; **73**: 133–40.
82. Pritikin JD, Jensen WA, Yenokida GG, Kirsch CM, Fainstat M. Respiratory failure due to a massive rheumatoid pleural effusion. *J Rheumatol* 1990; **17**: 673–5.
83. Joseph J, Sahn SA. Connective tissue diseases and the pleura. *Chest* 1993; **104**: 262–70.
●84. Ferrer JS, Munoz XG, Orriols RM, Light RW, Morell FB. Evolution of idiopathic pleural effusion: a prospective, long-term follow-up study. *Chest* 1996; **109**: 1508–13.
85. Faurschou P, Francis D, Faarup P. Thoracoscopic, histological, and clinical findings in nine case of rheumatoid pleural effusion. *Thorax* 1985; **40**: 371–5.
86. Salomaa ER, Viander M, Saaresranta T, Terho EO. Complement components and their activation products in pleural fluid. *Chest* 1998; **114**: 723–30.
●87. Pettersson T, Ojala K, Weber TH. Adenosine deaminase in the diagnosis of pleural effusions. *Acta Med Scand* 1984; **215**: 299–304.
88. Naylor B. The pathognomonic cytologic picture of rheumatoid pleuritis. *Acta Cytol* 1990; **34**: 465–73.
89. Aru A, Engel U, Francis D. Characteristic and specific histological findings in rheumatoid pleurisy. *Acta Pathol Microbiol Immunol Scand [A]* 1986; **94**: 57–62.
◆90. Sahn SA. Immunologic diseases of the pleura. *Clin Chest Med* 1985; **6**: 103–12.
91. Faurschou P. Decreased glucose in RA-cell-positive pleural effusion: correlation of pleural glucose, lactic dehydrogenase and protein concentration to the presence of RA-cells. *Eur J Respir Dis* 1984; **65**: 272–7.
92. Carr DT, McGuckin WF. Pleural fluid glycose. *Am Rev Resp Dis* 1968; **97**: 302–5.
93. Ferguson GC. Cholesterol pleural effusion in rheumatoid lung disease. *Thorax* 1966; **21**: 577–82.
94. Jones FL, Blodget RC. Empyema in rheumatoid pleuropulmonary disease. *Ann Intern Med* 1971; **74**: 665–71.
95. Dieppe PA. Empyema in rheumatoid arthritis. *Ann Rheum Dis* 1975; **34**: 181–5.
96. Anonymous. Pleural effusion in rheumatoid arthritis (Editorials). *Lancet* 1972; i: 480–1.
97. Faurschou P. Rheumatoid pleuritis and thoracoscopy. *Scand J Respir Dis* 1974; **55**: 277–83.
◆98. Ward R. Pleural effusion and rheumatoid disease. *Lancet* 1961; ii: 1336.
99. Russell ML, Gladman DD, Mintz S. Rheumatoid pleural effusion: lack of response to intrapleural corticosteroid. *J Rheumatol* 1986; **13**: 412–15.
100. Emerson RA. Pleural effusion complicating rheumatoid arthritis. *Br Med J* 1956; **1**: 428.
101. Walker WC, Wright W. Rheumatoid pleuritis. *Ann Rheum Dis* 1967; **26**: 467.
102. Brunk JR, Drash EC, Swineford O. Rheumatoid pleuritis successfully treated with decortication. *Am J Med* 1966; **251**: 545.
103. Yarbrough JW, Sealy WC, Miller JA. Thoracic surgical problems associated with rheumatoid arthritis. *J Thorac Cardiovasc Surg* 1975; **69**: 347–54.
104. Yigla M, Simsolo C, Goralnik L, Balabir-German A, Nahir AM. The

problem of empyematous pleural effusion in rheumatoid arthritis: report of two cases and review of the literature. *Clin Rheumatol* 2002; **21**: 180–3.
105. Chapman PT, O' Donnell JL, Moller PW. Rheumatoid pleural effusion: response to intrapleural corticosteroid. *Rheumatology* 1992; **19**: 478–80.
106. Light RW, Jenkinson SG, Minh Vea. Observations on pleural pressures as fluid is withdrawn during thoracentesis. *Am Rev Resp Dis* 1980; **121**: 799–804.
107. Funauchi M, Ikoma S, Yu H, *et al.* A case of progressive systemic sclerosis complicated by massive pleural effusion with elevated CA125. *Lupus* 2000; **9**: 382–5.
108. Hiramatsu K, Takeda N, Okumura S, Takuno H, Yasuda K. [Progressive systemic sclerosis associated with massive pleural and pericardial effusion in a 90-year-old woman]. *Nippon Ronen Igakkai Zasshi* 1996; **33**: 535–9.
109. Lee YH, Ji JD, Shim JJ, Kang KH, Song GG. Exudative pleural effusion and pleural leukocytoclastic vasculitis in limited scleroderma. *J Rheumatol* 1998; **25**: 1006–8.
110. Thompson AE, Pope JE. A study of the frequency of pericardial and pleural effusions in scleroderma. *Br J Rheumatol* 1998; **37**: 1320–3.
111. Takeda N, Teramoto S, Ihn H, *et al.* [A case of very late onset overlap syndrome of systemic sclerosis and systemic lupus erythematosus]. *Nippon Ronen Igakkai Zasshi* 2000; **37**: 74–9.
112. Lakhanpal S, Lie JT, Conn DL, Martin WJ. Pulmonary disease in polymyositis/dermatomyositis: a clinicopathological analysis of 65 autopsy cases. *Ann Rheum Dis* 1987; **46**: 23–9.
113. Ozawa Y, Kurosaka D, Hashimoto N. [An autopsy case of dermatomyositis with rapidly progressive interstitial pneumonia]. *Nihon Rinsho Meneki Gakkai Kaishi* 1995; **18**: 552–8.
114. Schwarz MI, Matthay RA, Sahn SA, *et al.* Interstitial lung disease in polymyositis and dermatomyositis: analysis of six cases and review of the literature. *Medicine (Baltimore)* 1976; **55**: 89–104.
115. Miyata M, Fukaya E, Takagi T, *et al.* Two patients with polymyositis or dermatomyositis complicated with massive pleural effusion. *Intern Med* 1998; **37**: 1058–63.
●116. Kawamata K, Haraoka H, Hirohata S, *et al.* Pleurisy in primary Sjogren's syndrome: T cell receptor beta-chain variable region gene bias and local autoantibody production in the pleural effusion. *Clin Exp Rheumatol* 1997; **15**: 193–6.
●117. Bloch KJ, Buchanan WW, Wohl MJ, Bunim JJ. Sjogren's syndrome. A clinical, pathological, and serological study of sixty-two cases. *Medicine (Baltimore)* 1992; **71**: 386–401.
●118. Constantopoulos SH, Papadimitriou CS, Moutsopoulos HM. Respiratory manifestations in primary Sjogren's syndrome. A clinical, functional, and histologic study. *Chest* 1985; **88**: 226–9.
●119. Papathanasiou MP, Constantopoulos SH, Tsampoulas C, Drosos AA, Moutsopoulos HM. Reappraisal of respiratory abnormalities in primary and secondary Sjogren's syndrome. A controlled study. *Chest* 1986; **90**: 370–4.
♦120. Strimlan CV, Rosenow EC III, Divertie MB, Harrison EG Jr. Pulmonary manifestations of Sjogren's syndrome. *Chest* 1976; **70**: 354–61.
121. Kashiwabara K, Kishi K, Narushima K, *et al.* [Primary Sjogren's syndrome accompanied by pleural effusion]. *Nihon Kyobu Shikkan Gakkai Zasshi* 1995; **33**: 1325–9.
122. Tanaka A, Tohda Y, Fukuoka M, Nakajima S. [A case of Sjogren's syndrome with pleural effusion]. *Nihon Kokyuki Gakkai Zasshi* 2000; **38**: 628–31.
♦123. Ogihara T, Nakatani A, Ito H, *et al.* Sjogren's syndrome with pleural effusion. *Intern Med* 1995; **34**: 811–14.
124. Alvarez-Sala R, Sanchez-Toril F, Garcia-Martinez J, Zaera A, Masa JF. Primary Sjogren syndrome and pleural effusion. *Chest* 1989; **96**: 1440–1.
125. Tanaka H, Itoh E, Shibusa T, *et al.* Pleural effusion in ankylosing spondylitis; successful treatment with intra-pleural steroid administration. *Respir Med* 1995; **89**: 509–11.
126. Dudley-Hart F, Bogdanovich A, Nichol WD. The thorax in ankylosing spondilitis. *Ann Rheum Dis* 1950; **9**: 116–31.
127. Kinnear WJ, Shneerson JM. Acute pleural effusions in inactive ankylosing spondylitis. *Thorax* 1985; **40**: 150–1.
128. Haslock I. Ankylosing spondylitis. *Baillieres Clin Rheumatol* 1993; **7**: 99–115.
♦129. Zorab PA. The lungs in ankylosing spondylitis. *Q J Med* 1962; **31**: 267–80.
130. Crompton GK, Cameron SJ, Langlands AO. Pulmonary fibrosis, pulmonary tuberculosis and ankylosing spondylitis. *Br J Dis Chest* 1974; **68**: 51–6.
●131. Spencer DG, Park WM, Dick HM, Papazoglou SN, Buchanan WW. Radiological manifestations in 200 patients with ankylosing spondylitis: correlation with clinical features and HLA B27. *J Reumatol* 1979; **6**: 305–15.
♦132. Rosenow E, Strimlan CV, Muhm JR, Ferguson RH. Pleuropulmonary manifestations of ankylosing spondylitis. *Mayo Clin Proc* 1977; **52**: 641–9.
♦133. Prakash UB. Respiratory complications in mixed connective tissue disease. *Clin Chest Med* 1998; **19**: 733–46, ix.
134. Battista G, Zompatori M, Poletti V, Canini R. Thoracic manifestations of the less common collagen diseases. A pictorial essay. *Radiol Med (Torino)* 2003; **106**: 445–1.
♦135. Bull TM, Fagan KA, Badesch DB. Pulmonary vascular manifestations of mixed connective tissue disease. *Rheum Dis Clin North Am* 2005; **31**: 451–64, vi.
♦136. Aiello M, Chetta A, Marangio E, Zompatori M, Olivieri D. Pleural involvement in systemic disorders. *Curr Drug Targets Inflamm Allergy* 2004; **3**: 441–7.
●137. Sullivan WD, Hurst DJ, Harmon CE, *et al.* A prospective evaluation emphasizing pulmonary involvement in patients with mixed connective tissue disease. *Medicine (Baltimore)* 1984; **63**: 92–107.
138. Beier JM, Nielsen HL, Nielsen D. Pleuritis-pericarditis – an unusual initial manifestation of mixed connective tissue disease. *Eur Heart J* 1992; **13**: 859–61.
139. Richard P, Sabouret P, Vayre F, Desrame J, Ollivier JP. [Pleuropericarditis complicated of tamponade disclosing mixed connective tissue disease. Remission with non-steroidal anti-inflammatory agents. Apropos of a case]. *Ann Cardiol Angeiol (Paris)* 1996; **45**: 513–15.
140. Hoogsteden HC, van Dongen JJ, van der Kwast TH, Hooijkaas H, Hilvering C. Bilateral exudative pleuritis, an unusual pulmonary onset of mixed connective tissue disease. *Respiration* 1985; **48**: 164–7.
141. Ilan Y, Ben Yehuda A, Okon E, Breuer R. Mixed connective tissue disease presenting as a left sided pleural effusion. *Ann Rheum Dis* 1992; **51**: 1157–8.
142. Swygert LA, Maes EF, Sewell LE, *et al.* Eosinophilia–myalgia syndrome. Results of national surveillance. *J Am Med Assoc* 1990; **264**: 1698–703.
●143. Williamson MR, Eidson M, Rosenberg RD, Williamson SL. Eosinophilia–myalgia syndrome: findings on chest radiographs in 18 patients. *Radiology* 1991; **180**: 849–52.
144. Killen JW, Swift GL, White RJ. Eosinophilic fasciitis with pulmonary and pleural involvement. *Postgrad Med J* 2000; **76**: 36–7.
145. Cullen MH, Stansfeld AG, Oliver RT, Lister TA, Malpas JS. Angio-immunoblastic lymphadenopathy: report of ten cases and review of the literature. *Q J Med* 1979; **48**: 151–77.
146. Sugiyama H, Kotajima F, Kamimura M, *et al.* [Pulmonary involvement in immunoblastic lymphadenopathy: case reports and review of literature published in Japan]. *Nihon Kyobu Shikkan Gakkai Zasshi* 1995; **33**: 1276–82.
●147. Guillevin L, Cohen P, Gayraud M, *et al.* Churg–Strauss syndrome. Clinical study and long-term follow-up of 96 patients. *Medicine (Baltimore)* 1999; **78**: 26–37.
♦148. Lanham JG, Elkon KB, Pusey CD, Hughes GR. Systemic vasculitis

with asthma and eosinophilia: a clinical approach to the Churg–Strauss syndrome. *Medicine (Baltimore)* 1984; **63**: 65–81.

●149. Choi YH, Im JG, Han BK, *et al.* Thoracic manifestation of Churg–Strauss syndrome: radiologic and clinical findings. *Chest* 2000; **117**: 117–24.

150. Erzurum SC, Underwood GA, Hamilos DL, Waldron JA. Pleural effusion in Churg–Strauss syndrome. *Chest* 1989; **95**: 1357–9.

●151. Hirasaki S, Kamei T, Iwasaki Y, *et al.* Churg–Strauss Syndrome with pleural involvement. *Intern Med* 2000; **39**: 976–8.

●152. Gonzalez L, Van Ordstrand HS. Wegener's granulomatosis. Review of 11 cases. *Radiology* 1973; **107**: 295–300.

153. Bambery P, Katariya S, Sakhuja V, *et al.* Wegener's granulomatosis in north India. Radiologic manifestations in eleven patients. *Acta Radiol* 1988; **29**: 11–13.

●154. Cordier JF, Valeyre D, Guillevin L, Loire R, Brechot JM. Pulmonary Wegener's granulomatosis. A clinical and imaging study of 77 cases. *Chest* 1990; **97**: 906–12.

●155. Fauci AS, Wolff SM. Wegener's granulomatosis: studies in eighteen patients and a review of the literature. *Medicine (Baltimore)* 1973; **73**: 315–24.

156. Lohrmann C, Uhl M, Schaefer O, *et al.* Serial high-resolution computed tomography imaging in patients with Wegener granulomatosis: differentiation between active inflammatory and chronic fibrotic lesions. *Acta Radiol* 2005; **46**: 484–91.

157. Blundell AG, Roe S. Wegener's granulomatosis presenting as a pleural effusion. *Br Med J* 2003; **327**: 95–6.

158. Weir IH, Muller NL, Chiles C, *et al.* Wegener's granulomatosis: findings from computed tomography of the chest in 10 patients. *Can Assoc Radiol J* 1992; **43**: 31–4.

159. Bosch X, Ramirez J. [Bilateral lung images and respiratory insufficiency in an 86-year-old man with polyarteritis nodosa]. *Med Clin (Barc)* 1999; **113**:189–97.

160. Romero S, Vela P, Padilla I, *et al.* Pleural effusion as manifestation of temporal arteritis. *Thorax* 1992; **47**: 398–9.

161. Turiaf J, Valere PE, Gubler MC. [Recurrent pleurisy during temporal arteritis]. *Poumon Coeur* 1967; **23**: 633–52.

162. Garcia-Alfranca F, Solans R, Simeon C, *et al.* Pleural effusion as a form of presentation of temporal arteritis. *Br J Rheumatol* 1998; **37**: 802–3.

163. Ramos A, Laguna P, Cuervas V. Pleural effusion in giant cell arteritis. *Ann Intern Med* 1992; **116**: 957.

164. Gur H, Ehrenfeld M, Izsak E. Pleural effusion as a presenting manifestation of giant cell arteritis. *Clin Rheumatol* 1996; **15**: 200–3.

165. Umezawa T, Saji T, Matsuo N, Odagiri K. Chest x-ray findings in the acute phase of Kawasaki disease. *Pediatr Radiol* 1989; **20**: 48–51.

●166. Tunaci A, Berkmen YM, Gokmen E. Thoracic involvement in Behcet's disease: pathologic, clinical, and imaging features. *AJR Am J Roentgenol* 1995; **164**: 51–6.

167. Walsh FW, Solomon DA, Espinoza LR, Adams GD, Whitelocke HE. Human adjuvant disease. A new cause of chylous effusions. *Arch Intern Med* 1989; **149**: 1194–6.

168. Pasteur M, Laroche C, Keogan M. Pleuropericardial effusion in a 50 year old woman. Pleuropericardial effusion caused by adult inset Still's disease. *Postgrad Med J* 2001; **77**: 346, 355–7.

169. Nishio J, Koike R, Iizuka H, *et al.* [A refractory case of adult-onset Still's disease]. *Nihon Rinsho Meneki Gakkai Kaishi* 1997; **20**: 191–8.

170. Cheema GS, Quismorio FP Jr. Pulmonary involvement in adult-onset Still's disease. *Curr Opin Pulm Med* 1999; **5**: 305–9.

33

Effusions caused by drugs

IOANNIS KALOMENIDIS

A variety of commonly used medications may cause pleural disorders, most commonly, pleural effusion. Pleural fibrosis and, rarely, hemothorax can be associated with the use of certain agents. The pathogenesis of drug-induced pleural disease is poorly understood in the majority of the cases. However, oxidant-induced mesothelial and/or endothelial cell injury, acute hypersensitivity-type reaction, direct dose-related toxic effect or chemically induced pleural inflammation, are among the possible mechanisms.[1,2]

Pleural disease can be the dominant or even the sole manifestation of an adverse drug reaction. Otherwise, it may appear in combination with drug-associated lung disease or even as a component of generalized syndromes. The most common symptom on patient presentation is dyspnea on exertion, which may be due to either underlying parenchymal disease or the accumulation of excessive amounts of pleural fluid, or even the progressive pleural fibrosis. Cough, thoracic pain and constitutional symptoms, such as fever, malaise and weight loss, are sometimes present.

The clinical importance of prompt recognition of an adverse drug reaction as the cause of pleural disease lies on the fact that in most cases, pleural disease resolves upon the withdrawal of the drug. For this reason, and although drug reactions account for a small percentage of pleural abnormalities, the clinician must consider the possibility of drug-induced pleural disease in all patients with pleural effusions or fibrosis and a detailed history of drug intake must be obtained. It should be remembered that a patient may not reveal the use of a drug unless asked specifically.[1] Treatment of drug-induced pleural disease mainly consists of discontinuation of the offending drug, a measure usually adequate to lead to partial or complete remission. Corticosteroids are sometimes administered, more commonly in patients with severe clinical manifestations, based on the belief that the underlying mechanism may include pleural inflammation. However, with the exception of certain conditions, the benefit of corticosteroids is uncertain.

In this chapter, I describe the clinical, radiographical and serological abnormalities that characterize pleural disease resulting from drug reactions. When available, information concerning the pathogenesis and the pathology, the clinical course and the response to the treatment of the diseases will be also provided. A drug is thought to be the cause of a pleural abnormality when the disease occurs after the administration of the drug, other usual or possible etiologies have been convincingly ruled out, and the disease resolves when the drug is discontinued. An even stronger proof is the recrudescence of the disorder when the drug is readministered. As will be noted, the clinical data presented by the authors of some case reports to support a casual relationship between the use of a drug and the subsequent pleural abnormalities are rather weak to definitely establish such a relationship. However, these cases will be presented to facilitate possible related future clinical observations, which may lead to outright conclusions.

NITROFURANTOIN

Nitrofurantoin is an antibiotic used in the prophylaxis and treatment of lower urinary tract infections. Since the mid-1960s, when the nitrofurantoin-associated pleuropulmonary toxicity was first recognized,[3] over 2000 cases have been reported.[4] Respiratory reactions to nitrofurantoin may be manifested in two distinct patterns characterized by the length of treatment prior to the development of the syndrome.[5]

The acute presentation (5–25 percent of the patients taking the drug) occurs within the first month of the onset of the treatment. The symptoms that may appear even within hours of the drug intake include dyspnea, non-productive cough and fever. The chest radiograph usually reveals alveolar and interstitial infiltrates that are more confluent at the lung bases. In one series of 335 patients,[6] 186 (56 percent) had infiltrates, 65 (19 percent) had infiltrates and effusion, 14 (3 percent) had only an effusion and 70 (21 percent) had a normal chest radiograph. Others have reported that the frequency of the effusions may be as high as 30 percent.[4] The majority of the patients with the acute syndrome have both peripheral eosinophilia (>350/mm^3) and lymphopenia (<1000/mm^3).[7] The only reported pleural fluid analysis showed 17 percent eosinophils in the pleural fluid.[7]

The chronic syndrome (5 percent of the patients taking the drug) occurs when the patient has been taking nitrofurantoin for 2 months to 5 years. The presentation is insidious, with the gradual onset of dyspnea and a non-productive cough.[5] Diffuse bibasilar infiltrates are the most common radiographic abnormality.[6] Pleural effusion occurs in fewer than 10 percent of patients and has never been reported in the absence of pulmonary infiltrates.[5] The pathogenesis of the acute syndrome may be related to a hypersensitivity reaction and is not dose-related,[8] while the pathogenesis of the chronic syndrome is thought to involve damage elicited by oxygen radicals.[5,8]

The diagnosis of nitrofurantoin pleuropulmonary reaction should be suspected in all patients with a pleural effusion who are taking nitrofurantoin. If the drug is discontinued, the patient with the acute syndrome usually improves clinically within 1–4 days, and the chest radiograph becomes normal within a week.[6] Symptoms and signs in patients with the chronic syndrome improve much more slowly and pulmonary function may remain permanently impaired.[3,6]

CARDIOVASCULAR AGENTS

Amiodarone

Amiodarone is a very effective antiarrhythmic drug, commonly prescribed for the prophylaxis and treatment of supraventricular and ventricular dysrhythmias. Pulmonary toxicity has been reported in up to 5–10 percent of the patients receiving the agent,[9] although others argue that this number may overestimate the real incidence.[10] It is speculated that the pathogenesis of adverse pulmonary and pleural reaction is most likely multifactorial and involves direct oxidant induced-damage and the participation of inflammatory or immunological responses in the disease process.[1] The toxicity is dose dependent, being clinically evident after the ingestion of more than 100 g of the drug, which accumulates in lung and pleural tissues.

The clinical manifestations of pulmonary toxicity may either have an acute or insidious onset and include non-productive cough, malaise, dyspnea, weight loss and occasionally fever, accompanied by either patchy alveolar or, most commonly, interstitial infiltrates.[8–10] Amiodarone withdrawal is the proposed treatment of parenchymal disease, even though the disease may progress after the discontinuation of the drug. Corticosteroids have been commonly used, but are of unproved efficacy.[10]

Pleural disease in the setting of amiodarone toxicity is rather uncommon and may be manifested as an exudative pleural effusion or pleural thickening.[8,11–13] Pleural effusion may be either unilateral or bilateral. In an initial report,[11] all of the 11 cases with pleural effusion were accompanied by parenchymal disease. However, pleural effusion in the absence parenchymal involvement may also occur.[12] The predominant cell population of the pleural fluid may be lymphocytes,[13] macrophages[12] or polymorphonuclear leukocytes.[11] Amiodarone-induced pleural disease has a benign course and should be expected to resolve when the drug is discontinued.

Beta-blockers

Practolol, a beta-blocker, was removed from the market in 1976 because it caused serious adverse effects including skin, eye, ear, renal, peritoneal and pleuropulmonary disorders.[1,8,14] Pleural effusions and pleuropulmonary fibrosis have been reported. There is weak evidence that another beta-blocker, oxyprenolol, may also cause pleural fibrosis.[15] Pleural fibrosis associated with beta-blockers may be progressive despite drug discontinuation and corticosteroid administration.

Minoxidil

Minoxidil, a potent vasodilator that is used in the treatment of severe arterial hypertension, has been associated with the development of pericardial effusion that may lead to tamponade.[1] There is only one report of a patient who developed exdutative bilateral pleural effusion and pericardial effusion, 2 months after the initiation of the drug.[16] Both the pericardial and the pleural effusion resolved upon the discontinuation of the drug. When minoxidil was readministered, only the pericardial effusion recurred, but again resolved after the cessation of the therapy.

Imidapril

Yoshida and associates reported on a patient with hypertension treated with imidapril for 6 years who developed low-grade fever and a left-sided pleural effusion[17] with pleural fluid and peripheral eosinophilia (38 and 28 percent, respectively) that did no respond to antibiotics.

CYTOKINES AND IMMUNOMODULATING AGENTS

Interleukin 2

Recombinant human interleukin 2 (rhIL-2), which has been used in the treatment of melanoma or renal cell carcinoma, is associated with a variety of reversible adverse effects, including fever, chills, lethargy, diarrhea, anemia, thrombocytopenia, eosinophilia, confusion and diffuse erythroderma.[18] Respiratory abnormalities include parenchymal infiltrates and pleural effusion. Two studies,[18,19] including a total of 108 patients, indicated that approximately half of those treated with rhIL-2 may develop pleural effusion. Diffuse infiltrates resembling pulmonary edema (41–80 percent) and focal infiltrates (22 percent) may also be present. Pleural effusion may be found in the absence of parenchymal abnormalities. The characteristics of the fluid were not reported. Patients receiving bolus rather than constant intravenous therapy were more likely to develop respiratory complications.[18] Severe respiratory failure was reported in 35 percent of the patients and some of them required intubation and mechanical ventilation. As reported in one of these studies, the pleural effusions tended to improve, but they persisted for 4 weeks following therapy cessation in 17 percent of patients.[18] Pleural effusions resolved later than the parenchymal infiltrates.

The respiratory adverse effects of the rhIL-2 are probably a manifestation of the generalized capillary leak syndrome that may occur after the administration of this cytokine. Berthianume *et al.*[20] proposed that pulmonary edema related to the rhIL-2 administration may be the combined result of increased permeability and hydrostatic pressure. Thus, it is possible that pleural fluid originates from the leaky capillaries in the lung.

Interleukin 11

Recombinant human interleukin 11 (rhIL-11) is used to prevent severe thrombocytopenia and to reduce the need for platelet transfusions following myelosuppressive chemotherapy in patients with non-myeloid malignancies. Fluid retention is a frequent adverse effect of rhIL-11 treatment and can manifest as peripheral and pulmonary edema as well as pleural effusions.[21] The frequency of pleural effusions in one study of patients with breast cancer patients was 42 percent.[22] Although all of these patients had distant metastases and thoracentesis was not performed in any, the fact that all the pleural effusions responded well to diuretic treatment suggests that the most probable explanation of the effusions is fluid overload.

Interferons

Interferons are used in the treatment of various malignancies and chronic hepatitis. Interferons can cause several significant adverse effects including depression, bone marrow suppression, interstitial pneumonitis, retinopathy, hearing loss, vitiligo and autoimmune diseases, as well as milder disorders including flu-like symptoms, headache, irritability and alopecia. Pleural effusion, possibly caused by recombinant human interferon-α, has been reported in a patient with chronic hepatitis C.[23] The patient developed an asymptomatic, moderate, right-sided exudative, lymphocytic pleural effusion 14 days after beginning the treatment. Although a slight increase of serum antinuclear antibody (ANA) titer was observed, the patient's symptoms and signs did not satisfy the criteria of any autoimmune disorders, including systemic lupus erythematosus (SLE), a disease that may either be exacerbated or induced by the drug. Tuberculus pleuritis, which is encountered with increased frequency in patients on interferon treatment, was ruled out. The pleural effusion gradually resolved upon the discontinuation of the interferon.

Granulocyte-colony stimulating growth factor

Busmanis *et al.*[24] reported a case of a 43-year-old woman with breast carcinoma who developed a pleural effusion after a cycle of chemotherapy supported by granulocyte-colony stimulating growth factor (G-CSF). Although infection and malignancy were ruled out, the possible role of the chemotherapeutic regimen in the development of the pleural effusion was not discussed. Subsequently, Nakamura *et al.*[25] reported a case of a 57-year-old man with rheumatoid arthritis and polycystic kidneys who received G-CSF for the treatment of methotrexate-induced pancytopenia. The patient was in a chronic hemodialysis program. He developed bilateral exudative pleural effusion 9 days after the end of a 10-day course of G-CSF. The effusion persisted for more than 20 days and resolved after the administration of prednisolone. In my opinion, other possible etiologies of the pleural effusion, such as rheumatoid pleuritis, uremia or hemodialysis, were not effectively ruled out. Thus, I do not think that this evidence linking the administration of G-CSF with the development of pleural effusion is convincing. However, deAvezo *et al.*[26] reported a life-threatening capillary leak syndrome after G-CSF was used for mobilization and collection of peripheral blood progenitor cells for allogeneic transplantation in a 37-year-old donor. During leukophoresis she suddenly developed hypotention, hypoxemia, ascites, pericardial and pleural effusions, edema, neurologic changes and hepatocellular injury. G-SCF was withdrawn and she was treated with the intravenous administration of fluid and methylprednizolone until she fully recovered.

Immunoglobulin

Bolanos-Meade *et al.*[27] reported a patient with recurrent pleural effusions attributed to the use of intravenous immunoglobulin (IVIG) for the treatment of idiopathic thrombocytopenic purpura. She was receiving a 2-day course of the IVIG every four to six weeks. On the second day of the seventh or the eighth course, bilateral exdutative lymphocytic pleural effusions developed, but resolved completely 2 weeks later. The effusions could not be attributed to infectious, malignant or autoimmune disease. The same thing happened with the next course of the IVIG. However, when a different preparation of IVIG was administered, there was no recurrence of the pleural effusions. Thus, I would suggest that pleural effusion could represent a reaction to a component of the first preparation and not of the IVIG itself.

ERGOT DERIVATIVES

Ergot derivatives have been used in the treatment and prophylaxis of migraine and cluster headaches (methysergide, ergotamine) and Parkinson's disease (bromocriptine, dihydroergotamine, nicergoline, pergolide, dopergine, lisuride, dihydroergocristine, dihydroergocryptine, cabergolide). The long-term administration of any of these drugs can lead to a distinctive pattern of pleuropulmonary abnormalities, consisting of pleural fibrosis with or without effusion, occasionally associated with parenchymal fibrosis. First described by Graham *et al.*[28] in 1966 in a patient receiving methysergide, the potential of ergot derivatives to produce these fibrosing abnormalities was subsequently confirmed and thoroughly characterized.[1,14,29–39] A variety of other fibrosing disorders of the retroperitoneum, mediastinum, pericardium and heart valves, either singly or, rarely, in combination with pleural disease has been also reported.[14,35,37,39,40]

The pathogenesis of the fibrosis which is induced by the ergot derivatives remains unclear. It has been suggested that fibrinogenesis may be related to the serotoninergic activity of the drugs, as similar fibrosing disorders may be seen in association with serotonin-secreting carcinoid tumors.[37] Serotonin can cause either pleural vasoconstriction[14] or stimulate fibroblast growth.[1] A rather rare mechanism could be fluid retention, as reported in a patient who was taking pergolide and developed bilateral pleural effusion and peripheral edema, both of which responded to diuretic therapy.[41] Furthermore, some authors proposed that prior exposure to asbestos represents a specific risk factor for the development of ergot-related pleural disease.[36,42]

Respiratory symptoms usually arise after a treatment period of more than 6 months, though latent periods of 3 weeks to 30 years have been reported.[37] Dyspnea develops insidiously and may be accompanied by dry cough, pleuritic or non-pleuritic chest pain, malaise and recurrent or chronic moderate to low-grade fever.[1,37] The radiographic abnormalities consist of unilateral or bilateral pleural thickening and/or effusion. Rounded atelectasis and occasional linear pleural calcification have been also observed.[37] Pleural thickening is often massive and irregular, resembling malignant mesothelioma. The pleural fluid is an exudate with predominantly lymphocytes and sometimes eosinophils.[32,37,43] Bloody effusion has been reported in a patient taking methysergide.[30] The erythrocyte sedimentation rate (ESR) and C-reactive protein (CRP) levels are frequently elevated[14,36,37] and normochromic anemia[35] as well as weakly positive serum ANA or rheumatoid factor (RF) have been reported.[37] Pleural biopsy reveals non-specific fibrosis of the parietal pleura with few inflammatory cells.[37]

A few patients on treatment with bromocryptine, ergotamine, cabergoline or dihydroergocristine develop parenchymal disease, usually but not always associated with pleural disease.[14,37] Chest X-ray revealed interstitial infiltrates in all patients and apical patchy fibrosis in one patient. Interestingly, in patients with pleural fibrosis with or without obvious parenchymal disease, bronchoalveolar lavage (BAL) discloses polymorphonuclear or lymphocytic alveolitis.

The vast majority of patients will experience gradual improvement of the symptoms upon the withdrawal of the drug. Classically, the pleural abnormalities will gradually clear over a period of months to 4 years often leaving residual pleural thickening.[14,37,44] Parenchymal infiltrates tend to resolve more rapidly and completely.[37] Corticosteroids are often used, but their necessity or their effectiveness are not established. Importantly, Ling *et al.*[35] reported a patient with pleuropulmonary fibrosis due to cabergoline who had persistent if not progressive disease, despite the discontinuation of the drug and the administration of long-term corticosteroid treatment. The patient died a few months after the diagnosis from respiratory insufficiency and, although the death was not attributed to the pleural thickening by the authors, this could be the only fatal case of pleuropulmonary fibrosis related to an ergot derivative.

Should the drug definitely be discontinued after it is recognized as the cause of pleuropulmonary fibrosis? Miller[14] reported that in seven of eight patients with pleuropulmonary disease caused by bromocriptine who continued the drug after the diagnosis was made had no clinical or radiographic evidence of progressive disease putting into question the necessity of drug withdrawal. However, Kok-Jensen *et al.*,[29] who followed-up 12 patients with pleural fibrosis caused by methysergide, reported that those who continued to take methysergide for the longest period after the onset had the worst disease after 6 months. Therefore, given the possibility that the disease is dose-related and related to the length of the time the patient has been on the drug, as well as the excellent outcome after the drug withdrawal, I would agree with the recommendation that patients who are taking ergot alkaloids on a long-term basis should have a radiograph annually; if there is evidence of pleural or parenchymal disease, strong consideration should be given to stopping the ergot alkaloids and using an alternative drug for the treatment of Parkinson's disease.[45]

RETINOIDS

Isotretinoin

Isoretinoin, a retinoid compound, has been used in the treatment of cystic acne and may be also useful as chemopreventive agent for various malignancies.[8] There are two case reports indicating that the drug can cause eosinophilic pleural effusion 1–6 months after the initiation of treatment.[46,47] Parenchymal disease or blood eosinophilia was absent. The effusion resolved 1–3 months after drug discontinuation. Fever and cough were reported in one of these patients, while the other experienced only dyspnea on exertion. The manufacturer of isotretinoin has on file three other cases of pleural effusion occurring in patients who took isotretinoin for acne.[47]

All-*trans*-retinoic acid

All-*trans*-retinoic acid (ATRA) is used in the treatment of acute promyelocytic leukemia.[48] Up to one-quarter of the patients taking the drug develop a life-threatening reaction that resembles capillary-leak syndrome which is attributed to IL-2.[49,50] Symptoms may develop 1–22 days after the initiation of the treatment and include fever, fluid retention, dyspnea, multiple organ failure and hemorrhagic and thrombotic manifestations. Leukocytosis is usually present. Chest X-ray reveals a combination any of the following: signs of fluid overload, ground glass opacities, nodules, consolidation and pericardial and pleural effusions. In one series, 11 of 15 patients with the syndrome developed either right-sided or bilateral pleural effusion. The characteristics of the pleural fluid were not reported.

Extreme respiratory manifestations of the syndrome, such as diffuse alveolar hemorrhage or acute respiratory distress syndrome (ARDS), may be fatal. In fact, among 148 patients with acute promyelocytic leukemia who were treated with ATRA, this syndrome was the reported reason of death in nine patients.[48,49] Early administration of high-dose corticosteroid treatment usually leads to prompt symptomatic improvement, while full radiographic recovery may require several days and residual pleural thickening may remain in an occasional patient.[49,50]

CHEMOTHERAPEUTIC AGENTS

The most common respiratory adverse effect caused by cytotoxic agents is interstitial pneumonitis that may present with fever, cough and progressive dyspnea, evolve into ARDS and be fatal.[1,8] Interstitial lung fibrosis, pleural effusion and pleural fibrosis may occur. Drug withdrawal and corticosteroids usually lead to resolution of the symptoms, although the radiographic clearance may be only partial. Pneumothorax has been rarely reported in patients with lung metastases treated with combination chemotherapy regimens.[14,51] The extent to which the drugs contribute in this complication is not defined. It is possible that the administration of the chemotherapeutic agent leads to the necrosis of a pleural metastases and a communication between the alveolus and the pleural space.

Methotrexate

The best known respiratory complication of methotrexate treatment is life-threatening pneumonitis, which occurs in patients who are taking long-term therapy for rheumatoid arthritis or other autoimmune diseases.[8,52] Lung histology reveals non-specific inflammatory findings. Pleural disease has not been reported in association with interstitial pneumonia. Two groups reported pleural disease associated with methotrexate in patients with malignancies who received high dose courses of methotrexate. Walden and co-workers[53] reported that 14 of 317 patients (4.5 percent) with trophoblastic tumors who had been treated with methotrexate developed pleuritic chest pain 2–5 days after the injection. Pleural effusions were found in four. Pleural disease was also reported in 18 of 210 patients (8.5 percent) who were treated for osteogenic sarcoma with weekly courses of methotrexate.[54] Most of the patients presented with severe pleuritic chest pain of sudden onset after the third or fourth course of the treatment. Chest X-ray revealed thickening of the interlobar pleura. There is no report of pleural effusion. The pain resolved after 3–5 days but the pleural thickening persisted, sometimes even for years.

Procarbazine

Procarbazine has been used in the treatment of Hodgkin's disease and lymphomas. Two case reports have described a hypersensitivity-like reaction related to procarbazine administration which is quite similar to the 'acute syndrome' caused by the nitrofurantoin. This reaction includes chills, cough, dyspnea, bilateral pulmonary infiltrates with pleural effusions and blood eosinophilia.[55,56] Pleural biopsy discloses eosinophilic infiltration. Rechallenge with procarbazine produced the same syndrome. When the drug was discontinued, the patients' symptoms and radiographic abnormalities resolved within days.[57,58]

Bleomycin

Bleomycin is a cytotoxic antibiotic that is used in the treatment of a variety of malignancies. Adverse pleuropulmonary effects occur in up to 10 percent of the patients treated with the drug and may be more common in older patients and in those receiving higher cumulative doses.[1] These include severe interstitial pneumonitis and fibrosis. Pleural effusions have been demonstrated in a small number of patients with acute pneumonitis.[1,8] Tissue damage associated with bleomycin appears to be induced by oxidant radicals. For this reason, the risk of respiratory complications increases when radiation or supplemental oxygen are administered.[2]

Mitomycin

Mitomycin is another antibiotic derived agent, often used in the treatment of adenocarcinomas. Mitomycin infrequently induces bilateral interstitial pneumonitis that can be life threatening.[1,8] Small pleural effusions or pleural thickening frequently coexist.[8,55]

Cyclophosphamide

Cyclophosphamide can cause interstitial pneumonitis and fibrosis that can be manifested years after exposure to the drug.[8] There is one report of an unusual acute pleural reaction in a patient with chronic myelogenic leukemia who received high-dose cyclophosphamide prior to bone transplantation.[56] Two days after the course, the patient developed painful, massive bilateral transudative effusions in the absence of heart dysfunction. After bilateral drainage, the effusions did not recur.

Docetaxel

It has been reported that patients may develop exudative pleural effusions of apparently indeterminate etiology after an average time of approximately 5 months from the first docetaxel administration.[2] The effusion gradually resolved over a period of several weeks after the end of the therapy.

Imatinib mesylate

Imatinib mesylate is a novel anti-neoplastic agent, most frequently used in the treatment of chronic myeloid leukemia and Philadelphia chromosome-positive acute lymphoblastic leukemia. Pleural effusions associated with the drug were initially reported in three pediatric patients but the authors did not clearly prove that the effusions should be attributed to the drug and not to the disease progression.[59] Unilateral or bilateral pleural effusions with or without associated pericardial effusions were subsequently reported in four adults with hematological malignancies 2 days to 54 weeks after the drug was first administered.[60,61] Edema and gain of body weight has been described in one patient.[60] The pathogenesis of the effusions in these patients is unknown though fluid retention has been proposed as a possible mechanism. The pleural fluid was characterized as an 'exudate' although in one case its characteristics were not described.[60] Interestingly, while the effusions resolved after the discontinuation of the drug with or without corticosteroids, when treatment with imatinib was restarted they relapsed in only one of seven patients.

MUSCLE RELAXANTS

Dantrolene sodium

Dantrolene sodium is a skeletal muscle relaxant with a chemical structure similar to that of nitrofurantoin.[62,63] Eosinophilic pleural effusion occurring 2 months to 12 years after the initiation of dantrolene[8,62–65] has been reported in patients treated with dantrolene for neurological disorders. The patients often experience fever and/or pleuritic chest pain but may also be asymptomatic.[14,63] The pleural effusions are always unilateral and peripheral blood eosinophilia (eosinophils ≥5 percent) is always present.[62] Pericarditis or pericardial effusion may coexist.[62] Parenchymal disease was not observed in any of the reported patients.

The pleural fluid is an exudate with more than 35 percent eosinophils.[62–65] When dantrolene is discontinued, the patients improve symptomatically within days, but it may take several months for the pleural effusions to resolve completely. Corticosteroid treatment may lead to rapid resolution of pleural effusion.

Tizanidine

Moufarrege and associates[66] reported on a patient who developed a right-sided pleural effusion that was incidentally found in a spinal computed tomography (CT), 3 months after the initiation of tizanidine was prescribed for persistent post-traumatic muscle and bone pain.[66] The fluid was an exhudate with 10 percent eosinophils. Other common etiologies were ruled out and the effusion disappeared over the first month after the discontinuation of the drug.

VITAMINS

A case of life-threatening eosinophilic pleural and pericardial effusion has been reported in a 76-year-old woman taking vitamins B_6 and H for alopecia.[67] The patient presented with chest pain and dyspnea, attributed to cardiac temponade and pleural effusion. Peripheral blood eosinophilia was detected. The pleural effusion relapsed despite pericardiotomy and serial thoracenteses. Infectious, allergic, autoimmune and malignant diseases were appropriately ruled out. Histological examination of both the pleura and the pericardium revealed eosinophilic infiltrate. Symptoms and eosinophilia resolved 1 week after the withdrawal of the vitamins and the patient was symptom-free at a 2-year follow-up visit.

ANTICOAGULANTS

Eosinophilic pleural effusion has been reported in a patient who presented with a dry cough and low-grade fever, 9 months after the initiation of warfarin treatment.[68] A right-sided exudative pleural effusion with 57 percent eosinophils, as well as blood eosinophilia, was found. No other etiologies for the syndrome were determined after extensive evaluation. The blood eosinophilia declined after the discontinuation of the drug. When warfarin was administered again, a left-sided pleural effusion appeared and the peripheral eosinophilia increased. Both the peripheral eosinophilia and the pleural effusions gradually resolved, after the final withdrawal of the drug.

Hemothorax can rarely happen in patients receiving anticoagulants or intrapleural fibrinolytics.[14,69] Most commonly (9 of 12 reported cases), hemothorax occur in patients being treated for pulmonary infarction. In all of those cases, the anticoagulant used was heparin and the complication occurred within the first week of the therapy.[14] In another patient who was treated with heparin, the bleeding source was pneumonia. The remaining two cases were taking warfarin and the hemothorax occurred contralaterally to the pulmonary embolus. Importantly, in the majority of the reported cases, the prothrombin time (PT) and partial thromboplastin time (PTT) were within 'safe' ranges.

MESALAMINE

Mesalamine, an anti-inflammatory drug used in the treatment of inflammatory bowel disease, has been associated with the development of pulmonary infiltrates with or without pleural effusion.[70] There is a case report of a 72-year-old woman who presented with cough, pleuritic chest pain, pink sputum, dyspnea and fever 2 months after mesalamine was first administered. She had bilateral pleural effusions and a pulmonary infiltrate. The effusion was said to be a 'transudate' but the characteristics of the fluid were not reported. The disease did not respond to empirical treatment and the symptoms finally resolved only after mesalamine discontinuation. Subsequently, Trisolini *et al.*[71] reported a patient with an eosinophilic pleural effusion associated with mesalamine treatment. There is also another case report of a patient who developed a pleuropericarditis 7 months after starting treatment with the drug.[72] The serological findings were thought to be suggestive of a lupus-like reaction and the syndrome remitted after the discontinuation of the drug.

CLOZAPINE

Clozapine, a commonly used antipsychotic agent, has been associated with the development of pleural effusions.[73–77] The pleural effusions develop within 7 days to 2 months of initial administration of the drug and are usually, but not always,[74] bilateral. Pericardial effusion[73,77] and even constrictive pericarditis[77] may accompany the pleural effusions. Pleuritic chest pain, fever, headache, skin rash or peripheral eosinophilia have also been observed in some of these patients. In one patient, the pleural effusions were part of a more generalized syndrome consisting of hepatitis, hyperglycemia and glomerular injury.[75] Pleural fluid analysis, reported in only one case, revealed a neutrophil predominant exudate.[73] Symptoms and radiographic abnormalities resolve within several days after the drug is discontinued. When two of the above patients underwent rechallenge, the symptoms and the effusions recurred.[73,74]

ANTIDIABETIC AGENTS

Gliclazide

A 52-year-old diabetic patient was reported, who developed a mild pneumonitis accompanied by an exudative eosinophilic (pleural fluid eosinophils were 80 percent) ipsilateral pleural effusion, accompanied by peripheral blood eosinophilia 2 weeks after beginning therapy with gliclazide, an oral hypoglycemic agent. The peripheral blood eosinophil count was 20 percent. The effusion and the blood eosinophilia resolved over the first month after the withdrawal of gliclazide.[78]

Troglitazone

A 47-year old man presented with cough and dyspnea 1 week after the first dose of troglitazone.[79] Small bilateral pleural effusions were evident 2 weeks later. The symptoms resolved within 24 hours after the discontinuation of the drug and no pleural fluid was found in a chest X-ray obtained 6 days later.

DRUG-INDUCED LUPUS PLEURITIS

With 15 000–20 000 new patients every year in the USA, drug-induced lupus (DIL) pleuritis is the most common cause of drug-associated pleural effusion.[8] While more than 80 drugs have been associated with the syndrome, definite evidence exists for a minority of them including procainamide, hydralazine, isoniazide, methyldopa, chlorpromazine, D-penicillamine and quinidine.[2,80] DIL differs from the idiopathic SLE in that: (i) it is reversible after drug withdrawal; (ii) it has a milder clinical course, with predominant arthralgias, myalgias, rash and serositis and infrequent renal and central nervous system involvement; (iii) it shows no sex predominance.

Pleural effusions, typically bilateral, are the most common radiographic abnormality. Pericardial effusions and, rarely, patchy infiltrates of acute onset may be seen. The patients with DIL pleuritis are usually symptomatic with fever and pleuritic chest pain.[1] Arthralgias and myalgias are very common.[8] The pleural fluid is exudate, with varying nucleated cell counts. The pleural fluid:serum ANA ratio may be ≥1. The presence of LE cells in the pleural fluid, although unusual, strongly suggests the diagnosis. The erythrocyte sedimentation rate and serum ANA titers are elevated. Among ANA, the anti-double-stranded DNA antibodies are very seldom detected while the anti-histone antibodies are suggestive, though not specific, for DIL.[2,14] Drug withdrawal typically leads to rapid patient improvement. However, non-steroid anti-inflammatory drugs or a short course of low-dose prednisolone may be beneficial when a patient is markedly symptomatic. A drug that is known to cause DIL pleuritis should never been given to a patient with SLE is because there is significant risk of aggravation of the symptoms.[1]

Procainamide

Approximately one-third of the patients taking the drug will develop DIL pleuritis within the first year of the therapy, although the disorder can appear anytime between the first month and the twelfth year of beginning treatment.[8] Pleural involvement occurs in more than half, while patchy parenchymal infiltrates may be seen in 40 percent of patients.[81]

Hydralazine

Although half of the patients taking hydralazine have positive ANA, only 2–20 percent, most commonly women, will develop DIL.[1,8] Pleural disease affects 30 percent of them, while parenchymal infiltrates are the sole respiratory manifestation in 5 percent. Arthralgias are the rule (85 percent) and fever is not uncommon (>40 percent), while renal disease may be more common compared with DIL caused by other agents.

Isoniazid

Isoniazid (INH) may induce ANA in one-quarter of the patients who take the drug, but INH-associated DIL is very rare.[82–84] However, an increase in the size of a tuberculous effusion or the development of a new pleural effusion 3–12 weeks after the initiation of anti-tuberculous treatment for pulmonary or pleural tuberculosis could be due to a poorly defined 'paradoxical response'.[84–90] It is speculated that this phenomenon represents an excessive response of the cell-mediated immunity to an increased antigen load resulting from the mycobacterial lysis. Gupta *et al.*[85] reported that pleural fluid was smear-positive in two, and culture positive in four of the 29 of patients who developed this 'paradoxical response'.[85] Pleural biopsy was negative for mycobacteria or tuberculous histology in 15 of the 20 biopsies carried out. The majority of these patients (83 percent), as well as all of the patients reported by others,[86–90] recovered without any modification in chemotherapy.[84] Hiroaka *et al.*[84] reported two patients who developed pleural effusion during anti-tuberculous treatment for pulmonary tuberculosis.[84] In both, the fluid was a lymphocytic exudate with normal glucose, high ANA titer, low CH50 and low ADA, thus resembling lupus effusion. The first patient had progressive rash and the INH was replaced with pyrazinamide. The INH-containing regimen was continued in the second patient. Pleural effusion disappeared in both. These two cases raise a question about the relationship of what is thought to be a 'paradoxical response' to anti-tuberculous treatment and INH-induced lupus pleuritis. Speaking practically, when should the clinician continue or withdraw INH, in the face of newly formed pleural effusion? The presence of pericarditis or generalized symptoms, such as rash and arthralgias, as well as positive serum ANA, makes the DIL pleuritis more likely. Furthermore, bilateral effusions are more likely due to DIL, while all the 43 pleural effusions, previously reported as the result of 'paradoxical response' were unilateral.[84–90] High pleural fluid ADA or the presence of granuloma in the pleural biopsy suggest a tuberculous origin. Pleural fluid ANA titers are not particularly useful, because 25 percent of the patients that take INH have elevated ANA[8] and pleural fluid ANA usually reflects the serum titers.[45] However, a negative serum ANA virtually rules out DIL. If DIL-associated symptoms are present, the INH should be changed to another effective drug. If DIL pleuritis is not clinically probable, the regimen should be continued and if the effusion is symptomatic, a therapeutic aspiration should be performed. If the effusions tend to relapse, a low dose, short-term course of corticosteroids usually hastens its resolution.[84]

OTHER DRUGS

Simvastatin

Simvastatin is an HMG-CoA reductase blocker used in the treatment of hypercholesterolemia. There is one case report of a patient who developed cough, progressive dyspnea and fatigue 6 months after the initiation of the therapy. Chest X-ray disclosed bilateral interstitial infiltrates and a moderate sized right-sided pleural effusion. Elevated liver function tests and serum IgE were detected. BAL revealed eosinophilia of 34 percent. The pleural fluid was described as darkish brown but analysis was not performed. Thoracoscopic biopsies revealed interstitial lung fibrosis and no pleural abnormalities. The discontinuation of simvastatin and prednisone administration led to clinical improvement, normalization of the liver tests and fall of the BAL eosinophil count.[91] Roncato-Saberan *et al.*[92] reported on a patient who presented with large bilateral pleural effusions and weight loss while being on simvastatin treatment for 13 years. He had peripheral and pleural fluid eosinophilia. The pleural effusions resolved and the patient regained weight within a month of the discontinuation of simvastatin with no relapse during a 2-year long follow-up period. In addition to the above, simvastatin has been reported to cause drug-induced lupus syndrome.[93,94]

L-Tryptophan

L-Tryptophan has been used as sleep-promoting drug. This drug is considered as the causal factor of vasculitis, which is clinically expressed as eosinophilia–myalgia syndrome.[8] The patients present with blood eosinophilia, myalgias and fatigue, progressive dyspnea and cough. The chest radiographs demonstrate bilateral interstitial/alveolar infiltrates and pleural effusions.[95] However, pleural fluid characteristics have not been reported. Drug withdrawal and corticosteroid administration were followed by clinical and radiographic resolution.

Acyclovir

Acyclovir is commonly used in the treatment of herpes virus disease. There is only one report of pleuropulmonary disease attributed to this drug.[96] A 71-year-old man who was being treated with acyclovir for ophthalmic herpes zoster developed fever and bilateral pulmonary infiltrates, 3 days after the initiation of the treatment. The next day he presented with a left-sided pleural effusion and hemoptysis. A ventilation-perfusion lung scan was 'not indicative' of pulmonary embolism and microbiological examination of BAL did not reveal any infective agent. Although one can notice that the hemoptysis suggests the presence of an underlying lung disease and that the results of the BAL and the lung scan do not completely rule out pulmonary embolism or pneumonia, the authors reported that acyclovir discontinuation was followed by fever remission. The pleural effusion and the pulmonary infiltrates resolved within 10 days of the drug withdrawal.

Metronidazole

There is one report[97] of a 42-year-old atopic woman who developed fever, skin rash and bilateral pneumonitis and pleural effusions within a day of starting of oral metronidazole. The drug was discontinued and she recovered completely over the next few days. Six months later, she developed a similar syndrome, without pneumonitis, with the first dose of metronidazole. Drug withdrawal again led to rapid improvement of the symptoms and complete recovery.

Valproic acid

Valproic acid, an antiepileptic drug, may cause pleural effusion. There is a report of a patient who developed exudative pleural effusion 9 months after the first administration of the drug.[98] The pleural fluid and the blood eosinophil percentages were 62 and 26 percent, respectively. The fluid gradually disappeared within several days after the withdrawal of valproic and did not recur during a 6-month follow-up period. However, the fact that the pleural fluid appeared a week after the onset of ipsilateral pneumonia makes it possible that it was really a post-pneumonia pleural effusion. Subsequently, eosinophilic pleural effusion and peripheral eosinophilia that resolved after valproic withdrawal was reported in another patient. More importantly, re-challenge with valproic acid produced recurrent symptoms.[99] Another patient who was taking valproic acid[100] developed a febrile lymphocyte predominant exudative pleural effusion. Microbiology studies, chest CT angiography and abdominal CT were normal and thoracoscopic biopsy revealed non-specific pleural inflammation. The effusion disappeared when valproic acid was substituted by another anticonvulsant. The authors did not state how long the patient had been in valproic acid treatment before the onset of pleuritis. More recently, Savvas and associates[101] attributed an episode of bilateral febrile eosinophilic pleural effusions that developed 20 days after cardiac surgery to the valproic acid that was administered because of seizures in the early postoperative period. However, other etiologies, including a post-traumatic pleural effusion and Dressler syndrome, were not considered in this case. Interestingly, the disease persisted after the discontinuation of the valproic acid and resolved only with systemic corticosteroids.

Dapsone

Dapsone causes a hypersensitivity reaction known as sulfone syndrome, consisting of fever, malaise, acute hepatitis, exfoliative dermatitis and hemolytic anemia.[102] Symptoms typically appear within 2–6 weeks after the institution of dapsone therapy. There is one report where a patient had a large unilateral exudative pleural effusion.[102]

D-Penicillamine

There is only one case report of a woman who developed an unexplained massive left-sided pleural effusion two years after D-penicillamine treatment was initiated for Wilson's disease.[103] Video-assisted thoracoscopic surgery (VATS) revealed white plaques over the parietal and visceral pleura, and the lung was encased within a thickened cortex. Talc pleurodesis was unsuccessful. Eventually, she underwent decortication and histology revealed changes of chronic non-specific inflammation. The drug was continued without further sequelae.

Propylthiouracil

There is an isolated case report of a man who developed pleuritic chest pain and an eosinophilic pleural effusion 3 weeks after starting propylthiouracil for treatment of Graves' disease.[104] Fluid analysis five weeks after starting therapy revealed 16 percent of eosinophils. As the treatment with propylthiouracil continued for two more weeks, the effusion enlarged and the eosinophils increased to 45 percent. Pleural biopsy revealed chronic inflammation with pronounced eosinophilia. The effusion resolved 3 months after drug withdrawal.

Itraconazole

Itraconazole is used in the treatment of systematic mycoses. A single patient was reported who may have developed itraconazole-associated exudative pleural and pericardial effusion, 2 months after the initiation of itraconazole treatment.[105]

Minocycline

Bando and associates[106] reported on a man who presented with bilateral interstitial eosinophilic pneumonitis, hilar adenopathy and pleural effusions (pleural fluid neutrophils 95 percent) 5 days after treatment with intravenous minocycline. The syndrome resolved with systemic corticosteroids but symptoms rapidly recurred when a provocation test with minocycline was attempted.

DIRECTION OF DEVELOPMENT

As new drugs will be continuously released in the market and some of the currently used ones will be administered to more patients, additional clinical observations concerning drug-induced pleural disease should be expected. Future reports should incorporate a thorough diagnostic work-up that convincingly rules out all the alternative etiologies, before the disease is attributed to the suspected drug. Future studies will also need to elucidate the pathogenesis of the drug-induced pleural abnormalities. Given the small number of the patients with these abnormalities, animal studies will be particularly useful in addressing this issue. Finally, even though drug withdrawal is a convenient treatment option for the majority of the patients, it may not be sufficient in the settings of a life-threatening drug-induced syndrome. Moreover, drug discontinuation is not desirable for some medications that are uniquely active against serious diseases. For these reasons, even given the relative scarcity of patients for the conduction of randomized-controlled studies, the role of the anti-inflammatory treatment, i.e. corticosteroids, should be further examined and new treatment modalities may need to be developed.

KEY POINTS

- A variety of widely used drugs, including anti-infectious, cardiovascular, cytotoxic, neuropsychiatric, anti-inflammatory and immunomodulating agents, may cause pleural disease.
- Drug-induced pleural disease should be considered in every patient with an undiagnosed pleural effusion or unexplained pleural fibrosis.
- Drug-induced pleural disease may be the sole manifestation of a drug toxicity or may coexist with pulmonary toxicity or even be part of generalized syndromes.
- The discontinuation of the drug leads to resolution of the pleural disease in the vast majority of the cases.

REFERENCES

● = Key primary paper
◆ = Major review article

◆1. Beck MJ. Drug-induced pleural disease. *Clin Chest Med* 1998; **19**: 341–50.

◆2. Huggins JT, Sahn SA. Drug-induced pleural disease. *Clin Chest Med* 2004; **25**:141–53.

3. Israel HL, Diamond P. Recurrent pulmonary infiltration and pleural effusion due to nitrofurantoin sensitivity. *N Engl J Med* 1962; **266**:1024–6.

4. Rosenow EC III. Drug-induced bronchopulmonary pleural disease. *J Allergy Clin Immunol* 1987; **80**: 780–7.
5. Cooper JA, White DA, Matthay RA. Drug-induced pulmonary disease. *Am Rev Respir Dis* 1986; **133**: 488–505.
●6. Holmberg L, Boman G. Pulmonary reactions to nitrofurantoin: 447 cases reported to the Swedish adverse drug reaction committee, 1966–1976. *Eur J Respir Dis* 1981; **62**: 180–9.
7. Geller M, Flaherty DK, Dickie HA, Reed CE. Lymphopenia in acute nitrofurantoin pleuropulmonary reactions. *J Allergy Clin Immunol* 1977; **59**: 445–8.
◆8. Morelock SY, Sahn SA. Drugs and the pleura. *Chest* 1999; **116**: 212–21.
9. Martin WJ II, Rosenow EC III. Amiodarone pulmonary toxicity. *Chest* 1988; **93**: 1067–74.
10. Pollak PT. Clinical organ toxicity of antiarrhythmic compounds: ocular and pulmonary manifestations. *Am J Cardiol* 1999 **84**: 37R–45R.
11. Gonzalez-Rothi RJ, Hannan SE, Hood I, Franzini DA. Amiodarone pulmonary toxicity presenting as bilateral exudative pleural effusions. *Chest* 1987; **92**: 179–82.
12. Stein B, Zaatari GS, Pine JR. Amiodarone pulmonary toxicity. Clinical, cytologic and ultrastructural findings. *Acta Cytol* 1987; **31**: 357–61.
13. Akoun GM, Cadranel JL, Blanchette G, Milleron BJ, Mayaud CM. Pleural T-lymphocyte subsets in amiodarone-associated pleuropneumonitis. *Chest* 1989; **95**: 596–7.
◆14. Miller WT. Pleural and mediastinal disorders related to drug use. *Semin Roentgenol* 1995; **30**: 35–48.
15. Page RL. Progressive pleural thickening during oxprenolol therapy. *Br J Dis Chest* 1979; **73**: 195–9.
16. Webb DB, Whale RJ. Pleuropericardial effusion associated with minoxidil administration. *Postgrad Med J* 1982; **58**: 319–20.
17. Yoshida H, Hasegawa R, Hayashi H, Irie Y. Imidapril-induced eosinophilic pleurisy. Case report and review of the literature. *Respiration* 2005; **72**: 423–6.
18. Vogelzang PJ, Bloom SM, Mier JW, Atkins MB: Chest roentgenographic abnormalities in IL-2 recipients. Incidence and correlation with clinical parameters. *Chest* 1992; **101**: 746–52.
●19. Saxon RR, Klein JR, Bar MH, *et al.* Pathogenesis of pulmonary edema during interleukin-2 therapy: correlation of chest radiographic and clinical findings in 54 patients. *AJR Am J Roentgenol* 1991; **156**: 281–5.
20. Berthianume Y, Boiteau P, Fick G, *et al.* Pulmonary edema during IL-2 therapy: Combined effect of increased permeability and hydrostatic pressure. *Am J Respir Crit Care Med* 1995; **152**: 329–35.
21. Smith JW. Tolerability and side-effect profile of rhIL-11. *Oncology (Williston Park)* 2000; **14**: 41s–7s.
22. Takeda A, Ikegame K, Kimura Y, *et al.* Pleural effusion during interferon treatment for chronic hepatitis C. *Hepatogastroenterology* 2000; **47**: 1431–5.
23. Isaacs C, Robert NJ, Bailey FA, *et al.* Randomized placebo-controlled study of recombinant human interleukin-11 to prevent chemotherapy-induced thrombocytopenia in patients with breast cancer receiving dose-intensive cyclophosphamide and doxorubicin. *J Clin Oncol* 1997; **15**: 3368–77.
24. Busmanis IA, Beaty AE, Basser RL. Isolated pleural effusion with hematopoietic cells of mixed lineage in a patient receiving granulocyte-colony-stimulating factor after high-dose chemotherapy. *Diagn Cytopathol* 1998; **18**: 204–7.
25. Nakamura M, Sakemi T, Fujisaki T, *et al.* Sudden death or refractory pleural effusion following treatment with granulocyte colony-stimulating factor in two hemodialysis patients. *Nephron* 1999; **83**: 178–9.
26. de Azevedo AM, Goldberg Tabak D. Life-threatening capillary leak syndrome after G-CSF mobilization and collection of peripheral blood progenitor cells for allogeneic transplantation. *Bone Marrow Transplant* 2001; **28**: 311–2.
27. Bolanos-Meade J, Keng YK, Cobos E. Recurrent lymphocytic pleural effusion after intravenous immunoglobulin. *Am J Hematol* 1999; **60**: 248–9.
●28. Graham JR, Suby HI, LeCompte PR, Sadowski NL. Fibrotic disorders associated with methysergide therapy for headache. *N Engl J Med* 1966; **274**: 350–68.
29. Kok-Jensen A, Lindeneg O. Pleurisy and fibrosis of the pleura during methysergide treatment of hemicrania. *Scand J Respir Dis* 1970; **51**: 218–222.
30. Hindle W, Posner E, Sweetnam MT, Tan RS. Pleural effusion and fibrosis during treatment with methysergide. *Br Med J* 1970; **1**: 605–6.
●31. Rinne UK. Pleuropulmonary changes during long-term bromocriptine treatment for Parkinson's disease. *Lancet* 1981; **i**: 44.
32. McElvaney NG, Wilcox PG, Churg A, Fleetham JA. Pleuropulmonary disease during bromocriptine treatment of Parkinson's disease. *Arch Intern Med* 1988; **148**: 2231–6.
33. Bhatt MH, Keenan SP, Fleetham JA, Calne DB. Pleuropulmonary disease associated with dopamine agonist therapy. *Ann Neurol* 1991; **30**: 613–16.
34. Frans E, Dom R, Demedts M. Pleuropulmonary changes during treatment of Parkinson's disease with a long-acting ergot derivative, cabergoline. *Eur Respir J* 1992; **5**: 263–5.
35. Ling LH, Ahlskog JE, Munger TM, Limper AH, Oh JK. Constrictive pericarditis and pleuropulmonary disease linked to ergot dopamine agonist therapy (cabergoline) for Parkinson's disease. *Mayo Clin Proc* 1999; **74**: 371–5.
36. De Vuyst P, Pfitzenmeyer P, Camus P. Asbestos, ergot drugs and the pleura. *Eur Respir J* 1997; **10**: 2695–8.
◆37. Pfitzenmeyer P, Foucher P, Dennewald G, *et al.* Pleuropulmonary changes induced by ergoline drugs. *Eur Respir J* 1996; **9**: 1013–19.
38. Oechsner M, Groenke L, Mueller D. Pleural fibrosis associated with dihydroergocryptine treatment. *Acta Neurol Scand* 2000; **101**: 283–5.
39. Graham JR. Cardiac and pulmonary fibrosis during methysergide therapy for headache. *Am J Med Sci* 1967; **254**: 1–12.
40. Shaunak S, Wilkins A, Pilling JB, Dick DJ. Pericardial, retroperitoneal, and pleural fibrosis induced by pergolide. *J Neurol Neurosurg Psychiatry* 1999; **66**: 79–81.
41. Varsano S, Gershman M, Hamaoui E. Pergolide-induced dyspnea, bilateral pleural effusion and peripheral edema. *Respiration* 2000; **67**: 580–2.
42. Knoop C, Mairesse M, Lenclud C, Gevenois PA, De Vuyst P. Pleural effusion during bromocriptine exposure in two patients with pre-existing asbestos pleural plaques: a relationship? *Eur Respir J* 1997; **10**: 2898–901.
43. Kinnunen E, Viljanen A. Pleuropulmonary involvement during bromocriptine treatment. *Chest* 1988; **94**: 1034–6.
44. Mohan K, Owen S, McCallum S, Magennis R. A patient with tremors and breathlessness. *Prim Care Respir J* 2005; **14**: 47–50.
◆45. Light RW. *Pleural diseases*, 4th edn. Philadelphia: Lippincott Williams & Wilkins, 2001: 265–70.
46. Bunker CB, Sheron N, Maurice PD, *et al.* Isotretinoin and eosinophilic pleural effusion. *Lancet* 1989; **1**: 435–6.
47. Milleron BJ, Valcke J, Akoun GM, Mayaud CM. Isotretinoin-related eosinophilic pleural effusion. *Chest* 1996; **110**: 1128.
48. Warrell RP Jr, Maslak P, Eardley A, *et al.* Treatment of acute promyelocytic leukemia with all-trans retinoic acid: an update of the New York experience. *Leukemia* 1994; **8**: 929–33.
●49. Jung JI, Choi JE, Hahn ST, *et al.* Radiologic features of all-*trans*-retinoic acid syndrome. *AJR Am J Roentgenol* 2002; **178**: 475–80.
50. Frankel SR, Eardley A, Lauwers G, Weiss M, Warrell RP Jr. The 'retinoic acid syndrome' in acute promyelocytic leukemia. *Ann Intern Med* 1992; **117**: 292–6.
51. Bini A, Zompatori M, Ansaloni L, *et al.* Bilateral recurrent pneumothorax complicating chemotherapy for pulmonary

metastatic breast ductal carcinoma: report of a case. *Surg Today* 2000; **30**: 469–72.

●52. Imokawa S, Colby TV, Leslie KO, Helmers RA. Methotrexate pneumonitis: review of the literature and histopathological findings in nine patients. *Eur Respir J* 2000; **15**: 373–81.

53. Walden PAM, Mitchell-Heggs PF, Coppin C, *et al.* Pleurisy and methotrexate treatment. *Br Med J* 1977; **2**: 867.

54. Urban C, Nirenberg A, Caparros B, *et al.* Chemical pleuritis as the cause of acute chest pain following high-dose methotrexate treatment. *Cancer* 1983; **51**: 34–7.

55. Gunstream SR, Seidenfield JJ, Sobonya RE, McMahon LJ. Mitomycin-associated lung disease. *Cancer Treat Rep* 1983; **67**: 301–4.

56. Schaap N, Raymakers R, Schattenberg A, *et al.* Massive pleural effusion attributed to high-dose cyclophosphamide during conditioning for MBT. *Bone Marrow Transplant* 1996; **18**: 247–8.

57. Jones SE, Moore M, Blank N, Castellino RA. Hypersensitivity to procarbazine (Matulane) manifested by fever and pleuropulmonary reaction. *Cancer* 1972; **29**: 498–500.

58. Ecker MD, Jay B, Keohane MF. Procarbazine lung. *AJR Am J Roentgenol* 1978; **131**: 527–8.

59. Goldsby R, Pulsipher M, Adams R, *et al.* Unexpected pleural effusions in 3 pediatric patients treated with STI-571. *J Pediatr Hematol Oncol* 2002; **24**: 694–5.

60. Ishii Y, Shoji N, Kimura Y, Ohyashiki K. Prominent pleural effusion possibly due to imatinib mesylate in adult Philadelphia chromosome-positive acute lymphoblastic leukemia. *Intern Med* 2006; **45**: 339–40.

●61. Breccia M, D'Elia GM, D'Andrea M, Latagliata R, Alimena G. Pleural-pericardic effusion as uncommon complication in CML patients treated with Imatinib. *Eur J Haematol* 2005; **74**: 89–90.

●62. Petusevsky ML, Faling J, Rocklin RE, *et al.* Pleuropericardial reaction to treatment with dantrolene. *J Am Med Assoc* 1979; **242**: 2772–4.

63. Mahoney JM, Bachtel MD. Pleural effusion associated with chronic dantrolene administration. *Ann Pharmacother* 1994; **28**: 587–9.

64. Felz MW, Haviland-Foley DJ. Eosinophilic pleural effusion due to dantrolene: resolution with steroid therapy. *South Med J* 2001; **94**: 502–4.

65. Le-Quang B, Camels P, Valayer-Caleat E, Fayolle-Minon I, Gautheron V. Dantrolene and pleural effusion: case report and review of literature. *Spinal Cord* 2004; **42**: 317–20.

66. Moufarrege G, Frank E, Carstens DD. Eosinophilic exudative pleural effusion after initiation of tizanidine treatment: a case report. *Pain Med* 2003; **4**: 85–90.

67. Debourdeau PM, Djezzar S, Estival JL, *et al.* Life-threatening eosinophilic pleuropericardial effusion related to vitamins B5 and H. *Ann Pharmacother* 2001; **35**: 424–6.

68. Kuwahara T, Hamada M, Inoue Y, Aono S, Hiwada K. Warfarin-induced eosinophilic pleurisy. *Intern Med* 1995; **34**: 794–6.

69. Bouros D, Schiza S, Siafakas N. Utility of fibrinolytic agents for draining intrapleural infections. *Semin Respir Infect* 1999; **14**: 39–47.

70. Sesin GP, Mucciardi N, Almeida S. Mesalamine-associated pleural effusion with pulmonary infiltration. *Am J Health Syst Pharm* 1998; **55**: 2304–5.

71. Trisolini R, Dore R, Biagi F, *et al.* Eosinophilic pleural effusion due to mesalamine. Report of a rare occurrence. *Sarcoidosis Vasc Diffuse Lung Dis* 2000; **17**: 288–91.

72. Pent MT, Anapathy S, Holdswotrth CD, *et al.* Mesalamine-induced lupus-like syndrome. *Br Med J* 1992; **305**:159.

73. Daly JM, Godber RJ, Braman SS. Polyserositis associated with clozapine treatment. *Am J Psychiatry* 1992; **149**: 1274–5.

74. Chatterjee A, Saffermaan A. Cellulitis, eosinophilia and unilateral pleural effusion associated with clozapine treatment. *J Clin Psychopharmacol* 1997; **17**: 323–33.

75. Thompson J, Chengappa KN, Good CB, *et al.* Hepatitis, hyperglycemia, pleural effusion, eosinophilia, hematuria and proteinuria occurring early in clozapine treatment. *Int Clin Psychopharmacol* 1998; **13**: 95–8.

76. Stanislav SW, Gonzalez-Blanco M. Papular rash and bilateral pleural effusion associated with clozapine. *Ann Pharmacother* 1999; **33**: 1008–9.

●77. Catalano G, Catalano MC, Frankel Wetter RL. Clozapine induced polyserositis. *Clin Neuropharmacol* 1997; **20**: 352–6.

78. Tzanakis N, Bouros D, Siafakas N. Eosinophilic pleural effusion due to gliclazide. *Respir Med* 2000; **94**: 94.

79. Koshida H, Shibata K, Kametani T. Pleuropulmonary disease in a man with diabetes who was treated with troglitazone. *N Engl J Med* 1998; **339**: 1400–1.

◆80. Yung RL, Richardson BC. Drug-induced lupus. *Rheum Dis Clin North Am* 1994; **20**: 61–85.

81. Cush JJ, Goldings EA. Drug-induced lupus; clinical spectrum and pathogenesis. *Am J Med Sci* 1985; **290**: 36–45.

82. Salazar-Paramo M, Rubin RL, Garcia-De La Torre I. Systemic lupus erythematosus induced by isoniazid. *Ann Rheum Dis* 1992; **51**: 1085–7.

83. Guleria R, Behera D, Jindal SK. Systemic lupus erythematosus during isoniazid therapy. *Indian J Chest Dis Allied Sci* 1990; **32**: 55–8.

●84. Hiraoka K, Nagata N, Kawajiri T, *et al.* Paradoxical pleural response to antituberculous chemotherapy and isoniazid-induced lupus. *Respiration* 1998; **65**:152–5.

85. Gupta RC, Dixit R, Purohit SD, Saxena A. Development of pleural effusion in patients during anti-tuberculous chemotherapy: analysis of twenty-nine cases with review of literature. *Indian J Chest Dis Allied Sci* 2000; **42**: 161–6.

86. Al-Ali MA, Almasri NM. Development of contralateral pleural effusion during chemotherapy for tuberculous pleurisy. *Saudi Med J* 2000; **21**: 574–6.

87. Puri MM, Arora VK. Contralateral pleural effusion during chemotherapy for tuberculous pleural effusion. *Med J Malaysia* 2000; **55**: 382–4.

88. Al-Majed SA.Study of paradoxical response to chemotherapy in tuberculous pleural effusion. *Respir Med* 1996; **90**: 211–14.

89. Vilaseca J, Lopez-Vivancos J, Arnau J, Guardia J. Contralateral pleural effusion during chemotherapy for tuberculous pleurisy. *Tubercle* 1984; **65**: 209–10.

90. Matthay RA, Neff TA, Iseman MD. Tuberculous pleural effusions developing during chemotherapy for pulmonary tuberculosis. *Am Rev Respir Dis* 1974; **109**: 469–72.

91. De Groot RE, Willems LN, Dijkman JH. Interstitial lung disease with pleural effusion caused by simvastin. *J Intern Med* 1996; **239**: 361–3.

92. Roncato-Saberan M, Hustache-Mathieu L, Hoen B. Eosinophilic pleural effusion caused by simvastatin after 13 years of exposure. *Eur J Intern Med* 2006; **17**: 450.

93. Khosla R, Butman A N, Hammer D F. Simvastatin-induced lupus erythematosus. *South Med J* 1998; **91**: 873–4

94. Bannwarth B, Miremont G, Papapietro P-M. Lupuslike syndrome associated with simvastatin. *Arch Intern Med* 1992; **152**: 1093–4.

95. Shore ET. L-tryptophane induced cough and pleural effusions associated with the eosinophelia–myalgia syndrome. *Chest* 1990; **98**: 1540.

96. Pusateri DW, Muder RR. Fever, pulmonary infiltrates and pleural effusion following acyclivir therapy for Herpes zoster opthalmicus. *Chest* 1990; **98**: 754–6.

97. Kristenson M, Fryden A. Pneumonitis caused by metronidazole. *J Am Med Assoc* 1988; **260**: 184.

98. Kaufman J, O'Shaughnessy IM. Eosinophilic pleural effusion associated with valproic acid administration. *South Med J* 1995; **88**: 881–2.

99. Kavetz JD, Federman DG. Valproic acid-induced eosinophilic pleural effusion. *South Med J* 2003; **96**: 803–6.

100. Andre S, Drowart A, De Bels D. Lymphocytic pleural effusion associated with valproic acid. *Eur J Intern Med* 2005; **16**: 535.

101. Savvas SP, Dimopoulou E, Koskinas J. Valproic acid-associated eosinophilic pleural effusion treated with corticosteroids. *Eur J Intern Med* 2006; **17**: 71.
102. Corp CC, Ghishan FK. The sulfone syndrome complicated by pancreatitis and pleural effusion in an adolescent receiving dapsone for treatment of acne vulgaris. *J Pediatr Gastroenterol Nutr* 1998; **26**: 103–5.
103. Karkos C, Moore A, Manche A, Thorpe JA. Pleural effusion associated with D-penicillamine therapy: a case report. *J Clin Pharm Therpeut* 1996; **21**: 15–17.
104. Middleton KL, Santella R, Couser JI. Eosinophilic pleuritis due to propylthiouracil. *Chest* 1993; **103**: 955–6.
105. Gonther J, Lode H, Raffenberg M, *et al.* Development of pleural and pericardial effusions during itraconazole therapy of pulmonary aspergillosis. *Eur J Clin Microbiol Inf Dis* 1993; **12**: 723–4.
106. Bando T, Fujimura M, Noda Y, *et al.* Minocycline-induced pneumonitis with bilateral hilar lymphadenopathy and pleural effusion. *Intern Med* 1994; **33**: 177–9.

34

Effusions after surgery

ONER DIKENSOY, RICHARD W LIGHT

INTRODUCTION

Pleural effusion after surgery can be defined as occurrence of a new pleural effusion following a recent surgical procedure. Although most of the pleural effusions occur within first couple of days following surgery, occurrence of late pleural effusions following coronary artery bypass graft (CABG) surgery has been reported.[1,2]

Most of the early studies concerning post-operative pulmonary complications were carried out in a population undergoing abdominal surgery and reported a very low prevalence of pleural effusions after surgery.[3–5] It is most likely that the low sensitivity of the diagnostic modalities utilized, and small sizes of the pleural effusions without clinical symptoms, were the main reasons for the low frequency of post-operative pleural effusions in these studies. The incidence of post-operative pleural effusions in more recent studies has been as high as 100 percent depending on the diagnostic modality used to detect the pleural effusion and the type of the surgical intervention.[6]

Although, any surgery can cause pleural effusion, abdominal and thoracic interventions such as splenectomy, cholecystectomy and CABG surgery are the most commonly reported surgical operations complicated by pleural effusion in the early post-operative period.[2–5] The causes of pleural effusion after surgery are shown in Table 34.1.

In this chapter, post-operative pleural effusions will be discussed in detail by reviewing the related literature to date.

Table 34.1 Causes of pleural effusion after different types of surgery

Causes
Trauma caused by surgery
Atelectasis
Pancreatitis
Pulmonary embolism
Subphrenic abscess (late >10 days)
Congestive heart failure
Pneumonia
Central line erosion through central venous structures
Chylothorax due to thoracic duct disruption
Hemothorax due to bleeding
Immunological mechanisms

EFFUSIONS AFTER ABDOMINAL SURGERY

Data on post-operative pleural effusions after abdominal surgery are limited. There have been several old series of pleural effusions after abdominal surgery and one recent study of pleural effusions after diaphragm peritonectomy or resection for advanced mullerian cancer.[3,5,7–10]

Incidence

In early reports, the frequency of pleural effusions after abdominal surgery was reported to be very low. Wightman[5] reviewed the pulmonary complications after 455 abdominal operations and found only one pleural effusion. Forthman and Shepard[3] reported no pleural effusions after 447 abdominal operations. Ti and Yong[8] found four pleural effusions after abdominal surgery in 346 patients. In none of these three series were routine post-operative chest roentgenograms obtained; however, Laszlo *et al.*[4] and Collins *et al.*[11] obtained chest X-rays on the second postoperative day after abdominal surgery in 44 and 132 patients, respectively, and neither study mentions the occurrence of pleural effusion.

More recently, two studies prospectively assessed patients undergoing abdominal surgery.[7,9] In the first study by Light *et al.*,[9] at a military hospital, all patients had posteroanterior, left lateral and bilateral decubitus radiographs 48–72 hours after surgery. Pleural effusions were found in 97 (49 percent) patients after abdominal surgery. The incidence of pleural effusions was higher after upper abdominal surgery in patients with postoperative atelectasis, and in patients with free abdominal fluid. Pleural effusions appeared to be more common in older patients. The mean age of patients with pleural effusion (33 years) was higher than the mean age of patients without effusions (27 years). They suggested that this was because older patients were more likely to have atelectasis.

In the second study by Nielsen *et al.*,[7] 128 patients who had undergone upper abdominal surgery were studied prospectively for the incidence of post-operative pleural effusions. Posterior and lateral chest radiographs were obtained preoperatively and on the second and fourth day after surgery. They found that 89 patients (69.5 percent) developed a post-operative pleural effusion: 33 unilateral and 56 bilateral. They concluded that patients with post-operative pleural effusions were older than those without effusion (median ages, 58.7 versus 50.4 years respectively). They found no correlation between the presence of post-operative pleural effusions and any of the following: type of the operation, site of the abdominal incision, gender, smoking habits or weight.

In the most recent study of pleural effusions after diaphragm peritonectomy or resection for advanced mullerian cancer, the records of all patients with stage IIIC–IV epithelial ovarian, fallopian tube or peritoneal cancer who had diaphragm peritonectomy or resection as part of optimal primary cytoreduction at their institution from 2000 to 2003 were reviewed.[10] All patients had preoperative and serial post-operative chest X-rays to detect and follow pleural effusions. Of the 215 patients who had primary cytoreduction during the study period, 59 (27 percent) underwent diaphragm peritonectomy or resection. In addition to standard cytoreduction, 31 (53 percent) of these 59 patients had diaphragm surgery alone, while 28 (47 percent) had diaphragm surgery in combination with other upper abdominal resections. Laterality of diaphragm surgery was as follows: right only, 43 (73 percent); left only, 2 (3 percent); and bilateral, 14 (24 percent). The overall rate of new or increased ipsilateral effusions was 58 percent; the overall rate of post-operative thoracentesis or chest tube placement was 15 percent. In 75 percent of these patients, thoracentesis or chest tubes were placed within 5 days of surgery (median, 3 days; range, 2–24 days).

Etiology

A number of hypothesis have been suggested for the etiology of pleural effusions after abdominal surgery.[7,9,12] Subphrenic abscess has been considered as the major cause of these pleural effusions;[12] however, the relation has been severely questioned by the findings of Light and George in the above-mentioned study.[9] The effusions likely to be associated with subphrenic abscess usually become apparent 10 or more days post-operatively, and are typically associated with signs and symptoms of systemic infection.[13]

In the studies by Light *et al.*[9] and Nielsen *et al.*,[7] similar factors such as pancreatitis, pulmonary emboli and peritoneal fluid were suggested to be occasional causes of pleural effusions after abdominal surgery. However, these two groups shared opposing views on the relative significance of atelectasis, diaphragmatic irritation and site of the incision with respect to the development of post-operative pleural effusions.

In the study by Eisenhauer *et al.*,[10] several hypotheses on the etiology of pleural effusions after diaphragm peritonectomy or resection for advanced mullerian cancer were suggested: (1) the large portion of diaphragm left uncovered by peritoneum after diaphragm peritonectomy or resection; (2) unrecognized disruption of the diaphragmatic muscle or underlying pleura in the process of diaphragm peritonectomy or resection may contribute to small defects that later connect to the pleural space; (3) large-volume ascites are seen in a larger proportion of their patients undergoing diaphragm peritonectomy or resection than are commonly reported in patients undergoing hepatectomy; or (4) the release of vascular endothelial growth factor (VEGF) or inflammatory mediators by resection of tumor or direct surgery on the diaphragm. In summary, one might suggest that multiple local or systemic factors play roles in the formation of pleural effusions after abdominal surgery. A subphrenic abscess should be considered when a pleural effusion develops 10 or more days post-operatively and is associated with signs and symptoms of systemic infection.

Clinical manifestations

Most of the effusions after abdominal surgery are found incidentally due to the fact that they are small in size and asymptomatic. In the study by Light *et al.*[9] the effusions were <4 mm on the decubitus film in 50 patients whereas it was between 4 and 10 mm in 26 patients, and >10 mm in 21 patients. However, a post-operative pleural effusion should be considered in cases that have an unexpected clinical deterioration following surgery. Although not common, large pleural effusions or infected pleural fluid can cause significant clinical symptoms and require interventions such as tube thoracostomy. In a case of acute dyspnea and a minimal pleural effusion, pulmonary embolus should also be considered.

Characteristics of pleural fluid

Only the study by Light *et al.*[9] reported the characteristics of the pleural fluid. They reported that 16 of the effusions were exudates while four were transudates. Transudates were attributed to congestive heart failure in two patients and volume overload in the other two. Pleural fluid cultures were positive for *Staphylococcus aureus* in one patient only.

Management

In most of the cases with pleural effusion following abdominal surgery, the effusion is self-limited and does not require any further intervention.[7,9] If the patient is febrile or has pleuritic chest pain and the size of the pleural effusion is more than minimal, a diagnostic thoracentesis should be performed. Chest tube drainage may be needed in occasional cases with a complicated clinical course, especially if the effusion is large and causes dyspnea or if the pleural infection occurs. Subphrenic abscess, pulmonary embolus, pleural infection and pancreatitis should always be considered in the differential diagnosis when evaluating patients with pleural effusion after abdominal surgery.[14]

EFFUSIONS AFTER CARDIAC SURGERY

Post-operative pleural effusions are common after cardiac surgery.[15,16] Most of these effusions are caused by the surgical procedure itself and follow a benign course. However, pleural effusions may also occur due to post-cardiac injury syndrome (PCIS) or as the initial manifestation of a potentially serious complicating event.

Three common cardiac procedures, CABG surgery, PCIS and heart transplantation, are often complicated by pleural effusions.[16–18]

Coronary artery bypass graft surgery

These effusions after CABG surgery are known as 'post-CABG pleural effusions'. Post-CABG pleural effusions can be categorized into two groups based on time course: 'early' and 'late'.[14] Early effusions are those that occur within 30 days of CABG surgery, and late effusions are those that occur after 30 days. Light *et al.*[16] graded these effusions between 0 and 5 based on the volume of fluid within the pleural space (Table 34.2).

Table 34.2 Quantification of size of pleural effusions after post-coronary artery bypass graft surgery

Grade of effusion	Characteristic of chest radiograph
0	No pleural fluid
1	Blunting of costophrenic angle
2	More than blunting of costophrenic angle but less than 25% of hemithorax occupied by pleural fluid
3	Pleural fluid occupying 25–50% of hemithorax
4	Pleural fluid occupying 50–75% of hemithorax
5	Pleural fluid occupying more than 75% of hemithorax

INCIDENCE

Pleural effusions are common after CABG surgery. The reported incidence ranges from 40 to 90 percent, depending on the diagnostic modality used to detect the presence of effusion.[15,19–22]

Early pleural effusions after CABG surgery are more common than late effusions.[21] Such effusions tend to occur on the left side of hemithorax. Vargas *et al.*[21] investigated the prevalence of pleural effusions in 47 patients who had undergone CABG surgery by performing ultrasonic examinations of the chest at 7, 14 and 30 days postoperatively. The prevalence of pleural effusion was 89 percent at 7 days, 77 percent at 14 days, and 57 percent at 30 days in this study.[21] They reported that most of the effusions were asymptomatic. However, in some patients the effusion enlarged and produced symptoms. A second study by Landymore and Howell[19] reported that at the time of discharge from the hospital, the prevalence of left-sided pleural effusion was 91 percent in 34 patients who had received an internal mammary artery (IMA) graft and had the pleura opened, whereas the prevalence of left-sided pleural effusion was 58 percent in 33 patients who had received an IMA graft but in whom the pleura was not opened.

A prospective study of late effusions noted that 63 percent of patients had a pleural effusion at 30 days after CABG surgery.[23] In contrast to early effusions, late effusion can be large, and 10 percent of the patients in the series described above had an effusion that occupied more than 25 percent of a hemithorax.[23] In another study,

Hurlbut *et al.*[20] obtained chest radiographs 8 weeks post-operatively on 76 patients who had received IMA grafts, and reported that five (9.1 percent) of 55 patients who underwent pleurotomy and three (14.5 percent) of 21 patients who had an IMA without pleurotomy had a pleural effusion. In a recent retrospective study of 410 patients who had undergone CABG surgery, the incidence of patients diagnosed with symptomatic newly developed large pleural effusions from 30 days to 6 months post-CABG was 3.1 percent.[24]

ETIOLOGY

Several potential causative factors have been suggested for early and late effusions, but their relative roles and importance have not been completely defined. The early effusions are usually bloody, with a median hematocrit above 5 percent.[25] The most likely underlying mechanism for these bloody effusions is trauma from the surgery and post-operative bleeding into the pleural space.[25]

Topical cardiac cooling with ice is another potential pathogenetic factor for early effusions.[2,26] In one retrospective study, pleural effusions occurred in 50 percent of patients who underwent topical cardiac cooling with ice but in only 14 and 18 percent of patients who received topical cold saline or no topical cardioplegia, respectively.[27] Similar results were reported in a different study of 191 patients.[26] The reason why iced slush is associated with an increased prevalence of pleural effusions is not known, but it has been speculated cold injury to the phrenic nerve may cause atelectasis which leads to development of pleural effusions.[28]

In contrast to the early effusions, late effusions tend to be serous in appearance with a predominance of lymphocytes in the pleural fluid.[1] Kim *et al.*[29] suggested that these late effusions might be a manifestation of the PCIS. However, the two main clinical manifestations of PCIS are chest pain and fever,[30] and both of these symptoms are uncommon in patients with pleural effusions more than 30 days after CABG surgery.[1]

Lymphocytic predominance with evidence of lymphocytic pleuritis found in the late effusions after CABG surgery suggests an immunological mechanism.[28] When immunohistochemical analysis is performed on the lymphocytes in the pleural specimens, there is a mixed population of lymphocytes with a predominance of B cells.[1] However, an autoimmune etiology has not yet been demonstrated.

It is not clear whether the type of the graft or pleurotomy contributes to the development of late pleural effusions after CABG surgery.[14] Pleurotomy is frequently performed in patients undergoing placement of an IMA coronary artery graft, and late pleural effusions have been suggested to be more common after IMA–CABG operations compared with those who had saphenous vein (SV) grafts alone.[19–21,31] In the study by Peng and colleagues,[15] 51 out of 122 patients developed pleural effusion after CABG surgery. The incidence of pleural effusion in the SV only group was 23/54 (43 percent) while the incidence in the IMA group was 28/68 (41 percent). The difference between the two groups was not statistically significant. Landymore and Howell[19] investigated the role of pleurotomy in 106 patients, including 34 patients that underwent IMA grafting with pleurotomy and 33 without pleurotomy. They included 39 patients undergoing valve replacement or revascularization with SV graft as controls. The patients were followed by chest X-rays that were performed prior to discharge and at 3 months post-operatively. The incidence of pleural effusion prior to discharge was 91 percent (31 out of 34) in the patients that had IMA grafting with pleurotomy, 58 percent (19 out of 33) in the patients that had IMA grafting without pleurotomy and 31 percent (12 out of 39) in the control patients. They concluded that pleurotomy has a role in the formation of pleural effusions after surgery and that the IMA should be exposed without pleurotomy.

Opening of the pericardium during surgery does not appear to be primarily responsible for the effusion because patients who have valve replacement have a lower prevalence of effusion than do patients who undergo CABG surgery.[7]

Patients who undergo CABG surgery off-pump (without cardiopulmonary bypass) (OP-CABG) have been reported to have a lower prevalence of large pleural effusion 4 weeks post-operatively than do those who undergo CABG surgery with cardiopulmonary bypass.[32] In the series by Mohamed *et al.*,[32] the prevalence of effusions at 30 days post-operatively that occupied more than 25 percent of the hemithorax was only 3 percent in the OP-CABG patients but was 10 percent in the CABG patients undergoing cardiopulmonary bypass. It is not clear whether the decreased prevalence of larger pleural effusion with OP-CABG surgery is caused by less trauma, omission of the iced slush hypothermia or omission of cardiopulmonary bypass, which is known to be associated with the systemic release of inflammatory mediators.[33]

CLINICAL MANIFESTATIONS

Small, usually left-sided, pleural effusions that typically encompass a radiographic area smaller than two intercostal spaces are common in the early post-operative course following CABG procedures, and such effusions are usually asymptomatic.[2,15] However, occasionally large pleural effusions causing significant symptoms may occur.[16] The primary symptom of patients with large pleural effusion after CABG is dyspnea. In the series of Light *et al.*,[23] 22 (75.9 percent) of 29 patients with an effusion occupying more than 25 percent of the hemithorax complained of dyspnea, but only three (10.3 percent) complained of chest pain, and only one (3.4 percent) complained of fever.

The early pleural effusions after CABG surgery are almost always small and unilateral on the left side.

Occasionally the effusion may be bilateral or unilateral on the right side.[1] In the study by Light *et al.*,[23] 62.4 percent of 349 patients had a pleural effusion 30 days after CABG surgery. The effusions were unilateral or larger on the left in 144 (73.4 percent), equal bilaterally in 38 (19.4 percent), and unilateral on the right or larger on the right in only 14 (7.2 percent).

CHARACTERISTICS OF PLEURAL FLUID

The characteristics of the pleural fluid after CABG surgery are dependent upon whether the effusion develops before or more than 30 days after surgery.[25,29] The pleural fluid from both types of effusions is exudative. The pleural fluid from the early effusions is bloody with a median hematocrit above 5 percent and a median red blood cell count of more than 700 000 cells/μL.[25] The pleural fluid is frequently eosinophilic, with a median eosinophil percentage of nearly 40.[25] The median pleural fluid lactic acid dehydrogenase (LDH) level is approximately twice the upper limit of normal for serum.[25] The pleural fluid protein is in the exudative range, and the pleural fluid glucose is not reduced.[25]

The characteristics of late effusions are quite different from the early effusions. The late effusion is usually a clear yellow exudate that contains predominantly lymphocytes. In one series of 26 pleural fluids from late effusions, the median lymphocyte percentage was 68, whereas the median eosinophil percentage was zero.[25] The median level of LDH approximates the upper normal limit for serum. The pleural fluid protein is in the exudative range, and the pleural fluid glucose is not reduced.[25]

MANAGEMENT

The majority of pleural effusions after CABG surgery are small and self-limited and are not associated with increased mortality or prolonged hospital stay.[34] Only symptomatic pleural effusions, predominantly effusions larger than 25 percent of the hemithorax, require therapeutic thoracentesis for relief of dyspnea. Patients who are febrile or have pleuritic chest pain should have a diagnostic thoracentesis because these symptoms are not usually seen in the typical post-CABG pleural effusion. Although most effusions resolve spontaneously, 73 percent of patients with an IMA–CABG and 29 percent with an SV CABG have persistent ultrasonographic evidence of pleural effusion 30 days after surgery,[6] and effusions may take 2–20 months to clear completely.[2,35] Symptomatic persistent effusions are best treated with serial thoracentesis. Although oral non-steroidal anti-inflammatory drugs (NSAIDs) and prednisone are frequently prescribed, there is no evidence of their efficacy. Chest tube drainage or pleurodesis is rarely required. If a symptomatic pleural effusion occurs after several thoracentesis, thoracoscopy with decortication appears to be effective.[2] Large effusions that require decortication for control are very rare.[2]

Post-cardiac injury syndrome

This is a condition associated with the occurrence of fever and pleuropericardial disease days or months after cardiac injury.[36–38] The syndrome is called 'postmyocardial infarction syndrome' when it follows a myocardial infarction and 'post-cardiotomy or post-pericardiotomy syndrome' when it follows cardiac surgery or trauma. PCIS is also a rare complication of pulmonary embolism, traumatic hemopericardium and implantation of pacemakers.[39]

INCIDENCE

The incidence of the syndrome has been reported to be 62 percent in Dressler's original series[40] and 83 percent in a later report.[41] Pleural effusions due to PCIS are most common following cardiac surgery compared to that following other conditions such as myocardial infarction.[1]

ETIOLOGY

Post-cardiac injury syndrome may be the consequence of an immunological response to damaged cardiac tissue. Evidence for autoimmunity includes the following:[42] (1) latent period; (2) antiheart antibodies; (3) preceding pericardial injury in many cases; (4) occurrence in patients with anatomically nontransmural infarctions, therefore without the direct visceral pericardial injury that causes epistenocardiac pericarditis; (5) frequent recurrences; (6) prompt response to anti-inflammatory agents; (7) frequent associated pleuritis with or without pneumonitis; (8) changes in cellular immunity suggested by altered lymphocyte subsets compared with control patients; and (9) evidence favoring immune complex formation incorporating antibody combined with myocardial antigen, complement pathway activation and evidence of cellular as well as humoral immunopathic responses. Antibodies – antiheart, antiactin and antimyosin – are provoked by both cardiac surgery and infarction; surgery is more immunostimulating than infarction.[43]

CLINICAL MANIFESTATIONS

Patients with PCIS present 1 week or more after myocardial injury. It has been reported that 65 percent of affected patients presented within 3 months and 100 percent within 12 months.[44]

Pericarditis almost always exists in patients with PCIS. These patients present with chest pain and fever.[1] On physical examination a pericardial rub may be found.[1] In addition, leukocytosis, an elevated erythrocyte sedimentation rate and combinations of pulmonary infiltrates and pleural effusions may be found on radiological examination.[1]

Typically, small and left-sided pleural effusion is present in almost 60 percent of patients, followed by bilateral, and rarely unilateral, right-sided effusions.[40] The effusion is hemorrhagic in 70 percent of cases and frankly bloody in 30 percent. The pleural fluid pH and glucose are normal in most cases and the predominant cells in the effusion are polymorphonuclear leukocytes during the acute phase and mononuclear cells later in the course.[40]

MANAGEMENT

The majority of patients with PCIS respond well to the initiation of anti-inflammatory agents such as aspirin or indomethacin.[1] Corticosteroids may be used in cases unresponsive to anti-inflammatory drugs.[45] Pleural effusion due to PCIS rarely requires invasive interventions such as therapeutic thoracentesis or any further procedure.

Pleural effusion after heart transplantation

INCIDENCE

Nearly 2300 heart transplants are performed each year in the USA.[16] While the prevalence of pleural effusions after CABG surgery and other cardiac surgeries has been well established, only two studies to date have described the prevalence of pleural effusions in the post-orthotopic heart transplant (OHT) population.[18,46] Lenner and associates[18] retrospectively evaluated the frequency of all pulmonary complications occurring after 159 orthotopic heart transplantation surgery. They reported 81 pulmonary complications in 47 heart recipients. Pleural effusions were accepted as complication of the surgery if seen on a chest radiograph or if an intervention, such as diagnostic thoracentesis, diuresis, antibiotic therapy or tube thoracostomy, was required. They reported effusions in only 10 (6.7 percent) subjects.

The first study evaluating specifically the prevalence of pleural effusions post-orthotopic heart transplantation was done in the authors' institution.[47] In this study, 81 patients who underwent OHT were screened by reviewing chest radiographs and chest computed tomography (CT) scans, and 72 patients were included in the study. Sixty-one patients (85 percent) developed an effusion at some time during the first 365 post-operative days.[47]

ETIOLOGY

The reported prevalence of post-OHT effusions is similar to that seen in the post-CABG patient population.[47] Misra *et al.*[47] hypothesized that the effusions post-OHT result from the actual surgical procedure of entering the chest cavity and disrupting the pleural space. While it is also possible that the occurrence of pleural effusions in the post-OHT population could be related to induction or maintenance immunosuppressive regimens, it seems less likely given the similarity in occurrence to the post-CABG population.

In the study by Misra *et al.*,[47] biochemical analysis for the pleural fluid was available for only four patients. Two of these four effusions were exudative, suggesting that congestive heart failure was not the primary underlying cause. However, it is likely that at least some of the effusions were due to cardiac dysfunction. In their series, none of the patients had any evidence for PCIS, such as pericarditis or pneumonitis. Other possible explanations suggested for these pleural effusions were interruption of the lymphatics that normally drain the pleural space, leakage of fluid from the mediastinum, damage from topical hypothermia or a hypersensitivity reaction to a drug.[47]

CLINICAL MANIFESTATIONS

The data on the clinical manifestations of pleural effusion after post-OHT surgery is limited to one study.[47] In this study, Misra *et al.* reported that pleural effusions were more common after OHT than pre-transplantation, despite the presence of severe cardiac dysfunction preoperatively. Sixty-one of the 72 patients (85 percent) had an effusion demonstrated at some point in the 12 months following transplantation. Ten of the 72 (14 percent) had a unilateral effusion on the left while only two (3 percent) had a unilateral effusion on the right. Forty-nine patients (68 percent) developed an effusion on each side at least once in the first 12 months after transplantation, and all of these patients also had concurrent bilateral pleural effusions noted at some point during that same time period.[47]

The majority of the post-operative effusions were small.[47] However, eight patients (13 percent) had 10 effusions occupying from 25 up to 50 percent of the hemithorax, and seven of those effusions were left-sided. Two different patients had an effusion occupying 50 percent or more of the hemithorax. Effusions were largest at median post-operative day 6.5 (5.0–7.0) on the left and 6.0 (5.0–9.0) on the right, expressed as mean day and 25th to 75th percentiles. The effusions tended to resolve with time.[47]

CHARACTERISTICS OF THE EFFUSIONS

Four patients with fluid studies were available for review in the study by Misra *et al.*[47] The fluid samples were obtained at a variety of times during the post-operative period, from post-operative day 12 to post-operative day 128. Two of the four effusions were exudates with LDH levels of 385 IU/L and 1623 IU/L (upper normal limit for LDH is 220 IU/L). The protein level was measured in only one of these exudates and it was 3.8 g/dL.[47]

MANAGEMENT

It appears from the very limited data that effusions after post-OHT tend to resolve with time and no intervention is necessary for the management of these effusions. In the study by Misra *et al.*[47] only eight patients (13 percent) had 10 effusions occupying from 25 up to 50 percent of the hemithorax, and two different patients had an effusion occupying 50 percent or more of the hemithorax. Effusions were largest at median post-operative day 6.5

(5.0–7.0) on the left and 6.0 (5.0–9.0) on the right, expressed as mean day and 25th to 75th percentile.[47]

PLEURAL EFFUSION AFTER LUNG TRANSPLANTATION

Incidence

Pleural effusion occurs in almost all lung transplant recipients in the early post-operative period (within 9 days).[6] Chiles *et al.*[6] reported a 100 percent incidence in 10 patients after heart–lung transplantation. Judson *et al.*[48] reported that nine patients underwent unilateral lung transplantation. All of these patients developed a pleural effusion. These effusions are usually bloody, exudative, neutrophil predominant and usually small to moderate in size. They tend to resolve spontaneously within 9 days of transplantation.[5] There are only two reports on late (more than 14 days) pleural effusions following lung transplantation.[46,49]

Herridge *et al.*[49] reviewed the pleural complications of unilateral and bilateral lung transplantation. They reported that none of the 53 single-lung transplant recipients had pleural effusions while 14 of 91 (15 percent) double lung transplant recipients did so. The effusions consisted of empyemas in seven patients, parapneumonic effusions that resolved spontaneously in four, hemothorax in two and chylothorax in one. Shitrit *et al.*[46] investigated the characteristics of late pleural effusions occurring 14–45 days in patients who underwent lung transplantation. Seven out of 35 patients (20 percent) had late pleural effusion. The median time for the appearance of pleural effusion was 23 days (range 14–34 days). It has been our observation that patients who experience rejection frequently had pleural effusions.

Etiology

Pulmonary lymphatics play a major role in the clearance of pleural fluid within the lung (almost 80 percent), whereas only 20 percent of the fluid is cleared through the pleural space.[50] Because the lymphatics are transected during surgery, the pleural space becomes the only route for fluid to exit from the lung. Two to four weeks are necessary for the reestablishment of the lymphatic integrity. This time-course corresponds with the observations of Judson *et al.*[48] who noted decreasing amounts of pleural fluid drainage by the ninth post-operative day.

Clinical manifestations and pleural fluid characteristics

There is limited data on the clinical manifestations and the characteristics of the pleural effusion after lung transplantation. Judson *et al.*[48] described the pleural fluid characteristics in nine single lung transplant recipients. Ipsilateral pleural fluid occurred immediately following the surgery and continued for up to 9 days. The effusions were exudative in all patients. The fluid was bloody in appearance with a high number of red blood cells (331 627 ± 122 583 mm^3, mean ± SEM). The white blood cell count in the fluid was 9803 ± 3470/mm^3 and decreased steadily after the first post-operative day. The initial LDH and protein values were approximately 3000 IU/L and 3.3 ± 0.2 g/dL, respectively. These values decreased by day nine.

Shtrit *et al.*[46] reported the characteristics of pleural fluids after single lung transplantation in seven patients. All the effusions were of medium size, with a median fluid volume of 700 mL (range 100–1300). Pleural fluids were exudative with lymphocyte predominance in all patients. In one patient, eosinophils were noted and in two patients, a bloody fluid was observed. LDH levels ranged between 322 and 560 IU/L (normal upper limit for LDH = 220 IU/L), and protein levels ranged between 4.9 and 6.3 g/dL.

Management

Because these effusions are usually either self-limited or easily treated systemically, it is seldom necessary to either examine or drain small to moderate pleural fluid collections in the first 10 days after transplantation.[48] When new or persistent pleural effusions are observed beyond the first few weeks after transplantation, the following etiologies should be considered: empyema or parapneumonic effusion, acute rejection, organizing pleural hematoma, lymphoproliferative disorder and cardiac or renal failure.[51] A diagnostic thoracentesis should be performed to help identify the etiology of the effusion.

PLEURAL EFFUSION AFTER LIVER TRANSPLANTATION

Incidence

Pleural effusions occur in 40–100 percent of the patients within 1 week after liver transplantation.[52–55] Afessa *et al.*[52] reported that 33 of 43 patients (77 percent) developed a pleural effusion in the first week, and four persisted beyond 6 weeks. Recently, Jiang *et al.*[56] reported that 11 out of 70 (16 percent) patients undergoing liver transplantation developed pleural effusion, which was the second most common complication following pneumonia.

Etiology

The exact mechanism responsible for the development of these effusions is not known. However, several possibilities have been suggested: (1) trauma to the right hemidiaphragm and lymphatics,[51] (2) blood component therapy, (3) atelectasis, (4) low protein levels, (5) hepatic hydrothorax,[57] (6) heart failure and (7) renal insufficiency.[46,58]

Clinical manifestations and pleural fluid characteristics

These effusions tend to be right-sided or bilateral in most cases.[46] One study reported that 34 out of 60 patients (57 percent) who developed pleural effusion after liver transplantation had pleural effusion on the right side and 26 (43 percent) had bilateral effusions.[57] Pirat *et al.*[59] investigated the risk factors for respiratory complications in 44 adult recipients undergoing liver transplantation. They reported that pleural effusion was the most frequent (40.9 percent) respiratory complication and patients who had pulmonary complications were significantly older (36 ± 14 versus 27 ± 12, $p = 0.039$) and required significantly more intraoperative transfusions ($p = 0.005$) compared with those who did not have any respiratory complications.

These effusions are generally transudative in nature.[54] Although they may persist for months, resolution occurs within 3–6 weeks in most cases.[52,53]

Management

These effusions are self-limited in most cases and thoracentesis is needed in less than 20 percent of the patients.[57,58,60] The usual course of these effusions is the development over the first several days to a week following surgery with resolution within 3–6 weeks.[52,53] The indications for thoracentesis are as follows: enlarging or persisting effusions or presence of evidence of pleural infection.[46] In case of respiratory insufficiency due to pleural effusion, chest tube thoracostomy may be needed.[58]

FUTURE DIRECTIONS

Pleural effusions after surgery are common. Several reasons have been suggested including trauma from the surgery itself, atelectasis, cardiac failure, etc. However, the exact mechanisms for the etiology of these pleural effusions are not clearly known. Further studies are needed to explain pathogenesis of pleural effusions following surgery. Understanding etiological mechanisms will help physicians to prevent or manage these effusions successfully in the future.

KEY POINTS

- Pleural effusions are common after surgery.
- Most of the effusions occur within first couple of days following surgery and are asymptomatic.
- Most of these effusions are self-limited.
- Trauma related to surgery itself is the most common mechanism producing the effusion.
- Late pleural effusions may occur, especially following post-CABG surgery.
- Effusions that are enlarging, persistent or causing respiratory compromise require interventions such as thoracentesis or tube thoracostomy.

REFERENCES

● = Key primary paper
◆ = Major review article

◆1. Light RW. *Pleural diseases*. Baltimore: Williams and Wilkins, 2007.
●2. Lee YCG, Vaz M, Ely K, *et al.* Symptomatic persistent post-coronary artery bypass graft pleural effusions requiring operative treatment: clinical and histologic features. *Chest* 2001; **119**: 795–800.
3. Forthman HJ, Shepard A. Postoperative pulmonary complications. *South Med J* 1969; **62**: 1198–200.
4. Laszlo G, Archer G, Darrell J, *et al.* The diagnosis and prophylaxis of pulmonary complications of surgical operation. *Br J Surg* 1973; **60**: 129–34.
5. Wightman JA. A prospective survey of the incidence of postoperative pulmonary complications. *Br J Surg* 1968; **55**: 85–91.
6. Chiles C, Guthaner D, Jamieson S, *et al.* Heart-lung transplantation: the postoperative chest radiograph. *Radiology* 1985; **154**: 299–304.
7. Nielsen PH, Jepsen SB, Olsen AD. Postoperative pleural effusion following upper abdominal surgery. *Chest* 1989; **96**: 1133–5.
8. Ti TK, Yong NK. Postoperative pulmonary complications – a prospective study in the tropics. *Br J Surg* 1974; **61**: 49–52.
9. Light RW, George RB. Incidence and significance of pleural effusion after abdominal surgery. *Chest* 1976; **69**: 621–5.
10. Eisenhauer EL, D'Angelica MI, Abu-Rustum NR, *et al.* Incidence and management of pleural effusions after diaphragm peritonectomy or resection for advanced mullerian cancer. *Gynecol Oncol* 2006; **103**: 871–7.
11. Collins CD, Darke CS, Knowelden J. Chest complications after upper abdominal surgery: their anticipation and prevention. *Br Med J* 1968; **1**: 401–6.
12. Sanders RC. Post-operative pleural effusion and subphrenic abscess. *Clin Radiol* 1970; **21**: 308–12.
13. Goodman LR. Postoperative chest radiograph: II. Alterations after major intrathoracic surgery. *AJR Am J Roentgenol* 1980; **134**: 803–13.
◆14. Light RW, Lee YCG. *Textbook of pleural diseases*. London: Arnold, 2003.
●15. Peng M, Vargas F, Cukier A, *et al.* Postoperative pleural changes after coronary revascularization. Comparison between saphenous vein and internal mammary artery grafting. *Chest* 1992; **101**: 327–30.
●16. Light RW, Rogers JT, Cheng D, *et al.* Large pleural effusions occurring after coronary artery bypass grafting. Cardiovascular Surgery Associates, PC. *Ann Intern Med* 1999; **130**: 891–6.

◆17. Light RW. Pleural effusions following cardiac injury and coronary artery bypass graft surgery. *Semin Respir Crit Care Med* 2001; **22**: 657–64.

●18. Lenner R, Padilla ML, Teirstein AS, *et al*. Pulmonary complications in cardiac transplant recipients. *Chest* 2001; **120**: 508–13.

19. Landymore RW, Howell F. Pulmonary complications following myocardial revascularization with the internal mammary artery graft. *Eur J Cardiothorac Surg* 1990; **4**: 156–61; discussion 161–2.

20. Hurlbut D, Myers ML, Lefcoe M, *et al*. Pleuropulmonary morbidity: internal thoracic artery versus saphenous vein graft. *Ann Thorac Surg* 1990; **50**: 959–64.

21. Vargas F, Cukier A, Hueb W, *et al*. Relationship between pleural effusion and pericardial involvement after myocardial revascularization. *Chest* 1994; **105**: 1748–52.

●22. Daganou M, Dimopoulou I, Michalopoulos N, *et al*. Respiratory complications after coronary artery bypass surgery with unilateral or bilateral internal mammary artery grafting. *Chest* 1998; **113**: 1285–9.

●23. Light R, Rogers J, Moyers J, *et al*. Prevalence and clinical course of pleural effusions at 30 days after coronary artery and cardiac surgery. *Am J Respir Crit Care Med* 2002; **166**: 1567–71.

●24. Peng M, Hou C, Li J, *et al*. Prevalence of symptomatic large pleural effusions first diagnosed more than 30 days after coronary artery bypass graft surgery. *Respirology* 2007; **12**: 122–6.

●25. Sadikot R, Rogers J, Cheng D, *et al*. Pleural fluid characteristics of patients with symptomatic pleural effusion after coronary artery bypass graft surgery. *Arch Intern Med* 2000; **160**: 2665–8.

26. Nikas D, Ramadan F, Elefteriades J. Topical hypothermia: ineffective and deleterious as adjunct to cardioplegia for myocardial protection. *Ann Thorac Surg* 1998; **65**: 28–31.

27. Allen B, Buckberg G, Rosenkranz E, *et al*. Topical cardiac hypothermia in patients with coronary disease. An unnecessary adjunct to cardioplegic protection and cause of pulmonary morbidity. *J Thorac Cardiovasc Surg* 1992; **104**: 626–31.

◆28. Light R. Pleural effusions after coronary artery bypass graft surgery. *Curr Opin Pulm Med* 2002; **8**: 308–11.

29. Kim Y, Mohsenifar Z, Koerner S. Lymphocytic pleural effusion in postpericardiotomy syndrome. *Am Heart J* 1988; **115**: 1077–79.

30. Mott A, Fraser CJ, Kusnoor A, *et al*. The effect of short-term prophylactic methylprednisolone on the incidence and severity of postpericardiotomy syndrome in children undergoing cardiac surgery with cardiopulmonary bypass. *J Am Coll Cardiol* 2001; **37**: 1700–6.

31. Jain U, Rao T, Kumar P, *et al*. Radiographic pulmonary abnormalities after different types of cardiac surgery. *J Cardiothorac Vasc Anesth* 1991; **5**: 592–5.

32. Mohamed KH JT, Rodriguez RM, Light RW. Pleural effusions post coronary artery bypass grafting performed with or without a bypass pump [Abstract]. *Am J Respir Crit Care Med* 2001; **163**: A901.

33. Ganapathy S, Murkin J, Dobkowski W, et al. Stress and inflammatory response after beating heart surgery versus conventional bypass surgery: the role of thoracic epidural anesthesia. *Heart Surg Forum* 2001; **4**: 323–7.

34. Cohen M, Sahn S. Resolution of pleural effusions. *Chest* 2001; **119**: 1547–62.

35. Paull D, Delahanty T, Weber F, *et al*. Thoracoscopic talc pleurodesis for recurrent, symptomatic pleural effusion following cardiac operations. *Surg Laparosc Endosc Percutan Tech* 2003; **13**: 339–44.

36. Jerjes-Sanchez C, Ibarra-Perez C, Ramirez-Rivera A, *et al*. Dressler-like syndrome after pulmonary embolism and infarction. *Chest* 1987; **92**: 115–17.

37. Tabatznik B, Isaacs JP. Postpericardiotomy syndrome following traumatic hemopericardium. *Am J Cardiol* 1961; **7**: 83–96.

38. Snow M, Agatston, AS, Kramer, HC, Samet, P The postcardiotomy syndrome following transvenous pacemaker insertion. *Pacing Clin Electrophysiol* 1987; **10**: 934.

39. Dressler W. The post-myocardial-infarction syndrome: a report on forty-four cases. *AMA Arch Intern Med* 1959; **103**: 28–42.

40. Stelzner TJ, King TE Jr, Antony VB, *et al*. The pleuropulmonary manifestations of the postcardiac injury syndrome. *Chest* 1983; **84**: 383–7.

41. Engle MA, Zabriskie JB, Senterfit LB, *et al*. Postpericardiotomy syndrome. A new look at an old condition. *Mod Concepts Cardiovasc Dis* 1975; **44**: 59–64.

42. Spodick DH. Decreased recognition of the post-myocardial infarction (Dressler) syndrome in the postinfarct setting: does it masquerade as 'idiopathic pericarditis' following silent infarcts? *Chest* 2004; **126**: 1410–11.

43. Spodick D. *The pericardium: a comprehensive textbook*. New York: Dekker, 1997.

44. Welin L, Vedin A, Wilhelmsson C. Characteristics, prevalence, and prognosis of postmyocardial infarction syndrome. *Br Heart J* 1983; **50**: 140–5.

45. Gregoratos G. Pericardial involvement in acute myocardial infarction. *Cardiol Clin* 1990; **8**: 601–8.

46. Shitrit D, Izbicki G, Fink G, *et al*. Late postoperative pleural effusion following lung transplantation: characteristics and clinical implications. *Eur J Cardiothorac Surg* 2003; **23**: 494–6.

●47. Misra H, Dikensoy O, Rodriguez RM, *et al*. The prevalence of pleural effusions post-orthotopic heart transplantation. *Respirology* 2007; **12**: 887–90.

●48. Judson MA, Handy JR, Sahn SA. Pleural effusions following lung transplantation. Time course, characteristics, and clinical implications. *Chest* 1996; **109**: 1190–4.

49. Herridge MS, de Hoyos AL, Chaparro C, *et al*. Pleural complications in lung transplant recipients. *J Thorac Cardiovasc Surg* 1995; **110**: 22–6.

50. Rodriguez RM MJ, Rogers JT, *et al*. Prevalence and clinical course of pleural effusion at 30 days post coronary artery bypass surgery. *Chest* 1999, **116**: 282S.

51. Marom EM, Palmer SM, Erasmus JJ, *et al*. Pleural effusions in lung transplant recipients: image-guided small-bore catheter drainage. *Radiology* 2003; **228**: 241–5.

●52. Afessa B, Gay PC, Plevak DJ, *et al*. Pulmonary complications of orthotopic liver transplantation. *Mayo Clin Proc* 1993; **68**: 427–34.

53. Spizarny DL, Gross BH, McLoud T. Enlarging pleural effusion after liver transplantation. *J Thorac Imaging* 1993; **8**: 85–7.

54. Olutola PS, Hutton L, Wall WJ. Pleural effusion following liver transplantation. *Radiology* 1985; **157**: 594.

55. Costello P, Williams CR, Jenkins RW, *et al*. The incidence and implications of chest radiographic abnormalities following orthotopic liver transplantation. *Can Assoc Radiol J* 1987; **38**: 90–5.

56. Jiang Y, Lv LZ, Cai QC, *et al*. Liver transplant for 70 patients with end-stage liver diseases. *Hepatobiliary Pancreat Dis Int* 2007; **6**: 24–8.

57. Golfieri R, Giampalma E, Sama C, *et al*. Pulmonary complications following orthotopic liver transplant: radiologic patterns and epidemiologic considerations in 100 cases. *Rays* 1994; **19**: 319–38.

58. Duran FG, Piqueras B, Romero M, *et al*. Pulmonary complications following orthotopic liver transplant. *Transpl Int* 1998; **11**(Suppl 1): S255–9.

59. Pirat A, Ozgur S, Torgay A, *et al*. Risk factors for postoperative respiratory complications in adult liver transplant recipients. *Transplant Proc* 2004; **36**: 218–20.

60. Bilik R, Yellen M, Superina RA. Surgical complications in children after liver transplantation. *J Pediatr Surg* 1992; **27**: 1371–5.

35

Hepatic hydrothorax

JOSÉ CASTELLOTE, XAVIER XIOL QUINGLES

DEFINITION

Hepatic hydrothorax is defined as the pleural effusion of patients with hepatic cirrhosis and portal hypertension without a primary cardiac, pulmonary or pleural disease.[1–3] Hepatic hydrothorax is an uncommon manifestation of portal hypertension and normally appears in patients with ascites, as the source of the pleural fluid is ascites that crosses the diaphragm. However, the presence of ascites is not necessary for the diagnosis as there have been many reports of hepatic hydrothorax in which ascites was not detectable even by ultrasonography.

Pleural fluid of cirrhotic patients can become infected, and spontaneous bacterial empyema (SBEM) is defined as an infection of a pre-existing hydrothorax without a subjacent pneumonia.[4,5] Generally, it is associated with spontaneous bacterial peritonitis (SBP), the infection of ascitic fluid, but as many as 40 percent of cases of SBEM are not associated with SBP.

Incidence

Hepatic hydrothorax accounts for 2–3 percent of all pleural effusions.[6–10] The incidence increases to 9.9 percent when only massive pleural effusions are considered.[10] In patients with cirrhosis the incidence of hepatic hydrothorax is low but depends on the severity of the cirrhosis and the presence of ascites. In a recent report of 862 Chinese cirrhotic patients,[11] 132 (15 percent) had pleural effusion although in most of them the effusion was only detectable by ultrasonography, and thoracentesis could only be performed in 56 (6.5 percent). The four larger series of cirrhotic patients with ascites,[12–15] including a total of 1155 cases, show a very similar incidence of hepatic hydrothorax: around 6 percent. Therefore, the incidence of hepatic hydrothorax is less than 5 percent if we consider all cirrhotic patients and 6 percent in cirrhotic patients with ascites. As many as 20 percent of patients with hepatic hydrothorax have no clinically detectable ascites.[16–18].

In a recompilation of 204 reported cases of hepatic hydrothorax in which the side of the effusion was specified, 162 (79.5 percent) were right-sided, 36 (17.5 percent) were left-sided and only six (3 percent) were bilateral.[12–14,18–20] It must be noted that the most frequent cause of all pleural effusions in developed countries is cardiac failure and accounts for the overwhelming majority of transudative pleural effusions.[21] Pleural effusions of cardiac origin are usually bilateral of relatively equal size; unilateral effusions are uncommon. Hepatic hydrothorax is the second cause in frequency of transudative effusions and should be suspected when a transudative pleural effusion is unilateral, especially if it is right-sided.[21]

ETIOLOGY

It is now broadly accepted that hepatic hydrothorax is secondary to transfer of peritoneal fluid directly via defects in the diaphragm: this mechanism was suggested by the observation of pneumothorax after injection of air into the peritoneal cavity, and confirmed by higher radioactivity in pleural fluid than in lymph or plasma after injection of albumin labeled with iodine-131 into ascitic fluid. Many other studies have proved that the injection of air, dyes or radiolabeled material into the peritoneal cavity of patients with hydrothorax is associated with the rapid movement of these materials into the pleural space.[1,22]

Many otherwise normal people probably have tiny congenital holes in the diaphragm. In patients with ascites, the increasing abdominal pressure and the diaphragmatic thinning secondary to malnutrition of cirrhotic patients enlarges the defects. Blebs of herniated peritoneum protrude through these defects and, if the blebs burst, a communication between peritoneal and pleural spaces is formed. There is a pressure gradient between peritoneal and pleural spaces that favors the unidirectional passage of ascitic fluid into the chest. A valvular mechanism may contribute to this unidirectional flow. The congenital diaphragmatic holes are frequently seen in the tendinous portion of the right diaphragm and less frequently in the left diaphragm, which is thicker and more muscular than the right. This fact, plus the piston effect of the liver, is why most hepatic hydrothoraces are right-sided. The diaphragmatic defects can also be secondary to previous trauma or surgery. Huang *et al.*[23] have classified the diaphragmatic defects associated with the development of hepatic hydrothorax on thoracoscopy into four morphological types: type I, no obvious defect; type II, blebs lying on the diaphragm; type III, broken defects (fenestrations) in the diaphragm and type IV, multiple gaps in the diaphragm.

In patients without ascites the mechanism of formation is the same. In these cases all the ascitic fluid formed rapidly crosses the diaphragm and becomes pleural fluid. This has been confirmed by scintigraphic studies.[24–26]

CLINICAL PRESENTATION

Hepatic hydrothorax should be suspected when a cirrhotic patient, especially with ascites, develops a pleural effusion. It should also be suspected in patients with an isolated right pleural effusion with transudative characteristics, especially if it is massive. Hepatic hydrothorax can be asymptomatic, or present with symptoms that can range from dyspnea on exertion to overt respiratory failure, depending on various factors such as the volume of the effusion, the amount of ascites present, the speed of the accumulation of pleural fluid and the presence of associated pulmonary disease, which is not infrequent in alcoholic patients. Life-threatening dyspnea secondary to an acute hepatic hydrothorax has been reported, probably secondary to a sudden increase in intra-abdominal pressure, such as straining or coughing that caused rupture of the pleuroperitoneal bleb.[27]

DIAGNOSIS

The diagnosis of hepatic hydrothorax is based on:

1. Presence of hepatic cirrhosis with portal hypertension;
2. Exclusion of a primary cardiac, pulmonary or pleural disease;
3. Eventual confirmation of the passage of ascites to the pleural space.

The diagnosis of hepatic cirrhosis is mainly histological but, in general practice, the diagnosis is based on clinical, analytical and ultrasonographic findings. The presence of ascites favors the diagnosis but its absence does not rule out hepatic hydrothorax.

To exclude a primary cardiac, pulmonary or pleural disease, a chest radiograph and thoracentesis with pleural fluid analysis should be performed.

A chest radiograph should always be obtained to confirm the effusion, rule out cardiomegaly and pulmonary or pleural pathology. In patients with massive pleural effusion the radiograph should be repeated when the effusion has decreased considerably (after diuresis or therapeutic thoracentesis) to evaluate pulmonary or pleural pathology that was masked by the effusion,[18] although this also can be evaluated by a thoracic scan.

Thoracentesis and pleural fluid study should be performed despite the appearance of a normal chest radiograph, because diagnostic thoracentesis with a fine needle (21 G) has very few complications and pleural fluid analysis is the best option to rule out pleural pathology and to detect the main complication of hepatic hydrothorax that is SBEM (the bacterial infection of a pre-existing hydrothorax). In 139 consecutive diagnostic thoracentesis performed with a fine needle, the most severe complication was pneumothorax that appeared in two cases (1.3 percent).[28] Despite a severe coagulation disorder in some patients, the incidence of bleeding complications was small (4 percent) and without clinical impact.[28] This observation confirms a previous report of the absence of increased bleeding after paracentesis and thoracentesis in patients with coagulation abnormalities.[29] There is a wide experience of paracentesis in cirrhotic patients with coagulation abnormalities,[30] and thoracentesis, if performed correctly avoiding the intercostal vessels, is a procedure very similar to paracentesis.

In a study of 60 consecutive cirrhotic patients admitted to the hospital with pleural effusion,[18] only 42 (70 percent) were considered to have uncomplicated hepatic hydrothorax based on pleural fluid analysis. Of the other 18 (30 percent), nine had spontaneous bacterial empyema, two had pleural tuberculosis, two had adenocarcinoma, two had parapneumonic empyema and three had undiagnosed exudates. In those cases in which the diagnosis was other than hydrothorax, the chest radiograph was only able to diagnose the patients with parapneumonic empyema. When the pleural effusion was right-sided, 37/46 (80 percent) were uncomplicated hydrothorax. Conversely, when it was left-sided only, 5/14 (35 percent) were hydrothorax and none of the five patients with left pleural effusion and absence of ascites had uncomplicated hepatic hydrothorax. Furthermore, according to this study, diagnosis other than hydrothorax often cannot be suspected by ascitic fluid analysis only.[18] This concurs with previous reports[20,31] that the presence of a pleural effusion in a cirrhotic patient should not automatically lead to the diagnosis of hepatic hydrothorax, especially if the effusion is left-sided. Pleural fluid analysis is mandatory and may add valuable information to ascitic fluid analysis for patients with ascites and pleural effusion. This approach has been recently emphasized by Light[32] who concluded in a recent review of pleural effusion that 'a thoracentesis should be performed in patients with a pleural effusion of unknown case unless the effusion is small (less than 10 mm on ultrasonography) or the patient has congestive heart failure and bilateral pleural effusions'.

Pleural fluid of hepatic hydrothorax has low protein and lactate dehydrogenase (LDH) concentration, very similar to those of ascitic fluid, and thus it has transudative characteristics,[33] although pleural fluid total proteins are greater than in ascites.[34] Light's criteria remain the best means of separating transudates from exudates.[35] However, it should be pointed out that a small number of patients with transudative pleural effusions are misclassified as having exudates when applying Light's criteria, mostly because total pleural fluid protein increases with diuresis.[36] In these cases, when hydrothorax is suspected and exudative criteria are met, a serum albumin gradient should be calculated (serum albumin minus pleural fluid albumin), and if it is above 12 g/L the effusion probably is a transudate,[35,37] although studies including a higher number of cirrhotic patients should be carried out to confirm the utility of albumin gradient in the diagnosis of hepatic hydrothorax.

In conclusion, the most advisable approach is to perform a chest radiograh, paracentesis if the patient has ascites and thoracentesis in all patients with suspected hepatic hydrothorax. Pleural fluid analysis should include protein and LDH determinations, polymorphonuclear count and culture in a blood culture bottle, in order to confirm that the fluid is transudate (applying Light criteria), to rule out SBEM and to rule out other causes of pleural effusion.[3,32] A smear to exclude malignancy, pleural fluid amylase (in alcoholic patients) and adenosine deaminase (ADA), especially in countries where tuberculosis is prevalent, should be considered when the fluid is an exudate or when the effusion is left-sided. In this last case, thoracic computed tomography (CT) can help to rule out pulmonary or pleural pathology.

The best way to confirm the communication between pleural and peritoneal space is with a scintigraphic study, although there has been a report of cases of hepatic hydrothorax in which the communication between peritoneal and pleural space was detected by ultrasonography or magnetic resonance.[38] These studies are not necessary for the diagnosis of hepatic hydrothorax in clinical practice. It can be used for confirming a hydrothorax when pleural fluid has exudative characteristics, or if is planned to close the communications between peritoneal and pleural spaces with video-assisted thoracoscopic surgery (VATS).

TREATMENT

Hepatic hydrothorax is secondary to the passage of ascites through a diaphragmatic defect, and ascites is secondary to portal hypertension and salt retention by the kidney. Treatment can be directed to improve salt retention (diuretics), to reduce portal hypertension (transjugular intrahepatic portosystemic shunt, TIPS), to close the diaphragmatic defects (through VATS, with concomitant talc pleurodesis) or to solve hepatic cirrhosis by liver transplantation. Therapeutic options and their relationship with the pathophysiological cascade of hepatic hydrothorax are shown in Table 35.1.

The first line of treatment is the same as for ascites: sodium restriction and diuretic therapy, spironolactone,

Table 35.1 Therapeutic options depending on the physiopathological steps of hepatic hydrothorax

Therapeutic options	
Liver cirrhosis	Liver transplantation
Portal hypertension	TIPS
Splanchnic vasodilatation	Vasoconstrictors:
	Octreotide
	Terlypressin
Ascites	Diuretics
	Peritoneo-venous shunts
	Large volume paracentesis
Diaphragmatic defects	Surgical closure
	Diaphragm reinforcement
	Videothoracoscopy
Transdiaphragmatic gradient pressure	CPAP
Hydrothorax	Therapeutic thoracentesis
	Pleurovenous shunts
	Chemical pleurodesis

CPAP, continuous positive airway pressure; TIPS, transjuglar intrahepatic portosystemic shunt.

and if there is no response to sequential increments or complications such as hyperkalemia, the addition of furosemide. In case of intolerance to spironolactone due to gynecomastia, triamterene or amiloride may be considered.

Those that do not respond to medical therapy are considered to have refractory hydrothorax (RH), that can be defined, using the same criteria for refractory ascites introduced in a Consensus Conference in 1996,[39] as a pleural effusion that cannot be mobilized (with diuretics, paracentesis or thoracentesis) or the early recurrence of which cannot be satisfactorily prevented by medical therapy. Similar definitions have been given recently: pleural effusion requiring repeated thoracenteses despite treatment with the highest tolerable doses of spironolactone and furosemide[17] or recurrent pleural effusion that, despite salt restriction and diuretic therapy, requires repeated therapeutic thoracenteses to control symptoms.[40] The incidence of refractory hydrothorax is not clearly established. In a retrospective study by our group,[14] 405 cirrhotic patients admitted over a 5 year period with ascites were studied. Seven out of 27 patients with hepatic hydrothorax (26 percent) were considered refractory to medical treatment. In a prospective study of 60 cirrhotic patients with hepatic hydrothorax,[34] 13 (22 percent) were considered refractory. Thus, we can estimate that the prevalence of refractory hepatic hydrothorax is 25 percent.

Management of refractory hydrothorax is a clinical challenge because most cirrhotic patients with RH have severely impaired liver function, frequently with associated renal insufficiency, and aggressive therapy in these very fragile patient results in high morbidity and mortality rates. With the exception of liver transplantation, no single therapy has been shown to be completely satisfactory because of associated morbidity or low efficacy. Controlled trials are lacking and therapeutic decisions must therefore be taken on the basis of anecdotal reports or small series of patients.

Thoracentesis is the most effective method for the rapid relief of dyspnea associated with hepatic hydrothorax. Owing to the fact that paracentesis has almost no side effects[41] and can improve dyspnea by decreasing intra-abdominal pressure, in patients with ascites and hydrothorax it is advisable to drain ascites first and only perform thoracentesis if there is no ascites or paracentesis does not ameliorate the dyspnea. Thoracentesis relieves patient symptoms easily, with few complications, except pneumothorax.[18] If performed correctly the risk of bleeding is small,[5,42] even without administering fresh frozen plasma. Protein depletion can be overcome by albumin administration. However, the risk of pneumothorax is not negligible. In 19 patients that were treated with 76 therapeutic thoracentesis, five patients had seven pneumothoraces (9 percent of the procedures, 26 percent of the patients). Although there was no mortality associated with pneumothorax, a chest tube had to be inserted because of dyspnea in four patients. A chest radiograph after therapeutic thoracentesis is advisable not only for detection of pneumothorax, but also to evaluate pulmonary or pleural pathology that was masked by the effusion. Re-expansion pulmonary edema, a very rare complication of thoracentesis, is associated with previous pulmonary disease and evacuation of a high pleural fluid volume in a short period of time.[43] In a series of 76 therapeutic thoracenteses in cirrhotic patients we did not have any post-evacuation pulmonary edema. It has been suggested that intravascular expansion with albumin may prevent this complication.[41] In any case, evacuation of more than 2000 mL of pleural fluid and use of vacuum is not advisable. Thus, for patients with refractory hydrothorax whose hepatic function is not expected to improve spontaneously, as occurs after variceal bleeding, bacterial infection or recent alcohol intake, repeated thoracenteses are not the treatment of choice and alternatives should be investigated.

Chest tube insertion should be avoided because it does not solve the problem and produces massive fluid loss that can lead to the death of the patient.[44] In a retrospective analysis, mortality of cirrhotic patients undergoing a chest tube placement mostly for hepatic hydrothorax and spontaneous bacterial empyema was 40 percent in patient with Child–Turcotte–Pugh (CTP) C and 16 percent in CTP B.[45] If a chest tube is placed, appropriate replacement of fluid losses and albumin of 6–8 g/L of pleural fluid removed, should be administered. It has been anecdotally reported that the concomitant administration of vasoconstrictor drugs (as usually used in hepatorenal syndrome) can decrease the output from the chest tube (Table 35.1).[46,47]

Pleural sclerosis with tetracycline or talc has been used in the past. The irritant is administered by a chest tube or thoracoscopy. Positive results were achieved in less than 50 percent of patients, although figures are better in the few cases without ascites.[48] Failure is caused by the continuous passage of ascitic fluid from abdominal cavity resulting in the irritant dilution. The results may be improved if irritant is administered by VATS.[49,50] To decrease this flood by decreasing the gradient pressure between pleural and peritoneal cavity, continuous positive airway pressure (CPAP) has been used in association with chemical pleurodesis[51] or alone.[52]

Peritoneovenous shunt was used in the past for refractory ascites and also for hepatic hydrothorax.[19] Problems associated with the shunt, such as obstruction or infection and lack of efficacy, limit its use. Anecdotal use of other shunts, such as the pleurovenous shunt, has been reported.[53]

Closure of transdiaphragmatic fenestrations can be performed by VATS with concomitant talc pleurodesis.[54–56] Mouroux *et al.*[54] found demonstrable diaphragmatic defects in six of eight patients (75 percent). The main duration of post-operative chest tube drainage was 7.6 days for the patients with demonstrable fenestrations and 16.5 days in the two patients without demonstrable pleural fenestrations. The pleural effusion did not recur in the six patients with fenestrations closed, but the other two patients had recurrent effusion and died 1 month and

2 months after the procedure, respectively. In the series reported by de Campos *et al.*[55] which included 18 patients, the main duration of the post-operative chest tube drainage was 13 days (range 4–38 days). Two patients developed empyema and six developed hyponatremia and hypoalbuminemia through chest tube drainage. Only in five patients could a suture be performed; three had a good response (60 percent), one died of post-operative pneumonia and liver failure and the other had empyema and drained fluid for 1 month. Ten of the 21 procedures, (47.6 percent) had a good response. Seven out of the 18 patients died 12–40 days after the procedure. Successful thoracoscopic pleura or Mersilene mesh onlay reinforcement of diaphragm in 10 cirrhotic patients with hepatic hydrothorax has been reported recently.[57]

In conclusion, VATS with concomitant talc pleurodesis for refractory hydrothorax is successful in 40–75 percent of patients, but may result in prolonged hospitalization and pleural space intubation with severe secondary effects (hyponatremia and empyema), and considerable mortality. Patients with demonstrable diaphragmatic defects treated with closure have better results than those without demonstrable fenestration. In patients with refractory ascites and refractory hydrothorax, closure of fenestration does not solve the refractory ascites. Its main indication are those patients with refractory hydrothorax without ascites or with low volume of ascites, or those with relatively good hepatic function in which TIPS is contraindicated because of advanced age, although more experience is needed to confirm its role in the management of refractory hydrothorax.

Transjugular intrahepatic portosystemic shunt is an interventional radiology technique that creates an anastomosis between portal and hepatic veins that behaves as a side-to-side portocaval shunt. It decompresses the hepatic and splanchnic vascular bed, causing the portal pressure to fall. Introduced for the treatment of variceal bleeding, it also works for ascites as portal hypertension is a prerequisite for ascites formation. It is useful for refractory ascites and for refractory hydrothorax. The main advantages of TIPS are the lack of post-operative complications related to laparotomy, it is effective in patients without ascites,[58] hepatic function may improve in long-term survivors and it does not preclude a future liver transplantation.

Although it can be successfully performed in patients with high post-operative risk, one of its main drawbacks is impairment of liver function due to the reduction of effective portal perfusion to the liver. This impairment can be dramatic for patients with poor liver function in whom it is contraindicated. Other problems are that it may induce or worsen hepatic encephalopathy. In addition, in most cases, stenosis or occlusion of the stents occurs in the medium or long term, although these complications are decreased with the new covered stents.

To date there have been seven reports of refractory hepatic hydrothorax treated by TIPS (Table 35.2). The first three series[16,59,60] included 41 patients and reported a high mortality. However, the last reports achieved a considerably better survival. Chalasani *et al.*[40] reported a survival of 80 percent at 6 months and 56 percent at 1 year. Factors influencing survival were bilirubin concentration, variceal

Table 35.2 Results of transjugular intrahepatic portosystemic shunt (TIPS) in refractory hydrothorax

Authors	*n*	Aetiology Child–Pugh	Response[a] Complete	Partial	No	Mortality 40 days	Survival 1 year	Enc[b]
Strauss *et al.*,[59] (1994)	5	60% alcohol 5 C	2/5 (40%)	2/5 (40%)	1/5 (20%)	0/5 (0%)		0%
Gordon *et al.*,[60] (1997)	24	54% alcohol 5 B, 19 C	14/24 (58%)	5/24 (21%)	5/24 (21%)	13/24 (54%)		37%
Jeffries *et al.*,[16] (1998)	12	0% alcohol 1 A, 5 B, 6 C	5/12 (42%)	2/12 (16%)	5/12 (42%)	4/12 (33%)		33%
Chalasani *et al.*,[40] (2000)	24	34% alcohol 30%B, 70%C					56%	20%
Siegerstetter *et al.*,[17] (2001)	40	70% alcohol 24 B, 16 C	21/40 (53%)	11/40 (27%)	8/40 (20%)	6/40 (15%)	64%	5%
Spencer *et al.*,[61] (2002)	21	7 B, 14 C	12/19 (63%)	2/19 (11%)	5/19 (11%)	6/21 (29%)		
Nuñez *et al.*,[62] (2002)	5	3 B, 2 C	3/5 (60%)	1/5 (20%)	1/5 (20%)	1/5 (20%)	60%	60%
Global	131	1 A, 51 B, 79 C 39% B, 60% C	57/105 (54%)	23/105 (22%)	25/105 (24%)	30/108 (28%)		

[a]Complete response: lack of pleural effusion. Partial response: persistence of some pleural fluid but no need for thoracentesis.
[b]Enc: New or worsening encephalopathy during follow-up.

hemorrhage requiring emergent TIPS, encephalopathy unrelated to bleeding previous to TIPS and an alanine aminotransferase (ALT) level of greater than 100 IU/L. In 2001, Siegerstetter *et al.*[17] reported a 1-year survival of 64 percent. The probability of being free of relapse was only 35 percent, although in most cases revision of TIPS solved the problem. Hydrothorax response and survival showed a significant inverse correlation with age over 60 years. Spencer *et al.*[61] reported a complete response of 63 percent but with an early mortality of 29 percent and Nuñez *et al.*[62] reported 60 percent encephalopathy.

In conclusion, in selected patients with refractory hepatic hydrothorax and a conserved hepatic function (especially those younger than 60 years old, with low levels of bilirubin and absence of encephalopathy), TIPS can be an effective treatment. It has been suggested that a 'model of end-stage liver disease' (MELD) <17 could be a good predictor of 3-month survival after TIPS.[63] It can be used as a bridge to hepatic transplantation or as definite therapy in those in whom hepatic transplantation is contraindicated.

Hepatic transplantation is the best treatment for decompensated hepatic cirrhosis and therefore for patients with hydrothorax. Most series reported few cases but the results are the same as those of patients with ascites.[16,40] It is indicated in refractory hydrothorax but also in patients with hydrothorax and poor hepatic function (CTP B or C) or after an episode of SBEM. In a retrospective study of our group we compared 28 patients with hepatic hydrothorax with 56 cirrhotic patients transplanted without hydrothorax.[64] There were no differences in peri- or post-operative complications, including transfusions, days of mechanical ventilation, intensive care unit (ICU) admission days or post-operative mortality. There were no differences in either long-term survival or graft survival. In conclusion, liver transplantation is the best therapy for patients with hepatic hydrothorax; there are no further complications related to pleural effusion and long-term survival is similar to that in patients without hydrothorax.

COMPLICATIONS: SPONTANEOUS BACTERIAL EMPYEMA

Spontaneous bacterial empyema is the infection of a preexisting hydrothorax in which a parapneumonic infection has been excluded. Spontaneous bacterial peritonitis is a well-known complication in cirrhotic patients with ascites[65] and SBEM is a very similar infection. In a prospective study of our group, nine of out 60 (15 percent) cirrhotic patients with pleural effusion had SBEM at admission. In a study from Taiwan,[11] the incidence of SBEM was 2 percent in cirrhotic patients and 13 percent in cirrhotic patients with hydrothorax.

In the cases prospectively studied in our center,[4,5,18] 53 percent were associated with spontaneous bacterial peritonitis, 30 percent had no ascites and 17 percent had non-infected ascites. In the Chinese series, SBEM were associated with SBP in 56 percent of cases.[11] Other cases of SBEM without infected ascites have been reported,[66–68] suggesting that SBEM is not necessarily secondary to spontaneous bacterial peritonitis. Probably, pathogens arrive in the pleural space through a bacteremia, in most cases originating in the gut, the same pathogenesis reported in spontaneous bacterial peritonitis,[65] although spreading of an infected ascitic fluid through diaphragmatic defects cannot be excluded in some cases. As SBEM can be present without a simultaneous SBP, both paracentesis and thoracentesis should be performed when an infection is suspected in a cirrhotic patient with ascites and hydrothorax. The fact that a thoracentesis is a procedure with low morbidity supports this approach.

Risk factors for developing SBEM have been defined. Sese *et al.*[34] found that low pleural protein and C3 levels and higher CTP score were associated with SBEM. Chen *et al.*[11] identified pleural fluid protein <12 g/L and a simultaneous SBP as independent risk factors for the development of SBEM.

Clinical manifestations of SBEM are shown in Table 35.3. It is noteworthy that thorax-related symptoms are scanty and thus, a high index of suspicion and a prompt diagnostic thoracentesis should be performed to diagnose SBEM when non-specific signs or symptoms are present such as renal insufficiency or hepatic encephalopathy. Criteria for diagnosis include: positive pleural fluid culture and a pleural fluid polymorphonuclear count greater than 250 cells/μL, and exclusion of parapneumonic infection; evidence of pleural fluid before infection or transudate characteristics during infection, and chest radiograph or CT scan without evidence of pneumonia.[4,5] Culture-negative SBEM is diagnosed when patients have a compatible clinical course, negative pleural fluid culture and a polymorphonuclear count greater than 500 cells/μL. Culture of pleural fluid should be carried out by inoculating 10 mL of pleural fluid into a blood culture bottle at the bedside because a causal bacteria is identified in 75 percent using

Table 35.3 Clinical manifestations in 65 reported cases of spontaneous bacterial empyema (SBEM)

	n	%
Temperature >38	40	61
Dyspnea	22	34
Abdominal pain	22	34
Encephalopathy	8	12
Septic shock	4	6
Mortality	19	29

this method while this rate is only 33 percent when conventional microbiological techniques are used.[5,11]

During the infectious episode, pleural fluid characteristics may change, although protein and glucose levels stay stable, LDH increases and in some cases the pleural fluid can be defined as an exudate by Light's criteria due to LDH increment.[5] It has been suggested that the serum–pleura albumin gradient >12 g/L accurately differentiate between hepatic hydrothorax or SBEM and other exudative pleural effusions.[37]

In the four series reported including 65 cases,[4,5,11,66] 34 were culture negative and 31 (48 percent) were culture positive, although etiological bacteria could be identified in 39 cases (60 percent): *Escherichia coli* in 21 cases, *Streptococcus* species in six, *Klebsiella pneumoniae* in five, *Enterococcus* species in four, *Clostridium perfringens* in one, *Pseudomonas stutzeri* in one and *Gemella morbillorum* in one. Due to the delay in culture results, pleural polymorphonuclear neutrophil (PMN) count is the cornerstone of the diagnosis. Recently, the use of reagent strips to detect leukocyte esterase in urine has been shown to be a very sensitive and specific method for a rapid diagnosis of SBP in cirrhotic patients with ascites[69] and has also been validated in pleural fluid to diagnose SBEM.[70]

Mortality in the four series was 29 percent (19 from 65). Intravascular expansion with albumin improves survival in cirrhotic patients with SBP,[71] although this approach has not been validated in patients with SBEM, it should improve prognosis because an impairment of systemic circulation after SBEM should be expected.

Treatment with a third-generation cephalosporin, cefotaxime or ceftriaxone, should be initiated without waiting for the pleural fluid culture when pleural fluid polymorphonuclear count is over 250 cells/μL. Aminoglycosides are contraindicated in cirrhotic patients because of significant side effects, especially renal insufficiency. None of the patients reported was treated with a chest tube, because pleural fluid did not meet the biochemical criteria for its insertion. Since most patients were cured of the infection without a chest tube and its insertion can be harmful in patients with hepatic hydrothorax,[44,45] a chest tube should not be used for treating SBEM. Owing to frequent recidivism of the infection, prophylaxis with norfloxacin is recommended to all survivors of an episode of SBEM. Long-term survival of patients with SBEM is poor. In a retrospective series from our hospital, median survival of cirrhotic patients with SBEM was 13 months; thus, a SBEM episode should be considered an indication for liver transplantation.[5]

FUTURE DIRECTIONS

The utility of albumin gradient in the diagnosis of hepatic hydrothorax has not been studied and should be investigated before recommending its application.

Because hydrothorax is secondary to ascites, the new treatments for ascites can be applied to hepatic hydrothorax. The introduction of selective vasoconstrictors to revert the splanchnic vasodilatation responsible of ascites in cirrhotic patients and the use of aquaretics may be future alternatives.[72] Video-assisted thoracoscopy with concomitant talc pleurodesis is useful therapeutically in the patients in which a communication between peritoneal and pleural cavity is detected. Identification of these patients before intervention can considerably improve the results of this technique.

KEY POINTS

- The presence of a pleural effusion in a cirrhotic patient should not automatically lead to the diagnosis of hepatic hydrothorax, especially if the effusion is left-sided. Because diagnostic thoracentesis is a safe procedure in patients with cirrhosis, pleural fluid analysis is mandatory and may add valuable information to ascitic fluid analysis for patients with ascites and pleural effusion.
- Patients with hydrothorax and poor hepatic function or those with refractory hydrothorax should be considered for liver transplantation.
- Transjugular intrahepatic portosystemic shunt is an effective treatment for refractory hydrothorax of selected patients with relatively conserved hepatic function, especially those with low levels of bilirubin and absence of encephalopathy. It can be used as a bridge to hepatic transplantation or as a definitive therapy in those in whom liver transplantation is contraindicated.
- Video-assisted thoracoscopy with concomitant talc pleurodesis can be an alternative, especially when no refractory ascites is associated.
- When a cirrhotic patient with pleural effusion is admitted to hospital or presents with fever, chills, encephalopathy or abdominal or chest pain, spontaneous bacterial empyema should be suspected. Thoracentesis with pleural fluid polymorphonuclear count and culture, inoculating 10 mL of pleural fluid to a blood culture bottle at bedside, should be performed in order to rule our SBEM, even when spontaneous bacterial peritonitis has been excluded. Antibiotic therapy with third-generation cephalosporins should be initiated without awaiting pleural fluid culture when the pleural fluid PMN count is over 250 cells/μL.

REFERENCES

● = Key primary paper
◆ = Major review article
∗ = Paper that represents the first formal publication of a management guideline

●1. Alberts WM, Salem AJ, Solomon DA, Boyce G. Hepatic hydrothorax. Cause and management. *Arch Intern Med* 1991; **151**: 2383–8.

◆2. Lazaridis KN, Frank JW, Krowka MJ, Kamath PS. Hepatic hydrothorax: pathogenesis, diagnosis and management. *Am J Med* 1999; **107**: 262–7

3. Xiol X, Guardiola J. Hepatic hydrothorax. *Curr Opin Pulm Med* 1998; **4**: 239–42.

●4. Xiol X, Castellote J, Baliellas C, *et al.* Spontaneous bacterial empyema in cirrhotic patients: analysis of eleven cases. *Hepatology* 1990; 11: 365–70.

5. Xiol X, Castellvi JM, Guardiola J, *et al.* Spontaneous bacterial empyema in cirrhotic patients: a prospective study. *Hepatology* 1996; **23**: 719–23.

6. Tinney WS, Olsen AM. The significance of fluid in pleural space: a study of 274 cases. *Proc Mayo Clin* 1945; **20**: 81–7.

7. Leuallen EC, Carr DT. Pleural effusion: a statistical study of 436 patients. *N Engl J Med* 1955; **255**: 79–83.

8. Light RW, MacGregor I, Luchsinger PC, Ball WC. Pleural effusions: the diagnostic separation of transudates and exudates. *Ann Intern Med* 1972; **77**: 507–13.

9. Romero S, Candela A, Martin C, *et al.* Evaluation of different criteria for the separation of pleural transudates from exudates. *Chest* 1993; **104**: 399–404.

10. Jimenez D, Díaz G, Gil D, *et al.* Etiology and prognostic significance of massive pleural effusions. *Respir Med* 2005; **99**: 1183–7.

11. Chen TA, Lo GH, Lai KH. Risk factors for spontaneous bacterial empyema in cirrhotic patients with hydrothorax. *J Chin Med Assoc* 2003; **66**: 579–85.

12. Jhonston RF, Loo RV. Hepatic hydrothorax. *Ann Intern Med* 1964; **61**: 385–401.

13. Lieberman FL, Peters RL. Cirrhotic hydrothorax. *Arch Intern Med* 1970; **125**: 114–17.

14. Esteve M, Xiol X, Fernadez F, *et al.* Treatment and outcome of hydrothorax in liver cirrhosis. *J Clin Nutr Gastroenterol* 1986; **1**: 139–44.

15. Giacobbe A, Facciorusso D, Barbano F, Andriulli A, Frusciante V. Hepatic hydrothorax. Diagnosis and management. *Clin Nucl Med* 1996; **21**: 56–60.

16. Jeffries MA, Kazanjian S, Wilson M, Punch J, Fontana RJ. Transjugular intrahepatic portosystemic shunts and liver transplantation in patients with refractory hepatic hydrothorax. *Liver Transpl Surg* 1998; **4**: 416–23.

17. Siegerstetter V, Deibert P, Ochs A, *et al.* Treatment of refractory hepatic hydrothorax with transjugular portosystemic shunt: long term results in 40 patients. *Eur J Gastroenterol Hepatol* 2001: **13**: 529–34.

18. Xiol X, Castellote J, Cortes-Beut R, *et al.* Usefulness and complications of thoracentesis in cirrhotic patients. *Am J Med* 2001; **111**: 67–9.

19. LeVeen HH, Piccone VA, Hutto RB. Management of ascites with hydrothorax. *Am J Surg* 1984; **148**: 210–13.

20. Ackerman Z, Reynolds TB. Evaluation of pleural fluid in patients with cirrhosis. *J Clin Gastroenterol* 1997; **25**: 619–22.

21. Kinasewitz GT. Transudative effusions. *Eur Respir J* 1997; **10**: 714–18.

22. Strauss RM, Boyer TD. Hepatic hydrothorax. *Sem Liv Dis* 1997; **17**: 227–32.

23. Huang PM, Chang YL, Yang CY, Lee YC. The morphology of diaphragmatic defects in hepatic hydrothorax. *J Thorac Cardiovasc Surg* 2005; **130**: 141–5.

24. Rubinstein D, McInnes IE, Dudley FJ. Hepatic hydrothorax in the absence of clinical ascites: diagnosis and management. *Gastroenterology* 1985; **88**: 188–91

25. Mentes BB, Kayhan B, Gorgul A, Unal S. Hepatic hydrothorax in the absence of ascites. Report of two cases and review of the mechanism. *Dig Dis Sci* 1997; **42**: 781–8.

26. Kataki S, Yoshinaga YT, Takayama OHT, *et al.* Hepatic hydrothorax in the absence of ascites. *Liver* 1998; **18**: 216–20.

27. Castellote J, Gornals J, López C, Xiol X. Acute tension hydrothorax: a life threatening complication of cirrhosis. *J Clin Gastroenterol* 2002; **34**: 588–9.

28. Castellote J, Xiol X, Cortés-Beut R, *et al.* Complicaciones de la toracentesis en pacientes cirróticos con derrame pleural. *Rev Esp Enferm Dig* 2001; **93**: 566–70.

29. McVay PA, Toy PTC. Lack of increased bleeding after paracentesis and thoracentesis in patients with mild coagulation abnormalities. *Transfusion* 1991; **31**: 164–71.

30. Runyon BA. Paracentesis of ascitic fluid. A safe procedure. *Arch Intern Med* 1986; **146**: 2259–61.

31. Mirouze D, Juttner HU, Reynolds TB. Left pleural effusion in patients with chronic liver disease and ascites. *Dig Dis Sci* 1981; **26**: 984–8.

32. Light R. Pleural effusion. *N Engl J Med* 2002; **346**: 1971–7.

33. Sahn S. The pleura. *Am Rev Respir Dis* 1988; **138**: 184–234

●34. Sese E, Xiol X, Castellote J, Rodríguez-Fariñas E, Tremosa G. Low complement levels and opsonic activity in hepatic hydrothorax. Its relationship with spontaneous bacterial empyema. *J Clin Gastroenterol* 2003; **36**: 75–7.

35. Light RW. Diagnostic principles in pleural disease. *Eur Respir J* 1997; **10**: 476–81.

36. Romero S, Fernandez C, Martin C, *et al.* Influence of diuretics on the concentration of proteins and other components of pleural transudates in patients with heart failure. *Am J Med* 2001; **110**: 681–6.

37. Tremosa G, Xiol X, Rodríguez E, *et al.* Valor del gradiente de albúmina en el diagnóstico diferencial de los derrames pleurales asociados a cirrosis hepática (abst). *Gastreonterologia y Hepatologia* 2002; **25**: 113–14.

38. Zenda T, Miyamoto S, Murata S, Mabuchi H. Detection of diaphragmatic defect as the cause of severe hepatic hydrothorax with magnetic resonance. *AJR Am J Roentgenol* 1998; **93**: 2288–9.

39. Arroyo V, Gines P, Gerbes AL, *et al.* Definition and diagnostic criteria of refractory ascites and hepatorenal syndrome in cirrhosis. *Hepatology* 1996; **23**: 164–73.

40. Chalasani N, Clark WS, Martin LG, *et al.* Determinants of mortality in patients with advanced cirrhosis after transjugular intrahepatic portosystemic shunting. *Gastroenterology* 2000; **118**: 138–44.

41. Runyon BA. Paracentesis of ascitic fluid. A safe procedure. *Arch Intern Med* 1996; **124**: 816–20.

42. McVay PA, Toy PTC. Lack of increased bleeding after paracentesis and thoracentesis in patients with mild coagulation annormalities. *Transfusion* 1991; **31**: 164–71.

43. Trachiotis GD, Vricella LA, Aaron BL, Hix WR. As originally published in 1988: Reexpansion pulmonary edema. Updated 1997. *Ann Thorac Surg* 1997; **4**: 1206–7.

44. Runyon BA, Greenblatt M, Ming HC. Hepatic hydrothorax is a relative contraindication to chest tube insertion. *Am J Gastroenterol* 1986; **7**: 566–7.

45. Liu LU, Haddadin HA, Bodian CA, *et al.* Outcome analysis of cirrhotic patients undergoing chest tube placement. *Chest* 2004; **126**: 142–8.

46. Dumortier J, Lepetre J, Scalone O, *et al.* Succesful treatment of hepatic hydrothorax with octreotide. *Eur J Gastroenterol Hepatol* 2000; **12**: 817–20.

47. Ibrisim D, Cakaloglu Y, Akyuz F, *et al.* Treatment of hepatic hydrothorax with terlipressin in a cirrhotic patient. *Scand J Gastroenterol* 2006; **41**: 862–5.
48. Cantó A, Gonzalez A, Moya J, *et al.* La pleurodesis con talco en los derrames pleurales masivos y recidivantes de las cirrosis hepáticas. *Arch Bronconeumol* 1989; **25**: 256–8.
49. Ferrante D, Arguedas M, Cerfolio RJ, *et al.* Video-assisted thoracoscopy surgery with talc pleurodesis in the management of symptomatic hepatic hydrothorax. *Am J Gastroenterol* 2002; **97**: 3172–5.
50. Cerfolio RJ, Bryant AS. Efficacy of video-assisted thoracocscopic surgery with talc pleurodesis for porous diaphragm syndrome in patients with refractory hepatic hydrothorax. *Ann Thorac Surg* 2006; **82**: 457–9.
51. Drohuin F, Fischer D, Law Koune D, *et al.* Traitement des hydrothorax des cirrhoses par pleurodèse chimique associeé à une ventilation avec pression positive continue. Résultats préliminaires. *Gastroenterol Clin Biol* 1991; **15**: 271–2.
52. Takahashi K, Chin K, Sumi K, *et al.* Resistant hepatic hydrothorax: a succesful case with treatmeny by nCPAP. *Respir Med* 2005; **99**: 262–4.
53. Hadsaitong D, Suttithawil W. Pleurovenous shunt in treating refractory nonmalignant hepatic hydrothorax: a case report. *Respir Med* 2005; **99**: 1603–5.
*54. Mouroux J, Perrin C, Venissac N, Blaive B, Richelme H. Management of pleural effusion of cirrhotic origin. *Chest* 1996; **109**: 1093–6.
55. De Campos JRM, Filho LO, Werebe EC, *et al.* Thoracoscopy and talc poudrage in the management of hepatic hydrothorax. *Chest* 2000; **118**: 13–17.
56. Kirsch CM. Cirrhotic hydrothorax and the law of unintended consequences. *Chest* 2000; **118**: 2–4.
57. Huang PM, Kuo SW, Lee JM. Thoracoscopic diaphragmatic repair for refractory hepatic hydrothorax: application of pleural flap and mesh onlay reinforcement. *Thorac Cardiov Surg* 2006; **54**: 47–50.
58. Andrade RJ, Martin-Palanca A, Fraile JM, *et al.* Transjugular intrahepatic portosystemic shunt for the management of hepatic hydrothorax in absence of ascites. *J Clin Gastroenterol* 1996; **22**: 305–7
*59. Strauss RM, Martin LG, Kaufman SL, Boyer TD. Transjugular intrahepatic portal systemic shunt for the management of symptomatic cirrhotic hydrothorax. *Am J Gastroenterol* 1994; **89**: 1520–2.
60. Gordon FD, Anastopoulos HT, Crenshaw W, *et al.* The successful treatment of symptomatic refractory hepatic hydrothorax with transjugular intrahepatic portosystemic shunt. *Hepatology* 1997; **25**: 1366–9.
61. Spencer EB, Cohen DT, Darcy MD. Safety and efficacy of transjugular intrahepatic portosystemic shunt creation for the treatment of hepatic hydrothorax. *J Vasc Interv Radiol* 2002; **13**: 385–90.
62. Nuñez O, Garcia A, Rincón D, *et al.* Derivación portosistémica percutanea intrahepática como tratamiento del hidrotórax hepático refractario. *Gastroenterol Hepatol* 2002; **25**: 143–7.
63. Salerno F, Merli M, Cazzaniga M, *et al.* MELD score is better than Child–Pugh score in predicting 3-month survival of patients undergoing transjugular intrahepatic portosystemic shunt. *J Hepatol* 2002; **36**: 494–500.
●64. Xiol X, Tremosa G, Castellote J, *et al.* Liver transplantation in patients with hepatic hydrothorax. *Transpl Int* 2005; **18**: 672–5.
◆65. Strauss RM, Boyer TD. Diagnosis and management of cirrhotic ascites. In: Zakim D, Boyer TD (eds). *Hepatology: a textbook of liver disease.* Philadelphia: WB Saunders Co, 1996: 764–88.
66. Chesta J, Ponichik J, Brahm J, *et al.* Spontaneous bacterial pleuritis in patients with liver cirrhosis. *Rev Med Chile* 1991; **119**: 295–8.
67. Malnick SDH, Somin M, Zimchoni SO, Sthoeger ZM. Spontaneous bacterial empyema in a patient with hepatitis C virus cirrhosis and sterile ascitic fluid. *Clin Infect Dis* 1996; **23**: 834–5.
68. Abba A, Laajam MA, Zargar SA. Spontaneous neutrocytic hepatic hydrothorax without ascites. *Respir* Med 1996; **90**: 631–4.
69. Castellote J, Lopez C, Gornals J, *et al.* Rapid diagnosis of spontaneous bacterial peritonitis by use of reagent strips. *Hepatology* 2003; **37**: 893–6.
70. Castellote J, Lopez C, Gornals J, *et al.* Use of reagent strips for the diagnosis of spontaneous bacterial empyema. *J Clin Gastroenterol* 2005; **39**: 278–81.
71. Sort P, Navasa M, Arroyo V, *et al.* Effect of intravenous albumin on renal imparment and mortality in patients with cirrhosis and spontaneous bacterial peritonitis. *N Eng J Med* 1999; **341**: 403–9.
72. Costello-Boerrigter LC, Boerrigter G, Burnett JC Jr. Revisiting salt and water retention: new diuretics, aquaretics and natriuretics. *Med Clin North Am* 2003; **87**: 475–91.

36

Effusions caused by gastrointestinal disease

CHARLIE STRANGE

INTRODUCTION

A variety of pleural effusions arise from diseases below the diaphragm. Usually caused by diseases of the upper abdomen, these effusions can provide diagnostic and prognostic assistance to disease management. The pleural space is anatomically only a few millimeters away from the abdomen, separated by the muscular and tendenous portions of the diaphragms. Since small lymphatics cross the diaphragm, any abdominal fluid collection that contacts the abdominal side of the diaphragm can cause pleural fluid to develop. In addition, any diaphragmatic disruption by surgery, catheters or trauma will allow fluid to reach the pleural space through the diaphragm.

Some effusions from abdominal diseases arise from above the diaphragm. Because the muscular portion of the diaphragm is richly vascularized, it may become inflamed. Therefore, abdominal events that affect the inferior aspect of the diaphragm can cause sufficient vascular inflammation on the thoracic side of the diaphragm to exude pleural fluid. These 'sympathetic' pleural effusions may result if pleural fluid production is high, resorption through parietal pleural lymphatics is low or if pain from the upper abdominal process produces pleuritic pain sufficient to cause atelectasis. Since small pleural effusions have been associated with atelectasis, the differentiation between pulmonary and diaphragmatic source of effusion in these patients remains unknown and clinically academic.

This chapter will focus on the gastrointestinal and abdominal illnesses that have been shown to produce pleural effusions. In an organ-by-organ approach, the infections and inflammatory disorders that arise will be addressed to describe the typical clinical presentation, diagnostic evaluation and therapeutic options. Hepatic hydrothorax and post-operative effusions have been addressed in another chapter.

PANCREATIC DISEASE

Pancreatitis is the most common gastrointestinal disease that causes pleural effusions. In acute pancreatitis, inflammatory pancreatic exudate enters the surrounding lymphatics that are part of the plexus of subperitoneal and subdiaphagmatic lymphatics that communicate with the pleural space through the diaphragm. Since pleural fluid amylase is higher than serum amylase in acute pancreatitis, these lymphatics must be participating in transfer of pancreatic exudate to the pleural space.

Pancreatitis is now known to occur from more than 50 causes and diagnosis can be extremely difficult, particularly in patients with chronic disease in which amylase elevations can be small or non-existent. The inflamed pancreas varies in the intensity of inflammation from mild disease to frank necrosis with intraglandular hemorrhage.

Clinically significant pleural effusions on chest radiography are seen in approximately 4–17 percent of cases of acute pancreatitis. However, pleural effusions are much more common if computed tomography (CT) is used, being found in 50 percent of a recent series of 133 patients within 72 hours of presentation.[1] Pleural effusions often are accompanied by peritoneal fluid or pericarditis.[2] These effusions are often too small to sample and resolve when the pancreatitis abates. They are invariably gone in 2 months or less.[2] These effusions are exudates with a neutrophil predominance and can have significant numbers of red blood cells. Pleural fluid amylase can be normal but as disease progresses usually becomes greater than two times the blood amylase.[3,4] Left-sided effusions are more common than bilateral or unilateral right effusions.

The presence of a pleural effusion has recently transitioned from being a marker of disease to becoming a key indicator of the severity of pancreatitis. Effusions are more commonly seen with pancreatic necrosis (Balthazar's score D and E).[5] By including the presence or absence of a pleural effusion, a newly proposed EPIC scoring system (ExtraPancreatic Inflammation on CT score)[6] has superior receiver operating characteristic scores to predict morbidity and mortality than other scoring systems that grade the severity of pancreatic injury alone. Although the effusions in acute pancreatitis are usually small, their importance is large since systemic inflammation, diaphragmatic inflammation, associated pulmonary atelectasis or early acute respiratory distress syndrome (ARDS) are the proposed mechanisms for pleural fluid formation.

The second form of pancreatic pleural effusion occurs with disruption of the pancreatic duct. Most commonly, this abnormality presents with chronic pancreatitis with ductal stenosis or stones but can also occur after pancreatic surgery, intraductal tumors[7] or trauma. Anterior fluid collections may rupture through the omentum and cause pancreatic ascites. Posterior rupture places fluid in the retroperitoneal space where it can reach the pleural space. Importantly, these fistulae continue to advance until pancreatic output is slowed, pancreatic ductal drainage is reestablished, or the area of abnormality is surgically resected. Pancreatograms performed during endoscopic retrograde cholangiopancreatography (ERCP) can demonstrate these fistulae and on occasion the contrast material can reflux into the pleural space. As would be expected, the amylase concentrations in the pleural fluid are extremely high with this condition, often reaching values greater than 100 000 IU/mL.

Occasionally, a pancreatic pseudocyst migrates toward the diaphragmatic surface without rupture. Although intact pseudocysts can migrate into the mediastinum, or rarely into the pleural space and present as mass lesions, more commonly the cyst leaks or ruptures into the subdiaphagmatic, mediastinal or pleural space. Rare ruptures into the airways have been described.[8,9] Because the pleural space is under negative pressure, migration of pseudocyst fluid into the pleural space is often the path of least resistance. Because the pseudocyst fluid is extremely caustic and impaired pancreatic drainage creates a continuous supply of pancreatic fluid, conditions are ripe for fistula formation.

A pleural effusion can be the initial manifestation of a pancreatopleural fistula.[10] Interestingly, many patients have few if any abdominal symptoms.[11] For that reason, the diagnosis can be missed if a pleural fluid amylase is not obtained. Although serum amylase is elevated in this condition, it may be only mildly so, since the majority of ductal drainage is released into the pleural space. Pleural fluid from pseudocysts or pancreatic fistulae is always exudative with a neutrophil-rich fluid. Bloody effusions can be associated with pleural fluid eosinophilia.[12]

Fistulae between the pancreatic body and the pleural space release large amounts of amylase-rich pancreatic fluid into the pleural space. The effusions are often large, filling one-half of the hemithorax. Right-sided pancreatopleural effusions have been described with fistulae that traverse the mediastinum where the esophagus penetrates the diaphragm before entry into the pleural space through the mediastinal pleura. Large bilateral effusions also have been seen.[13]

It should be remembered that other conditions cause pleural fluid to have high amylase levels. Benign conditions include esophageal rupture, tuberculosis and cirrhosis.[14] Rarely, pleural fluid amylase may be elevated in pneumonia.[15] Malignant effusions metastatic from many organs have been described that produce salivary amylase. In the setting of amylase-rich peritoneal fluid, the possibility of ovarian carcinoma or ectopic pregnancy should not be forgotten.[16]

Successful therapy of pancreatic fistulae with or without pseudocyst has most readily been obtained by 2–4 weeks of pancreatic rest, hyperalimentation and serial thoracentesis that is successful approximately 50 percent of the time.[17,18] No specific therapy is necessary for the pleural space. Endoscopic management by stenting of the pancreatic duct is possible in some cases.[19] Successful treatment series using nasopancreatic drains placed by ERCP have been reported. This modality allows for serial imaging by fistulograms through the nasal side of the tube.[20,21] Ligation of the fistula,[22] radiation of the fistula[23] and subtotal pancreatectomy have been used in some case series.

Pancreatic abscess is a rare complication of acute pancreatitis that occurs in approximately 4 percent of cases. Secondary infection of a pseudocyst can produce a similarly severe condition. Delays in abscess drainage may be fatal. Pleural effusions occurred in 39 percent of a series of 63 patients with pancreatic abscess and contributed to significant morbidity and mortality in these cases.[24]

SPLENIC DISEASES

Splenic infarctions, splenic hematomas and splenic abscesses often produce pleural effusions. These effusions are always left-sided and often accompanied by pleuritic pain. The effusions are usually small, neutrophil-rich exudates that require no specific therapy. Yet, recognition of the underlying diagnosis does make a difference. Rare presentations with tumors of the spleen, epidermoid cysts,[25] splenic vein thrombosis[26] and primary rupture of the spleen with amyloidosis have been associated with pleural effusions.

Splenic abscess is a rare condition that occurs in a variety of situations. *Clostridium perfringens* abscesses have been described in patients with sickle cell anemia and intravenous drug use.[27] Other causes have included trauma, infection in contiguous areas and endocarditis. Rare splenic abscesses with tuberculosis[28] have been described.

Splenic hematomas usually are formed from trauma. Yet, pleural effusions associated with a subphrenic hematoma may be distant from the time of trauma.[29] Some patients may not volunteer the trauma history since minor trauma can cause splenic hematomas. Rarely, splenic subcapsular hematomas from pancreatitis, associated with pleural effusions have been described.[30] Pleural fluid may or may not be hemorrhagic in this condition and usually resolves spontaneously over 2 weeks while the hematoma can persist for a longer time.[31]

Splenic infarctions result from vascular obstruction. The splenic arteries are single end arteries without significant collateral circulation. This anatomical arrangement makes the spleen particularly susceptible to sickle cell occlusion that may occur in unusual settings such as in sickle cell heterozygotes at altitude.[32] Therapeutic splenic infarction by embolization has been used to control the hypersplenism of cirrhosis. When 80 percent of the spleen is infarcted, pleural effusions are common.[33] Splenic infarction associated pleural effusions are usually small.

Other causes of splenomegaly may also be associated with pleural effusions. Castleman's disease, sarcoidosis and lymphomas would fit in this category.

ESOPHAGEAL RUPTURE

Esophageal rupture is usually associated with trauma, often from endoscopy or surgery. Spontaneous esophageal rupture is a rare disease usually seen after protracted vomiting but may be seen as a complication of esophageal carcinoma, perforation of Barrett's ulcer, intensive radiation therapy, esophageal Crohn's disease,[34] herpetic esophagitis[35] or tuberculous esophagitis.[36] Delayed recognition of this disease is common, accounting for significant morbidity and mortality.

Iatrogenic rupture following dilation procedures for esophageal stricture is the most common cause of rupture.[37] Other endoscopic procedures in which pleural effusions have been described include the removal of foreign bodies and sclerosis of esophageal varices.[38] The hallmark symptom of chest pain that is persistent for a few hours after the procedure should be followed by a contrast esophagram to establish the diagnosis, the discontinuation of oral feeding and the administration of antibiotics.

Traumatic or post-surgical esophageal perforation occurs from a variety of esophageal insults. Surgeries for esophageal carcinoma are prone to leakage at the primary anastamotic site; occasionally the esophagus is injured during other thoracic operations.[39] Rarely, blunt trauma may rupture the esophagus as may occur following a Heimlich maneuver[40] or automobile accidents.

The gastroesophageal junction lies adjacent to the mediastinal pleura. Esophageal rupture from any cause may allow esophageal fluids access to the mediastinum. Since the esophageal mucosa is not sterile, the introduction of bacteria into the mediastinum and pleural space is associated with mediastinitis and empyema, respectively. Although some case series have suggested that mediastinitis without pleural rupture carries a better prognosis, the difference in time to recognition and initiation of appropriate therapy is likely the most important factor in this observation. Most of the morbidity of esophageal perforation occurs as a consequence of infectious mediastinitis, usually with a combination of aerobic and anaerobic pathogens.[41] When pleural effusions develop, they usually need drainage since most qualify as empyemas.

Pleural fluid characteristics reflect the origin of the fluid. Pleural fluid amylase is elevated and, when fractionated, is of salivary origin. A rare case of normal pleural amylase in a patient with Sjögren's syndrome has been described.[42] Pleural fluid pH is low even if gastric pH is pharmacologically raised. This suggests that the low pH is from products of bacterial metabolism and polymorphonuclear neutrophil (PMN) sequestration in the pleural space.[43] Effusions can be large and either unilateral or bilateral; isolated right effusions are uncommon. When the etiology of pleural fluid is unclear, cytology for foodstuff can be helpful.[44]

Diagnosis should be made as quickly as possible. Any history of retching or esophageal procedures should prompt evaluation for esophageal rupture if any pulmonary symptoms are present. Corticosteroids may alter the clinical presentation by preventing fever and chest pain.[45] An upright chest radiograph should evaluate whether pleural fluid is present and whether air is in the mediastinum. Plain radiographs often give hints about the site of esophageal perforation. Left hydropneumothorax is commonly seen with perforation of the lower esophagus. Right-sided effusions usually occur after perforation of the mid-esophagus.[46] Plain films have been recorded as normal in 12 percent of cases in one series.[46] Computerized tomography is more sensitive and specific for mediastinal fluid collections and mediastinal air.[47]

The diagnostic test of choice is an esophagram. Small esophageal perforations can only be detected by contrast-enhanced swallowing studies. In larger perforations, operative planning can be aided by site-specific information. An initial esophagram should be performed with a water-soluble contrast agent since some esophageal leaks are quite large. If negative, a barium swallow should follow the water-soluble contrast study. The higher radiodensity of the barium allows for more sensitive detection of esophageal perforations. In one series of suspected esophageal perforation, 15 percent of perforations were missed by a water-soluble contrast agent.[48]

Therapy of this disorder remains controversial. For perforations that are small and recognized at the time of occurrence, antibiotics and strict avoidance of oral intake may allow primary closure. If pleural fluid is present it should receive chest tube drainage or complete thoracentesis. Following a dilation procedure and early diagnosis, a conservative treatment regimen is usually successful.

Late presentations with mediastinitis or empyema requires more intensive interventions.[49] The primary question is whether surgical resection of the involved esophagus is superior to esophageal repair. No randomized studies have been performed although retrospective series have suggested that resection is associated with higher survival rates.[50,51] In addition, surgical debridement, chest drains, esophageal wraps with omentum or muscle pedicles and T-tube drainage have been used.[52,53] Some patients with sepsis or significant co-morbidities may be candidates for covered stent placement, percutaneous drainage of large fluid collections and antibiotic therapy.[54]

Rarely, other diagnoses can present with esophageal rupture and need specific management. Esophageal carcinoma with fistulae may require surgery or stenting,[55] strangulated hiatal hernias require surgery and rare congenital malformations of the esophagus need targeted therapy. Anaerobic mediastinitis also occurs rarely after pharyngeal perforations or dental procedures.[56]

GASTRIC DISEASES

Abnormalities of the stomach rarely cause effusions. One exception is gastric lymphoma that may present with a lymphomatous effusion. The other gastric lesion that can present with a pleural empyema is gastric carcinoma. Since the stomach is immediately subjacent the left pleural space, carcinoma of the greater curvature can create a fistula to the pleural space. When sampled, the pleural fluid is acidic, discolored and may contain bacteria. Cases in which primary therapy has been initiated for empyema without recognizing the primary cause of this lesion have been described. Rarely, traumatic rupture of the stomach has been shown to produce amylase-rich pleural effusions.[57,58]

DISEASES OF THE SMALL AND LARGE INTESTINES

The few diseases of the intestines that are associated with pleural effusions are those that cause such significant hypoproteinemia that a transudative effusion develops. Clinically, an effusion rarely presents before albumin concentrations are <1.8 g/dL. Such diseases include Menetrier's disease,[59] HIV enteropathy and severe Crohn's disease.

Fistulae between the colon and the lung have been described rarely in Crohn's disease. Typically, these occur at the splenic flexure of the colon.[60]

DIAPHRAGMATIC RUPTURE

Rupture of the diaphragm usually occurs after trauma. The diagnosis is not often missed since bowel loops on radiography in the chest are prominent, particularly on chest CT. However, the surgeon evaluating the condition should recognize the potential for other disorders that are similar, such as hernias of the foramen of Bochdalek.[61]

GALLBLADDER DISEASES

Disease of the biliary tract is responsible for some pleural effusions. The most common pleural effusion from the gallbladder is a sympathetic effusion in the first 24 hours after cholecystectomy that has been found in one-third of patients.[62] Empyema of the gallbladder is often an indolent infection that can lead to both local and distant fluid collections. Fistulae that begin at the gallbladder bed can directly communicate with the pleural space. These biliopleural fistulae can be quite large with the most dramatic presentations being gallstones in the pleural space[63,64] or communicating with the airways with expectoration of gallstones.[65]

Biliopleural effusions also accompany transhepatic biliary drainage for biliary tract obstruction. Since transhepatic catheters invariably cross the pleural space in the costal recess, any catheter malfunction runs the risk of bile entering the pleural space. The diagnosis at time of bile leakage is established by pleural fluid bilirubin concentrations higher than serum values. Animal models have suggested that bilirubin is rapidly absorbed from the pleural space although a neutrophilic exudative inflammatory effusion persists.[66]

HEPATIC AND UPPER ABDOMINAL ABSCESSES

A number of infectious abscesses may complicate the upper abdomen. All are serious clinical problems with a high incidence of pleural fluid complicating disease. Subphrenic abscesses occur in the right subhepatic space, right suprahepatic space, left subdiaphragmatic space or lesser sac. In one series of 60 patients, abscesses that touched the diaphragm were associated with effusions 100 percent of the time.[67] These subphrenic abscesses are often of mixed bacterial flora with a prominent anaerobic complement of organisms including *Bacteroides* species.

Hepatic abscesses often cause pleural effusions. In the setting of diarrhea, the possibility of amebic liver abscess should be considered. The natural history of this infection begins with intestinal infection with *Entamoeba histolytica*. When the trophozoite traverses the intestinal wall, it travels through the portal system and lodges in the liver. Pleural effusions and pleuritic chest pain are common and may be the presenting manifestation of disease.[68] Cases of amebic empyema may result from rupture of liver abscess into the pleural space.

Pyogenic liver abscesses can occur with many organisms although *Escherichia coli* is the most frequent pathogen. Antibiotics alone are associated with mortality as high as 95 percent. Percutaneous drainage of abscesses under CT imaging allows for culture and improves survival.[69]

Pleural fluid analysis usually reveals a neutrophil predominant exudate without infectious organisms present. Effusions are typically small but may become large if the abscess ruptures into the pleural space creating an empyema.

INFLAMMATORY LIVER DISEASES

Exudative pleural effusions have been rarely seen with Hepatitis B infection. In a series of 2500 patients, effusions were documented in four cases.[70] Hepatitis B surface antigen and e-antigen have been detected in pleural fluid that is typically lymphocyte predominant.[71]

Effusions also accompany some rare infections of the liver. Hepatic hemorrhage occurs from dengue fever[72] where effusions are more common in severe disease.[73,74] Pleural effusions have also been noted in *Hantavirus* infections whose severity is correlated with gallbladder wall thickness.[75] Effusions have also been seen with chronic active *Epstein–Barr virus* infections that cause hepatomegaly and gallbladder wall thickening.[76] Non-infectious causes of inflammatory hepatic effusions include those following transhepatic catheter ablations of hepatomas.[77]

GENERALIZED APPROACH TO THERAPY

When pleural effusions are associated with pain in the abdomen at any location, both disorders should be evaluated. The pleural fluid evaluation begins with thoracentesis. Although pleural fluid amylase was rarely diagnostic in a large series of pleural effusions,[78] these studies did not select patients with concomitant abdominal disease. The pleural fluid characteristics of gastrointestinal disorders are shown in Table 36.1.

Table 36.1 Characteristics of common pleural effusions of gastrointestinal origin

	Characteristics	WBC (per μL)	Pleural amylase	Comments
Biliopleural fistula	PMN predominant exudate	1000–15 000 rarely pus	PF = serum	PF/serum bilirubin >1 while fistula is open; effusion becomes non-specific exudate when fistula closes
Esophageal rupture	Exudative, usually with pus or positive PF cultures	>10 000 occasionally pus	Elevated	Morbidity secondary to empyema. Pneumothorax seen in up to 25%. Surgical correction of esophageal leak often needed
Hepatitis	Mononuclear predominant exudate	<1000	PF = serum	Rare, spontaneously resolves. Consider unusual causes of hepatitis if effusion is significant in size
Pancreatitis	PMN predominant exudate	1000–50 000	>2× serum	Occasionally hemorrhagic. No specific therapy needed. Always resolves within 2 months
Pancreatic fistula	PMN predominant exudate	<10 000	Often >100 000	ERCP and abdominal CT indicated to determine site of fistula. Nasopancreatic catheter may allow serial fistulograms
Splenic infarction	PMN predominant exudate	<10 000	PF = serum	Usually associated with pleuritic chest pain. Occasionally hemorrhagic. Spontaneously resolves
Upper abdominal and hepatic abscesses	PMN predominant exudate	1000–50 000 occasionally pus	PF = serum	Anchovy paste pleural effusion has been described with amebic abscesses. Contrast-enhanced CT essential for site-specific localization of pathology

Abbreviations: CT, computed tomography; ERCP, endoscopic retrograde cholangiopancreatography; IU, international units; PF, pleural fluid; PMN, polymorphonuclear neutrophil; WBC, white blood cell count.

The differentiation of fluid collections in the upper abdomen, including peritioneal fluid from pleural fluid, requires a careful evaluation of the abdominal CT scan. One of the best differentiations occurs from an evaluation of the fluid interface at the diaphragmatic surface. Because of diaphragmatic movement, the interface between pleural effusions and the diaphragm is usually a hazy one. Alternatively, the interface between peritoneal fluid and the spleen is usually sharp.[79] In addition, pleural fluid is usually located posteromedially in the lower chest while peritoneal fluid is most often maximal in a posterolateral distribution, lateral to the liver and spleen.[80]

SUMMARY

The variety of causes of pleural effusions from gastrointestinal sources in the mediastinum and abdomen makes recognition of these disorders very difficult.[81] Once recognized, the therapy of each of these diseases usually requires specialty consultation from gastroenterologists and thoracic or general surgeons. Therapy of pleural effusions of gastrointestinal origin involves correcting the gastrointestinal problem. Although many disorders such as splenic infarctions or hepatitis B may be self-limited, others require specific therapy only recognized after establishing the correct diagnosis.

KEY POINTS

- Inflammation of most of the organs of the upper abdomen cause pleural effusions.
- Pleural fluid amylase should be obtained when an undiagnosed effusion persists.
- An esophagram is the diagnostic test of choice for suspected esophageal rupture. A water-soluble contrast agent should be followed by barium sulfate to definitively exclude the diagnosis.
- Gastrointestinal sources should be considered when empyema thoracis is diagnosed. A contrasted CT that includes the upper abdomen should be performed.
- Transhepatic biliary drainage catheters usually cross the pleural space. Catheter dysfunction may allow biliary fluid to leak into the pleural space. Pleural fluid bilirubin is higher than serum bilirubin transiently in this condition.
- Pancreatitis-associated pleural effusions are common and often respond to conservative therapy. Important diagnoses to exclude include pancreatic abscess and pancreatopleural fistula.

REFERENCES

● = Key primary paper
◆ = Major review article

1. Lankisch PG, Droge M, Becher R. Pleural effusions: a new negative prognostic parameter for acute pancreatitis. *Am J Gastroenterol* 1994; **89** 1849–51.
●2. Maringhini A, Ciambra M, Patti R, *et al.* Ascites, pleural, and pericardial effusions in acute pancreatitis. A prospective study of incidence, natural history, and prognostic role. *Dig Dis Sci* 1996; **41**: 848–52.
◆3. Lorch DG, Sahn SA. Pleural effusions due to diseases below the diaphragm. *Seminars Respir Med* 1987; **9**: 75–85.
4. Dewan NA, Kinney WM, O'Donahue WJ. Chronic massive pancreatic pleural effusion. *Chest* 1984; **85**: 497–500.
●5. Balthazar EJ, Ranson JH, Naidich DP, *et al.* Acute pancreatitis: prognostic value of CT. *Radiology* 198; **156**: 767–72.
●6. De Waele JJ, Delrue L, Hoste EA, *et al.* Extrapancreatic inflammation on abdominal computed tomography as an early predictor of disease severity in acute pancreatitis: evaluation of a new scoring system. *Pancreas* 2007; **34**: 185–90.
7. England DW, Kurrein F, Jones EL, Windsor CW. Pancreatic pleural effusion associated with oncocytic carcinoma of the pancreas. *Postgrad Med J* 1988; **64**: 465–6.
8. Christensen NM, Demling R, Mathewson C Jr. Unusual manifestations of pancreatic pseudocysts and their surgical management. *Am J Surg* 1973; **130**: 199–205.
9. Iglehart JD, Mansback C, Postlethwait R, Roberts L Jr, Ruth W. Pancreaticobronchial fistula. Case report and review of the literature. *Gastroenterology* 1986; **90**: 759–63.
10. Hyman PE, Brennan MF, Head G, McCarthy DM. Hyperamylasemia, duodenal duplication, and pleural effusions in hereditary spherocytosis. *Dig Dis Sci* 1981; **26**: 81–4.
11. Cameron JL. Chronic pancreatic ascites and pancreatic pleural effusions. *Gastroenterology* 1978; **74**: 134–40.
12. Masuda K, Ishioka S, Okusaki K, *et al.* A case of eosinophilic pleural effusion induced by pancreatothoracic fistula. *Hiroshima J Med Sci* 2000; **49**: 97–100.
13. Miridjanian A, Ambruoso VN, Derby BM, Tice DA. Massive bilateral hemorrhagic pleural effusions in chronic relapsing pancreatitis. *Arch Surg* 1969; **98**: 62–6.
●14. Villena V, Perez V, Pozo F, *et al.* Amylase levels in pleural effusions: a consecutive unselected series of 841 patients. *Chest* 2002; **121**: 470–4.
●15. Light RW, Ball WC. Glucose and amylase in pleural effusions. *J Am Med Assoc* 1973; **225**: 257–60.
16. Corlette MB, Dratch M, Sorger K. Amylase elevation attributable to an ovarian neoplasm. *Gastroenterology* 1978; **74**: 907–9.
17. Cameron JL, Kieffer RS, Anderson WJ, Zuidema GD. Internal pancreatic fistulas: pancreatic ascites and pleural effusions. *Ann Surg* 1976; **184**: 587–93.
18. Rockey DC, Cello JP. Pancreaticopleural fistula. Report of 7 patients and review of the literature. *Medicine (Baltimore)* 1990; **69**: 332–44.
19. Safadi BY, Marks JM. Pancreatic-pleural fistula: the role of ERCP in diagnosis and treatment. *Gastrointest Endosc* 2000; **51**: 213–5.
20. Brelvi ZS, Jonas ME, Trotman BW, *et al.* Nasopancreatic drainage: a novel approach for treating internal pancreatic fistulas and pseudocysts. *J Assoc Acad Minor Phys* 1996; **7**: 41–6.
21. Bhasin DK, Rana SS, Siyad I, *et al.* Endoscopic transpapillary nasopancreatic drainage alone to treat pancreatic ascites and pleural effusion. *J Gastroenterol Hepatol* 2006; **21**: 1059–64.
22. Greiner L, Prohm P. Pancreatico-pleural fistula with chronic pleural effusion-endoscopic- retrograde visualization and therapy by ultrasonically-guided drainage. *Endoscopy* 1983; **15**: 73–4.

23. Greenwald RA, Deluca RF, Raskin JB. Pancreatic–pleural fistula: demonstration by endoscopic retrograde cholangiopancreatography (ERCP) and successful treatment with radiation therapy. *Dig Dis Sci* 1979; **24**: 240–4.
24. Miller TA, Lindenauer SM, Frey CF, Stanley JC. Pancreatic abscess. *Arch Surg* 1974; **108**: 545–50.
25. Caillet B, Hakim F, Perol M, Bayle JY, Guerin JC. [A rare cause of pleurisy from subdiaphragmatic origin: epidermoid cyst of the spleen]. *Rev Pneumol Clin* 1990; **46**: 114–5.
26. Warren MS, Gibbons RB. Left-sided pleural effusion secondary to splenic vein thrombosis. A previously unrecognized relationship. *Chest* 1991; **100**: 574–5.
27. Gangahar DM, Delany HM. Intrasplenic abscess: two case reports and review of the literature. *Am Surg* 1981; **47**: 488–91.
28. Aubry P, Reynaud JP, Nbonyingingo C, Ndabaneze E, Mucikere E. [Ultrasonographic data of the solid organs of the abdomen in stage IV human immunodeficiency virus infection. A prospective study of 101 cases in central Africa]. *Ann Gastroenterol Hepatol (Paris)* 1994; **30**: 43–52.
29. Koehler PR, Jones R. Association of left-sided pleural effusions and splenic hematomas. *AJR Am J Roentgenol* 1980; **135**: 851–3.
30. Vitaux J, Theodore C, Molas G, *et al.* [Subcapsular haematoma of the spleen as complication of chronic pancreatitis. Contribution of echotomography to the diagnosis in two cases (author's transl)]. *Nouv Presse Med* 1981; **10**: 495–8.
31. Lupien C, Sauerbrei EE. Healing in the traumatized spleen: sonographic investigation. *Radiology* 1984; **151**: 181–5.
32. Cox RE. Splenic infarct in a white man with sickle cell trait. *Ann Emerg Med* 1982; **11**: 668–9.
33. Hirai K, Kawazoe Y, Yamashita K, *et al.* Transcatheter partial splenic arterial embolization in patients with hypersplenism: a clinical evaluation as supporting therapy for hepatocellular carcinoma and liver cirrhosis. *Hepatogastroenterology* 1986; **33**: 105–8.
34. Cosme A, Bujanda L, Arriola JA, Ojeda E. Esophageal Crohn's disease with esophagopleural fistula. *Endoscopy* 1998; **30**: S109.
35. Cronstedt JL, Bouchama A, Hainau B, *et al.* Spontaneous esophageal perforation in herpes simplex esophagitis. *Am J Gastroenterol* 1992; **87**: 124–7.
36. Ramo OJ, Salo JA, Isolauri J, Luostarinen M, Mattila SP. Tuberculous fistula of the esophagus. *Ann Thorac Surg* 1996; **62**: 1030–2.
37. Avanoglu A, Ergun O, Mutaf O. Management of instrumental perforations of the esophagus occurring during treatment of corrosive strictures. *J Pediatr Surg* 1998; **33**: 1393–5.
38. Bacon BR, Camara DS, Duffy MC. Severe ulceration and delayed perforation of the esophagus after endoscopic variceal sclerotherapy. *Gastrointest Endosc* 1987; **33**: 311–5.
39. Massard G, Ducrocq X, Hentz JG, *et al.* Esophagopleural fistula: an early and long-term complication after pneumonectomy. *Ann Thorac Surg* 1994; **58**: 1437–40; discussion 41.
40. Haynes DE, Haynes BE, Yong YV. Esophageal rupture complicating Heimlich maneuver. *Am J Emerg Med* 1984; **2**: 507–9.
●41. Maulitz RM, Good JT Jr, Kaplan RL, Reller LB, Sahn SA. The pleuropulmonary consequences of esophageal rupture: an experimental model. *Am Rev Respir Dis* 1979; **120**: 363–7.
42. Rudin JS, Ellrodt AG, Phillips EH. Low pleural fluid amylase associated with spontaneous rupture of the esophagus. *Arch Intern Med* 1983; **143**: 1034–5.
●43. Good JT Jr, Antony VB, Reller LB, Maulitz RM, Sahn SA. The pathogenesis of the low pleural fluid pH in esophageal rupture. *Am Rev Respir Dis* 1983; **127**: 702–4.
44. Drury M, Anderson W, Heffner JE. Diagnostic value of pleural fluid cytology in occult Boerhaave's syndrome. *Chest* 1992; **102**: 976–8.
45. Klygis LM, Jutabha R, McCrohan MB, Vanagunas AD. Esophageal perforations masked by steroids. *Abdom Imaging* 1993; **18**: 10–2.
46. Han SY, McElvein RB, Aldrete JS, Tishler JM. Perforation of the esophagus: correlation of site and cause with plain film findings. *AJR Am J Roentgenol* 1985; **145**: 537–40.
47. White CS, Templeton PA, Attar S. Esophageal perforation: CT findings. *AJR Am J Roentgenol* 1993; **160**: 767–70.
48. Tanomkiat W, Galassi W. Barium sulfate as contrast medium for evaluation of postoperative anastomotic leaks. *Acta Radiol* 2000; **41**: 482–5.
◆49. Kotsis L, Kostic S, Zubovits K. Multimodality treatment of esophageal disruptions. *Chest* 1997; **112**: 1304–9.
50. Tilanus HW, Bossuyt P, Schattenkerk ME, Obertop H. Treatment of oesophageal perforation: a multivariate analysis. *Br J Surg* 1991; **78**: 582–5.
51. Salo JA, Isolauri JO, Heikkila LJ, *et al.* Management of delayed esophageal perforation with mediastinal sepsis. Esophagectomy or primary repair? *J Thorac Cardiovasc Surg* 1993; **106**: 1088–91.
52. Larsson S, Pettersson G, Lepore V. Esophagocutaneous drainage to treat late and complicated esophageal perforation. *Eur J Cardiothorac Surg* 1991; **5**: 579–82.
◆53. Bufkin BL, Miller JI Jr, Mansour KA. Esophageal perforation: emphasis on management. *Ann Thorac Surg* 1996; **61**: 1447–51; discussion 51–2.
54. Serna DL, Vovan TT, Roum JH, Brenner M, Chen JC. Successful nonoperative management of delayed spontaneous esophageal perforation in patients with human immunodeficiency virus. *Crit Care Med* 2000; **28**: 2634–7.
55. Dougenis D, Petsas T, Bouboulis N, *et al.* Management of non resectable malignant esophageal stricture and fistula. *Eur J Cardiothorac Surg* 1997; **11**: 38–45.
56. Howell HS, Prinz RA, Pickleman JR. Anaerobic mediastinitis. *Surg Gynecol Obstet* 1976; **143**: 353–9.
57. Saugier B, Emonot A, Plauchu M, Galy P. [Effusions rich in amylase without pancreatitis. 14 cases]. *Nouv Presse Med* 1976; **5**: 2777–80.
58. Asch MJ, Coran AG, Johnston PW. Gastric perforation secondary to blunt trauma in children. *J Trauma* 1975; **15**: 187–9.
59. Baker A, Volberg F, Sumner T, Moran R. Childhood Menetrier's disease: four new cases and discussion of the literature. *Gastrointest Radiol* 1986; **11**: 131–4.
60. Domej W, Kullnig P, Petritsch W, *et al.* Colobronchial fistula: a rare complication of Crohn's colitis. *Am Rev Respir Dis* 1990; **142**: 1225–7.
61. Al-Emadi M, Helmy I, Nada MA, Al-Jaber H. Laparoscopic repair of Bochdalek hernia in an adult. *Surg Laparosc Endosc Percutan Tech* 1999; **9**: 423–5.
62. McAllister JD, D'Altorio RA, Snyder A. CT findings after uncomplicated percutaneous laparoscopic cholecystectomy. *J Comput Assist Tomogr* 1991; **15**: 770–2.
63. Cunningham LW, Grobman M, Paz HL, Hanlon CA, Promisloff RA. Cholecystopleural fistula with cholelithiasis presenting as a right pleural effusion. *Chest* 1990; **97**: 751–2.
64. Delco F, Domenighetti G, Kauzlaric D, Donati D, Mombelli G. Spontaneous biliothorax (thoracobilia) following cholecystopleural fistula presenting as an acute respiratory insufficiency. Successful removal of gallstones from the pleural space. *Chest* 1994; **106**: 961–3.
65. Chan SY, Osborne AW, Purkiss SF. Cholelithoptysis: an unusual complication following laparoscopic cholecystectomy. *Dig Surg* 1998; **15**: 707–8.
●66. Strange C, Allen ML, Freedland PN, Cunningham J, Sahn SA. Biliopleural fistula as a complication of percutaneous biliary drainage: experimental evidence for pleural inflammation. *Am Rev Respir Dis* 1988; **137**: 959–61.
67. DeCosse JJ, Poulin TL, Fox PS, Condon RE. Subphrenic abscess. *Surg Gynecol Obstet* 1974; **138**: 841–6.
68. Dietrick DB. Experience with liver abscess. *Am J Surg* 1984; **147**: 288–91.
●69. Perera MR, Kirk A, Noone P. Presentation, diagnosis and management of liver abscess. *Lancet* 1980; **ii**: 626–32.

●70. Katsilabros L, Triandafillow G, Kontoyiannis P, Katsilabros N. Pleural effusion and hepatitis. *Gastroenterology* 1972; **63**: 718–22.
71. Flacks LM, Lees D. A case of hepatitis B with pleural effusion. *Aust N Z J Med* 1977; **7**: 636–7.
72. Pramuljo HS, Harun SR. Ultrasound findings in dengue haemorrhagic fever. *Pediatr Radiol* 1991; **21**: 100–2.
73. Thulkar S, Sharma S, Srivastava DN, *et al.* Sonographic findings in grade III dengue hemorrhagic fever in adults. *J Clin Ultrasound* 2000; **28**: 34–7.
74. Setiawan MW, Samsi TK, Wulur H, Sugianto D, Pool TN. Dengue haemorrhagic fever: ultrasound as an aid to predict the severity of the disease. *Pediatr Radiol* 1998; **28**: 1–4.
75. Kim YO, Chun KA, Choi JY, *et al.* Sonographic evaluation of gallbladder-wall thickening in hemorrhagic fever with renal syndrome: prediction of disease severity. *J Clin Ultrasound* 2001; **29**: 286–9.
76. Moritani T, Aihara T, Oguma E, *et al.* Spectrum of Epstein–Barr virus infection in Japanese children: a pictorial essay. *Clin Imaging* 2001; **25**: 1–8.
77. Furui S, Otomo K, Itai Y, Iio M. Hepatocellular carcinoma treated by transcatheter arterial embolization: progress evaluated by computed tomography. *Radiology* 1984; **150**: 773–8.
●78. Branca P, Rodriguez RM, Rogers JT, *et al.* Routine measurement of pleural fluid amylase is not indicated. *Arch Intern Med* 2001; **161**: 228–32.
●79. Teplick JG, Teplick SK, Goodman L, Haskin ME. The interface sign: a computed tomographic sign for distinguishing pleural and intra-abdominal fluid. *Radiology* 1982; **144**: 359–62.
80. Griffin DJ, Gross BH, McCracken S, Glazer GM. Observations on CT differentiation of pleural and peritoneal fluid. *J Comput Assist Tomogr* 1984; **8**: 24–8.
◆81. Light RW. Exudative pleural effusions secondary to gastrointestinal diseases. *Clin Chest Med* 1985; **6**: 103–11.

37

Effusions of obstetric or gynecological origin

RICHARD W LIGHT

Pleural effusions can occur with a variety of gynecological and obstetrical conditions. Patients who are pregnant can have pleural effusions from common causes such as pneumonia, viral infections or pulmonary emboli. However, there are a few types of pleural effusions that are specific to obstetric and gynecological conditions, including the ovarian hyperstimulation syndrome, fetal pleural effusions and the pleural effusions that occur in the post-partum period.

OVARIAN HYPERSTIMULATION SYNDROME

Definition

The ovarian hyperstimulation syndrome (OHSS) is a serious complication of ovulation induction with human chorionic gonadotropin (hCG) and occasionally clomiphene. This syndrome is characterized by ovarian enlargement and fluid shifts resulting in intravascular volume depletion.[1] Severe OHSS is a life-threatening condition characterized by clinical and sonographic evidence of massive ascites or hydrothorax, as well as by breathing difficulties, increased blood viscosity, renal/hepatic dysfunction or anasarca. Critical OHSS includes, in addition, overt renal failure, thromboembolic phenomena, tense ascites or the acute respiratory distress syndrome (ARDS).[1]

Incidence and epidemiology

Severe OHSS occurs in approximately 3 percent of patients undergoing superovulation with gonadotropins.[2] Levin and coworkers[2] reviewed the medical charts and all available imaging studies of 771 women who had undergone induction of superovulation with gonadotropins during the period October 1990 to July 1992 at University Hospital in Western Ontario and reported that the incidence of severe OHSS was 3 percent. In another report, the medical records of all OHSS patients hospitalized between January 1987 and December 1996 in 16 of the 19 tertiary medical centers in Israel were reviewed.[3] The authors were able to find a total of 2902 patients (3305 hospitalizations) with OHSS of whom 196 (6.7 percent) had severe and 13 (0.4 percent) had critical OHSS. In this series, 27 of the 209 patients (12.9 percent) underwent thoracentesis,[3] while 130 patients were dyspneic and received chest radiographs. Thirty eight of the 130 patients (29 percent) had a pleural effusion.

Etiology and pathogenesis

The exact etiology of the pleural effusion seen with severe OHSS is not known. There are two primary components to OHSS: (a) enlargement of the ovaries accompanied by the formation of follicular, luteal and hemorrhagic ovarian cysts and edema of the stroma, and (b) an acute shift of fluid out of the intravascular space.[2] In patients undergoing ovulation induction, several risk factors have been reported to be associated with OHSS. These include young age (<35 years), asthenic habitus, patients with polycystic ovaries, pregnancy resulting from stimulation, hCG supplementation, high serum estradiol (>2500 pg/mL) and multiple follicles.[4]

At one time, it was thought that OHSS resulted from high local concentrations of estrogen in the ovaries causing altered capillary permeability and ascites which, in turn, led to the pleural effusion. This does not appear to be the complete explanation, however, since the syndrome can still be produced in rabbits when the ovaries are exteriorized.[5] Therefore, it is likely that systemic factors are also involved in the fluid shifts into the peritoneal and pleural cavity.

At present, the most likely explanation for OHSS is that the hyperstimulated ovary produces cytokines or other vasoactive substances that enter either the systemic circulation or the peritoneal cavity to produce the syndrome. The two most likely cytokines implicated in the pathogenesis of the OHSS are vascular endothelial growth factor (VEGF) and interleukin 6 (IL-6).[6]

Vascular endothelial growth factor is thought to be the major capillary permeability factor leading to ascites with the OHSS. VEGF is a potent vasoactive protein with a permeability enhancing capacity that is approximately 1000 times greater than that of histamine. Human - chorionic gonadotropin upregulates the expression of VEGF in granulosa cells from patients with the OHSS, but not in cells from control patients.[7] Both follicular fluid and peritoneal fluid from patients with OHSS induce a significant increase in the permeability of endothelial cells *in vitro*.[8] The addition of specific antibodies to VEGF neutralizes 70 percent of this capillary permeability activity.[9] When the VEGF levels are measured in follicular fluid, they are found to be 100-fold greater than those in the simultaneously obtained serum or peritoneal fluid.[10] The levels of VEGF in the ascitic fluid are greater than those in the pleural fluid in patients with severe OHSS.[11]

The levels of IL-6 are also markedly elevated in the follicular fluid, ascites, serum and pleural fluid of patients with severe OHSS.[4] IL-6 along with IL-1, IL-8 and tumor necrosis factor alpha (TNF-α), mediates systemic reactions characterized by leukocytosis, increased vascular permeability and increased concentrations of acute-phase proteins synthesized by the liver. The levels of these four cytokines are elevated in the pleural fluid and in the ascites of patients with severe OHSS.[11]

In patients with severe OHSS, there are probably two main mechanisms responsible for the accumulation of pleural fluid.[6] In patients with bilateral effusions, the probable mechanism is a generalized capillary leak syndrome. In patients with large right-sided pleural effusions, the fluid probably moves directly from the peritoneal space to the pleural space. Support for the second mechanism is provided by the observations in one case where the pleural fluid IL-6 level was more than 300 times higher than the simultaneously obtained serum level.[12] If fluid moved from the intravascular space to the pleural space, one would expect that the cytokine levels in the pleural fluid would not be higher than those in the serum. However, in another series there was not a close correlation between the cytokine levels in the pleural fluid and those in the ascitic fluid.[11]

Clinical presentation

Women who develop OHSS initially complain of abdominal discomfort and distention, followed by nausea, vomiting and diarrhea. If the syndrome worsens, the patients develop evidence of ascites and then hydrothorax and/or shortness of breath. The respiratory symptoms develop 7–14 days after the injection of the hCG.[13] In the most severe stages, the patients develop increased blood viscosity due to hemoconcentration, coagulation abnormalities and reduced renal function.[2]

When pleural effusions are present in patients with OHSS, they most commonly are right-sided. In the series of 38 patients reported by Abramov and coworkers, the pleural effusion was right-sided in 20 (53 percent), left-sided in 7 (18 percent) and bilateral in 11 (29 percent).[3] On rare occasions, a pleural effusion may be the sole manifestation of OHSS.[14] The pleural effusion may be a significant problem in patients with OHSS. In two different patients, 8500 mL[15] and 6800 mL,[14] respectively, were drained.

In patients with OHSS the pleural fluid is an exudates.[14] The mean pleural fluid protein level from 14 patients was 4.2 ± 3.6 gm/dL while the mean plasma protein in these patients was only 4.4 gm/dL.[16] The level of lactic acid dehydrogenase (LDH) is also in the exudative range.[13]

Investigations

The diagnosis is usually obvious in the patient with the complete syndrome. If the pleural effusion is the sole manifestation, the diagnosis may be missed if a complete history is not taken.

Treatment and management

The treatment of OHSS is primarily supportive. Since patients tend to have marked hypoproteinemia and hypovolemia, volume replacement is essential. In view of the hypoproteinemia, human albumin is frequently administered. However, one study of 16 patients demonstrated that 6 percent hydroxyethylstarch was superior to albumin as a colloid solution in the treatment of severe OHSS.[17] Patients who received the hydroxyethylstarch had higher urine output, needed fewer paracenteses and thoracenteses and had a shorter hospitalization.[17]

If the patient is short of breath and has a large pleural effusion, a therapeutic thoracentesis is indicated.[13] On occasion, two or three thoracenteses may be necessary for resolution of the syndrome.[14]

The incidence of OHSS can be reduced if the serum estrogen levels and the number of ovarian follicles are monitored. Injections of hCG should be withheld if the serum estradiol levels are very high or if there are more than 15 ovarian follicles with a high proportion of small and intermediate-sized follicles.[18] However, there is no universal agreement as to what level of estradiol should serve as an indication for cessation of the injections.

Complications

The two most common pulmonary complications (other than pleural effusion) of OHSS are pulmonary thromboembolism and pulmonary infiltrates. Abramov and associates[3] reported that four of 209 patients (2 percent) with severe OHSS had pulmonary thromboembolism. All presented with the acute onset of dyspnea, tachypnea and tachycardia. These same researchers reported that ARDS developed in five (2.4 percent) patients.[3] However, since all patients had received massive hydration (mean 5780 mL/24 hours) and all patients responded to fluid restriction and diuretics, it is likely that the pulmonary infiltrates were due to hypervolemia rather than ARDS.

Although the prognosis of patients with severe OHSS is excellent, there have been rare fatal cases. Semba and coworkers[19] reported that one patient's autopsy revealed massive pulmonary edema.

Future directions of development

In the future, it is probable that the exact mechanisms responsible for OHSS will be elucidated. Once the precise mechanisms are known, attempts to prevent and treat the syndrome will be more specific.

FETAL PLEURAL EFFUSIONS

A fetal pleural effusion is a pleural effusion which is diagnosed antenatally.

Incidence and epidemiology

The incidence of fetal pleural effusion is approximately one in 5–10 000 deliveries.[20] In a series reported from Portugal there were 20 cases of fetal pleural effusion complicating 112 000 deliveries over an 8-year period.[21] The incidence is approximately twice as high in boys as in girls.[22] There may be a genetic predisposition to fetal pleural effusions as there was one report of a lady who had three children with fetal pleural effusions.[23] Early in pregnancy, the incidence of pleural effusions is much higher. In one study in which 965 women were evaluated with ultrasound between 7 and 10 weeks gestation, the incidence of pleural effusion was 1.2 percent.[24] The presence of a pleural effusion early was bad prognostically as 86 percent of the women miscarried.[24] In this series the karyotype was abnormal in 9 of 11 instances (82 percent) in which it was performed.

Etiology and pathogenesis

The pathogenesis of the fetal pleural effusion is not known, and is probably multifactorial. It is likely that most fetal pleural effusions are actually chylothoraces. Evidence for this is as follows. (a) When the pleural fluid is analyzed, it contains predominantly lymphocytes. In one case there were primarily T-lymphocytes, while in a second case there were both T- and B-lymphocytes.[25] (b) Most congenital pleural effusions are chylothoraces[26] and congenital pleural effusions are probably a continuation of fetal pleural effusions. A definitive diagnosis of chylothorax cannot be made by pleural fluid analysis for triglycerides or chylomicrons because the fetuses are not ingesting any lipids.[6] There is one report that indicates that a pleural fluid/serum gamma globulin level above 0.60 is diagnostic of chylothorax.[27] The anatomical cause of fetal chylothorax has been recognized in only a few cases.[20]

A substantial proportion of fetuses with pleural effusions have other abnormalities. Polyhydramnios occurs in approximately 70 percent of patients with fetal pleural effusion.[20] The relationship between the fetal pleural effusion and the polyhydramnios is unclear. It has been suggested that the increased intrathoracic pressure with fetal pleural effusion may interfere with normal fetal swallowing.[20] Indeed, the intrathoracic pressure was measured in one fetus with a large pleural effusion and it was 39 mmHg.[28] This hypothesis is also supported by the observation that there is a lack of dye in the gastrointestinal tract after the intra-amniotic instillation of Urografin.[29] Other abnormalities in a review of 82 cases of fetal pleural effusion included cardiac defects (4.9 percent), Down syndrome (4.9 percent) and polydactyly (1.2 percent). Fetuses with pleural effusion have a high prevalence of chromosomal abnormalities. In one series, the prevalence of chromosomal abnormalities was 50 percent in 152 fetuses with other sonographic abnormalities and 12 percent in fetuses with isolated pleural effusion.[30]

Clinical presentation

The two most common reasons for ultrasound examination when cases of fetal pleural effusion are detected are polyhydramnios and preterm labor. The gestational age at the time of diagnosis varies between 15 and 39 weeks with a median gestational age of about 30 weeks.[20] In a review of the literature in 1998, 204 cases of isolated pleural effusion were found.[31] The effusions were bilateral in 74 percent, unilateral right-sided in 11 percent and unilateral left-sided in 14 percent.[31]

Treatment and management

The best way to manage patients with fetal pleural effusions is controversial.[20] If the pleural effusions are not treated, some will resolve spontaneously. Spontaneous regression of the effusion occurred in 22 percent of the 89 untreated patients in the series of Aubard *et al.*[31] Effusions which resolve spontaneously are more likely to be unilateral, the diagnosis made early in the second trimester, and are not associated with polyhydramnios or hydrops.[31] However, in others the effusion will increase in size and the fetus will develop generalized hydrops. If the effusion persists, the underlying lung will not develop and upon delivery the baby may die from pulmonary hypoplasia.[20]

A literature review of 204 cases of fetal hydrothoraces showed a mortality of 39 percent in 89 fetuses who received no *in utero* therapy. The mortality was higher if the fetus had hydrops (76 percent) or if the effusion was bilateral (47 percent).[31]

Therapeutic maneuvers had been attempted in the majority of patients. In Aubard's review 29 fetuses were treated with thoracentesis and the mortality was 45 percent.[31] The principal drawback of thoracentesis is the rapid reaccumulation of the effusion. Twenty-five of the 29 patients (86 percent) had either one or two thoracenteses. There is one report where the administration of medium chain triglycerides to the mother was thought to slow the reaccumulation of pleural fluid.[32] However, physiologically this is difficult to explain since the triglycerides ingested by the mother never get into the thoracic duct of the fetus.

Pleuroamniotic shunting, as described by Rodeck and coworkers,[33] is frequently used to treat fetal pleural effusions. With this technique a metal trocar with cannula is introduced through the maternal abdominal wall and through the fetal thorax as close as possible to the midaxillary line at the level of the base of the scapula. A double pigtail catheter is introduced through the trocar lumen. A short introducer rod is used to position the distal catheter loop inside the fetal thorax. The trocar is then used to position the proximal catheter loop in the amniotic cavity. Positioned in this manner, the catheter creates a permanent communication between the pleural space and the amniotic cavity.

In a review of 80 fetuses treated with pleuroamniotic shunts, the overall mortality was 26 percent.[31] In 43 fetuses where this information was specified, a pleuroamniotic shunt was placed bilaterally in 24 and unilaterally in 19 cases. The shunts become displaced intrathoracically in a significant percentage of fetuses, but since there appears to be no long-term pulmonary complications, such shunts need not be removed.[34]

Some have advocated creation of a pleurodesis in the fetus by the intrapleural injection of the immunostimulant OK-432[35] or maternal blood.[36] However, since the long-term side effects from a pleurodesis performed in a fetus remain to be determined, pleurodesis is not recommended.

In view of the above, the following approach to fetuses with a pleural effusion is recommended. When a fetus with hydrothorax develops acute fetal distress, a thoracentesis should be performed. At the time of thoracentesis, tests such as karyotype, fetal blood count, maternal serology and meticulous echography are performed in an attempt to ascertain if there are other congenital abnormalities. If there are abnormalities, then a decision must be made concerning the termination of the pregnancy. If there are no abnormalities and hydrops is present, a shunt is placed. One report suggested that the presence of a contralateral mediastinal shift and/or diaphragmatic inversion indicated that the intrathoracic pressure was high and should be indications for placement of the shunt.[28] Otherwise, if the effusion is well tolerated, the fetus is treated conservatively with a repeat ultrasound scan in 2 weeks. If upon repeat ultrasound scan, the effusion is shown to be enlarging and the fetus is less than 32 weeks gestation, a shunt is placed. If the fetus is more than 32 weeks gestation a thoracentesis is performed. If the effusion is not enlarging, repeat examinations are performed at 2-week intervals. Any fetus that has a significant effusion just prior to birth is subjected to a thoracentesis.[31]

The prognosis of fetuses that receive pleuroamniotic shunts and who survive appears to be good. Thompson *et al.*[37] studied 17 infants who had undergone pleuroamniotic shunting for a fetal pleural effusion at a median age of 12 months. They reported that respiratory symptoms and function were no different in these 17 infants than those in a control group.[37]

Complications

The placement of pleuroamniotic shunts is not without complication. Catheter migration occurred 10 times in 80 fetuses in one review, but this did not contraindicate the placement of a new shunt. Other complications include obstruction of the shunt and migration of the catheter into the maternal peritoneal cavity or the fetal thoracic cavity.[38]

Future directions of development

There are two areas for future development in the management of fetal pleural effusions. First, it would be important to develop indicators as to which fetuses with hydrothorax will progress and which ones will regress. Second, there needs to be improvements in the design of the catheters so that they are less likely to migrate and less likely to become occluded.

PLEURAL EFFUSIONS DURING PREGNANCY

There has never been a systematic study on the diseases causing pleural effusion in women that are pregnant.

Incidence and epidemiology

Pregnant women frequently have small pleural effusions demonstrable by ultrasonography. Kocijancic *et al.*[39] studied 47 women at a mean gestation of 24.4 weeks and reported that 28 (59.5 percent) had free pleural fluid that was bilateral in 18 (38.3 percent) and unilateral in 10 (21.2 percent). The mean thickness of the pleural fluid was 2.9 ± 1.1 mm and the patients were asymptomatic. The prevalence of demonstrable pleural fluid was 25 percent in 106 normal individuals studied by the same investigators.

Etiology and pathogenesis

When a woman develops a symptomatic pleural effusion early in pregnancy, the possibility of the ovarian hyperstimulation syndrome should be considered. This entity is discussed early in the chapter. The distribution of the diagnoses responsible for pleural effusions in pregnant women is probably similar to that in non-pregnant women of the same age.[40] Pulmonary embolism is probably the leading cause of pleural effusion in the pregnant woman[40] as the incidence of pleural embolism is higher in pregnant than in non-pregnant women.[41] The second leading cause is probably pneumonia.[40] In women with the HELLP syndrome (hemolysis, elevated liver enzymes and low platelet count) or with severe pre-eclampsia, the prevalence of pleural effusion is about 3 percent.[42] If a pregnant woman has a transudative pleural effusion, peripartum cardiomyopathy should be considered.

Clinical presentation and treatment

The clinical presentation and treatment for pregnant patients with pleural effusions is the same as that for non-pregnant patients with effusions of the same etiology.

POST-PARTUM PLEURAL EFFUSION (IMMEDIATE)

There are two types of post-partum pleural effusion. The first occurs in the immediate post-partum period and this effusion is small. The second occurs in the first few weeks after delivery and is associated with pulmonary infiltrates.

Incidence and epidemiology

The reported prevalence of small pleural effusions in the immediate post-partum period has varied from series to series. In a retrospective study Hughson and associates reported that the prevalence of pleural effusion in 112 patients who had delivered vaginally and had posteroanterior and lateral chest radiographs within 24 hours of delivery was 46 percent and the effusions were bilateral in 75 percent.[43] In a prospective study by the same researchers the prevalence of pleural effusion was 67 percent in a group of 30 patients and the effusions were bilateral in 55 percent.[43] Decubitus radiographs confirmed the effusion in seven of the ten women with effusions who had a decubitus radiograph. In contrast, Udeshi *et al.*[44] reported that the prevalence of pleural effusion was only 2 percent in a series of 50 patients who had ultrasonography of the chest. The one patient in this latter series who had a pleural effusion had severe pre-eclampsia with apparent pulmonary edema. An intermediate prevalence was reported by Wallis and coworkers[45] who prospectively studied 34 patients with moderate to severe pre-eclampsia with ultrasound and reported that six (17.6 percent) of the patients had a pleural effusion. The explanation for the marked discrepancy in the prevalence of pleural effusions in the different series is not clear.

Etiology and pathogenesis

The etiology of the post-partum pleural effusion is unknown. Hughson and coworkers[43] hypothesized that the following two factors were contributory. First, the colloid osmotic pressure is decreased during pregnancy and this decreased colloid osmotic pressure should lead to increased pleural fluid formation. Second, the Valsalva maneuvers typical of the second stage of labor could impair lymphatic drainage of the pleural space by elevating systemic venous pressure. In the study of Wallis and associates of patients with moderate to severe pre-eclampsia, the patients with pleural effusion did not have a greater degree of hypertension or proteinuria.[45]

Clinical presentation and treatment

Patients who develop these small effusions post-partum are asymptomatic and require no treatment.

POST-PARTUM PLEURAL EFFUSION (DELAYED)

In addition to the pleural effusion that occurs in the immediate post-partum period, there appears to be another distinct type of pleural effusion that occurs in the first few weeks post-partum. Patients with this syndrome present with pleural effusions and pulmonary infiltrates.

Incidence and epidemiology

The incidence of this syndrome is not known, but it must be extremely low since only four cases have been reported in the literature.[46,47] Another diagnosis that should be considered in patients with pleural effusions in the weeks to months after delivery is pulmonary embolism. The risk of pulmonary embolism is 15 times higher in the post-partum period than during pregnancy.[41]

Etiology and pathogenesis

The pathogenesis of the syndrome appears to be related to the presence of antiphospholipid antibodies. There are two different antiphospholipid antibodies: the lupus anticoagulant and the anticardiolipin antibody. The lupus anticoagulant was first discovered in patients who had systemic lupus erythematosus, but is now known to be found in other disease states, as well as in totally asymptomatic patients. It is a monoclonal antibody that reacts with platelet factor 3 to cause incomplete formation of the prothrombin activator complex. The lupus anticoagulant has been associated with the inhibition of prostacyclin production by endothelial cells. Other theories of its activity include interference with the anticoagulation system and inhibition of fibrinolysis. The anticardiolipin antibody also reacts with negatively charged phospholipids. Its mode of action is believed to be similar to that of the lupus anticoagulant.[47]

Clinical presentation

Patients with this syndrome typically present with fever, pleural effusions and pulmonary infiltrates within a few weeks of delivery.[46] The patients also frequently present with chest pain. Some of the patients also have evidence of myocarditis and/or of thrombosis of various vessels.[46] The patients have either lupus anticoagulant or anticardiolipin antibodies or both, but do not have antinuclear antibodies; neither do they fulfill the criteria for the diagnosis of systemic lupus erythematosus.[46] All of the reported patients reported had false-positive tests for syphilis.[46,47] It should be noted that the most well known complication of the antiphospholipid syndrome is spontaneous abortion, most commonly in the second trimester.

Investigations

The anticardiolipin antibody can be measured by enzyme-linked immunosorbent assay (ELISA). Currently, there is no definitive assay for the lupus anticoagulant. Its presence is suggested by any of several tests that show interference with phospholipid function. A prolonged activated partial thrombin time (aPTT) that does not become normal with the addition of an equal volume of normal plasma is strongly suggestive.[47]

Treatment and management

Pregnant patients known to have antiphospholipid antibodies should be carefully monitored in the post-partum period for early signs or symptoms of pleuropulmonary or cardiac disease or thrombotic episodes. When such post-partum complications are recognized, assays should be performed for antiphospholipid antibodies and, if they are positive, consideration should be given to immunosuppressive therapy after pulmonary embolus and infection have been carefully ruled out.[46]

Complications

The primary complications are myocarditis with congestive heart failure and venous thrombosis.

Future directions of development

It is unclear as to what is the true incidence of this syndrome. In the future, prospective studies will delineate the prevalence of this syndrome and its optimal treatment.

MEIGS' SYNDROME

When this syndrome was originally described by Meigs in 1937, the syndrome consisted of the presence of ascites and pleural effusions in patients with benign solid ovarian tumors.[48] Moreover, the syndrome required that when the ovarian tumor was removed, the ascites and the pleural effusion both had to resolve.[48] Subsequent to the initial description, it became apparent that a similar syndrome could occur with benign cystic ovarian tumors, benign tumors of the uterus (fibromyomata), low-grade ovarian malignant tumors without evidence of metastases[49] and endometriomas.[50] Although Meigs still prefers to reserve his name for only those cases in which the primary neoplasm is a benign solid ovarian tumor, I classify any patient with a pelvic neoplasm associated with ascites and pleural effusion in whom surgical removal of the tumor results in permanent disappearance of the ascites and pleural effusion as having had Meigs' syndrome.[6]

Incidence and epidemiology

Meigs' Syndrome is relatively uncommon. As of 1964, Majzlin and Stevens were able to find 128 cases in the literature.[51]

Etiology and pathogenesis

The reason that patients with Meigs' syndrome develop ascites appears to be the secretion of large amounts of fluid by the primary tumor. When tumors have been resected and placed in dry containers, the secretion of large amounts of fluid continues.[49] Larger tumors are more likely to be associated with free peritoneal fluid. Samanth and Black[52] reported that free peritoneal fluid was only found with tumors with a diameter greater than 11 cm.

It appears that the pathogenesis of the pleural effusion in patients with Meigs' syndrome is similar to that in patients with cirrhosis, ascites and a pleural effusion. It is thought that fluid passes from the peritoneal cavity into the pleural cavity through small holes in the diaphragm.[53] Supporting evidence for this theory includes the following: (a) the ascitic and the pleural fluid have similar characteristics, (b) the pleural fluid rapidly recurs following thoracentesis, and (c) some patients have ovarian tumors and ascites without pleural effusion. It should be noted, however, that some authors believe that the pleural fluid arises from the transdiaphragmatic transfer of ascitic fluid by the lymphatic vessels.[33,35,38]

It appears that the fluid secreted by the tumors into the peritoneal cavity has high levels of factors which may increase the permeability of vessels in the peritoneal and pleural cavities and lead to more fluid formation in these body cavities. The serum levels of IL-1, IL-6, IL-8, TNF-α and VEGF are all elevated in patients with Meigs' syndrome compared with controls. The levels of these factors are higher in the ascitic and pleural fluid than in the serum.[54–56]

The tumors most commonly responsible for Meigs' syndrome (my definition) are ovarian fibroma, followed by ovarian cysts, thecomas, granulosal cell tumors and leiomyomas of the uterus.[49]

Clinical presentation

Patients with Meigs' syndrome usually present with a chronic illness characterized by weight loss, a pleural effusion, ascites and a pelvic mass.[49] The only symptom related to the pleural effusion is shortness of breath. The ascites may not be detectable on physical examination. The most important aspect of Meigs' syndrome is to realize that not all patients who present with this picture have inoperable pelvic malignancy. It is also important to realize that some patients with Meigs' syndrome may have an elevated CA-125.[57,58]

The pleural effusion is unilateral right-sided in 70 percent, left-sided in 10 percent and bilateral in 20 percent.[51] Although it has been stated that the pleural fluid with Meigs' syndrome is a transudate,[49,59] this conclusion appears to be based on the gross appearance of the pleural fluid (clear yellow) rather than upon its chemical characteristics.[6] The pleural fluid with Meigs' syndrome meets the criteria for an exudate with protein levels above 3.0 g/dL.[59–62] The white blood cell (WBC) count of the pleural fluid is usually less than 1000 cells/mm^3. The pleural fluid is sometimes bloody. As mentioned above, the level of CA-125 in the pleural fluid may be elevated and this should not be taken as an indication of malignancy.[57,58]

Investigations and treatment

Before a female with a pelvic mass, ascites and a pleural effusion is labeled as having an inoperable malignancy, definite evidence of malignancy in a body fluid or a biopsy specimen should be obtained. The initial evaluation should include cytology on the ascitic and pleural fluid. If these cytologies are negative and there is no other evidence of malignancy elsewhere, exploratory laparotomy should be considered. If there is no evidence of malignancy, the primary neoplasm should be removed. The diagnosis is confirmed when the ascites and the pleural fluid resolve post-operatively and do not recur. The disappearance of these fluids post-operatively usually occurs within 2 weeks.[61]

Future directions of development

In the future, additional studies should reveal more precisely the role of various vasoactive substances and cytokines in the pathogenesis of Meigs' syndrome.

ENDOMETRIOSIS AND PLEURAL EFFUSIONS

On occasion, severe endometriosis is complicated by massive ascites[63] and a pleural effusion is present in approximately 30 percent of these patients.[63]

Incidence and epidemiology

Pleural effusions secondary to endometriosis are uncommon. In a review in 2000, only 13 cases were found and all were in conjunction with massive ascites.[64]

Etiology and pathogenesis

The pleural effusion is thought to be due to fluid flowing through small holes in the diaphragm from the peritoneal cavity to the pleural cavity. This same mechanism is responsible for the pleural effusions with hepatic hydrothorax and Meigs' syndrome.

Clinical presentation

Patients usually present with abdominal pain and distension, anorexia and nausea. The initial presumptive diagnosis is frequently malignancy because the patients usually have significant weight loss. Many patients also have clinical manifestations of endometriosis, such as progressive dysmenorrhea, and cul-de-sac and uterosacral ligament nodularity. Some patients have exacerbation of their symptoms with their menstrual periods.

The pleural fluid has not been systematically studied, but it is usually described as bloody or chocolate-colored.[64] Cytology of the fluid has shown numerous hemosiderin-laden macrophages with an elevated CA-125.[63] The pleural effusions have been unilateral right-sided in the majority of cases.[64]

Investigation

This diagnosis should be considered in any menstruating female who develops bloody or chocolate-colored pleural fluid. The diagnosis is usually definitively established at the time of laparotomy.

Treatment and management

The treatment of the massive ascites, pleural effusion and endometriosis is not easy. Hormonal therapy (progestational agents, danazol, or luprolide acetate [Lupron]) fails in more than 50 percent of cases. Most commonly, these patients are treated with total abdominal hysterectomy and bilateral salpingo-oophorectomy, but the presence of the pelvic endometriosis makes this surgery difficult.

Future directions of development

It is hoped that better treatment modalities will be developed for this condition, avoiding aggressive surgery.

CATAMENIAL HEMOTHORAX

Incidence and epidemiology

A review of the literature on catamenial hemothoraces in 1993 revealed a total of 16 cases.[65]

Etiology and pathogenesis

The majority of patients with catamenial hemothoraces have associated pelvic and abdominal endometriosis. The right hemithorax is almost always involved and some of the patients have diaphragmatic fenestrations. It has been hypothesized that the endometrial tissue enters the thorax through the diaphragmatic fenestrations. When the patient menstruates the endometrial tissue is shed into the pleural space and a hemothorax ensues.

Clinical presentation

Most patients who present with catamenial hemothorax are nulliparous and the average age has been 32 years.[65] The patients usually present with dyspnea or chest pain. The right hemithorax is universally involved.[65]

Investigations

Thoracentesis reveals a bloody pleural fluid. This finding, in conjunction with the history showing the relationship to menstruation and pelvic endometriosis, are usually sufficient to establish the diagnosis.

Treatment and management

The treatment of choice appears to be total hysterectomy and bilateral salpingo-oophorectomy because hormonal suppressive therapy appears to provide only temporary improvement. If the hemothorax is large, the patient should be treated with tube thoracostomy.

Future directions of development

Since this disease is so uncommon, it is difficult to know the future directions. A better therapy would be one that does not involve total hysterectomy and bilateral salpingo-oophorectomy in these young patients.

KEY POINTS

- Pleural effusions occur as a complication of the ovarian hyperstimulation syndrome which occurs in approximately 3 percent of patients who have undergone induction of superovulation with gonadotropins. The pleural effusions are secondary to a generalized capillary leak syndrome plus movement of ascitic fluid from the peritoneal cavity to the pleural cavity.
- Fetal pleural effusions which persist cause pulmonary hypoplasia at birth. Fetuses with persistent or recurrent pleural effusions are best managed with intra-uterine shunts.
- A sizeable fraction of patients have very small pleural effusions in the immediate post-partum period.
- The presence of a pelvic mass, ascites and a pleural effusion does not necessarily indicate disseminated malignancy – Meigs' syndrome should be considered.
- Pleural effusions at times complicate endometriosis with ascites or endometriosis of the pleura.

REFERENCES

● = Key primary paper
◆ = Major review article

1. Delvigne A, Rozenberg S. Review of clinical course and treatment of ovarian hyperstimulation syndrome (OHSS). *Hum Reprod Update* 2003; **9**: 77–96.
2. Levin MF, Kaplan BR, Hutton LC. Thoracic manifestations of ovarian hyperstimulation syndrome. *Can Assoc Radiol J* 1995; **46**: 23–6.
●3. Abramov Y, Elchalal U, Schenker JG. Pulmonary manifestations of severe ovarian hyperstimulation syndrome: a multicenter study. *Fertil Steril* 1999: **71**: 645–51.
4. Elchalal U, Schenker JG. The pathophysiology of ovarian hyperstimulation syndrome – views and ideas. *Hum Reprod* 1997; **12**: 1129–37.
5. Yarali H, Fleige-Zahradka BG, Yuen BH, McComb PF. The ascites in ovarian hyperstimulation syndrome does not originate from the ovary. *Fertil Steril* 1993; **59**: 657–61.
6. Light RW. *Pleural diseases*, 5th edn. Baltimore: Lippincott, Williams and Wilkins, 2007.
7. Wang TH, Horng SG, Chang CL, *et al.* Human chorionic gonadotropin-induced ovarian hyperstimulation syndrome is associated with up-regulation of vascular endothelial growth factor. *J Clin Endocrinol Metab* 2002; **87**: 3300–8.
●8. Goldsman MP, Pedram A, Dominguez CE, *et al.* Increased capillary permeability induced by human follicular fluid: a hypothesis for an ovarian origin of the hyperstimulation syndrome. *Fertil Steril* 1995; **63**: 268–72.
9. McClure N, Healy DL, Rogers PAW, *et al.* Vascular endothelial growth factor as capillary permeability agent in ovarian hyperstimulation syndrome. *Lancet* 1994; **344**: 235–6.
10. Krasnow JS, Berga SL, Gusick DS, *et al.* Vascular permeability factor and vascular endothelial growth factor in ovarian hyperstimulation syndrome: a preliminary report. *Fertil Steril* 1996; **65**: 552–5.
●11. Chen CD, Wu MY, Chen HF, *et al.* Prognostic importance of serial cytokine changes in ascites and pleural effusion in women with severe ovarian hyperstimulation syndrome. *Fertil Steril* 1999; **72**: 286–92.
12. Loret de Mola JR, Farredondo-Soberon F, Randle CP, *et al.* Markedly elevated cytokines in pleural effusion during the ovarian hyperstimulation syndrome: transudate or ascites? *Fertil Steril* 1997; **67**: 780–2.
13. Gregory WT, Patton PE. Isolated pleural effusion in severe ovarian hyperstimulation: A case report. *Am J Obstet Gynecol* 1999; **180**: 1468–71.
14. Rabinerson D, Shalev J, Royburt M, Ben-Rafael Z, Dekel A. Severe unilateral hydrothorax as the only manifestation of the ovarian hyperstimulation syndrome. *Gynecol Obstet Invest* 2000; **49**: 140–2.
15. Yuen BH, McComb P, Sy L, *et al.* Plasma prolactin, human chorionic gonadotropin, estradiol, testosterone, and progesterone in the ovarian hyperstimulation syndrome. *Am J Obstet Gynecol* 1979; **133**: 316–20.
16. Abramov Y, Elchalal U, Schenker JG. Febrile morbidity in severe and critical ovarian hyperstimulation syndrome: a multicentre study. *Hum Reprod* 1998; **13**: 3128–31.
17. Abramov Y, Fatum M, Abrahamov D, Schenker JG. Hydroxyethylstarch versus human albumin for the treatment of severe ovarian hyperstimulation syndrome: a preliminary report. *Fertil Steril* 2001; **75**: 1228–30.
18. Rizk B, Aboulghar M. Modern management of ovarian hyperstimulation syndrome. *Hum Reprod* 1991; **6**: 1082–7.
19. Semba S, Moriya T, Youssef EM, Sasano H. An autopsy case of ovarian hyperstimulation syndrome with massive pulmonary edema and pleural effusion. *Pathol Int* 2000; **50**: 549–52.
●20. Hagay Z, Reece A, Roberts A, Hobbins JC. Isolated fetal pleural effusion: a prenatal management dilemma. *Obstet Gynecol* 1993; **81**: 147–52.
21. Rocha G, Fernandes P, Rocha P, *et al.* Pleural effusions in the neonate. *Acta Paediatr* 2006; **95**: 791–8.
22. Eddleman KA, Levine AB, Chitkara U, Berkowitz RL. Reliability of pleural fluid lymphocyte counts in the antenatal diagnosis of congenital chylothorax. *Obstet Gynecol* 1991; **78**: 530–2.
23. Chang YL, Lien R, Wang CJ, *et al.* Congenital chylothorax in three siblings. *Am J Obstet Gynecol* 2005; **192**: 2065–6.
24. Hashimoto K, Shimizu T, Fukuda M, *et al.* Pregnancy outcome of embryonic/fetal pleural effusion in the first trimester. *J Ultrasound Med* 2003; **22**: 501–5.
25. Benacerraf BR, Frigoletto FD Jr, Wilson M. Successful midtrimester thoracentesis with analysis of the lymphocyte population in the pleural effusion. *Am J Obstet Gynecol* 1986; **155**: 398–9.
26. Chernick V, Reed MH. Pneumothorax and chylothorax in the neonatal period. *J Pediatr* 1970; **76**: 624–32.
27. Tsukimori K, Nakanami N, Fukushima K, *et al.* Pleural fluid/serum immunoglobulin ratio is a diagnostic marker for congenital chylothorax in utero. *J Perinat Med* 2006; **34**: 313–17.
28. Yamamoto M, Insunza A, Carrillo J, *et al.* Intrathoracic pressure in congenital chylothorax. Keystone for the rationale of thoracoamniotic shunting? *Fetal Diagn Ther* 2007; **22**: 169–171.
29. Murayama K, Jimbo T, Matsumoto Y, Mitsuishi C, Nishida H. Fetal pulmonary hypoplasia with hydrothorax. *Am J Obstet Gynecol* 1987; **157**: 119–20.
30. Waller K, Chaithongwongwatthana S, Yamasmit W, *et al.* Chromosomal abnormalities among 246 fetuses with pleural effusions detected on prenatal ultrasound examination: Factors associated with an increased risk of aneuploidy. *Genet Med* 2005; **7**: 417–21.
◆31. Aubard Y, Derouineau I, Aubard V, Chalifour V, Preux PM. Primary fetal hydrothorax: A literature review and proposed antenatal clinical strategy. *Fetal Diagn Ther* 1998; **13**: 325–33.
32. Bartha JL, Comino-Delgado R. Fetal chylothorax response to maternal dietary treatment. *Obstet Gynecol* 2001; **97** (5 Suppl 1): 820–3.
33. Rodeck CH, Fisk NM, Fraser DI, Nicolini U. Long-term *in utero* drainage of fetal hydrothorax. *N Engl J Med* 1988; **319**: 1135–8.
34. Sepulveda W, Galindo A, Sosa A, *et al.* Intrathoracic dislodgement of pleuro-amniotic shunt. Three case reports with long-term follow-up. *Fetal Diagn Ther* 2005; **20**: 102–5.
35. Chen M, Chen CP, Shih JC, *et al.* Antenatal treatment of chylothorax and cystic hygroma with OK-432 in nonimmune hydrops fetalis. *Fetal Diagn Ther* 2005; **20**: 309–15.
36. Parra J, Amenedo M, Muniz-Diaz E, *et al.* A new successful therapy for fetal chylothorax by intrapleural injection of maternal blood. *Ultrasound Obstet Gynecol* 2003; **22**: 290–4.
37. Thompson P, Greenough A, Nicolaides KH. Respiratory function in infancy following pleuro-amniotic shunting. *Fetal Diagn Ther* 1993; **8**: 79–83.
◆38. Wittman BK, Martin KA, Wilson RD, Peacock D. Complications of long-term drainage of fetal pleural effusion: case report and review of the literature. *Am J Perinatol* 1997; **14**: 443–7.
39. Kocijancic I, Pusenjak S, Kocijancic K, *et al.* Sonographic detection of physiologic pleural fluid in normal pregnant women. *J Clin Ultrasound* 2005; **33**: 63–6.
40. Light RW. Pleural diseases in pregnancy. *Int Pleural News* 2006; **4**: 6–7.
41. Heit JA, Kobbervig CE, James AH, *et al.* Trends in the indicence of venous thromboembolism during pregnancy or postpartum: a 30-year population-based study. *Ann Intern Med* 2005; **143**: 749–50.
42. Haddad B, Barton JR, Livingston JC, *et al.* HELLP (hemolysis, elevated liver enzymes, and low platelet count) syndrome versus severe preeclampsia: onset at ≤ 28 weeks' gestation. *Am J Obstet Gynecol* 2000; **183**: 1475–9.
●43. Hughson WG, Friedman PJ, Feigin DS, Resnick R, Moser KM.

Postpartum pleural effusion: a common radiologic finding. *Ann Intern Med* 1982; **97**: 856–8.

●44. Udeshi UL, McHugo JM, Selwyn CJ. Postpartum pleural effusion. *Br J Obstet Gynaecol* 1988; **95**: 894–7.

45. Wallis MG, McHugo JM, Carruthers DA, Selwyn Crawford J. The prevalence of pleural effusions in pre-eclampsia: an ultrasound study. *Br J Obstet Gynaecol* 1989; **96**: 431–3.

●46. Kochenour NK, Branch DW, Rote NS, *et al.* A new postpartum syndrome associated with antiphospholipid antibodies. *Obstet Gynecol* 1987; **69**: 460–8.

47. Ayres MA, Sulak PJ. Pregnancy complicated by antiphospholipid antibodies. *South Med J* 1991; **84**: 266–9.

●48. Meigs JV, Cass JW. Fibroma of the ovary with ascites and hydrothorax. *Am J Obstet Gynecol* 1937; **33**: 249–67.

49. Meigs JV. Pelvic tumors other than fibromas of the ovary with ascites and hydrothorax. *Obstet Gynecol* 1954; **3**: 471–86.

50. Yu J, Grimes DA. Ascites and pleural effusions associated with endometriosis. *Obstet Gynecol* 1991; **78**: 533–4.

51. Majzlin G, Stevens FL. Meigs' syndrome: case report and review of literature. *J Int Coll Surg* 1964; **42**: 625–30.

52. Samanth KK, Black WC III. Benign ovarian stromal tumors associated with free peritoneal fluid. *Am J Obstet Gynecol* 1970; **107**: 538–45.

53. Kirschner PA. Porous diaphragm syndromes. *Chest Surg Clin N Am* 1998; **8**: 449–72.

54. Ishiko O, Yoshida H, Sumi T, Hirai K, Ogita S. Vascular endothelial growth factor levels in pleural and peritoneal fluid in Meigs' syndrome. *Eur J Obstet Gynecol Reprod Biol* 2001; **98**: 129–30.

●55. Abramov Y, Anteby SO, Fasouliotis SJ, Barak V. Markedly elevated levels of vascular endothelial growth factor, fibroblast growth factor, and interleukin 6 in Meigs' syndrome. *Am J Obstet Gynecol* 2001; **184**: 354–5.

56. Abramov Y, Anteby SO, Fasouliotis SJ, *et al.* The role of inflammatory cytokines in Meigs' syndrome. *Obstet Gynecol* 2002; **99** (5 Suppl 1): 917–9.

57. Patsner B. Meigs' syndrome and "false positive" preoperative serum CA-125 levels: analysis of ten cases. *Eur J Gynaecol Oncol* 2000; **21**: 362–3

58. Loizzi V, Cormio G, Resta L, *et al.* Pseudo-Meigs syndrome and elevated CA125 associated with struma ovarii. *Gynecol Oncol* 2005; **97**: 282–4.

59. O'Flanagan SJ, Tighe BF, Egan TJ, Delaney PV. Meigs' syndrome and pseudo-Meigs' syndrome. *J R Soc Med* 1987; **80**: 252–3.

60. Hurlow RA, Greening WP, Krantz E. Ascites and hydrothorax in association with stroma ovarii. *Br J Surg* 1976; **63**: 110–2.

61. Jimerson SD. Pseudo-Meigs' syndrome: an unusual case with analysis of the effusions. *Obstet Gynecol* 1973; **42**: 535–7.

62. Neustadt JE, Levy RC. Hemorrhagic pleural effusion in Meigs' syndrome. *J Am Med Assoc* 1968, **204**: 179–80.

63. Muneyyirci-Delale O, Neil G, Serur E, *et al.* Endometriosis with massive ascites. *Gynecol Oncol* 1998; **69**: 42–6.

◆64. Bhojawala J, Heller DS, Cracchiolo B, Sama J. Endometriosis presenting as bloody pleural effusion and ascites – report of a case and review of the literature. *Arch Gynecol Obstet* 2000; **264**: 39–41.

65. Shepard MK, Mancini MC, Campbell GD, George RB. Right-sided hemothorax and recurrent abdominal pain in a 34-year-old woman. *Chest* 1993; **103**: 1239–40.

38

Benign fibrous tumor of the pleura

MARC DE PERROT

INTRODUCTION

There are approximately 800 cases of solitary fibrous tumors of the pleura (SFTP) reported in the literature. Most of them are pedunculated mass and harbor benign histological features.[1] Although they may be relatively large, these tumors are usually treated by simple excision and do not recur if their resection is microscopically complete.[2] Approximately 12 percent of SFTP, however, have malignant behavior and eventually lead to death due to local recurrence or metastastic disease.[3] The malignant form of SFTP still remains enigmatic. The behavior is often unpredictable and does not always correlate with histological findings.[1] In addition, in some cases benign SFTP may remain silent for several years before degenerating into a malignant type.[4]

HISTORICAL BACKGROUND

The first report of a primary localized pleural tumor is attributed to Wagner in 1870.[5] However, it was only in 1931 that Klemperer and Rabin[6] published the first accurate pathological description, and classified mesothelioma as either 'localized' or 'diffuse'. Since tissue culture[7] and ultrastructural analysis[8,9] demonstrated the presence of epithelial-like cells in localized mesotheliomas, in 1942 Stout and Murray[7] claimed that localized mesothelioma had a mesothelial origin. However, other investigators have shown that the mesothelial layer covering the tumor was intact and they postulated that the epithelial cells seen could have been trapped within growing fibrous mesenchymal tumors.[8,10] The controversy over the origin of these tumors persisted for several decades and is reflected by the variety of terms given to the neoplasm (Table 38.1).

Over the last 20 years, immunohistochemical studies have provided strong evidence for a mesenchymal origin of these tumors. Indeed, as opposed to the diffuse mesothelioma type, localized tumors have been shown to lack expression of cytoplasmic keratins and to express vimentin, a marker of mesenchymal cells.[11,12] In addition, some authors have recently shown that localized tumors of the pleura express CD34.[13,14] CD34 is a transmembrane cell surface glycoprotein (originally described as a marker of human hematopoietic stem cells) that is ubiquitously observed on a novel family of interstitial spindle cells involved in antigen presentation and characterized by slender dendritic prolongation of their cytoplasm.[15,16] van

Table 38.1 Terms given to solitary fibrous tumors of the pleura (SFTP) over the years

Given terms
Localized mesothelioma
Localized fibrous mesothelioma
Localized fibrous tumors
Solitary fibrous mesothelioma
Fibrous mesothelioma
Pleural fibroma
Submesothelial fibroma
Subserosal fibroma

de Rijn and Rouse[17] have described this distinctive group of cells as 'dendritic interstitial cells' and have raised the possibility that solitary fibrous tumors seen in the lung and in other sites may originate from such cells.

CLINICAL FEATURES

Solitary fibrous tumors of the pleura have been described in all age groups from 5 to 87 years, but they peak in the sixth and seventh decade of life with an even distribution between men and women.[1,3,18] The majority of benign tumors are small and pedunculated, whereas most malignant SFTP are large and symptomatic.[1,4,19,20] Symptoms usually include cough, chest pain, and dyspnea (Table 38.2). More rarely, hemoptysis and obstructive pneumonitis are observed as a result of airway obstruction.[1,4]

Table 38.2 Approximate incidence of symptoms

Approximate incidence	%
Asymptomatic	60
Chest pain	18
Dyspnea	15
Cough	12
Weight loss	2
HPO	2
Hypoglycemia[a]	1
Fever	1

[a]Doege–Potter syndrome.
HPO, hypertrophic pulmonary osteoarthropathy.

Digital clubbing and hypertrophic pulmonary osteoarthropathy (HPO, Pierre–Marie–Bamberg syndrome) have been described in patients with either benign or malignant SFTP.[1,19,21,22] Patients with HPO commonly complain of bilateral arthritic symptoms including stiffness of the joints, edema of the ankles, arthralgias and pain along the long bones, especially in the tibias from periosteal elevation. HPO can resolve immediately after the tumor is removed. Digital clubbing usually improves within 2–5 months or sometimes longer after removal of the tumor, but may reappear with recurrence of the tumor.[1,20–23]

In less than 5 percent of the patients, SFTP can also secrete an insulin-like growth factor II (IGF II), which causes refractory hypoglycemia (Doege–Potter syndrome).[1,3,24] A high serum level of IGF II is typically associated with low levels of insulin. Refractory hypoglycemia will disappear within 3–4 days after resection of the tumor.[22,23,25,26]

RADIOLOGICAL FEATURES

Benign and malignant SFTP usually appear as a well-defined, homogeneous and rounded mass on the initial chest radiograph.[1,19–21] Rarely, a pleural effusion is associated with malignant SFTP.[1,20,21] While small tumors arising from the parietal pleura classically form obtuse angles with the chest wall, large or pedunculated SFTP may form acute angles and be confused with intrapulmonary masses.[27,28] Pedunculated SFTP have occasionally been reported to be moving on successive chest radiographs because of their pedunculated attachment in the fissure of the lung.[29,30]

Computed tomography (CT) scan usually demonstrates a well delineated, homogeneous and occasionally lobulated mass of soft tissue attenuation.[31] Although no specific CT features have been described for the diagnosis of SFTP, the tumors typically appear in contact with the pleural surface and show displacement or invasion of the surrounding structures.[20] Heterogeneity may be observed with benign and malignant variants of SFTP because of myxoid degeneration, hemorrhage or necrosis (Figure 38.1). Tumors arising in an interlobar fissure may be more difficult to differentiate from an intraparenchymal mass, because the lesion appears to be surrounded by lung parenchyma.[32] Calcifications may be observed in a few tumors regardless of their benign or malignant histological features.[1,4,20]

Magnetic resonance imaging (MRI) has limited use in the assessment of pleural disease.[33] However, the morphology and relationship of large SFTP to adjacent mediastinal and major vascular structures may be better appreciated with MRI than with CT.[34] MRI is helpful in differentiating the tumor from other structures and in confirming intrathoracic localization when the tumor abuts the

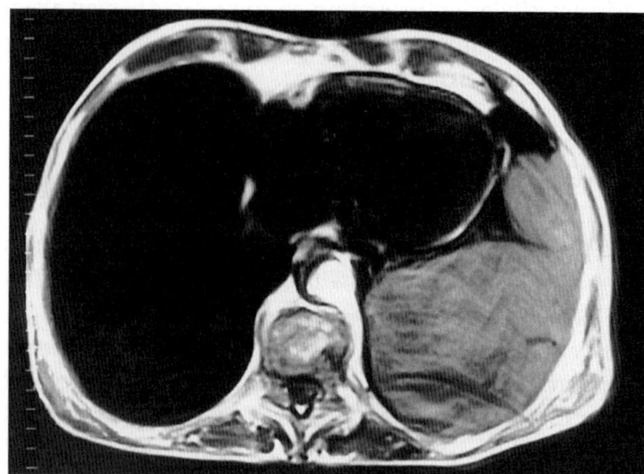

Figure 38.1 Magnetic resonance imaging (MRI) showing a large solitary fibrous tumor of the pleura situated on the left hemidiaphragm with heterogenous zones due to hemorrhage and necrosis of the tumor.

diaphragm.[4,31,35] Fibrous tissue as seen in both benign and malignant SFTP has low signal intensity on T1-weighted images.[34,36,37] On T2-weighted images, however, mature fibrous tissue containing few cells and abundant collagen stroma has a low intensity, whereas malignant fibrosis invariably appears with high signal intensity because of increased vascularity, edema and cellularity.[34,36,37] Unfortunately, benign SFTP can often also have areas of high signal intensity on T2-weighted images because of intratumoral necrosis or myxoid degeneration and thus may not be differentiable from malignant SFTP.[34,38,39]

Positron-emission tomography (PET) scan has minimal utility in the evaluation of these tumors. Few cases have been reported in the literature and the tumor showed no or minimal uptake on PET.[40,41]

HISTOPATHOLOGY

Benign and malignant SFTP are widely distributed in the chest. While most of the benign SFTP are small pedunculated tumors, the malignant variants are often larger than 10 cm and grow beneath the parietal pleura of the chest wall, diaphragm or mediastinum.[1,4,20,42]

Macroscopically, benign and malignant tumors appear as firm, smoothly lobulated masses. Most of them are encapsulated by a thin, translucent membrane, containing a reticulated vascular network. Firm adhesion without signs of invasion may be present between visceral and parietal pleura at the surface of the tumor. The cut surface appears gray-white to tan with a whorled pattern, and may disclose areas of hemorrhage and necrosis.[1,43] Hemorrhagic and necrotic areas may be present in benign tumors, but they usually predominate in the malignant form, most likely because of their larger size.[1]

Microscopically, SFTP are characterized by a proliferation of uniform elongated spindle cells intimately intertwining with various amounts of connective tissue. Zones of hypercellularity may alternate with hypocellular or fibrous areas within the same tumor. Typically, fibroblasts and connective tissue are arranged in a so-called 'patternless pattern' or 'storiform pattern', characterized by a haphazard distribution of spindle cells and collagen fibrils.[44,45] Occasionally, an increased amount of blood vessels within the tumor cause a hemangiopericytoma-like pattern.[1,44] More rarely, other patterns such as herringbone and neural palisading are also observed inside the tumor.[1]

Histological signs of malignancy include:

1. high mitotic counts defined as more than four mitoses per 10 high-power field (HPF);
2. mild to marked pleomorphism based on nuclear size, irregularity and nuclear prominence;
3. bundles of high cellularity with crowding and overlapping of nuclei;
4. presence of necrotic and/or hemorrhagic zones;
5. stromal and/or vascular invasion.

The presence of occasional large bizarre cells or focal high cellularity in the absence of cellular atypia or mitosis is usually not sufficient to categorize the tumor as malignant.[1,43,46]

The use of immunohistochemistry has been an extremely useful tool to differentiate SFTP from mesotheliomas and sarcomas over the last few years. Indeed, SFTP by definition is vimentin positive and keratin negative. In addition, CD34 is positive in most benign and malignant SFTP, whereas it remains negative for most other pulmonary tumors. Occasionally, malignant SFTP may be CD34 negative.[13,43] The expression of bcl-2 can be a useful marker to confirm the diagnosis of SFTP if CD34 is negative.[47,48]

Recently, some authors have demonstrated that CD99 and factor XIIIa could be expressed by solitary fibrous tumors located in the pleura and in other locations.[48–51] However, in contrast to CD34 and bcl-2, CD99 and factor XIIIa are not strongly expressed by SFTP and can also frequently be positive with other tumors such as synovial sarcomas or neural tumors and, thus, are less specific for the diagnosis of SFTP.[52]

MANAGEMENT

Complete *en bloc* surgical resection is the mainstay of therapy for all benign and malignant SFTP. A distance of 1–2 cm from the tumor is usually recommended to have adequate margins. While pedunculated tumors can be safely resected with a wedge resection of the lung, large sessile tumors can be difficult to resect because of extensive adhesions and may occasionally require a lobectomy or a pneumonectomy in order to achieve complete resection.[53–55] Frozen sections can be helpful to demonstrate that the resection margins are free of tumors, but are not routinely required.

Tumors adherent to the parietal pleura require an extra-pleural dissection.[22,53] However, concomitant chest wall resection can be necessary if the tumor densely adheres to or invades the chest wall.[19] In 3 percent or less of cases the tumor can be 'inverted' and grow inside the lung parenchyma (Figure 38.2).[56,57] These tumors often require a lobectomy or a sleeve lobectomy.[43,53,58,59] In our experience in Toronto, a sleeve lobectomy was required in one case for a solitary fibrous tumor growing from the left lower lobe bronchus inside the left main bronchus. Interestingly, the tumor was growing without invading the main bronchus and could be simply pulled back from the main bronchus.[52]

Thoracoscopic approaches can be safely used to remove small pedunculated tumors located on the visceral pleura.[53,60] Some authors have also recommended the assistance of a video-camera to obtain a more precise view of the resection margins in some large broad-based tumors of the parietal pleura.[53] Extreme caution should be used to avoid contact between the tumor and the thoracoscopic

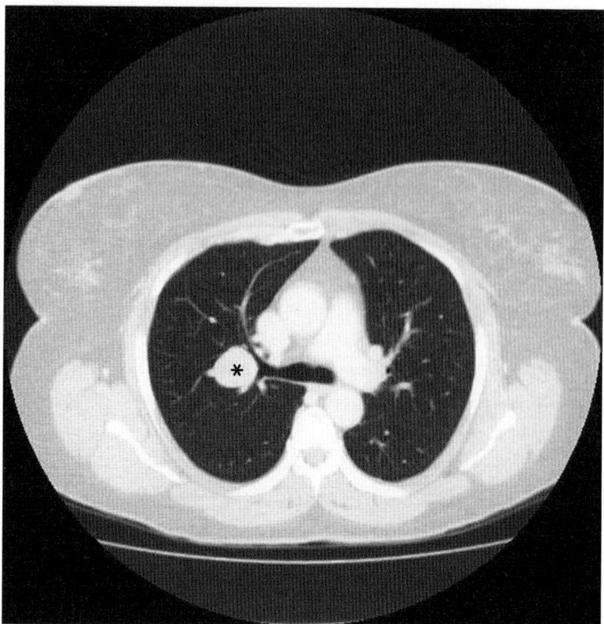

Figure 38.2 Solitary fibrous tumor growing inside the lung parenchyma and located at the bifurcation between the segmental bronchi of the right upper lobe (*). A lobectomy was required to remove this tumor. Histological evaluation demonstrated a benign solitary fibrous tumor of the pleura. The risk of recurrence of benign intraparenchymal tumors is estimated to be approximately 8 percent.

sites, since contact metastasis and local recurrence at the port sites have been reported.[53,54]

ADJUVANT THERAPY

The role of adjuvant therapy in SFTP has not been systematically explored because of the limited number of patients.[61] However, evidence suggests that radiotherapy and chemotherapy could be beneficial in some patients. Suter and colleagues[19] have reported one patient who is alive with no evidence of disease more than 20 years after subtotal resection of the tumor followed by radiotherapy, and Veronesi and colleagues[62] have observed significant reduction of an inoperable recurrent SFTP with ifosfamide and adriamycine. Although neoadjuvant therapy could be helpful in large malignant tumors, its use is limited by the difficulty to obtain a precise preoperative diagnosis even with an open biopsy.[62] Currently, we would recommend the administration of adjuvant therapy after resection of malignant sessile tumors, in particular if they are recurrent.

Additional therapies such as brachytherapy and photodynamic therapy have been developed for malignant mesothelioma and could be applied for other pleural tumors. However, their use in SFTP has rarely been reported and their utility remains unproven.[61,63]

PROGNOSIS

Morphological and histological parameters are important predictors of outcome.[64] In 1981, Briselli and coworkers[3] presented eight new cases and reviewed 360 cases from the literature. Twelve percent of the tumors followed a malignant course and led to death. The authors observed that the growth pattern of the tumor was more important for prognosis than the histological characteristics. More recently, England and coworkers[1] reported 223 cases from the files of the Armed Forced Institute of Pathology, of which 82 were described as histologically malignant. While none of the patients with a histologically benign disease died, 55 percent of those with a malignant form died because of recurrences and/or metastases. The authors observed that among the malignant variants, complete resection was the single most important predictor of outcome.

In order to stratify the risk of recurrence, a staging system was developed after reviewing all publications with adequate follow-up for patients with a diagnosis of SFTP proven by histology and immunohistochemistry.[52] Among a total of 185 reported cases, 35 (19 percent) presented with recurrence and 16 of them died (Table 38.3). Of the 35 patients who presented with recurrent tumor, 27 had a primary sessile tumor with histological sign of malignancy, whereas five presented with a primary sessile histologically benign tumor and two with a primary pedunculated histologically malignant tumor. One patient with a pedunculated histologically benign tumor presented a recurrence (or a new primary tumor) and died 10 years after the initial resection.[43]

The risk of recurrence was therefore observed to be the highest in patients with malignant sessile tumors (estimated to be approximately 63 percent) and this type of SFTP were classified as stage III. Patients with malignant pedunculated tumor were found to have a 14 percent risk of recurrence and were classified as stage II. Patients with benign sessile tumor had an 8 percent risk of recurrence and were classified as stage I. Patients presenting with benign pedunculated tumor were found to have a risk of recurrence of less than 2 percent and were considered as benign, therefore classified as stage 0 (Table 38.4).

Some authors observed that tumors larger than 10 cm had a worse prognosis than smaller tumors.[65,66] However, the worse prognosis is related to the higher frequency of malignant histological characteristics present in these large tumors and to the higher rate of incomplete resection in this group of patients. In our review of the literature,[52] we observed that all patients with a histologically benign tumor larger than 10 cm that was completely resected had a good clinical outcome, whereas 16 out of the 28 tumors larger than 10 cm with malignant characteristics were associated with recurrence. Hence, although the majority of malignant tumors are larger than 10 cm, histological characteristics and resectability rather than size are the principal indicators of clinical outcome.

Table 38.3 Summary of recent publications on solitary fibrous tumors of pleura (SFTP)[a]

	Malignant sessile	Malignant pedunculated	Benign sessile	Benign pedunculated
Total number of patients	43	15	62	65
Number of patients without recurrence	16 (37%)	13 (86%)	57 (92%)	64 (98%)
Number of patients with recurrence	27 (63%)	2 (14%)	5 (8%)	1 (2%)
Number of deaths related to the tumor	13 (30%)	1 (7%)	1 (2%)	1 (2%)

[a]Includes all series reporting adequate follow-up for patients with a diagnosis of SFTP proven by histology and immunohistochemistry (adapted from reference 52).

Table 38.4 Classification of solitary fibrous tumors of the pleura

Stage		Estimated risk of recurrence (%)
Stage 0	Pedunculated tumor without signs of malignancy[a]	<2
Stage I	Sessile or intraparenchymal tumor without signs of malignancy[a]	8
Stage II	Pedunculated tumor with histological signs of malignancy[a]	14
Stage III	Sessile or intraparenchymal tumor with histological signs of malignancy[a]	63
Stage IV	Multiple synchronous metastatic tumors	>95

[a]Malignancy is recognized by the presence of the following features: high cellularity with crowding and overlapping of nuclei, cellular pleomorphism; high motitic count (>4/10 high-power field), necrosis or stromal/vascular invasion.

FOLLOW-UP

Recurrence after surgical resection is most often located in the same hemithorax and has been reported up to 17 years after resection.[21] Intrathoracic recurrence may be fatal because of mediastinal compression and inferior vena cava obstruction.[3,67] Metastases, if present, are usually blood-borne and located by order of frequency, in the liver, central nervous system, spleen, peritoneum, adrenal gland, gastrointestinal tract, kidney and bone.[1]

The risk of recurrence is high after resection of malignant sessile SFTP. However, most of the recurrences are initially located inside the pleural cavity and distant metastasis seems to be a late event in the evolution of the disease. Recurrences are often associated with a progression in the degree of malignancy.[19,43] The majority of recurrence after resection of malignant sessile tumors occurs within the first 24 months after the initial resection. Hence, half-yearly radiological control with chest X-ray or CT scan during the initial 2 years after the resection and yearly thereafter seems warranted and may help to reduce the mortality from malignant SFTP. In case of recurrence, aggressive surgical resection remains the treatment of choice and may lead to long-term survival.[20] Adjuvant therapy should be considered if the tumor appears histologically malignant.

CONCLUSIONS

Solitary fibrous tumor of the pleura is a mesenchymal tumor that has been increasingly recognized over the past few years. The tumor was initially described in the pleura but has been reported in many other sites lately. Although the majority of these tumors have a benign course, the malignant form still remains enigmatic. Their behavior is often unpredictable and does not always correlate with histological findings. In addition, benign tumors may remain silent for several years before degenerating into a malignant form. Complete *en bloc* surgical resection is the mainstay of therapy for all benign and malignant SFTP. Histological and morphological characteristics are the principal indicators of clinical outcome.

FUTURE DIRECTIONS OF DEVELOPMENT

Better understanding of the molecular mechanisms leading to the malignant form of solitary fibrous tumors will be important in the future. This may help to develop novel targeted therapy for patient at risk of recurrence or with advanced disease.

KEY POINTS

- Solitary fibrous tumor of the pleura is a mesenchymal tumor growing along the pleura or within the lung parenchyma.
- Solitary fibrous tumor of the pleura can be benign or malignant.
- Histological signs of malignancy include: high cellularity with crowding and overlapping of nuclei, cellular pleomorphism, high mitotic count (>4/10 HPF), necrosis or stromal/vascular invasion.
- Complete *en bloc* surgical resection is the mainstay of therapy for all benign and malignant solitary fibrous tumors of the pleura.
- Histological and morphological characteristics are the principal indicators of outcome.
- Benign pedunculated tumors are considered benign with a risk of recurrence of less than 2 percent.
- Benign sessile or intraparenchymal tumors have an estimated risk of recurrence of 8 percent.
- Malignant pedunculated tumors have an estimated risk of recurrence of 14 percent.
- Malignant sessile tumors have the highest rate of recurrence with an estimated risk of recurrence of 63 percent.

REFERENCES

● = Key primary paper
◆ = Major review article
∗ = Paper that represents the first formal publication of a management guideline

●1. England DM, Hochholzer L, McCarthy MJ. Localized benign and malignant fibrous tumors of the pleura. A clinicopathologic review of 223 cases. *Am J Surg Pathol* 1989; **13**: 640–58.
2. Watts DM, Jones GP, Bowman GA, Olsen JD. Giant benign mesothelioma. *Ann Thorac Surg* 1989; **48**: 590–1.
●3. Briselli M, Mark EJ, Dickersin GR. Solitary fibrous tumors of the pleura: eight new cases and review of 360 cases in the literature. *Cancer* 1981; **47**: 2678–89.
4. de Perrot M, Kurt AM, Robert JH, Borisch B, Spiliopoulos A. Clinical behavior of solitary fibrous tumors of the pleura. *Ann Thorac Surg* 1999; **67**: 1456–9.
5. Wagner E. Das tuberkelahnliche Lymphadenom (Der cytogene oder reticulirte Tuberkel). *Arch Heilk (Leipzig)* 1870; **11**: 497.
6. Klemperer P, Rabin CB. Primary neoplasm of the pleura. A report of five cases. *Arch Pathol* 1931; **11**: 385–412.
7. Stout AP, Murray MR. Localized pleural mesothelioma. *Arch Pathol* 1942; **34**: 951–64.
8. Foster EA, Ackerman LV. Localized mesotheliomas of the pleura. *Am J Clin Pathol* 1960; **34**: 349–64.
9. Luse SA, Spjut HJ. An electron microscopic study of solitary pleural mesothelioma. *Cancer* 1964; **17**: 1546–54.
10. Scharifker D, Kaneko M. Localized fibrous mesothelioma of pleura (submesothelial fibroma). A clinicopathologic study of 18 cases. *Cancer* 1979; **43**: 627–35.
11. Hernandez FJ, Hernandez BB. Localized fibrous tumors of pleura: A light and electron microscopic study. *Cancer* 1974; **34**: 1667–74.
12. Al-Azzi M, Thurlow NP, Corrin B. Pleural mesothelioma of connective tissue type, localized fibrous tumor of the pleura, and reactive submesothelial hyperplasia. An immunohistochemical comparison. *J Pathol* 1989; **158**: 41–4.
13. van de Rijn M, Lombard CM, Rouse RV. Expression of CD34 by solitary fibrous tumors of the pleura, mediastinum, and lung. *Am J Surg Pathol* 1994; **18**: 814–20.
14. Flint A, Weiss SW. CD-34 and keratin expression distinguishes solitary fibrous tumor (fibrous mesothelioma) of pleura from desmoplastic mesothelioma. *Hum Pathol* 1995; **26**: 428–31.
15. Weiss SW, Nickoloff BJ. CD34 is expressed by a distinctive cell population in peripheral nerve, nerve sheath tumours, and related lesions. *Am J Surg Pathol* 1993; **17**: 747–53.
16. Nickoloff J. The human progenitor cell antigen (CD34) is localized on endothelial cells, dermal dendritic cells, and perifollicular cells in formalin-fixed normal skin, and on proliferating endothelial cells and stromal spindle shaped cells in Kaposi's sarcoma. *Arch Dermatol* 1991; **127**: 523–9.
17. van de Rijn M, Rouse RV. CD34, a review. *Appl Immunohistochem* 1994; **2**: 71–80.
18. Robinson LA, Reilly RB. Localized pleural mesothelioma. The clinical spectrum. *Chest* 1994; **106**: 1611–5.
19. Suter M, Gebhard S, Boumghar M, Peloponisios N, Genton CY. Localized fibrous tumours of the pleura: 15 new cases and review of the literature. *Eur J Cardiothorac Surg* 1998; **14**: 453–9.
20. Saifuddin A, Da Costa P, Chalmers AG, Carey BM, Robertson RJ. Primary malignant localized fibrous tumours of the pleura: clinical, radiological, and pathological features. *Clin Radiol* 1992; **45**: 13–7.
21. Okike N, Bernatz PE, Woolner LB. Localized mesothelioma of the pleura. Benign and malignant variants. *J Thorac Cardiovasc Surg* 1978; **75**: 363–72.
22. Rena O, Filosso PL, Papalia E, *et al.* Solitary fibrous tumour of the pleura: surgical treatment. *Eur J Cardiothorac Surg* 2001; **19**: 185–9.
23. Chaugle H, Parchment C, Grotte GJ, Keenan DJM. Hypoglycemia associated with a solitary fibrous tumour of the pleura. *Eur J Cardiothorac Surg* 1999; **15**: 84–6.
24. Chamberlain MH, Taggart DP. Solitary fibrous tumor associated with hypoglycemia: an example of the Doege–Potter syndrome. *J Thorac Cardiovasc Surg* 2000; **119**: 185–7.
25. Cole FH Jr, Ellis RA, Goodman RC, Weber BC, Courington DP. Benign fibrous pleural tumor with elevation of insulin-like growth actor and hypoglycemia. *South Med J* 1990; **83**: 690–4.
26. Sakamoto T, Kaneshige H, Takeshi A, Tsushima T, Hasegawa S. Localized pleural mesothelioma with elevation of high molecular weight insulin-like growth factor II and hypoglycemia. *Chest* 1994; **106**: 965–7.
27. Theros EG, Feigin DS. Pleural tumors and pulmonary tumors: differential diagnosis. *Semin Roentgenol* 1977; **12**: 239–47.
28. Mendelson DS, Meary E, Buy JN, Pigeau I, Kirschner PA. Localized fibrous pleural mesothelioma: CT findings. *Clin Imag* 1991; **15**: 105–8.
29. Lewis MI, Horak DA, Yellin A, *et al.* The case of the moving intrathoracic mass. *Chest* 1985; **88**: 897–8.
30. Karabulut N, Goodman LR. Pedunculated solitary fibrous tumor of the interlobar fissure: a wandering chest mass. *AJR Am J Roentgenol* 1999; **173**: 476–7.
31. Lee KS, Im J, Choe KO, Kim CJ, Lee BH. CT findings in benign fibrous mesothelioma of the pleura. *Am J Radiol* 1992; **158**: 983–6.
32. Spizarny DL, Gross BH, Shepard JAO. CT findings in localized fibrous mesothelioma of the pleural fissure. *J Comput Assist Tomogr* 1986; **10**: 942–4.
33. Muller NL. Imaging of the pleura. *Radiology* 1993; **186**: 297–309.

34. Ferretti GR, Chiles C, Cox JE, Choplin RH, Coulomb M. Localized benign fibrous tumors of the pleura: MR appearance. *J Comput Assist Tomogr* 1997; **21**: 115–20.
35. Norton SA, Clark SC, Sheehan AL, Ibrahim NBN, Jeyasingham K. Solitary fibrous tumour of the diaphragm. *J Cardiovasc Surg* 1997; **38**: 685–6.
36. Arrive L, Hricak H, Tavares NJ, Miller TR. Malignant versus nonmalignant retroperitoneal fibrosis: differentiation with MR imaging. *Radiology* 1989; **172**: 139–43.
37. Falaschi F, Battolla L, Mascalchi M, *et al.* Usefullness of MR signal: intensity in distinguishing benign from malignant pleural disease. *AJR Am J Roentgenol* 1966; **166**: 963–8.
38. Verluis PJ, Lamers RJ. Localized pleural fibroma: radiological features. *Eur J Radiol* 1994; **18**: 124–5.
39. Harris GN, Rozenstein A, Schiff MJ. Benign fibrous mesothelioma of the pleura: MR imaging findings. *AJR Am J Roentgenol* 1995; **165**: 1143–4.
40. Alexander M, Yang S, Yung R, Brasic JR, Pannu H. Diagnosis of benign solitary fibrous tumors by positron emission tomography. *South Med J* 2004; **97**: 1264–7.
41. Kramer H, Pieterman RM, Slebos DJ, *et al.* PET for the evaluation of pleural thickening observed on CT. *J Nucl Med* 2004; **45**: 995–8.
42. Witkin GB, Rosai J. Solitary fibrous tumor of the mediastinum. A report of 14 cases. *Am J Surg Pathol* 1989; **13**: 547–57.
43. Yokoi T, Tsuzuki T, Yatabe Y, *et al.* Solitary fibrous tumour: significance of p53 and CD34 immunoreactivity in its malignant transformation. *Histopathology* 1998; **32**: 423–32.
44. Moran CA, Suster S, Koss MN. The spectrum of histologic growth patterns in benign and malignant fibrous tumours of the pleura. *Semin Diagn Pathol* 1992; **9**: 169–80.
45. Stout AP. Tumors of the pleura. *Harlem Hosp Bull* 1971; **5**: 54–7.
46. Hanau CA, Miettinen M. Solitary fibrous tumor: histological and immunohistochemical spectrum of benign and malignant variants presenting at different sites. *Hum Pathol* 1995; **26**: 440–9.
47. Chilosi M, Facchetti F, Dei Tos AP, *et al.* bcl-2 expression in pleural and extrapleural solitary fibrous tumours. *J Pathol* 1997; **181**: 362–7.
48. Suster S, Fisher C, Moran CA. Expression of bcl-2 oncoprotein in benign and malignant spindle cell tumors of soft tissue, skin, serosal surfaces, and gastrointestinal tract. *Am J Surg Pathol* 1998; **22**: 863–72.
49. Vallat-Decouvelaere AV, Dry SM, Fletcher CDM. Atypical and malignant solitary fibrous tumors in extrathoracic locations. Evidence of their comparability to intra-thoracic tumors. *Am J Surg Pathol* 1998; **22**: 1501–11.
50. Mentzel T, Bainbridge TC, Katenkamp D. Solitary fibrous tumour: clinicopathological, immunohistochemical, and ultrastructural analysis of 12 cases arising in soft tissues, nasal cavity and nasopharynx, urinary bladder and prostate. *Virchows Arch* 1997; **430**: 445–53.
51. Alawi F, Stratton D, Freedman PD. Solitary fibrous tumor of the oral soft tissues. A clinicopathologic and immunohistochemical study of 16 cases. *Am J Surg Pathol* 2001; **25**: 900–10.
◆52. de Perrot M, Fischer S, Brundler MA, Sekine Y, Keshavjee S. Solitary fibrous tumors of the pleura. *Ann Thorac Surg* 2002; **74**: 285–93.
53. Cardillo G, Facciolo F, Cavazzana AO, *et al.* Localized (solitary) fibrous tumors of the pleura: an analysis of 55 patients. *Ann Thorac Surg* 2000; **70**: 1808–12.
54. Nomori H, Horio H, Fuyuno G, Morinaga S. Contacting metastasis of a fibrous tumor of the pleura. *Eur J Cardiothorac Surg* 1997; **12**: 928–30.
55. Sung SH, Chang JW, Kim J, *et al.* Solitary fibrous tumors of the pleura: surgical outcome and clinical course. *Ann Thorac Surg* 2005; **79**: 303–7.
56. Yousem SA, Flynn SD. Intrapulmonary localized fibrous tumor. Intraparenchymal so-called localized fibrous mesothelioma. *Am J Clin Pathol* 1988; **89**: 365–9.
57. Patsios D, Hwang DM, Chung TB. Intraparenchymal solitary fibrous tumor of the lung: an uncommon cause of a pulmonary nodule. *J Thorac Imaging* 2006; **21**: 50–3.
58. Khalifa M, Montgomery EA, Azumi N, *et al.* Solitary fibrous tumors: a series of lesions, some in unusual sites. *South Med J* 1997; **90**: 793–9.
59. Aufiero TX, McGary SA, Campbell DB, Phillips PP. Intrapulmonary benign fibrous tumor of the pleura. *J Thorac Cardiovasc Surg* 1995; **110**: 549–51.
60. Sanguinetti CM, Marchesani F, Ranaldi R, Pela R, Cecarini L. Localized fibrous pleural tumour of the interlobular pleura. *Eur Respir J* 1996; **9**: 1094–6.
*61. de Perrot M. Fibrous tumors of the pleura. *Curr Treat Options Oncol* 2000; **1**: 293–8.
62. Veronesi G, Spaggiari L, Mazzarol G, *et al.* Huge malignant localized fibrous tumor of the pleura. *J Cardiovasc Surg* 2000; **41**: 781–4.
63. Martini N, McCormack PM, Bains MS, *et al.* Pleural mesothelioma. *Ann Thorac Surg* 1987; **43**: 113–20.
64. Chan JKC. Solitary fibrous tumour – everywhere, and a diagnosis in vogue. *Histopathology* 1997; **31**: 568–76.
65. Brozzetti S, D'Andrea N, Limiti MR, *et al.* Clinical behavior of solitary fibrous tumors of the pleura. An immunohistochemical study. *Anticancer Res* 2000; **20**: 4701–6.
66. Chang YL, Lee YC, Wu CT. Thoracic solitary fibrous tumor: clinical and pathological diversity. *Lung Cancer* 1999; **23**: 53–60.
67. Dalton WT, Zolliker AS, McCaughey WTE, Jacques J, Kannerstaein M. Localized primary tumors of the pleura. An analysis of 40 cases. *Cancer* 1979; **44**: 1465–75.

39

Undiagnosed pleural effusions

NICK A MASKELL

INTRODUCTION

Despite a full work up, approximately 15 percent of pleural effusions elude a definite diagnosis.[1] All respiratory physicians therefore face this problem in their clinical practice. This chapter discusses an approach to this problem. The principle aims are to exclude any treatable causes of the effusion, avoid subjecting frail patients to unnecessary interventions and at the same time manage patients' expectations.

IS THE PLEURAL EFFUSION A TRANSUDATE OR EXUDATE?

In practice, many of us will often simply rely on the pleural protein level to establish whether a pleural effusion is a transudate or exudate. However, in cases where the pleural protein is close to the arbitrary cut off of 30 g/L, and in all cases of a persistent undiagnosed effusion, it is the authors opinion that this needs to be revisited and that Light's criteria should be used (see Table 39.1).[2] This will then help triage further investigations accordingly (see also Chapter 17, Pleural fluid analysis).

It is worth noting that Light's criteria has the weakness of occasionally labeling an effusion in a patient with congestive heart failure on diuretics, as an exudate. This is important as these effusions are also likely to be lymphocytic and so if the clinical suspicion is one of heart failure, then a trial of increased diuretics may be useful. Tables 39.2 and 39.3 list the common cases of both transudates and exudates.

Table 39.1 Modified Light's criteria[a]

Pleural fluid is an exudate if one or more of the following criteria are met:
Pleural fluid protein divided by serum protein greater than 0.5
Pleural fluid LDH divided by serum LDH greater than 0.6
Pleural fluid LDH >0.45 the upper limits of normal serum LDH

[a]Modified from Heffner JE. *Clin Chest Med* 1998; **19**: 277–93.
LDH, lactate dehydrogenase.

REVISITING THE PATIENTS' HISTORY

It is good practice to revisit the patients' drug history for possible causative drugs. A useful resource in this regard is the web site www.pneumotox.com. Important pointers in the history are significant weight loss which suggests underlying malignancy and a history of sweats and fevers, which would be in keeping with pleural infection.

Table 39.2 Causes of transudative pleural effusions

Causes	
Left ventricular failure	Constrictive pericarditis
Mitral stenosis	Urinothorax
Liver cirrhosis	Peritoneal dialysis
Nephrotic syndrome	Superior vena cava obstruction
Hypoalbuminemia	
Trapped lung (remote from inflammatory process)	

Table 39.3 Some of the common conditions causing an exudative pleural effusion

Common conditions	
Parapneumonic effusion	Pulmonary infarction
Malignancy	Connective tissue diseases
Tuberculosis	Fungal infections
Drugs	Benign asbestos effusion
Post-cardiac injury syndrome (PCIS)	Yellow nail syndrome
Rheumatoid arthritis	Pancreatitis
Trapped lung (when inflammatory process not remote)	

EXCLUDING TREATABLE DISEASE

The next step is to try and rule out any disease process which is potentially amenable to treatment. Figure 39.1 shows a suggested algorithm for this process. Each of these conditions will also be discussed in the text below.

Pulmonary embolus

Pulmonary embolism is the fourth leading cause of pleural effusion.[3,4] It always needs to be considered in cases of persistent undiagnosed effusions because they are both life-threatening and treatable. The effusions are usually unilateral and occupy less than one-third of the hemithorax.[3] In 80 percent of cases they are exudates, 20 percent transudates and the pleural fluid is often blood stained. The pleural fluid is often lymphocytic, but there are no characteristic features which enable pulmonary embolus to be completely ruled out. Common presenting features include pleuritic chest pain with associated shortness of breath.[5] If suspected, a D-dimer measurement is a useful starting point, followed by a computer tomography pulmonary angiogram (CTPA) if the D-dimer test is positive.[6] (Further discussion can be found in Chapter 30, Effusions from vascular causes.)

Effusion after coronary artery bypass surgery

Effusions are common after coronary artery bypass surgery. These are commonly left-sided. Approximately 10 percent of patients have a pleural effusion that occupies more than 25 percent of their hemithorax, within the first 4 weeks of surgery. These effusions are exudates and usually predominantly lymphocytic. A small percentage of these can reaccumulate after drainage for periods in excess of 1 year after surgery.[7]

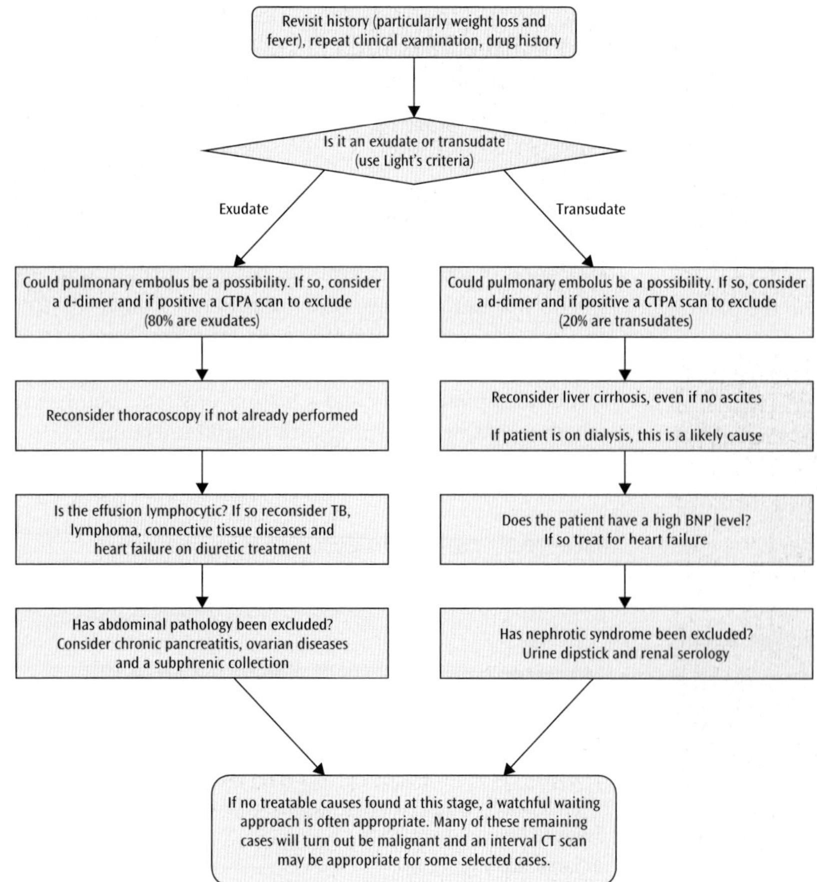

Figure 39.1 Algorithm for a persistent undiagnosed pleural effusion. BNP, brain natriuetic protein; CTPA, computed tomography pulmonary angiogram; TB, tuberculosis.

Meigs' syndrome

Meigs' syndrome was initially reported in 1937 in a small group of women with ovarian fibromas associated with ascities and pleural effusions.[8] A hallmark of this condition is the resolution of both the pleural effusion and ascites once the tumour has been surgically removed. It is postulated that fluid probably moves into the pleural space through small diaphragmatic defects and possibly through diaphragmatic lymphatics moving from the peritoneal cavity to the pleural cavity. In 70 percent of cases the effusion is right-sided, in 20 percent it is bilateral and is left-sided in the remaining 10 percent.[9–11] The pleural fluid is usually an exudate and the diagnosis should be thought of in female patients presenting with an effusion and ascites. It is most common in women in their fifth to seventh decades. Figure 39.2 shows two chest radiographs of a patient with Meigs' syndrome before and after surgery.

Lymphoma

Often pleural effusions secondary to lymphoma are accompanied with mediastinal lymphadenopathy. However, this is not always the case and primary pleural lymphoma is a recognized disease entity. The incidence of lymphoma is currently increasing in the western world and therefore a diagnosis of lymphoma should be entertained in patients presenting with a lymphocytic effusion. Flow cytometry and cytogenetics can be extremely helpful in this setting but often pleural tissue or lymph node sampling will be required to obtain a definitive diagnosis.

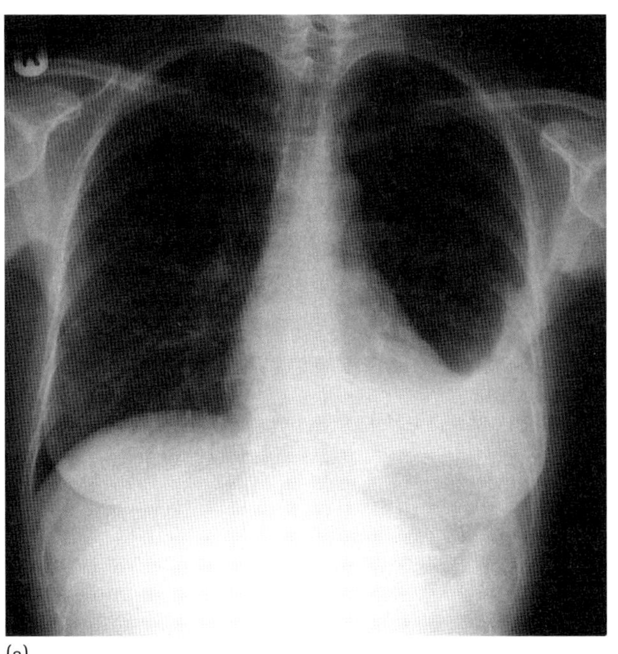

(a)

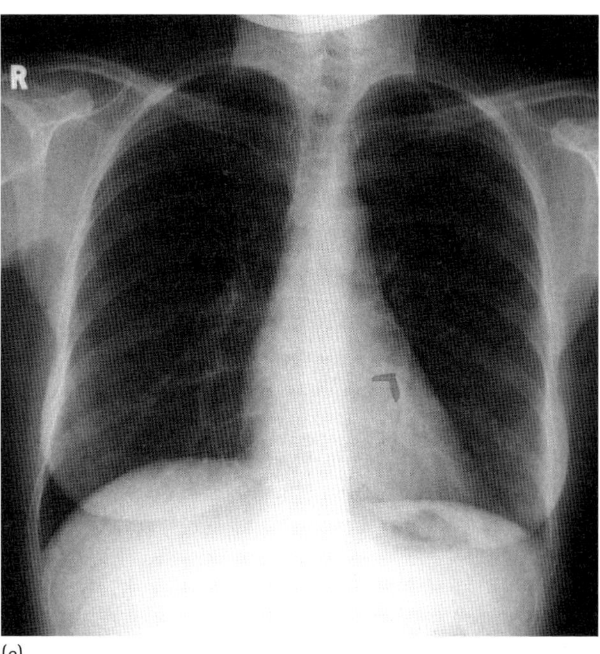

(c)

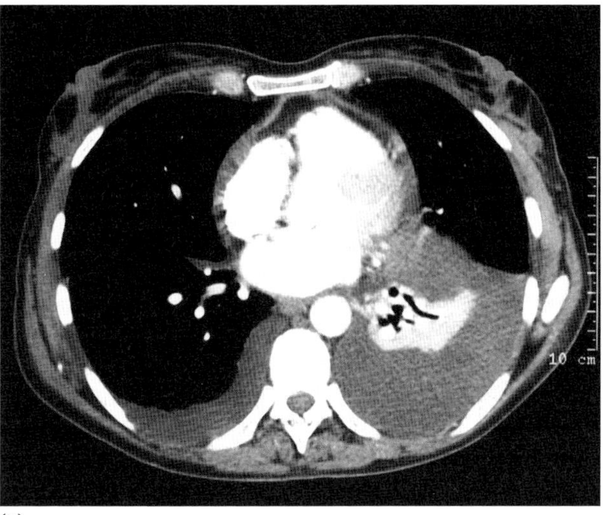

(b)

Figure 39.2 Chest radiography in a patient with Meigs' syndrome. (a) Chest radiograph showing left pleural effusion. (b) Computed tomography thorax one week later showing bilateral pleural effusions. (c) Chest radiograph 2 weeks after surgical removal of benign ovarian tumor.

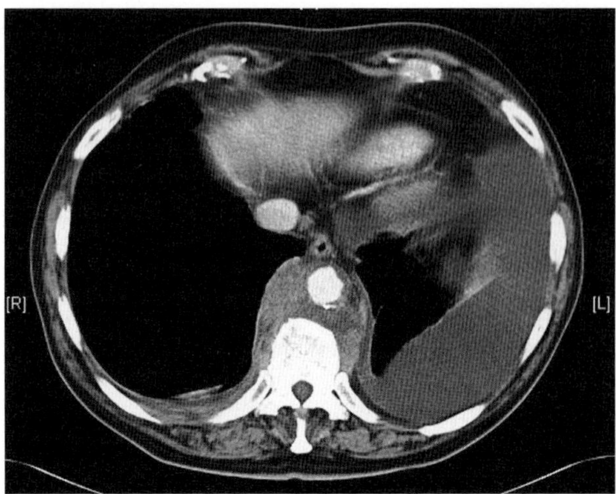

Figure 39.3 Computed tomography image of a man with non-Hodgkins lymphoma with a paraspinal mass and unilateral pleural effusion.

Figure 39.3 shows a CT image of a man with non-Hodgkins lymphoma who presented with a unilateral pleural effusion.

Benign asbestos pleural disease

Benign asbestos pleural effusion can occur following asbestos exposure (see also Chapter 40). Their occurrence is unusual beyond 25 years after first exposure. This contrasts with malignant mesothelioma where the incidence increases with increasing time after initial exposure to asbestos.[12] Because malignant mesothelioma cannot be fully excluded careful follow-up is required in such cases.

Pleural effusions in acquired immunodeficiency syndrome

Pleural effusions are common in patients with acquired immunodeficiency syndrome (AIDS; discussed further in Chapter 31). *Human immunodeficiency virus* (HIV) testing always needs to be considered in cases of persistent effusions. Most of these are due to infection which may be bacterial or tuberculosis. There is a high incidence of parapneumonic effusions in AIDS patients. The most common causative organisms, however, are common community-acquired organisms such as *Streptococcus* spp.[13]

Trapped lung

Trapped lung occurs when a thick layer of fibrous tissues encases part of the visceral pleura preventing the lung from full expansion to the chest wall. This results in recurrent pleural effusion as the intrapleural pressure will be more negative than usual. These usually occur as part of a malignant process, but can occur after a parapneumonic illness that has not been treated adequately or in a timely manner. It therefore needs to be considered in difficult-to-diagnose cases and not assumed to be definitely malignant in origin.[14,15] If the patient is fit enough, decortication is the treatment of choice, in symptomatic and non-malignant cases. It also allows extensive sampling of the visceral pleura to exclude underlying malignancy.

Tuberculous pleurisy

Smears for acid-fast bacilli are only positive in 10–20 percent of tuberculous effusions and only 25–50 percent are positive on pleural fluid culture.[16,17] The addition of pleural biopsy histology and culture improves the diagnostic rate to approximately 90 percent.[17] Although not widely available, high adenosine deaminase (ADA) levels can be useful in adding weight to a clinical suspicion of tuberculosis (TB) pleuritis, particularly if the effusion is lymphocytic. Unfortunately, it is also often elevated with pleural infection and rheumatoid pleurisy and so must be interpreted with caution. In one study of 405 pleural fluids including 91 that were due to tuberculosis, all cases had an ADA level above 45 units/mL.[18] The management of TB pleural effusions is discussed in Chapter 27.

Pleural effusions caused by abdominal pathologies

It is also important to consider abdominal pathology in persistent undiagnosed pleural effusions. Causes include cirrhosis of the liver, which causes a pleural transudate often accompanied by ascites. Chronic pancreatitis can also cause pleural effusions without any abdominal symptoms. If this is suspected, pleural fluid amylase levels will usually be elevated. Subphrenic abscesses can also cause sterile effusions in the early stages of this disease process. There is often a history of recent abdominal surgery in these cases.[9,19]

Pleural effusion secondary to collagen vascular disease

Pleural inflammation mediated through compliment activation and vasculitis causing increased capillary permeability is largely responsible for these pleural effusions (see also Chapter 32, Effusions from connective tissue diseases). Collagen vascular disease needs to be considered, particularly when there are bilateral exudative effusions with a history of other suggestive problems such as Raynold's phenomenon. Often the serum autoimmune profile is suggestive, e.g. a positive anti-nuclear antibody

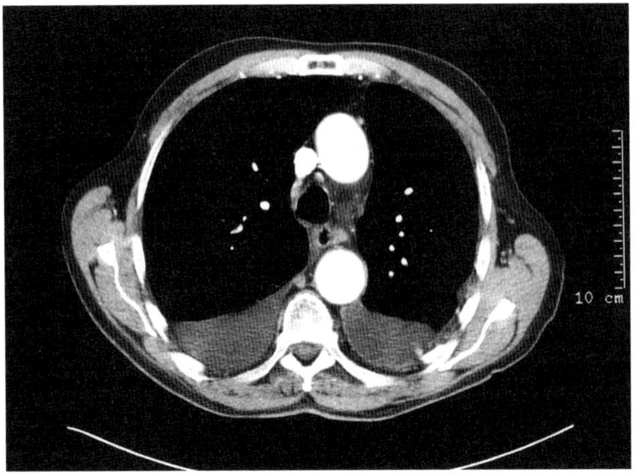

Figure 39.4 Computed tomography showing bilateral pleural effusions in a man with an undifferentiated connective tissue disorder.

(ANA), but non-diagnostic. Figure 39.4 shows a CT image of one such case who presented with bilateral exudates, effusions and a history of Raynold's phenomenon and a positive ANA, and went on to develop a pericardial effusion because of a undifferentiated connective tissue disorder.

Pleural involvement occurs in 5 percent of patients with rheumatoid arthritis. In these cases the most common thoracic manifestation is pleurisy. There tends to be a male predominance and it tends to occur in older men with rheumatoid nodules. Appearance of pleural fluid in rheumatoid arthritis is variable. It can be serous, turbid, yellowish green, milky, bloody or chylous. Figure 39.5 shows the chest radiograph and pseudochylous effusion of a man with rheumatoid arthritis. The fluid contained cholesterol crystals and a high cholesterol level with low levels of triglycerides.

Up to 50 percent of patients with systemic lupus erythematosus (SLE) will have pleural disease at some time in the course of their disease. Here, pleural biopsies tend to show nonspecific inflammation and infiltration with lymphocytes and plasma cells. When pleural fluid ANA exceeds 1:160 and the pleural fluid:serum ANA ratio >1, the diagnosis of lupus is likely. Drugs that are most commonly incriminated in drug-induced lupus are hydralozine, phenytoin and chlorpromazine.[20–22]

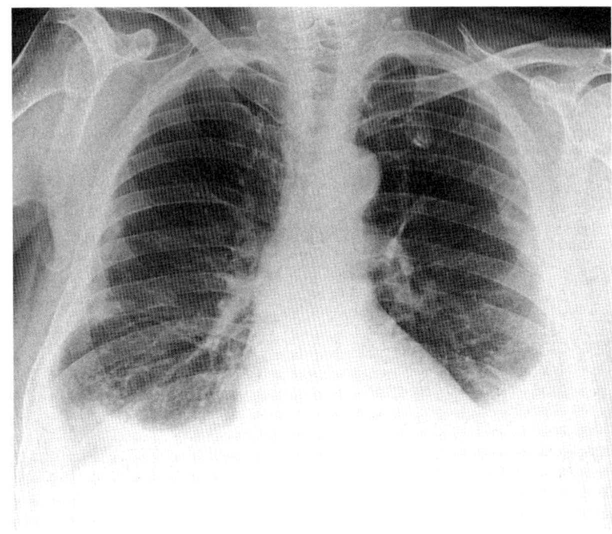

(a)

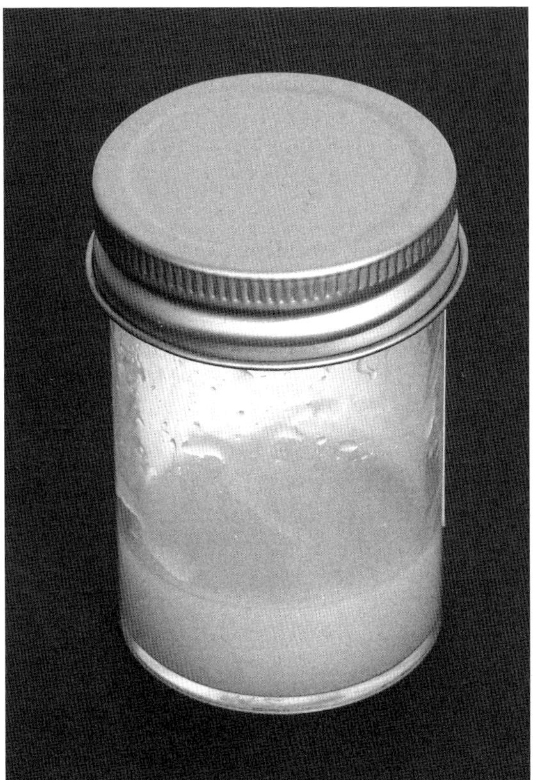

(b)

Figure 39.5 Chest radiograph (a) and pseudochylous effusion (b) in a man with rheumatoid arthritis. (For (b), see also Color Plate 48.)

Chylous and pseudochylous effusions

True chylous effusions result from disruption of the thoracic duct or its tributaries. This leads to the presence of chyle in the pleural space. Approximately 50 percent are due to malignancy (particularly lymphoma), 25 percent trauma (especially during surgery) and the rest are miscellaneous causes such as TB, sarcoid, amyloidosis, aneurysm of the thoracic aorta, lymphangioleiomyomatosis and tuberous sclerosis.[23] The pleural fluid contains high levels of triglycerides. Chylothorax must be distinguished from pseudochylothorax or 'cholesterol pleurisy' which is due to the accumulation of cholesterol crystals in a long-standing pleural effusion. In these cases the pleura is usually markedly thickened and fibrotic.[24]

In the past, the most common causes of a pseudochylous effusion were tuberculosis and artificial pneumothorax. Chronic rheumatoid pleurisy is now the usual cause.

These two types of effusion can be discriminated by lipid analysis of the fluid. A true chylothorax will usually have a pleural fluid triglyceride level of >1.24 mmol/L (110 mg/dL), and can usually be excluded if the triglyceride is <0.56 mmol/L (50 mg/dL). Asking the laboratory to look for the presence of chylomicrons is useful to confirm the diagnosis of chylothorax. In a pseudochylothorax the cholesterol level is greater than 5.18 mmol/L (200 mg/dL), chylomicrons are not found and cholesterol crystals are often seen at microscopy.[25] Effusions from disruption of the lymphatics are discussed in Chapter 29.

Pleural malignancy

Many undiagnosed effusions will eventually turn out to be a malignant process. As cytology alone has a sensitivity of only 60 percent and often the CT thorax does not reveal an area of focal pleural thickening to undertake a percutaneous biopsy, the clinician will often find himself in the position where malignancy is suspected but the patient is too frail for thoracoscopy. In these situations, watchful waiting in the outpatient setting is often appropriate.

Thoracoscopy remains the diagnostic tool of choice for undiagnosed effusions where malignancy is suspected. Harris *et al.*[26] described 182 consecutive patients who underwent thoracoscopy over a 5-year period and showed it to have a diagnostic sensitivity of 95 percent for malignancy. Malignancy was shown by thoracoscopy in 66 percent of patients who had previously had a non-diagnostic closed pleural biopsy and in 69 percent of patients who had had two negative pleural cytological specimens.[26] A similar sensitivity for malignant disease was described by Page *et al.*[27] in 121 patients with undiagnosed effusion. In addition, it has a very low complication rate. In patients with a prior asbestos history, mesothelioma should always be considered. In this setting the yield from cytology alone can be as low as 25 percent and thoracoscopy improves this to 95 percent in some series.[27] In addition to obtaining a tissue diagnosis, several liters of fluid can be removed during the procedure and the opportunity is also provided for talc pleurodesis. Thoracoscopy may therefore be therapeutic as well as diagnostic[28] (see also Chapters 47 and 48).

Parapneumonic effusions

The vast majority of these cases present with classical symptoms of infection and cause no diagnostic difficulty. The patient will often have a fever, high inflammatory markers and a chest radiograph showing consolidation and an effusion. The management and investigation of these have been covered in Chapter 26.

It is, however, important to state that occasionally the presentation will be much less clear cut. There may be no fever or sweats, just a history of generalized lethargy and mild weight loss. The pleural fluid aspirated may also not reveal any clues as it might still be straw colored even it is has been present for some time. The diagnostic problems do not stop there as up to 40 percent of pleural fluid cultures are negative. Sometimes the diagnosis is only made at the time of video-assisted thoracoscopic surgery (VATS) where biopsies show evidence of a chronic empyema rather than the malignancy. The key message here is to keep an open mind and always ask the question 'could this be due to infection?'

Cardiac failure

Cardiac failure is the most common cause of a transudative effusion (Chapter 24). Usually, this diagnosis is made clinically and the chest X-ray reveals bilateral effusions. However, they can occur unilaterally, and when they do they are twice as common on the right side.[29]

Although these effusions are usually transudates, they occasional present as exudates, particularly in patients already on diuretics. The predominant cell count can be lymphocytic and the fluid often also contains mesothelial cells. Plasma brain natriuretic peptide (BNP) level can be very useful in diagnosing these less obvious cases. Measuring pleural fluid BNP level does not convey any additional benefit to the plasma level alone.[30,31]

Hepatic hydrothorax

Some patients present with a hepatic hydrothorax without ascites and, therefore, needs to be thought about in persistently undiagnosed pleural effusions. In one series 27 of the 28 cases were right-sided. The explanation of the pleural effusion in the absence of overt ascites is that patients have defects in their diaphragm and the fluid flows into the pleural space because of negative pleural pressure. Hepatic hydrothorax is secondary to the passage of ascites through diaphragmatic defects and the ascites is secondary to portal hypertension and salt retention. First-line treatment is sodium restriction and spironolactone.

Nephrotic syndrome

This causes bilateral transudative effusions in 25 percent of patients. Checking the patients' renal function, serum protein and urine for protein is important if this condition is suspected. In addition patients with nephrotic syndrome are at increased risk of pulmonary embolus so a low threshold for CTPA is needed.[32]

Table 39.4 summarizes some useful additional tests to order in selected cases of persistent undiagnosed pleural effusions.

Table 39.4 Some useful tests to consider

Test	Suspected problem
Pro-brain natriuretic peptide (BNP)	Cardiac failure
D-dimer and if positive CTPA[a]	Pulmonary embolus
Amylase	Chronic pancreatitis, esophageal rupture
Flow cytometry	Pleural lymphoma
Adenosine deaminase (ADA)	Tubeculous pleuritis
Ultrasound/computed tomography abdomen and pelvic	Meigs' syndrome or subphrenic collection, cirrohosis
Cholesterol/triglycerides, chylomicrons and cholesterol crystals	Chylous/pseudochylous effusion
Thyroid function	Hypothyroidism
Urine dipstick for proteinuria	Nephrotic syndrome

[a]CTPA, computed tomography pulmonary angiogram.

WHAT TO DO IF TESTS REMAIN PERSISTENTLY NEGATIVE – A SUGGESTED MANAGEMENT PLAN

For a large proportion of patients, periodic outpatient follow-up is the correct management strategy. This would typically be three monthly follow-ups with chest radiographs. Over time the underlying cause will usually evolve. Many will unfortunately turn out to have underlying malignancy but some will have less sinister causes such as a chronically trapped lung or chronic heart failure.

An interval CT thorax is another useful investigation in some of these patients. This is largely performed looking for evidence of new pleural nodularity or new mediastinal pleural thickening, both of which suggest underlying malignancy.

If the undiagnosed effusion is causing recurrent symptoms of breathlessness then relief may be needed by performing pleural fluid drainage. In these cases, it may be appropriate to attempt a chemical pleurodesis (even without a diagnosis of malignancy) or to insert an indwelling pleural catheter.

SUMMARY

After the standard initial workup for undiagnosed pleural effusions, the cause is undetermined in around 15 percent of cases. When faced with this problem it is sensible to first revisit the history (including drugs) and clinical examination. The next step is to re-evaluate whether it is a transudate or exudate by Light's criteria. This will help channel further investigations.

All treatable causes of pleural effusions need to be considered and ruled out. These include pulmonary embolus where a CTPA scan needs to be performed if suspected.

Serum BNP levels are another useful investigation where congestive heart failure is thought possible. Special tests to exclude TB and lymphoma may also be necessary.

Unfortunately, many of the remaining effusions will eventually turn out to be due to malignancy. Often these patients are frail and watchful waiting is usually appropriate.

KEY POINTS

- When reviewing a patient with a pleural effusion, where the underlying cause remains obscure, it is useful to revisit the patient's full (including drug) history and whether it is a transudate or exudate. This will help streamline further investigations.
- Revisiting treatable causes of the pleural effusion is a key management step, in cases of diagnostic uncertainty. These causes include: pulmonary embolus, lymphoma, cardiac failure, tuberculosis and connective tissue disorders.
- Sometimes, 'watchful waiting' is appropriate management, particularly when dealing with frail patients or those who are happy to live with a degree of diagnostic uncertainty.

REFERENCES

● = Key primary paper
◆ = Major review article

1. Turton CW Troublesome pleural fluid. *Br J Dis Chest* 1987; **81**: 217–23.
2. Light RW, MacGregor MI, Luchsinger PC, Ball WCJ. Pleural effusions: the diagnostic separation of transudates and exudates. *Ann Intern Med* 1972; **77**: 507–13.

◆3. Light RW Pleural effusion due to pulmonary emboli. *Curr Opin Pulm Med* 2001; **7**: 198–201.

●4. Marel M, Arusiova M, Stasny B, *et al.* Incidence of pleural effusion in a well defined region: epidemiologic study in Central Bohemia. *Chest* 1993: **104**: 1466–99.

5. Fedullo PF. Pulmonary thromboembolism. In: Murray JF, Nadel JA (eds). *Textbook of respiratory medicine.* Philadelphia: WB Saunders, 2000: 1503–31.
6. Goodman PC. Spiral CT for pulmonary embolism. *Semin Resp Crit Care Med* 2000; **21**: 508–10.

7. Light RW, Rogers JT, Moyers JP, *et al.* Prevalance and clinical course of pleural effusions at 30 days post coronary artery bypass surgery. *Am J Respir Crit Care Med* 2002: **166**: 1563–6.
8. Meigs JV, Cass JW. Fibroma of the ovary with ascities and hydrothorax. *Am J Obstet Gynecol* 1937; **33**: 249–67.
◆9. Sahn SA. The pleura – state of the art. *Am Rev Respir Dis* 1988; **138**: 184–23.
10. Majzlin G, Stevens FL. Meigs' syndrome: case report and review of literature. *J Int Coll Surg* 1964: **42**: 625–30.
11. Meigs JV. Fibroma of the ovary with ascities and hydrothorax – Meigs' syndrome. *Am J Obstet Gynecol* 1954: **67**: 962–87.
12. Robinson BWS, Musk AW. Benign asbestos pleural effusion: diagnosis and course. *Thorax* 1981; **36**: 896–90.
●13. Joseph J, Strange C, Shan SA. Pleural effusions in hospitalised patients with AIDS. *Ann Intern Med* 1983; **118**: 856–859.
14. Moore PJ, Thomas PA. The trapped lung with chronic pleural space, a cause of recurring pleural effusion. *Military Med* 1967; **132**: 998–1002.
15. Farber JE, Lincoln NS. The unexpandable lung. I. Statement of the problem. *Am Rev Tuberc* 1939: **40**: 704–9.
16. Berger HW, Mejia E. Tuberculous pleurisy. *Chest* 1973; **63**: 88–92.
17. Idell S. Evaluation of perplexing pleural effusions. *Ann Intern Med* 1994; **110**: 567–9.
18. Ocana IM, Martinez Vazquez JM, Seguna R, *et al.* Adenosine deaminase in pleural fluids. *Chest* 1983; **84**: 51–3.
19. Idell S. Granulomatous disease of the pleura. *Semin Respir Med* 1994; **6**: 31–9.
20. Good JT Jr, King TE, Antony VB, *et al.* Lupus pleuritis. Clinical features and pleural fluid characteristics with special reference to pleural fluid antinuclear antibodies. *Chest* 1983; **84**: 714–18.
21. Leechawengwong M, Berger HW, Sukumaran M. Diagnostic significance of antinuclear antibodies in pleural effusion. *Mt Sinai J Med* 1979: **46**: 137–9
●22. Joseph J, Sahn SA. Connective tissue diseases and the pleura. *Chest* 1993; **104**: 262–70.
23. Turton CW. Troublesome pleural fluid. *Br J Dis Chest* 1987; **81**: 217–24.
24. Hillerdal G. Chylothorax and pseudochylothorax. *Eur Respir J* 1997; **10**: 1157–62
25. Romero S, Martin C, Hernandez L, *et al.* Chylothorax in cirrhosis of the liver: analysis of its frequency and clinical characteristics. *Chest* 1998; **114**: 154–9.
26. Harris RJ, Kavuru MS, Rice TW, Kirby TJ. The diagnostic and therapeutic utility of thoracoscopy. A review. *Chest* 1995; **108**: 828–41.
◆27. Page RD, Jeffrey RR, Donnelly RJ. Thoracoscopy: a review of 121 consecutive surgical procedures. *Ann Thorac Surg* 1989; **48**: 66–8.
28. Loddenkemper R. Thoracoscopy – state of the art. *Eur Respir J* 1998; **11**: 213–21.
29. Race GA, Scheifley CH, Edwards JE. Hydrothorax in congestive heart failure. *Am J Med Sci* 1947; **214**: 243–7.
30. Gegenhuber A, Muller T, Dieplinger B, *et al.* Plasma B-type natriuretic peptide in patients with pleural effusions. *Chest* 2005; **128**: 1003–9.
●31. Muller T, Haltmayer,M. Natriurectic peptide measurements as part of the diagnostic work up in pleural effusions. *Eur Resp J* 2006; **28**: 7–9.
◆32. Light RW The undiagnosed pleural effusion. *Clin Chest Med* 2006; **27**: 309–19.

40

Asbestos-related pleural diseases

A WILLIAM MUSK, NICHOLAS H DE KLERK

INTRODUCTION

Asbestos is a term used for a number of fibrous silicates with particular properties, which occur in deposits large enough to be of commercial interest. Thus, the origin of the term is geological as well as commercial. There are other fibrous minerals, which have some similar biological effects, particularly tremolite (a non-commercial amphibole), erionite (a fibrous silicate found in volcanic rock and implicated in mesothelioma and pulmonary fibrosis in Turkey) and wollastonite (a silicate used in ceramics) and some forms of talc.[1] Most (>90 percent) of the world's production of asbestos has been of chrysotile, which is of the serpentine group of minerals. The remainder of production has been of crocidolite, amosite and anthophyllite, which are amphiboles.[2]

Asbestos fibers are generally strong, easily separable (splitting longitudinally rather than transversely), long and thin (aspect ratio >3:1), flexible and heat and fire resistant. Whereas chrysotile fibers tend to be feathery and curved, the amphiboles are straight and thin, and more durable. Crocidolite has very long thin fibers, anthophyllite has the thickest fibers and amosite fibers are of intermediate dimensions. The amphiboles also differ in their chemical composition and the properties of these same minerals obtained from different places are also slightly different.[1]

Variability in the biological activity of these four main types of asbestos appears to be determined more by physical shape and durability than by chemical properties. The entry of (fibrous) particles into the gas-exchanging regions of the lungs from where they may gain access to the pleura is determined by their aerodynamic diameter as they 'line up' with the laminar flow of the inspired air so that penetration is much less determined by their length than by their physical diameter. The conducting airways have an efficient mucocilliary transport process. However, when the fibers penetrate beyond the conducting airways, their removal is dependent on cellular clearance, which is much slower. The longer the fibers, the less amenable they are to phagocytosis by cellular transport up to the mucocilliary escalator of the conducting airways or into the lymphatics of the interstitium and pleura. Also, the more durable the fibers the less likely they are to be digested within the defence cells of the airspaces of the lungs. The more persistent they are within the tissues, the more inflammation they appear to incite (and the more carcinogenic they appear to be). Thus, of all the forms of asbestos, crocidolite is the most toxic to the pleura (and peritoneum) and the lungs.[3]

Pleural changes are common with all the amphiboles but also occur with chrysotile exposure. However, much commercial chrysotile has been contaminated with amphiboles (particularly with tremolite), so it has been difficult to determine which particular fibers are responsible for the diseases seen. Also, most manufacturing plants using asbestos have used different varieties at different times depending on market conditions, so this contributes to the same confusion in attributing cause, especially when dealing with individuals. Man-made mineral fibers now widely used as asbestos substitutes have not been implicated in pleural diseases.[4]

The benign pleural effects of exposure to asbestos can be classified into:

- circumscribed pleural plaques (CPP);
- diffuse pleural thickening (DPT);
- benign asbestos pleural effusion (BAPE);
- rolled atelectasis (RA);
- transpulmonary bands (TPB).

Solitary fibrous tumor of the pleura, previously called benign fibrous mesothelioma, is not related to asbestos exposure and is not further considered here (see Chapter 38, Benign fibrous tumor of the pleura).

DEFINITIONS

Circumscribed pleural plaques are discrete areas of hyaline or calcified pleural fibrosis which are nearly always bilateral and localized on the parietal pleura of the chest wall, diaphragm or mediastinum but may also occur in the interlobular fissures when they simulate pulmonary neoplasms radiographically.[5] Pleural plaques which occur on the visceral pleura are associated with abnormality in the underlying lung with interstitial fibrotic lines radiating out and giving rise to the term 'hairy plaques'.[6]

Diffuse pleural thickening is a condition of more extensive, active and progressive pleural fibrosis which involves the visceral pleura (Figure 40.1). Calcification may also occur in longstanding DPT. It is less specific for asbestos exposure because other causes of exudative effusions (e.g. empyema, hemothorax) may also cause it.[6]

Benign asbestos pleural effusion is a term applied to an exudative pleural effusion occurring in a subject with asbestos exposure (for which no alternative cause can be identified).

Rolled atelectasis is a process that occurs within the lung parenchyma adjacent to an area of diffuse pleural thickening in which the lung tissues are drawn in to the pleural or subpleural fibrosis.

Transpulmonary bands are coarse bands of fibrosis which also occur in the lung parenchyma in the presence of diffuse pleural thickening.

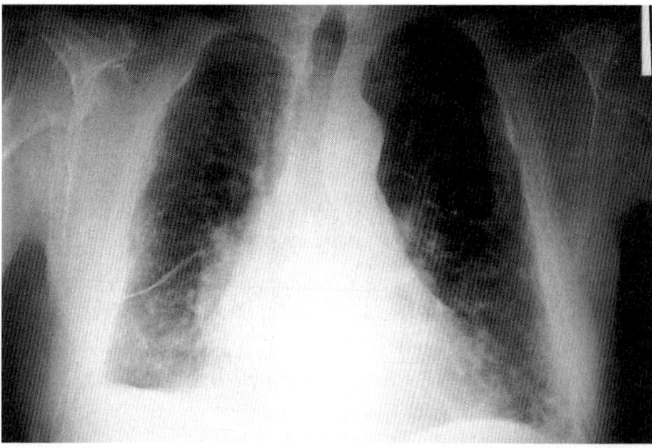

Figure 40.1 Standard plain chest X-ray showing diffuse pleural thickening with characteristic loss of the costophrenic angles and face-on as well as extensive in-profile changes, especially in the mid and lower zones. There is some pleural calcification in the upper zones and the transverse fissure is thickened reflecting involvement of visceral pleura.

EPIDEMIOLOGY

All varieties of asbestos may be responsible for the various manifestations of benign pleural disease[7] although Hillerdal *et al.*[8,9] have shown that subjects exposed to crocidolite or erionite are more likely to have diffuse pleural thickening and benign asbestos pleural effusion (as well as a greater risk of malignant mesothelioma) than those exposed to Finnish anthophyllite in whom circumscribed plaques are relatively more common.

Pleural plaques

Plaques are the most common manifestation of asbestos exposure, especially in subjects with previous environmental or household exposure. They mainly occur posteriorly and laterally following the contours of the eighth to tenth ribs and rarely in the apices or costophrenic angles.[10] The distribution of pleural plaques in the general population is related to the frequency of opportunities for asbestos exposure and age.[11,12] Plain X-ray studies underestimate the frequency of plaques by orders of magnitude: more sensitive radiographic techniques (such as computed tomography [CT] scanning), surgical and post-mortem studies show them to be much more frequent (Figure 40.2).[13] Pleural plaques are more common in subjects with higher asbestos fiber counts in lung tissue (ie. they are dose-related).[14] Also, plaques are more common in people living in urban than in rural areas.[15] Tobacco smoking does not appear to influence the occurrence of pleural plaques.

The natural history of circumscribed pleural plaques following crocidolite exposure is that they appear to

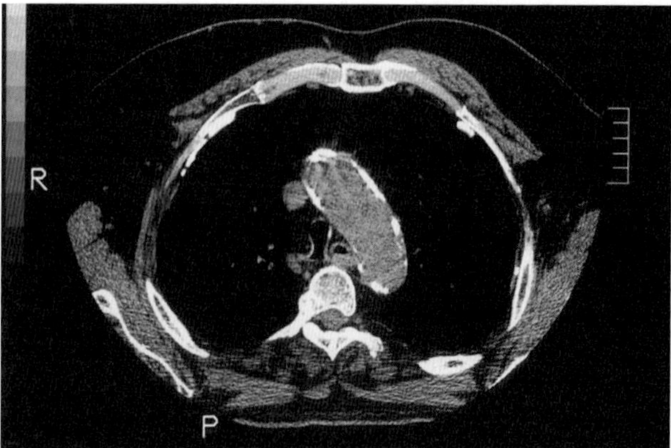

Figure 40.2 Chest computed tomography showing extensive circumscribed pleural plaques with calcification (as well as aortic calcification).

become visible on plain chest x-rays within the first 10 years following initial exposure to asbestos but do not subsequently progress in size/extent. However, they may become more easily seen on radiographs due to increasing calcification.[16,17] Initially the calcification is punctate but becomes denser with time.

Talc and kaolin exposure may also cause pleural plaques although with talc this may be a result of asbestos contamination.

Benign asbestos pleural effusion

Benign asbestos pleural effusions tend to occur earlier following asbestos exposure than mesothelioma, at least in crocidolite exposed subjects.[16,18] Their average latency is also shorter than is the development of pleural plaques or asbestosis. The incidence of benign asbestos pleural effusions[16,19] also increases with the dose of asbestos exposure.

Cookson *et al.*[16] showed that the occurrence of benign asbestos pleural effusion in the Wittenoom cohort was uncommon beyond 25 years after first exposure to amphibole asbestos (the median time following first exposure was 16 years). This contrasts with malignant mesothelioma, the incidence of which rises exponentially with increasing time after initial exposure to asbestos (mainly if not exclusively the amphibole varieties).[20]

Diffuse pleural thickening

Diffuse pleural thickening appears more closely related to amphibole than chrysotile exposure.[8] It is more common in those more heavily exposed and increases in incidence with increasing time since first exposure.[17,21] There is no consistent relationship between smoking status and diffuse pleural thickening.

Rolled atelectasis

There is no consistent epidemiological data on the distribution and determinants of rolled atelectasis apart from the clinical observation of its association with other manifestations of asbestos exposure, including asbestosis, plaques and diffuse pleural thickening (Figure 40.3).

AETIOLOGY/PATHOGENESIS

With the exception of airborne exposure to one or other of the varieties of asbestos, erionite, wollastonite or talc, other factors do not appear to be important in the aetiology of benign asbestos-induced pleural disease: smoking does not appear to be related to any of the diagnostic entities and *Simian Virus 40* (SV40), which appears to have been exonerated as a cause of malignant mesothelioma,[22] has not been implicated (although not specifically sought).

It is widely accepted that circumscribed plaques form as a direct result of the presence of asbestos fibers inciting an inflammatory response in the parietal pleura, possibly as a result of fibers protruding from the visceral pleural surface causing mechanical irritation during the movement of the lung during respiration,[23] even though pathological data has not shown that there are fibers projecting from the visceral pleura or even that fibers are long enough to be anchored in the visceral pleura to cause this process to occur. It has also been suggested that fibers reach the pleural space by a transpleural route and enter the parietal pleura through (hypothetical) stomata in the pleural surface or by retrograde drainage from and intercostal lymphatics.[23]

Many cases of diffuse pleural thickening appear to follow benign asbestos pleural effusion[16] and it is thought that this is the most likely inflammatory pathway for all cases.[23]

Pleural fibrosis (hyaline or diffuse) appears to resemble fibrosis in other tissues with excessive deposition of matrix components and destruction of normal architecture.[24] Complex interactions have been demonstrated between resident and imported inflammatory cells, mediators, coagulant and fibrinolytic pathways etc (see also Chapter 10, Pleural reactions to mineral dusts).

Rolled atelectasis has been postulated as most likely to occur as a result of a localized low-grade inflammatory reaction in the pleura involving both pleural surfaces with progressive thickening and contraction of the fibrosis resulting in retraction and contraction of the underlying lung tissue. The indrawn lung takes its airway and vessels with it producing a characteristic (almost diagnostic) 'comet tail' appearance radiographically.[25]

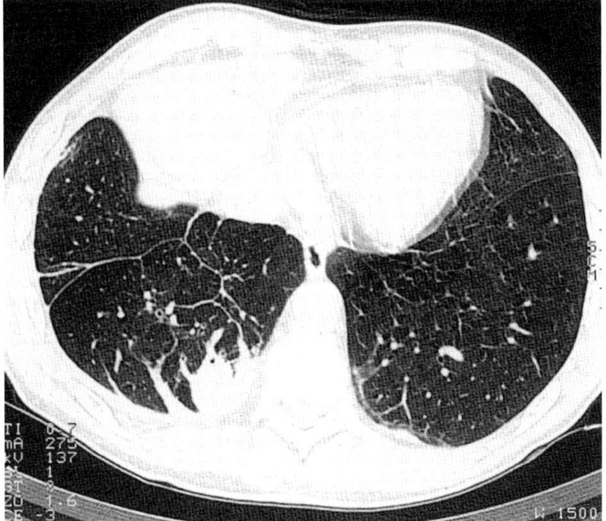

Figure 40.3 Chest computed tomography showing rolled atelectasis with characteristic features, nevertheless justifying fine needle biopsy to exclude the presence of malignancy and justify follow-up.

PATHOLOGY

Circumscribed pleural plaques characteristically appear macroscopically as shining white elevations with sharp borders on the parietal pleura, most commonly on the mid to lower zones of the costal pleura, the dome of the diaphragm and the mediastinal (including the pericardial) pleura. They are usually multiple, up to several centimeters across and tend to lie parallel to the ribs. Microscopically they consist of dense sparsely cellular (hyaline) fibrous tissue covered with normal mesothelium. Asbestos fibers are rarely found within the plaques with light microscopy but small fibers may be seen occasionally with electron microscopy. Calcification is seen microscopically quite early but radiologically only late in the natural history of CPP.[26]

CLINICAL FEATURES

Circumscribed pleural plaques are most commonly found incidentally when plain chest X-rays or CT of the chest are performed for some other reason (except if radiography is being used to identify abnormality in subjects known to have been exposed to asbestos). Although people with plaques are frequently asymptomatic, there is an association of plaques with chest pain which is most likely to have the characteristics of angina.[27] Hence they may be found when chest pain is being investigated. There is no guideline to help determine if the pain is caused by the plaques so that attribution to plaques is by careful exclusion of other possible causes. Pleural plaques are associated with minor changes in lung function (particularly vital capacity[28]) when large groups of subjects with plaques are compared with similar subjects without plaques.[29] It is generally conceded that circumscribed plaques themselves are not responsible for sufficient physiological abnormality to cause exertional breathlessness. Thus other explanations for breathlessness should be sought in dyspnoeic subjects with plaques and it is not usually considered that the mere presence of plaques entitles a person to workers' compensation for disablement (with the proviso that they constitute an independent indicator of previous asbestos exposure in an applicant with diffuse interstitial lung disease, pleural effusion or lung cancer).[30]

Diffuse pleural thickening, in contrast to plaques, may result in significant reductions in lung volumes and cause exertional dyspnoea especially when it is bilateral (see further below). No association with chest pain has been described so the presence of chest pain should raise the issue of malignancy.

Benign asbestos pleural effusion usually presents with exertional dyspnoea (or worsening dyspnoea if there is associated disease) if it is of sufficient size. Pleuritic pain may be a feature initially and this pain may persist or recur. The presence of fever, sweating or other constitutional symptoms raises the index of suspicion that some other inflammatory or neoplastic process is responsible for the effusion.[18] BAPE should not be diagnosed on the basis of a single aspiration with no specific diagnostic outcome, especially as repeated or more invasive diagnostic procedures may be needed before malignant cells are identified in malignant mesothelioma. BAPE may remit and recur ipsilaterally or occur later on the other side.[18] It may be followed by DPT.

Pleural rubs heard on auscultation of the chest are sometimes found in subjects with asbestos exposure with plaques or with diffuse pleural thickening. The rubs may be palpable. They are often evanescent but may be recurrent for months and sometimes years.

INVESTIGATIONS

Plain chest radiography

The standard plain postero-anterior chest radiograph is still the most common means of identifying all the benign asbestos-induced pleural diseases. It has often been performed for other indications and the benign disease found incidentally, especially CPP. Lateral and oblique views increase the likelihood of finding abnormality but are rarely carried out because, if being specifically sought, CPP are much better demonstrated with CT of the chest: when compared with autopsy or thoracotomy only about 15 percent of CPP are diagnosed by the radiologist.[31] On plain film CPP are best seen tangentially and when calcified. If of sufficient thickness, non-calcified plaques may be seen face-on on the plain film as faint, sharply delineated relatively homogeneous shadowing/infiltrates. The International Labour Organization's classification of radiographs of pneumoconioses[32] includes a systematic means of recording the presence of benign asbestos-induced pleural diseases which is useful for epidemiological purposes but not of much value clinically. It does, however, include a convenient definition of the extent of thickening of the pleura constituting a plaque as opposed to diffuse thickening which serves as a useful arbitrary guide for descriptive purposes.

Circumscribed smooth non-calcified pleural shadowing bilaterally and mainly in the mid zones on the lateral chest walls is likely to be due to subpleural fat as it is seen more commonly in subjects with high body mass indices[33] and does not of itself usually warrant further investigation, although CT will demonstrate that the density of the shadowing is that of fat. Calcification within pleural plaques is also much more readily and elegantly demonstrated by CT. Healed rib fractures, metastases in the chest wall and myeloma deposits need to be considered in the differential diagnosis of CPP. Soft tissue shadowing from the serratus anterior muscle and 'companion shadows' (thin lines parallel to the upper ribs) also need to be recognized. Visceral pleural plaques in the inter-lobar fissures need to be differentiated from pulmonary neoplasms.

Benign asbestos-induced pleural effusion may be free within the pleural cavity, which can be demonstrated with decubitus films or loculated, especially when it is recurrent and associated with diffuse pleural thickening.

Computed tomography

Computed tomography of the chest provides a much more elegant means of demonstrating the type, distribution and extent of all the benign asbestos induced pleural diseases. Technical recommendations for the performance of high-resolution computed tomography (HRCT) scans to provide highest quality images of the pleura are soft tissue windows of approximately (height/width) 50/350 Hounsfield Units.[34]

Magnetic resonance imaging

Patients with pleural plaques show low signal intensity on both unenhanced and enhanced T1-weighted and proton density and T2-weighted images contrasting with malignant mesothelioma which shows high signal intensity on the proton density and T2-weighted images and inhomogeneous contrast enhancement in the post-contrast T1-weighted images. The sensitivity, specificity and diagnostic accuracy of magnetic resonance imaging (MRI) in classifying a lesion as suggestive of malignancy in one study[35] were 100, 95 and 95 percent, respectively. Depending on the population being examined, this is probably not much different from CT. For the purposes of clinical management of a patient with pleural thickening and of satisfying compensation authorities that a mesothelioma is present, histological or cytological proof of malignancy is usually required so that MRI, which is much less readily available and much more expensive than CT and still provides only indirect evidence of the nature of the process, is rarely undertaken in clinical practice.

Positron emission tomography

Qualitative assessment of pleural thickening with positron emission tomography (PET) has been claimed to accurately discriminate between benign and malignant pleural thickening with high negative predictive value.[36] However, infections, talc pleurodesis and uraemic pleurisy may result in high isotope 18-flourodeoxyglucose (FDG) avidity and give false positive results.[36–38] A negative PET scan highly favors benign thickening.

Ultrasound

Ultrasound is frequently and advisedly used to guide pleural aspiration and intercostal catheter insertion in patients with pleural thickening and effusion seen radiographically. It is not of diagnostic value *per se*.[10]

Pulmonary function

Circumscribed pleural plaques have a negligible effect on lung function,[28,39,40] although in population studies they can be shown to have a small effect on lung volumes (total lung capacity and vital capacity). They are not considered to be disabling unless accompanied by other abnormality.

Diffuse pleural thickening in contrast to CPP may markedly reduce lung volumes which in turn may result in exertional breathlessness in the absence of asbestosis (i.e. asbestos-induced diffuse interstitial lung disease).[41] This may result from inflammatory involvement of the costal surfaces of the diaphragms and lower costal pleura causing a pleurodesis which limits the excursion of the diaphragm and appears as loss of the costophrenic angle on the plain chest X-ray as well as from reduced distensibility of the pleura and the space-occupying effect of the thickened pleura. Gas transfer measured by the single breath diffusing capacity for carbon monoxide (DL_{CO}) is well preserved (if there is no co-existing asbestosis) and the diffusion constant may be increased as a result of a disproportionately reduced lung volume as measured by alveolar volume (VA).[42] The degree of breathlessness and limitation of exercise capacity may be demonstrated by exercise testing as in all the occupational lung disorders.[43] DPT appears to be associated with an increased ventilatory response to exercise without oxygen desaturation (oxygen desaturation usually indicates interstitial disease) such that the subject's maximum performance may be determined by their ventilatory ability rather than by cardiovascular limitation.

Exhaled nitric oxide

Sandrina *et al.*[44] have shown that the concentration of nitric oxide (NO) in exhaled breath is elevated in patients with asbestosis. This observation is plausible as asbestos is known to induce reactive oxygen and nitrogen species as part of an inflammatory response. The observation is interesting and the advantage of this test is that it is non-invasive. However, the diagnostic and epidemiological value has not been established.

MANAGEMENT

Circumscribed pleural plaques

There are no specific management issues relating to CPP beyond the recognition of their significance as indicators of asbestos or occasionally talc exposure in the past.[45] Their presence therefore assists in attributing other abnormalities such as interstitial lung disease or pleural effusion to past asbestos exposure, especially as some subjects seem to not recall their exposure and some reporting radiologists seem to require their presence before conceding that observed interstitial fibrosis may result from asbestos exposure. It is therefore important to recognize that the converse does not apply, i.e. the absence of plaques does not exclude asbestos as the agent responsible for some abnormality of interest. As CPP does not significantly impair lung function, other causes of impairment need to be sought when a subject with impairment and plaques is being investigated.

Diffuse pleural thickening

The main specific management issue with DPT is its diagnostic differentiation from primary or secondary malignancy of the pleura, especially desmoplastic malignant mesothelioma. It is important to be precise as management is determined by the cause of the pleural thickening. Mesothelioma is increasingly attracting treatment with chemotherapy (despite an abysmal response rate) and even surgery (despite the absence of any scientifically valid evidence that it improves quality of life or survival). Also, secondary tumors (especially breast and prostate cancers) in the pleura may require specific treatment measures.

Decortication of the lung to improve lung volumes and ventilatory capacity has not been a useful procedure. Unlike pleural thickening in tuberculosis or other infective causes of pleural thickening following empyema, a plane of dissection/cleavage does not exist, making hemostasis difficult and the response of lung volume unsatisfactory.

Benign asbestos pleural effusion

The main management issues with BAPE relate to establishing its diagnosis by exclusion of other disease processes, the control of dyspnea by pleural aspiration or drainage, and very occasionally the need to perform some form of pleurodesis to prevent further recurrence. The pleurodesis may be performed surgically at open thoracotomy (pleurectomy, pleural abrasion or talc – or other agent – insufflation), at pleuroscopy (now usually video-assisted), also with talc insufflation or simply with talc slurry following tube drainage.

ROLLED ATELECTASIS AND TRANSPULMONARY BANDS

There are no specific management issues relating to these entities. The main issue with RA is the exclusion of a peripheral lung cancer. While the radiological features are often sufficiently characteristic to permit confidence in the diagnosis, fine needle aspiration biopsy may be indicated if there is doubt and follow-up radiographic (usually CT) examination is usually suggested for reassurance of the patient and the physician.

COMPLICATIONS

None of the asbestos-related benign pleural diseases is associated with particular complications, other than those which may arise from diagnostic procedures or efforts to control symptoms, although it has been suggested that both plaques and diffuse thickening increase the risk of future peritoneal (but not pleural) mesothelioma, in addition to the increased risk from asbestos exposure alone.[46]

FUTURE DIRECTIONS

The banning of the use of amphibole asbestos worldwide would significantly reduce the future occurrence of asbestos-related pleural diseases if the ban were observed. The ongoing use of chrysotile, however, means that such cases will still present in future. The study of molecular biology has provided some hints to the etiology of asbestos-related pleural diseases. Recently, early evidence from genetic studies suggest that genetic predisposition to the effects of asbestos exposure may exist and, in future, may serve as a way to identify individuals at risk.

KEY POINTS

- The main significance of circumscribed pleural plaques is that they are indicators of past asbestos exposure. They cause minor impairment of lung function and are statistically associated with chest pain which has features of angina.
- Diffuse pleural thickening involves the visceral and parietal pleura and may thereby cause significant impairment of lung function and give rise to exertional breathlessness.
- Benign asbestos pleural effusion is an exudative effusion which follows asbestos exposure but which has no specific diagnostic features and is therefore a diagnosis of exclusion.
- Benign asbestos pleural effusion may be recurrent and may be followed by diffuse pleural thickening.

REFERENCES

● = Key primary paper
◆ = Major review article

1. Pooley F. Asbestos mineralogy. In: Autman K, Aisner J (eds). *Asbestos-related malignancy.* Orlando: Grune and Stratton 1987: 3–30.
2. World Health Organization. *Asbestos and other mineral fibers.* Geneva: WHO 1986.
3. Davis J. *Mineral fiber carcinogenesis: experimental data relating to*

the importance of fiber type, size, deposition, dissolution and migration. Lyon: IARC Scientific Publications, 1989: 33–45.

4. Oberdorster G. Determinants of the pathogenicity of man-made vitreous fibers (MMVF). *Int Arch Occup Environ Health* 2000; **73** (Suppl): S60–8.
5. Rockhoff SD, Chu J, Rubin LJ. Special report: asbestos induced pleural plaques; a disease process associated with ventilatory impairment and respiratory symptoms. *Clin Pulm Med* 2002; **9**: 113–24.
6. Roach HD, Davies GJ, Attanoos R, *et al.* Asbestos: when the dust settles an imaging review of asbestos-related disease. *Radiographics* 2002; **22**: S167–84.
●7. Albelda SM, Epstein DM, Gefter WB, Miller WT. Pleural thickening: its significance and relationship to asbestos dust exposure. *Am Rev Respir Dis* 1982; **126**: 621–4.
●8. Hillerdal G, Musk AW. Pleural lesions in crocidolite workers from Western Australia. *Br J Ind Med* 1990; **47**: 782–3.
●9. Hillerdal G, Zitting A, van Assendelft AH, Kuusela T. Rarity of mineral fiber pleurisy among persons exposed to Finnish anthophyllite and with low risk of mesothelioma. *Thorax* 1984; **39**: 608–11.
10. Evans AL, Gleeson FV. Radiology in pleural disease: state of the art. *Respirology* 2004; **9**: 300–12.
11. Hillerdal G. Pleural changes and exposure to fibrous minerals. *Scand J Work Environ Health* 1984; **10**: 473–9.
12. Craighead JE, Abraham JL, Churg A, *et al.* The pathology of asbestos-associated diseases of the lungs and pleural cavities: diagnostic criteria and proposed grading schema. Report of the Pneumoconiosis Committee of the College of American Pathologists and the National Institute for Occupational Safety and Health. *Arch Pathol Lab Med* 1982; **106**: 544–96.
13. Hillerdal G, Lindgren A. Pleural plaques: correlation of autopsy findings to radiographic findings and occupational history. *Eur J Respir Dis* 1980; 61: 315–19.
14. Karjalainen A, Karhunen PJ, Lalu K, *et al.* Pleural plaques and exposure to mineral fibers in a male urban necropsy population. *Occup Environ Med* 1994; **51**: 456–60.
15. Zitting AJ, Karjalainen A, Impivaara O, *et al.* Radiographic small lung opacities and pleural abnormalities in relation to smoking, urbanization status, and occupational asbestos exposure in Finland. *J Occup Environ Med* 1996; **38**: 602–9.
●16. Cookson WO, De Klerk NH, Musk AW, *et al.* Benign and malignant pleural effusions in former Wittenoom crocidolite millers and miners. *Aust N Z J Med* 1985; **15**: 731–7.
●17. de Klerk NH, Cookson WO, Musk AW, Armstrong BK, Glancy JJ. Natural history of pleural thickening after exposure to crocidolite. *Br J Ind Med* 1989; **46**: 461–7.
●18. Robinson BW, Musk AW. Benign asbestos pleural effusion: diagnosis and course. *Thorax* 1981; **36**: 896–900.
●19. Epler GR, McLoud TC, Gaensler EA. Prevalence and incidence of benign asbestos pleural effusion in a working population. *J Am Med Assoc* 1982; **247**: 617–22.
◆20. De Klerk NH, Armstrong BK. The epidemiology of asbestos and mesothelioma. In: Henderson DW, Shilkin KB, Langlois SL, Whitaker D (eds). *Malignant mesothelioma.* New York: Hemisphere, 1992: 223–50.
◆21. Rudd R. Benign pleural disease. In: Hendrick DJ, Burge PS, Beckett WS, Churg A (eds). *Occupational disorder of the lung recognition, management and prevention.* London: WB Saunders and Co, 2002: 343–57.
◆22. Rizzo P, Bocchetta M, Powers A, *et al.* SV40 and the pathogenesis of mesothelioma. *Semin Cancer Biol* 2001; **11**: 63–71.
23. Huggins JT, Sahn SA. Causes and management of pleural fibrosis. *Respirology* 2004; **9**: 441–7.
24. Mutsaers SE, Prele CM, Brody AR, Idell S. Pathogenesis of pleural fibrosis. *Respirology* 2004; **9**: 428–40.
◆25. Cugell DW, Kamp DW. Asbestos and the pleura: a review. *Chest* 2004; **125**: 1103–17.
26. Hillerdal G. The pathogenesis of pleural plaques and pulmonary asbestosis: possibilities and impossibilities. *Am Rev Respir Dis* 1980; **61**: 129–38.
●27. Mukherjee S, de Klerk N, Palmer LJ, *et al.* Chest pain in asbestos-exposed individuals with benign pleural and parenchymal disease. *Am J Respir Crit Care Med* 2000; **162**: 1807–11.
●28. Kilburn KH, Warshaw R. Pulmonary functional impairment associated with pleural asbestos disease. Circumscribed and diffuse thickening. *Chest* 1990; **98**: 965–72.
29. Hilt B, Lien JT, Lund-Larsen PG. Lung function and respiratory symptoms in subjects with asbestos-related disorders: a cross-sectional study. *Am J Ind Med* 1987; **11**: 517–28.
30. Peacock C, Copley SJ, Hansell DM. Asbestos-related benign pleural disease. *Clin Radiol* 2000; **55**: 422–32.
31. Ameille J, Brochard P, Brechot JM, *et al.* Pleural thickening: a comparison of oblique chest radiographs and high-resolution computed tomography in subjects exposed to low levels of asbestos pollution. *Int Arch Occup Environ Health* 1993; **64**: 545–8.
32. International Labour Office. *Guidelines for the use of ILO international classification of radiographs of pneumoconiosis.* Revised 1980. Geneva: ILO, 1980.
●33. Lee YC, Runnion CK, Pang SC, de Klerk NH, Musk AW. Increased body mass index is related to apparent circumscribed pleural thickening on plain chest radiographs. *Am J Ind Med* 2001; **39**: 112–16.
34. Webb WR, Muller NL, Naidich DP. Standardized terms for high-resolution computed tomography of the lung: a proposed glossary. *J Thorac Imaging* 1993; **8**: 167–75.
35. Boraschi P, Neri S, Braccini G, *et al.* Magnetic resonance appearance of asbestos-related benign and malignant pleural diseases. *Scand J Work Environ Health* 1999; **25**: 18–23.
36. Kramer H, Pieterman RM, Slebos DJ, *et al.* PET for the evaluation of pleural thickening observed on CT. *J Nucl Med* 2004; **45**: 995–8.
37. Duysinx B, Nguyen D, Louis R, *et al.* Evaluation of pleural disease with 18-fluorodeoxyglucose positron emission tomography imaging. *Chest* 2004; **125**: 489–93.
38. Kwek BH, Aquino SL, Fischman AJ. Fluorodeoxyglucose positron emission tomography and CT after talc pleurodesis. *Chest* 2004; **125**: 2356–60.
39. Van Cleemput J, De Raeve H, Verschakelen JA, *et al.* Surface of localized pleural plaques quantitated by computed tomography scanning: no relation with cumulative asbestos exposure and no effect on lung function. *Am J Respir Crit Care Med* 2001; **163**: 705–10.
40. Broderick A, Fuortes LJ, Merchant JA, Galvin JR, Schwartz DA. Pleural determinants of restrictive lung function and respiratory symptoms in an asbestos-exposed population. *Chest* 1992; **101**: 684–91.
41. Cotes JE, King B. Relationship of lung function to radiographic reading (ILO) in patients with asbestos related lung disease. *Thorax* 1988; **43**: 777–83.
42. Cookson WO, Musk AW, Glancy JJ. Pleural thickening and gas transfer in asbestosis. *Thorax* 1983; **38**: 657–61.
43. Cotes JE, Steel J. *Work-related lung disorders.* London: Blackwell, 1987.
44. Sandrini A, Johnson AR, Thomas PS, Yates DH. Fractional exhaled nitric oxide concentration is increased in asbestosis and pleural plaques. *Respirology* 2006; **11**: 325–9.
◆45. American Thoracic Society. Diagnosis and initial management of nonmalignant diseases related to asbestos. *Am J Respir Crit Care Med* 2004; **170**: 691–715.
●46. Reid A, de Klerk N, Ambrosini G, *et al.* The additional risk of malignant mesothelioma in former workers and residents of Wittenoom with benign pleural disease or asbestosis. *Occup Environ Med* 2005; **62**: 665–9.

41

Malignant mesothelioma

BRUCE WS ROBINSON

INTRODUCTION

Mesothelioma is a malignant tumor of the serosal surfaces, mostly of the pleura and peritoneum, almost always caused by asbestos.[1] Whilst there is a benign form of the disease, that is rare and the term 'mesothelioma' almost always refers to the malignant form of the disease. Mesothelioma was a rare disease but has become common over the past few decades. It is now approximately as common a cause of death as cancers of the liver, bone, cervix, ovary and bladder in many countries.[2] Its incidence is expected to continue to increase for the next decade or so (see below). Almost everyone who lives in the western world, and increasing numbers in the developing world, have asbestos fibers in their lungs and many individuals recall incidental asbestos exposure, e.g. plumbers, carpenters, insulation installers, home renovators, military personnel, school teachers plus students who handled asbestos mats or blankets, and in many other situations.[3] Indeed, the word 'mesothelioma' is becoming well known in the public arena due to the widespread publicity that asbestos has received over the past 15 years and since the death from mesothelioma of some famous individuals such as actor Steve McQueen.

Media interest has produced awareness, even anxiety, about mesothelioma. The complex medico-legal aspects of the disease, plus this awareness, have led to a lot of interest in mesothelioma.

EPIDEMIOLOGY

Whilst most common cancers do not have clearly defined single carcinogens (even cigarette smoke has many potential carcinogens), the link between asbestos as a single carcinogen and mesothelioma is clearly established.[3] There are not many diseases with such a close link between the occurrence in the community of the disease and exposure to the carcinogen as defined as they are for mesothelioma. In fact, mesothelioma is essentially a disease that would still be rare but for the widespread use of asbestos. That link was first recognized by J.C. Wagner, a pathologist working in South Africa.[4]

Mesothelioma is linked to exposure to asbestos but not to cigarette smoking.[3] Other generally recognized causes of mesothelioma include endemic erionite exposure in Turkey,[5] ionizing radiation and chest injuries.[6] There is a potential role for *Simian virus 40* (SV40) (discussed below).

Males are more likely to get mesothelioma than females through occupational exposure. The sporadic background rate of mesothelioma is around one per million. This rises to over 40 per million in some countries.[2] As expected, industrialized countries have higher rates than non-industrialized countries, relating to production and utilization of asbestos[7].

The post-war mesothelioma 'epidemic'[7] (Figure 41.1), resulted from a rapid increase in asbestos use worldwide, though the long incubation period between the onset of the disease and time since first exposure (usually over 30 years) means that the peak incidence of mesothelioma is yet to be reached. Whereas cessation of exposure to tobacco smoke reduces the risk of developing lung cancer and approaches that of a 'never-smoker' after 25–30 years, the risk of mesothelioma which is almost nil in the first 10–12 years following first exposure, progressively increases with increasing time.[8]

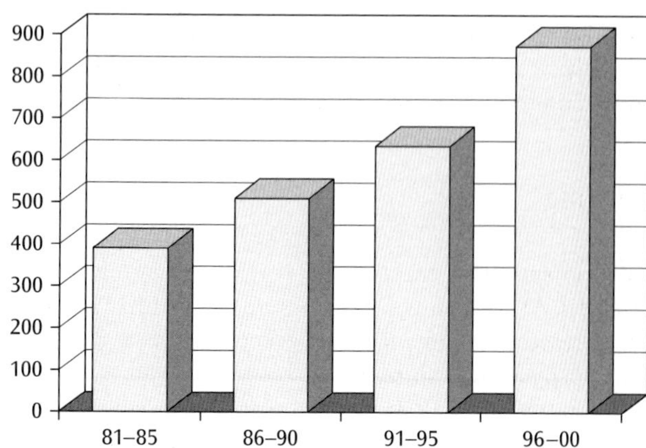

Figure 41.1 Increasing incidence of mesothelioma. Mesothelioma death rates in England, 1981 and 2000. (Source UK Health and Safety Executive. http://www.hse.gov.uk/statistics/causdis/area8100.pdf).

PATHOGENESIS

There are several ways in which a mineral fiber such as asbestos induces cancer:

1. *Pleural irritation* – fiber shape and length-to-width ratio are the main attributes that determine penetration and capacity to irritate the pleural space.[9] Long and thin fibers penetrate the lung and scratch the mesothelial surface, inducing multiple cycles of damage, repair and local inflammation, leading either to scarring ('plaques') or cancer ('mesothelioma').
2. *Mitosis interference* – asbestos fibers can interfere with the mitotic spindle by piercing the mitotic spindle causing disruption to mitosis. This can lead to aneuploidy and the other forms of chromosome damage seen in mesothelioma.[10]
3. *Toxic oxygen radicals* – asbestos-induced DNA damage is partly mediated by iron-related reactive oxygen species (ROS) – this can also lead to strand breakage.[11]
4. *Kinase-mediated signaling* – asbestos induces the phosphorylation of the mitogen-activated protein (MAP) kinases and extracellular signal-regulated kinases (ERK) 1 and 2 and this is associated with expression of early response proto-oncogenes (fos/jun or activator protein 1 family members).[12] Many growth factors drive mesothelioma proliferation but the only factors whose blockade has been shown to slow mesothelioma growth are transforming growth factor beta (TGF-β) and platelet-derived growth factor (PDGF) A chain.[13]

Simian virus 40 40 and mesothelioma

Simian virus 40 has been suggested to be a 'cofactor' in the causation of mesothelioma.[14,15] A small double-stranded DNA virus, SV40 blocks tumor suppressor genes and is a potent oncogenic virus for human and rodent cells. SV40 DNA sequences are present in tumor tissues of selected types, e.g. brain and bone tumors, lymphomas and malignant mesotheliomas.[14] In microdissection experiments, SV40 is present in the tumor cells but not in normal adjacent cells, or in lung cancer tissue.[15]

The virus was present in polio vaccines used throughout the world in the 1950s and 1960s and may be transmitted horizontally in humans. Evidence connecting vaccine-derived infection and the occurrence of mesothelioma is scanty and unconfirmed. A role for SV40 in mesothelioma remains unclear.

The molecular basis of mesothelioma

Mesotheliomas have abnormal karyotypes, with aneuploidy and structural rearrangements common.[16] Loss of chromosome 22 is the most common gross change, but structural rearrangement of 1p, 3p, 9p and 6q are seen. Loss of heterozygosity (LOH) of neurofibromatosis type 2 (NF2) at 22q12 has been reported in most mesothelioma cell lines.[17] The most common genetic abnormalities seen are loss of $p16^{INK4A}$, $p14^{ARF}$ and NF2. This implies that a pattern of tumor-suppressor gene loss is required for mesothelioma to occur (see also Chapter 11, Genetic alterations in mesothelioma pathogenesis).

CLINICAL PRESENTATION

Pleural effusion, usually with breathlessness and often with chest wall pain, is the most common presentation in mesothelioma patients.[18] Unexplained pleural effusion with chest wall pain should evoke a detailed clinical history of possible asbestos exposure. Weight loss and fatigue usually occur later in the course of disease and are associated with a poor prognosis.[18] Mesothelioma can occasionally be discovered on chest X-ray as asymptomatic pleural effusions or pleural masses. Peritoneal mesothelioma presents with abdominal distension, abdominal pain and sometimes bowel obstruction.[19] Mesotheliomas do occur in the pericardium or tunica vaginalis, though rarely, and present with features of pericardial effusion/tamponade or blood-stained hydrocoele.[20,21]

A fixed hemithorax clinically, i.e. unilateral lack of expansion, is usually a late sign. Clubbing is rare.

Peritoneal mesothelioma manifests as ascites, tenderness and, later in their course, palpable masses.[19] Subcutaneous masses are almost always associated with surgery or the insertion of intercostal drainage tubes.[18]

Local invasion of superior vena cava (presenting as obstruction), the spinal cord (resulting in back pain and paralysis), the pericardium (resulting in pericardial effusions and tamponade), the contralateral lung (presenting as contralateral pleural effusion) or sympathetics (presenting as Horner's Syndrome) do occur, but rarely at presentation.[18]

Metastatic deposits of mesothelioma are common at post mortem but are not usually detected clinically.[22] Hilar, mediastinal, internal mammary and supraclavicular lymph node spread is common. Metastases to major organs and occasionally miliary spread have been reported.[23]

DIAGNOSIS

Pathology

Differentiation of mesothelioma from adenocarcinoma in tissues and from reactive mesothelial cells in effusion samples are the major issues for pathologists.[24]

CYTOPATHOLOGY

The quality of current immunohistochemical and ultrastructural methods of cytological assessment make cytological diagnosis alone quite accurate in experienced hands with the appropriate antibodies.[25] Closed needle biopsy using Abrams' needle often produces inconclusive results.

Ultrastructural examination is helpful. Fine needle aspiration cytology is useful for sampling pulmonary, chest wall or lymph node masses, when there is no effusion present in particular. Core biopsy samples are used for large pleural-based lesions, especially in the absence of an effusion.[26]

The immunocytochemical stains used to distinguish mesothelioma from adenocarcinoma and other diseases are listed below but, importantly, calretinin identifies cells as being of mesothelial origin and epithelial membrane antigen (EMA) staining in cytological samples in a thick membrane distribution using the correct antibody is highly suggestive of mesothelioma.[27]

HISTOPATHOLOGY

Distinguishing adenocarcinoma from mesothelioma can be difficult[28] – adenocarcinoma resembles mesothelioma macroscopically and microscopically and both tumors can form papillary structures. Epithelioid mesothelioma cells are more uniform, cuboidal and less crowded than adenocarcinoma but a suite of immunohistochemical markers usually has to be used to aid the differential diagnosis of mesothelioma. Staining with calretinin can reveal if the tissue is of mesothelial origin, and EMA expression on the luminal aspects of the tumor can help determine if it is a malignant mesothelioma. Cytokeratin stains help distinguish mesothelioma from sarcomas and melanoma.[29] Wilm's tumor suppressor gene (WT1), cytokeratin 5/6, HBME-1 (human mesothelial cell 1) and mesothelin stains are also used. Mesothelioma must be distinguished from adenocarcinoma using carcinoembryonic antigen (CEA), CD15, thyroid transcription factor 1 (TTF-1) and B72.3.

Mesothelioma *in situ* (atypical mesothelial proliferation) has been described.[30] Electron microscopy can distinguish mesothelioma from adenocarcinoma and is occasionally necessary to distinguish desmoplastic/sarcomatoid mesothelioma from fibrous pleuritis.

Imaging

The conventional chest X-ray typically shows a pleural effusion. An encircling rind of tumor and/or extensive lobulated pleural-based tumor masses can be seen early but are usually a late feature.[31]

Computed tomography (CT) scanning usually shows a pleural effusion only. Pleural-based masses with or without thickening of interlobular septae can also be seen at presentation.[32,33] A CT scan can help identify signs of asbestos exposure, e.g. plaques. With progression, encirclement of lung with restriction of expansion is seen (Figure 41.2). CT scanning in peritoneal mesothelioma shows ascites and sometimes scattered mesothelioma masses.

Magnetic resonance imaging (MRI) can determine invasion of local structures such as rib and diaphragm but is not widely used.[34,35]

Positron emission tomography (PET) may lend support towards a diagnosis of pleural malignancy, but is most useful for staging, particularly in identifying extrathoracic mesothelioma and lymph node involvement.[36] Sometimes extensive tumor outside the lung can be detected by PET scanning when not suspected clinically (Figure 41.3).

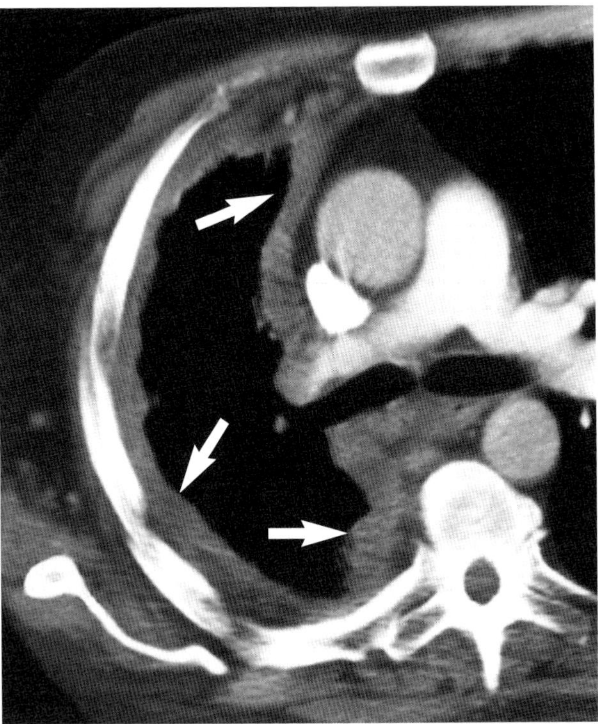

Figure 41.2 Computed tomography of a patient with mesothelioma showing tumor (gray tissue – arrowed) encasing and restricting expansion of the lung (black).

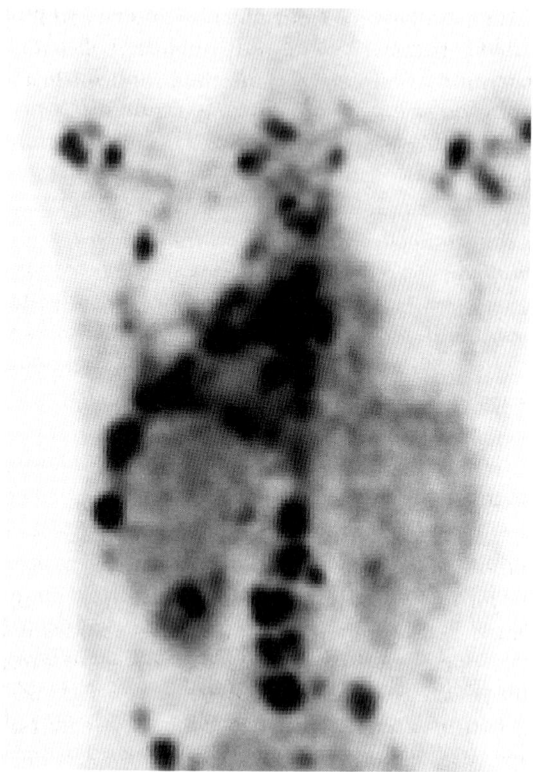

Figure 41.3 Positron emission tomography (PET) in mesothelioma. Mesothelioma patient showing multiple metastatic deposits (black spots) with only small amounts of tumor in the involved lung (right side). (Image courtesy of Dr A van der Schaff).

Use of serum biomarkers for diagnosis

Recently, several serum markers of mesothelioma have been published. Soluble mesothelin-related protein (SMRP) is the circulating product of mesothelin, a surface protein thought to be important in mesothelial cell adhesion and possibly signaling.[37] In mesothelioma patients, 84 percent have elevated levels of SMRP at late stages of disease compared with less than 2 percent of patients with other pleural or pulmonary inflammatory or malignant diseases and this figure is around 55 percent at diagnosis[38] (Figure 41.4). The specificity of SMRP is over 80 percent compared with other lung tumors/pleural diseases and healthy individuals exposed to asbestos. There are also data suggesting that SMRP may prove useful in the early detection of mesothelioma in at-risk individuals.

Recent studies have shown that measurement of SMRP in pleural effusions or ascites may be even more sensitive for the presence of mesothelioma than serum measurements.[38]

Osteopontin is another serum biomarker for mesothelioma, although its specificity for mesothelioma is lower than SMRP.[39]

DNA microarray and mesothelioma diagnosis

There have been several studies of microarray findings in mesothelioma,[40,41] with one study comparing expression levels of a small number of genes reportedly able to accu-

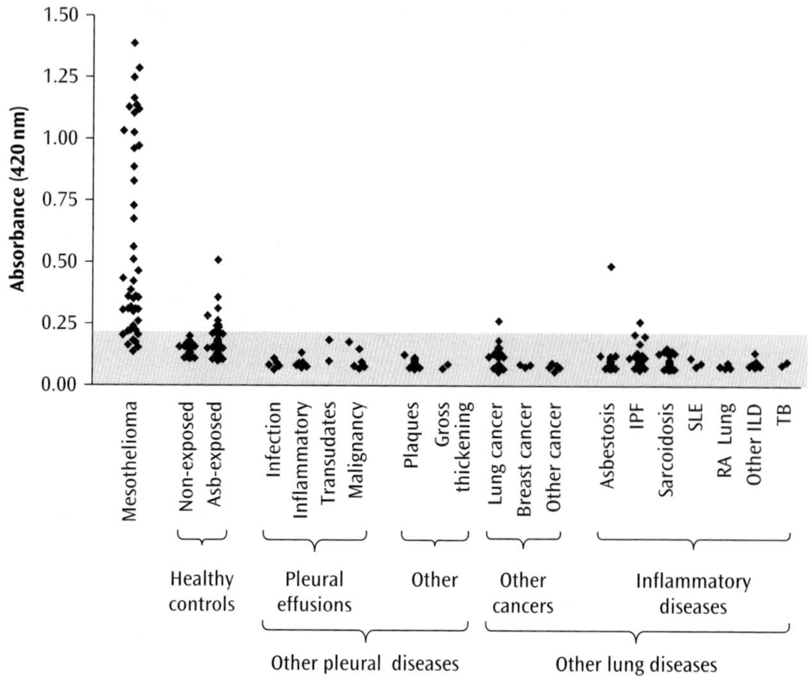

Figure 41.4 Serum mesothelin/soluble mesothelin-related protein (SMRP) levels in mesothelioma. Levels of serum mesothelin in 44 patients with mesothelioma, 68 healthy adults (28 non-asbestos exposed, 40 asbestos exposed) plus 92 patients with lung inflammatory diseases, 30 patients with non-mesothelioma cancers without pleural involvement, 20 patients with non-mesothelioma pleural effusions and 18 patients with other non-malignant pleural diseases without effusions. Shaded area represents the 'normal range' healthy subjects. ILD, interstitial lung disease; IPF, idiopathic pulmonary fibrosis; SLE, systemic lupus erythematosus; TB, tuberculosis. (Figure reprinted with permission from Elsevier: Robinson B, Creany J, Lake R *et al.* Mesothelin-family proteins and diagnosis of mesothelioma. *Lancet* 2003; **362**: 1612–16).

rately discriminate between mesothelioma and lung cancer. The method depends upon quantitative polymerase chain reaction (PCR) to measure gene expression ratios of paired markers.[42] In another study, a panel of 15 genes was able to distinguish these two tumors, partly because the authors subtracted genes from reactive mesothelial cells in their analysis.[43]

Staging and prognosis

Staging has implications for surgical management if the latter is being considered. The International Mesothelioma Interest Group (IMIG) staging system is the most widely used.[44] Although accurate preoperative assessment requires CT, PET and often thoracoscopy and mediastinoscopy, final staging only occurs at surgery.[44]

Mesothelioma remains a universally fatal disease of increasing incidence worldwide. Median survival from the time of presentation is 9–12 months.[45–47] Prognostication for mesothelioma is currently dependent on relatively crude criteria, such as tumor extension and differentiation, rather than on genetic information.[48] Poor prognosis is associated with a poor performance status, a high white blood cell (WBC) count, a probable/possible histological diagnosis of mesothelioma, male gender and having the sarcomatoid histological subtype.[49] A better prognosis is essentially the opposite and the absence of pain in the previous 6 months.[50]

A small microarray study in mesothelioma identified four genes which were predictive of outcome.[30]

MANAGEMENT

More effective chemotherapies and new approaches to surgery have occurred in recent years.

Surgery

Diagnostic surgery includes video thoracoscopy, open pleural biopsy and/or mediastinoscopy or laparoscopy to establish a diagnosis of mesothelioma.[51] Palliative surgery includes partial pleurectomy with pleurodesis, thoracoscopy with pleurodesis and pleuroperitoneal shunting.[52] 'Potentially curative' surgery, which is only used in a limited number of centres, involves extrapleural pneumonectomy usually followed by some form of adjuvant therapy. The difficulty of the surgery and peri-operative mortality rate combined to make the role of radical surgery controversial.[53–56]

Chemotherapy

Cures are rare with chemotherapy regimes but recently several regimes have been shown to be of value for palliation. They decrease tumor burden, improve symptoms and prolong survival. Pemetrexed (or raltitrexed) plus cisplatin, a combination of a multi-targeted anti-folate and a platinum compound, improved overall survival by nearly 3 months with an objective response rate of 41 percent.[57] Gemcitabine plus cisplatin has objective response rates of 48 and 33 percent in a total of 74 patients, with symptomatic improvement and quality of life benefits.[54]

Although PDGF and epidermal growth factor (EGF) signaling paths may always be involved in mesothelioma, imatinib mesylate (Gleevec) and gefitinib (Iressa), which block each of these pathways, have demonstrated no convincing evidence of response.[55]

Radiotherapy

Radiotherapy results have been disappointing except for local post-surgical radiotherapy to prevent seeding of tumor cells.[56] The diffuse nature of the tumor makes it difficult to undertake radical radiotherapy without causing pneumonitis. Intensity modulated radiotherapy (IMRT) is being used in some centers with benefit.[57] Local radiotherapy, e.g. radioactive colloids and other forms of brachytherapy, have been disappointing.

Immunotherapy

Mesothelioma appears to be sensitive to destruction by immunotherapies though none have entered routine clinical use.[58] Anti-mesothelioma immune responses can be detected in many patients.[59] Recombinant interferon alpha given systemically produced response rates of around 10–15 percent, and although that approach is complicated by lethargy, weight loss and fevers, some patients exhibit long-lasting responses.[60]

Gene therapy

Gene therapy using either 'suicide gene' therapy or 'immunogene' therapy have been used clinically in mesothelioma. These pioneering approaches are reviewed elsewhere (see Chapter 49, Gene therapy in pleural disease).

Other therapies

Photodynamic therapy, involving the generation of toxic oxygen radicals in mesothelioma cavities, is laborious and time-consuming and is an effective form of cytoreduction.[61] Clinical trials using other novel agents (e.g. the anti-angiogenic agents SU5416, bevacizumab, thalidomide and PTK/ZK 787) have been or currently are being tried.[62,63]

Inhibitors of histone deacetylase superoylanilide and hydroxamic acid (SAHA), a proteosome inhibitor (PS-341), another histone deacetyalase inhibitor (PXD101), and another vascular endothelial growth factor (VEGF) antagonist (AZD2171) are also being studied.[64,65] Immunotoxin trials using monoclonal antibodies labeled with toxins are also underway.[66]

PALLIATION

Recurrent pleural effusions are best controlled by pleurodesis, e.g. talc instillation or occasionally surgery. Invasion of the chest wall can cause localized somatic pain, intercostal nerve invasion or vertebral invasion can cause neuropathic pain and lung invasion can cause diffuse visceral pain.[67] There is no limit of dose for opioids to control this pain, e.g. use liquid morphine plus sustained release morphine in doses that do not cause unnecessary side effects. Somatic pain responds to non-steroidal anti-inflammatory drugs and neuropathic pain requires an anti-convulsant such as carbamazepine or sodium valproate.[68] Some patients require procedural pain relief, e.g. intrathecal analgesia or nerve block.[67] Weight loss and anorexia respond to dietary advice and to drug therapy, e.g. dexamethasone. Dyspnea due to pleural effusion, or more commonly tumor spread, is also common.

Psychosocial care is also important in palliation given the fear, anger and suffering associated with this disease.

KEY POINTS

- Asbestos is almost always the causative agent.
- A role for SV40 remains uncertain.
- Most patients present with pleural effusion plus chest wall pain.
- New biomarkers such as SMRP are useful for diagnosis.
- Pemetrexed, or gemcitabine, plus cisplatin are useful chemotherapy regimes.
- Positron-emission tomography is essential for preoperative staging if resection is planned.

REFERENCES

● = Key primary paper
◆ = Major review article

◆1. Robinson BWS, Lake RL. Advances in malignant mesothelioma. *New Eng J Med* 2005; **353**: 1591–603.
2. Cancerstats Incidence. UK. *Mesothelioma.* www.cancerresearchuk.org/statistics
3. Greenberg AK, Lee TC, Rom WN. The North American experience with malignant mesothelioma. In: Robinson BWS, Chahinian AP (eds). *Mesothelioma.* London: Martin Dunitz, 2002; 1–27.
●4. Wagner JC, Sleggs CA, Marchand P. Diffuse pleural mesothelioma. *Br J Ind Med* 1960; **17**: 260–71.
●5. Baris YL, Simonato L, Artvinli M, *et al.* Epidemiological and environmental evidence of the health effects of exposure to erionite fibers. *Int J Cancer* 1987; **39**: 10–17.
6. Comin CE, de Klerk NH, Henderson DW. Malignant mesothelioma. *Ultrastruct Pathol* 1997; **21**: 315–20
7. de Klerk NH, Musk AW. Epidemiology of mesothelioma. In: Robinson BWS, Chahinian AP (eds). *Mesothelioma.* London: Martin Dunitz, 2002: 339–50.
8. de Klerk NH, Musk AW, Williams VM, *et al.* Comparison of measures of exposure to asbestos in former crocidolite workers from Wittenoom Gorge, W. Australia. *Am J Ind Med* 1996; **30**: 579–87.
9. Sebastien P, Janson X, Gaudichet A, Hirsch A, Bignon J. Asbestos retention in human respiratory tissues: comparative measurements in lung parenchyma and in parietal pleura. *IARC Sci Publ* 1980; **30**: 237–46.
10. Ault, JG, Cole RW, Jensen CG, *et al.* Behavior of crocidolite asbestos during mitosis in living vertebrate lung epithelial cells. *Cancer Res* 1995; **55**: 792–8.
11. Shatos, MA, Doherty JM, Marsh JP, Mossman BT. Prevention of asbestos-induced cell death in rat lung fibroblasts and alveolar macrophages by scavengers of active oxygen species. *Environ Res* 1987; **44**: 103–16.
12. Zanella CL, Posada J, Tritton TR, Mossman, BT. Asbestos causes stimulation of the extracellular signal-regulated kinase 1 mitogen-activated protein kinase cascade after phosphorylation of the epidermal growth factor receptor. *Cancer Res* 1996; **56**: 5334–8.
13. Marzo AL, Fitzpatrick DR, Robinson BWS, Scott B. Antisense oligonucleotides specific for transforming growth factor beta 2 inhibit the growth of malignant mesothelioma both *in vitro* and *in vivo*. *Cancer Res* 1997; **57**: 3200–7.
14. Gazdar AF, Carbone M. Molecular pathogenesis of mesothelioma and its relationship to Simian Virus 40. *Clin Lung Cancer* 2003; **5**: 177–81.
15. Shivapurkar N, Wiethege T, Wistuba II, *et al.* Presence of simian virus 40 sequences in malignant mesotheliomas and mesothelial cell proliferations. *J Cell Biochem* 1999; **76**: 181–8.
16. Murthy SS, Testa JR. Asbestos, chromosomal deletions, and tumor suppressor gene alterations in human malignant mesothelioma. *J Cell Physiol* 1999; **180**: 150–7.
17. Pylkkanen L, Sainio M, Ollikainen T, *et al.* Concurrent LOH at multiple loci in human malignant mesothelioma with preferential loss of NF2 gene region. *Oncol Rep* 2002; **9**: 955–9.
18. Scott B, Mukherjee S, Lake R, Robinson BWS. Malignant mesothelioma. In: Hanson H (ed.). *Textbook of lung cancer.* London: Martin Dunitz, 2000; 273–93.
19. Berry G, de Klerk NH, Reid A, *et al.* Malignant pleural and peritoneal mesotheliomas in former miners and millers of crocidolite at Wittenoom, Western Australia. *Occup Environ Med* 2004; **61**: 14.
20. Hirano H, Maeda T, Tsuji M, *et al.* Malignant mesothelioma of the pericardium: case reports and immunohistochemical studies including Ki-67 expression. *Pathol Int* 2002; **52**: 669–76.
21. Abe K, Kato N, Miki K, *et al.* Malignant mesothelioma of testicular tunica vaginalis. *Int J Urol* 2002; **9**: 602–3.
22. Lumb PD, Suvarna SK. Metastasis in pleural mesothelioma. Immunohistochemical markers for disseminated disease. *Histopathology* 2004; **44**: 345–52.
23. Musk AW. More cases of miliary mesothelioma. *Chest* 1995; **108**: 587.
24. Segal A, Whitaker D, Henderson D, Shilkin K. Pathology of

mesothelioma. In: Robinson BWS, Chahinian AP (eds). *Mesothelioma.* London: Martin Dunitz, 2002: 143–184.

◆25. Whitaker D, Shilkin KB. Diagnosis of pleural malignant mesothelioma in life – a practical approach. *J Pathol* 1984; **143**: 147–75.

26. Sterrett GF, Whitaker D, Shilkin KB, Walters MN. Fine needle aspiration cytology of malignant mesothelioma. *Acta Cytol* 1987; **31**: 185–93.

●27. Wolanski KD, Whitaker D, Shilkin KB, Henderson DW. The use of epithelial membrane antigen and silver-stained nucleolar organizer regions testing in the differential diagnosis of mesothelioma from benign reactive mesothelioses. *Cancer* 1998; **82**: 583–90.

28. Nguyen GK, Akin MR, Villanueva RR, Slatnik J. Cytopathology of malignant mesothelioma of the pleura in fine-needle aspiration biopsy. *Diagn Cytopathol* 1999; **21**: 253–9.

29. Segal A, Whitaker D, Henderson D, Shilkin K. Pathology and mesothelioma. In: Robinson BWS, Chahinian AP (eds). *Mesothelioma.* London: Martin Dunitz, 2002: 143–84.

30. Whitaker D, Henderson DW, Shilkin KB. The concept of mesothelioma *in situ*: implications for diagnosis and histogenesis. *Semin Diagn Pathol* 1992; **9**: 151–61.

31. Rabinowitz JG. Imaging in mesothelioma. In: Robinson BWS, Chahinian AP (eds). *Mesothelioma.* London: Martin Dunitz, 2002: 201–8.

◆32. Wang ZJ, Reddy GP, Gotway MB, *et al.* Malignant pleural mesothelioma: evaluation with CT, MR imaging, and PET. *Radiographics* 2004; **24**: 105–19.

33. Kebapci M, Vardareli E, Adapinar B, Acikalin M. CT findings and serum CA125 levels in malignant peritoneal mesothelioma: report of 11 new cases and review of the literature. *Eur Radiol* 2003; **13**: 2620–6.

◆34. Marom EM, Erasmus JJ, Pass HI, Patz EF Jr. The role of imaging in malignant pleural mesothelioma. *Semin Oncol* 2002; **29**: 26–35.

35. Weber MA, Bock M, Plathow C, *et al.* Asbestos-related pleural disease: value of dedicated magnetic resonance imaging techniques. *Invest Radiol* 2004; **39**: 554–64.

36. Flores RM, Akhurst T, Gonen M, Larson SM, Rusch VW. Positron emission tomography defines metastatic disease but not locoregional disease in patients with malignant pleural mesothelioma. *J Thorac Cardiovasc Surg* 2003; **126**: 11–16.

●37. Robinson BWS, Creaney J, Lake RA, *et al.* Mesothelin-family proteins and diagnosis of mesothelioma. *Lancet* 2003; **362**: 1612–16.

●38. Creaney J, Yeoman D, Naumoff L, *et al.* Soluble mesothelin in effusions – a useful tool for the diagnosis of malignant mesothelioma. *Thorax* 2007; **62**: 569–76.

39. Pass HI, Lott D, Lonardo F, *et al.* Asbestos exposure, pleural mesothelioma, and serum osteopontin levels. *N Engl J Med* 2005; **353**: 1564–73.

40. Ramos-Nino ME, Scapoli L, Martinelli M, Land S, Mossman BT. Microarray analysis and RNA silencing link fra-1 to cd44 and c-met expression in mesothelioma. *Cancer Res* 2003; **63**: 3539–45.

41. Singhal S, Wiewrodt R, Malden LD, *et al.* Gene expression profiling of malignant mesothelioma. *Clin Cancer Res* 2003; **9**: 3080–97.

●42. Gordon GJ, Jensen RV, Hsiao LL, *et al.* Translation of microarray data into clinically relevant cancer diagnostic tests using gene expression ratios in lung cancer and mesothelioma. *Cancer Res* 2002; **62**: 4963–7.

●43. Holloway AJ, Diyagama DS, Opeskin K, *et al.* A molecular diagnostic test for distinguishing lung adenocarcinoma from malignant mesothelioma using cells collected from pleural effusions. *Clin Cancer Res* 2006; **12**: 5129–35.

44. Rusch VW. A proposed new international TNM staging system for malignant pleural mesothelioma. From the International Mesothelioma Interest Group. *Chest* 1995; **108**: 1122–8.

45. Leigh J, Robinson BWS. The history of mesothelioma in Australia 1045–2001. In: Robinson BWS, Chahinian AP (eds). *Mesothelioma.* London: Martin Dunitz, 2002: 55–110.

46. de Klerk NH, Olsen N, Threlfall T, *et al. Mesothelioma survival in Western Australia.* Perth: 1st Perth Mesothelioma Centre Symposium 2004.

47. Armstrong BK, Musk AW, Baker JE, *et al.* Epidemiology of mesothelioma in Western Australia. *Med J Aust* 1984; **141**: 86–8.

48. di Muzio M, Spoletini L, Strizzi L, *et al.* Prognostic significance of presence and reduplication of basal lamina in malignant pleural mesothelioma. *Hum Pathol* 2000; **31**: 1341–5.

49. Curran D, Sahmoud T, Therasse P, *et al.* Prognostic factors in patients with pleural mesothelioma: the European Organization for Research and Treatment of Cancer experience. *J Clin Oncol* 1998; **16**: 145–52.

50. Boutin C, Schlesser M, Frenay C, Astoul P. Malignant pleural mesothelioma. *Eur Respir J* 1998; **12**: 972–81.

51. Waller DA.. Malignant mesothelioma – British surgical strategies. *Lung Cancer* 2004; **45**: S81–4.

52. Sugarbaker DJ, Jaklitsch MT, Bueno R, *et al.* Prevention, early detection, and management of complications after 328 consecutive extrapleural pneumonectomies. *J Thorac Cardiovasc Surg* 2004; **128**: 138–46.

53. Stewart DJ, Martin-Ucar A, Pilling JE, *et al.* The effect of extent of local resection on patterns of disease progression in malignant pleural mesothelioma. *Ann Thorac Surg* 2004; **78**: 245–52.

54. Rusch VW. Indications for pneumonectomy. Extrapleural pneumonectomy. *Chest Surg Clin N Am* 1999; **9**: 327–38.

55. Pass HI, Kranda K, Temeck BK, Feuerstein I, Steinberg SM. Surgically debulked malignant pleural mesothelioma: results and prognostic factors. *Ann Surg Oncol* 1997; **4**: 215–22.

56. Treasure T, Sedrakyan A. Pleural mesothelioma: little evidence, still time to do trials. *Lancet* 2004; **364**: 1183–5.

57. Kindler HL. Malignant pleural mesothelioma. *Curr Treat Options Oncol* 2000; **1**: 313–26.

●58. Vogelzang NJ, Rusthoven JJ, Symanowski J, *et al.* Phase III study of pemetrexed in combination with cisplatin versus cisplatin alone in patients with malignant pleural mesothelioma. *J Clin Oncol* 2003; **21**: 2636–44.

●59. Nowak AK, Byrne MJ, Williamson R, *et al.* A multicentre phase II study of cisplatin and gemcitabine in malignant mesothelioma. *Br J Cancer* 2002; **87**: 491–6.

60. Nowak A, Lake RA, Kindler HL, Robinson BWS. New approaches for mesothelioma: biologics, vaccines, gene therapy, and other novel agents. *Semin Oncol* 2002; **29**: 82–96.

61. Baldini EH. External beam radiation therapy for the treatment of pleural mesothelioma. *Thorac Surg Clin* 2004; **14**: 543.

62. Ahamad A, Stevens CW, Smythe WR, *et al.* Intensity-modulated radiation therapy: a novel approach to the management of malignant pleural mesothelioma. *Int J Radiat Oncol Biol Phys* 2003; **55**: 768–75.

63. Mukherjee S, Robinson BWS. Immunotherapy of malignant mesothelioma. In: Robinson BWS, Chahinian AP (eds). *Mesothelioma.* London: Martin Dunitz, 2002: 325–38.

64. Kindler HL. Moving beyond chemotherapy: novel cytostatic agents for malignant mesothelioma. *Lung Cancer* 2004; **45**: S125–7.

65. Kindler HL. Malignant pleural mesothelioma. *Curr Treat Options Oncol* 2000; **1**: 313–26.

66. Hassan R, Bera T, Pastan I. Mesothelin: a new target for immunotherapy. *Clin Cancer Res* 2004; **10**: 3937–42.

67. Lee, YC, Thompson RI, Dean A, Robinson BWS. Clinical and palliative care aspects of malignant mesothelioma. In: Robinson BWS, Chahinian AP (eds). *Mesothelioma.* London: Martin Dunitz, 2002: 111–26.

68. Finnerup NB, Gottrup H, Jensen TS. Anticonvulsants in central pain. *Expert Opin Pharmacother* 2002; **3**: 1411–20.

42

Spontaneous pneumothorax

ANDREW C MILLER

HISTORICAL BACKGROUND

In 1903 Emerson[1] published a compilation of all previous literature on pneumothorax, including the first examples of its naming (Itard 1803), use of needle aspiration (B. Bell 1804), full clinical description (Laennec 1819), a primary case – with blebs – (McDowell 1856), the coin sign (Trouseau 1857), underlying physics (J. Bell 1857), pleural reabsorption of air (Skoda 1857), fatal tension (Medsel 1859), treatment by indwelling catheter (Orlebar 1882), and the value of oxygen therapy (Rodet and Nicholas 1895). Both before and since then, cavitatory tuberculosis was thought to be the main cause, as in 78 percent of cases in Vienna in 1880.[2] This perspective changed following publication of a landmark doctoral thesis by Kjærgaard in 1932.[3] Until then only 200 cases of primary pneumothorax, mainly as single case reports, had been identified. Kjærgaard considered 'pneumothorax simplex' to be 'comparatively rare', but recognized that many minor cases were being overlooked; hence all but 18 percent of his 51 cases had complete lung collapse, the reverse of subsequent experience.

DEFINITIONS

'Spontaneous' pneumothorax by definition occurs unexpectedly. It is traditional to subdivide it into 'secondary' and 'primary' depending upon whether or not the patient has significant underlying lung disease (Table 42.1). Semantically, this is not an accurate distinction because the great majority of primary cases do have identifiable underlying pathology (see section Primary pneumothorax).

The usual causes of secondary pneumothorax are shown in Table 42.1. Most have either (1) known widespread generalized lung disease causing chronic respiratory symptoms, impaired lung function tests and bilateral abnormalities on chest radiograph, or (2) a localized abnormality where the patient may be otherwise well. An intriguing example which defies neat classification is catamenial pneumothorax in which patients are otherwise asymptomatic with normal lung function, one lung is abnormal and pneumothorax occurs during menstruation. Some cases of lymphangioleiomyomatosis first present as pneumothorax with no apparent parenchymal disease on chest radiograph. The important clinical differences between primary and secondary pneumothorax are summarized in Table 42.2.

The term 'closed' pneumothorax refers to one in which the pleural defect has sealed, whereas in an 'open' pneumothorax air leak is continuing; this distinction has a major bearing on the success of initial management and treatment options.

EPIDEMIOLOGY

Incidence

The incidence of pneumothorax in those presenting as an emergency to hospital has been calculated to be 8–12 per 100 000 per year.[4–7] This was confirmed in a much large study for a 5-year period,[8] with an additional 17 per 100 000 annually presenting first to their family doctor – an overall incidence of 40.7 (men) and 15.6 (women) per 100 000 per year. The latter report is of particular importance because most published series underestimate the

Table 42.1 Classification of spontaneous pneumothorax

Classification	Definition	Example	
Primary	'Normal' lungs		Young otherwise healthy patients
Secondary	Generalized: chronic disease	Bullous	Emphysema
			Cystic fibrosis
		Fibrotic	Cryptogenic fibrosing alveolitis
			Fibrotic sarcoid
			Pneumoconiosis
		Miscellaneous	Acquired immune deficiency syndrome
			Connective tissue disorders
			Histiocytosis-X
			Lymphangioleiomyomatosis
Other	Localized: subacute or acute disease	Cavitatory	Tuberculosis
			Pneumonia (e.g. staphylococcal)
			Wegener's granulomatosis
			Rheumatoid nodules
			Hydatid disease
		Malignant	Bronchial carcinoma
			Mesothelioma
			Pulmonary metastases
		Miscellaneous	Catamenial

Table 42.2 Differences between primary and secondary pneumothorax

		Primary	Secondary
Presentation	Age	Usually <35 years	Usually >45 years
	Chest pain	Usual, may be severe	Occasional
	Dyspnoea	Usually mild/moderate	Often severe
Chest radiograph	Degree of collapse	Any size, often small	Usually small or moderate
	Pleural reaction	Common, may suggest diagnosis	Occasional
	Other findings	Often mediastinal shift in complete collapse	Changes of underlying disease
Resolution on medical management	Observation alone	Often possible, outpatient	Usually inappropriate, requires admission
	Preferred initial intervention	Simple aspiration	Simple aspiration or indwelling catheter
	Persistent air leak	Occasional, surgery indicated	Common, but 20% eventually resolve
Prevention of recurrence	Medical pleurodesis	Not appropriate	If high surgical risk
	Operative approach	Thoracoscopy	Thoracotomy may be needed

true incidence by being skewed towards those either referred to chest clinics from family doctors, or who self-refer to hospital but may not be admitted, or who are transferred to specialist thoracic units.

Gender

The above male:female ratio of 2.5:1, similar to that in large series from tertiary centers,[9] is likely to be more accurate than the male preponderance of 80–95 percent in other studies.[4,10–14] Catamenial cases account for about 3 percent of those in young women, in whom smoking and body shape are less relevant than in men.[15] There are few reports of pneumothorax in pregnancy,[16] half of these women having other attacks outside pregnancy; half of the episodes occurred during or shortly after labor. Another cause exclusive to females is lymphangioleiomyomatosis.[17–20]

Age

Primary pneumothorax is mainly a disease of young adults with a unimodal age distribution for the first episode peaking in the early twenties;[10,21–25] therefore, it is not unusual for patients to present in early adolescence.[26–29] As expected, most cases of secondary pneumothorax due to emphysema and pulmonary fibrosis occur in the second half of life whereas Langerhans-cell histiocytosis,[30] lymphangioleiomyomatosis, cystic fibrosis and acquired immune deficiency syndrome (AIDS) usually affect young adults.

Body shape

It has long been recognized that pneumothorax and its recurrence are particularly common in young men with an ectomorphic build.[24,25,31,32] Such individuals are already taller than controls at age 6 years with a particularly rapid increase at puberty;[33] this may accentuate the known pressure differential between the lung apex and base which accounts for the upper lobe alveoli being larger.[34] This is cited as the reason for such pathological changes being particularly common at the apices. A contributing factor might be abnormal connective tissue, since there seems to be an association between primary pneumothorax and both mitral valve prolapse[35,36] and Ehlers–Danlos syndrome.[37]

Familial

There have been occasional reports on families with several members having pneumothorax, with a probable autosomal dominant inheritance;[38–45] in one large cohort 3 percent had affected close relatives.[41] In some this seems to be due to mutations in the folliculin gene, as in the autosomal dominant Birt–Hogg–Dube syndrome which causes pneumothorax due to thin-walled subpleural cysts.[45,46]

Smoking

As well as being an important factor in secondary pneumothorax due to emphysema, it has long been known that current smoking is usual in those with primary pneumothorax. The strength of the association is directly related to the amount smoked,[5,11,24,38,47] with heavy smokers having a 12 percent lifetime risk of developing pneumothorax compared with 0.1 percent for 'never smokers'.[5] However, in two large cohorts of mainly young patients a third were non-smokers.[25,26]

Exercise

Despite what patients assume, there is no theoretical reason to suppose that lung collapse would occur during vigorous exercise, and such a history is unusual.[12,21,23,38,48–53] Patients find such information reassuring, since many otherwise assume that they must henceforth avoid straining their chest to avoid recurrence.

Environmental factors

Although various claims have been made that the incidence of pneumothorax is related to seasons of the year, changes in barometric pressure, thunderstorms, humidity and phases of the moon,[54–57] the suggested mechanisms seem unconvincing and evidence is very weak.[25,27,58–60] Equally surprising is a suggested association with proximity to loud music.[61]

Geographical variations

In parts of the world where pulmonary tuberculosis remains common, there continue to be reports[62–66] of patients with pneumothorax secondary to advanced cavitatory disease, often with associated pleural fluid (see section Persistent air leak). An occasional cause in Mediterranean countries is pulmonary hydatid disease.[67]

PATHOGENESIS

Studies on artificially inflated animal[68] and human[69] lungs demonstrate that the visceral pleura is very resistant to rupture, as Kjærgaard recognized.[3] In fatal cases of barotrauma due to diving, those with pneumothorax all had pleural adhesions and lung bullae.[70] Cases have been described after the rapid and high intrathoracic pressure changes in weightlifting,[71] obstetric delivery,[16,72,73] cannabis use[74] and even vomiting[75] and lung function testing.[76] Most of these are secondary to pneumomediastinum which is uncommon at presentation in spontaneous pneumothorax. Pneumothorax is a recognized hazard of the rapid G-force changes in military aviation[51,58,77,78] and of bungee-jumping,[79] but it is likely that most of these patients have the same underlying pathology found in other cases of primary pneumothorax.[51]

Primary pneumothorax

Although only occasionally visible on standard chest radiographs,[50,80] the great majority of patients have subpleural blebs, bullae and/or localized emphysematous changes on computed tomography (CT),[81–84] inspection at surgery,[22,38,50,80,85–89] pathology of resection specimens,[38,90–95] and at autopsy.[70] Despite recent alternative views,[96–98] there is no reason to modify the 'generally accepted concept that the ruptured bled is the etiological factor';[50] indeed, in some cases the site of air leak can be identified at surgery.[99] Resected lung tissue frequently shows combinations of cystic changes, atelectasis, fibrosis, chronic inflammation, reactive alveolar cell proliferation and endarteritis.[38,90] Identical pathology is seen in dogs with pneumothorax, both macroscopically and microscopically.[100] The presence of inflammatory, vascular, granulomatous and degenerative changes may account for the higher incidence of pneumothorax in smokers. Patients with normal chest radiographs have normal spirometry[38,50] but may have abnormalities on more sophisticated testing suggestive of localized or mild generalized disease.[98,101]

Such changes would be expected to be bilateral, as has been observed both clinically[12,21,102] and on CT scanning;[82,84,103] one team operated on both sides in 26 patients with unilateral pneumothorax and found bilateral blebs in all but one.[85] Most contralateral episodes occur independently, but occasionally bilateral simultaneous pneumothorax may occur ranging in severity from being asymptomatic to fatal.[104–110] Despite the conclusions of some investigators, analysis of all reports shows no predilection for either lung.

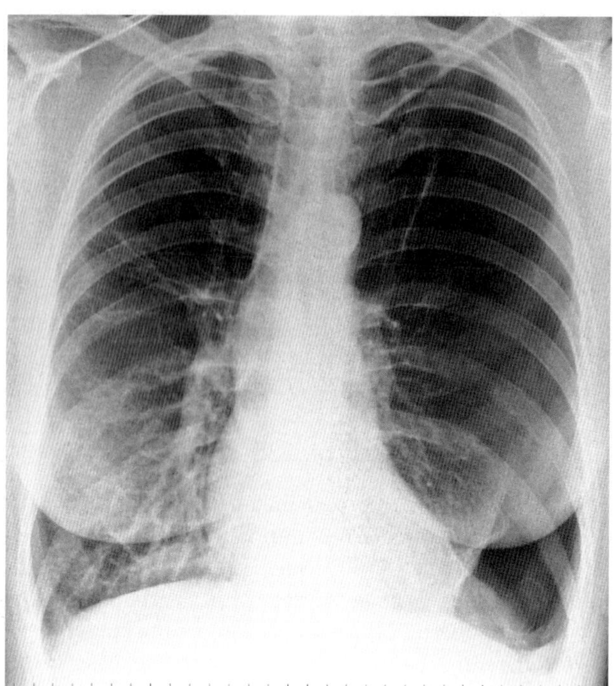

Figure 42.1 Partial left pneumothorax in a woman with bullous emphysema.

Airways disease

Pneumothorax is a well-recognized, potentially lethal and often hard to treat complication of emphysema. However, chronic obstructive pulmonary disease is common and the risk of this complication is very low, occurring in only 1 in 400 of Mayo Clinic patients.[111] Clinical experience suggests that incidence increases with severity of emphysema, particularly in those with sizeable bullae (Figure 42.1). In cystic fibrosis extensive subpleural pathology is common;[91] otherwise pneumothorax is rare in airway diseases such as bronchiectasis. Likewise, it occurs in less than 1 percent of patients with bronchial carcinoma[112] (which is only occasionally subpleural, and where associated emphysema might instead explain pneumothorax[113]). So, does asthma (which does not affect the lung parenchyma) really predispose to pneumothorax, as is widely assumed and taught?[12,23] Asthma is very common and some patients will happen to have subpleural blebs that might rupture during an acute attack;[114] in most cases where the two conditions coexist the asthma is mild and pneumothorax occurs outside an exacerbation.[12,115] Chest radiography reveals pneumothorax in under 2 percent of adults with acute asthma,[116,117] although in up to 8 percent of those that subsequently need assisted ventilation.[118]

Other malignant disease

Again, pulmonary metastatic disease only causes pneumothorax when the visceral pleura is involved, as has been documented in a wide variety of tumors arising from the breast, bowel, uterus as well as sarcomas and germ-call tumors; it may be induced by tissue death due to chemotherapy.[119] Such cases are rare, but if a patient with known malignant disease presents with a pneumothorax, such an association should be seriously considered even when chest radiography appears normal.[120–123] Likewise, malignant mesothelioma involving the visceral pleura may rarely present as spontaneous pneumothorax.[124–126] Although such cases are present in most large series and in individual reports, no comprehensive review has been published.

Interstitial disease

Pneumothorax secondary to interstitial lung disease (Table 42.1) is common, often complicated by persistent air leak and has a high risk of recurrence. An instructive example is sarcoidosis – in one series from a specialist unit this was the cause of pneumothorax in 26 of 505 patients[127] – where pneumothorax can occur both in the active form if granulomata involve the pleura[128] (the same explanation as for the occasional pleural effusion in this disease) and in the chronic form if fibrosis leads to the development of subpleural bullae or cavities (Figure 42.2).[129,130]

Acquired immune deficiency syndrome

Spontaneous pneumothorax is a common – and ominous – complication of AIDS, several specialist units reporting more than 25 such cases.[131–137] Major associations are

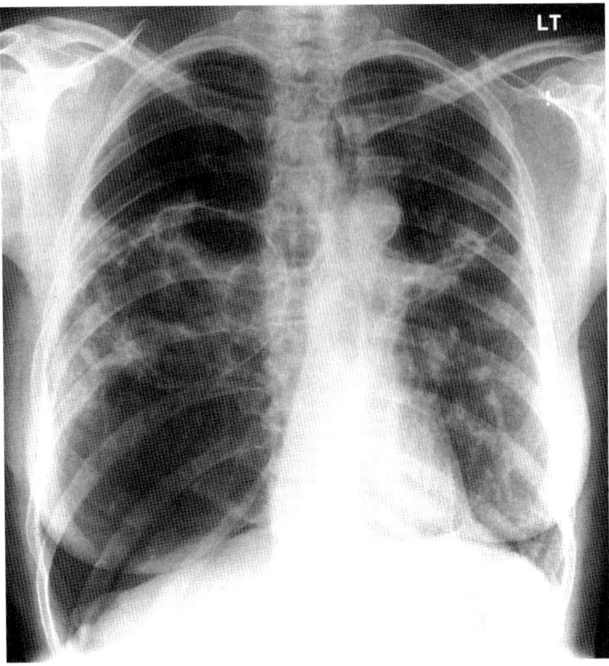

Figure 42.2 Pneumothorax in a woman with cavitatory fibrotic sarcoid; she has also needed repeated bronchial artery embolization for mycetoma-related hemoptysis.

active or previous infection with *Pneumocystis* or tuberculosis, and radiographic evidence of bullae and cysts; CT scans show that the latter are very common,[138] probably resulting from recurrent lung infection.

Catamenial pneumothorax

The authors of the first case report[139] suggested that this was due to transperitoneal migration of endometrial tissue from the pelvis through small defects that are known to be common in the right (rarely the left[140]) diaphragm, a view largely confirmed since.[141–144] One case with life-threatening hemopneumothorax has been reported.[145]

CLINICAL FEATURES

Occasionally, spontaneous pneumothorax, even bilateral, may be detected in an asymptomatic patient;[108,109,146] in a survey of 994 Air Force personnel 7 percent were only detected on routine chest radiography.[58] However, most patients present because of chest pain and/or dyspnea. Pain is almost always the main presenting symptom in primary pneumothorax;[22,25–28,115] in secondary cases, which includes most elderly patients with pneumothorax, the dominant symptom is dyspnea.[111,118,147,148] In primary cases symptoms usually come on suddenly and subside after several hours, but many present several days after onset.[21,22,149]

Pain

It seems remarkable that, until recently,[150] no explanation for this frequent symptom in primary cases has been clearly documented. It has long been known that intrapleural air is painless and causes no pleural reaction,[151] and that a significant hemopneumothorax (resulting from rupture of a pleural adhesion or a vascular abnormality[152]) only occasionally occurs.[153] It seems likely that as bleb rupture occurs, inflammatory agents are released into the pleural cavity irritating the very sensitive parietal pleura. This leads to 'eosinophilic pleuritis',[154] associated with rapid appearance of eosinophils, neutrophils and inflammatory mediators in the pleural cavity;[155,156] it explains the common finding of a pleural reaction on radiography[157] and the occasional appearance of clear yellow fluid in the syringe at the end of successful aspiration. The above theory[150] considers the possibility of bleb rupture without air leak, explaining why attacks of similar pain without demonstrable pneumothorax are often reported. Although pain arises from the parietal pleura, it is rarely 'pleuritic' because the two pleural surfaces are separated by air.

There is no correlation between severity of pain and degree of lung collapse.[25] Although the pain is often described as like a stitch, patients may imagine that they are having a heart attack. In others symptoms can easily be attributed to pleurisy, pneumonia or a musculo-skeletal problem, all of which conditions are much more common reasons for attending the emergency room. Since a small pneumothorax can easily be overlooked on chest radiograph if the film quality is poor and the doctor inexperienced, and the chest pain may be affected by movement rather than by respiration, it is not surprising that an incorrect diagnosis is commonly made.[49,158,159] However, a patient who has already experienced one episode is usually immediately able to recognize any recurrence.[3,50]

Dyspnea

Allowing for the severity of chest pain, the degree of breathlessness in primary pneumothorax is variable; it is frequently minimal,[22,26–28] and otherwise is often only mild or moderate even in complete collapse, so that many are not tachypneic.[115] On the other hand, dyspnea (worse than usual) is a prominent symptom in secondary pneumothorax, where even a small degree of collapse can be life-threatening; it is often assumed that such patients are suffering an exacerbation of their known lung disease, and the pneumothorax is often hard to detect clinically, so misdiagnosis here is common.[111,115,159]

Other

Of the classical clinical signs, the most common are reduced ipsilateral chest expansion[21] and breath sounds,[25] hyper-resonance being found mainly in moderate or complete collapse. Chest examination is unhelpful in some primary and most secondary[118] cases. An occasional auscultatory finding with shallow left-sided collapse is a clicking, crunching or crackling sound at the cardiac apex in time with the pulse,[160,161] distinct from those described in mediastinal emphysema.[162] Some with 'noisy pneumothorax' are themselves aware of these sounds.[160] Although not widely known, commonly patients with resolving pneumothorax (whether right- or left-sided) describe or admit to bubbling sounds in that lung, particularly on lying down and varying with posture, disappearing when the lung fully re-inflates. Some even have electrocardiographic changes leading to a mistaken diagnosis of pericarditis, myocardial infarction or pulmonary embolism.

Although subcutaneous emphysema and pneumomediastinum may occur in traumatic pneumothorax and with barotrauma, they are rare in spontaneous pneumothorax at presentation although they commonly complicate drainage procedures;[13] in experimental or artificial pneumothorax air cannot be forced into the mediastinum. Where they are associated, the pneumothorax is small and complicates the pneumomediastinum rather than the other way round.[69,162,163] The pathogenesis of mediastinal emphysema differs in that rupture occurs in alveoli contiguous with connective tissue in the pulmonary vasculature and then spreads towards the mediastinum,[69] which requires much less pressure to rupture than visceral pleura. Spontaneous pneumomediastinum is a benign condition which can nearly always be diagnosed on clinical grounds and good-quality chest radiography; management is conservative[164] and a good clinician will not request CT scanning[165] or tests to exclude esophageal perforation.

CHEST RADIOGRAPHY

Technical considerations

Since expiratory films exaggerate the radiographic changes of pneumothorax, standard practice was to request paired films in suspected cases, a practice that is now discouraged,[166] and in reality only inspiratory films are routinely requested for patients presenting with chest pain or dyspnea. Apparent justification for inspiratory-only films comes from two studies in which the only errors were in two (out of 138) patients with minimal collapse,[167,168] but these films were reported by experienced radiologists, whereas in most emergency rooms decisions are based on those viewed by junior doctors. The latter are less accurate in recognizing pneumothorax than their seniors,[169] and the error rate is halved when paired expiratory films are available.[158] The variable quality of emergency room radiographs can make a small pneumothorax easy to overlook, but a closer scrutiny of the film may be prompted by identifying a basal pleural reaction, a change found in two-thirds of patients with primary pneumothorax, often with an air–fluid level.[38,157] With careful inspection small blebs or larger bullae may be apparent.[80,157] The latter can be mistaken for pneumothorax by the unwary, with potentially adverse consequences if drainage is attempted; a suggestive sign is air surrounding both walls of the bulla,[170] and CT is useful where uncertainty remains.[171] Lateral radiographs occasionally demonstrate a small pneumothorax not detected on a standard film, but have a high false-negative rate[172] and are not recommended.

In secondary pneumothorax, chest radiography usually also reflects the underlying pathology (Figures 42.1 and 42.2); exceptions include early cases of lymphangioleiomyomatosis and pleural-based malignancy.

Size of pneumothorax

Although attempts have been made to calculate the percentage of lung collapse from standard radiographs,[173–177] only the simplest (the 'Light index'[176]) correlates well with the volume of air that can be aspirated.[178] The latter is predicted best by CT, probably because the lung collapses asymmetrically; in any case the authors[179] also concluded 'perhaps more emphasis should be placed on the clinical status of the patient when making a decision of treatment strategy'. This latter premise is reflected in the 1993 British Thoracic Society (BTS) guidelines, which instead used three defined categories ('small', 'moderate' and 'large'). However, in line with others, [157,180] the BTS now prefers two groupings only, using a plain film rim of air of 2 cm (equivalent to 50 percent collapse) as cut-off.[166] Some studies refer to patients with 'complete' or 'total' pneumothorax even though semantically these terms should be reserved for those with an airless lung. In any case, initial management depends not only upon the size of pneumothorax but also its cause and degree of associated breathlessness.

Tension

The BTS also redefined tension as 'any pneumothorax with cardio-respiratory collapse', because of the widespread misunderstanding that the presence of mediastinal shift plus depression and flattening of the diaphragm on radiography represents a medical emergency. Such changes have been recorded in 19 percent of all cases of pneumothorax;[181] they are very common in large pneumothorax,[38,53,157] and many such patients are not unduly distressed (Figure 42.3).[181,182] In contrast with true tension (discussed in Chapter 43, Non-spontaneous pneumotho-

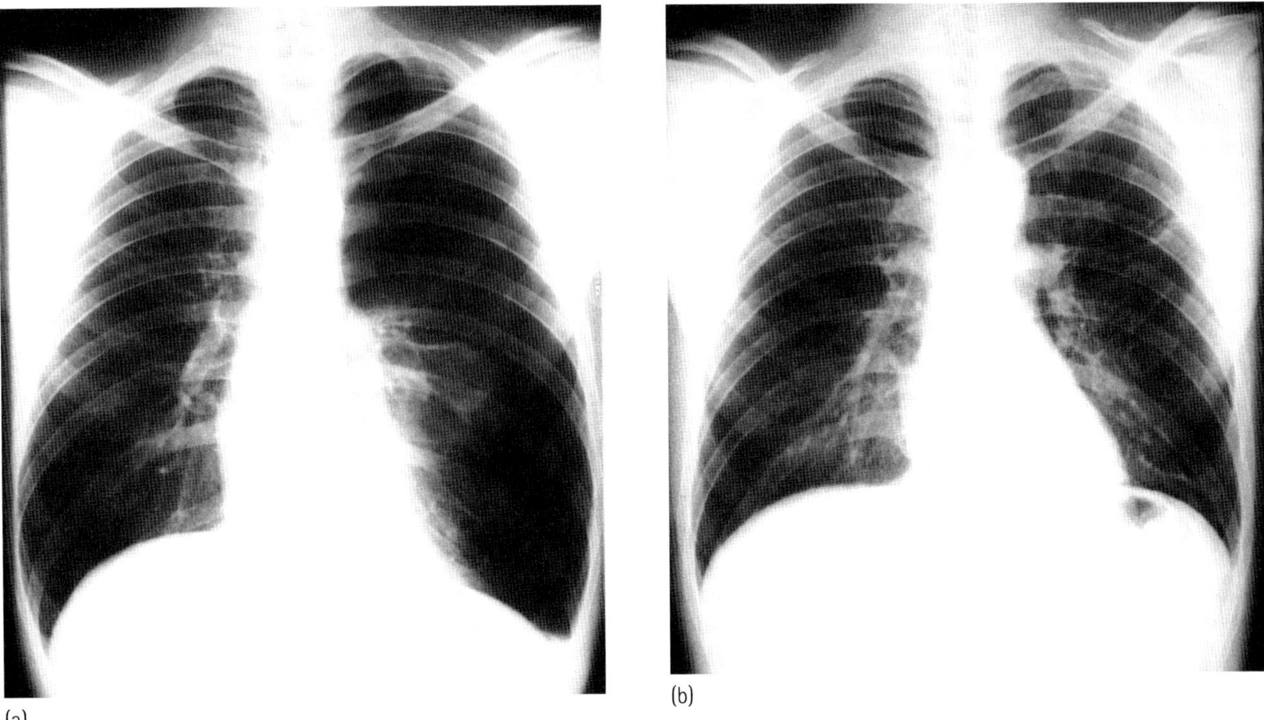

(a) (b)

Figure 42.3 This is not a tension pneumothorax. A 51-year-old man referred with a week of mild dyspnea. Radiograph (a) showed a large left pneumothorax with displacement of heart and hemidiaphragm, fully resolving after simple aspiration in clinic (b). He was not admitted and has had no recurrence.

rax), fluoroscopic screening shows that these shifts disappear during deep inspiration.[183]

Cardiovascular collapse is rare in primary pneumothorax;[180,184] yet even recently it has been stated that patients with *radiographic* tension 'are at risk of sudden deterioration and possibly cardiac arrest… potentially life-threatening situation'. However, only one of the four patients described was unstable,[185] and this was due to hemopneumothorax, as in one of two previously reported who were severely ill.[21] Kjærgaard did describe eight such patients, but these were collected from a large area over 20 years and only three were sufficiently ill to require urgent drainage.[3] There seems no reason to dissent from the view of Nissen[180] that untreated pneumothorax in otherwise healthy people is 'very seldom fatal'. Conversely, a patient with secondary pneumothorax who rapidly deteriorates even when radiological collapse is small should be decompressed by immediate cannulation.

MEDICAL MANAGEMENT

Only one national guideline has been introduced, by the BTS in 1993, which 10 years later was updated, modified and expanded.[6,166] The BTS approach is now included in all UK textbooks of general, respiratory and emergency medicine, and has been introduced elsewhere.[7,186]

Otherwise, there is widespread variation in practice with little agreement on fundamental issues such as the place of outpatient observation, initial drainage method, size of intercostal tube, value of suction, clamping chest drains and indications for surgery.[187–189] The American College of Chest Physicians developed a consensus document on these issues from recognized international authorities,[190] but on several of these issues there was a wide range of views, and its effect on standardizing American practice is unclear. In that document simple aspiration, although recommended by some of its contributors,[6,191] was nevertheless strongly discouraged, a view that is no longer tenable.

Historical

In the early part of the last century most cases, even with major lung collapse, were treated with bed rest because it was assumed that they had underlying tuberculosis. As spontaneous pneumothorax was increasingly recognized, some physicians familiar with inducing artificial pneumothorax in tuberculosis (often in outpatients who continued at work) used the same apparatus for aspirating pneumothorax,[49,192] which others avoided because of fear that the metal needles available might puncture the lung.[3,86,115,193] Increasing thoracic surgical experience with rubber tube drains (originally used mainly in post-operative cases) led to their adoption by other specialists for pneumothorax, and references to metal needles were withdrawn in later editions of medical textbooks.[192,194] The degree of collapse for which tube drainage was indicated dropped from 50 percent[195] to 30 percent,[196] and eventually the arbitrary figure of 15 percent became generally accepted.[176] Even so, many surgeons had for years been operating on most cases of pneumothorax,[86] while at the same time many of their physician colleagues were encouraging those with minor collapse to continue at work with outpatient observation.[10,192,197] In one hospital where pneumothorax patients were admitted equally between physicians and thoracic surgeons, the former were over three times more likely to adopt a conservative approach.[48]

The increasing vogue for large-bore intercostal tubes was challenged by a Michigan physician in 1965, anticipating current thinking: 'The vast majority of patients recover completely without any intervention… A small polyethylene catheter inserted through a needle is easier to handle, evokes much less chest discomfort when left in place, and in many hands is equally as effective as a large catheter'.[198] Small catheters had already been used with encouraging results in Connecticut.[48,102] The advantages over underwater drainage of a flutter valve, originally introduced in 1965 for war trauma cases[124] and later for post-operative patients, became recognized both for large-bore tubes[199] and fine-bore catheters;[200] as early as 1973 a French surgical group were using these as a means of outpatient management, and were successful in 74 percent of 167 patients.[199] In 1979 two junior hospital doctors in England[201] conceived the technique of simple aspiration, merely using a standard cannula, 50 mL syringe and three-way tap (Figure 42.4); the value of this was confirmed by others in the UK[197,202,203] stimulating a randomized trial[204] and leading to national guidelines.[6]

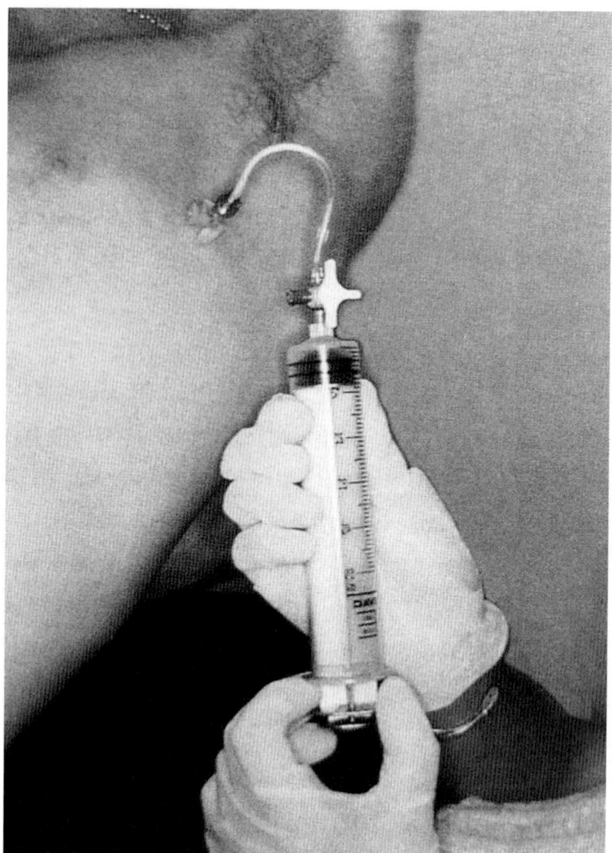

Figure 42.4 Simple aspiration being performed for the first time by a newly-qualified doctor, with success. Note that the three-way tap has a flexible extension arm, so that the cannula is not easily dislodged.

Observation

It is widely accepted that a primary pneumothorax of less than 15 percent does not require intervention, but the BTS documents agree with earlier clinical practice that observation is appropriate in greater degrees of collapse provided that the patient is only mildly breathless. In the UK this can be carried out as an outpatient procedure because much of the population live relatively near their district general hospital. The great majority of patients with minor lung collapse have a closed pneumothorax. It has been known since the nineteenth century that intrapleural air is rapidly reabsorbed; early animal experiments showed this to be accelerated by breathing an oxygen-rich mixture.[205,206] This has been confirmed by more sophisticated recent research in rabbits[207,208] as well as in human studies.[209,210] An early study calculated that air reabsorbs at a rate of approximately 1.25 percent of the lung volume per day,[211] but a more accurate figure is 2.2 percent (95 percent confidence interval 1.4–3.0 percent).[212] The suggestion that patients with primary pneumothorax may not need hospitalization has been criticized as being potentially dangerous,[213] but this has been widely practiced for years in Britain with no recorded fatalities. Where death has been recorded in primary pneumothorax, either it occurred during inpatient observation,[214] was a complication of treatment,[215] diagnosis had been overlooked[104] or was due to concomitant bleeding.[3] Overnight observation is indicated if the patient lives remote from the hospital; all agree that this is mandatory in secondary pneumothorax, although many of these can be discharged if stable.[9]

Drainage

If the pneumothorax is closed then any method of draining the air will be successful. Although it has long been assumed, and taught, that the presence of a large-bore intercostal drain for a few days promotes pleural adherence, thus allegedly reducing the risk of recurrence,[86] a randomized controlled trial showed that in this respect it was no better than simple aspiration.[204] This British study has since been confirmed by two larger trials from Belgium[216] and Kuwait,[217] as well as in a French comparison of indwelling catheter with large-bore drains.[218]

Compiling available information from all studies on primary pneumothorax, the immediate success rate for simple aspiration is 73 percent (440/606 – 16 studies[217,219,220]) and for indwelling catheter 80 percent (441/560 – 12 studies[53,219,221,222]). The advantage of the latter is that it allows time for a continuing small air leak to heal, which is why its success rates approach the 83 percent (938/1134 – 11 studies[217,219,221,222]) for large-bore drains. The pros and cons of these three procedures are outlined in Table 42.3. The high success rate of simple aspiration suggests that the initial pleural tear has already sealed by the time of diagnosis, and such rapid healing is even seen in traumatic pneumothorax where most chest drains can be removed within a day.[223] It is often assumed that complete lung collapse suggests an open pneumothorax, but in one study where three-quarters of patients had complete collapse, simple aspiration was highly effective.[216] With the exception of hemopneumothorax, there is now little justification for using large-bore tubes for initial drainage of either primary or secondary pneumothorax; one French group switched over entirely to indwelling catheters in 1977.[224] Harvey, co-author of the BTS guidelines, has calculated that adoption of simple aspiration throughout Europe and the USA would avoid 75 000 intercostal drains per annum in patients with primary pneumothorax.

There are three reasons why simple aspiration should be considered as the first-line intervention in such patients. First, it requires minimal training, an important consideration when many are initially seen by non-specialist junior doctors, who often have never inserted a chest tube,[225] have inadequate technique,[226] use an inappropriate site[227,228] and may cause major complications.[229,230] Second, hospital admission is often unnecessary; even in patients with complete collapse it is successful in over 60 percent,[203,216,231] and yet many are reluctant to attempt aspiration in such patients.[25,189] Third, it can usually predict both the existence and size of an air-leak: (1) if air continues to be easily aspirated a large air leak is present; (2) should the lung appear to re-inflate but then after a few minutes further air can again be aspirated there is a small air leak;[232] and (3) if after coughing, no more air can be aspirated after several minutes, it is a closed pneumothorax and after confirmatory chest radiograph the patient can be discharged or the cannula can be secured in place for a few hours.[233] The accepted approach if aspiration is unsuccessful is insertion of an indwelling catheter; whether this is always necessary is discussed later (see section Persistent air leak). Unlike catheters, plastic cannulae (which are very cheap, readily available and extremely easy for inexperienced doctors to use) are easily dislodged from the pleural cavity if left *in situ* for the effect of aspiration to be assessed. Also, the cannula must be at least 5 cm long to be sure of penetrating the pleura[234] and is perhaps preferably inserted using an axillary rather than an anterior approach.[235]

There is less information on simple aspiration in secondary pneumothorax, where it is successful in 47 percent (32/68 – 4 studies[219]); the latest of these was the largest, in which an indwelling drain was only required in 19 of 35.[236] As well as being effective in many, in those who fail the size of the air leak can be inferred, as above. Although standard practice has been to use a large-bore drain (at least 16 FG), usually an indwelling catheter is effective,[222] although less advisable in those who clearly have a large air leak and who are likely to require prolonged drainage. BTS guidelines no longer advocate large-bore bore tube drains, and catheter drainage instead is recommended.[166]

Management of chest drains

Since experience has shown that small-bore catheters may become displaced, blocked, kinked or are poorly positioned,[7,200,224,237] it is advisable to choose one 12–14 FG size and relatively stiff. Those introduced by a Seldinger technique are marketed by several manufacturers and are becoming increasingly popular; they have proved successful in various types of pleural drainage with few complications.[238]

Table 42.3 Comparison of different drainage techniques

	Advantages	Disadvantages
Simple aspiration	Minimal experience needed Rapid detection of air leak May avoid admission	Needs to be removed Ineffective if air leak
Indwelling catheter	Useful if small air leak Flutter valve allows discharge Talc pleurodesis possible	Some experience required Catheter tip may shear May become kinked/blocked
Large bore drain	Only if large air leak Blockage very unusual Talc pleurodesis possible	Operator must be experienced Restricts mobility Often painful Major complications possible

The traditional method of attaching the drain to an underwater seal allows bubbling of air to be easily recognized. However, using a flutter valve instead has the major advantage of allowing the option of outpatient management[199,239] and there is some evidence that it is more effective;[240] however, care is needed to ensure it is connected the correct way.[241] Newer devices have been developed to simplify outpatient drainage;[242–245] although effective, these are expensive and are unlikely to replace catheter plus flutter valve.

The widespread practice of applying suction to a chest drain derives from thoracic surgical practice of draining viscous secretions in post-resection, empyema and trauma cases, but its logic in drainage of air is dubious and early textbooks had polarized views.[194,246] Some imagine that air leak is more likely to stop if the lung can be brought into apposition against the chest wall, but this is no more convincing than the argument that a collapsed lung is more likely to heal. The clinical impression that applying suction increases the risk of rare[247] but potentially fatal re-expansion pulmonary edema, particularly if the lung has been collapsed for several days (Figure 42.5),[157,248,249] has been elegantly confirmed in a monkey model.[250] Three groups who compared standard suction with none found no advantage either in sealing air leaks or reducing hospital stay;[237,251,252] they disagreed about whether, once the lung re-expands with no further air leak, the drain can be removed immediately, and many practitioners still prefer delayed removal.[188] Randomized studies following pulmonary resection[253] and video-assisted surgery[254] show that applying suction to chest drains delays tube removal and lengthens hospital stay. An important implication of this is that deferring such a decision by clamping is unnecessary, a practice which most British pulmonologists abandoned following advice from thoracic surgeons and the 1993 BTS guidelines. If air leakage has ceased, clamping confers no advantage, but if not a dangerous situation may develop unrecognized. Such a consensus has not been reached elsewhere.[190] It makes no difference whether the drain is removed in expiration or inspiration.[255]

In the absence of a persistent air leak, failure of the lung to re-expand is nearly always due to the drain having becoming blocked, displaced (Figure 42.6), disconnected or clamped; occasionally it results from lung fibrosis or bronchial obstruction.[256]

OPERATIVE MANAGEMENT

Urgent surgical intervention is required in those with spontaneous hemo-pneumothorax who are hemodynamically compromised, although milder cases can be managed conservatively.[153,257] Non-urgent cases may be treated either by medical thoracoscopists (Chapter 47) or thoracic surgeons (Chapter 48), who strongly disagree about which procedure is best. Different practices both between and within countries are largely governed by who admits the patient: (1) thoracic surgeon, or (2) non-interventional pulmonologists with established surgical links, or (3) pulmonologist experienced at medical thoracoscopy. Whichever is preferred, patients can be reassured that this will have no long-term effect on lung function or physical fitness.[258,259] However, there is a significant incidence of chronic troublesome post-operative pain and paraesthesia,[103,260,261] sometimes not mentioned in ongoing debates about indications for, timing of and technique of operative intervention.

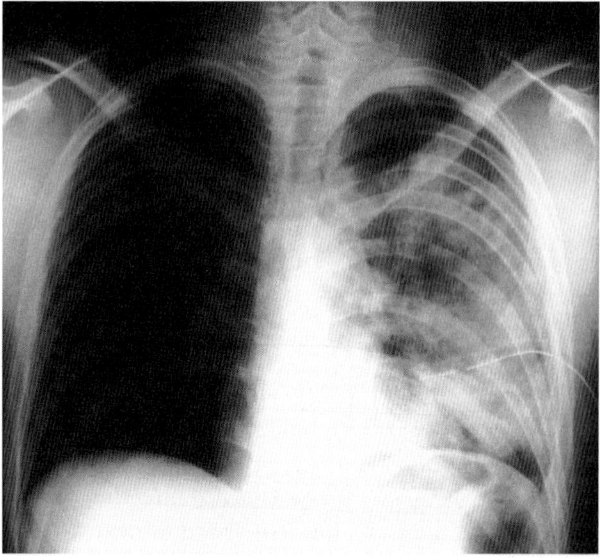

Figure 42.5 Pulmonary edema during intercostal tube drain. The left lung had been fully collapsed for at least a week. Suction had not been used. The patient had minimal symptoms and an uncomplicated recovery.

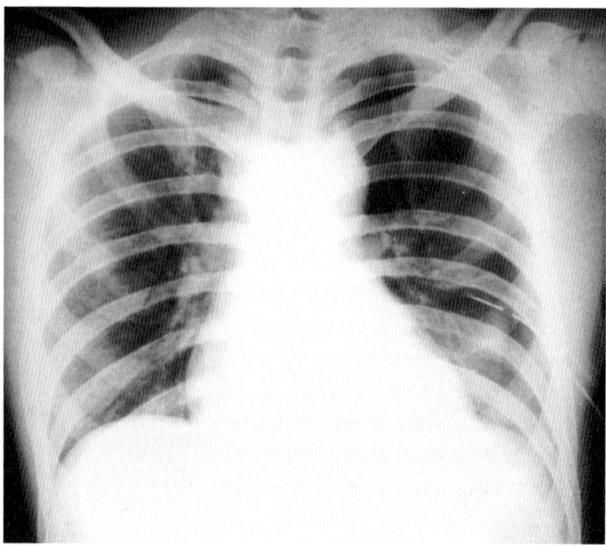

Figure 42.6 Partial pneumothorax, yet chest drain was not bubbling. Examination showed that it had become subcutaneous.

At presentation

In a 1992 survey two-thirds of Dutch specialists in large institutions perform thoracoscopy for the first episode,[187] and others have suggested that all such patients should be referred for surgical repair;[262–265] a variation on this approach is described by a Russian team who perform thoracoscopy in all patients before deciding who should proceed to surgery.[266] The great majority of experts[190] consider this inappropriate both because it is occasionally harmful but mainly because most patients respond to conservative treatment and never have recurrence. Nevertheless there is an intermediate, and increasingly popular, surgical approach: early video-assisted thoracoscopic surgery (VATS) in the minority who fail initial aspiration. The arguments for such an interventional approach, designed to reduce hospital stay, seem less compelling in the light of the following discussion.

Persistent air leak

Continuing air leak can be detected either at presentation by simple aspiration or following catheter drainage. Although more accurate methods of identifying open pneumothorax have been described, these require specialist equipment and experience and are rarely used. One is based on measuring intrapleural pressures,[267] another involves an inhaled marker gas.[236] The principle behind the latter was used in 1928 in a patient breathing oxygen, when it was shown that the gas coming out of the chest drain caused a lighted match to flare,[3] a fascinating observation that it is easily reproducible – but not recommended!

Although initial assessment may show that the pneumothorax is open, the defect may seal within the next few days. In two studies of primary pneumothorax [216,217] 37 percent had an open pneumothorax at presentation, yet two-thirds of these sealed within a week, by which time, therefore, only 12 percent of the whole cohort had persistent air leak. This makes the above case for early VATS less convincing, especially since there is an increasing trend to allow patients home with an indwelling catheter plus flutter valve. Indeed, it could be argued that in selected cases of failed initial aspiration but only minor breathlessness, discharge without drainage but with early clinic review may be an option. Allowing a patient home with an open pneumothorax could only be considered if there is easy access to hospital in the unlikely event of deterioration, and planned review at 1 week will determine whether re-expansion has occurred (in which case the patient can be discharged) or air leak is still present (in which case intervention is indicated as below).

In primary pneumothorax, an air leak that is going to seal does so within the first few days, whereas in secondary cases[268,269] more prolonged drainage may obviate surgery, which otherwise might require full thoracotomy. Persistent air leak is much more common in secondary cases,[9] particularly in the elderly;[148] and this group of patients include many with poor respiratory reserve who would tolerate full thoracotomy poorly. Catheter/flutter valve drainage with early mobilization is often preferable, as in those in whom it is desirable (although there are exceptions[270]) not to obliterate the pleural space prior to possible lung transplantation, as in lymphangioleiomyomatosis and cystic fibrosis.[271,272] In the latter, pneumothorax often occurs late in the disease and so is a marker of poor long-term prognosis,[273,274] similar to the situation in AIDS[131–136] where again good results can be obtained by catheter/flutter valve outpatient treatment.[275] One patient with prolonged air leak due to severe bullous disease was successfully treated by radiotherapy targeted to the identified pleural defect.[276]

In secondary cases, where recurrence may be particularly undesirable, successful intercostal drainage should lead to consideration of pleurodesis before the catheter is removed. Pleurodesis is discussed fully in Chapter 46.

There is no agreed approach to the management of catamenial pneumothorax, since some require hormone manipulation enough to prevent menstruation, others surgery, and some both;[143,144,277,278] pelvic endometriosis itself has a very variable response to treatment. Development of pneumothorax in pulmonary tuberculosis usually heralds prolonged air leak with weeks of pleural drainage while chemotherapy takes effect, surgery only occasionally being necessary.[62,66]

Prevention of recurrence

Where the initial episode resolves with conservative management, most specialists wait until a second episode before advising operative intervention; even then only half the patients will have a further recurrence, and if each occasion was managed without hospitalization, many prefer further conservative management.

The likelihood of further episodes is independent of whether management is conservative or by drainage without pleurodesis, and is not affected by the drainage method used.[7,12,49,164,216–218,279] Several studies[280] give a wide spread of recurrence rates (16–52 percent, mean 30 percent). In the most methodologically sound report,[281] the 1-, 5- and 10-year recurrence rates for primary pneumothorax were 15, 23 and 29 percent, respectively. Recurrence appeared more common in secondary pneumothorax, but numbers in this group were low, and other publications disagree.[9,282] The Dutch finding that recurrence rate decreases with time confirmed those of a much larger series,[58] most further episodes occurring within the first year. Ectomorphic build and continued smoking are independent risk factors for recurrence,[281,283] although such information leads to smoking cessation in few.[38,83,98] Although CT scanning may predict which patients are most likely to have a contralateral episode,[284] it may not be useful in forecasting ipsilateral recurrence.

Occupational and recreational considerations

As well as in those with persistent air leak, there are three other indications for surgery after the first episode: (1) those expecting to spend some time without access to medical care either for occupational or recreational reasons; (2) professional and amateur divers – particularly important with the widespread popularity of scuba diving; and (3) military aviators, who are at increased risk because of breathing pure oxygen with forced expiration, marked changes in gravitational force and rapid decompressions[51] (in many countries it is policy that a pilot with a documented pneumothorax requires pleurectomy before resuming flying duties). It is possible that future recommendations, which currently vary between countries, will advise CT scanning to identify which of these should have bilateral preventative surgery.[284]

Because the reduced cabin pressure in commercial aircraft causes a closed pneumothorax to enlarge at altitude – although by less than 25 percent – most airlines suggest a delay of 6 weeks before flying after resolution of a pneumothorax because of the risk of early recurrence. This is an arbitrary figure and it is rare for those who already have, or develop, spontaneous pneumothorax during flight to run into problems.[51,285]

KEY POINTS

- Initial management should be guided primarily by symptoms and whether significant underlying lung disease is present.
- Complete lung collapse on chest radiograph is not in itself an emergency.
- Simple aspiration is the preferred initial method of drainage, particularly if the attending doctor is not a trained pulmonologist. It is easy to learn, very cheap, allows evaluation of the presence and size of air leak, and may avoid hospital admission.
- In experienced hands, medium-bore (12–16 FG) indwelling catheters are an equally appropriate form of drainage. They allow time for small air leaks to seal, and attachment of a flutter valve allows patient mobility and the option of outpatient management.
- The use of large-bore intercostal tubes as an initial method of drainage should now be considered unacceptable medical practice.
- In primary pneumothorax, air leak has already ceased in two-thirds on presentation and in 88% within the next week.
- Intervention should be considered where air leak persists at 5 days in primary pneumothorax. A more conservative approach should be considered in secondary cases, depending upon the severity of underlying lung disease; frail patients with persistent air leak may be managed successfully by prolonged drainage catheter plus flutter valve; where drainage is successful talc pleurodesis can be considered.
- Recurrence rate after first episode in primary pneumothorax is only 30%. The current increasing trend towards early surgery in primary cases should be discouraged.
- Effective definitive treatment of pneumothorax (persistent air leak, prevention of recurrence) can usually be performed thoracoscopically, preferably by a thoracic surgeon.
- It is not yet clear whether the increasing use of computed tomography materially improves patient management.
- The previously accepted theory that primary pneumothorax is due to rupture of subpleural blebs remains valid.
- Early advice from pulmonologists by non-specialists, and from thoracic surgeons by pulmonologists, should always be sought, especially in patients with poor respiratory reserve.

REFERENCES

● = Key primary paper
◆ = Major review article
$*$ = Paper that represents the first formal publication of a management guideline

◆1. Emerson C. Pneumothorax: a historical, clinical, and experimental study. *John Hopkins Hosp Rep* 1903; **11**: 1–450.
2. Biach A. On the etiology of pneumothorax in Vienna [German]. *Med Wohnschr* 1880; **30**: 431.
●3. Kjærgaard H. Spontaneous pneumothorax in the apparently healthy. *Acta Med Scand* 1932; Suppl 43: 1–159.
4. Melton LJ, Hepper NGG, Offord KP. Incidence of spontaneous pneumothorax in Olmsted County, Minnesota: 1950–1974. *Am Rev Respir Dis* 1979; **120**: 1379–82.
5. Bense L, Eklund G, Odont D, Wiman L-G. Smoking and the increased risk of contracting spontaneous pneumothorax. *Chest* 1987; **92**: 1009–12.
*6. Miller AC, Harvey JE. Guidelines for the management of spontaneous pneumothorax. *Brit Med J* 1993; **307**: 114–6.
7. Hernandez Ortiz C, Zugasti Garcia K, Emparanza Knorr J, *et al.* Idiopathic spontaneous pneumothorax: treatment by small-caliber catheter aspiration compared to drainage through a chest tube [Spanish]. *Arch Bronconeumol* 1999; **35**: 179–82.
●8. Gupta D, Hansell A, Nichols T, *et al.* Epidemiology of pneumothorax in England. *Thorax* 2000; **55**: 666–71.
9. Ferraro P, Beauchamp G, Lord F, Emond C, Bastien E. Spontaneous primary and secondary pneumothorax: a 10-year study of management alternatives. *Can J Surg* 1994; **37**: 197–202.

●10. Stradling P, Poole G. Conservative management of spontaneous pneumothorax. *Thorax* 1966; **21**: 145–9.

11. Jansveld CAF, Dijkman JH. Primary spontaneous pneumothorax and smoking. *Br Med J* 1975; **4**: 559–60.

12. Hart GJ, Stokes TC, Couch AH. Spontaneous pneumothorax in Norfolk. *Br J Dis Chest* 1983; **77**: 164–70.

13. Teixidor Sureda J, Estrada Salo G, Sole Montserrat J, *et al.* Spontaneous pneumothorax: a review of 2,507 cases [Spanish]. *Arch Bronconeumol* 1994; **30**: 131–5.

14. Ji Woong Son, Jae Yong Park, Kwan Young Kim, *et al.* Clinical analysis of spontaneous pneumothorax. *Tubercul Respir Dis* 1999; **47**: 374–82.

15. Nakamura H, Konishiike J, Sugamura A, Takeno Y. Epidemiology of spontaneous pneumothorax in women. *Chest* 1986; **89**: 378–82.

16. Van Winter JT, Nichols IIIFC, Pairolero PC, Ney JA, Ogburn PL Jr. Management of spontaneous pneumothorax during pregnancy: case report and review of the literature. *Mayo Clin Proc* 1996; **71**: 249–52.

17. Cohen MM, Pollock-Barziv S, Johnson S. The emerging clinical picture of lymphangioleiomyomatosis. *Thorax* 2005; **60**: 875–9.

18. Almoosa KF, Ryu JH, Mendez J, *et al.* Management of pneumothorax in lymphangioleiomyomatosis: effects on recurrence and lung transplantation complications. *Chest* 2006; **129**: 1274–81.

19. Ryu JH, Moss J, Beck GJ, *et al.* The NHLBI lymphangioleiomyomatosis registry: characteristics of 230 patients at enrollment. *Am J Respir Crit Care Med* 2006; **173**: 105–11.

20. Taveira-DaSilva AM, Steagall WK, Moss J. Lymphangioleiomyomatosis. *Cancer Control* 2006; **13**: 276–85.

21. Myers JA. Simple spontaneous pneumothorax. *Dis Chest* 1954; **26**: 420–41.

22. Seremetis MG. The management of spontaneous pneumothorax. *Chest* 1970; **57**: 65–8.

23. Watt AG. Spontaneous pneumothorax: a review of 210 consecutive admissions to Royal Perth Hospital. *Med J Austr* 1978; **1**: 186–8.

24. Nakamura H, Izuchi R, Hagiwara T, *et al.* Physical constitution and smoking habits of patients with idiopathic spontaneous pneumothorax. *Jpn J Med* 1983; **22**: 2–8.

25. Abolnik IZ, Lossos IS, Gillis D, Breuer R. Primary spontaneous pneumothorax in men. *Am J Med Sci* 1993; **305**: 297–303.

26. Getz SB, Beasley WE. Spontaneous pneumothorax. *Am J Surg* 1983; **145**: 823–7.

27. Escribano Montaner A, Herrejon Silvestre A, Simo Mompo M, Blanquer Olivas J. Spontaneous idiopathic pneumothorax in adolescents [Spanish]. *Ana Espan Ped* 1995; **42**: 261–4.

28. Wilcox DT, Glick PL, Karamanoukian HL, Allen JE, Azizkhan RG. Spontaneous pneumothorax: a single-institution, 12-year experience in patients under 16 years of age. *J Pediatr Surg* 1995; **30**: 1452–4.

29. Wong KS, Liu HP, Yeow KM. Spontaneous pneumothorax in children. *Acta Paediatr Taiwan* 2000; **41**: 263–5.

30. Vassallo R, Ryu JH, Schroeder DR, Decker PA, Limper AH. Clinical outcomes of pulmonary Langerhans'-cell histiocytosis in adults. *N Engl J Med* 2002; **346**: 484–90.

31. Melton LJ 3rd, Hepper NG, Offord KP. Influence of height on the risk of spontaneous pneumothorax. *Mayo Clin Proc* 1981; **56**: 678–82.

32. Kawakami Y, Irie T, Kamishima K. Stature, lung height, and spontaneous pneumothorax. *Respiration* 1982; **43**: 35–40.

33. Fujino S, Inoue S, Tezuka N, *et al.* Physical development of surgically treated patients with primary spontaneous pneumothorax. *Chest* 1999; **116**: 899–902.

●34. West JB. Distribution of mechanical stress in the lung: a possible factor in localisation of pulmonary disease. *Lancet* 1971; i: 839–41.

35. Margaliot SZ, Barzilay J, Bar-David M, *et al.* Spontaneous pneumothorax and mitral valve prolapse. *Chest* 1986; **89**: 93–4.

36. Bitar ZI, Ahmed S, Amin AE, Jamal K, Ridha M. Prevalence of mitral valve prolapse in primary spontaneous pneumothorax. *Prim Care Respir J* 2006; **15**: 342–5.

37. Lopes C, Manique A, Sotto-Mayor R, *et al.* Ehlers-Danlos syndrome – a rare cause of spontaneous pneumothorax [Portuguese]. *Rev Port Pneumol* 2006; **12**: 471–80.

38. Hallgrimsson JG. Spontaneous pneumothorax in Iceland with special reference to idiopathic type: a clinical and epidemiological investigation. *Scand J Thorac Cardiovasc Surg* 1978; **Suppl 21**: 1–85.

39. Lenler-Petersen P, Grunnet N, Jespersen TW, Jaeger P. Familial spontaneous pneumothorax. *Eur Respir J* 1990; **3**: 342–5.

40. Nickoladze GD. Surgical management of familial spontaneous pneumothorax. *Respir Med* 1990; **84**: 107–9.

41. Abolnik IZ, Lossos IS, Zlotogora J, Brauer R. On the inheritance of primary spontaneous pneumothorax. *Am J Med Genet* 1991; **40**: 155–8.

42. Yellin A, Shiner RJ, Lieberman Y. Familial multiple bilateral pneumothorax associated with Marfan syndrome. *Chest* 1991; **100**: 577–8.

43. Cheng YJ, Chou SH, Kao EL. Familial spontaneous pneumothorax: report of seven cases in two families [Chinese]. *Kao J Med Sci* 1992; **8**: 390–4.

44. Morrison PJ, Lowry RC, Nevin NC. Familial primary spontaneous pneumothorax consistent with true autosomal dominant inheritance. *Thorax* 1998; **53**: 151–2.

45. Chiu HT, Garcia CK. Familial spontaneous pneumothorax. *Curr Opin Pulm Med* 2006; **12**: 268–72.

46. Toro JR, Pautler SE, Stewart L, *et al.* Lung cysts, spontaneous pneumothrorax and genetic associations in 89 families with Birt-Hogg-Dube syndrome. *Am J Respir Crit Care Med* 2007; **22**: 22.

47. Elfeldt RJ, Schroder D, Schroeder P, Schaube H, Nissen R. Relation between smoking and idiopathic spontaneous pneumothorax: a case-control study. *Theor Surg* 1993; **8**: 131–5.

48. Lindskog GE, Halasz NA. Spontaneous pneumothorax. *Arch Surg* 1957; **75**: 693–8.

49. Lenox-Smith I. Spontaneous pneumothorax: a study of 94 cases. *Br J Dis Chest* 1962; **56**: 1–10.

50. Klassen KP, Meckstroth CV. Treatment of spontaneous pneumothorax: prompt expansion with controlled thoracotomy tube suction. *J Am Med Assoc* 1962; **182**: 111–5.

51. Voge VM, Anthracite R. Spontaneous pneumothorax in the USAF aircrew population: a retrospective study. *Aviat Space Environ Med* 1986; **57**: 939–49.

52. Bense L, Wiman LG, Hedenstierna G. Onset of symptoms in spontaneous pneumothorax: correlations to physical activity. *Eur J Respir Dis* 1987; **71**: 181–6.

53. Marquette CH, Marx A, Leroy S, *et al.* Simplified stepwise management of primary spontaneous pneumothorax: a pilot study. *Eur Respir J* 2006; **27**: 470–6.

54. Bense L. Spontaneous pneumothorax related to falls in atmospheric pressure. *Eur J Respir Dis* 1984; **65**: 544–6.

55. Ozenne G, Poignie P, Lemercier JP, Nouvet G, Grancher G. Meteorological conditions and spontaneous pneumothorax: a retrospective study of 165 cases in the Rouen region. *Rev Pneumol Clin* 1984; **40**: 27–33.

56. Smit HJM, Deville WL, Schramel FMNH, *et al.* Atmospheric pressure changes and outdoor temperature changes in relation to spontaneous pneumothorax. *Chest* 1999; **116**: 676–81.

57. Sok M, Mikulecky M, Erzen J. Onset of spontaneous pneumothorax and the synodic lunar cycle. *Med Hypotheses* 2001; **57**: 638–41.

58. Cran IR, Rumball CA. Survey of spontaneous pneumothorax in the Royal Air Force. *Thorax* 1967; **22**: 462–5.

59. Morales Suarez-Varela M, Martinez-Selva MI, Llopis-Gonzalez A, Martinez-Jimeno JL, Plaza-Valia P. Spontaneous pneumothorax related with climatic characteristics in the Valencia area. *Eur J Epidem* 2000; **16**: 193–8.

60. Ayed AK, Bazerbashi S, Ben-Nakhi M, *et al.* Risk factors of spontaneous pneumothorax in Kuwait. *Med Princ Pract* 2006; **15**: 338–42.
61. Noppen M, Verbanck S, Harvey J, *et al.* Music: a new cause of primary spontaneous pneumothorax. *Thorax* 2004; **59**: 722–4.
62. Blanco-Perez J, Bordon J, Pineiro-Amigo L, *et al.* Pneumothorax in active pulmonary tuberculosis: resurgence of an old complication? *Respir Med* 1998; **92**: 1269–73.
63. Javaid A, Amjad M, Khan W, *et al.* Pneumothorax: aetiology, complications and outcome. *J Coll Phys Surg Pakistan* 1998; **8**: 14–16.
64. Hussain SF, Aziz A, Fatima H. Pneumothorax: a review of 146 adult cases admitted at a university teaching hospital in Pakistan. *J Pakistan Med Assoc* 1999; **49**: 243–6.
65. Gupta D, Mishra S, Faruqi S, Aggarwal AN. Aetiology and clinical profile of spontaneous pneumothorax in adults. *Indian J Chest Dis Allied Sci* 2006; **48**: 261–4.
66. Mezghani S, Abdelghani A, Njima H, *et al.* Tuberculous pneumothorax: retrospective study of 23 cases in Tunisia [French]. *Rev Pneumol Clin* 2006; **62**: 13–18.
67. Darwish B. Clinical and radiological manifestations of 206 patients with pulmonary hydatidosis over a ten-year period. *Prim Care Respir J* 2006; **15**: 246–51.
68. West S. The Bradshawe lecture: on pneumothorax. *Br Med J* 1887; ii: 393–400.
●69. Macklin CC. Pneumothorax with massive collapse from experimental over-inflation of the lung substance. *Can Med J* 1937; **36**: 414–20.
70. Calder IM. Autopsy and experimental observations on factors leading to barotrauma in man. *Undersea Biomed Res* 1985; **12**: 165–81.
71. Marnejon T, Sarac S, Cropp AJ. Spontaneous pneumothorax in weightlifters. *J Sports Med Phys Fitness* 1995; **35**: 124–6.
72. Reeder SR. Subcutaneous emphysema, pneumomediastinum, and pneumothorax in labor and delivery. *Am J Obstet Gynecol* 1986; **154**: 487–9.
73. Nieboer B, Aboosy N, Verschoor L, Huisman A. Pneumomediastinum as a cause of acute chest pain postpartum. *J Matern Fetal Neonatal Med* 2006; **19**: 243–5.
74. Heppner HJ, Sieber C, Schmitt K. 'Usual' cannabis abuse producing unusual consequences [German]. *Deutsch Med Wochenschr* 2007; **132**: 560–2.
75. Reddymasu S, Borhan-Manesh F, Jordan PA. Spontaneous pneumomediastinum due to achalasia: a case report. *South Med J* 2006; **99**: 892–3.
76. Manco JC, Terra-Filho J, Silva GA. Pneumomediastinum, pneumothorax and subcutaneous emphysema following the measurement of maximal expiratory pressure in a normal subject. *Chest* 1990; **98**: 1530–2.
77. Dermskian G, Lamb LE. Spontaneous pneumothorax in apparently healthy flying personnel. *Ann Intern Med* 1959; **51**: 39–51.
78. Robb DJ. Cases from the aerospace medicine residents' teaching file: Case H57 – complete spontaneous pneumothorax in-flight in an F-16 pilot during a high-G maneuver. *Aviat Space Environ Med* 1994; **65**: 170–2.
79. Pedersen MN, Jensen BN. Pneumothorax after 'reversed bungee jump' [Danish]. *Ugeskr Laeger* 1999; **161**: 5547–8.
80. Jordan KG, Kwong JS, Flint J, Muller NL. Surgically treated pneumothorax: radiologic and pathologic findings. *Chest* 1997; **111**: 280–5.
81. Lesur O, Delorme N, Fromaget JM, Bernadac P, Polu JM. Computed tomography in the etiologic assessment of idiopathic spontaneous pneumothorax. *Chest* 1990; **98**: 341–7.
82. Mitlehner W, Friedrich M, Dissmann W. Value of computer tomography in the detection of bullae and blebs in patients with primary spontaneous pneumothorax. *Respiration* 1992; **59**: 221–7.
83. Smit HJ, Chatrou M, Postmus PE. The impact of spontaneous pneumothorax, and its treatment, on the smoking behaviour of young adult smokers. *Respir Med* 1998; **92**: 1132–6.
84. Van Belle AF, Lamers RJ, ten Velde GP, Wouters EF. Diagnostic yield of computed tomography and densitometric measurements of the lung in thoracoscopically-defined idiopathic spontaneous pneumothorax. *Respir Med* 2001; **95**: 292–6.
85. Baranofsky ID, Warden HG, Kaufman JL, Whately J, Hanner JM. Bilateral therapy for unilateral spontaneous pneumothorax. *J Thorac Cardiovasc Surg* 1957; **34**: 1767–9.
86. Mills M, Baisch BF. Spontaneous pneumothorax: a series of 400 cases. *Ann Thorac Surg* 1965; **1**: 286–97.
87. Radomsky J, Becker HP, Hartel W. Pleural porosity in idiopathic spontaneous pneumothorax [German]. *Pneumologie* 1989; **43**: 250–3.
88. Janssen JP, Schramel FM, Sutedja TG, Cuesta MA, Postmus PE. Videothoracoscopic appearance of first and recurrent pneumothorax. *Chest* 1995; **108**: 330–4.
89. Ayed AK, Chandrasekaran C, Sukumar M. Video-assisted thoracoscopic surgery for primary spontaneous pneumothorax: clinicopathological correlation. *Eur J Cardiothorac Surg* 2006; **29**: 221–5.
90. Lichter I, Gwynne JF. Spontaneous pneumothorax in young subjects: a clinical and pathological study. *Thorax* 1971; **26**: 409–17.
91. Tomashefski JF, Dahms B, Bruce M. Pleura in pneumothorax: comparison of patients with cystic fibrosis and idiopathic spontaneous pneumothorax. *Arch Pathol Lab Med* 1985; **109**: 910–16.
92. Becker HP, Weidringer JW, Willy C, Hartel W, Blumel G. Light and scanning electron microscopy studies of the pleura: a contribution to the pathogenesis of spontaneous pneumothorax in young patients [German]. *Langenbecks Arch Chir* 1991; **376**: 295–301.
93. Haraguchi S, Fukuda Y. Histogenesis of abnormal elastic fibers in blebs and bullae of patients with spontaneous pneumothorax: ultrastructural and immunohistochemical studies. *Acta Pathol Jpn* 1993; **43**: 709–22.
94. Luna E, Tomashefski JF Jr, Brown D, Clarke RE, Kleinerman J. Reactive eosinophilic pulmonary vascular infiltration in patients with spontaneous pneumothorax. *Am J Surg Pathol* 1994; **18**: 195–9.
95. Cyr PV, Vincic L, Kay JM. Pulmonary vasculopathy in idiopathic spontaneous pneumothorax in young subjects. *Arch Pathol Lab Med* 2000; **124**: 717–20.
96. Smit HJ, Wienk MA, Schreurs AJ, Schramel FM, Postmus PE. Do bullae indicate a predisposition to recurrent pneumothorax? *Br J Radiol* 2000; **73**: 356–9.
97. Noppen M. CT scanning and bilateral surgery for unilateral primary pneumothorax? *Chest* 2001; **119**: 1293–4.
98. Smit HJM, Golding RP, Schramel FMNH, *et al.* Lung density measurements in spontaneous pneumothorax demonstrate air trapping. *Chest* 2004; **125**: 2083–90.
99. Ayed AK, Chandrasekaran C, Sukumar M. Video-assisted thoracoscopic surgery for primary spontaneous pneumothorax: clinicopathological correlation. *Eur J Cardiothorac Surg* 2006; **29**: 221–5.
100. Lipscomb VJ, Hardie RJ, Dubielzig RR. Spontaneous pneumothorax caused by pulmonary blebs and bullae in 12 dogs. *J Am Anim Hosp Assoc* 2003; **39**: 435–45.
101. De Troyer A, Yernault JC, Rodenstein D, Englert M, de Coster A. Pulmonary function in patients with primary spontaneous pneumothorax. *Bull Eur Physiopathol Respir* 1978; **14**: 31–9.
102. Gobbel WG. Spontaneous pneumothorax. *J Thorac Cardiovasc Surg* 1963; **46**: 331–45.
103. Sihoe AD, Au SS, Cheung ML, *et al.* Incidence of chest wall paresthesia after video-assisted thoracic surgery for primary spontaneous pneumothorax. *Eur J Cardiothorac Surg* 2004; **25**: 1054–8.
104. Simonsen K. Sudden death due to bilateral spontaneous

pneumothorax caused by rupture of congenital lung cysts. *Z Rechtsmed* 1990; **103**: 379–83.
105. Hay E, Sternfeld M, Rashid A, Kunichevsky S, Eliraz A. Simultaneous bilateral spontaneous pneumothorax: case report. *Am J Emerg Med* 1992; **10**: 50–2.
106. Kendall IG, Harborne DJ, Premswarup I. Beware spontaneous bilateral pneumothorax. *Arch Emerg Med* 1992; **9**: 51–3.
107. Hatta T, Mastuda S, Kuris S, *et al.* A case of simultaneous bilateral spontaneous pneumothorax. *Jpn J Thorac Surg* 1993; **46**: 287–9.
108. Kadokura M, Yamamoto S, Nonaka M, *et al.* Asymptomatic bilateral spontaneous pneumothorax [Japanese]. *Kyobu Geka* 1994; **47**: 215–18.
109. Ohara K, Yamazaki T, Sakaguchi K, Nakayama M, Kobayashi A. A case of simultaneous bilateral spontaneous pneumothorax [Japanese]. *Jpn J Thorac Surg* 1994; **47**: 1110–11.
110. Sayar A, Turna A, Metin M, *et al.* Simultaneous bilateral spontaneous pneumothorax report of 12 cases and review of the literature. *Acta Chir Belg* 2004; **104**: 572–6.
111. Dines DE, Clagett OT, Payne WS. Spontaneous pneumothorax in emphysema. *Mayo Clin Proc* 1970; **45**: 481–7.
112. Lai RS, Perng RP, Chang SC. Primary lung cancer complicated with pneumothorax. *Jpn J Clin Oncol* 1992; **22**: 194–7.
113. Sakai S, Matsuoka H, Tsuwano S, *et al.* Lung cancer associated with bulla found during an operation of pneumothorax; report of a case [Japanese]. *Kyobu Geka* 2006; **59**: 1209–12.
114. Houacine S, Belhamri A, Damache MB, Ihaddaden A, Drif M. Recurrent pneumothorax during asthma attacks. *Rev Pneumol Clin* 1986; **42**: 204–6.
115. Hyde L. Benign spontaneous pneumothorax. *Ann Intern Med* 1962; **56**: 746–51.
116. Burke GJ. Pneumothorax complicating acute asthma. *S Afr Med J* 1979; **55**: 508–10.
117. Pickup CM, Nee PA, Randall PE. Radiographic features in 1016 adults admitted to hospital with acute asthma. *J Accid Emerg Med* 1994; **11**: 234–7.
118. Limthongkul S, Wongthim S, Udompanich V, Charoenlap P, Nuchprayoon C. Status asthmaticus: an analysis of 560 episodes and comparison between mechanical and non-mechanical ventilation groups. *J Med Assoc Thai* 1990; **73**: 495–501.
119. Srinivas S, Varadhachary G. Spontaneous pneumothorax in malignancy: a case report and review of the literature. *Ann Oncol* 2000; **11**: 887–9.
120. Ouellette D, Inculet R. Unsuspected metastatic choriocarcinoma presenting as unilateral spontaneous pneumothorax. *Ann Thorac Surg* 1992; **53**: 144–5.
121. Stein ME, Haim N, Drumea K, Ben-Itzhak O, Kuten A. Spontaneous pneumothorax complicating chemotherapy for metastatic seminoma: a case report and a review of the literature. *Cancer* 1995; **75**: 2710–3.
122. Furrer M, Althaus U, Ris HB. Spontaneous pneumothorax from radiographically occult metastatic sarcoma. *Eur J Cardiothorac Surg* 1997; **11**: 1171–3.
123. Sakurai H, Hada M, Miyashita Y, *et al.* Simultaneous bilateral spontaneous pneumothorax secondary to metastatic angiosarcoma of the scalp: report of a case. *Surg Today* 2006; **36**: 919–22.
●124. Heimlich HJ. Valve drainage of the pleural cavity. *Dis Chest* 1968; **53**: 282–7.
125. Kolber C, Souquet PJ, Geriniere L, *et al.* Spontaneous pneumothorax revealing malignant mesothelioma. *Rev Pneumol Clin* 1996; **52**: 42–4.
126. Alkhuja S, Miller A, Mastellone AJ, Markowitz S. Malignant pleural mesothelioma presenting as spontaneous pneumothorax: a case series and review. *Am J Ind Med* 2000; **38**: 219–23.
127. Weissberg D, Refaely Y. Pneumothorax: experience with 1,199 patients. *Chest* 2000; **117**: 1279–85.
128. Froudarakis ME, Bouros D, Voloudaki A, *et al.* Pneumothorax as a first manifestation of sarcoidosis. *Chest* 1997; **112**: 278–80.
129. Akelsson IG, Eklund A, Skold CM, Tornling G. Bilateral spontaneous pneumothorax and sarcoidosis. *Sarcoidosis* 1990; **7**: 136–8.
130. Fraticelli A, Picat-Joossen D, Astoul P. Pneumothorax and multiple lung masses: unusual manifestations of sarcoidosis [French]. *Rev Mal Respir* 2000; **17**: 885–7.
131. Byrnes TA, Brevig JK, Chin Bor Y. Pneumothorax in patients with acquired immunodeficiency syndrome. *J Thorac Cardiovasc Surg* 1989; **98**: 546–50.
132. Pellerin M, Lafontaine E, Toma E, Bard C. Surgical treatment of pneumothorax in patients with AIDS. *Ann Chir* 1993; **47**: 844–7.
133. Metersky ML, Colt HG, Olson LK, Shanks TG. AIDS-related spontaneous pneumothorax: risk factors and treatment. *Chest* 1995; **108**: 946–51.
134. Pastores SM, Garay SM, Naidich D, Rom WN. Review: pneumothorax in patients with AIDS-related *Pneumocystis carinii* pneumonia. *Am J Med Sci* 1996; **312**: 229–34.
135. Spivak H, Keller S. Spontaneous pneumothorax in the AIDS population. *Am Surg* 1996; **62**: 753–6.
136. Trachiotis GD, Vricella LA, Alyono D, Aaron BL, Hix WR. Management of AIDS-related pneumothorax. *Ann Thorac Surg* 1996; **62**: 1608–13.
137. Tumbarello M, Tacconelli E, Pirronti T, Cauda R, Ortona L. Pneumothorax in HIV-infected patients: role of *Pneumocystis carinii* pneumonia and pulmonary tuberculosis. *Eur Respir J* 1997; **10**: 1332–5.
138. Kuhlman JE, Knowles MC, Fishman EK, Sigelman SS. Premature bullous damage in AIDS: CT diagnosis. *Radiology* 1989; **173**: 23–6.
●139. Maurer ER, Schaal JA, Mendez FL. Chronic recurrent spontaneous pneumothorax due to endometriosis of the diaphragm. *J Am Med Assoc* 1958; **168**: 2013–14.
140. Suzuki S, Yasuda K, Matsumura Y, Kondo T. Left-side catamenial pneumothorax with endometrial tissue on the visceral pleura. *Jpn J Thorac Cardiovasc Surg* 2006; **54**: 225–7.
141. Stern H, Toole AL, Merino M. Catamenial pneumothorax. *Chest* 1980; **78**: 480–2.
142. Guerin JC, Champel F, Martinat Y, Boniface E. Thoracoscopic study of 6 cases of catamenial pneumothorax [French]. *Rev Mal Respir* 1987; **4**: 167–71.
◆143. Joseph J, Sahn SA. Thoracic endometriosis syndrome: new observations from an analysis of 110 cases. *Am J Med* 1996; **100**: 164–70.
144. Bagan P, le Pimpec Barthes F, Assouad J, Souilamas R, Riquet M. Catamenial pneumothorax: retrospective study of surgical treatment. *Ann Thorac Surg* 2003; **75**: 378–81.
145. Morcos M, Alifano M, Gompel A, Regnard JF. Life-threatening endometriosis-related hemopneumothorax. *Ann Thorac Surg* 2006; **82**: 726–9.
146. Kadokura M, Nonaka M, Yamamoto S, *et al.* Five cases of asymptomatic spontaneous pneumothorax. *Ann Thorac Cardiovasc Surg* 1999; **5**: 187–90.
147. Liston R, McLoughlin R, Clinch D. Acute pneumothorax: a comparison of elderly with younger patients. *Age Ageing* 1994; **23**: 393–5.
148. Loscertales J, Garcia Diaz F, Jimenez Merchan R, *et al.* Treatment of spontaneous pneumothorax in patients over 70 years of age [Spanish]. *Arch Bronconeumol* 1994; **30**: 344–7.
149. Hagen RH, Reed W, Solheim K. Spontaneous pneumothorax. *Scand J Thorac Cardiovasc Surg* 1987; **21**: 183–5.
●150. Miller AC. Hypothesis: chest pain in primary spontaneous pneumothorax. *Int J Clin Pract* 2007; **61**: 290–2.
151. Forlanini C. Early results of artificial pneumothorax in pulmonary phthisis [Italian]. *Gazz med Torina* 1894; **45**: 381–4, 401–3.
152. Wu YC, Lu MS, Yeh CH, *et al.* Justifying video-assisted thoracic surgery for spontaneous hemopneumothorax. *Chest* 2002; **122**: 1844–7.
◆153. Hsu NY, Shih CS, Hsu CP, Chen PR. Spontaneous hemopneumothorax revisited: clinical approach and systemic review of the literature. *Ann Thorac Surg* 2005; **80**: 1859–63.

154. Askin FB, McCann BG. Reactive eosinophilic pleuritis. *Arch Pathol Lab Med* 1977; **101**: 187–91.
155. De Smedt A, Vanderlinden E, Demanet C, *et al.* Characterisation of pleural inflammation occurring after primary spontaneous pneumothorax. *Eur Respir J* 2004; **23**: 896–900.
156. Noppen M. Normal volume and cellular contents of pleural fluid. *Paediatr Respir Rev* 2004; **5**: (Suppl A):S201–3.
●157. Vincent M, Celard P, Pinet F, *et al.* Radiology of spontaneous pneumothorax in young patients: a study of 200 cases [French]. *Sem Hop* 1984; **60**: 759–65.
158. Aitchison F, Bleetman A, Munro P, McCarter D, Reid AW. Detection of pneumothorax by accident and emergency officers and radiologists on single chest films. *Arch Emerg Med* 1993; **10**: 343–6.
159. Bulynin VI, Red'kin AN, Solod NV. Prehospital diagnostic errors and therapeutic policy in spontaneous pneumothorax [Russian]. *Klin Med* 1997; **75**: 41–3.
●160. Scadding JG, Wood P. Systolic clicks due to left-sided pneumothorax. *Lancet* 1939; **ii**: 1208–11.
161. Semple T, Lancaster WM. Noisy pneumothorax: observations based on 24 cases. *Br Med J* 1961; **2**: 1342–6.
162. Hamman L. Spontaneous mediastinal emphysema. *Bull John Hopkins Hosp* 1939; **64**: 1–21.
163. Aisner M, Franco J. Mediastinal emphysema. *New Engl J Med* 1949; **241**: 818–25.
164. Freixinet J, Garcia F, Rodriguez PM, *et al.* Spontaneous pneumomediastinum: long-term follow-up. *Respir Med* 2005; **99**: 1160–3.
165. Koullias GJ, Korkolis DP, Wang XJ, Hammond GL. Current assessment and management of spontaneous pneumomediastinum: experience in 24 adult patients. *Eur J Cardiothorac Surg* 2004; **25**: 852–5.
166. Henry M, Arnold T, Harvey J. BTS guidelines for the management of spontaneous pneumothorax. *Thorax* 2003; **58** (Suppl 2): 39S–52S.
167. Bradley M, Williams C, Walshaw MJ. The value of routine expiratory films in the diagnosis of pneumothorax. *Arch Emerg Med* 1991; **8**: 115–16.
168. Schramel FM, Wagenaar M, Sutedja TG, Golding RP, Postmus PE. Diagnosis of pneumothorax not improved by additional roentgen pictures of the thorax in the expiration phase [Dutch]. *Ned Tijdschr Geneeskd* 1995; **139**: 131–3.
169. Eisen LA, Berger JS, Hegde A, Schneider RF. Competency in chest radiography: a comparison of medical students, residents, and fellows. *J Gen Intern Med* 2006; **21**: 460–5.
170. Waitches GM, Stern EJ, Dubinsky TJ. Usefulness of the double-wall sign in detecting pneumothorax in patients with giant bullous emphysema. *Am J Roentgenol* 2000; **174**: 1765–8.
171. Bourgouin P, Cousineau G, Lemire P, Hebert G. Computed tomography used to exclude pneumothorax in bullous lung disease. *J Can Assoc Radiol* 1985; **36**: 341–2.
172. Glazer HS, Anderson DJ, Wilson BS, Molina PL, Sagel SS. Pneumothorax: appearance on lateral chest radiographs. *Radiology* 1989; **173**: 707–11.
173. Axel L. A simple way to estimate the size of a pneumothorax. *Invest Radiol* 1981; **16**: 165–6.
174. Rhea J, de Luca S, Greene R. Determining the size of pneumothorax in the upright patient. *Radiology* 1985; **144**: 733–6.
175. Collins CD, Lopez A, Mathie A, *et al.* Quantification of pneumothorax size on chest radiographs using interpleural distances: regression analysis based on volume measurements from helical CT. *Am J Roentgenol* 1995; **165**: 1127–30.
176. Light RW. Pneumothorax. In: Light RW (ed). *Pleural diseases*, 3rd edn. Baltimore: Williams & Wilkins, 1995: 242–77.
177. Choi BG, Park SH, Yun EH, Chae KO, Shinn KS. Pneumothorax size: correlation of supine anteroposterior with erect posteroanterior chest radiographs. *Radiology* 1998; **209**: 567–9.
178. Noppen M, Alexander P, Driesen P, Slabbynck H, Verstraete A. Quantification of the size of primary spontaneous pneumothorax: accuracy of the Light index. *Respiration* 2001; **68**: 396–9.
179. Engdahl O, Toft T, Boe J. Chest radiograph – a poor method for determining the size of a pneumothorax. *Chest* 1993; **103**: 26–9.
180. Nissen H. Spontaneous pneumothorax: a clinical and histological study of aetiological factors, pathogenesis and management [Danish]. Copenhagen (Thesis); 1969.
181. Clark S, Ragg M, Stella J. Is mediastinal shift on chest X-ray of pneumothorax always an emergency? *Emerg Med* 2003; **15**: 429–33.
182. Kupferschmid JP, Carr T, Fonger JD, Aldea GS, Vosburgh E. Chronic tension pneumothorax mimicking tension bullae: use of video-assisted thoracoscopy for diagnosis. *Chest* 1993; **104**: 1913–14.
183. Teplick SK, Clark RE. Various faces of tension pneumothorax. *Postgrad Med* 1974; **56**: 87–92.
◆184. Gilbert TB, McGrath BJ. Tension pneumothorax: aetiology, diagnosis, pathophysiology, and management. *J Intensive Care Med* 1994; **9**: 139–50.
185. Holloway VJ, Harris JK. Spontaneous pneumothorax: is it under tension? *J Accid Emerg Med* 2000; **17**: 222–3.
186. Chan SS. Current opinions and practices in the treatment of spontaneous pneumothorax. *J Accid Emerg Med* 2000; **17**: 165–9.
187. Janssen JP, Cuesta MA, Postmus PE. Treatment of spontaneous pneumothorax: survey among Dutch pneumonologists [Dutch]. *Ned Tijdschr Geneeskd* 1994; **138**: 661–4.
188. Baumann MH, Strange C. The clinician's perspective on pneumothorax management. *Chest* 1997; **112**: 822–8.
189. Sutherland M, Burdon J, Hart D. Primary spontaneous pneumothorax: treatment practices in Australia. *Respirology* 2000; **5**: 277–80.
*190. Baumann MH, Strange C, Heffner JE, *et al.* Management of spontaneous pneumothorax: an American College of Chest Physicians Delphi Consensus Statement. *Chest* 2001; **119**: 590–602.
191. Light RW. Disorders of the pleura. In: Fauci AS, Braunwald E, Isselbacher KJ, *et al.* (eds). *Harrison's principles of internal medicine*, 14th edn. New York: McGraw Hill, 1998: 1472–5.
192. Crofton J, Douglas A. *Respiratory diseases*, 1st edn. Oxford: Blackwell Scientific Publications, 1969.
193. Coope R. *Diseases of the chest.* Edinburgh: Livingstone, 1944.
194. Crofton J, Douglas A. *Respiratory diseases.* 3rd ed. Oxford: Blackwell Scientific Publications; 1981.
195. Rubin EH, Rubin M. *Thoracic disease.* Philadelphia: Saunders, 1961.
196. Cumming G, Semple SJ. *Disorders of the respiratory system.* Oxford: Blackwell Scientific Publications, 1973.
197. Jones JS. A place for aspiration in the treatment of spontaneous pneumothorax. *Thorax* 1985; **40**: 66–7.
198. Green RA. Pneumothorax. In: Baum GL (ed.). *Textbook of pulmonary diseases.* London: Churchill, 1965: 694–5.
199. Mercier C, Page A, Verdant A, *et al.* Outpatient management of intercostal tube drainage in spontaneous pneumothorax. *Ann Thorac Surg* 1976; **22**: 163–5.
200. Conces DJ, Tarver RD, Gray WC, Pearcy EA. Treatment of pneumothoraces utilizing small caliber chest tubes. *Chest* 1988; **94**: 55–7.
201. Raja OG, Lalor AJ. Simple aspiration of spontaneous pneumothorax. *Br J Dis Chest* 1981; **75**: 207–8.
202. Flint K, Hillawi AH, Johnson AM. Conservative management of spontaneous pneumothorax. *Lancet* 1984; **i**: 687–8.
203. Archer GJ, Hamilton AA, Upadhyay R, Finlay M, Grace PM. Results of simple aspiration of pneumothoraces. *Br J Dis Chest* 1985; **79**: 177–82.
204. Harvey JE, Prescott RJ. Simple aspiration versus intercostal tube drainage for spontaneous pneumothorax in patients with normal lungs. *Br Med J* 1994; **309**: 1338–9.
205. Skoda J. Pneumothorax [German]. *Allgem Wiener Med Zeitung* 1857: 113.

206. Rodet N. Experimental research in pneumothorax [French]. *Congres Franc Med* 1895: 894.
207. Hill RC, DeCarlo DP, Jr., Hill JF, *et al.* Resolution of experimental pneumothorax in rabbits by oxygen therapy. *Ann Thorac Surg* 1995; **59**: 825–7; discussion 7–8.
208. England GJ, Hill RC, Timberlake GA, *et al.* Resolution of experimental pneumothorax in rabbits by graded oxygen therapy. *J Trauma* 1998; **45**: 333–4.
209. Northfield TC. Oxygen therapy for spontaenous pneumothorax. *Br Med J* 1971; **4**: 86–8.
210. Chadha TS, Cohn MA. Noninvasive treatment of pneumothorax with oxygen inhalation. *Respiration* 1983; **44**: 147–52.
●211. Kircher LT, Swartzel RL. Spontaneous pneumothorax and its treatment. *J Am Med Assoc* 1954; **153**: 24–9.
212. Kelly AM, Loy J, Tsang AY, Graham CA. Estimating the rate of re-expansion of spontaneous pneumothorax by a formula derived from computed tomography volumetry studies. *Emerg Med J* 2006; **23**: 780–2.
213. Baumann MH, Strange C. Treatment of spontaneous pneumothorax: a more aggressive approach? *Chest* 1997; **112**: 789–804.
214. O'Rourke JP, Yee ES. Civilian spontaneous pneumothorax: treatment options and long-term results. *Chest* 1989; **96**: 1302–6.
215. Peatfield RC, Edwards PR, Johnson NM. Two unexpected deaths from pneumothorax. *Lancet* 1979; i: 356–8.
216. Noppen M, Alexander P, Driesen P, Slabbynck H, Verstraeten A. Manual aspiration versus chest tube drainage in first episodes of primary spontaneous pneumothorax: a multicenter, prospective, randomized pilot study. *Am J Respir Crit Care Med* 2002; **165**: 1240–4.
217. Ayed AK, Chandrasekaran C, Sukumar M. Aspiration versus tube drainage in primary spontaneous pneumothorax: a randomised study. *Eur Respir J* 2006; **27**: 477–82.
218. Andrivet P, Djedaini K, Teboul JL, Brochard L, Dreyfuss D. Spontaneous pneumothorax: comparison of thoracic drainage vs immediate or delayed needle aspiration. *Chest* 1995; **108**: 335–9.
219. Miller AC. Spontaneous pneumothorax. In: Light RW, Lee YCG. (eds). *Textbook of pleural diseases*, 1st edn. London: Arnold, 2003: 445–63.
220. Camuset J, Laganier J, Brugiere O, *et al.* Needle aspiration as first-line management of primary spontaneous pneumothorax. *Presse Med* 2006; **35**: 765–8.
221. Vedam H, Barnes DJ. Comparison of large- and small-bore intercostal catheters in the management of spontaneous pneumothorax. *Intern Med J* 2003; **33**: 495–9.
222. Tsai WK, Chen W, Lee JC, *et al.* Pigtail catheters vs large-bore chest tubes for management of secondary spontaneous pneumothoraces in adults. *Am J Emerg Med* 2006; **24**: 795–800.
223. Knottenbelt JD, van der Spuy JW. Traumatic pneumothorax: a scheme for rapid patient turnover. *Injury* 1990; **21**: 77–80.
224. Burgaud JC, Offenstadt G, Bencharif G, Hericord P, Amstutz P. Spontaneous pneumothorax: drainage by catheter or drain? *Rev Pneumol Clin* 1985; **41**: 317–19.
225. Lee P, Chee CB, Wang YT. Questionnaire survey on management of spontaneous pneumothorax. *Singapore Med J* 2000; **41**: 538–41.
226. Courtney PA, McKane WR. Audit of the management of spontaneous pneumothorax. *Ulster Med J* 1998; **67**: 41–3.
227. Baldt MM, Bankier AA, Germann PS, *et al.* Complications after emergency tube thoracostomy: assessment with CT. *Radiology* 1995; **195**: 539–43.
228. Griffiths JR, Roberts N. Do junior doctors know where to insert chest drains safely? *Postgrad Med J* 2005; **81**: 456–8.
229. Burge TS. Complications of prophylactic intercostal tube drainage – including tension pneumothorax. *J R Army Med Corps* 1992; **138**: 138–9.
230. Landay M, Oliver Q, Estrera A, *et al.* Lung penetration by thoracostomy tubes: imaging findings on CT. *J Thorac Imaging* 2006; **21**: 197–204.
231. Ng AW, Chan KW, Lee SK. Simple aspiration of pneumothorax. *Singapore Med J* 1994; **35**: 50–2.
232. Mark JBD, p344 in Gobbel WG. Spontaneous pneumothorax. *J Thorac Cardiovasc Surg* 1963; **46**: 331–45.
233. Light RW. Management of spontaneous pneumothorax. *Am Rev Respir Dis* 1993; **148**: 245–8.
234. Britten S, Palmer SH, Snow TM. Needle thoracocentesis in tension pneumothorax: insufficient cannula length and potential failure. *Injury* 1996; **27**: 321–2.
235. Rawlins R, Brown KM, Carr CS, Cameron CR. Life threatening haemorrhage after anterior needle aspiration of pneumothoraces. A role for lateral needle aspiration in emergency decompression of spontaneous pneumothorax. *Emerg Med J* 2003; **20**: 383–4.
236. Kiely DG, Ansari S, Davey WA, *et al.* Bedside tracer gas technique accurately predicts outcome in aspiration of spontaneous pneumothorax. *Thorax* 2001; **56**: 617–21.
237. So SY, Yu DY. Catheter drainage of spontaneous pneumothorax: suction or no suction, early or late removal? *Thorax* 1982; **37**: 46–8.
238. Horsley A, Jones L, White J, Henry M. Efficacy and complications of small-bore, wire-guided chest drains. *Chest* 2006; **130**: 1857–63.
239. Choi SH, Lee SW, Hong YS, *et al.* Can spontaneous pneumothorax patients be treated by ambulatory care management? *Eur J Cardiothorac Surg* 2007; **8**: 8.
240. Waller DA, Edwards JG, Rajesh PB. A physiological comparison of flutter valve drainage bags and underwater seal systems for postoperative air leaks. *Thorax* 1999; **54**: 442–3.
241. Mainini SE, Johnson FE. Tension pneumothorax complicating small-caliber chest tube insertion. *Chest* 1990; **97**: 759–60.
242. Samelson SL, Goldberg EM, Ferguson MK. The thoracic vent: clinical experience with a new device for treating simple pneumothorax. *Chest* 1991; **100**: 880–2.
243. Martin T, Fontana G, Olak J, Ferguson M. Use of pleural catheter for the management of simple pneumothorax. *Chest* 1996; **110**: 1169–72.
244. Roggla M, Wagner A, Brunner C, Roggla G. The management of pneumothorax with the thoracic vent versus conventional intercostal tube drainage. *Wien Klin Wochenschr* 1996; **108**: 330–3.
245. Dernevik L, Roberts D. Mini-drainage in pneumothorax is expensive, but still beneficial [Swedish]. *Lakartidningen* 2000; **97**: 3726–8.
246. Holman CW, Muschenheim C. *Bronchopulmonary diseases and related disorders.* Baltimore: Harper & Row, 1972.
247. Rozenman J, Yellin A, Simansky DA, Shiner RJ. Re-expansion pulmonary oedema following spontaneous pneumothorax. *Respir Med* 1996; **90**: 235–8.
248. Mahfood S, Hix WR, Aaron BL. Re-expansion pulmonary edema. *Ann Thorac Surg* 1988; **45**: 340–4.
249. Matsuura Y, Nomimura T, Nurikami H. Clinical analysis of re-expansion pulmonary edema. *Chest* 1991; **100**: 1562–6.
250. Miller WC, Toon R, Palat H, Lacroix J. Experimental pulmonary edema following re-expansion of pneumothorax. *Am Rev Respir Dis* 1973; **108**: 664–6.
251. Sharma TN, Agnihotri SP, Jain NK, Madan A, Deopura G. Intercostal tube thoracostomy in pneumothorax: factors influencing re-expansion of lung. *Indian J Chest Dis Allied Sci* 1988; **30**: 32–5.
252. Reed MF, Lyons JM, Luchette FA, Neu JA, Howington JA. Preliminary report of a prospective, randomized trial of underwater seal for spontaneous and iatrogenic pneumothorax. *J Am Coll Surg* 2007; **204**: 84–90.
253. Marshall M, Deeb M, Bleier J, *et al.* Suction vs water seal after pulmonary resection. *Chest* 2002; **121**: 831–5.
254. Ayed AK. Suction versus water seal after thoracoscopy for primary spontaneous pneumothorax: prospective randomized study. *Ann Thorac Surg* 2003; **75**: 1593–6.

255. Bell RL, Ovadia P, Abdullah F, Spector S, Rabinovici R. Chest tube removal: end-inspiration or end-expiration? *J Trauma Injury Infect Crit Care* 2001; **50**: 674–7.
256. Tanaka F, Ezaki H, Isobe J, *et al.* Four cases of spontaneous pneumothorax with no reexpansion of collapsed lung despite chest tube drainage [Japanese]. *Jpn J Thorac Surg* 1992; **45**: 515–18.
257. Kakaris S, Athanassiadi K, Vassilikos K, Skottis I. Spontaneous hemopneumothorax: a rare but life-threatening entity. *Eur J Cardiothorac Surg* 2004; **25**: 856–8.
258. Fackeldey V, Franke A, Schachtrupp A, Becker HP, Schwab R. Physical fitness after apical resection for the treatment of primary spontaneous pneumothorax. *Mil Med* 2005; **9**: 760–3.
259. Cardillo G, Carleo F, Carbone L, *et al.* Long-term lung function following videothoracoscopic talc poudrage for primary spontaneous recurrent pneumothorax. *Eur J Cardiothorac Surg* 2007; **28**: 28.
260. Passlick B, Born C, Sienel W, Thetter O. Incidence of chronic pain after minimal-invasive surgery for spontaneous pneumothorax. *Eur J Cardiothor Surg* 2001; **19**: 355–8.
261. Ben-Nun A, Soudack M, Best LA. Video-assisted thoracoscopic surgery for recurrent spontaneous pneumothorax: the long-term benefit. *World J Surg* 2006; **30**: 285–90.
262. Schramel FM, Sutedja TG, Braber JC, van Mourik JC, Postmus PE. Cost-effectiveness of video-assisted thoracoscopic surgery versus conservative treatment for first time or recurrent spontaneous pneumothorax. *Eur Respir J* 1996; **9**: 1821–5.
263. Abdala OA, Levy RR, Bibiloni RH, *et al.* Advantages of video assisted thoracic surgery in the treatment of spontaneous pneumothorax. *Medicina* 2001; **61**: 157–60.
264. Torresini G, Vaccarili M, Divisi D, Crisci R. Is video-assisted thoracic surgery justified at first spontaneous pneumothorax? *Eur J Cardiothorac Surg* 2001; **20**: 42–5.
265. Sawada S, Watanabe Y, Moriyama S. Video-assisted thoracoscopic surgery for primary spontaneous pneumothorax: evaluation of indications and long-term outcome compared with conservative treatment and open thoracotomy. *Chest* 2005; **127**: 2226–30.
266. Iablonskii PK, Atiukov MA, Pishchik VG, El'kina EA. Diagnostic and treatment strategy for patients with the first episode of primary spontaneous pneumothorax [Russian]. *Vestn Khir Im I I Grek* 2005; **164**: 11–14.
267. Herrejon A, Inchaurraga I, Vivas C, Custardoy J, Marin J. Initial pleural pressure measurement in spontaneous pneumothorax. *Lung* 2000; **178**: 309–16.
268. Mathur R, Cullen J, Kinnear WJ, Johnston ID. Time course of resolution of persistent air leak in spontaneous pneumothorax. *Respir Med* 1995; **89**: 129–32.
269. Chee CB, Abisheganaden J, Yeo JK, *et al.* Persistent air-leak in spontaneous pneumothorax: clinical course and outcome. *Respir Med* 1998; **92**: 757–61.
270. Curtis HJ, Bourke SJ, Dark JH, Corris PA. Lung transplantation outcome in cystic fibrosis patients with previous pneumothorax. *J Heart Lung Transplant* 2005; **24**: 865–9.
271. Noyes BE, Orenstein DM. Treatment of pneumothorax in cystic fibrosis in the era of lung transplantation. *Chest* 1992; **101**: 1187–8.
272. Edenborough FP, Hussain I, Stableforth DE. Use of a Heimlich flutter valve for pneumothorax in cystic fibrosis. *Thorax* 1994; **49**: 1178–9.
273. Spector ML, Stern RC. Pneumothorax in cystic fibrosis: a 26-year experience. *Ann Thorac Surg* 1989; **47**: 204–7.
274. Flume PA, Strange C, Ye X, *et al.* Pneumothorax in cystic fibrosis. *Chest* 2005; **128**: 720–8.
275. Vricella LA, Trachiotis GD. Heimlich valve in the management of pneumothorax in patients with advanced AIDS. *Chest* 2001; **120**: 15–18.
●276. Ong YE, Sheth A, Simmonds NJ, *et al.* Radiotherapy: a novel treatment for pneumothorax. *Eur Respir J* 2006; **27**: 427–9.
277. Tripp HF, Thomas LP, Obney JA. Current therapy of catamenial pneumothorax. *Heart Surg Forum* 1998; **1**: 146–9.
278. Marshall MB, Ahmed Z, Kucharczuk JC, Kaiser LR, Shrager JB. Catamenial pneumothorax: optimal hormonal and surgical management. *Eur J Cardiothorac Surg* 2005; **27**: 662–6.
279. Alfageme I, Moreno L, Huertas C, *et al.* Spontaneous pneumothorax: long-term results with tetracycline pleurodesis. *Chest* 1994; **106**: 347–50.
◆280. Schramel FM, Postmus PE, Vanderschueren RG. Current aspects of spontaneous pneumothorax. *Eur Respir J* 1997; **10**: 1372–9.
281. Lippert HL, Lund O, Blegvad S, Larsen HV. Independent risk factors for cumulative recurrence rate after first spontaneous pneumothorax. *Eur Respir J* 1991; **4**: 324–31.
282. Videm V, Pillgram-Larsen J, Ellingsen O, Andersen G, Ovrum E. Spontaneous pneumothorax in chronic obstructive pulmonary disease: complications, treatment and recurrences. *Eur J Respir Dis* 1987; **71**: 365–71.
283. Sadikot RT, Greene T, Meadows K, Arnold AG. Recurrence of primary spontaneous pneumothorax. *Thorax* 1997; **52**: 805–9.
284. Sihoe ADL, Yim APC, Lee TW, *et al.* Can CT scanning be used to select patients with unilateral primary spontaneous pneumothorax for bilateral surgery? *Chest* 2000; **118**: 380–3.
285. Haid MM, Paladini P, Maccherini M, *et al.* Air transport and the fate of pneumothorax in pleural adhesions. *Thorax* 1992; **47**: 833–4.

43

Non-spontaneous pneumothorax

MICHAEL H BAUMANN

INTRODUCTION

Pneumothorax references continue to subdivide pneumothorax into spontaneous and traumatic.[1–3] The preceding chapter (Chapter 42) dealt with spontaneous pneumothoraces. Spontaneous pneumothoraces occur without preceding trauma or obvious underlying precipitating cause and are classified as primary (no clear underlying lung disease) and secondary (an underlying causal lung disease present). This chapter will focus upon traumatic and tension pneumothoraces. Traumatic pneumothoraces occur as a result of direct or indirect trauma and can be subdivided into non-iatrogenic and iatrogenic. Non-iatrogenic pneumothoraces occur as a result of direct or indirect trauma, generally to the chest, unrelated to any medical procedure. Traumatic pneumothoraces resulting from medical interventions are termed iatrogenic pneumothoraces. Tension pneumothorax may occur with any of the aforementioned categories of pneumothorax.

NON-IATROGENIC TRAUMATIC PNEUMOTHORAX

Incidence and epidemiology

Trauma related deaths exceed 50 000 per year in the USA. Chest trauma is causal in 25 percent of these deaths and plays a significant role in an additional 50 percent. Pneumothorax ranks second to rib fractures as the most common manifestation of chest injury and may be noted in 40–50 percent of patients with chest trauma.[4–6] Traumatic pneumothorax may also present after blunt trauma to the abdomen.[4,6] At least 20 percent of traumatic pneumothoraces have an accompanying hemothorax.[7]

Classification

Traumatic pneumothoraces may be classified by mechanism of injury into penetrating and non-penetrating (blunt).[2] The object penetrating the chest disrupts the visceral pleural surface prompting pleural air entry or allows air entry through the breached chest wall. The etiology of pneumothorax arising from blunt chest trauma is less immediately apparent in the absence of a rib fracture lacerating the visceral pleura. Blunt chest trauma may prompt abrupt alveolar pressure elevations causing alveolar rupture. Air may then dissect into the lung interstitium and then to the visceral pleural or the mediastinal pleural surface. Rupture of either the visceral or mediastinal pleura may then cause a pneumothorax.

Clinical presentation

Up to 6 percent of traumatic pneumothoraces present with tension.[8] Alternatively, a substantial number of traumatic pneumothoraces may be occult, not seen on an initial chest radiograph but found by additional imaging. The proportion of trauma-related pneumothoraces that are occult compared with those seen on chest radiography ranges from 29 to 72 percent,[9,10] emphasizing the need for a high index of suspicion and incorporating early routine computed tomography (CT) in all chest and multi-trauma patients.[7] Subcutaneous emphysema, pulmonary contusion, and rib fracture(s) are independent predictors of an occult pneumothorax (Table 43.1).[10] CT imaging detects other abnormalities in addition to pneumothorax, including lung contusion, diaphragmatic rupture and hemothorax leading to an alteration in patient care in up to 41 percent of cases.[7] Pneumothorax detection is critical given concerns for progression, particularly if the patient is

Table 43.1 Independent predictors of occult traumatic pneumothorax[10]

Predictor	Sensitivity (%)	Specificity (%)	PPV (%)	NPV (%)	Odds ratio	*p*-value
Subcutaneous emphysema	16	98	57	86	5.47	0.005
Pulmonary contusion	45	81	32	88	3.25	0.001
Rib fracture(s)	59	73	30	90	2.65	0.005

PPV = positive predictive value; NPV = negative predictive value.

mechanically ventilated or anesthesia becomes necessary.[5,6,9,10] Consideration and evaluation for disruption of major airways should be considered in the traumatic pneumothorax patient, often with a persistent air leak, where their condition deteriorates out of proportion to the findings on the chest radiograph or physical examination.[11,12]

Treatment and management

Generally, traumatic pneumothoraces have been treated with placement of a chest tube.[5,13] This approach remains the subject of debate and scrutiny in the setting of both non-occult and occult traumatic pneumothoraces.[5,8–10,13,14]

NON-OCCULT TRAUMATIC PNEUMOTHORACES

Conservative management, i.e. observation without chest tube placement, has been reported in selected patients sustaining non-occult traumatic pneumothoraces with a failure rate of 7 to 9 percent.[8,13] Johnson[13] retrospectively reported 29 patients with minimal, small or moderate sized traumatic pneumothoraces managed without drainage; two patients (6.9 percent) required chest tube drainage due to asymptomatic radiographic pneumothorax enlargement. Johnson emphasized that drainage is mandatory when positive pressure ventilation is required or the patient sustains respiratory compromise from lung collapse.[13] Knottenbelt and van der Spuy[8] prospectively limited chest tube placement in 804 traumatic pneumothorax patients ($n = 645$, penetrating knife wounds) to the following: those with a significant pneumothorax by chest radiograph (>1.5 cm lung collapse, arbitrarily selected); smaller pneumothoraces if bilateral; patients requiring mechanical ventilation; and if the patient's respiratory reserve was limited for any reason. Forty-one percent ($n = 329$) of patients met criteria for conservative management; 29 of these 329 patients (8.8 percent) treated conservatively required chest tube placement for an enlarging pneumothorax.[8] Only four of the 804 patients suffered a gunshot wound and all patients were observed in hospital.

OCCULT TRAUMATIC PNEUMOTHORACES

Occult pneumothoraces may also be successfully treated conservatively, arguably, even in the setting of positive-pressure mechanical ventilation. However, the risk of failure with a conservative approach appears significant. Bridges and colleagues[6] noted that of 25 patients with occult traumatic pneumothoraces treated conservatively (none intubated), five (20 percent) required chest tube placement due to respiratory distress, hemodynamic instability or pneumothorax progression. Further, in this retrospective study, all occult pneumothorax patients requiring intubation (an additional 10 patients) were, by preference, treated with a chest tube.[6] Enderson and colleagues'[5] prospective study of 40 trauma patients sustaining occult pneumothorax randomized to chest tube placement ($n = 19$) or observation ($n = 21$) noted that 8 of the 21 (38 percent) patients conservatively managed had pneumothorax progression with mechanical ventilation with three of the eight (38 percent) developing a tension pneumothorax. The authors conclude that patients with traumatic occult pneumothoraces requiring positive-pressure ventilation should have a chest tube placed.

By contrast, a retrospective study of occult pneumothorax promotes the safety of withholding immediate chest tube placement in 13 of 26 patients treated conservatively.[14] Six of these conservatively managed patients received intubation and positive-pressure ventilation with one (17 percent) requiring chest tube placement. An additional patient initially receiving immediate chest tube placement removed his chest tube during mechanical ventilation and required emergent replacement due to recurrent pneumothorax. Despite a nearly 20 percent complication rate in pneumothorax patients without chest tubes on mechanical ventilation, the authors conclude that their data do not support the use of prophylactic chest tube placement before mechanical ventilation in patients with occult traumatic pneumothoraces.[14]

Brasel and colleagues[15] also provide evidence regarding conservative management of CT diagnosed occult pneumothoraces even during mechanical ventilation. The authors note no difference in complication rates in 39 patients with 44 pneumothoraces prospectively randomized to chest tube placement ($n = 18$) versus observation ($n = 21$). Nine patients in each group were mechanically ventilated. Interestingly, the four patients in the chest tube group having pneumothorax progression (three on mechanical ventilation) were not on pleural suction and had suction reinstituted as therapy for pneumothorax progression. Lack of suction may account for the reported pneumothorax progression. Three of the observation group had pneumothorax progression, including two on mechanical ventilation. If the three patients in the chest tube group on mechanical ventilation had been maintained on suction and had no pneumothorax progression, the authors' reported lack of difference in complication rates between the two groups would disappear. Hence, this study does not provide definitive evidence for superiority of conservative management of occult traumatic pneumothoraces, particularly in the presence of mechanical ventilation.

Ball and colleagues[10] provide the largest prospective study of occult traumatic pneumothoraces revealing a preference for chest tube placement in occult pneumothorax patients that are mechanically ventilated. Paired chest radiographs and CT scans were available in 338 of 761 trauma patients (44 percent) (98.5 percent blunt trauma). One-hundred and three pneumothoraces were present in 89 patients and 57 (55 percent) of these pneumothoraces were occult. Independent risk factors for occult pneumothorax were identified (see above, Table 43.1). In this single institution study, no specific protocol was in place prompting chest tube placement. Twenty-three of 49 patients (47 percent) with an occult pneumothorax received a chest tube (28 French in 33 percent and 32 French in 57 percent, $p = 0.02$). Occult pneumothoraces were found to be treated differently if the patients required mechanical ventilation. In the occult pneumothorax non-ventilated patient subgroup, 10 of 32 (31 percent) received a chest tube compared with 13 of 17 (76 percent) of the subgroup being mechanically ventilated ($p = 0.03$). No differences in complications rate were noted between the ventilated and non-ventilated chest tube groups. Of four of 17 (24 percent) ventilated patients and of 22 of 32 (69 percent) nonventilated patients who were observed without chest tube insertion, two (8 percent) later required tube placement due to pneumothorax progression (one patient each in the ventilated and nonventilated group).

Classification of the size of CT classification of size may be useful in determining the need for chest tube placement. A prospective utilization of CT classification of 44 traumatic pneumothoraces (36 patients), by size from minuscule to limited anterior to anterolateral (smallest to largest), touts the safety of close inpatient observation in the first two groups.[4] Eighty-nine percent, or 24 of 27 patients in the minuscule and anterior pneumothorax size groups, did not require tube thoracostomy. Chest tubes were placed in all anterolateral pneumothoraces based on the preference of the institution's surgeons and chest tubes were preferentially placed in all anterior pneumothoraces receiving mechanical ventilation.[4] A similar but retrospective study incorporating CT size classification of occult traumatic pneumothoraces suggests that small occult pneumothoraces may be managed by observation even in the presence of positive-pressure ventilation. Larger pneumothoraces and those associated with two rib fractures may require early chest tube placement.[16]

Assimilating this information, chest tube placement in patients with traumatic pneumothoraces seems a reasonable approach in many but not all patients (Figure 43.1). Such tubes may serve to treat not only the pneumothorax but also the accompanying hemothorax found in 20 percent of cases.[7] After initial chest radiographic and CT assessment of the chest, if the patient has a large pneumothorax (arbitrarily, greater than 1.5 cm collapse of the lung from the parietal pleura seen by chest radiograph), hemodynamic or respiratory instability, or the presence of an accompanying hemothorax, a large-bore chest tube (28–32 F) should be strongly considered. If only a chest radiograph is available, the presence of subcutaneous emphysema, pulmonary contusion or rib fracture(s) should prompt consideration of an occult pneumothorax (Table 43.1). A large-bore tube is suggested to effectively drain any potential blood or large air leak. If the pneumothorax is small (less than 1.5 cm collapse by chest radiograph) or occult by CT (minuscule or anterior) and the patient is hemodynamically and respiratory stable, very close in-hospital observation with a series of chest

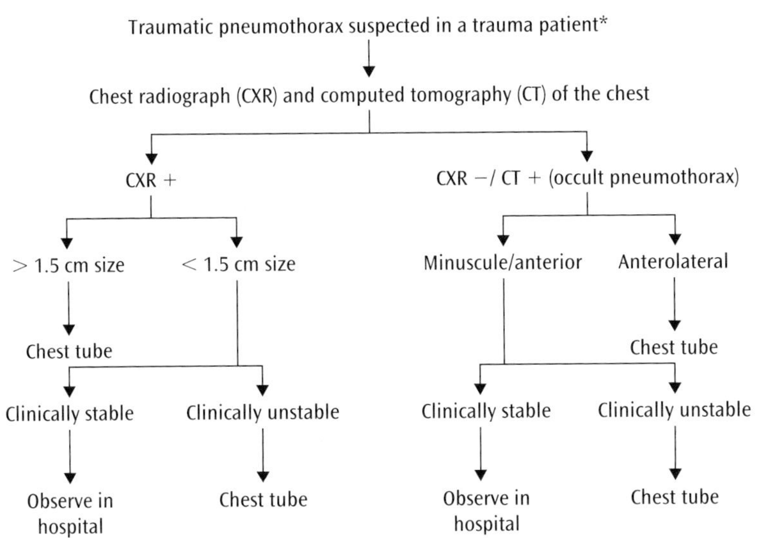

Figure 43.1 Management algorithm for suspected traumatic pneumothorax. *See text for details; +, positive; −, negative. Any patient requiring intubation and mechanical ventilation should prompt strong consideration for chest tube placement.

radiographs may be pursued. However, if observation is used, significant confidence in those providing the monitoring is necessary. If any patient with an occult or non-occult traumatic pneumothorax requires intubation and mechanical ventilation, prophylactic chest tube placement is likely prudent given an up to 38 percent likelihood of pneumothorax progression.

Persistent air leaks and surgical management

Air leaks accompanying a traumatic pneumothorax stop within 12 hours in approximately 80 percent of patients having a chest tube placed. Of 504 traumatic pneumothoraces receiving chest tube drainage, one patient required urgent thoracotomy for massive air leak, six underwent thoracotomy for persistent air leak while in hospital and another two patients required readmission and thoracotomy due to recurrent pneumothorax (9 of 504, 1.8 percent).[8] Twenty of 379 patients (5.3 percent) suffering traumatic chest injury required chest tube replacement after tube removal due to pneumothorax recurrence in Etoch and colleagues retrospective review.[17] Helling and colleagues[18] retrospectively report traumatic pneumothorax recurrence after chest tube removal requiring tube replacement in 10 of 216 patients (4.6 percent). Using only the appearance of a recurrent pneumothorax after chest tube removal as a marker of persistent air leak, persistent air leak occurrence appeared higher in the preceding two studies, 33 of 379 (8.7 percent) and 51 of 216 (23.6 percent) patients, respectively.[17,18] The necessity of replacing a chest tube after its initial removal is more likely a reflection of a persistent air leak as opposed to entry of air into the pleural space upon removal of the tube. In the latter situation drainage is not indicated.

The type and timing of surgical intervention for a persistent air leak in traumatic pneumothorax are not absolutely established. Carrillo and colleagues[12] demonstrated the success of early video-assisted thoracoscopic surgery (VATS). Eleven traumatic pneumothorax patients with failure of lung re-expansion from an associated air leak and failure of radiographic pneumothorax resolution, within 72 hours, prospectively underwent bronchoscopic assessment for associated tracheobronchial injury and therapeutic VATS. Findings at operation contributing to persistent pneumothorax included retained hemothorax and lacerated lung ($n = 5$), lung herniation ($n = 2$), ruptured congenital blebs ($n = 2$), cavitation injury ($n = 1$) and unknown ($n = 1$). The authors conclude, based on presumed cost savings, reduced complications, improved patient comfort and reduced hospital time, that early VATS should be the treatment of choice for traumatic pneumothoraces with a persistent air leak (>72 hours). More recently, Divisi and colleagues[19] similarly advocate early VATS as an alternative to chest tube placement in stable trauma patients, especially in the setting of hemothorax and hemopneumothorax.

Follow-up issues

The most common findings upon prospective outpatient follow-up of 530 traumatic pneumothorax patients in descending order of frequency are chest pain ($n = 70$, 13.2 percent), residual air ($n = 56$, 10.6 percent), pyrexia (≥ 38°C, $n = 54$, 10.2 percent), and atelectasis ($n = 25$, 4.7 percent). All other findings were ≤ 2.5 percent. Notably, on discharge, 119 patients receiving chest tubes had minor residual air not requiring drainage after chest tube removal. Ten of the 56 patients seen during outpatient follow-up demonstrated air requiring drainage, with two requiring thoracostomy.[8] In contrast, a retrospective review builds the case for not obtaining follow-up chest radiographs in selected patients during outpatient reassessment. One-hundred and fifty-five hospitalized trauma patients requiring chest tube placement for traumatic pneumothorax ($n = 79$, 51 percent), hemothorax ($n = 28$, 18 percent) or hemopneumothorax ($n = 34$, 22 percent) were reviewed. Of the 61 patients seen in outpatient follow-up with an accompanying chest radiograph, 92 percent ($n = 56$) were found to have no pneumothorax, 5 percent ($n = 3$) a small pneumothorax and 3 percent ($n = 2$) a resolving pneumothorax.[20] The authors conclude that a chest radiograph is not necessary in the asymptomatic trauma patient during follow-up if the pre-discharge chest radiograph is negative for pneumothorax or hemothorax.[20] However, patients with minor blunt chest trauma treated as outpatients (two or less rib fractures, <65 years of age, no lung or other system injury) require close follow-up. Of 709 such patients, 14 (1.8 percent) developed a delayed pneumothorax within 48 hours and 52 (7.3 percent) developed a delayed hemothorax within 2 weeks. No surgical management for the delayed pneumothoraces was required; however, 42 (81 percent) of the delayed hemothoraces required chest tube placement.[21]

Air travel

What advice should be given to a patient requesting to pursue air travel after a traumatic pneumothorax? Cheatham and Safcsak's published prospective evaluation of 12 consecutive patients with recent traumatic pneumothorax notes that air travel appears safe 14 days following radiographic resolution of their pneumothorax.[22] Of 10 patients waiting at least 14 days after radiographic resolution before commercial air travel, all were asymptomatic in flight. One of two patients who flew earlier than 14 days developed respiratory distress suggestive of pneumothorax recurrence.[22] These findings support the earlier recommendations by the Aerospace Medical Association Air Transport Medicine Committee suggesting that air travel should be safe 2–3 weeks after successful drainage of unspecified types of pneumothoraces.[23] Commercial airlines have adopted a 6-week 'no fly' rule between pneumothorax occurrence and air travel.[24] The British Thoracic

Society notes that this rule seems arbitrary without accounting for type of pneumothorax, underlying disease, therapeutic interventions or demographic factors but ultimately suggests that patients may travel safely 6 weeks after a definitive surgical recurrence prevention procedure or chest radiographic resolution of unspecified types of pneumothoraces.[24]

IATROGENIC PNEUMOTHORAX

Incidence and epidemiology

Iatrogenic pneumothoraces (IP) occur commonly and their incidence is likely on the rise due to the ever-growing adoption of and evolution in invasive diagnostic and supportive modalities. Steier and colleagues[25,26] noted such an increase in IP in the early 1970s and attributed it to the use of volume-controlled ventilation and subclavian vein catheterization. With rising use of invasive diagnostic and therapeutic interventions involving the neck, thorax and abdomen, IP incidence continues to climb with ever increasing possible etiologies.[27] Such diversity in etiology places a significant responsibility on the physician to be suspicious for pneumothorax in any patient recently subjected to a diagnostic or therapeutic procedure involving the mouth, neck, chest or abdomen.

Reported IP incidence and proportion in relation to traumatic and spontaneous pneumothoraces varies widely. Weissber and Refaely[28] reported only 6 percent of hospitalized patients with pneumothorax as iatrogenic in origin with 60 percent being spontaneous, and 34 percent being traumatic, at a metropolitan medical center. In contrast, IP (106 of 204 pneumothoraces, 52 percent) exceeded spontaneous (98 of 204 pneumothoraces, 48 percent) at the Long Beach Veterans Administration Hospital.[29] The experience of the physicians performing various procedures also affects the IP, as noted in central vein catheterization.[30] The variable incidence is also likely due to reporting institution type (academic or non-academic institution, trauma or non-trauma center), institutional utilization of various invasive procedures and in- or out-patient management.

Despite the variability in reports, the six most common causes in 535 patients suffering an IP in the Veterans Administration patient population in the early 1990s were transthoracic needle lung biopsy (24 percent), subclavian vein catheterization (22 percent), thoracentesis (20 percent), transbronchial biopsy (10 percent), pleural biopsy (8 percent) and positive-pressure ventilation (7 percent).[31] Reported occurrence rates vary from ≤10 to 50 percent for transthoracic needle lung biopsy, <1 to >13 percent for central line placement and 5–20 percent for thoracentesis and pleural biopsy. Mechanical ventilation and transbronchial lung biopsy are other frequently reported causes[2] with reported occurrence rates of 1–40 percent and <1 to 3 percent, respectively.[32] IP may be associated with significant morbidity, occasional mortality and increased hospital stay and cost.[29,32] Unfortunately, despite increased national emphasis and interest in patient safety,[33] recent measures to reduce iatrogenic complications have not reduced the occurrence of IP. Resident work-hour limits have not reduced the incidence of IP.[34] Also, the Veteran's Administration system-wide implementation of patient safety indicators, including those for IP, actually resulted in increased rates of IP.[35] This may not reflect worse care but increased reporting of IP.[35]

Clinical presentation and diagnosis

The patient's clinical presentation depends upon the patient's underlying lung health, the inciting mechanism and other surrounding circumstances prompting the development of the IP. The poorer the patient's underlying lung health, the greater the symptoms will be, even with a smaller size pneumothorax. Positive-pressure ventilation may drive the rapid enlargement of an IP and predispose the patient to the development of a tension pneumothorax. Any signs or symptoms of respiratory difficulty after a procedure should prompt an investigation for the development of an IP.

The Veteran's Administration large cooperative study[31] of 535 IP found that, in most cases (96 percent), the clinical diagnosis was established by a chest radiograph. The diagnosis was made by chest radiograph alone in 68 percent of patients. In 5 percent of patients the pneumothorax was an incidental finding on a chest radiograph obtained unrelated to the procedure precipitating the pneumothorax. The remaining 27 percent were diagnosed from a combination of a chest radiograph and symptoms or physical findings suggestive of a pneumothorax. Symptoms included pleuritic chest pain and acute onset of dyspnea; physical findings included tracheal shift, decreased breath sounds and cutaneous crepitation. The size of the pneumothorax appeared to be related to the procedure causing it. Transthoracic needle aspiration, pleural biopsy, thoracentesis and transbronchial biopsy were associated primarily with minimal to moderate sized pneumothoraces. Nearly half the patients suffering an IP due to positive-pressure ventilation developed large or tension pneumothorax.

The chest radiograph remains the key to diagnosis. However, initial post-procedure chest radiographs may not demonstrate an IP.[31,36,37] In the setting of central line related IP, delayed chest radiographic diagnosis of an IP ranges from 0.36[37] to 4 percent.[38] Plaus reports a delay of 8–96 hours in diagnosis. Such a delay may be related to poor quality of the initial post-procedure radiograph, small size of initial pneumothorax, slow pleural leak or later introduction of positive-pressure ventilation in the face of earlier unrecognized pleural damage.[36]

In the setting of transthoracic needle aspiration, the role of a post-procedure chest radiograph is debatable but potentially important in detecting delayed pneumothoraces. Prospectively, each of 64 patients underwent a CT reimaging with two additional views immediately after needle biopsy, and an expiratory chest radiograph was obtained 4 hours post procedure.[39] Only 2 of 64 patients (3 percent) developed a delayed pneumothorax detected by the 4-hour post-procedure chest radiograph. Only one of these two patients required chest tube drainage (1.5 percent). The authors conclude that post-procedure chest radiographs should be omitted and instead state that patients should be instructed on signs and symptoms of pneumothorax and seek medical attention if any of these occur.[39] By contrast, Choi and colleagues[40] report that 15 of 458 patients (3.3 percent) undergoing transthoracic needle biopsy under fluoroscopic ($n = 280$), CT (n=21) or ultrasound ($n = 157$) guidance developed a delayed pneumothorax (occurring ≥3 hours post procedure, range 5–120 hours) not detected on an immediate post-procedure chest radiograph. Three of these 15 patients (20 percent) required tube drainage.[40] The authors considered the incidence of delayed pneumothorax and subsequent need for tube drainage clinically important.[40]

Risk factors for iatrogenic pneumothorax

Transthoracic needle aspiration and intensive care setting related IP have associated variables that may predict pneumothorax risk. Multiple studies have assessed potential risk factors associated with the development of a pneumothorax after transthoracic needle biopsy (Table 43.2).[40–46] Greater lesion depth is consistently associated with a higher likelihood of an associated pneumothorax.[41–46] Smaller lesions size also appears to be a risk factor for pneumothorax.[40,41,44,46] Less consistently, the presence of or severity of emphysema is reported as a risk factor for pneumothorax.[40,41,45] Paradoxically, the number of needle passes[41,44–46] and needle size[41,45,46] are not associated with pneumothorax development. The percentage of patients with a pneumothorax subsequently having a drainage tube placed or simple aspiration ranges from 5[46] to 53 percent.[43] The incidence of post-biopsy pneumothorax does not appear to differ whether using CT or fluoroscopy guidance.[47] Finally, placing the patient in the lateral decubitus position with biopsy side down does not reduce the incidence of transthoracic needle biopsy related IP.[48–50]

The value of preoperative lung function predicting IP occurrence is debatable.[39,51–54] Three studies,[39,42,53] including one likely suffering beta error,[39] have found no correlation between lung function findings compatible with obstructive lung disease and CT-directed needle biopsy IP rates. An early study by Poe and colleagues[54] of fluoroscopically directed needle biopsy of lung lesions found a correlation between increased total lung capacity (a potential measure of obstruction) and pneumothorax occurrence. The same data published in two venues noted a correlation of obstructive lung function changes and CT-guided needle biopsy related pneumothorax.[51,52] Obstructive lung disease predicted a 46 percent pneumothorax event rate compared with a 19 percent rate in patients with normal lung function;[51] the FEV_1 (forced expiratory volume in one second) was the most predictive single variable.[52] Notably the later two studies obtained pulmonary function in only 35 percent of reported patients,[51,52] raising the issue of study bias. However, a more recent study supported the thought that a lower FEV_1 is predictive of iatrogenic pneumothorax occurrence in univariant but not multiple regression analysis.[43]

The incidence of mechanical ventilation related pneumothorax has declined,[29,31] likely secondary to newer modes of mechanical ventilation[29] and lung protective ventilation strategies in acute respiratory distress syndrome (ARDS).[55,56] However, pneumothorax remains one of the most common iatrogenic complications in the intensive care unit (ICU).[57] IP in the ICU occurs primarily as a complication of volutrauma from mechanical ventilation or after a procedure.[57] A large prospective observational study of 3430 patients in the ICU for more than 24 hours recently identified associated risks for the development of IP in the ICU (Table 43.3).[57] IP was seen in 94

Table 43.2 Potential risk factors associated with the development of a pneumothorax after transthoracic needle biopsy

Author	Study type	*n* (biopsies or patients)	Iatrogenic pneumothorax (*n*, %)	Lesion depth	Small lesion size	Emphysema	Number of needle passes	Needle size
Cox *et al.*[41]	Unclear	356	144 (40%)	+	+	+	–	–
Laurent *et al.*[42]	Prospective	307	61 (20%)	+	–	–	NA	NA
Saji *et al.*[43]	Retrospective	289	77 (27%)	+	–	NA	NA	NA
Yamagami *et al.*[44]	Prospective	134	46 (34%)	+	+	–	–	NA
Topal and Ediz[45]	Unclear	453	85 (19%)	+	NA	+	–	–
Yeow *et al.*[46]	Unclear	660	155 (23%)	+	+	–	–	–
Choi *et al.*[40]	Prospective	458	85 (19%)	NA	+	+	NA	NA

+, Statistically significant positive correlation with iatrogenic pneumothorax occurrence; –, no statistically significant correlation with iatrogenic pneumothorax occurrence; NA, not assessed.

Table 43.3 Statistically significant risk factors (multivariate analysis) associated with the occurrence of an iatrogenic pneumothorax in the intensive care unit setting[57]

Risk	Hazard ratio	95% CI, *p*
Weight <80 kg	2.4	1.3–4.2, 0.004
History of AIDS	2.8	1.2–6.4, 0.02
Diagnosis of ARDS on admission	5.3	2.6–11, <0.001
Diagnosis of cardiogenic edema on admission	2.0	1.1–3.6, 0.03
Central vein or PA catheter insertion, first 24 hours	1.7	1.0–2.7, 0.04
Inotrope, first 24 hours	2.1	1.3–3.4, 0.002

CI, confidence interval; AIDS, acquired immunodeficiency syndrome; ARDS, acute respiratory distress syndrome; PA, pulmonary artery.

patients (2.7 percent) within the first 30 days. The most common causes of IP, in descending order, were volutrauma ($n = 42$), and invasive procedures including central venous catheter insertion ($n = 28$), thoracentesis ($n = 21$), and other procedures in three. Mortality risk was 2.6 times greater in patients with IP versus those without (95 percent confidence interval, 1.3–4.9). The simplified acute physiologic score (SAPS II) on the first ICU day was greater in patients suffering an IP ($p = 0.001$).

Treatment and management

Current management of patients suffering iatrogenic pneumothoraces is variable, with the development of treatment protocols complicated by inadequate monitoring and reporting of these iatrogenic events.[32] As opposed to spontaneous pneumothorax,[1,58] pneumothorax recurrence considerations are not an issue with patients suffering an iatrogenic pneumothorax. Instead, treatment focuses upon the least invasive intervention appropriate to the patient's underlying lung health and associated clinical circumstances (Figure 43.2).

A recent text recommends observation and oxygen supplementation for patients not mechanically ventilated with minimal symptoms and a limited (<15 percent) pneumothorax. If a patient has more than minimal symptoms or a larger pneumothorax (>15 percent), simple aspiration is recommended.[2] Given that the chest radiograph may be a poor guide to predicting pneumothorax size[59] and the formulae to calculate percent pneumothorax size can be cumbersome, a simpler approach may be useful. A measurement from the visceral to parietal pleural surface as used in traumatic pneumothorax[8] may be easier. Suggested size cut points outlined in the American College of Chest Physicians (ACCP) statement on management of spontaneous pneumothorax[58] may be used: <3 cm and ≥3 cm lung collapse, for <15 percent and >15 percent pneumothorax size, respectively.

Observation and simple aspiration may be successful in managing selected patients with an IP.[44] However, given the variety of commercially available small-bore catheters[60] that can be attached to a Heimlich valve or similar one-way valve device, incorporating a versatile small-bore catheter instead of a simple aspiration is recommended where drainage is deemed necessary. Other commercially packaged alternatives containing a catheter and one-way valve system in one unit are also available and noted to be successful in iatrogenic pneumothoraces (TRU-CLOSE™ Thoracic Vent; Davis and Geck, Wayne, NJ, USA).[61] Caution is urged when incorporating a Heimlich valve, or similar one-way valve device, particularly for patients discharged to home. Clear instructions regarding device orientation to ensure airflow out of the chest and device maintenance are requisite to prevent complications, including tension pneumothorax.[62,63]

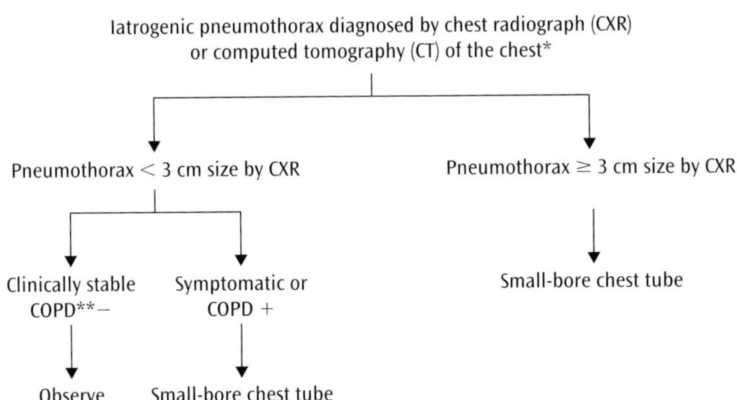

Figure 43.2 Management algorithm for iatrogenic pneumothorax. *See text for details; **COPD, chronic obstructive pulmonary disease; +, positive; –, negative. Any patient on mechanical ventilation requires a large-bore chest tube.

The presence of obstructive lung disease predicts the need for chest tube placement in patients undergoing a needle biopsy of the lung[39,41,51,53] and for longer duration of treatment post pneumothorax compared with patients without a history of obstructed lung disease.[31] Cox and colleagues[41] reported a significantly greater need for chest tube placement in patients with underlying computed tomographic evidence of emphysema (27 percent with evidence versus 9 percent without, $p < 0.01$) sustaining a needle lung biopsy related iatrogenic pneumothorax.[41] Hence, initial placement of a small-bore catheter and foregoing observation is preferred in such patients.

Safe outpatient management utilizing a small-bore catheter attached to a Heimlich valve has been reported in central venous catheter related iatrogenic pneumothoraces patients.[37] This retrospective study notes only 60 percent success (resolution of pneumothorax with no subsequent air leak or pneumothorax enlargement) with observation and a 40 percent failure rate requiring placement of a chest catheter. Alternatively, 85 percent success accompanies the initial placement of a small-bore catheter (8.5 F) attached to a Heimlich valve with a mean catheter residence time of only 1.6 days. Similar reports of successful and safe management of iatrogenic pneumothoraces with small-bore catheters, including in outpatients, placed initially or after short periods of unsuccessful observation have been published.[64,65]

All mechanically ventilated patients developing an iatrogenic pneumothorax from any cause should receive a chest tube. Iatrogenic pneumothoraces resulting directly from positive-pressure mechanical ventilation may be accompanied by bronchopleural fistula and the development of tension pneumothorax.[66,67] Air leaks in this setting may be quite large and variably contribute to alteration in physiological gas exchange including increased carbon dioxide excretion and decreased utilization of inspired oxygen due to escape of carbon dioxide and oxygen through the fistula.[66] Mechanically ventilated patients with an iatrogenic pneumothorax require prompt chest tube placement, often large bore,[66–69] and foregoing consideration of observation. In addition to the placement of an appropriate size chest tube, adjusting the ventilator mode to limit the amount of positive pressure delivered to the patient may assist in minimizing the air leak and healing the fistula.[66,67]

Surgical management and persistent air leaks

The incidence of iatrogenic pneumothorax related air leaks appears related to the underlying etiology of the pneumothorax and any associated lung disease. The Veterans Administration cooperative study does not clearly delineate the treatment modalities incorporated in patients with an iatrogenic pneumothorax. However, using duration of treatment as a rough surrogate for presumed accompanying air leak, 288 of 385 patients (75 percent) in the Veterans Administration cooperative study completed treatment in 1–7 days.[31] Patients with chronic obstructive pulmonary disease (COPD) required significantly longer treatment times than those without COPD. Thoracotomy had to be performed in one of 535 (0.2 percent) patients because of a persistent air leak.

Schoenenberger and colleagues[70] retrospective review of 47 patients provides more direct information regarding the occurrence of persistent air leaks and the role and timing of surgical intervention in patients suffering an iatrogenic pneumothorax. Patients with at least a 20 percent iatrogenic pneumothorax and placement of a 20 to 24 F chest tube were analyzed. Percent air leak resolution was 100 percent at 72 hours after chest tube placement for patients without underlying lung disease and 71 percent for those with an underlying lung disease. Air leak resolution reached a plateau at 72 hours for those with underlying lung disease; no statistically significant increase in air leak resolution occurred after 72 hours.[70] Hence, use of an invasive intervention including VATS or thoracotomy should be strongly considered for patients suffering an iatrogenic pneumothorax with an air leak persisting at 72 hours after chest tube placement.

TENSION PNEUMOTHORAX

Incidence, epidemiology and pathophysiology

Both spontaneous and traumatic (non-iatrogenic and iatrogenic) pneumothoraces may present with or develop into tension pneumothorax. Tension pneumothorax is present when the intrapleural pressure exceeds atmospheric pressure throughout expiration and frequently during inspiration.[2] Many patients suffering a tension pneumothorax have positive pressure applied to their airways during mechanical ventilation[71] or during resuscitation.[72] Seventy-one of 74 patients developing pneumothorax during mechanical ventilation had a tension component in Steier and colleagues review.[26] Presentation is particularly abrupt in patients receiving mechanical ventilation and may carry a particularly high mortality rate.[26] Intra- and post-cardiopulmonary resuscitation (CPR) patients should receive special scrutiny for the possibility of tension of pneumothorax, particularly if positive-pressure ventilation is administered. Unsuspected or untreated tension pneumothoraces were found in 12 of 3500 autopsies. Ten of these 12 patients were receiving some form of endotracheal positive pressure. Eight of these 10 patients were mechanically ventilated; two were receiving intermittent positive pressure. Seven of these 10 patients had also received CPR.[72] Successful diagnosis and treatment of intra- and post-resuscitation tension pneumothorax could mean the difference between successful and unsuccessful CPR. Tension may also develop in spontaneously breathing patients but inherent is the presumed presence of a one-way valve process permitting air to enter the pleural space during inspiration but not exit during expiration.

The dramatic clinical presentation of tension marked by cardiopulmonary compromise is likely multifactorial in etiology. The decrease in the partial pressure of arterial oxygen (PaO_2) and increase in alveolar–arterial oxygen difference that may be seen with any pneumothorax results from alterations in ventilation–perfusion relationships, anatomic shunt and dead space.[73,74] Anatomic shunt may in fact increase secondary to worsening ventilation–perfusion relationships after pleural air drainage with improvement delayed up to 90 minutes emphasizing the need for supplemental oxygen in pneumothorax patients.[73]

Decreased PaO_2 and impaired cardiac output, alone or in combination, play a role in the clinical decompensation noted in tension pneumothorax. Earlier studies performed in goats and monkeys with induced tension pneumothorax note no fall in cardiac output in goats and a minimal drop in monkeys. The animals' clinical distress was attributed to the precipitous fall in PaO_2.[75] Subsequent reports in sheep found a similar lack of cardiac output compromise with induced tension pneumothorax.[76] More recent animal investigations in sheep note a drop in cardiac output accompanied by a fall in PaO_2. The abnormalities in gas exchange persisted for up to 60–90 minutes after recovery.[77] Similarly, Barton[78] found a drop in cardiac output and PaO_2 in ventilated pigs with hypoxemia developing early and preceding the development of hypotension. In four documented cases of tension pneumothorax in three patients on pressure control ventilation, significant decreases in cardiac index were observed.[79] Similarly, Connolly[80] reported a drop in cardiac index in a mechanically ventilated patient with tension pneumothorax.

Clinical presentation and diagnosis

Patients with tension pneumothorax typically present with severe distress, displaying cyanosis, diaphoresis, tachycardia, hypotension and labored respirations.[2,26] Unusually, patients may present quiescently even during mechanical ventilation.[80,81] The diagnosis should and can be made clinically in the majority of cases based on the usual dramatic presentation. Treatment should generally not be delayed for radiographic confirmation, particularly in the mechanically ventilated patient. Such a delay can increase mortality more than fourfold. Twelve of 74 (16 percent) mechanically ventilated patients with pneumothorax died in Steier and colleagues' review.[26] Seventy-one of these 74 patients had a tension component. Treatment was delayed from 30 minutes to 8 hours in 29 patients awaiting chest radiographic confirmation. Nine of these 29 (31 percent) patients died of pneumothorax compared with a 7 percent mortality rate in the 45 patients with a clinical diagnosis and immediate treatment.[26] A clue to the development of a pneumothorax including tension pneumothorax is worsening dynamic and static lung compliance (increasing peak and plateau pressures, respectively) while on volume cycle ventilation. Worsening in both dynamic and static compliance can also be found in pulmonary edema, ARDS, pneumonia and atelectasis.[82] The rapidity of deterioration in lung compliance may be a clue to tension pneumothorax over the other possibilities. If the patient is on pressure-cycled ventilation, decreasing delivered tidal volumes is noted.

The chest radiograph itself may be a misleading tool to diagnose tension. The classic radiographic findings of tension may indeed not represent tension.[2] Classic radiographic findings include a shift of the mediastinum to the contralateral side, ipsilateral enlargement of the hemithorax and depressed hemidiaphragm. Such findings may occur due to the natural recoil properties of the chest wall and the lung when air enters the pleural space without intrapleural pressures exceeding the surrounding atmospheric pressure throughout the expiratory cycle.[2] Further, radiographic findings of pneumothorax may be altered in the supine patient, as is often the case for critically ill patients on mechanical ventilation. This may be further compounded by extensive pulmonary parenchymal disease and accompanying alterations in pulmonary compliance not allowing ready collapse of the lung upon air entry into the pleural space. A chest radiographic change found in supine patients wherein pleural air tracks anteriorly and inferiorly creating a deep lateral costophrenic sulcus is the 'deep sulcus sign'.[83]

Treatment

Urgent treatment of tension pneumothorax is key. As noted, mortality may be considerably increased awaiting chest radiographic confirmation. Treatment provides confirmation of the diagnosis. Prompt drainage by placement of an intravenous needle (14–16 F) in the pleural space will usually elicit an audible rush of air due to air rushing out of the pressurized pleural space. Alternatively, the needle may be fitted with a partially water (sterile) filled syringe and introduced into the pleural space until air is aspirated. Marked bubbling after the syringe plunger is removed confirms pleural air under pressure. Needle placement through the second anterior intercostal space has been advocated,[2] however, placement of the needle through the lateral fifth intercostals space may be safer.[84] Prompt subsequent placement of a chest tube is required regardless of whether an audible air rush or water syringe bubbling is noted, given the potential for having induced a pneumothorax in an already compromised patient by placing a needle into the chest. Placement of a larger-bore chest tube in the setting of a tension pneumothorax in a mechanically ventilated patient is preferred.

FUTURE DIRECTIONS

Additional prospective studies of all aspects of the management of both spontaneous and non-pneumothorax are required for the more effective and less costly care of patients at risk for, and who sustain, a pneumothorax. For both non-iatrogenic and iatrogenic pneumothoraces, additional studies should include more accurately discerning the risk factors for patients requiring placement of a chest tube versus those who can be safely observed. Such knowledge will limit the need to place chest tubes with their attendant potential morbidity, hospitalization and cost. More refined knowledge regarding the risk factors for iatrogenic pneumothorax will lead to appropriate interventions (including alternative procedures to reduce pneumothorax risk and management options) mitigating or preventing their occurrence. Such information will also lead to more completely informed patients and families regarding the risks of pneumothorax during the consent process and during the care of patients in high-risk settings such as the intensive care environment. More accurate and transparent reporting, in a non-punitive environment, of iatrogenic pneumothorax occurrence will assist in developing such risk predictions.

KEY POINTS

Non-iatrogenic traumatic pneumothorax

- Pneumothorax ranks second to rib fractures as the most common manifestation of chest injury.
- Twenty-nine to 72 percent of traumatic pneumothoraces may be occult emphasizing the need for a chest CT for diagnosis that may reveal other abnormalities including hemothorax.
- The presence of subcutaneous emphysema, pulmonary contusion or rib fracture(s) in a trauma patient should prompt consideration of an occult pneumothorax.
- Traumatic pneumothoraces usually require placement of a chest tube although carefully selected patients may be observed closely.
- A traumatic pneumothorax in a mechanically ventilated patient should prompt placement of a chest tube in most patients

Iatrogenic pneumothorax

- The most common causes of iatrogenic pneumothorax are transthoracic needle lung biopsy, subclavian vein catheterization, thoracentesis, transbronchial lung biopsy, pleural biopsy and mechanical ventilation
- Iatrogenic pneumothorax should be considered in any patient with deteriorating cardiopulmonary status after a procedure, even several days after the procedure.
- Smaller targeted lung lesions and greater lesion depth during transthoracic lung biopsy pose increased risks for an iatrogenic pneumothorax.
- Mortality risk is 2.6 times greater in patients sustaining an iatrogenic pneumothorax in the ICU setting versus those without an iatrogenic pneumothorax. Associated risk factors for developing an iatrogenic pneumothorax in the ICU include a history of AIDS, diagnosis of ARDS or cardiogenic pulmonary edema on admission, and placement of a central venous catheter or use of an inotropic agent within the first 24 hours of admission.
- Simple observation or the placement of a small-bore chest tube may be used to treat iatrogenic pneumothorax. Use of a chest tube for iatrogenic pneumothorax treatment is preferred for larger pneumothoraces, symptomatic patients, in patients with underlying COPD and in mechanically ventilated patients.

Tension pneumothorax

- Tension pneumothorax may occur with spontaneous and traumatic pneumothoraces. However, mechanically ventilated patients more commonly have tension pneumothorax.
- Tension pneumothorax is an emergent problem preferably diagnosed clinically and treated promptly by placement of a drainage catheter. Waiting for a confirmatory chest radiograph increases mortality.

REFERENCES

● = Key primary paper
◆ = Major review article
* = Paper that represents the first formal publication of a management guideline

◆1. Baumann M. Management of spontaneous pneumothorax. *Clin Chest Med* 2006; **27**: 369–81.

2. Light RW, Lee YCG. Pneumothorax, chylothorax, hemothorax, and fibrothorax. In: Mason RJ, Broaddus VC, Murray JF, *et al.* (eds). *Textbook of respiratory medicine.* Philadelphia: WB Saunders Company, 2005: 1961–88.

◆3. Sahn SA, Heffner JE. Spontaneous pneumothorax. *N Engl J Med* 2000; **342**: 868–74.

4. Wolfman NT, Myers WS, Glauser SJ, *et al.* Validity of CT classification on management of occult pneumothorax: a prospective study. *AJR Am J Roentgenol* 1998; **171**: 1317–20.

●5. Enderson BL, Abdalla R, Frame SB, *et al.* Tube thoracostomy for occult pneumothorax: a prospective randomized study of its use. *J Trauma* 1993; **35**: 726–30.

6. Bridges KG, Welch G, Silver M, *et al.* CT detection of occult pneumothorax in multiple trauma patients. *J Emerg Med* 1993; **11**: 179–86.

●7. Trupka A, Waydhas C, Hallfeldt K, *et al.* Value of thoracic computed tomography in the first assessment of severely injured patients with blunt chest trauma: results of a prospective study. *J Trauma* 1997; **43**: 405–11.

●8. Knottenbelt JD, van der Spuy JW. Traumatic pneumothorax: a scheme for rapid patient turnover. *Br J Accident Surg* 1990; **21**: 77–80.

◆9. Ball C, Hameed S, Evans D, *et al.* Occult pneumothorax in the mechanically ventilated trauma patient. *Can J Surg* 2003; **46**: 373–9.

●10. Ball C, Kirkpatrick A, Laupland K, *et al.* Incidence, risk factors, and outcomes for occult pneumothoraces in victims of major trauma. *J Trauma* 2005; **59**: 917–25.

11. Guest JL, Anderson JN. Major airway injury in closed chest trauma. *Chest* 1977; **72**: 63–6,

12. Carrillo EH, Schmacht DC, Gable DR, *et al.* Thoracoscopy in the management of postraumatic persistent pneumothorax. *J Am Coll Surg* 1998; **186**: 636–40.

13. Johnson G. Traumatic pneumothorax: is a chest drain always necessary? *J Accid Emerg Med* 1996; **13**: 173–4.

14. Collins JC, Levine G, Waxman K. Occult traumatic pneumothorax: immediate tube thoracostomy versus expectant management. *Am Surg* 1992; **58**: 743–6.

15. Brasel KJ, Stafford RE, Weigelt JA, *et al.* Treatment of occult pneumothoraces from blunt trauma. *J Trauma* 1999; **46**: 987–91.

16. Garramone RR, Jacobs LM, Sahdev P. An objective method to measure and manage occult pneumothorax. *Surg Gynecol Obstet* 1991; **173**: 257–61.

17. Etoch SW, Bar-Natan MF, Miller FB, et al. Tube thoracostomy. Factors related to complications. Arch Surg 1995; 130: 521–6.

18. Helling TS, Gyles NR, Eisenstein CL, *et al.* Complications following blunt and penetrating injuries in 216 victims of chest trauma requiring tube thoracostomy. *J Trauma* 1989; **29**: 1367–70.

19. Divisi D, Battaglia C, De Berardis B, *et al.* Video assisted thoracoscopy in thoracic injury: early or delayed indication? *Acta Biomed Ateneo Parmense* 2004; **75**: 158–63.

20. Golden P. Follow-up chest radiographs after traumatic pneumothorax or hemothorax in the outpatient setting: a retrospective review. *Int J Trauma Nurs* 1999; **5**: 88–94.

21. Misthos P, Kakaris S, Sepsas E, *et al.* A prospective analysis of occult pneumothorax, delayed pneumothorax and delayed hemothorax after minor blunt thoracic trauma. *Eur J Cardiothorac Surg* 2004; **25**: 859–64.

●22. Cheatham ML, Safcsak K. Air travel following traumatic pneumothorax: when is it safe? *Am Surg* 1999; **65**: 1160–4.

*23. Committee AMAATM. Medical guidelines for air travel. *Aviat Space Environ Med* 1996; **67** (Supplement): B1–16.

24. British Thoracic Society Standards of Care Committee. Managing passengers with respiratory disease planning air travel: British Thoracic Society recommendations. *Thorax* 2002; **57**: 289–304.

●25. Steier M, Ching N, Bonfils-Roberts E, *et al.* Iatrogenic causes of pneumothorax: increasing incidence with advances in medical care. *N Y State J Med* 1973; **173**: 1296–8.

26. Steier M, Ching N, Bonfils Roberts E, *et al.* Pneumothorax complicating continuous ventilatory support. *J Thoracic Caridiovasc Surg* 1974; **67**: 17–23.

27. Janmeja A, Tandon S, Gupta K, *et al.* Uncommon iatrogenic pneumothorax. *J Assoc Physicians India* 1999; **47**: 560–1.

28. Weissberg D, Refaely Y. Pneumothorax. Experience with 1,199 patients. *Chest* 2000; **117**: 1279–85.

●29. Despars JA, Sassoon CSH, Light RW. Significance of iatrogenic pneumothoraces. *Chest* 1994; **105**: 1147–50.

30. Sznajder JI, Zveibil FR, Bitterman H, *et al.* Central vein catheterization. Failure and complication rates by three percutaneous approaches. *Arch Intern Med* 1986; **146**: 259–61.

●31. Sassoon CSH, Light RW, O'Hara VS, *et al.* Iatrogenic pneumothorax: etiology and morbidity. *Respiration* 1992; **59**: 215–20.

32. Berger R. Iatrogenic pneumothorax. *Chest* 1994; **105**: 980–2.

33. Committee on data standards for patient safety. *Patient safety. Achieving a new standard for care.* Washington, DC: National Academies Press, 2004.

●34. Poulose BK, Ray WA, Arbogast PG, *et al.* Resident work hour limits and patient safety. *Ann Surg* 2005; **241**: 847–56.

●35. Rosen AK, Zhao S, Rivard P, *et al.* Tracking rates of patient safety indictors over time. Lessons from the Veterans Administration. *Med Care* 2006; **44**: 850–61.

36. Thomas C, Butler C. Delayed pneumothorax and hydrothorax with central venous migration. *Anaesthesia* 1999; **54**: 987–90.

37. Laronga C, Meric F, Truong MT, *et al.* A treatment algorithm for pneumothoraces complicating central venous catheter insertion. *Am J Surg* 2000; **180**: 523–7.

38. Plaus WJ. Delayed pneumothorax after subclavian vein catheterization. *J Parenter Enter Nutr* 1990; **14**: 414–15.

39. Byrd RP, Fields-Ossorio C, Roy TM. Delayed chest radiographs and the diagnosis of pneumothorax following CT-guided fine needle aspiration of pulmonary lesions. *Respir Med* 1999; **93**: 379–81.

●40. Choi C-M, Um S-W, Yoo C-G, *et al.* Incidence and risk factors of delayed pneumothorax after transthoracic needle biopsy of the lung. *Chest* 2004; **126**: 1616–21.

●41. Cox JE, Chiles C, McManus CM, *et al.* Transthoracic needle aspiration biopsy: variables that affect risk of pneumothorax. *Radiology* 1999; **212**: 165–8.

●42. Laurent F, Michel P, Latrabe V, *et al.* Pneumothoraces and chest tube placement after CT-guided transthoracic lung biopsy using coaxial technique: incidence and risk factors. *AJR Am J Roentgenol* 1999; **172**: 1049–53.

●43. Saji H, Nakamura H, Tsuchida T, *et al.* The incidence and the risk of pneumothorax and chest tube placement after percutaneous CT-guided lung biopsy. The angle of the needle trajectory is a novel predictor. *Chest* 2002; **121**: 1521–6.

●44. Yamagami T, Nakamura T, Iida S, *et al.* Management of pneumothorax after percutaneous CT-guided lung biopsy. *Chest* 2002; **121**: 1159–64.

●45. Topal U, Ediz B. Transthoracic needle biopsy: factors affecting risk of pneumothorax. *Eur J Radiol* 2003; **48**: 263–7.

●46. Yeow K-M, Su I-H, Pan K-T, *et al.* Risk factors of pneumothorax and bleeding. Multivariant analysis of 660 CT-guided coaxial cutting needle lung biopsies. *Chest* 2004; **126**: 748–54.

47. Bungay H, Berger J, Traill Z, *et al.* Pneumothorax post CT-guided lung biopsy: a comparison between detection on chest radiographs and CT. *Br J Radiol* 1999; **72**: 1160–3.

48. Tanisaro K. Patient positioning after fine needle lung biopsy-effect on pneumothorax rate. *Acta Radiologica* 2003; **44**: 52–5.

49. Masterson AV, Haslam P, Logan PM, *et al.* Patient positioning after lung biopsy: influence on the incidence of pneumothorax. *Can Assoc Radiol J* 2003; **54**: 31–4.

50. Berger R, Smith D. Efficacy of the lateral decubitus position in preventing pneumothorax after needle biopsy of the lung. *South Med J* 1988; **81**: 1140–3.

51. Fish G, Stanley J, Miller KS, *et al.* Postbiopsy pneumothorax: estimating the risk by chest radiography and pulmonary function tests. *AJR Am J Roentgenol* 1988; **150**: 71–4.

52. Miller K, Fish G, Stanley J, *et al.* Prediction of pneumothorax rate in percutaneous needle aspiration of the lung. *Chest* 1988; **93**: 742–5.

53. Anderson CLV, Crespo JC, Lie Th. Risk of pneumothorax not increased by obstructive lung disease in percutaneous needle biopsy. *Chest* 1994; **105**: 1705–8.

54. Poe RH, Kallay MC, Wicks CM, *et al.* Predicting risk of pneumothorax in needle biopsy of the lung. *Chest* 1984; **85**: 232–5.

55. Amato M, Barbas C, Medeiros D, *et al.* Effect of protective-ventilation strategy on mortality in the acute respiratory distress syndrome. *N Engl J Med* 1998; **338**: 347–54.

56. Network ARDS. Ventilation with lower tidal volumes as compared with traditional tidal volumes for acute lung injury and the acute respiratory distress syndrome. *N Engl J Med* 2000; **342**: 1301–8.

●57. de Lassence A, Timsit J-F, Tafflet M, *et al.* Pneumothorax in the intensive care unit. Incidence, risk factors, and outcome. *Anesthesiology* 2006; **104**: 5–13.

*58. Baumann MH, Strange C, Heffner JE, *et al.* Management of spontaneous pneumothorax. An American College of Chest Physicians Delphi consensus statement. *Chest* 2001; **119**: 590–602.

59. Engdahl O, Toft T, Boe J. Chest radiograph – a poor method for determining size of a pneumothorax. *Chest* 1993; **103**: 26–9.

●60. Baumann MH, Patel PB, Roney CW, *et al.* Comparison of function of commercially available pleural drainage units and catheters. *Chest* 2003; **123**: 1878–86.

61. Roggla M, Wagner A, Brunner C, *et al.* The management of pneumothorax with the thoracic vent versus conventional intercostal tube drainage. *Wien Klin Wochenschr* 1996; **108**: 330–3.

62. Mainini SE, Johnson FE. Tension pneumothorax complicating small-caliber chest tube insertion. *Chest* 1990; **97**: 759–60.

63. Crocker HL, Ruffin RE. Patient-induced complications of a Heimlich flutter valve. *Chest* 1998; **113**: 838–9.

64. Delius RE, Obeid F, Horst M, *et al.* Catheter aspiration for simple pneumothorax. *Arch Surg* 1989; **124**: 833–6.

65. Brown KT, Brody LA, Getrajdman GI, *et al.* Outpatient treatment of iatrogenic pneumothorax after needle biopsy. *Radiology* 1997; 205: 249–52.

66. Baumann MH, Sahn SA. Medical management and therapy of bronchopleural fistulas in the mechanically ventilated patient. *Chest* 1990; **97**: 721–8.

◆67. Lois M, Noppen M. Bronchopleural fistuals. An overview of the problem with special focus on endoscopic management. *Chest* 2005; **128**: 3955–65.

68. Baumann MH, Strange C. Treatment of spontaneous pneumothorax. A more aggressive approach? *Chest* 1997; **112**: 789–804.

69. Baumann MH, Strange C. The clinician's perspective on pneumothorax management. *Chest* 1997; **112**: 822–8.

●70. Schoenenberger R, Haefeli W, Weiss P, *et al.* Evaluation of conventional chest tube therapy for iatrogenic pneumothorax. *Chest* 1993; 104: 1770–2.

71. Barton E, Rhee P, Hutton K. The pathophysiology of tension pneumothorax in ventilated swine. *J Emerg Med* 1997; **15**: 147–53.

72. Ludwig J, Kienzle GD. Pneumothorax in a large autopsy population. *Am J Clin Pathol* 1978; **70**: 24–6.

73. Norris RM, Jones JG, Bishop JM. Respiratory gas exchange in patients with spontaneous pneumothorax. *Thorax* 1968; **23**: 427–33.

74. Moran JF, Jones RH, Wolfe WG. Regional pulmonary function during experimental unilateral pneumothorax in the awake state. *J Thorac Cardiovasc Surg* 1977; **74**: 396–402.

75. Rutherford RB, Hurt HH, Brickman RD, *et al.* The pathophysiology of progressive, tension pneumothorax. *J Trauma* 1968; **8**: 212–27.

76. Gustman P, Yerger L, Wanner A. Immediate cardiovascular effects of tension pneumothorax. *Am Rev Respir Dis* 1983; **127**: 171–4.

77. Carvalho P, Hilderbrandt J, Charan NB. Changes in bronchial and pulmonary arterial blood flow with progressive tension pneumothorax. *J Appl Physiol* 1996; **81**: 1664–9.

◆78. Barton ED. Tension pneumothorax. *Curr Opin Pulm Med* 1999; 5: 269–74.

79. Beards S, Lipman J. Decreased cardiac index as an indicator of tension pneumothorax in the ventilated patient. *Anaesthesia* 1994; **49**: 137–41.

80. Connolly J. Hemodynamic measurements during tension pneumothorax. *Crit Care Med* 1993; **21**: 294–6.

81. Baumann MH, Sahn SA. Tension pneumothorax: diagnostic and therapeutic pitfalls. *Crit Care Med* 1993; **21**: 177–9.

82. Pilbeam SP. *Basic patient assessment and methods to improve ventilation. Mechanical ventilation. Physiological and clinical applications.* St Louis: Mosby, 1998; 244–61.

●83. Gordon R. The deep sulcus sign. *Radiology* 1980; **136**: 25–7.

84. Rawlins R, Brown KM, Carr CS, *et al.* Life threatening haemorrhage after anterior needle aspiration of pneumothoraces. A role for lateral needle aspiration in emergency decompression of spontaneous pneumothorax. *Emerg Med J* 2003; **20**: 383–4.

44

Pediatric pleural diseases

ELIZABETH A PERKETT, PAUL E MOORE

INTRODUCTION

The overall anatomy and physiology of the pleural space in children is the same as in adults.[1] Many of the past reports of pediatric pleural effusions have been retrospective and include small numbers of patients and data from adult studies were extrapolated to pediatrics. However, several recent studies highlight the differences in pediatric and adult patients with pleural disease.[2] Not only is the differential diagnosis of pediatric pleural effusions different from that for adults, but pediatric co-morbid conditions are different which likely influences outcomes. For example, a prospective study of fibrinolytic therapy for parapneumonic effusions in adults concluded no benefit[3] while a study of pediatric patients suggested advantages to fibrinolytic therapy.[4] In 2005, The British Thoracic Society (BTS) published the first pediatric specific guidelines for the management of pleural infection children.[5] While this is a very useful document and provides an extensive review of the literature, the authors highlight the need for additional pediatric data.

FETAL PLEURAL EFFUSION

The exact incidence of pleural effusion in the fetus is unknown, but even with the increasing use of sonography in pregnancies, it is a rare disorder, occurring in approximately one per 15 000 pregnancies.[6] Fetal pleural effusions are usually detected during routine ultrsonograhy but some cases may not be detected if the fetus aborts.[6,7] Primary fetal pleural effusions are the most common and are usually chylous, which is diagnosed by finding a predominance of lymphocytes. Viral infections may result in increased numbers of lymphocytes in the effusion, and manifestations of infection in other organs may support the viral diagnosis. In one retrospective review of pleural fluid samples, the prevalence of chromosome abnormalities in isolated pleural effusions was 12 percent – highlighting the importance of thorough evaluation of the fetus.[8]

Primary chylous effusions may be caused by congenital lymphangiectasis, a rare condition, with abnormal development of the lymphatics, which can present in the fetal period.[9,10] In most cases the etiology of the chylous effusion is unknown and prognosis is good, particularly if the effusion is not large. Management of primary effusions is not standardized, but small effusions are usually followed with simple observation and some show spontaneous resolution.[11] Large effusions can result in pulmonary hypoplasia and significant respiratory distress at birth. To avoid pulmonary hypoplasia, effusions are aspirated and when repeated drainage is needed, pleural amniotic shunts are put in place.[11,12] The outcome of a simple effusion is good and now, with aggressive management of large effusions, outcomes have improved with one retrospective study of fetus pleural amniotic shunts reporting a survival rate of 48 percent.[12]

Secondary fetal pleural effusions are secondary to generalized edema in immune or non-immune hydrops. Secondary effusions are associated with a wide variety of disorders including chromosomal anomalies, cardiac, gastrointestinal, hematological, pulmonary, infectious, and metabolic and malformations of the umbilical cord and placenta. With the high incidence of underlying anomalies, it is important to have a careful evaluation of the fetus not only by sonography but also including karyotyping and fetal echocardiogram. If a major underlying congenital anomaly is diagnosed, no further evaluation may be indicated, but in many cases a fetal thoracentesis is needed to distinguish primary from secondary effusions. The underlying condition is the most important factor in determining overall outcome.

Pleural effusions detected *in utero* may persist into the newborn period. Significant accumulations will cause respiratory distress at birth, both by limiting lung expansion and by causing underlying pulmonary hypoplasia. At the time of delivery, personnel should be present to provide resuscitation and drainage to relieve respiratory distress. Additional therapies may be indicated if an underlying disorder, such as congenital heart disease, was also detected *in utero*.

DIAGNOSIS OF PLEURAL EFFUSIONS IN INFANTS AND CHILDREN

Effusions may be detected on upright chest radiographs with blunting of the costrophrenic angles if the effusions are large, a fluid line is identifiable. Lateral decubitus films are frequently more useful to demonstrate the presence of an effusion, in particular in small infants where chest radiographs are rarely taken in an upright position. Total opacification of the hemithorax makes it difficult to determine whether fluid is present on either upright or decubitis radiographs so other imaging modalities are frequently used. Ultrasonography is very useful in the evaluation of effusions to distinguish between non-aerated lung and pleural fluid, in identifying loculations and in providing assistance in directed thoracentesis or placement of a chest tube. Ultrasound has the additional advantage of not requiring sedation and can be carried out at the bedside. Early reports suggested that ultrasound might be useful for grading effusions, but several studies have not found ultrasound to provide prognostic information.[4,13,14] If there is concern about a mediastinal mass or tumor, a computed tomography (CT) scan needs to be carried out. Areas of aeration can be detected on CT, but it may be impossible to differentiate proteinous fluid from consolidated parenchyma, unless vascular contrast is used, where the tissue will have some enhancement from its vasculature.[15] The presence of a thickened peel is thought to suggest empyema, however, CT cannot always differentiate an empyema from a parapneumonic effusion. As CT scanning has become more readily available, increased numbers of CT scans are being performed, although there are little data to support its routine use in children with pleural effusions.[5] CT has the disadvantage of increased radiation exposure and in infants and young children, sedation is required. In centers where video-assisted thoracoscopic surgery (VATS) is used in the management of pleural effusions, CT scans are frequently carried out although, again, there are limited data to support this use.

In adults, thoracentesis is recommended for every patient with an undiagnosed pleural effusion. In pediatrics, thoracentesis is frequently performed and is definitely needed for diagnostic studies of acute infectious effusion, malignancies and chylothorax. Pediatric parapneumonic effusions are sometimes detected when the patient is in the recovery phase of an infection and the effusion is not causing any symptoms. In such patients, diagnostic thoracentesis is often not necessary, but close follow-up is indicated to determine that there has been resolution of the effusion.

CHYLOTHORAX

The exact incidence of neonatal effusions is not known. A retrospective review of neonates admitted to six referral centers found that 32 percent were congenital and 68 percent acquired.[16] The most common form of pleural effusion in the newborn is a chylothorax which occurs most frequently on the right side.[17] With congenital idiopathic chylothorax, symptoms may be present at birth or develop in the first week of life. Secondary chylothorax may present at birth or later, depending on the underlying cause. The diagnosis of chylothorax is made by thoracentesis and examination of the fluid, keeping in mind that if enteral feedings have not been initiated, the fluid will be clear and yellow, not milky. Cellular analysis will reveal a predominance of lymphocytes (90 percent) which are predominantly T lymphocytes. The etiology may be idiopathic or secondary to trauma to the thoracic duct during thoracic surgery or repair of congenital heart diseases.[17] Blunt trauma, including non-accidental trauma, has been associated with chylothorax.[18] Secondary chylothorax can occur secondary to increased venous pressure associated with congenital heart disease or thrombosis (e.g. from central lines). Treatment of the underlying condition is important in the management of patients with chylothorax but, if the effusion is large, drainage will be needed to relieve respiratory distress. Although simple chest tube drainage may relieve the respiratory distress, loss of large volumes of fluid, including proteins and lymphocytes, may result in the risk of infection from immunosuppresssion and metabolic disturbances, and replacement of proteins may be indicated. Initial conservative management is aimed at decreasing lymph flow by restricting dietary fats to medium chain triglycerides or total parental nutrition (TPN). There are several case reports of successful therapy with octreotide, a synthetic analogue of somatostatin, which is thought to reduce lymph flow.[19] Patients with direct trauma to the thoracic duct frequently have spontaneous resolution with conservative management. In one series, patients with elevated venous pressure had longer duration and higher volume of drainage. Overall, 80 percent of the patients responded to conservative management.[17] There are various criteria for failure of conservative management, but most suggest 2–3 weeks before considering surgical intervention. VATS allows a less invasive approach for ligation of the thoracic duct, but in the very small infant the technology may be limited, particularly if there has been prior thoracic surgery.

Pulmonary lymphangiectasis

Pulmonary lymphangiectasis is associated with abnormal pulmonary lymphatics in the pleura and interstitium of the lung.[20] The overall incidence is unknown and scattered cases continue to be reported, but pulmonary lymphangiectasis is very rare. Esther and Barker[21] proposed categorizing pulmonary lymphangiectasis as primary or secondary (which is related to pulmonary venous or lymphatic obstruction). Diagnosis may be suspected by the presence of increased interstitial markings that are apparent on chest radiograph secondary to the dilated lymphatics throughout the pleural and connective tissue. Open lung biopsy is usually required for definitive diagnosis. Patients with pulmonary lymphangiectasis who present with respiratory distress in the newborn period had previously been thought to have a very poor prognosis, but with aggressive supportive care pleural effusions seem to subside, and infants are surviving beyond the neonatal period.

PEDIATRIC EFFUSIONS

Pleural effusions are uncommon findings on pediatric radiographs. Beyond the newborn period, a newly detected pleural effusion is most likely secondary to infection – a parapneumonic effusion. The true incidence of pleural effusions in the pediatric population is not known because most studies are retrospective and based on hospitalized children. Alkrinawi and Chernick[22,23] reviewed charts of 127 pediatric patients (<18 years of age) admitted with pleural effusions from 1987 to 1995. Fifty percent of the patients had pneumonia with a parapneumonic effusion. Other etiologies included congenital heart disease (17 percent – mostly post-operative, 2 percent congestive heart failure), malignancy (10 percent), renal (9 percent) and trauma (7 percent). As in other studies, pleural fluid was more than twice as likely to occur in boys.

Congenital heart disease

In pediatrics, congestive heart failure is not common, although it can occur with congenital heart disease. One of the challenging pediatric pleural effusions is that associated with single ventricle congenital heart disease and post-operatively with the Fontan procedure. The precise etiology of the post-Fontan pleural effusion is not clear, and is likely multifactorial – including fluids, pressures, arrhythmias and inflammatory cytokines. Management has been frustrating and conventional therapy with chest tube drainage, dietary interventions or pleurodesis have variable success.[24] Aggressive attention to fluid management, oxygen therapy and other medical therapies has been reported to decrease the duration of the effusions.[25] Octreotide has been reported to have benefit for the chylothorax following congenital heart surgery,[26] however, no prospective randomized controlled trials have been carried out.

Malignancies

Although a small percentage of pediatric pleural effusions are associated with malignancies, it is a very important category. Malignancy must be considered in a child who presents with an effusion, without symptoms or history suggesting infection or trauma. Lymphomas are common childhood cancers and frequently present with a mediastinal mass and pleural effusion.[27,28] One report found 71 percent of patients with lymphoblastic lymphoma had a pleural effusion at presentation while only 11 percent of patients with Hodgkin's disease presented with effusions.[27] A large effusion may result in respiratory compromise, necessitating drainage, but pleural fluid analysis can also provide a definitive diagnosis in most cases.[29] Pleural effusions have been seen with other intrathoracic malignancies including leukemia, neuroblastoma, Wilm's tumor, sarcomas and mesothelioma (extremely rare in pediatrics).[30,31]

Pleurodesis is used in adult oncology patients but there is little information about its usefulness in pediatric patients. In a report of seven end-stage pediatric oncology patients with intractable pleural effusions, pleurodesis with doxycycline provided significant relief of respiratory symptoms.[32]

Infections

Tuberculous pleural effusions occur in children, but less frequently than in adults. A review of 175 children <18 years of age with primary pulmonary tuberculosis (TB) revealed that 22 percent had an effusion identified on the chest radiograph.[33] The average age of the children with effusions was significantly greater – 13.5 years versus 7.0 years – than the age of patients with parenchymal TB. The effusion was unilateral and was the only radiographic finding in 41 percent. TB should be considered in cases of pleural effusions where other etiologies are not clearly identified. TB workup would include a thorough history for contacts and skin testing. In older children workup would be similar to adults, including assessment of sputum and pleural fluid. In young children, induced sputum or gastric aspirate may be needed.

In pediatric patients infections with *Mycoplasma pneumoniae* and viruses are very common. Pleural effusions may occur with *M. pneumoniae* pneumonia, but the effusions are generally small and do not cause respiratory symptoms.[34] The incidence of pleural effusions in association with viral pneumonia is not known, since most patients with viral respiratory disease are seen as outpatients and chest radiographs are not routinely obtained. There are anecdotal reports of the discovery of large parapneumonic effusions on chest radiographs taken after resolution of an acute respiratory illness. It is presumed that these effusions are the result of a viral pneumonia, but since the patients are asymptomatic, no specific intervention is performed. Viral infections can be associated with large effusions which result in respiratory distress and thoracentesis may be needed both for diagnostic and therapeutic reasons.

Bacterial pneumonia is the most common cause of pleural effusions in children and there are some reports which suggest that the incidence of empyema in children is increasing.[35] Historically, three specific organisms have been associated with pleural effusions: *Staphylococcus aureus*, *Haemophilus influenzae* and *Streptococcus pneumoniae*. Over the past decade, universal vaccination against *H. influenzae* and *S. pneumoniae* has reduced the importance of these pathogens, although in most reports *S. pneumoniae* is still the most common pathogen. A recent retrospective review of empyema suggested that *Staphylococcus aureus*, particularly methicillin-resistant *S. aureus*, was becoming more prevalent.[36] However, in that report, causative organisms were detected in only 43 percent of the cases, perhaps related to previous antibiotic therapy. Anaerobic organisms are rarely isolated in children, but infrequent use of anaerobic culture media may have reduced the detection of anaerobes.

The emergence of antibiotic resistant organisms, including methicillin-resistant *S. aureus* and *S. pneumoniae*, may be associated with more complicated effusions and empyema. However, overall, patients still respond well if treated with appropriate antibiotics.[37,38] The increase in antibiotic resistant infections secondary to *S. aureus* and *S. pneumoniae* underscores the importance of a diagnostic tap in children who present with a pleural effusion. Identification of an organism with accompanying drug susceptibilities allows the clinician to tailor antibiotic therapy and may prevent the need for more invasive procedures. Although the prior use of antibiotics may limit the ability to recover an organism from culture, even its presence on Gram stain may help guide therapy. The use of polymerase chain reaction (PCR) and pneumococcal antigen detection in pleural fluid specimens can be helpful for more rapid diagnosis of *S. pneumoniae* when culture results are negative.[39]

As additional PCR-based detection studies become available they will improve the ability to rapidly detect other organisms. Analyses of protein, lactate dehydrogenase (LDH), glucose and pH play important roles in the management of pleural effusions in adult. These studies are not always routinely performed in pediatrics, and with only a few reports available, their role in pediatrics is not yet clear.[35]

Management of parapneumonic effusions and empyemas in children is controversial. Sonographic evaluation is carried out to define whether loculations are present and provide guidance for the thoracentesis. Intravenous antibiotics should be started, with coverage for the common organisms *S. aureus* and *S. pneumoniae,* with consideration given to the pattern of antibiotic resistance in the community. Therapy can be adjusted once an organism has been identified from either pleural fluid or blood culture. After adequate antibiotic coverage, there is significant debate about additional therapies of pleural infections, in particular about surgical intervention with chest tube drainage, fibrinolytic therapy and VATS. All these therapies have been reported to be successful. Most clinicians agree that if the fluid accumulation is large enough to cause significant respiratory symptoms, then the fluid should be drained with a chest tube; many would suggest that chest tubes are needed for all empyemas.

Studies of intrapleural fibrinolytic therapy in adults do not support its use for the treatment of pleural infection.[40,41] In contrast, a randomized trial of intrapleural urokinase in children was associated with shorter hospital stay.[4] A prospective study comparing urokinase and VATS found no difference in outcomes, and recommended urokinase as the treatment option.[42] A retrospective report of primary VATS versus non-operative therapy[43] and a small prospective study of VATS[44] suggested that primary VATS therapy was superior. There is a paucity of data on simple medical therapy. In a report of 14 patients treated with intravenous antibiotics and simple chest tube drain, all patients completely recovered without aggressive surgical intervention.[45] Routine chest tubes for all empyemas in children was challenged in study of 65 patients.[46] In the conservatively managed group, the patients received a chest tube only if there was significant mediastinal shift, respiratory distress or uncontrolled infection. These patients did just as well as the patients who had chest tubes placed for large pleural effusions and/or fibrinopurulent effusion.

All agree that appropriate antibiotic therapy is the mainstay of therapy. While the controversy continues regarding other aspects of care, the good news is that children do well with all the currently proposed therapies.[35] There are several factors that likely contribute to the conflicting results. Many studies are small and retrospective. There is no consistent definition of the patients in the studies. Many patients are referred after failure of primary antibiotic therapy. Not all studies utilized similar diagnostic studies, including analyses of pleural fluid. Studies are not consistent in the outcome measures, should it be length of stay or pulmonary outcomes. In pediatrics, one of the goals of therapy is not to just maintain lung function, but also not to interfere with future lung growth.

There is little information about the long term consequences of empyema in children. A small studied looked at the results of spirometry and exercise testing in children following recovery from empyema.[47] No differences were found in children who had chest tube drainage and those who only received antibiotics. Another report measured lung function 3–24 months after discharge and found no evidence of restrictive lung disease in children with antibiotics and simple chest tube drainage.[45] Yet another study found a restrictive defect in patients at 3 months after treatment for empyema but most had normalized in 1 year.[48]

FUTURE THERAPIES

Improved diagnostic testing is needed to better characterize pediatric pleural effusions. A better characterization of patients, and the nature of their effusions, will result in improved understanding of the natural history of the effusions and optimal management.

SUMMARY

The incidence of pleural disease and effusions is uncommon in children when compared with that in adults and, in general, pediatric outcomes are better than that in adults which may reflect less severe co-morbidities. The underlying etiologies in the fetus and young children are frequently related to other congenital conditions. In the neonate, chylothorax is the most common pleural effusion. As children progress from infancy to childhood, parapneumonic effusions become more frequent. Pediatric-specific diagnostic and therapeutic approaches need to be developed.

KEY POINTS

- Pleural effusions in the fetus are frequently related to underlying congenital anomalies.
- Chylothorax is the most common pleural effusion in newborns.
- Parapneumonic effusions are the most common pleural effusions in children.
- Management of parapneuomic effusions in children is controversial.

REFERENCES

● = Key primary paper
◆ = Major review article
∗ = Paper that represents the first formal publication of a management guideline

●1. Montgomery MSD. Air and liquid in the pleural space. In: Chernick VBT, Wilmott RW, Bush A (eds). *Kendig's disorders of the respiratory tract in children*, 7th edn. Phildelphia: Saunders, 2006: 368–87.
2. Bush A. Update in pediatric lung disease 2006. *Am J Respir Crit Care Med* 2007; **175**: 532–40.
3. Maskell NA, Davies CW, Nunn AJ, *et al.* U.K. Controlled trial of intrapleural streptokinase for pleural infection. *N Engl J Med*; **352**: 865–74.
●4. Thomson AH, Hull J, Kumar MR, Wallis C, Balfour Lynn IM. Randomised trial of intrapleural urokinase in the treatment of childhood empyema. *Thorax* 2002; **57**: 343–7.
∗5. Balfour-Lynn IM, Abrahamson E, Cohen G, *et al.* BTS guidelines for the management of pleural infection in children. *Thorax*; **60** (Suppl 1): i1–21.
6. Longaker MT, Laberge JM, Dansereau J, *et al.* Primary fetal hydrothorax: natural history and management. *J Pediatr Surg* 1989; **24**: 573–6.
7. Bianchi D. Hydrothorax. In: Bianchi DW, Crombleholm TM, D'Alton ME (eds). *Fetology: Diagnosis and management of the fetal patient.* New York: McGraw-Hill, 2000; 313–21.
8. Waller K, Chaithongwongwatthana S, Yamasmit W, Donnenfeld AE. Chromosomal abnormalities among 246 fetuses with pleural effusions detected on prenatal ultrasound examination: factors associated with an increased risk of aneuploidy. *Genet Med* 2005; **7**: 417–21.
9. Bellini C, Boccardo F, Campisi C, Bonioli E. Congenital pulmonary lymphangiectasia. *Orphanet J Rare Dis* 2006; **1**: 43.
10. Jacquemont S, Barbarot S, Boceno M, Stalder JF, David A. Familial congenital pulmonary lymphangectasia, non-immune hydrops fetalis, facial and lower limb lymphedema: confirmation of Njolstad's report. *Am J Med Genet* 2000; **93**: 264–8.
11. Klam S, Bigras JL, Hudon L. Predicting outcome in primary fetal hydrothorax. *Fetal Diagn Ther* 2005; **20**: 366–70.
12. Smith RP, Illanes S, Denbow ML, Soothill PW. Outcome of fetal pleural effusions treated by thoracoamniotic shunting. *Ultrasound Obstet Gynecol* 2005; **26**: 63–6.
13. Kalfa N, Allal H, Lopez M, *et al.* Thoracoscopy in pediatric pleural empyema: a prospective study of prognostic factors. *J Pediatr Surg* 2006; **41**: 1732–7.
14. Kearney SE, Davies CWH, Davies RJO, Gleeson FV. Computed tomography and ultrasound in parapneumonic effusions and empyema. *Clin Radiol* 2000; **55**: 542–7.
15. Heller RM, Hernanz-Schulman M. Applications of new imaging modalities to the evaluation of common pediatric conditions. *J Pediatr* 1999; **135**: 632–9.
16. Rocha G, Fernandes P, Rocha P, *et al.* Pleural effusions in the neonate. *Acta Paediatr* 2006; **95**: 791–8.
17. Beghetti M, La Scala G, Belli D, *et al.* Etiology and management of pediatric chylothorax. *J Pediatr* 2000; **136**: 653–8.
18. Geismar SL, Tilelli JA, Campbell JB, Chiaro JJ. Chylothorax as a manifestation of child abuse. *Pediatr Emerg Care* 1997; **13**: 386–9.
19. Siu SL, Lam DS. Spontaneous neonatal chylothorax treated with octreotide. *J Paediatr Child Health* 2006; **42**: 65–7.
20. Noonan JA, Walters LR, Reeves JT. Congenital pulmonary lymphangiectasis. *Am J Dis Child* 1970; **120**: 314–19.
21. Esther CR Jr, Barker PM. Pulmonary lymphangiectasia: diagnosis and clinical course. *Pediatr Pulmonol* 2004; **38**: 308–13.
22. Alkrinawi S, Chernick V. Pleural fluid in hospitalized pediatric patients. *Clin Pediatr (Phil)* 1996; **35**: 5–9.
23. Alkrinawi S, Chernick V. Pleural infection in children. *Semin Respir Infect* 1996; **11**: 148–54.
24. Kiziltepe U, Eyileten ZB, Uysalel A, Akalin H. Prolonged pleural effusion following Fontan operation: effective pleurodesis with talc slurry. *Int J Cardiol* 2002; **85**: 297–9.
25. Cava JR, Bevandic SM, Steltzer MM, Tweddell JS. A medical strategy to reduce persistent chest tube drainage after the fontan operation. *Am J Cardiol* 2005; **96**: 130–3.

26. Chan SY, Lau W, Wong WH, *et al.* Chylothorax in children after congenital heart surgery. *Ann Thorac Surg* 2006; **82**: 1650–6.
27. Chaignaud BE, Bonsack TA, Kozakewich HP, Shamberger RC. Pleural effusions in lymphoblastic lymphoma: a diagnostic alternative. *J Pediatr Surg* 1998; **33**: 1355–7.
28. Pietsch JB, Whitlock JA, Ford C, Kinney MC. Management of pleural effusions in children with malignant lymphoma. *J Pediatr Surg* 1999; **34**: 635–8.
29. Wong JW, Pitlik D, Abdul-Karim FW. Cytology of pleural, peritoneal and pericardial fluids in children. A 40-year summary. *Acta Cytol* 1997; **41**: 467–73.
30. Easa D, Balaraman V, Ash K, Thompson B, Boychuk R. Congenital chylothorax and mediastinal neuroblastoma. *J Pediatr Surg* 1991; **26**: 96–8.
31. Goyal M, Swanson KF, Konez O, Patel D, Vyas PK. Malignant pleural mesothelioma in a 13-year-old girl. *Pediatr Radiol* 2000; **30**: 776–8.
32. Hoffer FA, Hancock ML, Hinds PS, *et al.* Pleurodesis for effusions in pediatric oncology patients at end of life. *Pediatr Radiol* 2007; **37**: 269–73.
33. Merino JM, Carpintero I, Alvarez T, *et al.* Tuberculous pleural effusion in children. *Chest* 1999; **115**: 26–30.
34. Ward MA. Lower respiratory tract infections in adolescents. *Adolesc Med* 2000; **11**: 251–62.
●35. Jaffe A, Balfour-Lynn IM. Management of empyema in children. *Pediatr Pulmonol* 2005; **40**: 148–56.
36. Schultz KD, Fan LL, Pinsky J, *et al.* The changing face of pleural empyemas in children: epidemiology and management. *Pediatrics* 2004; **113**: 1735–40.
37. Hardie WD, Roberts NE, Reising SF, Christie CD. Complicated parapneumonic effusions in children caused by penicillin-nonsusceptible *Streptococcus pneumoniae*. *Pediatrics* 1998; **101**: 388–92.
38. Tan TQ, Mason EO Jr, Barson WJ, *et al.* Clinical characteristics and outcome of children with pneumonia attributable to penicillin-susceptible and penicillin-nonsusceptible *Streptococcus pneumoniae*. *Pediatrics* 1998; **102**: 1369–75.
39. Le Monnier A, Carbonnelle E, Zahar JR, *et al.* Microbiological diagnosis of empyema in children: comparative evaluations by culture, polymerase chain reaction, and pneumococcal antigen detection in pleural fluids. *Clin Infect Dis* 2006; **42**: 1135–40.
40. Maskell N, Nunn A, Davies RJ. Intrapleural streptokinase for pleural infection. *Br Med J* 2006; **332**: 552.
41. Cameron R, Davies HR. Intra-pleural fibrinolytic therapy versus conservative management in the treatment of parapneumonic effusions and empyema. *Cochrane Database Syst Rev* 2004; **2**: CD002312.
42. Sonnappa S, Cohen G, Owens CM, *et al.* Comparison of urokinase and video-assisted thoracoscopic surgery for treatment of childhood empyema. *Am J Respir Crit Care Med* 2006; **174**: 221–7.
43. Avansino JR, Goldman B, Sawin RS, Flum DR. Primary operative versus nonoperative therapy for pediatric empyema: a meta-analysis. *Pediatrics* 2005; **115**: 1652–9.
44. Kurt BA, Winterhalter KM, Connors RH, Betz BW, Winters JW. Therapy of parapneumonic effusions in children: video-assisted thoracoscopic surgery versus conventional thoracostomy drainage. *Pediatrics* 2006; **118**: e547–53.
45. Satish B, Bunker M, Seddon P. Management of thoracic empyema in childhood: does the pleural thickening matter? *Arch Dis Child* 2003; **88**: 918–21.
46. Epaud R, Aubertin G, Larroquet M, *et al.* Conservative use of chest-tube insertion in children with pleural effusion. *Pediatr Surg Int* 2006; **22**: 357–62.
47. Redding GJ, Walund L, Walund D, *et al.* Lung function in children following empyema. *Am J Dis Child* 1990; **144**: 1337–42.
48. Kohn GL, Walston C, Feldstein J, *et al.* Persistent abnormal lung function after childhood empyema. *Am J Respir Med* 2002; **1**: 441–5.

45

Drainage techniques

HENRI COLT

INTRODUCTION

Health care providers today must do their best to choose the most appropriate diagnostic or therapeutic drainage procedure among those available for a particular patient. This is not always a simple task, demanding thought, expertise and experience. Indications should be individualized. Ideally, operators should be aware of or experienced in several methods of drainage so that choices are based upon what is best for the patient and not on what is simply available within a single physician's personal procedural arsenal. In the next paragraphs a step-by-step approach to several drainage techniques used to diagnose and treat patients with pleural diseases is described.

THORACENTESIS

Definition, indications and contraindications

Thoracentesis is defined as a drainage technique during which a needle is inserted into the pleural cavity in order to remove fluid. The major indication for a diagnostic thoracentesis is when a patient has a first episode pleural effusion unless fluid overload is the obvious cause. Such a procedure is safely performed at the bedside, in a special procedure unit or operating theater, in the intensive care unit or in a radiology suite using a variety of instruments.

The major contraindication is found in patients with bleeding disorders. Although caution is obviously necessary in patients receiving anticoagulants or thrombolytic agents,[1] using small needles, thoracentesis is safe even in these individuals. Several studies have demonstrated no increased risk of bleeding despite presence of a low platelet count (25 000 per mm^3 or less). As in procedures such as flexible bronchoscopy, patients with uremia and elevated creatinine levels are at potential risk for bleeding. Careful technique and the use of pleural ultrasonography further increase the safety of thoracentesis. Care is always taken to avoid the intercostal vascular bundle, the perforation of which, even in a patient who is not anticoagulated, can result in significant blood loss into the pleural cavity. Another contraindication to thoracentesis is a severely infected chest wall or overlying skin (pyoderma or herpes zoster). In this situation, thoracentesis should be performed in an area adjacent to but not part of the infected region.

Today, it is also well accepted that this procedure is also safe in critically ill or mechanically ventilated patients. In these patients, the major risk is that of procedure-related pneumothorax. Although the introduction of a small amount of air into the pleural cavity is usually without consequence, iatrogenic penetration or perforation of the lung parenchyma resulting in a visceral pleural tear and air leak frequently prompts chest tube insertion in mechanically ventilated patients.

Positioning patient for thoracentesis

Several positions are possible for patients undergoing thoracentesis. Most important is the overall comfort of the patient, operator and assistants. The patient might sit on the bed, or on a stool with their back straight and upright. The arms may rest on a pillow placed on a gurney or table in front of them. Behind the patient, a rotating or swivel stool is placed for the operator. To the operator's left or right, depending on whether the operator is left or right handed, a small procedure table holds all the necessary instrumentation. Once set up as a sterile procedure, additional nursing

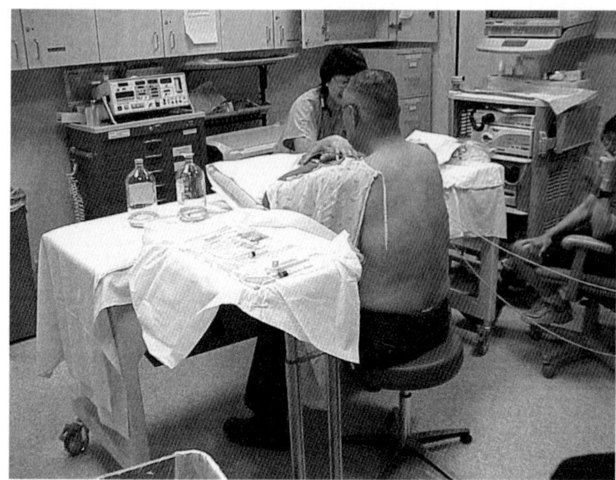

Figure 45.1 Patient position during preparation for thoracentesis.

or technician assistance is not actually required. Thus, a single operator without assistance readily performs thoracentesis. The object is for the operator to have ready access to all instrumentation, as well as to be able to comfort the patient during the entire procedure (Figure 45.1). The operator's assistant, rather than handle instruments, can monitor patients' vital signs, and provide verbal and physical reassurance to the patient during the procedure.

The patient is positioned sitting with their back vertical so that the lowest part of the hemithorax is posterior. Indeed, if the patient leans forward too far, the lowest part of the hemithorax moves anteriorly and no fluid flows posteriorly. In patients with small pleural effusions collecting in the costophrenic or cardiophrenic angles, patients can be asked to lean slightly to the right or to the left depending on the situation. When ultrasound guidance is used for thoracentesis, fluid is readily withdrawn using this posterior approach. Here too, although the patient maintains the same sitting position, the patient can be rotated slightly to the left or to the right, or be asked to lean to the left or to the right to identify ultrasonographically a small or loculated effusion.

On some occasions, patients are too ill to assume a sitting position. In other cases, patients are unable to come to a procedure suite and procedures must be performed at the bedside. When performed at the bedside, it is best is to have a small footstool placed on the floor for the patient to have a place to rest their feet. The bed should be elevated so that the operator does not have to stoop. The operator may sit on the bed behind the patient, or remain standing. I find it most comfortable for the patient to sit on the side of the bed with their arms and head resting on one or more pillows placed on a bedside table. Often, a family member is present to help support and reassure the patient. In other instances, procedures are performed with patients lying in a lateral decubitus position, lying on the side of the pleural effusion. In other instances, particularly in the intensive care unit with mechanically ventilated or unstable patients, the procedure must be must be carried out with the patient sitting upright. In these instances, the rolled bedsheet technique described later in this chapter is readily employed.

Selecting the area for thoracentesis

Physical examination will reveal decreased breath sounds in the area of pleural fluid and loss of tactile fremitous. Light percussion will become dull. It is generally taught that thoracentesis should be attempted one interspace below the spot where tactile fremitous is lost and percussion note becomes dull. One must recognize, however, the position of the diaphragm, which, in the lateral decubitus position might ride as high as the fourth intercostal space: failed thoracenteses are usually the result of inserting the needle too low in the hemithorax. A low thoracentesis attempt also increases the potential risk for hepatic or splenic perforation. Chest radiographs and or computed tomography scans should be reviewed.

Thoracentesis is usually performed through the posterior chest, several inches lateral to the spine in an area where the ribs are easily palpated. Posteriorly, the intercostal bundle is still near the middle of the intercostal space for a distance approximately 12–13 cm from the spine. It is only here that the intercostal bundle truly runs directly behind the rib in the intercostal notch. This intercostal bundle includes arteries, veins and nerves. It is also traditionally taught, therefore, that the thoracentesis needle should be introduced 'above the rib below', so that the needle is inserted just superior to the rib itself, substantially decreasing potential injury to the intercostal vascular bundle. I have often found that my selected site is three fingerbreadths below the tip of the scapula, slightly medial or slightly lateral to the mid-scapular line.

Pleural ultrasonography is a safe and simple non-invasive technique for determining the presence of pleural fluid when physical examination is unclear, or when radiographs and computed tomography scans suggest that the effusion is small or loculated. Pleural ultrasonography can be performed at the patient's bedside, as well as on fully sedated individuals, and requires no cooperation or effort on the part of the patient. In addition, pleural ultrasonography yields information about the quantity and quality of the pleural fluid, including the presence or absence of loculations and the precise locations of loculated pockets of fluid. Associated pleural masses and lung parenchymal abnormalities such as consolidation are also seen.

Most studies show that complications are decreased in patients undergoing thoracentesis with pleural ultrasonography compared with those performed without ultrasound guidance.[2–5] Practically speaking though, most thoracenteses can be safely performed without it. Should it be impossible to obtain pleural fluid, patients can then be referred to interventional radiology or to an interventional pulmonologist with expertise in pleural ultrasonography.

Usually, I recommend that most thoracenteses be attempted without ultrasound guidance, unless pleural ultrasonography is readily available within the operator's interventional suite. On the other hand, if the amount of pleural fluid is very small, or if the patient is critically ill and mechanically ventilated in the intensive care unit, pleural ultrasonography can be used initially.[6–13]

Thoracentesis instrumentation

Several needles and thoracentesis kits are commercially available. Examples include the Pharmaseal needle-catheter kit, distributed by Allegiance Healthcare Corp (McGaw Park, IL, USA), the Argyle–Turkel needle previously distributed by Sherwood, Davis and Geck, and the Arrow–Clark thoracentesis kits distributed by Arrow (Reading, PA, USA). Other needles include the Wang thoracentesis needle, and the Garg thoracentesis needle, each distributed by Bard Interventional Products, Melrose Laboratories (Melrose, NJ, USA). There is also a reusable stainless steel needle available called the Boutin pleural needle, manufactured and distributed by the Richard Wolf Medical Instrumentation Corporation (Vernon Hills, IL, USA) (Figures 45.2–45.4).

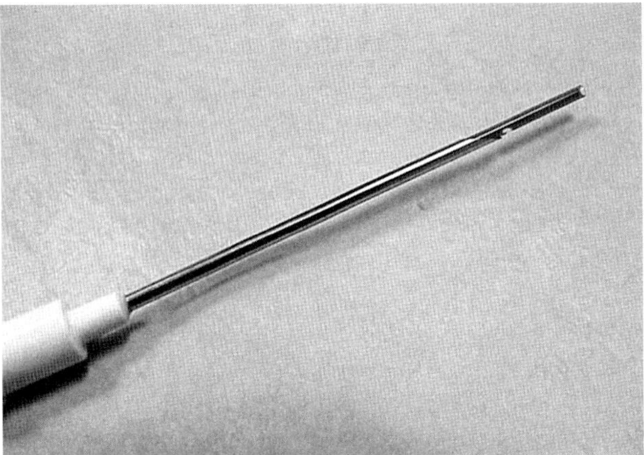

Figure 45.2 Pharmaseal thoracentesis needle and catheter (Allegiance Healthcare Corporation, McGaw Park, IL, USA).

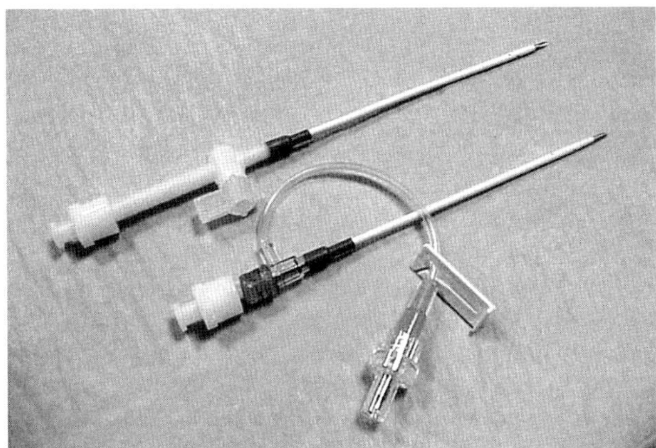

Figure 45.3 Wang and Garg thoracentesis needles (Meditech, Watertown, MA, USA).

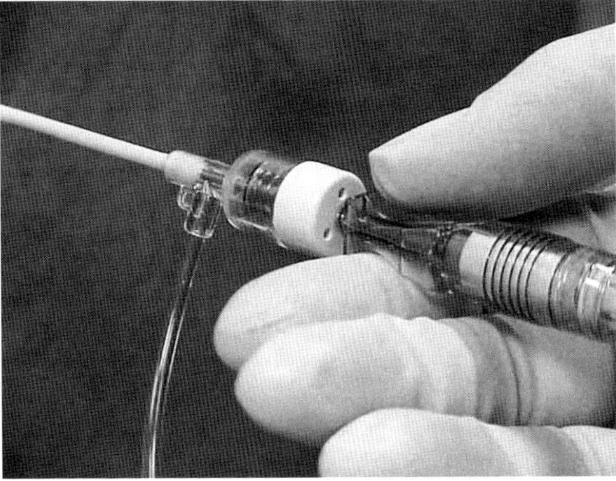

Figure 45.4 Turkel thoracentesis needle (Sherwood, Davis and Geck, St Louis, MO, USA).

General techniques

After having carefully explained the procedure to the patient and obtaining informed consent, the procedure can be started. Atropine 1.0 mg need not be administered, but should be available for potential subcutaneous or intramuscular injection, should patients become hypotensive and sweaty or develop other signs suggestive of a vasovagal reaction. Most patients do not require anti-anxiety medication, although those who request it might receive a small amount (most often less than 2 mg) of intravenous midazolam. With the patient seated, the physical examination identifies the site for thoracentesis. The site is cleaned thoroughly with antiseptic solution, which may include Betadine swab, gel or liquid solution. The area covered should be up to 5 cm around the selected site. I keep my sterile field extremely small – there is no need to prep the patient's entire back!

It is essential to anesthetize the skin and intercostal space with satisfactory amounts of anesthetic solution. Often, 5 mg of lidocaine is included in thoracentesis kits. Thoracentesis should and can almost always be a painless procedure. It is often taught to anesthetize the skin, the periosteum of the rib, as well as the parietal pleural. I find that anesthetizing the periosteum is painful and usually unnecessary. Once the site (intercostal space) has been selected, it can be maintained using two fingers of one hand placed onto the patient's posterior chest. Holding the syringe in the other hand, a small wheal is raised using 1 percent lidocaine and a short 25 gauge needle. Additional injections of lidocaine are performed through this wheal. The 25-gauge needle is replaced by a 22-gauge 1 or 1½ inch (2.5 or 3.8 cm) long needle, which is inserted through the wheal and into the intercostal space, directly above the rib.

Additional lidocaine is instilled as the needle is advanced. It has also been advocated that as the needle is advanced, aspiration should be followed by injection of small amounts of lidocaine every 1–2 mm (Figure 45.5).

I usually advance the needle rapidly through the intercostal space into the parietal pleura, injecting lidocaine as I go. With some experience, one 'feels' the needle traversing all the different tissues. I then aspirate when I feel that I am inside the pleural cavity, and once I have a small amount of pleural fluid coming up into the syringe, I pull my needle back slightly and then inject additional lidocaine into the parietal pleura. I withdraw the needle, and maintaining my thoracentesis site in position using two fingers of my left hand, I proceed to make a small stab incision with a #11 scalpel, which allows me to easily insert my thoracentesis trocar or needle and catheter ensemble. Regardless of the instrument used, the goal is to introduce the catheter along the same needle track. Once 50 mL pleural fluid is withdrawn into a 50 mL syringe attached to the catheter, the needle is then retracted up into the catheter so that there is no sharp object remaining within the pleural space during fluid removal and eventual lung re-expansion.[14] The pleural catheter is then advanced as additional pleural fluid is aspirated into the 50 cc syringe.

There are occasions when pleural fluid is not readily obtained. In these cases, it is possible that: (1) the needle was too short (this is often the case when patients have abundant subcutaneous tissue or extensive pleural thickening; thoracentesis in obese patients can be particularly difficult); (2) the needle itself or catheter was not inserted exactly along the track that allowed initial identification of pleural fluid; (3) the catheter may have been kinked or bent on insertion; (4) the small rim of pleural fluid is too thin and may have been missed as the needle was inserted; or (5) no pleural fluid is present in the hemithorax. Personally, I have found that it is extremely rare that a 1½ inch (3.8 cm) needle need be replaced with a longer needle.

What if all does not go smoothly? Lung perforation will usually be identified when air bubbles are obtained during the thoracentesis, particularly when local anesthetic is still present within a syringe and the needle is inserted into the chest cavity. Should this occur, and thoracentesis still needs to be performed, it may be necessary to change the site for needle entry, usually dropping down one intercostal space. Most lung perforations do not result in clinically significant pneumothorax, but one should always obtain a post-procedure chest radiograph if lung perforation is suspected. In general, I do not obtain a post-procedure chest radiograph unless I need to document the evacuation of all fluid as a baseline film in case of recurrent symptoms, or if symptoms are encountered suggestive of pneumothorax, hemothorax, or trapped lung. Should a dry tap occur and neither fluid nor air bubbles be obtained on the initial thoracentesis, it is possible that the needle was inserted an intercostal space too low. In this case, it may be necessary to repeat the procedure one intercostal

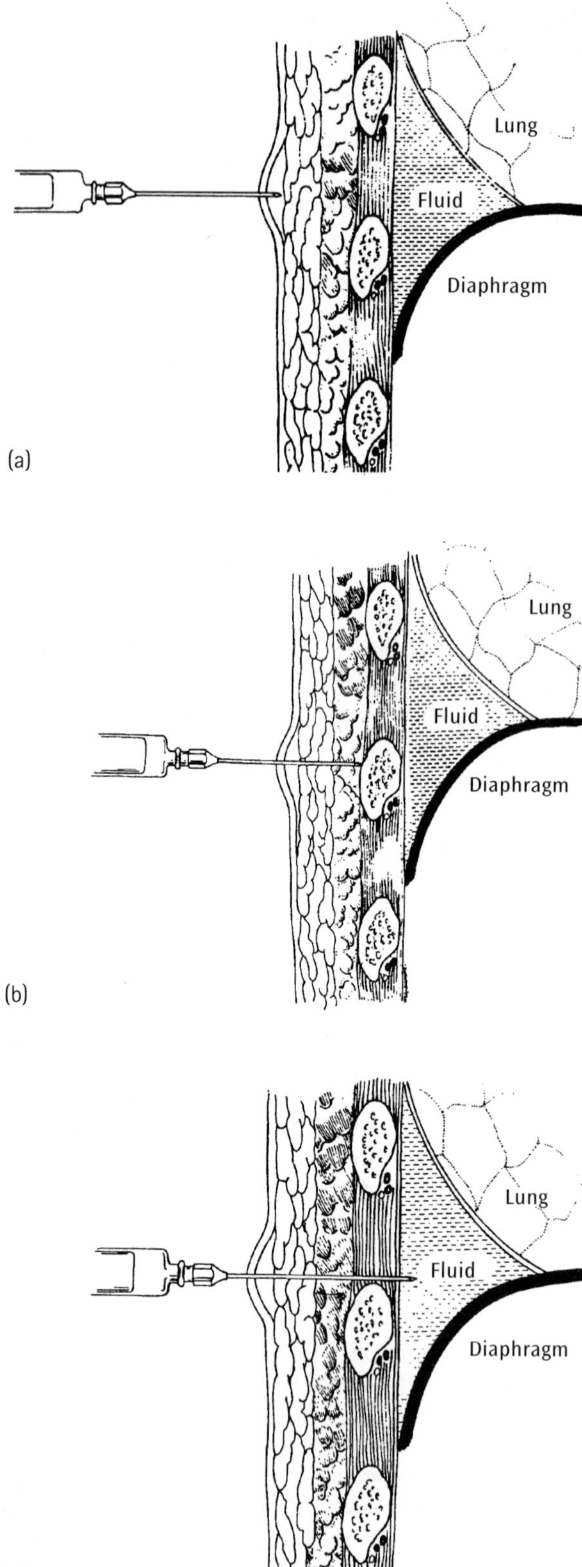

Figure 45.5 Diagnostic thoracentesis. (a) The skin is injected using a 25-gauge needle with a local anesthetic agent. (b) The periosteum is injected with the local anesthetic. (c) The pleural space is entered, and pleural fluid is obtained. (From Light RW, *Pleural diseases*, 3rd edn. Lippincott, Williams and Wilkins, 1995, Figure 23.2, with permission.)

space above the initial insertion site. In general, it is almost always safe to use a small fine needle of 22 or 25 gauge.

Examples of specific techniques

BEDSIDE THORACENTESIS IN CRITICALLY ILL PATIENTS USING 'THE ROLLED BED SHEET TECHNIQUE'

The rolled bed sheet technique allows for the placement of the seated patient into an optimum position for thoracentesis or for ultrasound guided thoracentesis.[15] I have found this technique to be particularly helpful because the risks of patient positioning, which in the intensive care unit may be associated with accidental extubation, loss of central venous access or deterioration of hemodynamic status, are diminished. A bedsheet is rolled lengthwise and then placed gently behind the patient's back. The head of the bed is raised, as the bedsheet is easily slid down behind the patient's back to the level of the scapula before lowering the head of the bed again. While each end of the bedsheet is held by an assistant and pulled forward toward the foot of the bed, the operator has room to work behind the patient, who is kept in the sitting position throughout the procedure (Figure 45.6).

THE REUSABLE BOUTIN PLEURAL PUNCTURE NEEDLE

The Boutin pleural needle manufactured by the Richard Wolf Company (Vernon Hills, IL, USA) is a stainless steel reusable needle designed for performing thoracentesis. It is a large-bore 2.8 mm diameter three-part instrument with an 80 mm working length. It is comprised of an outer cannula with a open–shut tab at one end, a blunt trochar and a sharp inner trochar (Figure 45.7). After making a small stab incision with a #11 scalpel, the Boutin needle is assembled with the sharp trochar inside the outer cannula. The shaft of the needle is held between the thumb and index finger while the proximal end of the needle is braced against the palm of the hand. The needle is then advanced through the subcutaneous tissue above the rib below and up to the parietal pleura.[16] The sharp trochar is replaced by the blunt trochar just before traversing the parietal pleural.

The advantages of this needle are less risk of traumatic puncture of the lung, simple use of accessory suction systems or manometers and the relatively large bore of the needle, which facilitates removal of large amounts of fluid as well as fibrin, blood or pus. Because the needle is reusable, there is an initial non-recurring cost for the instrument, but the cost of each subsequent use is nil. Disadvantages include possible air entry at the time of the exchange between sharp and blunt pleural trochars and the potential laceration of an intercostal vessel because the sharp trochar itself has a cutting, pyramidal tip design.

THORACENTESIS USING THE ARGYLE–TURKEL SAFETY THORACENTESIS SET

The system consists of a blunt multisided spring-loaded inner cannula coaxilly housed within a 16 gauge conventional sharp beveled hollow needle. While the needle is advanced through the skin and intercostal tissues, the blunt cannula is forced into the shaft of the needle. When the tip of the needle encounters low resistance, such as pleural effusion or loss of tissue resistance, the spring-loaded cannula automatically extends beyond the bevel, protecting underlying tissue from further penetration. Although the procedure requires some feel, a great advantage for some operators is a green indicator on the needle housing which identifies the position of the blunt cannula. If resistance is being felt such that the sharp tip of the needle is exposed, the indicator is red. When resistance is lost, the indicator turns green. Therefore, once the needle is in pleural space, the indicator turns green. A one-way valve prevents any air entry after the needle is removed (Figure 45.4).

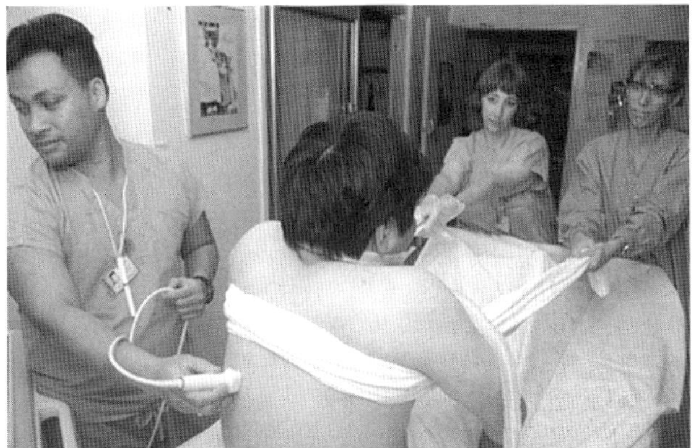

Figure 45.6 Bedside ultrasound-guided thoracentesis using the 'rolled bedsheet' technique.

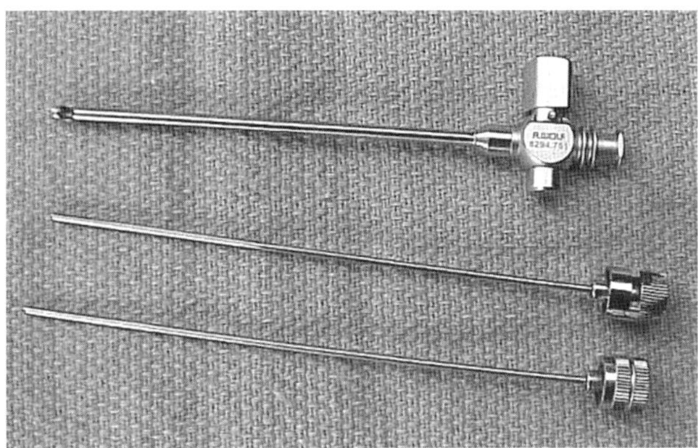

Figure 45.7 Boutin pleural puncture needle (Richard Wolf Corp, Bloomington, IN, USA).

THORACENTESIS USING THE BARD MILROSE WANG AND GARG THORACENTESIS NEEDLES AND KITS

Each of these needles is 17 gauges, with a catheter sheath diameter of 2.3 mm and length of 8 cm (Figure 45.3). Needles are available individually or in a procedural kit intended for single use. A small side port catheter is attached to the Wang needle sheath to facilitate fluid removal into Vacutainer bottles. The sheath septum allows for multiple insertions of the needle without passage of air. Rather than a small-attached tubing, this Garg needle comes with a stopcock feature, which prevents passage of air and also permits multiple insertions of the needle into the sheath.

Complications from thoracentesis

Complications from thoracentesis are the same as those from closed needle pleural biopsy or even chest tube drainage. The most common complication is a pneumothorax.[17–22] It appears, however, that the incidence of pneumothorax is reduced if experienced individuals perform the procedure. Iatrogenic pneumothorax is also decreased when pleural ultrasonography is used for guidance. In general, there are three reasons why a pneumothorax may occur following thoracentesis. The first, and potentially most consequential, is that of an accidental laceration of the lung parenchyma. This is easily recognized at the time of thoracentesis by air bubbles coming up into the pleural fluid. A second reason for air in the pleural space is that air was accidentally entered the pleural space through the catheter and needle at the time of thoracentesis. This rarely results in a large pneumothorax and air can be readily removed by attaching the catheter to a suction device or syringe. If left in the hemithorax, air will spontaneously be absorbed at a rate of approximately 1 percent per day. A third reason is the presence of a trapped lung.[23] This might occur in patients with chronic pleural effusions, empyema or pleural thickening, or malignancy and malignant mesothelioma. A thick pleural peel is present over the parietal and visceral pleura. The lung is not fully expanded, so after fluid is removed, the chest radiograph reveals a pneumothorax.

Other complications from thoracentesis include vasovagal reactions, cough, chest pain and hemothorax. Cough most frequently complicates a thoracentesis when large amounts of pleural fluid are removed. If a patient begins to cough excessively, the procedure should be stopped. Chest pain is infrequent, but might be related to anesthetic technique, needle insertion or evacuation of pleural fluid. Sometimes, chest discomfort can be decreased by decreasing the rapidity with which pleural fluid is withdrawn, or by removing pleural fluid using manual syringe suction techniques rather than a high negative-pressure Vacutainer bottle.

Vasovagal reactions are characterized by decreased stroke volume, fallen cardiac output, bradycardia and hypotension. Anxiety, pain, sight of blood and apprehension are promoting factors. When the reaction is noted, the procedure should be terminated and the patient should be placed in the reverse Trendelenburg position while vital signs are assessed. Recuperation usually occurs within 15 minutes.

Hemothorax is an extremely infrequent complication, but can result from laceration of an intercostal vein or artery. Hemothorax is probably more frequent after closed needle pleural biopsy than after thoracentesis but, regardless of etiology, may require thoracoscopic exploration and even open thoracotomy for additional diagnosis and management. A hemothorax should be suspected when a follow-up chest radiograph reveals an immediate reaccumulation of pleural fluid. Hemothorax should also be suspected if bright red blood suddenly appears within the syringe during fluid removal.

In patients with fever, new pleural effusions or symptoms suggestive of lung or pleural infection, and who have had a recent history of thoracentesis, bacterial contamination of the pleural space should be suspected. In these cases, I suggest repeating the thoracentesis in order to identify a new etiology for the pleural effusion. Other potential complications from thoracentesis include liver or spleen laceration. Soft tissue infection is also a possibility. Potential seeding of the needle track with tumor cells has been rarely reported in patients undergoing percutaneous lung biopsy, but is a feared complication of pleural procedures in patients with malignant mesothelioma.

Comments are warranted regarding the risk for hepatitis or *Human immunodeficiency virus* (HIV) infection due to operator injury. Needles should never be recapped during a procedure. Neither should needles should be placed onto gauze pads or back into the procedure tray because one might inadvertently pick up the gauze pad and thus stick oneself. When discarding sharps, they should be grasped using a hemostat, rather than one's hands.

In view of increasing concerns regarding patient safety, a few comments are warranted pertaining to the use of pleural ultrasonography for thoracentesis. This technology is frequently used in training programs, even for many routine thoracenteses, and helps decrease the frequency of thoracentesis-related complications, improve physical diagnostic skills and examine the pleural space for multiloculations that might impact management decisions, particularly for malignant effusions being considered for pleurodesis, and parapneumonic effusions being considered for drainage. However, ultrasound units are not always readily accessible from radiology departments and the cost of a portable ultrasound machine is currently more than $10 000. Certainly, if pleural ultrasonography is not needed routinely, patients can at the least be risk-stratified so that high-risk blind thoracenteses are avoided, and ultrasound can be desirable when effusions are noted to be small (on chest radiograph or computed tomography scan), multiloculated or in patients with poor lung function or significant bullous disease.

CLOSED NEEDLE PLEURAL BIOPSY

Definition, indications and contraindications

Closed needle pleural biopsies consist of percutaneous sampling of parietal pleura using a needle inserted through the posterior chest wall. These procedures are usually performed after one or two thoracenteses have been nondiagnostic. The primary advantage to obtaining parietal pleural tissue is that specimens can be examined by surgical pathologists as well as submitted for culture, special immunohistochemical staining or tumor markers. In addition, thorough drainage of the pleural effusion can be performed at the time the pleural biopsy is obtained.[24] Although closed needle pleural biopsy can be performed anytime a pleural effusion remains unexplained after thoracentesis, its yields are highest when parietal pleural thickening or an unexplained exudative pleural effusion is present in patients with suspected pleural carcinomatosis or tuberculosis. In these instances, closed needle pleural biopsy is an excellent alternative to thoracoscopy or repeat thoracentesis.[25–30]

There are few contraindications to closed needle pleural biopsy. However, the procedure should be avoided in any patient who is unable to sit quietly and cooperate or consent. In inexperienced hands, this procedure can be extremely painful, and often only muscle or fibrin without representative parietal pleura are obtained. In addition, because closed needle pleural biopsy is a blind procedure, inadvertent laceration of intercostal vessels is always possible. Therefore, patients with uncorrected coagulopathies, and patients with known bleeding diatheses, uremia, thrombocytopenia or anticoagulant use, should also be avoided. Percutaneous introduction of needles through areas of pyoderma, herpes zoster or cutaneous infiltration with neoplasm is contraindicated. Finally, patents with uncontrollable cough should also be avoided because a sharp inner trochar is often introduced into the pleural cavity during the initial insertion of the biopsy needle.

General techniques, patient positioning and selecting the right area

Closed needle pleural biopsy is performed similarly to a thoracentesis. Procedures are most likely to be successful and without complications when there is ample, nonloculated fluid in the pleural cavity. Biopsies are best performed with the patient seated, with the arms well raised so that the scapula are pulled upwards and outwards and the intercostal spaces are widened posteriorly. Before inserting the biopsy needle, abundant local anesthesia should be administered to the skin, intercostal tissues and parietal pleura. A wider and larger field of local anesthesia is warranted than for simple thoracentesis because biopsies might be obtained from several quadrants surrounding the initial needle insertion site, all through the initial needle tract. I often administer a narcotic intramuscularly or intravenously as well.[31–34]

The cope needle

The cope needle consists of four separate components: These are an 11 gauge 3 mm diameter outer cannula, a 13 gauge hooked biopsy trochar, a hollow beveled trochar and an inner stylet. Procedures are relatively straightfoward. After placing a syringe on the hooked biopsy trochar, the inner stylet is inserted through the beveled trochar and both of these are inserted through the hollow cannula into the pleural cavity. This is carried out as if performing a thoracentesis, although it will be simpler if a small stab incision using a #11 scalpel is made prior to inserting the trochar–cannula ensemble. Once the pleural cavity is entered and pleural fluid is obtained on aspiration, the patient should be asked to hum or hold their breath. The beveled trochar and inner stylet are then removed simultaneously. The operator places a thumb over the outer cannula to prevent inadvertent air entry should the patient inhale during this time. As the patient hums again the hooked biopsy trochar (with the syringe attached) is inserted through the cannula into the pleural cavity.

Pleural fluid is once more aspirated to confirm position. A perpendicular tab on the biopsy trochar indicates the direction of the distal biopsy hook. The ensemble is then gently withdrawn as the distal tip of the needle is tilted up to 45° downward. Pressure should be maintained on the needle tip and pleural tissues so that constant contact with the parietal pleura is assured. In order to obtain a parietal pleural biopsy, the entire ensemble should be withdrawn with the hook directed inferiorly. Some resistance will be felt as the hooked biopsy instrument engages the parietal pleura. While maintaining gentle traction on the biopsy trochar, the outer cannula is then rotated and advanced into the pleural cavity. Simultaneously, using the other hand which is holding the engaged hook needle, the operator must pull slightly but continuously. As the outer cannula is rotated and advanced, a small piece of parietal pleural specimen will be sheared off into the curetted biopsy hook. The biopsy trochar is then removed, and once more care is immediately taken to rapidly place the thumb or index finger over the outer cannula. This procedure is repeated three or four times in order to obtain specimens. At the end of the procedure, the needle is withdrawn and a small sterile dressing is placed on the wound (Figures 45.8 and 45.9).

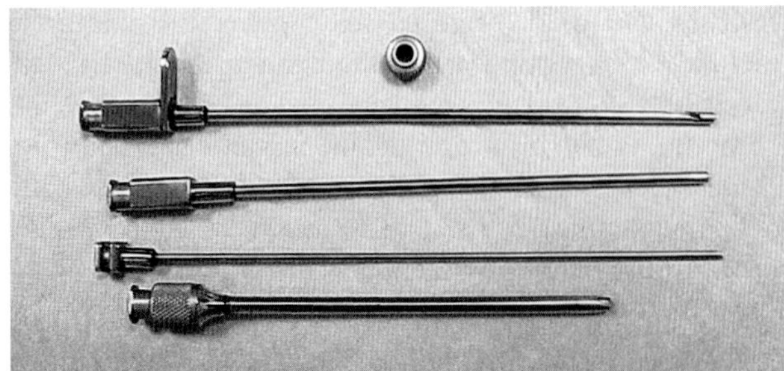

Figure 45.8 Cope closed pleural biopsy needle.

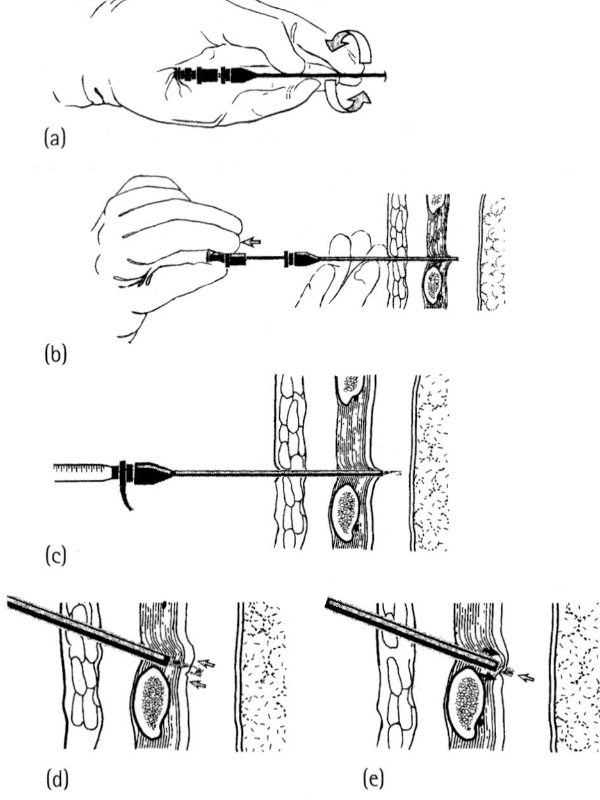

Figure 45.9 Cope needle biopsy technique. (a) The needle is inserted through a small stab incision using a rotating forward pushing motion. (b) Once in the pleural space, the inner trocar is removed while the patient hums or exhales. (c) Pleural fluid can be aspirated by attaching a syringe to the outer canula. (d) A small amount of fluid is again aspirated, and the entire ensemble is withdrawn as traction is maintained on the biopsy curette as it hooks onto parietal pleura. (e) While maintaining traction on the biopsy curette, the outer cannula is rotated and gently pushed back into the pleural space, shearing off the biopsy specimen caught on the curette. (From Colt HG, *Manual of pleural procedures*, Lippincott, Williams and Wilkins, 1999', Figure 10.2, with permission.)

The Abrams needle

The Abram's biopsy needle is a three-part needle consisting of a 4 mm diameter outer cannula with a beveled notch proximal to its tip, a hollow inner cannula and an inner stylet. The outer cannula's tip is blunt and usually will not damage the lung. The stylet is inserted into the inner cannula, which is then inserted through the outer cannula and locked into place by twisting it clockwise. The entire assembly is inserted through a small stab incision through the intercostal tissues and into the pleural space. As the stylet is removed, a 20 mL syringe can be attached in its place to the outer cannula. The hexagonal proximal tip of the inner cannula is then twisted counter-clockwise so that the beveled notch is pointing downwards. The entire ensemble is then withdrawn. Constant pressure should be maintained while tilting the distal tip of the needle up to 45° downward. When resistance is felt, parietal pleura has hopefully been caught inside the notch. The hexagonal proximal tip is then rotated clockwise. This closes the beveled opening. Thus, the cutting action of the rotating inner cannula samples the pleura. Once the specimen is obtained, the entire ensemble is removed from the chest. Obviously, more samples increase yield for representative tissue. (Figures 45.10 and 45.11).

Complications from closed needle pleural biopsy

Closed needle pleural biopsy should be a painless procedure. Abundant local anesthesia to the skin, intercostal tissues and parietal pleura is mandatory. Procedure-related complications include pneumothorax, both from introduction of a small amount of air during the procedure (which might be expected in up to 15 percent of cases), or by causing laceration of lung parenchyma. A chest radiograph is almost always warranted after closed needle pleural biopsy.

Other procedure-related complications include subcutaneous emphysema, pneumomediastinum, vasovagal reactions and hemothorax.[35,36] On rare occasions, a closed

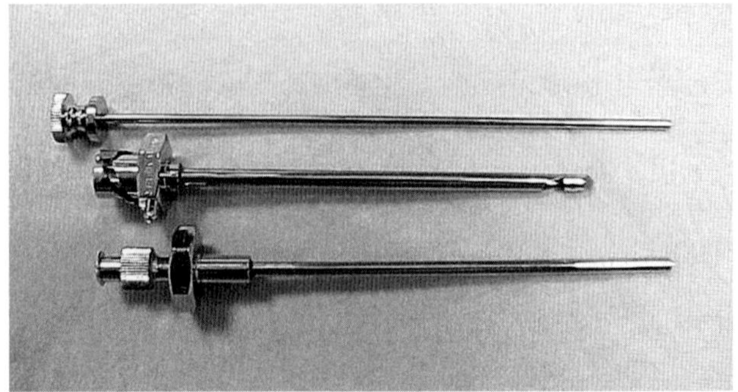

Figure 45.10 Abrams pleural biopsy needle.

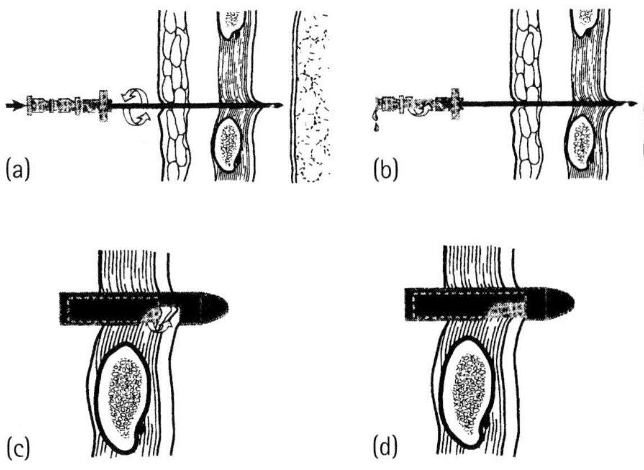

Figure 45.11 Abrams needle biopsy technique. (a) The needle is inserted through a stab incision into the pleural space using a gentle rotating forward movement. (b) If the patient hums as the stylet is removed, pleural fluid will be evacuated. (c) To avoid pneumothorax from air entry during inspiration, place a syringe onto the inner cannula. The hexagonal grip of the inner cannula is twisted counterclockwise so that the beveled notch is oriented downward. The ensemble is then gently withdrawn until resistance is felt and the parietal pleura is caught in the notch. (d) By rotating the hexagonal grip clockwise, the beveled opening is closed, shearing the specimen off into the cannula. The entire needle is then withdrawn from the pleural space. (From Colt HG, *Manual of pleural procedures*, Lippincott, Williams and Wilkins, 1999, Figure 10.3, with permission.)

pleural biopsy needle samples the liver, spleen or kidney. One should therefore be particularly careful to never perform closed needle pleural biopsy too low.

A comment is warranted pertaining to the apparent decline in the number of closed-needle pleural biopsies being performed in Europe, Asia and the USA. Thoracoscopy and flex-rigid pleuroscopy[37,38] are excellent alternatives to blind sampling, and provide the added benefit of removing all pleural fluid, evaluating the visceral and parietal pleural surfaces, breaking down adhesions to enhance lung expansion, and obtain forceps biopsies. In addition, increasingly, measurements of adenosine deaminase assist in making a diagnosis of tuberculous pleurisy, and increased use of computed tomography helps with differential diagnosis of malignant and nonmalignant effusions. Only time will tell whether closed needle biopsy becomes an antiquated technique.[39]

CHEST TUBES

Definition, indications and contraindications

Chest tube drainage consists of a percutaneous insertion of a small- or large-bore tube, usually made of silicone or polyurethane, into the pleural cavity.[40] This procedure is warranted in certain patients with pleural and pulmonary diseases. Major indications for chest tube placement include patients with pneumothorax, empyema, recurrent pleural effusions, complicated parapneumonic effusions, hemothorax, patients undergoing pleurodesis and after thoracic surgery.

Patients requiring chest tubes are often acutely ill.[41–50] Comorbidities might include coagulopathy, hemodynamic compromise, chronic or terminal illness, malignancy, cardiac dysfunction, sepsis and malnutrition. Although risks of chest tube drainage must always be considered, usually if there is an indication for chest tube placement, the procedure is performed regardless of risk. These risks include bleeding at the incision site, hemorrhage or pneumothorax related to inadvertent tearing of pleural adhesions or lung tissue, insertion of the tube into the heart, abdomen or pulmonary arteries, and hypersensitivity or allergy to medications used for analgesia or anesthesia. Difficulties are sometimes encountered if the patient has abnormal body habitus or cannot be positioned in such a way that allows proper chest tube insertion. Risks can be diminished by correcting coagulopathies, using ultrasound or CT guidance in selected instances (such as loculated pleural effusions or loculated pneumothoraces), maintaining platelet counts greater than 25 000 and serum creatinine below 6 mg/dL, or referring for thoracoscopy, rib resection or open thoracotomy.

Insertion techniques

INSERTING SMALL-BORE CHEST TUBES

Small-bore chest tubes (less than 20 French) are usually placed to evacuate small or loculated pleural effusions and to evacuate air in case of iatrogenic pneumothorax.[51–53] This might also be necessary when pneumothorax occurs after a transbronchial lung biopsy. Small-caliber tubes are inserted using catheter systems such as the catheter over/through needle technique and the catheter over guide wire (Seldinger) technique (Figure 45.12). When using the catheter over/through needle technique, procedures are begun just as if performing a thoracentesis. With the needle attached to a syringe, the needle is pointed towards the intrapleural location of interest. A catheter sheath is usually inserted over or through the needle while holding an introducer. In case of pneumothorax, these catheters are directed towards the apex, whereas in case of pleural effusions, catheters are directed inferiorly and posteriorly into the costal diaphragmatic recess. The catheter is connected to either a bag or negative pressure suction system and is tied to the skin using non-absorbable sutures.

When using the Seldinger technique, an 18-gauge needle is usually advanced into the pleural space attached to a syringe. The syringe is disconnected while pointing the needle in the desired direction and a guide wire is passed through the needle into the pleural space. After removal, a

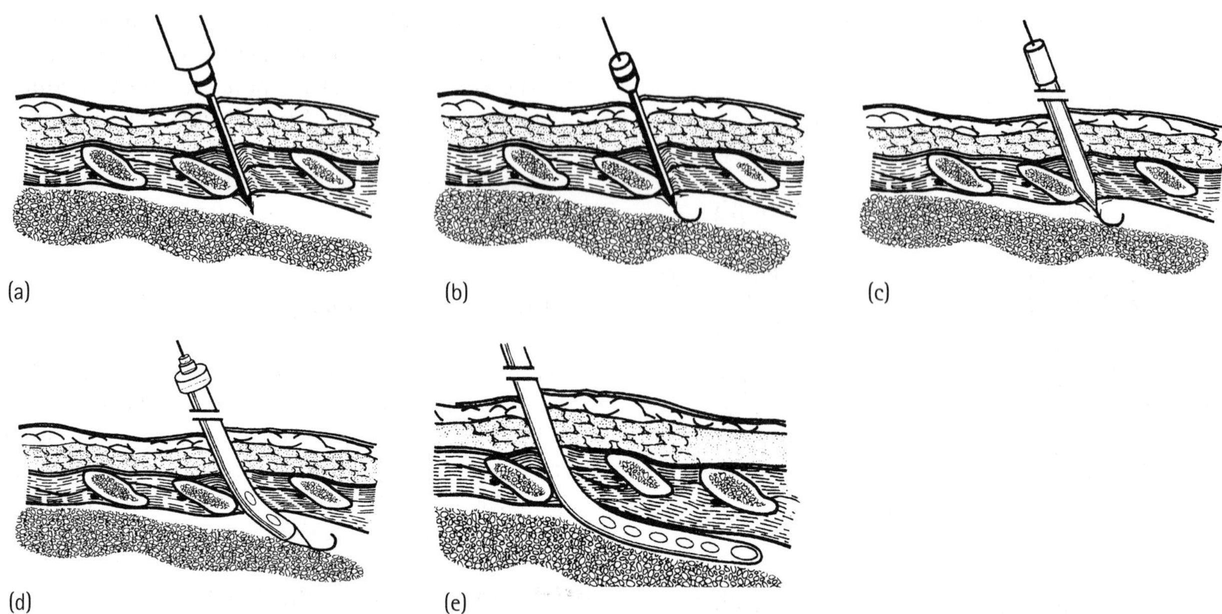

Figure 45.12 Catheter over guidewire (Seldinger technique) of a small-bore chest tube insertion. (a) The pleural space is accessed. (b) The guidewire is threaded through the needle. (c) The dilator is threaded over the guidewire, then removed. (d) The chest tube is threaded over the guidewire. (e) The guidewire is removed, leaving the chest tube in position. The chest tube will be secured using a simple stitch tied down onto the chest tube using a surgeon's knot. (From Colt HG, *Manual of pleural procedures*, Lippincott, Williams and Wilkins, 1999, Figure 12.5, with permission.)

small stab incision is made with a #11 scalpel. A dilating catheter is threaded over the guide wire and advanced through the chest wall and intercostal space using a rotating twisting movement of the hand. Small-bore chest tubes inserted using the above techniques include those manufactured by Cook Critical Care, Arrow International Inc, and Meditech[54] (Figure 45.13). Chest tubes have different characteristics in regard to shape, softness, firmness, curvature (some of them are curved at their end like a pig's tail) and size (from 8.0 to 36.0 French).

A third technique is used for inserting chest tubes mounted on a sharp-tipped pleural trochar. Most often, a 1–3 cm incision is made through the intercostal space after which the trochar is inserted. Once in place, an inner stylet is removed, and the tube is advanced into the chest. The trochar is removed by sliding it back over the chest tube. The chest tube is then clamped between the trochar and the chest wall. The tube remains clamped until it is attached to a drainage device.

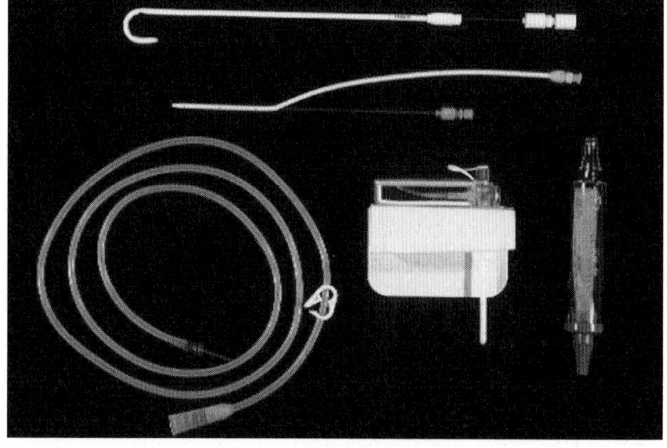

Figure 45.13 Small-bore chest tubes (from top to bottom: 12 F J-tip tube by Meditech, Watertown MA, USA; Cook CPT tube by Cook Inc, Bloomington IN, USA; Truclose 10F Thoracic Vent by Davis and Geck, Wayne NJ, USA; and One-way Heimlich valve by Becton Dickinson, Franklin lakes, NJ, USA).

INSERTING LARGE-BORE CHEST TUBES (BLUNT DISSECTION TECHNIQUE)

The advantage of the blunt dissection technique is that it allows the introduction of a finger into the pleural space in order to insure proper placement of the chest tube within the pleural cavity and to avoid adhesions. The technique is straightforward but not always easy, particularly in patients with abundant subcutaneous tissues, or when satisfactory analgesia has not been obtained. The skin is incised enough to allow introduction of the index finger into the pleural cavity. Intercostal tissues are dissected bluntly using Kelly forceps, allowing access to the pleural space (Figure 45.14). In case of pneumothorax, air will immediately be heard to exit the wound. In case of pleural effusion, it is common that fluid spurts forth through the wound. A finger placed through the incision site seeks pleural adhesions that might misdirect the tube towards the lung, apex or base. If adhesions are found, the probing finger can gently break them

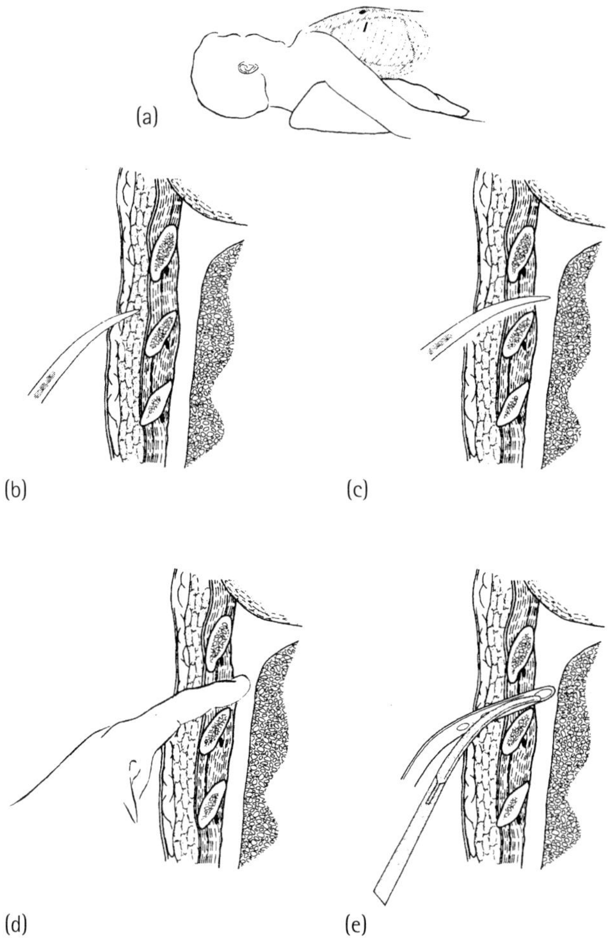

Figure 45.14 Chest tube insertion techniques using blunt dissection. (a,b) The 2–4 cm long skin incision should be parallel to the intercostals space and made smoothly through the dermis, subcutaneous tissues and fascia overlying the intercostals muscles. The intercostals muscle fibers are spread apart using the jaws of the scissors or hemostat. By placing an index finger in the incision, the space between the muscle fibers is enlarged and the ribs are easily felt. (c) Staying close to the upper margin of the lower rib, the intercostals fascia is sectioned, the intercostals muscles are spread further using the hemostat, and the parietal pleura is gently penetrated. (d) An index finger will make the hole bigger and allow one to gently push the lung out of the way. (e) After grasping the chest tube in the jaws of the clamp, guide it gently through the incision into the pleural space. Advance the tube well into the pleural space before releasing the clamp. (From Colt HG, *Manual of pleural procedures*, Lippincott, Williams and Wilkins, 1999, Figure 13.3, with permission.)

down. The large-bore chest tube (usually 20–36 French) is then clamped using a large Kelly forceps, placed through the site, and released from the clamp as it is directed into its appropriate position inside the chest. With the most proximal chest tube hole at least 2 cm within the pleural cavity, the incision is closed and the tube firmly secured to the chest wall. This technique has several advantages. These include the ability to manually palpate the pleura, palpate the lung, avoid adhesions and control the direction of the tube as it is inserted into the pleural cavity. This technique also allows placement of large-bore chest tubes in order to enhance the evacuation of blood, thick pleural fluid, or large quantities of air. The disadvantages of this technique are that it requires experience and has potentially greater risk of bleeding.

Suturing and dressing

There are several ways of suturing a chest tube in order to secure it to the chest wall.[41–54] For large-bore tubes, the method I prefer is to first place a mattress suture through each lateral margin of the skin incision. This is performed before the chest tube is inserted. An additional mattress suture is placed through the midportion of the incision. The two ends of this suture are kept free and can be used to close the incision when the chest tube is removed. After the tube is in, I tie each lateral suture down to the skin using a double knot, which is laid down flat, then secured with a surgeon's knot. The free end of each lateral suture is then brought up and wrapped around the chest tube, and tied in such a way to secure the chest tube firmly in place. When wrapping the suture around the chest tube, the free ends are wrapped tightly around the tube in opposite directions (Figure 45.15). When the chest tube is removed, these lateral sutures are unwound from around the chest tube. The chest tube is pulled while the patient exhales. An assistant pinches closed the insertion site using two fingers while the operator ties down the midline suture[55] (Figure 45.16).

Complications from chest tube insertion

Several complications can be associated with chest tube insertion.[56–63] These may be due to operator inexperience,

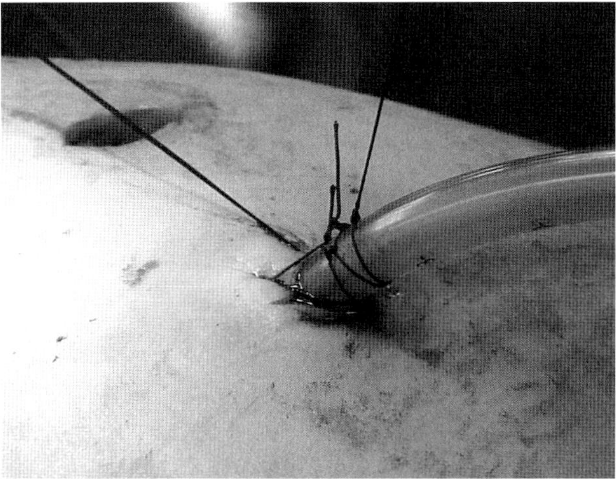

Figure 45.15 Example of sutured large-bore chest tube.

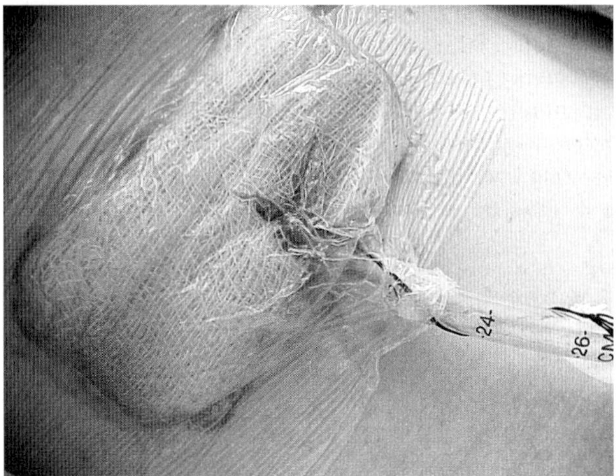

Figure 45.16 Transparent dressings allow rapid inspection of dressing sites.

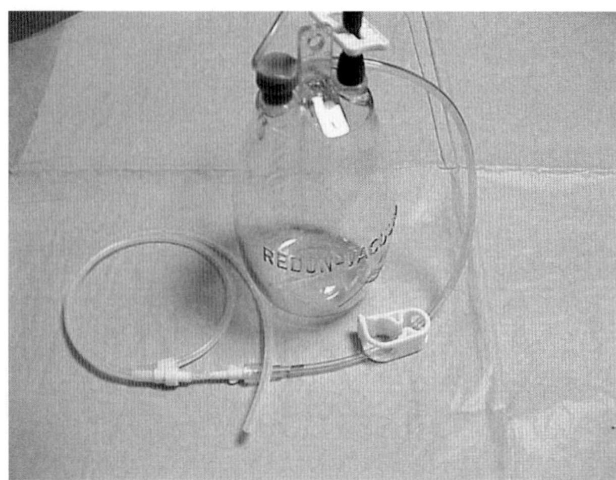

Figure 45.17 Home drainage apparatus (disposable suction bottle) by Denver Biomedical, Boulder CO, USA, for use with indwelling pleural catheters (hospital or home aspiration and pleurodesis).

the type of chest tube used or the patient's underlying disease. The risks of pain, bleeding and infection decrease with careful technique and careful observation, and intelligent use of analgesics. Almost all chest tubes cause some intrapleural adhesion formation. This can occasionally result in lung entrapment, particularly in patients with chronic pleural effusions or empyema. An inadvertent laceration of the lung at the time of chest tube insertion might result in persistent bronchopleural fistula.[64] This happens most frequently when tube-over-trocars are used, and might even require thoracoscopy or thoracotomy for repair. Chest radiographs should be obtained after tube insertion to confirm tube position. Tubes may be inadvertently placed into fissures, into the lung or even into adjacent organs such as the esophagus or liver. Tubes may be inadvertently tunneled into subcutaneous tissue and not even enter the pleural space. This occurs more frequently in obese patients. Sometimes, chest tubes may also induce temporary intercostal nerve damage from pressure within the intercostal space, or even cardiogenic shock when compression of the right ventricle occurs.

The Denver 'Pleurx' pleural catheter and shunts

Another drainage method that warrants description is the novel Denver Pleurx Catheter.[65–68] This is a 66 cm long, 15.5 French soft silicone catheter with a radio opaque stripe and side holes. Its proximal shaft has a single polyester cuff designed to promote fibrosis and prevent catheter migration. There is also a hub that contains a valve at the proximal tip of the catheter. The valve prevents inadvertent leakage of fluid or air into the pleural space. When the tube is not being used for drainage, a cap can be placed over it. Fluid drainage is accomplished using an attached vacuum bottle with a preconnected tube that contains a dilator at its other end and a clamp along its shaft. The dilator is inserted through the valve of the catheter. When the clamp is opened, aspiration of pleural fluid is possible. Drainage is performed independently by the patient as needed into small single-use collection containers (Figure 45.17).

The Denver Pleurx catheter has been approved by the Food and Drug Administration since October 1997. It allows safe, long-term outpatient control of selected patients with recurrent malignant pleural effusions regardless of whether pleurodesis is achieved. It is an excellent alternative for patients who have failed pleurodesis as well as in patients with trapped lung. In one study, 43 percent of catheters inserted required only a 24-hour hospital admission.[67] The tunneled catheter can be an excellent alternative to standard chest tube insertion and hospitalization. It is usually well tolerated, though some patients report chest wall discomfort. Complications include pneumothorax, subcutaneous emphysema and tumor growth along the catheter tract. Potential outpatient management of patients with recurrent malignant pleural effusions could substantially reduce healthcare-related costs in the individuals. In a retrospective review of 100 patients undergoing pleural catheter insertion between 1994 and 1998, outpatient pleural catheter charges up to 7 days after catheter insertion (including initial insertion charges) were an average of $3300.00, compared with inpatient charges of approximately $11 000.00.[68]

Catheters are placed through a small incision made on the mid-axillary line overlying the pleural effusion. Some operators use fluoroscopic guidance. Procedures are performed using conscious sedation. The skin and intercostal tissues are anesthetized with 1 percent lidocaine and the pleural space is entered using a small 18 gauge needle. A 0.03-inch (0.76-mm) guide wire is advanced into the pleural cavity. Additional anesthetic is administered locally

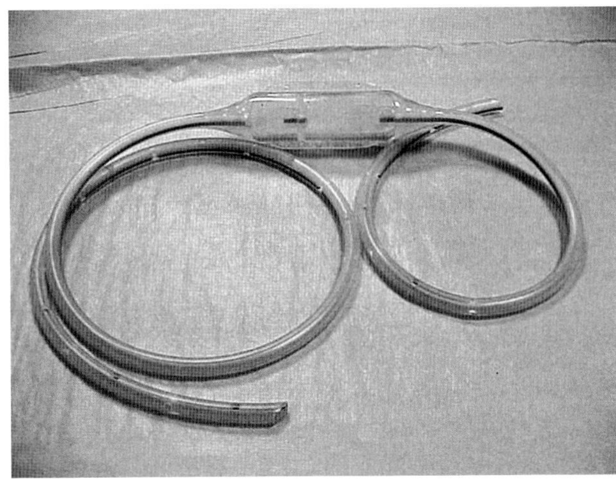

Figure 45.18 Denver indwelling pleuroperitoneal, or pleural-external shunt (Denver Biomedical, Boulder CO, USA).

to subcutaneous tissues along a route 5–8 cm anterior and inferior to this insertion site. The distal end of the catheter is tunneled through the subcutaneous tissue to the pleural entry site. The needle within the pleural space is exchanged for a 16 French peel away sheath. The catheter is advanced through the peel away sheath and the sheath is removed. The catheter is secured to the skin at its exit site and the pleural entry site is also closed using absorbable sutures.

Another mode of drainage includes placement of a similar pleural effusion catheter that is indwelling between the pleural space and the peritoneal cavity (the Denver shunt). With this shunt, inserted using a technique similar to that described previously, pleural fluid is manually pumped from the pleural cavity into the peritoneal cavity (Figure 45.18). Two devices are available for insertion. One includes a pump chamber that is approximately 7 cm long. This chamber is connected to a 15.5 French 49-cm long peritoneal catheter on one end, and to a 15.5 French 27-cm long pleural catheter on the other. The two catheters and the pump chamber can be completely implanted subcutaneously. A similar device can be placed using an external pump chamber, in which case pleural fluid is transferred into from the pleural space to the peritoneal cavity by pumping the shunt manually by grasping it between two fingers of one hand.

Results of tunneled pleural catheters have been promising. In one study, 250 procedures were performed for malignant pleural effusions in 223 patients during a 3-year period. Spontaneous pleurodesis occurred in 43 percent of the procedures and, overall, catheters could be kept in place within the pleural cavity for a median duration of 56 days, prompting authors to suggest that insertion of a tunneled catheter should be considered as a first-line treatment option.[69] In another study,[70] however, chronic indwelling PleurX catheters were placed in 17 patients with malignant effusions. Although catheter use was uneventful in 80 percent of cases and provided symptomatic relief with a mean duration of catheter drainage of two months, infections occurred in two patients (12 percent) and catheters became dislodged in three (18 percent). Attention to dislodgment, obstruction and infection certainly warrant close supervision, consideration for home nursing care and specific catheter-related education of patients, and family members and home care givers.

CHEST DRAINAGE DEVICES

Definitions, indications and contraindications

Chest drainage devices come in many forms. The objective is to collect pleural fluid, or to allow safe evacuation of air. Suction tubing is attached to the proximal end of a chest tube and connected to the drainage apparatus. This might consist of a simple collection bag, a bottle system or a single-use water column or valve-controlled Pleurevac-type apparatus. All chest tubes should be connected to a drainage apparatus of some sort. If suction is not required, a simple drainage bag might suffice for fluid removal using gravity drainage alone, or, in the absence of fluid, a one-way valve which allows expulsion of air from the pleural space might be desirable. Decisions regarding which type of apparatus depend on availability, physician biases, need for hospitalization or outpatient care, and desire for patient autonomy and ambulation.

The one-, two- and three-bottle systems

Many different drainage systems are available. Each can be attached to the chest tube in order to allow application of negative pressure to the pleural space, facilitate lung re-expansion and remove air or fluid from the pleural cavity. Usually, suction is placed at a fixed level of −5 to −20 cm of H_2O. Early collection systems were made of glass and consisted of one, two or three bottles placed in series. Using a one bottle system, the bottle served as both a collection container and a water seal, thereby preventing air from entering the pleural space on inspiration. The chest tube was connected to a rigid cannula inserted through a rubber stopper into the sterile bottle. Enough sterile saline solution or water was instilled into the bottle so that the tip of the rigid cannula was approximately 2 cm below the surface of the saline solution. When the patient exhaled, air in the pleural space would flow into the bottle and be evacuated through the 'waterseal', then out of the bottle through a stopper which contained a hole or vent. This avoided pressure from increasing inside the bottle. Of course, if fluid were also draining out of the chest, this fluid would accumulate inside the bottle, also 'raising' the level of the waterseal.

In order to circumvent some the disadvantages of the single-bottle system, a two-bottle system was developed using one bottle as a collection chamber for drained fluid, and another bottle connected serially to it, serving as a water seal chamber. Fluid accumulates in this first bottle, and air passes through the first bottle into a shorter cannula and into a second bottle, which is the water seal chamber. A suction pump such as an Emerson pump (which is a regulated negative pressure device) can be attached to the bottles. The amount of negative pressure applied during aspiration can be most readily controlled. However, a third suction control bottle can be added to the two-bottle system. In this case, a vent (cannula) in the suction control bottle is connected to a vent in the water seal bottle. When suction is applied, air enters the bottle through the rigid cannula if the pressure in the bottle is more negative than the depth of the cannula below the fluid. The three-bottle system was used for many years, but has the inconveniences of spillage, tubing, possible disconnection, fragility and decreased mobility because of multiple bottles on the floor at a patient's bedside (Figure 45.19).

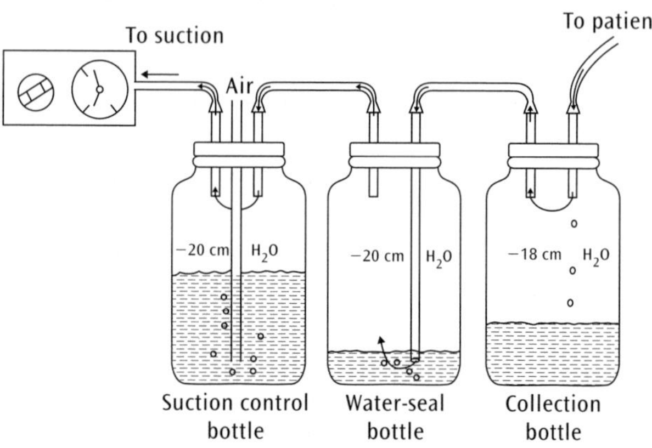

Figure 45.19 Three-bottle chest tube system. (From Light RW, *Pleural diseases*, Lippincott, Williams and Wilkins, 1995, Figure 24.7, with permission.)

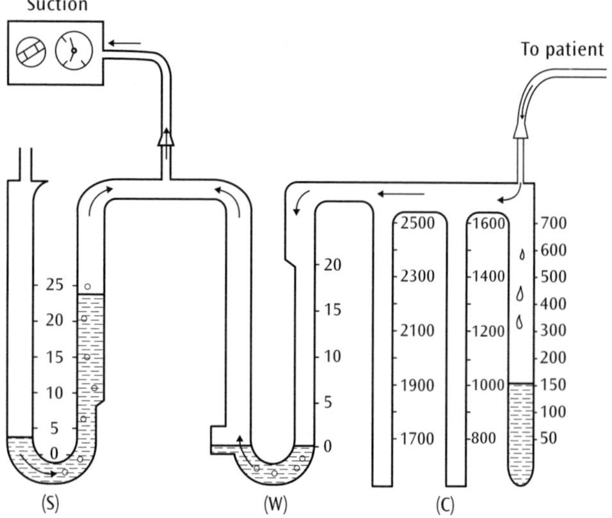

Figure 45.20 Inner workings of the Pleurevac system. (From Light RW, *Pleural diseases*, Lippincott, Williams and Wilkins, 1995, Figure 24.9, with permission.)

COMMERCIALLY AVAILABLE DRAINAGE SYSTEMS

These systems consist of disposable molded plastic units with three chambers duplicating the classic three-bottle system (Figure 45.20). These initially used water columns in order to regulate the amount of negative pressure exerted upon the pleural cavity. More recently they use dry suction units in which a valve replaces the water column. The advantage of these 'dry' units is their silence, and relative absence of spillage of fluid if tipped over. In addition, pleural fluid can be removed from the system for analysis, and patient ambulation is facilitated (Figure 45.21).

It is noteworthy that in both dry and water column systems, the water seal chamber always contains approximately 2 cm of colored fluid. This is the chamber reflecting the pleural pressures within the pleural cavity. Using these systems, negative suction can be applied at levels ranging from 0 to −40 cmH_2O of suction. Intermittent or constant bubbling within the water seal chamber is indicative of an air leak. This leak could be occurring from anywhere within the system, from the lung and pleural space to the suction tubing to connections to cracks within the plastic containers themselves. Patency of the chest tube is verified by observing inspiratory and expiratory fluctuation of the fluid in the water seal chamber when the patient is taken off suction. If there is no fluctuation of this fluid column with the patient off suction, the tube is said to be occluded. This means that there is no communication with the pleural space and that pleural pressures are not being communicated to the chest tube drainage device. Either (1) the chest tube is kinked or obstructed by clot or fibrinous debris inside the pleural cavity; (2) the chest tube catheter or rubber tubing going to the chest drainage device is kinked or crushed, perhaps by the wheel of a bed or a chair; (3) the lung is completely expanded, obliterating the drainage holes of the chest tube inside the chest; or (4) the chest tube or chest tube tubing outside the pleural cavity is obstructed by fibrin or blood.

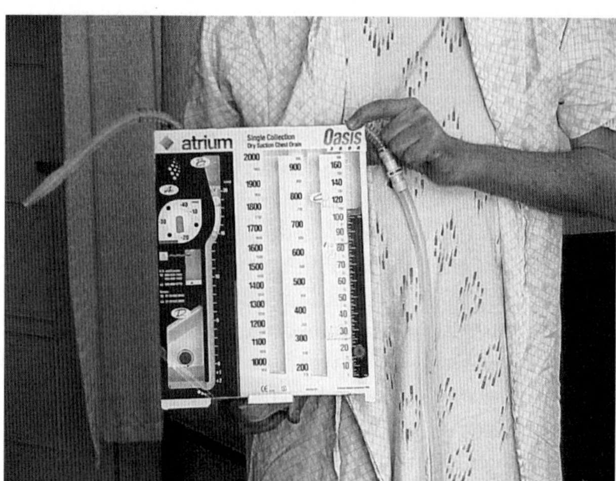

Figure 45.21 Patient holding commercially available negative-pressure pleural drainage apparatus.

When monitoring chest drainage devices, it is essential that the amount and character of drainage fluid or air be assessed regularly. On daily inspection, the height of the fluid column should be marked with a magic marker. The presence or absence of an air leak should be ascertained. The presence of bubbling in the water sealed chamber does not necessarily mean that there is communication between the lung and the pleural space. For example, if the chest tube is not inserted far enough into the pleural cavity, and one of its drainage holes is outside the pleural cavity and within the chest wall, dressing or beyond the skin, air can be suctioned from the atmosphere into the drainage tubing and through the drainage apparatus to the water seal chamber. The presence of an intermittent or constant air leak within the water seal chamber should prompt one to obtain a chest radiograph, examine all connections of rubber tubing, search for potential cracks within the drainage apparatus system itself and inspect the chest tube insertion site searching for drainage holes outside the skin. Tubes can easily migrate externally if they are not securely sutured into place and in patients who are obese, debilitated or restless.

The one-way Heimlich valve

The Heimlich valve is used most frequently in patients with pneumothorax who are going to be managed as outpatients. The chest tube is attached to a plastic one-way flutter valve using a five-in-one connector. As inspiration occurs, the thin flexible rubber tubing within the plastic container of the Heimlich valve collapses. This is because pressure outside the tubing is greater than pressure inside the tubing. During expiration, pleural pressure becomes positive, so the flexible rubber tubing inside the container is kept open, allowing air to escape from the pleural cavity, through the container and into the atmosphere. Because some patients with pneumothorax may also have small amounts of fluid draining from their chest, it is reasonable to attach the one-way Heimlich valve to a bag collection system that can then be taped to the patient's chest or abdomen. One of the upper corners of the collection bag should be cut so that any air accompanying the fluid can be easily evacuated (Figure 45.22).

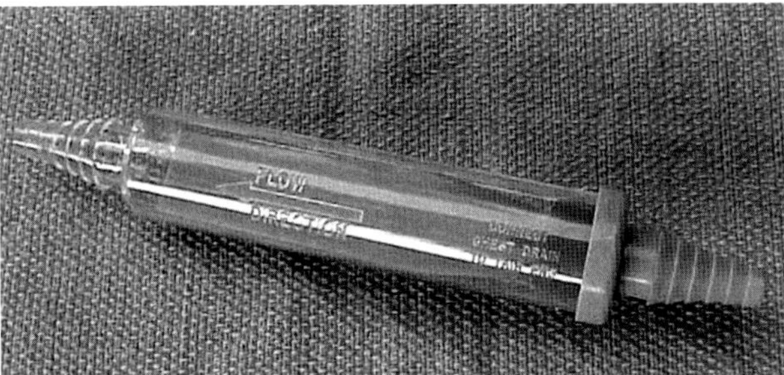

Figure 45.22 One-way Heimlich valve.

FUTURE DIRECTIONS

As new technologies become available, drainage procedures should become even more safe, and comfortable for patients. Novel devices might improve the efficiency of drainage techniques and pleurodesis, allowing operators to expand indications and improve curative or palliative care to patients with trapped lung, persistent pneumothorax or chylothorax, for example. Increased availability of Flex-rigid pleuroscopy, performed as readily as flexible bronchoscopy, might enhance the way chest physicians work up and manage patients with pleural effusions.[71] Regardless of advances, however, it is unlikely that any innovations will replace a careful physical examination and review of imaging studies prior to chest drainage. For many patients with complex pleural and pulmonary disease, a multidisciplinary approach involving medical physicians, surgeons and radiologists always warrants consideration.

KEY POINTS

- Drainage techniques of the pleural cavity are based on the premise of safe access, sterile technique, satisfactory re-expansion of underlying lung and avoidance of pleural or pulmonary injury, and adequate evacuation of fluid or air.
- A variety of needles, tubes and catheters are used. Each requires specific expertise and manual dexterity.
- Closed needle biopsy, although still performed for diagnosis of cancer or tuberculosis, is being increasingly replaced by thoracoscopy in many centers.
- There is no clear cut demonstrated advantage for small- or large-bore chest tubes. Therefore, operators should be aware of the advantages and disadvantages of each.
- New catheters and indwelling tubes that allow permanent evacuation of fluid, particularly in patients suffering from recurrent effusion and trapped lung, warrant greater attention and increased use.

REFERENCES

● = Key primary paper
◆ = Major review article

1. McVay PA, Toy PT. Lack of increased bleeding after paracentesis and thoracentesis in patients with mild coagulation abnormalities. *Transfusion* 1991; 31: 164–71.

2. O'Moore PV, Mueller PR, Simone JF. Sonographic guidance in diagnostic and therapeutic interventions in the pleural space. *AJR Am J Roentgenol* 1987; **149**: 1–5.
3. Petersen S, Freitag M, Albert W, Tempel S, Ludwig K. Ultrasound-guided thoracentesis in surgical intensive care patients [letter] [see comments]. *Intensive Care Med* 1999; **25**: 1029.
4. Sheth S, Hamper UM, Stanley DB, Wheeler JH, Smith PA. US guidance for thoracic biopsy: a valuable alternative to CT. *Radiology* 1999; **210**: 721–6.
5. Yang PC. Ultrasound-guided transthoracic biopsy of peripheral lung, pleural, and chest-wall lesions. *J Thorac Imag* 1997; **12**: 272–84.
6. Gervais DA, Petersein A, Lee MJ, *et al.* US-guided thoracentesis: requirement for postprocedure chest radiography in patients who receive mechanical ventilation versus patients who breathe spontaneously. *Radiology* 1997; **204**: 503–6.
7. Godwin JE, Sahn SA. Thoracentesis: a safe procedure in mechanically ventilated patients [see comments]. Ann Intern Med 1990; **113**: 800–2.
8. Hsu WH, Chiang CD, Hsu JY, *et al.* Value of ultrasonically guided needle biopsy of pleural masses: an under-utilized technique. *J Clin Ultrasound* 1997; **25**: 119–25.
9. Keske U. Ultrasound-aided thoracentesis in intensive care patients [editorial; comment]. *Intensive Care Med* 1999; **25**: 896–7.
10. Lichtenstein D, Hulot JS, Rabiller A, Tostivint I, Mezière G. Feasibility and safety of ultrasound-aided thoracentesis in mechanically ventilated patients. *Intensive Care Med* 1999; **25**: 955–8.
●11. McCartney JP, Adams JWD, Hazard PB. Safety of thoracentesis in mechanically ventilated patients. *Chest* 1993; **103**: 1920–1.
◆12. Moulton JS. Image-guided drainage techniques. *Semin Respir Infect* 1999; **14**: 59–72.
◆13. Strange C. Pleural complications in the intensive care unit. *Clin Chest Med* 1999; **20**: 317–27.
14. Schachner A, Aisenberg R, Levy MJ. Retrograde embolization of a detached polyethylene catheter. *Chest* 1981; **79**: 600–1.
15. Mahon RT, Colt HG. Bedside thoracentesis in critically ill patients: the 'rolled bedsheet' technique. *J Bronchol* 2000; **7**: 340–2.
16. Clark SJ, Vanselow CHG. Use of the reusable Boutin pleural needle for thoracentesis. *Bronchol*, 1999; **6**: 207–10.
17. Alemán C, Alegre J, Armadans L, *et al.* The value of chest roentgenography in the diagnosis of pneumothorax after thoracentesis. *Am J Med* 1999; **107**: 340–3.
18. Bartter T, Mayo PD, Pratter MR, *et al.* Lower risk and higher yield for thoracentesis when performed by experienced operators. *Chest* 1993; **103**: 1873–6.
19. Collins TR, Sahn SA. Thoracocentesis: clinical value, complications, technical problems, and patient experience. *Chest* 1987; **91**: 817–22.
●20. Colt HG, Brewer N, Barbur E. Evaluation of patient-related and procedure-related factors contributing to pneumothorax following thoracentesis. *Chest* 1999; **116**: 134–8.
21. Grogan DR, Irwin RS, Channick R *et al.* Complications associated with thoracentesis. A prospective, randomized study comparing three different methods. *Arch Intern Med* 1990; **150**: 873–7.
●22. Capizzi SA, Prakash UB. Chest roentgenography after outpatient thoracentesis. *Mayo Clin Proc* 1998; **73**: 948–50.
23. Villena V, Lopez-Encuentra A, Pozo F, De-Pablo A, Martin-Escribano P. Measurement of pleural pressure during therapeutic thoracentesis. *Am J Respir Crit Care Med* 2000; **162**: 1534–8.
24. Walsh LJ, Macfarlane JT, Manhire AR, Sheppard M, Jones JS. Audit of pleural biopsies: an argument for a pleural biopsy service. *Respir Med* 1994; **88**: 503–5.
25. Kirsch CM, Kroe DM, Azzi RL, *et al.* The optimal number of pleural biopsy specimens for a diagnosis of tuberculous pleurisy. *Chest* 1997; **112**: 702–6.
26. Chen NH, Hsieh IC, Tsao TC. Comparison of the clinical diagnostic value between pleural needle biopsy and analysis of pleural effusion. *Chang-Keng i Hsueh Tsa Chih* 1997; **20**: 11–16.
27. Emad A, Rezaian GR. Diagnostic value of closed percutaneous pleural biopsy vs. pleuroscopy in suspected malignant pleural effusion or tuberculous pleurisy in a region with a high incidence of tuberculosis: a comparative, age-dependent study. *Respir Med* 1998; **92**: 488–92.
28. Nance KV, Shermer RW, Askin FB. Diagnostic efficacy of pleural biopsy as compared with that of pleural fluid examination. *Modern Pathol* 1991; **4**: 320–4.
29. Roggli VL. Role of closed-needle biopsy in the diagnosis of malignant mesothelioma of the pleura [letter; comment]. *Chest* 1994; **105**: 321–2.
30. Suri JC, Goel A, Gupta DK, Bhatia A. Role of serial pleural biopsies in the diagnosis of pleural effusions. *Indian J Chest Dis Allied Sci* 1991; **33**: 63–7.
31. Kirsch CM, Kroe DM, Jensen WA *et al.* A modified Abrams needle biopsy technique. *Chest* 1995; **108**: 982–6.
32. O'Connor S, Yung T. A comparison of Abrams and Raja pleural biopsy needles. *Austr N Z J Med* 1992; **22**: 237–9.
33. Screaton NJ, Flower CD. Percutaneous needle biopsy of the pleura. *Radiol Clin North Am* 2000; **38**: 293–301.
34. Ogirala RG, Agarwal V, Vizioli, Pinsker KL, Aldrich TK. Comparison of the Raja and the Abrams pleural biopsy needles in patients with pleural effusion. *Am Rev Respir Dis* 1993; **147**: 1291–4.
35. Eng P, Colt HG. Fracture of Cope's needle in closed pleural biopsy [letter]. *Chest* 1994; **106**: 977–8.
36. Bhandari S, Sellars L. Splenic hematoma complicating pleural biopsy [letter]. *Postgrad Med J* 1995; **71**: 319.
37. Lee P, Colt HG. Rigid and semirigid pleuroscopy: the future is bright. *Respirology* 2005; **10**: 418–25.
38. Lee P, Hsu A, Lo C, Colt HG. Prospective evaluation of flex-rigid pleuroscopy for indeterminate pleural effusion: accuracy, safety and outcome. *Respirology* 2007; **12**: 881–6.
39. Silviestri GA, Strange C. Rest in peace: the decline on training and use of the closed pleural biopsy. *J Bronchol* 2005; **12**: 131–32.
40. Tomlinson MA, Treasure T. Insertion of a chest drain: how to do it. *Br J Hosp Med* 1997; **58**: 248–52.
41. Rashid MA, Wikström T, Ortenwall P. A simple technique for anchoring chest tubes. *Eur Respir J* 1998; **12**: 958–9.
42. Smith L, Baker F, McDougall C, Stead L. Removal of chest drains. *Nursing Times* 1999; **95**: 1–2.
40. Palesty JA, McKelvey AA, Dudrick SJ. The efficacy of X-rays after chest tube removal. *Am J Surg* 2000; **179**: 13–6.
43. Pacanowski JP, Waack ML, Daley BJ, *et al.* Is routine roentgenography needed after closed tube thoracostomy removal? *J Trauma* 2000; **48**: 684–8.
◆44. Carroll P. What's new in chest-tube management. *RN* 1991; **54**: 34–8, 40.
◆45. Carroll P. Exploring chest drain options. *RN* 2000; **63**: 50–4; quiz 56.
46. Collop NA, Kim S, Sahn SA. Analysis of tube thoracostomy performed by pulmonologists at a teaching hospital. *Chest* 1997; **112**: 709–13.
47. Gordon P, Norton JM. Managing chest tubes: what is based on research, and what is not? *Dimens Crit Care Nurs* 1995; **14**: 14–16.
48. Gross SB. Current challenges, concepts, and controversies in chest tube management. *AACN Clin Iss Crit Care Nurs* 1993; **4**: 260–75.
49. Martino K, Merrit S, Boyakye, *et al.* Prospective randomized trial of thoracostomy removal algorithms. *J Trauma* 1999; **46**: 369–71; discussion 372–3.
50. Altman E, Ben-Nun A, Curtis W Jr, Best LA. Modified Seldinger technique for the insertion of standard chest tubes. *Am J Surg* 2001; **181**: 354–5.
51. Tattersall DJ, Traill ZC, Gleeson FV. Chest drains: does size matter? *Clin Radiol* 2000; **55**: 415–21.
52. Gammie JS, Banks MC, Fuhrman, *et al.* The pigtail catheter for pleural drainage: a less invasive alternative to tube thoracostomy. *J Soc Laparoendosc Surg* 1999; **3**: 57–61.

53. Grodzin CJ, Balk RA. Indwelling small pleural catheter needle thoracentesis in the management of large pleural effusion. *Chest* 1997; **111**: 981–8.
54. Bell RL, Ovadia P, Abdullah F, Spector S, Rabinovici R. Chest tube removal: end-inspiration or end-expiration? *J Trauma*, 2001; **50**: 674–7.
55. Bailey RC. Complications of tube thoracostomy in trauma. *J Accid Emerg Med* 2000; **17**: 111–14.
56. Baldt MM, Bankier A, Germann PS, *et al.* Complications after emergency tube thoracostomy: assessment with CT. *Radiology* 1995; **195**: 539–43.
57. Chan L, Reilly KM, Henderson C, Kahn F, Salluzzo RF. Complication rates of tube thoracostomy. *Am J Emerg Med* 1997; **15**: 368–70.
58. Desai AV, Phipps PR, Barnes DJ. Shock and ipsilateral pulmonary oedema after tube thoracostomy for spontaneous pneumothorax. *J Accid Emerg Med*, 1999; **16**: 454–5.
59. Foresti V, Villa A, Casati O, Parisio E, De Filippi G. Abdominal placement of tube thoracostomy due to lack of recognition of paralysis of hemidiaphragm. *Chest* 1992; **102**: 292–3.
60. Etoch SW, Bar-Natan MF, Miller FB, Richardson JD. Tube thoracostomy. Factors related to complications. *Arch Surg* 1995; **130**: 521–5; discussion 525–6.
61. Shapira OM, Aldea GS, Kupferschmid J, Shemin RJ. Delayed perforation of the esophagus by a closed thoracostomy tube. *Chest* 1993; **104**: 1897–8.
62. Zieren J, Enzweiler C, Müller JM. Tube thoracostomy complicates unrecognized diaphragmatic rupture. *Thoracic Cardiovasc Surg* 1999; **47**: 199–202.
63. Cloutier R, Gignac MA. Pneumothorax following tube thoracostomy and water seal drainage. *Can J Surg* 2001; **44**: 387.
●64. Pien GW, Gant MJ, Washam CI, Sterman DH. Use of an implantable pleural catheter for trapped lung syndrome in patients with malignant pleural effusion. *Chest* 2001; **119**: 1641–6.
65. Pollak JS, Burdge CM, Rosenblatt M, *et al.* Treatment of malignant pleural effusion with tunneled long-term drainage catheters. *J Vasc Interv Radiol* 2001; **12**: 201–8.
66. Putnam JB Jr, Light RW, Rodriguez RM, *et al.* A randomized comparison of indwelling pleural catheter and doxycycline pleurodesis in the management of malignant pleural effusion. *Am Cancer Soc* 1999; **86**: 1992–9.
67. Putnam JB Jr, Walsh GL, Swisher SG, *et al.* Outpatient management of malignant pleural effusion by chronic indwelling pleural catheter. *Ann Thorac Surg* 2000; **69**: 369–75.
68. Vricella LA, Trachiotis GD. Heimlich valve in the management of pneumothorax in patients with advanced AIDS. *Chest* 2001; **120**: 15–18.
69. Tremblay A, Michaud G. Single center experience with 250 tunneled pleural catheter insertions for malignant pleural effusions. *Chest* 2006; **129**: 362–8.
70. Van den Toorn LM, Schaap E, Surmont VFM, *et al.* Management of recurrent malignant pleural effusions with a chronic indwelling pleural catheter. *Lung Cancer* 2005; **50**: 123–7.
71. Lee P, Colt HG. *Flex-rigid pleuroscopy step-by-step.* Singapore: CMP Medica, 2005.

46

Pleurodesis

HELEN E DAVIES, YC GARY LEE

Pleurodesis is the iatrogenic induction of symphysis of the visceral and parietal pleura. The aim of pleurodesis is to obliterate the pleural space and prevent the accumulation of fluid or air.

INDICATIONS FOR PLEURODESIS

The main indications for pleurodesis are recurrent, symptomatic malignant pleural effusion or pneumothorax. In selected cases pleurodesis is performed for benign, recurrent pleural effusion.

In the future there is likely to be a rise in the number of potential candidates for pleurodesis reflecting the increased incidence of malignant effusion in an ageing population and cases of secondary pneumothorax related to underlying chronic obstructive pulmonary disease.

Malignant pleural effusion

Malignant pleural effusions are common and affect 660 patients per million population per year.[1] In 20 percent of patients they represent the initial presentation of malignancy. Up to 50 percent of patients with breast cancer, a quarter of those with bronchogenic carcinoma and over 95 percent of patients with mesothelioma will develop a pleural effusion during their disease course.[2–4] Symptomatic fluid reaccumulation following drainage occurs in 70–90 percent of patients[5] and can significantly reduce quality of life. Pleurodesis may provide effective control of fluid reaccumulation (see also Chapter 25).

Pneumothorax

Pleurodesis in pneumothorax is indicated primarily to prevent recurrence (see also Chapter 42).

For patients with primary spontaneous pneumothorax, recurrence rates increase with successive events[6] and the risk of contralateral pneumothorax is also higher.[7] Pleurodesis is indicated in patients with a second ipsilateral pneumothorax, first contralateral pneumothorax, synchronous pneumothoraces, a continuous air leak or a spontaneous hemopneumothorax as well as in those with job restrictions, e.g. divers and airline staff.[8] No study has directly compared surgical and bedside pleurodesis in the setting of pneumothoraces. Based on results from observational studies, surgical pleurodesis is generally preferred over bedside pleurodesis via a chest tube, the latter usually being reserved for patients unwilling or unsuitable for surgery.

In those with secondary pneumothorax who have failed conservative therapy, pleurodesis is advocated as 45–67 percent of patients with a secondary pneumothorax will suffer recurrence[9–11] which are often symptomatic and may be life threatening.

Other

Benign, recurrent, symptomatic pleural effusions may also be treated with pleurodesis should conservative management fail (see below).

HOW PLEURODESIS WORKS

Pleurodesis is the obliteration of the pleural space through induction of pleural fibrosis. Pleurodesis is usually performed by the intrapleural injection of a chemical agent or by mechanical abrasion during surgery. These processes directly injure the pleura, causing acute pleural inflammation and denudement of mesothelial cells.[12] The mesothelial layer is later restored by cell migration and proliferation. The inflammation elicited may resolve (failed pleurodesis) or progress to chronic inflammation and fibrosis. If sufficient fibrosis is produced, symphysis develops between the visceral and parietal surfaces and the pleural space is obliterated (successful pleurodesis).

The coagulation cascade is also important in pleural fibrosis/pleurodesis (see Chapter 9). It is generally believed that fibrinous adhesions form a skeleton upon which collagen is deposited, to produce mature adhesions. Interestingly, nerve fibers have recently been demonstrated within adhesions.[13] Also, data suggest that angiogenesis is important in pleurodesis, and that antagonizing vascular endothelial growth factor (VEGF), a potent inducer of vascular formation, significantly reduces vascular density on pleural tissues and pleural fibrosis.[14] Similar observations have been made in pulmonary fibrosis models.[15]

The cellular source of the collagen deposition and fibrosis has been much debated. Myofibroblasts migrate into the pleural surface and deposit matrix proteins following talc pleurodesis.[16] Although fibroblasts are important, mesothelial cells significantly outnumber other cell types in the pleural setting. It is now recognized that mesothelial cells can undergo epithelial–mesenchymal transformation and become fibroblast-like. Mesothelial cells are known to produce collagen and some believe that an intact mesothelium plays a significant role in successful pleurodesis.[17]

Traditionally, the pleural inflammatory response is believed to be necessary for pleurodesis, as co-administration of corticosteroids inhibits the inflammation and the subsequent pleurodesis.[18] The levels of pro-inflammatory mediators, e.g. interleukin (IL)-8, tumor necrosis factor (TNF)-α and nitric oxide, in the pleural fluid are significantly elevated following chemical pleurodesis.[19,20] Neutrophils are attracted, via an IL-8 mediated mechanism, into the pleural space, followed by macrophages.[20] The activated macrophages also release IL-8 and monocyte chemoattractant protein (MCP)-1 and, together with the adhesion molecules on the mesothelial cells, serve to amplify the inflammatory response.[21] Pleurodesis is often associated with chest pain and fever,[22] which is likely the result of acute pleural injury and intense pleural inflammation. For instance, fever occurred in up to 62 percent of patients following talc pleurodesis[22] and severe pain was reported by >50 percent of patients who received tetracycline pleurodesis for pneumothorax.[11]

Efforts have focused on identifying the key mediators that promote pleural fibrosis downstream to the pleurodesis-induced inflammatory process, which can potentially induce fibrosis without causing pain and fever. Transforming growth factor-beta (TGF-β) is one of the most potent pro-fibrotic cytokines, and pleural fluid levels of active TGF-β increase in patients following talc pleurodesis (YCG Lee, unpublished data). Direct intrapleural administration of human recombinant TGF-β induces a significant increase in collagen deposition, and excellent pleurodesis in rabbits[23,24] and sheep,[25] at a rate faster than talc slurry.[23] In animal studies of TGF-β pleurodesis, no significant acute physiological disturbance or extra-pleural histological abnormalities were detected.[25,26] In addition, TGF-β has immunomodulatory properties: following the intrapleural injection of TGF-β, the pleural fluid levels of inflammatory markers (e.g. leukocyte, lactate dehydrogenase [LDH] and IL-8 levels),[23,24,27] are significantly lower than those following the injection of talc or doxycycline. Co-administration of systemic corticosteroids did not impair TGF-β-induced pleurodesis.[28] These results challenge the necessity of pleural inflammation in creating pleurodesis. It has been suggested that other growth factors, such as basic fibroblast growth factor, play a role in pleurodesis.[29]

WHAT IS A SUCCESSFUL PLEURODESIS?

No universally recognized criteria exist to define pleurodesis success. However, response to pleurodesis has been subdivided in many trial settings into complete, partial or failure. Complete response or 'success' is often considered if no reaccumulation of pleural fluid within the same hemithorax is seen during the designated period of follow up (usually 30 days). This is determined either on clinical examination or plain chest radiography. 'Partial success' is present if radiographically pleural fluid recurrence is exhibited but clinically the patients' symptoms are relieved and further pleural intervention is not required. This group of patients has not been identified by all investigators adding to the difficulty in interpretation of studies evaluating pleurodesis agents. Failure is accepted when the pleural effusion persists with no change in fluid accumulation rate or patient symptoms following the procedure.

Measurement of the patients' overall quality of life and relief of symptoms may be a more appropriate way of assessing the impact of pleurodesis.

PRACTICAL ASPECTS OF PLEURODESIS

Types of pleurodesis

MECHANICAL PLEURODESIS

Mechanical pleurodesis may be accomplished by pleural abrasion or parietal pleurectomy. Video-assisted thoracoscopic surgery (VATS) is now the procedure of choice amongst surgeons and is associated with a shorter hospital stay and recovery time than open thoracotomy and transaxillary mini-thoracotomy.

Pleural abrasion is technically easier to perform but pleurectomy had a slightly lower recurrence rate in one large series; 0.4 percent ($n = 752$) versus 2.3 percent ($n = 301$).[30] Total parietal pleurectomy is associated with higher post-operative morbidity than apical pleurectomy alone or pleural abrasion. Hemothorax occurs in approximately 4 percent of cases.[31]

CHEMICAL PLEURODESIS

The instillation of pleurodesing agents is usually via a chest tube, except for talc which may also be administered thoracoscopically. Pleurodesis via tube thoracostomy has comparable success rates to surgical pleurodesis, is potentially cheaper and does not involve general anesthetic risks (which can be significant in elderly patients with malignant effusions or secondary spontaneous pneumothoraces).

TECHNICAL ASPECTS OF PLEURODESIS

Choice of pleurodesis agent

Over 30 pleurodesis agents have been proposed since 1935 yet none is ideal. In a survey of over 800 pulmonologists, physicians were only 'somewhat satisfied' with available preparations.[32,33]

All pleurodesis agents have differing degrees of efficacy and side effect profiles, and suggested newer alternatives to date have not been rigorously compared with conventional agents.

Current practice is largely anecdotal. Success rates quoted are often over-inflated by selection bias and the rates are much lower in 'real life' clinical practice. Over 30 randomized controlled trials comparing different agents have been performed but patient numbers are small and few results reach statistical significance.[34] Pleurodesis success rates of different sclerosing agents vary (Table 46.1).

TALC

Talc is the most commonly used agent worldwide. It is a heterogeneous group of minerals rather than a pure compound and has the chemical formula $Mg_3(Si_2O_5)_2(OH)_2$. It is mined from different deposits throughout the world, each with their own unique composition. Modern talc supplies are asbestos-free although mineral dusts such as calcite, quartz, dolomite and others may be present. Sterilization is achieved using dry heat, ethylene oxide or γ irradiation, although potential contamination with mediators such as endotoxin or other materials may occur.

During the preparatory process commercial talc is sifted through mesh of varying pore size; smaller particles are commonly selected for use in the USA (11–20 μm) whereas in France larger talc particles are chosen (mean 34 μm). This difference may explain why talc-related acute respiratory distress syndrome (ARDS) is more frequently reported in the USA (see below).

Talc can be administered as a powder (poudrage) insufflated at thoracoscopy or thoracotomy (Figure 46.1) or as 'talc slurry' (talc powder mixed with normal saline and agitated to form a suspension) via a chest tube.[35–37] Dosages previously used have ranged from 1 to 14 g, however, less than 5 g is advised as adverse effects seem to be more common with higher talc doses. Success rates for pleurodesis are similar for both thoracoscopic talc

Table 46.1 Success rates and relative efficacy of commonly used pleurodesis agents[22,38,51,56,57,60,61,70,129]

Pleurodesing agent	Success rate (CR) (%)	Dose
Talc poudrage	68–97	2.5–10 g
Talc slurry	72–94	2.5–10 g
Doxycycline	61–88	500 mg (1 to 3 instillations required)
Tetracycline	47–67	500 mg–20 mg/kg (1 dose or multiple: no difference)
Bleomycin	42–70	15–240 units
Quinacrine	64–91	500 mg (1 or 2 treatments required)
Iodopovidone	64–92	100 mL of 2%
Corynebacterium parvum	32–76	3.5–14 mg
Silver nitrate	75–90	20 mL of 0.5%

CR, complete response.

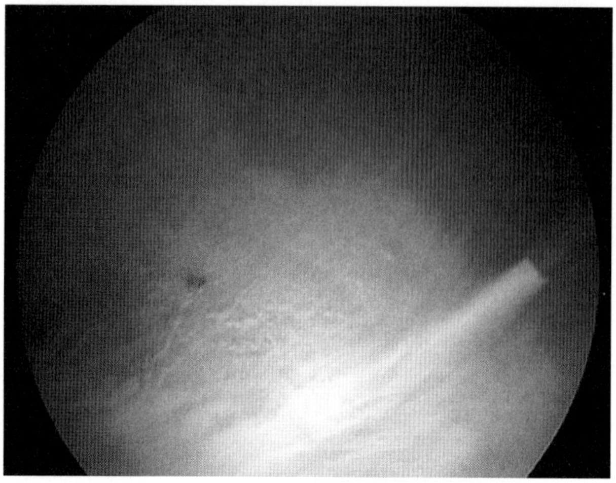

Figure 46.1 Thoracoscopic view of talc insufflation demonstrating the parietal pleural surface.

poudrage and talc slurry instillation. Two randomized trials to date have demonstrated no difference in 30-day freedom from radiological effusion recurrence ($n = 501$[38] and $n = 57$[37]).

The effectiveness of talc has been comprehensively documented,[39–50] as it has shown superiority in most randomized trials over chest tube drainage, tetracycline derivatives and bleomycin (Table 46.2). Talc, however, has been associated with potentially lethal side effects (see below).

CYCLINES

Tetracycline (1500 mg or 20 mg/kg), doxycycline (500 mg) and minocycline (300 mg) have all been used as pleurodesing agents. In the International Survey of Pleurodesis Practice (ISPP, 2003), 26 percent of participating pulmonologists rated cyclines as their agent of choice.[33]

Parenteral tetracycline is now unavailable in many countries due to cessation of its production, and parenteral doxycycline is difficult to acquire in many coun-

Table 46.2 Prospective randomized trials comparing talc with other agents

Authors	Number of patients	Outcome measure	Results
Talc slurry versus pleural drainage alone			
Sorensen *et al.*[130]	31	Complete resolution of effusion and subjective improvement	Favored talc 100% versus 58%
Thoracoscopic talc poudrage versus tetracycline			
Fentiman *et al.*[43]	41	Radiological control	Favored talc (92% versus 48%, $p = 0.022$)
Thoracoscopic talc poudrage versus bleomycin			
Hamed *et al.*[45]	29	Radiological control ≥ 1 month	Favored talc (0% reaccumulation versus 33%, $p = 0.057$)
Diacon *et al.*[41]	36	Radiological recurrence rate and cost effectiveness	Favored talc at 30 days ($p = 0.12$), 90 days ($p = 0.01$) and 120 days ($p = 0.005$) Cost estimation favored talc
Talc slurry versus bleomycin			
Noppen *et al.*[48]	26	Recurrent pleural fluid ≥50% of initial volume or requiring pleurocentesis	No significant difference between groups
Zimmer *et al.*[50]	35	Radiological control	Favored talc (90% versus 79%, $p = 0.388$) Significant cost advantage with talc ($12.36 versus $955.83)
Ong *et al.*[49]	50	Radiological control ≥ 1 month Cost analysis	Favored talc (89% versus 70%, $p = 0.168$) Cost analysis favored talc
Haddad *et al.*[44]	71	No recurrence of pleural effusion or asymptomatic recurrence of small effusion. Cost analysis	No difference seen between groups at 30, 60 or 180 days ($p = 0.724$) Talc significantly cheaper ($p < 0.001$)
Thoracoscopic talc poudrage versus mustine			
Fentiman *et al.*[42]	46	Radiological control	Favored talc (90% versus 56%, $p < 0.025$)

tries.[51] However, oral forms of doxycycline dissolved in normal saline demonstrated similar efficacy in rabbits and may offer a less expensive, safe alternative to the parenteral forms in humans (not yet tested).[52]

CYTOTOXIC AGENTS

Nitrogen mustard (mechlorethamine hydrochloride) was one of the first pleurodesis agents used in the 1950s. Numerous cytotoxic agents (mitoxantrone, bleomycin, mitomycin, thiotepa, cytarabine and others) have since been tested with variable success rates (25–85 percent).[53] The mechanism of action of the cytotoxic agents remains unknown but is probably through a direct inflammatory pleural insult rather than a local anti-neoplastic effect. Nowadays, bleomycin (1 unit/kg, 15–240 units) is the only agent in regular use.[33] It has lower success rates in randomized trials versus talc and is expensive, limiting its widespread use.

OK432

OK432 is a preparation of *Streptococcus pyogenes* type A3 originally developed as an immunotherapeutic anti-tumor agent. It is widely used in Japan where talc is not commercially available. The exact mechanism of action is unclear although it is postulated to have a direct cytotoxic effect as well as irritant action.[54]

SILVER NITRATE

Silver nitrate was first utilized in the 1940s to control recurrent pneumothorax.[55,56] Its use was subsequently abandoned, probably because of intense pain and development of large pleural effusions associated with silver nitrate preparations of 1–10 percent concentrations. However, a recent study comparing lower concentrations (0.5 percent) of silver nitrate with sterile talc pleurodesis showed few short-term side effects and similar efficacy rates; although patient numbers were small and long-term success rates await evaluation.[57]

IODOPOVIDONE

Iodopovidone (100 mL of 2 percent) is an inexpensive iodine-derived topical antiseptic which should be avoided in iodine allergic patients. Several small studies evaluating its potential as a pleurodesing agent report promising pleurodesis rates although pleuritic chest pain and hypotension were experienced by some patients.[51,58] No large controlled trials have yet been performed and its routine use is not advocated.

QUINACRINE

Quinacrine, an anti-malarial agent, has been used routinely in Scandinavia for decades.[59] Ukale *et al.*[59] reported pleurodesis success rates of 89 percent with quinacrine (500 mg) compared with 96 percent with talc (5 g) recently.[59] However, case reports of patients experiencing temporary confusion, hallucinations and convulsions following intrapleural administration rendered it unpopular in large parts of Europe and the USA and serious central nervous system toxicity has been described in rabbits.[60]

CORYNEBACTERIUM PARVUM

Use of *C. parvum* was previously favored in Europe but ceased when its commercial production was discontinued. Unlike other sclerosing agents, administration directly into the pleural cavity without an intercostal tube was possible.[61]

OTHER AGENTS

Intrapleural administration of methylprednisolone acetate is postulated to work by reducing permeability of the pleural membrane and by exerting a local anti-tumor effect. Although early data suggested a possible benefit this has not been borne out in larger studies.[62,63]

Use of *Staphylococcal aureus* superantigen (SSAg) in humans was assessed by Ren *et al.*[64] following demonstrable tumoricidal effects in animal models and potential to induce regression of malignant effusions. In this study ($n = 14$), intrapleural SSAg controlled pleural fluid production in 100 percent of patients at 30 days and 86 percent at 90 days, and the median survival was 7.9 months. These results have not yet been verified in controlled trials.

Autologous ‘blood patch’ pleurodesis using 50–100 mL of venous blood taken from the same patient has been used, usually in patients with non-resolving pneumothorax who are not suitable for surgery.[65] It is a simple, painless procedure presumably acting by generating fibrogenesis, but its success rate has not been thoroughly assessed. Adverse effects are uncommon but pleural infection or tension pneumothorax may occur.[66]

Kinoshita *et al.*[67] instilled diluted fibrin glue and reported a success rate of 87.5 percent for intractable pneumothoraces and post lung-resection dead space in patients not fit for thoracotomy. In their study, intrapleural contrast medium was used to ensure adequate spread of the glue and identify persistent air leaks. Fibrin glue is less effective as a pleurodesing agent for pleural effusion with a recurrence rate of up to 25 percent[68] and overall success has been limited by chest tube blockage following administration.

COMBINATIONS OF AGENTS

Combinations of different sclerosing agents, including uniting surgical and chemical pleurodesis methods, to exploit a potential synergistic action have been evaluated in few published studies.[54,69–72] These have failed to show conclusive benefit over single-agent pleurodesis.

Randomized trials are required to determine optimal combinations and compare with current practice.

TIMING OF PLEURODESIS

Malignant pleural effusion

No consensus exists regarding the timing of pleurodesis. Some pulmonologists advise pleurodesis as soon as a malignant pleural effusion is diagnosed whereas others delay until symptomatic recurrence. The reported success rate of pleurodesis between these groups is similar;[33] however more advanced pleural malignancy reduces the likelihood of success.[73] Delay also increases the risk of eventual development of a 'trapped lung' which will preclude pleurodesis.

Timing of pleurodesis in chemotherapy-sensitive tumor is controversial. In ISPP, two-thirds favored waiting to see if chemotherapy is effective in controlling effusion accumulation, but one-third would pleurodese. Oncologists often favor the former option.[74] No data exist on how often these chemotherapy-sensitive tumors recur, and no definitive strategy is known. Risks of not pleurodesing include a potential site of infection during neutropenic sepsis and third spacing of chemotherapeutic drugs with resultant toxicity.[75] The Food and Drug Administration (FDA) body recommends that pleural effusions secondary to malignant pleural mesothelioma be drained prior to chemotherapy with Pemetrexed.

After the chest tube insertion, instillation of the pleurodesis agent is traditionally delayed until the daily pleural fluid drainage rate is <150 mL. This practice is supported by the majority of pulmonologists,[33] but increases the period of drainage, prolongs hospital stay and has not been shown to be more effective. The amount of fluid drained, when the X-ray shows no residual fluid, likely represents the amount of fluid formation and may not be further reduced by prolonged drainage. There is an equal chance of success if pleurodesis is performed when radiographic lung re-expansion is achieved and this practice is recommended.[76]

Pneumothorax

Debate surrounding the optimal timing and type of pleurodesis in patients with primary spontaneous pneumothorax continues. Historical series suggest that surgical intervention with pleurectomy or mechanical abrasion is superior, however, little evidence-based justification exists for this approach over chemical pleurodesis in primary pneumothoraces.

Discussion and referral for surgical intervention is generally recommended at day five to seven in patients with a persistent air leak despite tube drainage, although this cut-off time is arbitrary.[11,77,78] VATS allows identification and control of the source of the air leak as well as mechanical pleurodesis which carries a recurrence rate of <5 percent. Talc poudrage via VATS demonstrates comparable efficacy and is favored by some surgeons.

Traditionally, chemical pleurodesis via the chest drain is advocated only if the patient is unsuitable for surgery. However, in certain centers, patients with spontaneous pneumothorax for whom chest drainage is required undergo first-line medical thoracoscopy. This allows pneumothorax evacuation, assessment and coagulation of accessible blebs or bullae, as well as pleurodesis by talc poudrage without the risk of general anesthesia.

In patients with secondary pneumothorax and a persistent air leak, early referral (day two to four) is recommended. Video-assisted thoracoscopy is superior to chemical pleurodesis via chest tube with recurrence rates of <5 percent and approximately 20 percent respectively. However, if the patient is not fit for general anesthesia, e.g. because of poor lung functions, chemical pleurodesis via a chest drain may be appropriate.

Congestive cardiac failure

In selected patients with congestive cardiac failure and pleural effusion(s) refractory to conventional therapy, pleurodesis may be considered.[78,79] Pleural fluid accumulates as an escape route for interstitial fluid in congestive cardiac failure and pleurodesis carries a theoretical risk of worsening contralateral fluid accumulation or alveolar edema,[80,81] but this has not been demonstrated clinically.

Hepatic hydrothorax

Often, hepatic hydrothoraces form, in part, by the transdiaphragmatic migration of ascitic fluid. Caution should be exercised against routine chest drain placement in such patients as massive fluid loss may occur associated with secondary loss of electrolytes and protein. If medical treatment fails and repeated therapeutic thoracenteses for symptomatic relief are required, pleurodesis may be attempted. The concomitant application of continuous positive airway pressure ventilation to decrease the peritoneopleural pressure gradient (and reduce passage of ascitic fluid into the pleural cavity via diaphragmatic stomata) showed promising initial results but these have not been validated in larger studies.[82] Video-assisted thoracoscopy with closure of demonstrable diaphragmatic defects and simultaneous talc pleurodesis offers a potential therapeutic strategy although identification of patients with such defects is not yet possible.[83,84]

Chylothorax

After conservative measures have failed, and/or ligation of the thoracic duct is not suitable, pleurodesis should be considered.[85–87] It was previously believed that successful chemical pleurodesis for chylothorax was difficult to achieve: this has been attributed to normal underlying pleura or chemical composition of chyle. In recent years, however, large series have shown that pleurodesis can work for recurrent chylothoraces but ongoing medical management to lessen chyle production should continue following all attempts.[73]

PATIENT SELECTION

Performance status reflects the predicted survival of patients with malignant pleural effusion and should be assessed in all patients prior to pleurodesis.[88–90] If the expected survival is short (arbitrary suggestion, less than 3 months), less invasive procedures are appropriate (e.g. therapeutic thoracentesis). Patients with a good performance status are more likely to derive benefit from pleurodesis.[89,90]

Pleurodesis is only recommended in malignant pleural effusion if symptomatic improvement from thoracentesis is exhibited.[91,92] Dyspnea is often multi-factorial and up to 50 percent of patients do not have demonstrable symptomatic relief following fluid evacuation.[93] In this group, alternative causes for dyspnea should be addressed, e.g. obstructive airways disease, lymphangitis, pulmonary embolism or 'trapped lung'. The presence of 'trapped lung', when lung expansion is restricted either by visceral pleura tumor encasement or by endobronchial obstruction, prohibits effective pleurodesis as the pleural surfaces do not oppose. Pleurodesis may also precipitate fibrosis of the visceral pleura exacerbating restriction of the underlying lung.

In patients with metastatic malignant disease involving serosal surfaces, pleural, pericardial and ascitic fluid collections may concomitantly occur. Clinical management of such patients is often difficult. Statistically, patients with extensive disease have a very short prognosis (e.g. weeks) particularly if other treatment modalities (e.g. chemotherapy) are not a viable option. Repeated therapeutic aspiration may be more appropriate. Insertion of an ambulatory indwelling pleural catheter may also provide relief in such cases. Ascitic fluid should be drained prior to attempted pleurodesis to reduce the transdiaphragmatic migration of fluid, which may reduce likelihood of success.

The identification of clinical or biochemical parameters to guide selection of patients for pleurodesis has been the focus of much previous research. Several measures have been suggested including patients' performance status, size of effusion on chest X-ray and pleural fluid LDH (>2× upper normal limit for serum), glucose (<60 mg/dL) or pH (<7.20).[90,94,95] Low pleural fluid glucose (and pH) appears to arise secondary to tumor infiltration, which decreases glucose transport into the pleural space, as well as via increased glucose utilization by cancer cells and reduced efflux of acidic byproducts from the pleural cavity.[96,97] Cytological examination is frequently positive. A direct correlation has been observed between low pleural fluid pH (<7.30) and reduced survival rates;[98] however, data only weakly supports its use (pH <7.20) as a discriminative tool to determine likelihood of pleurodesis success.[94] Therefore, although low pleural pH may indicate patients in whom the likelihood of pleurodesis success may be lower, it should not be used in isolation and this group should not be denied pleurodesis on this basis alone.

TRANSPLANT CONSIDERATIONS

Many patients who eventually require lung transplantation encounter complications which raise the question of the appropriateness of pleurodesis, e.g. recurrent pneumothoraces in chronic obstructive pulmonary disease (COPD), cystic fibrosis or lymphangioleiomyomatosis (LAM). Previously, pleurodesis was seen as a contraindication to transplantation and avoidance of pleurodesis with postponement of definitive preventative measures was recommended in any potential future transplant candidate. However, recent evidence from patients with recurrent pneumothoraces and underlying lymphangioleiomyomatosis suggests pleural adhesion/fibrosis does not preclude successful transplantation, although it does increase the rate of perioperative bleeding and technical difficulty.[10] Liaison with a specialist transplantation unit is recommended prior to pleurodesis in any potential future lung transplant candidate.

CLINICAL CONSIDERATIONS AT PLEURODESIS

Size of chest tube for pleurodesis

No adequately powered randomized trials define an optimal chest drain size to maximize pleurodesis efficacy. Traditionally, large-bore chest tubes have been employed; however, pleurodesis via small-bore tubes (<16 F) is associated with comparable success rates and a large number of non-randomized studies suggest they are better tolerated than larger bore drains.[94,99–106] Interestingly, despite this evidence, small-bore drains are still under-utilized with larger (28–32 F) tubes preferred in the USA and Canada, and 20–24 F favored in UK and Australasia.[33] Ambulatory small-bore catheters enable pleurodesis to be performed on an outpatient basis obviating the need for hospital admission and associated costs.[107,108] This has been successfully applied with most pleurodesing agents, including talc slurry.

Patient rotation

Whether rotation of the patient following administration of the pleurodesing agent aids its distribution and improves success remains debatable. The success rate of pleurodesis and distribution of talc throughout the pleural cavity appear independent of rotation in small studies.[109,110] Concerns, however, have been expressed for talc slurry as it is not soluble and particles gravitate towards the bases of the pleural cavity. As rotation is a safe procedure, there is little to contradict its use.

Clamping time

Whether prolonged contact of a pleurodesing agent with the pleural surface is required to induce inflammation and successful pleural union has not been assessed, and no studies address the optimal chest tube clamping time. Significant variations in practice occur and most pulmonologists clamp the tube for 1–4 hours.[33]

Suction

In order to achieve opposition of the pleural membranes, suction is applied in some centers following release of tube clamping. No universal guideline exists but some advocate suction until tube drainage is less than 100 mL daily. If used, careful graded suction should be initiated to prevent re-expansion pulmonary edema.

Chest tube removal

The optimal duration for drainage following pleurodesis is unknown, though most chest drains can be taken out at 48 hours. Some pulmonologists use daily fluid drainage to guide removal whereas others remove the drain at a specific time after pleurodesis regardless of fluid volume.[33] A recent study ($n = 41$) showed no difference in pleurodesis success rates in patients randomized to drain removal at 24 hours compared with those whose drain was removed at 72 hours. However, length of hospital stay was significantly reduced in the former group (4 days versus 8 days; $p < 0.01$).[111]

Best analgesia

Pleurodesis can be painful, presumably from the intense pleural inflammation provoked. Instillation of intrapleural analgesia is recommended before administration of the pleurodesing agent[99] but evidence supporting this practice is scant and questions remain on whether the effectiveness of the anesthetic is maintained following dilution when the pleurodesing agent is subsequently introduced. Only one small non-randomized ($n = 20$) study has compared 250 mg versus 200 mg of intrapleural lidocaine and the result was difficult to interpret.[112] Further randomized, blinded trials are needed.

Narcotic analgesia and/or conscious sedation should be used as pre-medication provided that no contraindications exist. There are no clinical studies evaluating efficacy of different analgesic agents following pleurodesis.

Effect of non-steroidal anti-inflammatory drugs and prednisolone

Modulation of the inflammatory cascade, theorized to play a salient role in effective pleurodesis, may limit pleurodesis efficacy. Experimental animal studies have shown that concomitant administration of corticosteroids or non-steroidal anti-inflammatory drugs (NSAIDs) reduces formation of talc- and doxycycline-induced pleural adhesions.[18,113,114] Conflicting evidence exists; in another animal study using short-term NSAIDs no effect was seen, and the systemic use of these agents did not influence the outcome of silver nitrate- or TGF-β-induced pleurodesis.[28,114] Until adequate human studies have been performed, it is recommended that wherever possible these agents should be avoided prior to, and in the immediate period following, pleurodesis. A randomized trial is underway to assess pleurodesis efficacy with either NSAIDs or opiate analgesia used at the time of pleurodesis.

Effect of heparin

Activation of the coagulation cascade has been shown to play an important role in organ fibrosis and stimulation of systemic and pleural coagulation pathways have been demonstrated following talc poudrage. The use of prophylactic heparin (or its derivatives) to prevent thromboembolic disease is common in clinical practice, however, it has been postulated that their use may reduce pleurodesis efficacy via an inhibitory action on pleural coagulation.[115,116] Further study to address the significance of this effect is needed.

SIDE EFFECTS/COMPLICATIONS OF PLEURODESIS

Common side effects of all sclerosing agents include chest pain and fever, presumably from the intense pleural inflammation provoked.

Talc and its safety

Whilst talc is effective, concerns regarding potential lethal side effects persist.

Talc-induced ARDS has been widely reported,[115,117–124] and its incidence ranges from 0–9 percent in different studies. The mechanism remains poorly understood.

Acute respiratory distress syndrome has been seen after both talc slurry instillation and talc poudrage,[122] and with low (2 g) and high (10 g) talc doses.[118] It is hypothesized that acute lung inflammation secondary to the systemic distribution of talc particles occurs and a resultant pneumonitis precipitates respiratory failure. To date, many ARDS cases have been reported from the USA where, interestingly, commercial preparations used have predominantly smaller (<20 μm) size talc particles.[125] Randomized controlled trials support the theory that talc preparations consisting of mainly small particle sizes are absorbed in higher concentrations systemically in animals, possibly through parietal pleural pores, and induce more lung and systemic inflammation.[74] Further studies demonstrate deposition of talc in extra-pleural tissues following pleurodesis and in rabbit models there is a dose-dependent effect.[115,120] However, in all the animal and human studies, few (if any) actually developed ARDS despite the demonstration of extrapleural talc deposition and raised systemic inflammation.

In addition to small-size talc particles, impurities and other contaminants of talc preparations may also be contributing causes of ARDS. A large prospective study of over 550 patients in continental Europe failed to identify any cases of ARDS after pleurodesis using graded talc of mainly large particle size.[126]

At present, the evidence is not sufficient to discourage the use of talc, but small particle size talc preparations should be avoided. Special care should be exercised in patients with pre-existing hypoxia or advanced lung disease who need pleurodesis. An alternative agent (e.g. tetracycline) should be considered in such circumstances.

LONG-TERM EFFECTS OF PLEURODESIS

The long-term outlook in patients following pleurodesis for pneumothorax is good. Lange *et al.*[127] showed that talc pleurodesis in 114 patients with primary spontaneous pneumothoraces was associated with only mild and clinically insignificant restriction in lung function and total lung capacity. Györik and colleagues[128] concurred with these findings observing normal lung function at a median follow up of 118 months in patients who did not smoke. Although pleural thickening may be evident radiographically, there is no increased risk of pleural malignancy.

ALTERNATIVES – WHAT TO DO IF PLEURODESIS FAILS

No good data exist to guide the management of patients who have failed pleurodesis, but the following options can be considered.

Repeat pleurodesis

Repeated talc pleurodesis may be appropriate in patients with good performance status, although anecdotally it is associated with lower success rates. One comparison study between 500 mg quinacrine ($n = 54$) and 5 g talc slurry ($n = 56$) reported the need for repeat administration in 31 versus 7 percent of patients respectively following initial treatment. Repeat talc instillation was successful in 50 percent of patients (2/4), increasing the overall success rate by only 3.6 percent.[51]

A different agent may be used but quality evidence to support this practice is lacking.

Ambulatory indwelling pleural catheter

The insertion of a long term indwelling tunneled pleural catheter allows outpatient management of refractory malignant pleural effusion (Figure 46.2). It is also indicated in patients with a symptomatic effusion and underlying 'trapped lung'. The catheters can be inserted as a day case obviating hospital admission and their presence induces a complete or partial pleurodesis in up to 58 percent of patients.[104,108] The patient (or carer) can drain the effusion as guided by symptoms avoiding hospitalization, and the catheters are generally well tolerated. Recognized complications include local tumor invasion at the insertion site, pleural infection and catheter displacement.

Pleuroperitoneal shunt

Insertion of a pleuroperitoneal shunt may be considered if pleurodesis fails. Shunt occlusion (approximately 10 percent), pain, and infection are potential complications.

Parietal pleurectomy

Parietal pleurectomy aims to create uniform adhesions between the visceral pleura and chest wall. For recurrent spontaneous pneumothorax, failure rates of <0.5 percent are quoted (although this rate is not for patients who have already failed pleurodesis).[31,77] Parietal pleurectomy is effective in patients with refractory malignant pleural effusions, however, case selection is important as it is not suitable for patients with a trapped lung and should be reserved for patients with exceptionally good performance status and prognosis.

Repeated thoracentesis

Serial therapeutic thoracenteses to relieve breathlessness should be considered in patients with a poor performance status, a short predicted life expectancy (e.g. less than

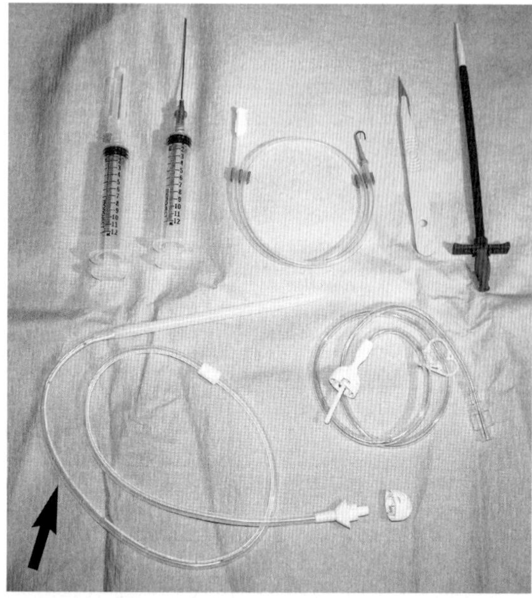

(a)

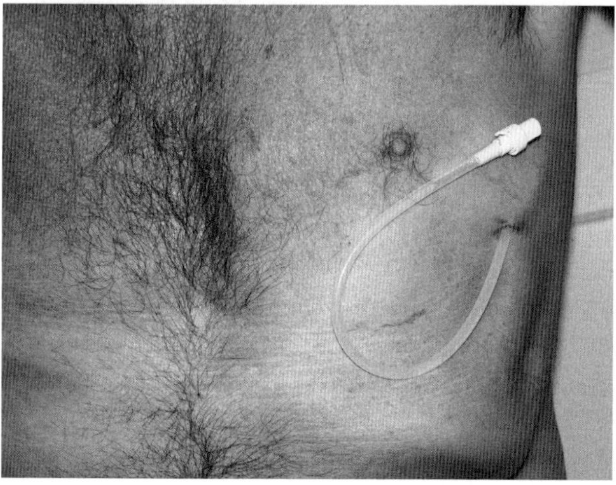

(b)

Figure 46.2 (a) Equipment for insertion of ambulatory indwelling pleural catheter. The distal end of the catheter (arrow) is inserted into the pleural cavity using a standard Seldinger technique. It is then tunneled subcutaneously, the proximal end remaining visible (image (b)). A Dacron cuff (*) secures the catheter in position at the midpoint of the subcutaneous tract. The catheter has a one-way valve (A) into which the drainage tubing, attached to a collecting bottle, is placed for drainage as required. (b) Indwelling pleural catheter *in situ.*

3 months) or trapped lung. However, repeated aspirations are not usually recommended as they are uncomfortable for the patient, exacerbate protein loss[73] and introduce the risk of pleural infection and pneumothorax.

Heimlich valve

The one-way Heimlich valve enables patients with recurrent persistent pneumothorax to be treated as outpatients.

Non-invasive palliation

Opiates to alleviate the sensation of dyspnea, and supplementary oxygen therapy may be appropriate in terminally ill patients with symptomatic effusions. Other possible contributory factors for the dyspnea should be addressed.

FUTURE DIRECTIONS

The incidence of pleural disease is rising as a result of an ageing population at risk of developing diseases associated with pleural effusion (e.g. malignancy) and pneumothorax (e.g. chronic respiratory disease).

Little data exist on the best selection of patients who will have successful pleurodesis. Recommendations given by professional societies are often based on expert opinions. More research is required on the role of pleurodesis to substantiate advice given to fellow physicians and in particular to address the following:

1. Determine the target outcome. In patients with recurrent malignant pleural effusion most previous studies have chosen the development or amount of pleural fluid reaccumulation as the primary outcome. For the patient with a malignant pleural effusion and an average life span of 6 months, the prime aim should be to improve quality of life by reducing morbidity. Measurements of quality of life may therefore be more appropriate as endpoints in future studies of management of malignant pleural effusions. A randomized trial recently started in the UK comparing conventional inpatient talc pleurodesis against ambulatory indwelling pleural catheter drainage (without chemical pleurodesis) as first-line management of malignant effusions, using quality of life and symptoms of breathlessness as endpoints, is an important first step towards symptom-based outpatient management.
2. Identify and characterize those patients who are likely to benefit from pleurodesis. Dependable predictors for pleurodesis failure would allow identification of patients who are unlikely to benefit from pleurodesis and hence reduce unnecessary exposure of this cohort to potentially serious side effects of sclerosing agents. Initial determination of pleural fluid pH may give a clue towards the chance of pleurodesis success but more accurate and repeatable markers would be invaluable.
3. Assessment of novel agents as clinical pleurodesis agents is required. Recent manipulation of cytokines, such as TGF-β, to generate effective pleurodesis in animals is exciting but further research to determine applicability in humans is crucial. Randomized trials to assess optimal application of current pleurodesis agents and re-evaluate ones previously discounted, e.g. silver nitrate, would be valuable, as well as evaluating combination therapies for a potential synergistic effect.

4. A deeper understanding of the process by which pleural fluid initially develops is required and would allow primary prevention of malignant pleural effusion rather than secondarily addressing the fluid once it has accumulated.

The potential role of intrapleural therapy with chemotherapeutic agents, immune modulators and gene therapy offers a novel approach. Gene therapy is the subject of exciting ongoing research and although still in its infancy, may provide a future treatment of pleural malignancies (see Chapter 49).

KEY POINTS

- Pleurodesis is an effective therapeutic option for recurrent pleural effusions and pneumothoraces. It should be considered in patients with recurrent effusions who have symptomatic relief of dyspnea upon fluid removal.
- Various surgical and chemical pleurodesing methods/agents exist, each with its advantages and side effect profiles.
- Talc is the most commonly used and effective agent, though it carries potentially lethal complications. Talc poudrage and slurry are of similar efficacy in randomized studies.
- The best protocol of administration of chemical pleurodesis (e.g. tube size, analgesia, use of suction etc.) remains poorly defined.
- Indwelling pleural catheters should be considered for ambulatory drainage in patients who are unsuitable for, or have failed, pleurodesis.
- Success of pleurodesis should be defined by best symptomatic relief to the patients rather than by radiographic measures.

REFERENCES

1. Marel M, Zrustova M, Stasny B, Light RW. The incidence of pleural effusion in a well-defined region. Epidemiologic study in central Bohemia. *Chest* 1993; **104**: 1486–9.
2. Lee YCG, De Clerk NH, Henderson DW, Musk AW. Malignant mesothelioma. In Hendrick DJ, Burge PS, Beckett WS, Churg A (eds). *Occupational disorders of the lung. Recognition, management and prevention.* London: WB Saunders & Co., 2002: 359–79.
3. Lee YCG, Dean A, Thompson RI, Robinson BWS. Clinical and palliative care aspects of malignant mesothelioma. In Robinson BWS, Chahinian P (eds). *Mesothelioma.* London: Martin Dunitz, 2002: 111–26.
4. Sahn SA. Malignancy metastatic to the pleura. *Clin Chest Med* 1998; **19**: 351–61.
5. Anderson CB, Philpott GW, Ferguson TB. The treatment of malignant pleural effusions. *Cancer* 1974; **33**: 916–22.
6. Gobbel WGJ, Rhea WGJ, Nelson IA. Spontaneous pneumothorax. *J Thorac Cardiovasc Surg* 1963; **46**: 331–45.
7. Sadikot RT, Greene T, Meadows K, Arnold AG. Recurrence of primary spontaneous pneumothorax. *Thorax* 1997; **52**: 805–9.
8. Henry M, Arnold T, Harvey J. BTS guidelines for the management of spontaneous pneumothorax. *Thorax* 2003; **58** (Suppl 2): ii39– 52.
9. Lippert HL, Lund O, Blegvad S, Larsen HV. Independent risk factors for cumulative recurrence rate after first spontaneous pneumothorax. *Eur Respir J* 1991; **4**: 324–31.
10. Almoosa KF, Ryu JH, Mendez J, *et al.* Management of pneumothorax in lymphangioleiomyomatosis: effects on recurrence and lung transplantation complications. *Chest* 2006; **129**: 1274–81.
11. Light RW, O'Hara VS, Moritz TE, *et al.* Intrapleural tetracycline for the prevention of recurrent spontaneous pneumothorax. Results of a Department of Veterans Affairs cooperative study. *J Am Med Assoc* 1990; **264**: 2224–30.
12. Kennedy L, Harley RA, Sahn SA, Strange C. Talc slurry pleurodesis. Pleural fluid and histologic analysis. *Chest* 1995; **107**: 1707–12.
13. Montes JF, Garcia-Valero J, Ferrer J. Evidence of innervation in talc-induced pleural adhesions. *Chest* 2006; **130**: 702–9.
14. Guo YB, Kalomenidis I, Hawthorne M, *et al.* Pleurodesis is inhibited by anti-vascular endothelial growth factor antibody. *Chest* 2005; **128**: 1790–7.
15. Tzouvelekis A, Anevlavis S, Bouros D. Angiogenesis in interstitial lung diseases: a pathogenetic hallmark or a bystander? *Respir Res* 2006; **7**: 82.
16. Genofre EH, Vargas FS, Antonangelo L, *et al.* Ultrastructural acute features of active remodeling after chemical pleurodesis induced by silver nitrate or talc. *Lung* 2005; **183**: 197–207.
17. Marchi E, Vargas FS, Acencio MM, *et al.* Evidence that mesothelial cells regulate the acute inflammatory response in talc pleurodesis. *Eur Respir J* 2006; **28**: 929–32.
18. Xie C, Teixeira LR, McGovern JP, Light RW. Systemic corticosteroids decrease the effectiveness of talc pleurodesis. *Am J Respir Crit Care Med* 1998; **157**: 1441–4.
19. Agrenius V, Gustafsson LE, Widstrom O. Tumour necrosis factor-alpha and nitric oxide, determined as nitrite, in malignant pleural effusion. *Respir Med* 1994; **88**: 743–8.
20. van den Heuvel MM, Smit HJ, Barbierato SB, *et al.* Talc-induced inflammation in the pleural cavity. *Eur Respir J* 1998; **12**: 1419–23.
21. Nasreen N, Hartman DL, Mohammed KA, Antony VB. Talc-induced expression of C-C and C-X-C chemokines and intercellular adhesion molecule-1 in mesothelial cells. *Am J Respir Crit Care Med* 1998; **158**: 971–8.
22. Walker-Renard PB, Vaughan LM, Sahn SA. Chemical pleurodesis for malignant pleural effusions. *Ann Intern Med* 1994; **120**: 56–64.
23. Lee YCG, Teixeira LR, Devin CJ, *et al.* Transforming growth factor-beta2 induces pleurodesis significantly faster than talc. *Am J Respir Crit Care Med* 2001; **163**: 640–4.
24. Light RW, Cheng DS, Lee YC, *et al.* A single intrapleural injection of transforming growth factor-beta(2) produces an excellent pleurodesis in rabbits. *Am J Respir Crit Care Med* 2000; **162**: 98–104.
25. Lee YC, Lane KB, Parker RE, *et al.* Transforming growth factor beta(2) (TGF beta(2)) produces effective pleurodesis in sheep with no systemic complications. *Thorax* 2000; **55**: 1058–62.
26. Lee YC, Yasay JR, Johnson JE, *et al.* Comparing transforming growth factor-beta2, talc and bleomycin as pleurodesing agents in sheep. *Respirology* 2002; **7**: 209–16.
27. Lee YCG, Lane KB, Zoia O, *et al.* Transforming growth factor-beta induces collagen synthesis without inducing IL-8 production in mesothelial cells. *Eur Respir J* 2003; **22**: 197–202.
28. Lee YC, Devin CJ, Teixeira LR, *et al.* Transforming growth factor beta2 induced pleurodesis is not inhibited by corticosteroids. *Thorax* 2001; **56**: 643–8.

29. Mutsaers SE, Kalomenidis I, Wilson NA, Lee YC. Growth factors in pleural fibrosis. *Curr Opin Pulm Med* 2006; **12**: 251–8.
30. Weeden D, Smith GH. Surgical experience in the management of spontaneous pneumothorax, 1972–82. *Thorax* 1983; **38**: 737–43.
31. Thomas P, Le Mee F, Le Hors H, *et al.* [Results of surgical treatment of persistent or recurrent pneumothorax]. *Ann Chir* 1993; **47**: 136–40.
32. Bethune N. Pleural poudrage: a new technique for the deliberate production of pleural adhesions as a preliminary to lobectomy. *J Thorac Surg* 1935; **4**: 251–61.
33. Lee YC, Baumann MH, Maskell NA, *et al.* Pleurodesis practice for malignant pleural effusions in five English-speaking countries: survey of pulmonologists. *Chest* 2003; **124**: 2229–38.
34. Tan C, Sedrakyan A, Browne J, Swift S, Treasure T. The evidence on the effectiveness of management for malignant pleural effusion: a systematic review. *Eur J Cardiothorac Surg* 2006; **29**: 829–38.
35. Antony VB, Loddenkemper R, Astoul P, *et al.* Management of malignant pleural effusions. *Eur Respir J* 2001; **18**: 402–19.
36. Kennedy L, Sahn SA. Talc pleurodesis for the treatment of pneumothorax and pleural effusion. *Chest* 1994; **106**: 1215–22.
37. Yim AP, Chan AT, Lee TW, Wan IY, Ho JK. Thoracoscopic talc insufflation versus talc slurry for symptomatic malignant pleural effusion. *Ann Thorac Surg* 1996; **62**: 1655–8.
38. Dresler CM, Olak J, Herndon JE, *et al.* Phase III intergroup study of talc poudrage vs talc slurry sclerosis for malignant pleural effusion. *Chest* 2005; **127**: 909–15.
39. Webb WR, Ozmen V, Moulder PV, Shabahang B, Breaux J. Iodized talc pleurodesis for the treatment of pleural effusions. *J Thorac Cardiovasc Surg* 1992; **103**: 881–5.
40. Adler RH, Sayek I. Treatment of malignant pleural effusion: a method using tube thoracostomy and talc. *Ann Thorac Surg* 1976; **22**: 8–15.
41. Diacon AH, Wyser C, Bolliger CT, *et al.* Prospective randomized comparison of thoracoscopic talc poudrage under local anesthesia versus bleomycin instillation for pleurodesis in malignant pleural effusions. *Am J Respir Crit Care Med* 2000; **162**: 1445–9.
42. Fentiman IS, Rubens RD, Hayward JL. Control of pleural effusions in patients with breast cancer. A randomized trial. *Cancer* 1983; **52**: 737–9.
43. Fentiman IS, Rubens RD, Hayward JL. A comparison of intracavitary talc and tetracycline for the control of pleural effusions secondary to breast cancer. *Eur J Cancer Clin Oncol* 1986; **22**: 1079–81.
44. Haddad FJ, Younes RN, Gross JL, Deheinzelin D. Pleurodesis in patients with malignant pleural effusions: talc slurry or bleomycin? Results of a prospective randomized trial. *World J Surg* 2004; **28**: 749–53.
45. Hamed H, Fentiman IS, Chaudary MA, Rubens RD. Comparison of intracavitary bleomycin and talc for control of pleural effusions secondary to carcinoma of the breast. *Br J Surg* 1989; **76**: 1266–7.
46. Hartman DL, Gaither JM, Kesler KA, *et al.* Comparison of insufflated talc under thoracoscopic guidance with standard tetracycline and bleomycin pleurodesis for control of malignant pleural effusions. *J Thorac Cardiovasc Surg* 1993; **105**: 743–7.
47. Lynch T, Kalish L, Mentzer SJ, *et al.* Optimal therapy of malignant pleural effusions: report of a randomised trial of bleomycin, tetracycline, and talc and a meta-analysis. *Int J Oncol* 1996; **8**: 183–90.
48. Noppen M, Degreve J, Mignolet M, Vincken W. A prospective, randomised study comparing the efficacy of talc slurry and bleomycin in the treatment of malignant pleural effusions. *Acta Clin Belg* 1997; **52**: 258–62.
49. Ong KC, Indumathi V, Raghuram J, Ong YY. A comparative study of pleurodesis using talc slurry and bleomycin in the management of malignant pleural effusions. *Respirology* 2000; **5**: 99–103.
50. Zimmer PW, Hill M, Casey K, Harvey E, Low DE. Prospective randomized trial of talc slurry vs bleomycin in pleurodesis for symptomatic malignant pleural effusions. *Chest* 1997; **112**: 430–4.
51. Dikensoy O, Light RW. Alternative widely available, inexpensive agents for pleurodesis. *Curr Opin Pulm Med* 2005; **11**: 340–4.
52. Bilaceroglu S, Guo Y, Hawthorne ML, *et al.* Oral forms of tetracycline and doxycycline are effective in producing pleurodesis. *Chest* 2005; **128**: 3750–6.
53. Marchi E, Vargas FS, Teixeira LR, *et al.* Comparison of nitrogen mustard, cytarabine and dacarbazine as pleural sclerosing agents in rabbits. *Eur Respir J* 1997; **10**: 598–602.
54. Kishi K, Homma S, Sakamoto S, *et al.* Efficacious pleurodesis with OK-432 and doxorubicin against malignant pleural effusions. *Eur Respir J* 2004; **24**: 263–6.
55. Brock RC. The use of silver nitrate in the production of aseptic obliterative pleuritis. *Guys Hosp Rep* 1942; **91**: 99–103.
56. Brock RC. Recurrent and chronic spontaneous pneumothorax. *Thorax* 1948; **3**: 88–91.
57. Paschoalini MS, Vargas FS, Marchi E, *et al.* Prospective randomized trial of silver nitrate vs talc slurry in pleurodesis for symptomatic malignant pleural effusions. *Chest* 2005; **128**: 684–9.
58. Olivares-Torres CA, Laniado-Laborin R, Chavez-Garcia C, *et al.* Iodopovidone pleurodesis for recurrent pleural effusions. *Chest* 2002; **122**: 581–3.
59. Ukale V, Agrenius V, Hillerdal G, Mohlkert D, Widstrom O. Pleurodesis in recurrent pleural effusions: a randomized comparison of a classical and a currently popular drug. *Lung Cancer* 2004; **43**: 323–8.
60. Bjorkman S, Elisson LO, Gabrielsson J. Pharmacokinetics of quinacrine after intrapleural instillation in rabbits and man. *J Pharm Pharmacol* 1989; **41**: 160–3.
61. Foresti V. Corynebacterium parvum for malignant pleural effusions. *Thorax* 1995; **50**: 104.
62. Bartal AH, Gazitt Y, Zidan G, Vermeulen B, Robinson E. Clinical and flow cytometry characteristics of malignant pleural effusions in patients after intracavitary administration of methylprednisolone acetate. *Cancer* 1991; **67**: 3136–40.
63. North SA, Au HJ, Halls SB, Tkachuk L, Mackey JR. A randomized, phase III, double-blind, placebo-controlled trial of intrapleural instillation of methylprednisolone acetate in the management of malignant pleural effusion. *Chest* 2003; **123**: 822–7.
64. Ren S, Terman DS, Bohach G, *et al.* Intrapleural staphylococcal superantigen induces resolution of malignant pleural effusions and a survival benefit in non-small cell lung cancer. *Chest* 2004; **126**: 1529–39.
65. Dumire R, Crabbe MM, Mappin FG, Fontenelle LJ. Autologous "blood patch" pleurodesis for persistent pulmonary air leak. *Chest* 1992; **101**: 64–6.
66. Williams P, Laing R. Tension pneumothorax complicating autologous "blood patch" pleurodesis. *Thorax* 2005; **60**: 1066–7.
67. Kinoshita T, Miyoshi S, Katoh M, *et al.* Intrapleural administration of a large amount of diluted fibrin glue for intractable pneumothorax. *Chest* 2000; **117**: 790–5.
68. Guerin JC, Van Derschueren RG. [Treatment of recurrent pneumothorax applying fibrin adhesive under endoscopy]. *Rev Mal Respir* 1989; **6**: 443–5.
69. Chen JS, Hsu HH, Kuo SW, *et al.* Effects of additional minocycline pleurodesis after thoracoscopic procedures for primary spontaneous pneumothorax. *Chest* 2004; **125**: 50–5.
70. Dikensoy O, Zhu Z, Donnelly E, *et al.* Combination therapy with intrapleural doxycycline and talc in reduced doses is effective in producing pleurodesis in rabbits. *Chest* 2005; **128**: 3735–42.
71. Rusch VW, Figlin R, Godwin D, Piantadosi S. Intrapleural cisplatin and cytarabine in the management of malignant pleural effusions: a Lung Cancer Study Group trial. *J Clin Oncol* 1991; **9**: 313–9.
72. Tanaka A, Sato T. [Adhesion therapy for malignant pleural effusion (intrapleural administration of OK-432 with minocycline)]. *Nihon Kokyuki Gakkai Zasshi* 1999; **37**: 531–7.

73. Rodriguez-Panadero F, Antony VB. Pleurodesis: state of the art. *Eur Respir J* 1997; **10**: 1648–54.
74. Maskell NA, Lee YC, Gleeson FV, *et al.* Randomized trials describing lung inflammation after pleurodesis with talc of varying particle size. *Am J Respir Crit Care Med* 2004; **170**: 377–82.
75. Li J,.Gwilt P. The effect of malignant effusions on methotrexate disposition. *Cancer Chemother Pharmacol* 2002; **50**: 373–82.
76. Villanueva AG, Gray AW Jr, Shahian DM, Williamson WA, Beamis JF Jr. Efficacy of short term versus long term tube thoracostomy drainage before tetracycline pleurodesis in the treatment of malignant pleural effusions. *Thorax* 1994; **49**: 23–5.
77. O'Rourke JP, Yee ES. Civilian spontaneous pneumothorax. Treatment options and long-term results. *Chest* 1989; **96**: 1302–6.
78. Sudduth CD, Sahn SA. Pleurodesis for nonmalignant pleural effusions. Recommendations. *Chest* 1992; **102**: 1855–60.
79. Glazer M, Berkman N, Lafair JS, Kramer MR. Successful talc slurry pleurodesis in patients with nonmalignant pleural effusion. *Chest* 2000; **117**: 1404–9.
80. Davidoff D, Naparstek Y, Eliakim M. The use of pleurodesis for intractable pleural effusion due to congestive heart failure. *Postgrad Med J* 1983; **59**: 330–1.
81. Glazer M, Berkman N, Lafair JS, Kramer MR. Successful talc slurry pleurodesis in patients with nonmalignant pleural effusion. *Chest* 2000; **117**: 1404–9.
82. Boiteau R, Tenaillon A, Law Koune JD, *et al.* Treatment for cirrhotic hydrothorax with CPAP on mask and tetracycline pleural sclerosis (abstract). *Am Rev Respir Dis* 1990; **A770**: 141.
83. De Campos, Filho LO, Werebe EC, *et al.* Thoracoscopy and talc poudrage in the management of hepatic hydrothorax. *Chest* 2000; 13–7.
84. Mouroux J, Perrin C, Venissac N, Blaive B, Richelme H. Management of pleural effusion of cirrhotic origin. *Chest* 1996; **109**: 1093–6.
85. Fogli L, Gorini P, Belcastro S. Conservative management of traumatic chylothorax: a case report. *Intensive Care Med* 1993; **19**: 176–7.
86. Mares DC, Mathur PN. Medical thoracoscopic talc pleurodesis for chylothorax due to lymphoma: a case series. *Chest* 1998; **114**: 731–5.
87. Norum J, Aasebo U. Intrapleural bleomycin in the treatment of chylothorax. *J Chemother* 1994; **6**: 427–30.
88. Bernard A, de Dompsure RB, Hagry O, Favre JP. Early and late mortality after pleurodesis for malignant pleural effusion. *Ann Thorac Surg* 2002; **74**: 213–17.
89. Burrows CM, Mathews WC, Colt HG. Predicting survival in patients with recurrent symptomatic malignant pleural effusions: an assessment of the prognostic values of physiologic, morphologic, and quality of life measures of extent of disease. *Chest* 2000; **117**: 73–8.
90. Martinez-Moragon E, Aparicio J, Sanchis J, *et al.* Malignant pleural effusion: prognostic factors for survival and response to chemical pleurodesis in a series of 120 cases. *Respiration* 1998; **65**: 108–13.
91. Lee YCG, Rodrigues RM, Lane KB, Light RW. Pleurodesis for recurrent pleural effusions in the new millennium. *Recent Adv Res Updates* 2001; **2**: 81–9.
92. Light RW. *Pleural diseases.* Baltimore: Lippincott, Williams & Wilkins, 2001.
93. Shinto RA, Stansbury DW, Fischer CE, Light RW. Does therapeutic thoracentesis improve the exercise capacity of patients with pleural effusion? *Am Rev Respir Dis* 1988; **A244**: 135.
94. Heffner JE, Nietert PJ, Barbieri C. Pleural fluid pH as a predictor of pleurodesis failure: analysis of primary data. *Chest* 2000; **117**: 87–95.
95. Loddenkemper R. Are prognostic factors helpful in determining the indication for pleurodesis in malignant pleural effusions? *Respiration* 1998; **65**: 106–7.
96. Clarkson B. Relationship between cell type, glucose concentration, and response to treatment in neoplastic effusions. *Cancer* 1964; **17**: 914–28.
97. Good JT Jr, Taryle DA, Sahn SA. The pathogenesis of low glucose, low pH malignant effusions. *Am Rev Respir Dis* 1985; **131**: 737–41.
98. Sahn SA, Good JT Jr. Pleural fluid pH in malignant effusions. Diagnostic, prognostic, and therapeutic implications. *Ann Intern Med* 1988; **108**: 345–9.
99. Antunes G, Neville E, Duffy J, Ali N. BTS guidelines for the management of malignant pleural effusions. *Thorax* 2003; **58** (Suppl 2): ii29–38.
100. Bloom AI, Wilson MW, Kerlan RK Jr, Gordon RL, LaBerge JM. Talc pleurodesis through small-bore percutaneous tubes. *Cardiovasc Intervent Radiol* 1999; **22**: 433–6.
101. Marom EM, Patz EF Jr, Erasmus JJ, *et al.* Malignant pleural effusions: treatment with small-bore-catheter thoracostomy and talc pleurodesis. *Radiology* 1999; **210**: 277–81.
102. Morrison MC, Mueller PR, Lee MJ, *et al.* Sclerotherapy of malignant pleural effusion through sonographically placed small-bore catheters. *AJR Am J Roentgenol* 1992; **158**: 41–3.
103. Musani AI, Haas AR, Seijo L, Wilby M, Sterman DH. Outpatient management of malignant pleural effusions with small-bore, tunneled pleural catheters. *Respiration* 2004; **71**: 559–66.
104. Saffran L, Ost DE, Fein AM, Schiff MJ. Outpatient pleurodesis of malignant pleural effusions using a small-bore pigtail catheter. *Chest* 2000; **118**: 417–21.
105. Spiegler PA, Hurewitz AN, Groth ML. Rapid pleurodesis for malignant pleural effusions. *Chest* 2003; **123**: 1895–8.
106. Walsh FW, Alberts WM, Solomon DA, Goldman AL. Malignant pleural effusions: pleurodesis using a small-bore percutaneous catheter. *South Med J* 1989; **82**: 963–5, 972.
107. Putnam JB Jr, Light RW, Rodriguez RM, *et al.* A randomized comparison of indwelling pleural catheter and doxycycline pleurodesis in the management of malignant pleural effusions. *Cancer* 1999; **86**: 1992–9.
108. Putnam JB Jr, Walsh GL, Swisher SG, *et al.* Outpatient management of malignant pleural effusion by a chronic indwelling pleural catheter. *Ann Thorac Surg* 2000; **69**: 369–75.
109. Dryzer SR, Allen ML, Strange C, Sahn SA. A comparison of rotation and nonrotation in tetracycline pleurodesis. *Chest* 1993; **104**: 1763–6.
110. Mager HJ, Maesen B, Verzijlbergen F, Schramel F. Distribution of talc suspension during treatment of malignant pleural effusion with talc pleurodesis. *Lung Cancer* 2002; **36**: 77–81.
111. Goodman A, Davies CW. Efficacy of short-term versus long-term chest tube drainage following talc slurry pleurodesis in patients with malignant pleural effusions: a randomised trial. *Lung Cancer* 2006; **54**: 51–5.
112. Sherman S, Ravikrishnan KP, Patel AS, Seidman JC. Optimum anesthesia with intrapleural lidocaine during chemical pleurodesis with tetracycline. *Chest* 1988; **93**: 533–6.
113. Teixeira LR, Wu W, Chang DS, Light RW. The effect of corticosteroids on pleurodesis induced by doxycycline in rabbits. *Chest* 2002; **121**: 216–9.
114. Teixeira LR, Vargas FS, Acencio MM, *et al.* Influence of antiinflammatory drugs (methylprednisolone and diclofenac sodium) on experimental pleurodesis induced by silver nitrate or talc. *Chest* 2005; **128**: 4041–5.
115. Rodriguez-Panadero F, Segado A, Torres I, *et al.* Thoracoscopy and talc poudrage induce an activation of the systemic coagulation system. *Am J Respir Crit Care Med* 1995; **151**: 785–90.
116. Rodriguez-Panadero F, Segado A, Martin J, *et al.* Activation of systemic coagulation in talc poudrage can be (partially) controlled with prophylactic heparin. *Am J Respir Crit Care Med* 1996; **152**: A458.
117. Bouchama A, Chastre J, Gaudichet A, Soler P, Gibert C. Acute pneumonitis with bilateral pleural effusion after talc pleurodesis. *Chest* 1984; **86**: 795–7.

118. Campos JR, Werebe EC, Vargas FS, Jatene FB, Light RW. Respiratory failure due to insufflated talc. *Lancet* 1997; **349**: 251–2.
119. Marel M, Skacel Z, Bednar M, Julak J, Light RW. Corynebacterium parvum, bleomycin and talc in the treatment of malignant pleural effusions. *J BUON* 1998; **1**: 165–70.
120. Migueres J, Jover A. [Indications for intrapleural talc under pleuroscopic control in malignant recurrent pleural effusions. Based on 26 cases (author's transl)]. *Poumon Coeur* 1981; **37**: 295–7.
121. Nandi P. Recurrent spontaneous pneumothorax; an effective method of talc poudrage. *Chest* 1980; **77**: 493–5.
122. Rehse DH, Aye RW, Florence MG. Respiratory failure following talc pleurodesis. *Am J Surg* 1999; **177**: 437–40.
123. Rinaldo JE, Owens GR, Rogers RM. Adult respiratory distress syndrome following intrapleural instillation of talc. *J Thorac Cardiovasc Surg* 1983; **85**: 523–6.
124. Todd TR, Delarue NC, Ilves R, Pearson FG, Cooper JD. Talc poudrage of malignant pleural effusion. *Chest* 1980; **78**: 542–3.
125. Ferrer J, Villarino MA, Tura JM, Traveria A, Light RW. Talc preparations used for pleurodesis vary markedly from one preparation to another. *Chest* 2001; **119**: 1901–5.
126. Janssen JP, Collier G, Astoul P, *et al.* Safety of pleurodesis with talc poudrage in malignant pleural effusion: a prospective cohort study. *Lancet* 2007; **369**: 1535–9.
127. Lange P, Mortensen J, Groth S. Lung function 22–35 years after treatment of idiopathic spontaneous pneumothorax with talc poudrage or simple drainage. *Thorax* 1988; **43**: 559–61.
128. Gyorik S, Erni S, Studler U, *et al.* Long term follow up of thoracoscopic talc pleurodesis for primary spontaneous pneumothorax. *Eur Respir J* 2006.
129. Vargas FS, Teixeira LR, Vaz MA, *et al.* Silver nitrate is superior to talc slurry in producing pleurodesis in rabbits. *Chest* 2000; **118**: 808–13.
130. Sorensen PG, Svendsen TL, Enk B. Treatment of malignant pleural effusion with drainage, with and without instillation of talc. *Eur J Respir Dis* 1984; **65**: 131–5.

47

Medical thoracoscopy

ROBERT LODDENKEMPER

INTRODUCTION

Thoracoscopy was first used almost 100 years ago, primarily as a diagnostic procedure,[1] but soon also as a therapeutic technique for lysis of pleural adhesions by means of thoracocautery ('Jacobaeus operation') to facilitate pneumothorax treatment of tuberculosis.[2] Later, the addition of the term 'medical' was necessary[3] in order to distinguish this procedure from 'surgical' thoracoscopy which is much more invasive, using general anesthesia, a double-lumen endotracheal tube and multiple points of entry.[4] Surgical thoracoscopy is better described as video-assisted thoracic surgery (VATS), whereas medical thoracoscopy can be performed under local anesthesia or conscious sedation, in an endoscopy suite, using non-disposable rigid or semi-rigid instruments. It is therefore considerably less invasive and less expensive.[5]

Medical thoracoscopy is today primarily a diagnostic method, but it can also be applied for therapeutic purposes. Pleural effusions are by far the leading indication for medical thoracoscopy, both for diagnosis – mainly in exudates of unknown etiology and for staging in diffuse malignant mesothelioma or lung cancer – and for treatment by talc pleurodesis in malignant or other recurrent effusions, or in cases of empyema. An excellent indication for medical thoracoscopy is pneumothorax, for staging as well as for local treatment. For those familiar with the technique, other mainly diagnostic indications are biopsies from the diaphragm, the lung, the mediastinum and the pericardium. In addition, medical thoracoscopy is a remarkable tool for research as a 'gold standard' in the study of pleural effusions.[5]

In Europe, medical thoracoscopy is part of the training program of pneumology,[6] but it is also becoming more popular in the USA, where according to a national survey in 1994 medical thoracoscopy was applied frequently by 5 percent of all pneumologists.[7] In an Amercan College of Chest Physicians (ACCP) survey of 2002/2003, on US pulmonary/critical care fellowship programs, only 12 percent of the directors stated that medical thoracoscopy/pleuroscopy were offered in their programs,[8] although the interest in this procedure seems to be much larger.[9] In the UK, where medical thoracoscopy was under-utilized when compared with the rest of Europe, there is also now growing interest.[10]

Medical thoracoscopy as well as rigid bronchoscopy are parts of the field of interventional pulmonology.[11] In order to avoid confusion with surgical thoracoscopy, it can be discussed whether the term 'pleuroscopy', as already used in 1923 in the French literature,[12] should be substituted for the term 'medical thoracoscopy'.

HISTORICAL BACKGROUND

Hans-Christian Jacobaeus, an internist working in Stockholm/Sweden, in 1910 introduced thoracoscopy at the same time as laparoscopy in a paper entitled 'Concerning the possibility of using cystoscopy in the examination of serous cavities'.[1] However, it has to be mentioned that Francis

Richard Cruise in Ireland most probably was the first who in 1866 performed a binocular thoracoscopy.[13,14] After the report by Jacobaeus, thoracoscopy was used for diagnostic purposes by some other pulmonary specialists, mainly in Scandinavia, Germany, Italy and other European countries.[15] Jacobaeus published his vast diagnostic experiences in 1925, describing in detail his studies of the etiology and staging of tuberculous pleurisy, of malignant effusion, rheumatoid effusion, empyema, parapneumonic effusion, as well as idiopathic pneumothorax.[16]

However, Jacobaeus himself initiated the therapeutic application of thoracoscopy for lysis of pleural adhesions by means of thoracocautery to facilitate pneumothorax treatment of tuberculosis (Jacobaeus' operation).[2] During the ensuing 40 years, his technique of using one entry for the thoracoscope and another for the electrocautery was applied worldwide for this specific therapeutic purpose,[12] until antibiotic therapy of tuberculosis was introduced and proved much more successful. However, during these times thoracoscopy was also used by several authors, again mainly in Europe, as a therapeutic tool in non-tuberculous diseases, especially in the treatment of patients with idiopathic spontaneous pneumothorax.[17] Later, in 1963, the first report on talc poudrage during thoracoscopy for pleurodesis in chronic, mainly malignant pleural effusions was published.[18] This technique is now frequently applied because of its high success rate.[19] Between 1950 and 1960, a generation of chest physicians already familiar with the therapeutic application of thoracoscopy began to use the technique on a much broader basis in pleuropulmonary biopsy diagnosis, even for localized and diffuse lung diseases and, in the following years, the technique became popular mainly in continental Europe,[20,21] and later in other parts of the world.[22–24]

The excellent results of laparoscopic surgery and the tremendous advances in endoscopic technology stimulated many thoracic surgeons almost simultaneously in Europe and the USA to develop minimally invasive techniques which were termed 'therapeutic' or 'surgical thoracoscopy' as well as 'video-controlled' or 'video-thoracoscopic surgery' or 'video-assisted thoracic surgery' (VATS).[4,25,26]

Particularly in the USA, where thoracoscopy was performed only by few pulmonary physicians, a heated debate was started whether thoracoscopy should be the domain of the pulmonologists or of the thoracic surgeon,[26,27] while in most parts of Europe this was not a controversial issue as many pneumologists had been performing thoracoscopy for several years before the introduction of VATS.[28,29] Today, American thoracic surgeons agree that medical thoracoscopy (pleuroscopy) is in the domain of pulmonologists, but correctly claim that adequate training is needed.[30,31]

TECHNIQUES

Medical thoracoscopy is an invasive technique, which should be used only when other simple methods fail. As with all technical procedures, there is a learning curve before full competence is achieved.[32] Appropriate training is therefore mandatory. The technique is actually very similar to chest-tube insertion by means of a trocar, the difference being that the pleural cavity can be visualized in addition and biopsies can be taken from all areas of the pleural cavity including the chest wall, diaphragm, mediastinum and lung. If indicated, talc poudrage can be performed prior to chest-tube insertion. In our experience, medical thoracoscopy is easier to learn than flexible bronchoscopy, if sufficient expertise in thoracentesis and chest-tube placement has already been gained.[5]

Jacobaeus[1] in his pioneering paper defined three main prerequisites for the examination of serous cavities. First, the possibility to introduce a trocar (or puncture needle) into the respective cavity without lacerating the inner organs and without causing too much pain. Second, the introduction of a transparent medium into the cavity – he used filtered air for this purpose. Third, an endoscope of such small dimensions that it can be introduced through the trocar. He felt that these three main prerequisites were fulfilled even better by thoracoscopy than by laparoscopy.

An absolute prerequisite for thoracoscopy is the presence of an adequate pleural space, which should be at least 6–10 cm in diameter. If not already present, a pneumothorax is induced, immediately before thoracoscopy under fluoroscopic/sonographic control or the day before under radiographic control. If extensive pleuropulmonary adhesions exist, 'extended' thoracoscopy without creating a pneumothorax can be carried out, but this requires special skills and should not be undertaken without special training.[33] The use of mini-thoracoscopy may be a less invasive alternative in patients with loculated effusions.[34]

The main advantage of medical thoracoscopy compared with VATS is that the examination can be performed under local anesthesia or conscious sedation (neuroleptic analgesia) after adequate premedication, and thus without the support of an anesthetist. Furthermore, medical thoracoscopy is also less expensive because it may be safely performed with non-disposable instruments and in an appropriate endoscopy room.

There are two different techniques of diagnostic and therapeutic thoracoscopy, as performed by the pneumologist. The one method, very similar to the technique first described by Jacobaeus for diagnostic purposes, uses a single entry with a rigid 9 mm thoracoscope (Storz Company/Olympus) with a working channel for accessory instruments and an optical biopsy forceps under local anesthesia[3,20,35] (Figure 47.1).

The single entry technique has now been modified by the introduction of an autoclavable semi-rigid pleuroscope (Olympus) which has the advantage that handling is very simple, similar to a flexible bronchovideoscope (Figure 47.2).[24,36,37]

The other technique, as used by Jacobaeus for lysis of adhesions, uses two entries, one with a 7 mm trocar for the rigid examination telescope and the other with a 5 mm

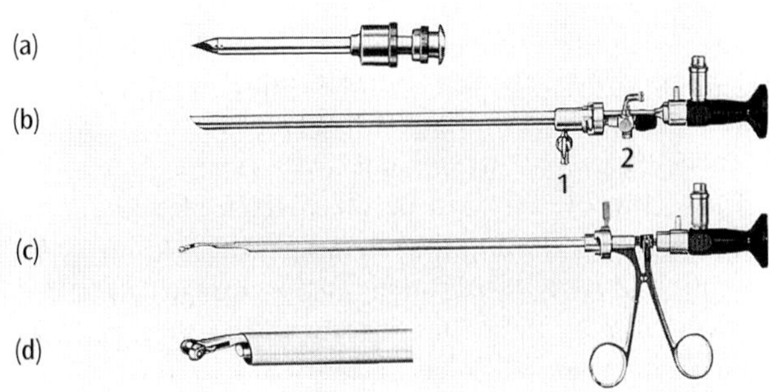

Figure 47.1 Thoracoscopy instruments (Storz Company): (a) trocar and cannula; (b) single-entry thoracoscope for adults (c) biopsy forceps with straight optics, which fit through the thoracoscope shaft; (d) forceps in the thoracoscope shaft ready for biopsy.

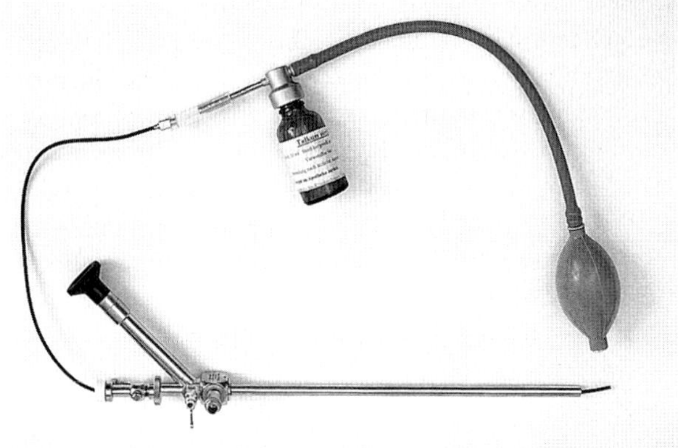

Figure 47.3 Thoracoscope with angled optic and a flexible suction catheter, which is connected to a small bottle containing talc, and to a pneumatic atomizer, is introduced through the working channel of the thoracoscope.

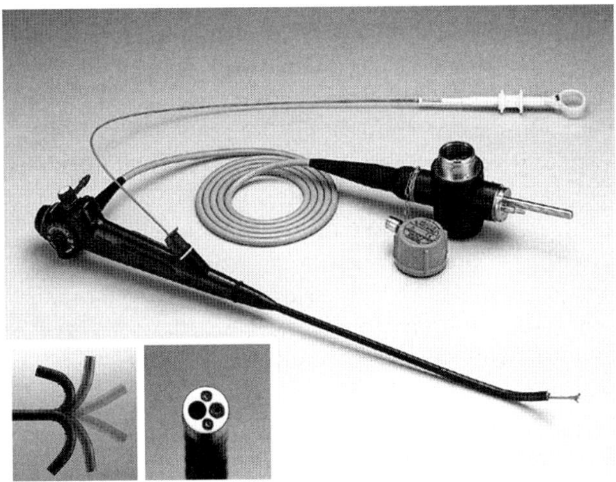

Figure 47.2 Semi-rigid videothoracoscope (Olympus).

trocar for accessory instruments, including the biopsy forceps (Wolf Company). For this technique, neuroleptic or general anesthesia is preferred.[21]

Endoscopy can be performed either under direct visual control through the endoscopic optique or indirectly by video transmission, which allows a magnified view, better teaching by demonstration to assistants and others, as well as appropriate documentation.[38] Video transmission is not a prerequisite for rigid thoracoscopy in this setting, but only a modification of the technique, whereas VATS (or 'surgical thoracoscopy') definitely requires video equipment and thereby the aid of an assistant and the use of (disposable) instruments such as staplers.[4]

For cauterization of adhesions and blebs, or in case of bleeding after biopsy, electrocoagulation (or laser coagulation) should be available. For pleurodesis of effusions, 8–10 mL of sterile, dry asbestos-free talc is insufflated through a rigid or flexible suction catheter with a pneumatic atomizer[19,21] (Figure 47.3). In pneumothorax patients, 2–3 mL of talc is sufficient.[39,40] After thoracoscopy, a chest tube is introduced through which immediate suction is started carefully.

The one-entry technique is easy to perform under local anesthesia[20,23,24,35] but some premedication (midazolam/hydrocodon or others) should be routinely administered. Thoracoscopy is usually carried out in the lateral decubitus position, with the hemithorax to be studied facing upwards. Fluoroscopy allows evaluation of adhesions between the lung and chest wall, which might complicate introduction of the thoracoscope. It should be recalled that the diaphragm is positioned much higher than when the patient is upright. The site of induction of the thoracoscope depends on the location of radiographically detected abnormalities, while avoiding potentially hazardous areas such as that of the internal mammary artery, the axillary region with the lateral thoracic artery and the infraclavicular region with the subclavian artery. The region of the diaphragm is unsuitable, not only because adhesions are frequent, but also because the liver or spleen may be accidentally injured. Insertion of the cannula in the lateral thoracic region between the mid- and anterior axillary lines in the sixth or seventh intercostal space is preferred.

After introducing the trocar, the pleural effusion – if present – should be removed as completely as possible. This can be done without risk because, by using a suction tube which does not completely occlude the cannula, air rapidly enters the pleural space to provide pressure equilibration. After removing the effusion, the thoracoscope is introduced and the entire cavity inspected (Figures 47.4 and 47.5). In case of a pleural effusion, biopsies are taken from several suspicious areas, including the anterior and posterior chest wall and the diaphragm (Figure 47.6). Biopsies from the lung are not taken routinely, but only when the parietal pleura appears normal but the lung surface shows abnormal lesions, to avoid creation of a fistula. Biopsies are taken for histologic evaluation and, if suspicious, for tuberculosis culture.

Following thoracoscopy, a chest tube should be introduced and connected to a suction system. Suction should be applied carefully, especially in cases of trapped lung, long-standing effusion or pneumothorax, in order to avoid re-expansion pulmonary edema, or creation of a fistula.

If indicated, talc poudrage is performed by uniform distribution of talc to all pleural surfaces under direct visual control (Figures 47.7 and 47.8). Additional pain medication should be given as necessary.[41]

The two-entry technique is usually performed under general or neuroleptic anesthesia, if biopsies are taken through the second point of entry. Details are given in the

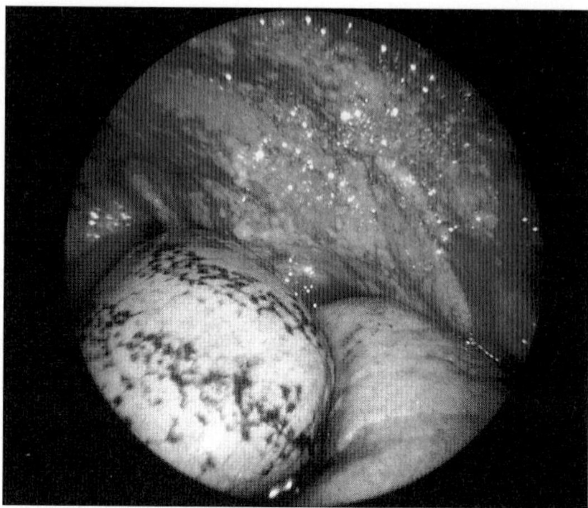

Figure 47.4 Thoracoscopic view into the left pleural cavity with normal upper and lower lobes of the lung. The chest wall pleura is covered by a whitish layer of small tumor nodules (diffuse malignant pleural mesothelioma). (See also Color Plate 49.)

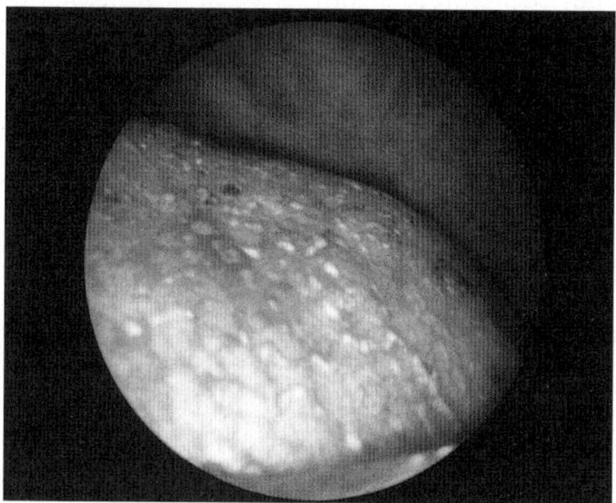

Figure 47.5 Lymphangiosis carcinomatosis of the lower lobe in a patient with right-sided pleural effusion. No tumor growth on the parietal pleura. (See also Color Plate 50.)

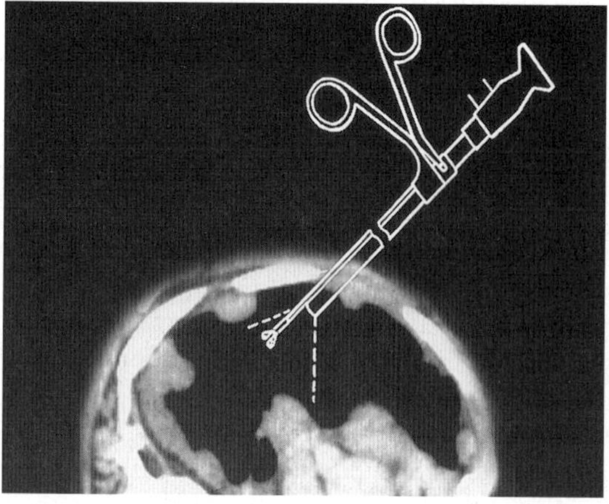

Figure 47.6 Computed tomography simulation of medical thoracoscopy in the lateral position. Biopsies are taken under visual control from different areas.

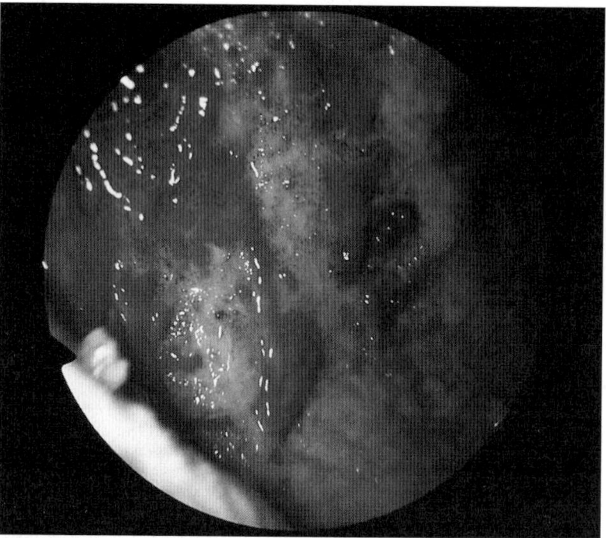

Figure 47.7 Larger hemorrhagic tumor nodules on the chest wall pleura (metastatic adenocarcinoma). (See also Color Plate 51.)

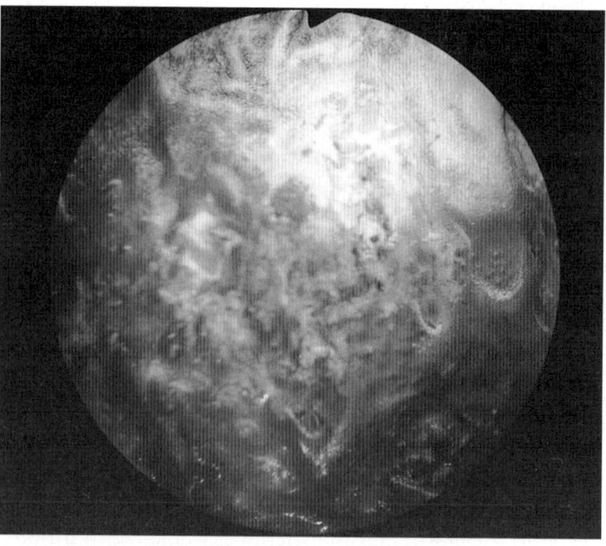

Figure 47.8 Same patient as in Figure 45.7 after talc poudrage. (See also Color Plate 52.)

book *Practical Thoracoscopy* by Boutin, Viallat and Aelony.[21]

CONTRAINDICATIONS AND PREVENTION OF COMPLICATIONS

Medical thoracoscopy is safe if the contraindications are observed, and if certain standard criteria are fulfilled.[20,21,41] An obliterated pleural space is an absolute contraindication. Relative contraindications include bleeding disorders, hypoxemia and an unstable cardiovascular status, as well as persistent uncontrollable cough.

Cardiorespiratory functions should be monitored during the procedure by electrocardiogram (ECG), measurement of blood pressure and continuous oximetry. Complications such as benign cardiac arrhythmias, low-grade hypertension or hypoxemia can be almost completely prevented by nasal administration of oxygen.[38,42] Since significant hypoventilation has been observed under sedation-assisted local anaesthesia, the additional measurement of cutaneous carbon dioxide tension ($PcCO_2$) is recommended.[43]

The most serious, but fortunately least frequent, complication is severe hemorrhage due to blood vessel injury during the procedure. This, and pulmonary perforations, can be avoided by using safe points of entry and a cautious biopsy technique. In case of persistent bleeding, electrocoagulation may be necessary. In our experience of almost 7000 thoracoscopies, surgical intervention was never necessary to stop bleeding caused by medical thoracoscopy. The most serious complication of pneumothorax induction is air or gas embolism, which occurs very rarely (<0.1 percent), provided that the necessary precautionary measures are taken.[14]

The reported mortality rates (<0.01 percent) are very low.[38,44] Even several liters of fluid can be completely removed during thoracoscopy with little risk of pulmonary re-expansion edema because immediate equilibration of pressures is provided by direct entrance of air through the cannula into the pleural space. If the re-expansion potential of the lung appears to be diminished, at most only low-pressure suction should be applied through the intrapleural drainage tube, which is always placed at the end of thoracoscopy. Following lung biopsy, a bronchopleural fistula may result. This may require longer than the usual suction periods of 3–5 days, particularly in cases with stiff lungs. After talc poudrage, fever may occur. Local site infection is, however, uncommon, and empyema has been reported only very rarely,[44] often as sequelae of long-term drainage with bronchopleural fistula.[20]

In cases of mesothelioma, radiotherapy should be carried out after medical thoracoscopy to prevent the late complications of tumor growth at the sites of entry:[45] 10–12 days after thoracoscopy, once the incision has healed, Boutin and co-workers in a randomized trial applied electron therapy between 12.5 and 15 MeV to the thoracic wall over all puncture sites. None of the 20 mesothelioma patients who received radiotherapy developed malignant outgrowths from the chest wall, whereas of the 20 who were not irradiated, nine (45 percent, $p < 0.05$) developed nodules. However, tumor growth may occur even after diagnostic thoracentesis with small needles, or after closed needle biopsy. The usefulness of prophylactic radiotherapy in mesothelioma was confirmed in a report from the UK.[46]

INDICATIONS

Medical thoracoscopy is primarily a diagnostic procedure.[3,5] The indications for its use include evaluation of exudative effusions of unknown cause, staging of malignant mesothelioma or lung cancer, and treatment of malignant or other recurrent effusions with talc pleurodesis. The procedure is not only the gold standard in the diagnosis of pleural effusions, but it is also a remarkable tool for research as a gold standard in the study of pleural effusions. It can also be useful in the management of early empyema and of pneumothorax. If placement of a chest tube is indicated anyhow, and if the facilities are available, medical thoracoscopy should be performed at the time of chest-tube insertion by the trocar technique. For those familiar with the technique, other, mainly diagnostic indications are biopsies from the diaphragm, the lung, the mediastinum and the pericardium, but today there is a definite trend towards its use almost exclusively in pleural effusions and pneumothorax.

The changed indications for medical thoracoscopy are reflected by the development at our own institution, Lungenklinik Heckeshorn in Berlin/Germany.[15] Pleural effusions are by far the most frequent application of medical thoracoscopy (over 90 percent). A decline in the other indications is explained by several factors. Medical thoracoscopy for diagnostic purposes in localized lung and chest wall lesions has been almost abandoned since imaging techniques such as computed tomography (CT) or magnetic resonance imaging (MRI) very often deliver the diagnosis or allow differentiation between malignant and benign disease. Furthermore, VATS or surgical thoracoscopy has the advantage that the lesion can be removed simultaneously. Our indications for lung biopsies in diffuse lung disease have decreased, too. This is due to the improved diagnostic results of bronchoscopy using transbronchial lung biopsies and bronchoalveolar lavage, as well as to the development of high-resolution CT (HRCT), which has considerably improved the diagnostic evaluation of diffuse lung diseases. At our institution, for many years, the department of thoracic surgery has been responsible for almost all patients with spontaneous pneumothorax. However, the thoracic surgeons today routinely apply medical thoracoscopy at the time of chest-tube insertion through the cannula, under local anesthesia, in their cases with spontaneous pneumothorax.[47] They also use this approach frequently for cases of empyema, where the medical thoracoscopic technique is applied at the time of chest-tube placement.[48]

The absolute number of pleural effusions at our institution has risen markedly because more and more cases of pleural effusion are referred for diagnostic and therapeutic purposes, more than two-thirds are malignant effusions. The number of tuberculous pleurisies fell considerably due to the decrease in incidence, and pleural effusions of other origin now comprise about 25 percent. Here, medical thoracoscopy was performed mainly for differential diagnosis, in particular to exclude malignancy or tuberculosis (TB), in a few cases also for talc pleurodesis in cases of recurrent pleural effusion of non-malignant etiology. If one takes the estimate of Light for the annual incidences of 750 000 non-cardiac and non-parapneumonic pleural effusions in the USA, one would, by that rationale, expect about 6000 pleural effusions annually in our catchment area, which comprises mainly the western part of Berlin with approximately two million inhabitants. Of these, approximately 2000 would be of malignant origin, and less than 5–10 percent of these would finally undergo medical thoracoscopy.[5]

PLEURAL EFFUSIONS

Conservative estimates suggest that approximately 25 percent of the cases seen in a general pulmonologist's practice demonstrate pleural effusions.[49,50] In approximately 25 percent of these cases, a specific diagnosis cannot be made, even after thoracentesis and closed pleural biopsy.[51] In a series by Boutin *et al.*[32] of 1000 consecutive patients with pleural effusion, 215 cases remained undiagnosed even after repeated pleural fluid analysis and performance of pleural biopsies. This is in agreement with the results of several other authors, who report that without thoracoscopy, at least 20–25 percent of pleural effusions remain undiagnosed, although this certainly depends strongly on patient populations.

Several studies have tried to determine the diagnostic accuracy of medical thoracoscopy in the setting of undiagnosed pleural effusion, but the results vary widely, with a range of 69 to 90 percent. Closer evaluation of the study designs reveals that the duration of follow-up was occasionally short and frequently not mentioned at all. One well-designed study reported by Menzies[52] with follow-up periods between 1 and 2 years found a sensitivity of 91 percent, specificity of 100 percent, accuracy of 96 percent, and negative predictive value of 93 percent. Boutin *et al.*[32] reported a false-negative rate of 15 percent within 1 year of follow-up, while Enk and Viskum[53] reported a diagnostic accuracy of 69 percent with a 5-year follow-up period. A retrospective study of 709 patients with pleural effusion showed that 29 percent remained inconclusive after thoracoscopy.[54] After long-term follow-up, a malignancy was found in 4.3 percent and a true benign disease in 24.7 percent of the whole group. In 15 percent of the patients, the diagnosis of non-specific pleuritis after thoracoscopy appeared to be false-negative. The authors calculated a positive predictive value of 100 percent and a negative predictive value of 92 percent. In another retrospective study of 75 patients diagnosed with non-specific pleuritis after thoracoscopy, follow-up revealed a malignant origin in 8.3 percent (three cases with lung cancer, two cases with mesothelioma).[55] The authors conclude that a histological diagnosis of non-specific pleuritis does not necessarily imply a clinical diagnosis of idiopathic pleuritis. They recommend a close follow-up, particularly in patients with a history of asbestos exposure. Autofluorescence videothoracoscopy may help in the future to avoid some of the false-negative results.[56]

In comparison, even in a study on thoracotomy in patients with pleural effusion of undetermined etiology after a pathological diagnosis of a benign pleural process, 25 percent of patients were still diagnosed with a malignancy within 6 months.[57]

Because of its high diagnostic accuracy, we perform diagnostic medical thoracoscopy in almost all cases of exudates in which the etiology remains undetermined after pleural fluid analysis. Due to the low additional diagnostic yield of closed blind needle biopsy, we recommend medical thoracoscopy after inconclusive diagnostic work-up of the pleural fluid if the facilities for medical thoracoscopy are available.[19] The procedure allows fast and more definite biopsy diagnosis, including a high yield in tuberculosis cultures, and determination of hormone receptors in some malignancies. Furthermore, staging in lung cancer and diffuse mesothelioma is possible. The exclusion of malignancy or TB is provided with high probability. Furthermore, medical thoracoscopy allows complete fluid removal and evaluation of the re-expansion potential of the lung. Fibrinous loculations in tuberculosis and empyema are easily removed, thus creating a single pleural cavity, which allows more efficient treatment.[5]

MALIGNANT PLEURAL EFFUSIONS

Malignant pleural effusions are today the leading diagnostic and therapeutic indication for medical thoracoscopy.[27,28,58,59] In a prospective intrapatient comparison, the diagnostic yield of non-surgical biopsy methods in malignant pleural effusions was studied simultaneously in 208 patients, including 58 diffuse malignant mesotheliomas, 29 cancers of the lung, 116 metastatic pleural effusions with 28 breast cancers, 30 cancers of various other organs, 58 of undetermined origin and 5 malignant lymphomas.[60] The diagnostic yield was 62 percent by pleural fluid cytology, 44 percent by closed pleural biopsy and 95 percent by medical thoracoscopy (Table 47.1). The sensitivity of medical thoracoscopy was higher than that of cytology and closed pleural biopsy combined (95 versus 74

Table 47.1 Sensitivity (%) of non-surgical biopsy methods in malignant pleural effusions. Prospective simultaneous comparison ($n = 206$)

Method	Sensitivity (%)
Fluid cytology (FC)	62
Closed needle (CN)	44
FC + CN	74
Medical thoracoscopy (MT)	95
MT + FC	96
MT + FC + CN	97

Taken from Loddenkemper *et al.*[60]

percent, $p > 0.001$). The combined non-surgical methods were diagnostic in 97 percent of malignant pleural effusions. In six of the 208 cases (2.8 percent), an underlying neoplasm was suspected at thoracoscopy, but confirmed only by thoracotomy or autopsy. Similar results have been reported by other investigators.[32,52,61]

The reasons for false-negative results of medical thoracoscopy include insufficient and non-representative biopsies that depend largely on the experience of the thoracoscopist and the presence of adhesions preventing access to the neoplastic tissue.[28,32] An additional reason could be that early lesions are not detected by normal, but only by autofluorescence light.[56]

The diagnostic sensitivity of medical thoracoscopy is similar for all types of malignant effusion (Table 47.2). The overall yield in 287 cases was 62 percent for cytology and 95 percent for medical thoracoscopy; the yield for cytology and in particular medical thoracoscopy did not vary greatly between lung carcinomas ($n = 67$) with 67 versus 96 percent, extrathoracic primaries ($n = 154$) with 62 versus 95.5 percent, and diffuse malignant mesotheliomas ($n = 66$) with 58 versus 92 percent.[5,19]

Medical thoracoscopy may be useful in staging lung cancer, diffuse malignant mesothelioma (Figure 47.4) and metastatic cancer (Figures 47.7 and 47.8). In lung cancer patients, thoracoscopy can help to determine whether the effusion is malignant or paramalignant.[28] As a result, it may be possible to avoid exploratory thoracotomy for tumor staging. Weissberg *et al.*[62] performed thoracoscopies in 45 patients with lung cancer and pleural effusion. In 37, they found pleural invasion; three patients had mediastinal disease, the remaining five had no evident metastatic disease, and, therefore, no contraindication for tumor resection. Canto *et al.*[63] found no thoracoscopic evidence of pleural involvement in 8 of 44 patients, six proceeded to resection with no pleural involvement found.[63]

In diffuse malignant mesothelioma, medical thoracoscopy can provide an earlier diagnosis and better histologic classification than closed pleural biopsy because of larger and more representative biopsies, and more accurate staging.[64,65] This may have important therapeutic implications, since much better responses to local immunotherapy or local chemotherapy have been observed in the early stages (I and II).[66–68] The technique is also helpful in the diagnosis of benign asbestos-related pleural effusion (BAPE) by excluding mesothelioma or malignancies. Fibrohyaline or calcified, thick and pearly white pleural plaques may be found, indicating possible asbestos exposure.[68] Thoracoscopic pulmonary biopsies and even biopsies from special lesions on the parietal pleura may demonstrate high concentrations of asbestos fibers and thereby provide further support for a diagnosis of asbestos-induced disease.[69]

A further advantage of medical thoracoscopy in metastatic pleural disease is that biopsies of the visceral and diaphragmatic pleura are possible under direct observation. In addition, because of the larger size of thoracoscopic biopsies, these may provide easier identification of primary tumor, including hormone receptor determination in breast cancer,[70,71] and improved morphological classification in lymphomas.[72] In addition, the extent of intrapleural tumor spread can be semiquantified using a scoring system which has been shown to correlate quite closely with survival,[73] and with the success of talc pleurodesis.[74]

The main advantage in using thoracoscopy to diagnose malignancy is that talc poudrage can be performed during medical thoracoscopy (Figures 47.7 and 47.8), which is probably the best conservative option today for pleurodesis, with success rates of more than 80 percent.[28,75] These high success rates may be due to the more even distribution of talc powder to all parts of the pleura. It has also proven very efficient in the treatment of lymphomatous

Table 47.2 Sensitivity (%) of medical thoracoscopy and pleural fluid cytology in different malignant etiologies. Prospective simultaneous comparison at Lungenklinik Heckeshorn, Berlin, Germany

Method	Bronchial carcinoma ($n = 67$)	Extrathoracic primaries ($n = 154$)	Diffuse malignant mesothelioma ($n = 66$)	All ($n = 287$)
Pleural fluid cytology	67	62	58	62
Medical thoracoscopy	96	95.5	92	95

chylothorax, even after all other treatment options have failed.[76]

TALC POUDRAGE

Talc poudrage is the most widely reported method of talc instillation into the pleural space.[19] It can be easily performed at medical thoracoscopy (Figure 47.3) under local anesthesia with some additional pain medication, if necessary.

As a prerequisite for successful pleurodesis, all pleural fluid must be removed before spraying talc. Removal can be easily accomplished during thoracoscopy, as air is entering the pleural cavity, thus creating the desired equilibrium in pressures. Complete collapse of the lung is desirable, because it permits wide and uniform distribution of the talc.[28,75]

The optimal dose of talc for poudrage is not known, but usually about 4–6 g (8–12 mL) are recommended for malignant effusions.[39,77] Thoracoscopic inspection of the pleural cavity should be done during talc insufflation to ensure that talc is uniformly distributed over pleural surfaces (Figures 47.7 and 47.8).

After talc poudrage, an 8–11 mm (24–30 French) chest tube should always be inserted. Suction should be applied carefully and progressively to avoid creation of air leaks which can be caused by necrotic tissue in the visceral pleura. The chest tube can be removed when the daily amount of fluid production is lower than 100 mL. Pleurodesis success rates with talc poudrage are usually above 80 percent, but there are only few prospective studies comparing talc with other pleurodesis agents.[78–83]

The advantage of talc poudrage compared with slurry is probably the more even distribution over the whole pleural surface, which can be achieved under visual control.[75] In our own experience, we observe fewer loculations than with talc slurry. In a large randomized trial of talc poudrage versus talc slurry with 501 patients, an advantage of poudrage was seen only in those patients (whether they lived 30 days or not) who had more than 90 percent lung re-expansion (78 versus 71 percent efficacy of sclerosis with prevention of recurrence, $p = 0.045$).[84] If the two most common etiologies (breast and lung cancer) for malignant pleural effusion were examined, there was also a statistical difference favoring poudrage ($p = 0.022$) in patients living 30 days with more than 90 percent re-expansion. The authors concluded that prevention of recurrence of malignant pleural effusions from breast or lung cancers can be achieved with a success rate of 82 percent with poudrage versus 67 percent with slurry.

Talc is inexpensive and highly effective. Its most common short-term adverse effects include fever, due to systemic inflammatory reaction,[85] and pain. Cardiovascular complications such as arrhythmias, cardiac arrest, chest pain, myocardial infarction or hypotension have been noted; whether these complications result from the procedures or are related to talc *per se* has not been determined.[19] Acute respiratory distress syndrome (ARDS), acute pneumonitis and respiratory failure have also been reported to occur after both talc poudrage and slurry.[84,86,87] The development of respiratory failure most likely is related to dose and, in particular, particle size.[88–90] It is remarkable that several large series from Europe and from Israel did not observe ARDS after thoracoscopic talc insufflations.[28,75,91–93] This was also found in a large multicenter, open-label, prospective cohort study of 558 patients with malignant pleural effusions who underwent medical thoracoscopy and talc poudrage with 4 g of calibrated French graded large-particle talc. No patient developed acute respiratory distress syndrome, proving that the use of large-particle talc for pleurodesis is safe.[77,94]

In vitro studies suggest that talc induces apoptosis in human malignant mesothelioma cells and might therefore have an anti-tumorous effect.[95] One explanation may be that talc mediates angiostasis in malignant pleural effusion via endostatin induction.[96]

TUBERCULOUS PLEURAL EFFUSIONS

Although the diagnostic yield of pleural fluid TB culture and of closed needle biopsy combined is quite high, there may be indications for medical thoracoscopy in otherwise uncertain pleural effusions.[5] The diagnostic accuracy of thoracoscopy is almost 100 percent because the pathologist is provided with multiple, selected biopsies and because the cultural proof of tubercle bacilli growth is more frequent.

In a prospective intrapatient comparison, the immediate diagnosis in 100 TB cases was established histologically by medical thoracoscopy in 94 percent, compared with only 38 percent with needle biopsy.[97] This may be of clinical importance, because anti-tuberculous chemotherapy can be started without delay. The combined yield of histology and bacteriological culture was 99 percent for medical thoracoscopy and 51 percent for needle biopsy, and 61 percent when culture results from effusions were added (Table 47.3). The percentage of positive TB cultures was twice as high from thoracoscopic biopsies, including cultures from fibrinous membranes (78 percent), as the percentage from pleural fluid and needle biopsies combined (39 percent), allowing bacteriological confirmation of the diagnosis and, furthermore, susceptibility tests. In 5 of the 78 positive cases (6.4 percent), resistance to one or multiple anti-tuberculous drugs was found, which influenced therapy and prognosis. The chance for positive TB cultures was much higher (78 percent) in cases with fibrin production. This type, with a diffusely thickened pleura, multiple adhesions, and sometimes formation of encapsulated membranes with fluid loculations, was present in 75 percent of cases (Figure 47.9). By comparison, the typical picture of sago-like early pleuritis with miliary tuberculous granulomas and without fibrin layers was seen in only 25

Table 47.3 Sensitivity (%) of non-surgical biopsy methods in tuberculous pleural effusions (histological and bacteriological results). Prospective simultaneous comparison (*n* = 100)

Method	Histology positive	Culture positive	Histology and/ or culture
Effusion (E)	–	28	28
Closed needle (N)	38	25	51
E + N	38	39	61
Medical thoracoscopy (MT)	94	76	99
MT + N	95	76	99
MT + E	94	78	100

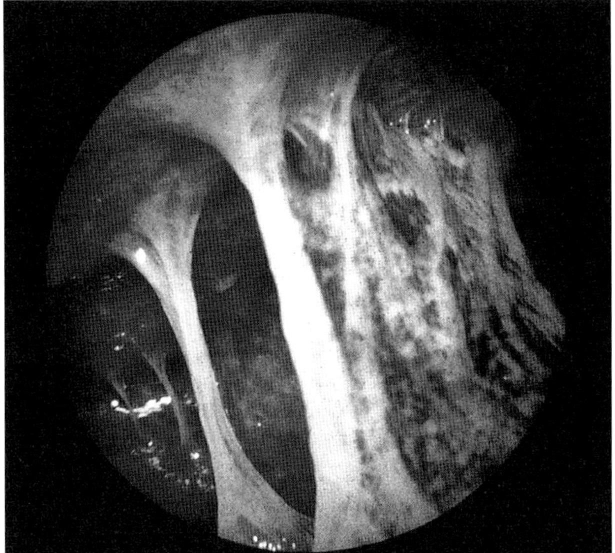

Figure 47.9 Tuberculous pleural effusion with fibrinous adhesions between the lung and the chest wall. (See also Color Plate 53.)

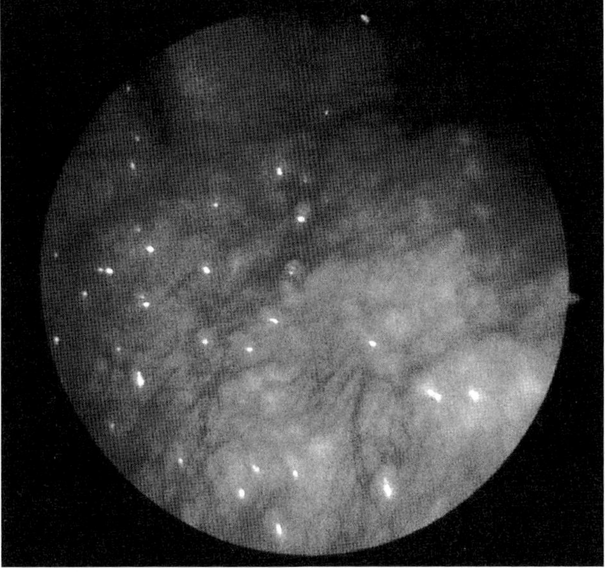

Figure 47.10 Tuberculous pleural effusion with typical sago-like nodules on the inflamed pleura. (See also Color Plate 54.)

percent (Figure 47.10). Here, positive TB cultures were obtained from all materials in only 50 percent, giving a highly significant difference ($p > 0.0005$). Interestingly, this study also showed that the chance of positive TB cultures from pleural effusion alone was statistically much better in cases with a low pleural glucose level (<50 mg per dL), indicating an increased metabolism by TB bacilli and/or higher degree of inflammation (59 percent positive versus 25 percent with glucose levels above 50 mg per dL, $p > 0.005$).

In another prospective study, medical thoracoscopy in 40 cases from South Africa had a diagnostic yield of 98 percent in comparison with an 80 percent diagnostic yield with Abram's needle biopsies.[98] This led to the conclusion that in areas with a high prevalence of TB, Abram's closed needle biopsy (in this case three biopsies were obtained and each examined histologically and microbiologically) can contribute significantly to a diagnosis. However, in a further study on the effect of corticosteroids in the treatment of TB pleurisy, the authors found that the initial complete drainage of the effusion, performed during and after thoracoscopy, was associated with greater symptomatic improvement than any subsequent therapy.[99] No studies are known which compare the influence of thoracoscopy with its early diagnosis and complete drainage and subsequent early drug treatment to a group with drug treatment alone. In our institution, Lungenklinik Heckeshorn, no single case has been observed during the last decade which needed decortication because of development of fibrothorax, perhaps a result of routine medical thoracoscopy with evacuation of all pleural fluid and opening of intrapleural loculations during medical thoracoscopy.[5] In a recent study from the same institution in South Africa, 51 patients with undiagnosed exudative pleural effusion were recruited for a prospective, direct comparison between bronchial wash, pleural fluid microbiology, and biochemistry (adenosine deaminase [ADA] and cell count), closed needle biopsy and medical thoracoscopy.[100] The final diagnosis was TB in 41 patients (82 percent). Sensitivity of histology, culture and combined histology/culture was 66, 48 and 79 percent, respectively, for closed needle biopsy and 100, 76 and 100 percent respectively, for thoracoscopy. Since the combination of ADA, lymphocyte/neutrophil ratio ≥0.75 plus closed needle biopsy reached 93 percent sensitivity and 100 percent specificity, the authors concluded that this high diagnostic accuracy is sufficient in areas with a high incidence of tuberculosis. However, if this test is negative despite a high clinical suspicion of tuberculous pleurisy, if antibiotic resistance is of concern or if other possible diagnoses are considered, they recommend medical thoracoscopy as the method of choice.

It is our policy not to treat patients with anti-tuberculous drugs merely on the suspicion of tuberculous pleurisy. At least in countries with a low prevalence of TB, where even other laboratory tests may not be very distinctive, medical thoracoscopy should be performed when needle biopsies show negative histological results, in order to prove or exclude TB. In addition, the high yield in positive TB cultures from thoracoscopic biopsies gives rise to the possibility of obtaining susceptibility tests which, in particular in patients born in countries with high rates of multidrug resistance (MDR) or extensive drug resistance (XDR),[101] may have a considerable impact on treatment and prognosis. In a study from Japan using the semi-rigid thoracoscope under local anaesthesia, 30 out of 32 patients (94 percent) were successfully diagnosed by histology of the pleural biopsy, whereas bacteriological examination of the pleural fluid was positive only in 11 cases (eight culture-positive, three PCR-positive).[102] Twenty-one of the cases (66 percent) were diagnosed by histology alone. The low yield of bacteriological confirmation (compared with the results of the other studies mentioned[97,98,100]) is explained by the fact that biopsy specimens were not taken for bacteriological examination. The finding of only five positive thoracoscopic TB cultures was surprisingly low compared with the results of the other studies.[97,98,100]

OTHER PLEURAL EFFUSIONS

In cases with effusions that are neither malignant nor tuberculous, thoracoscopy may give macroscopic clues to the etiology (e.g. in rheumatoid effusions, effusions following pancreatitis, liver cirrhosis, extension from the abdominal cavity or trauma).[20] Although in these entities history, pleural fluid analysis, physical and other examinations are usually diagnostic,[50] thoracoscopy may be indicated in those cases without a definite diagnosis.[59,103,104] If pleural effusion is secondary to underlying lung diseases such as pulmonary infarct or pneumonia, the diagnosis can frequently be made on macroscopic examination and be confirmed microscopically from a biopsy of the lung.[20] As already mentioned, thoracoscopy is well suited for diagnosis of benign asbestos-related pleural effusions, which, by definition, are a diagnosis of exclusion.[68]

In other pleural effusions, when the origin is unknown, the main diagnostic value of medical thoracoscopy lies in its ability to exclude, with high probability, malignant and tuberculous disease.[5,59] By means of thoracoscopy, the proportion of so-called idiopathic pleural effusions usually falls markedly below 10 percent, whereas studies which have not used thoracoscopy report failure to obtain a diagnosis in over 20 percent.[51] However, this certainly also depends on the selection of patients and on the definition of 'idiopathic'.[54,55]

It is occasionally impossible to perform thoracoscopy in the presence of effusion because of dense pleuropulmonary adhesions. In these cases, multiple closed needle biopsies should be performed, or more invasive surgical procedures should be considered.[4]

In some selected cases of recurrent pleural effusion of non-malignant etiology including chylothorax, pleurodesis may be induced by applying talc poudrage during medical thoracoscopy.[75,76,105]

EMPYEMA

Medical thoracoscopy can also be used in the management of early empyema.[48,106–108] In cases with multiple loculations, it is possible to open these spaces to remove the fibrinopurulent membranes (Figure 47.11) by forceps and to create one single cavity, which can be drained and irrigated much more successfully. This was demonstrated in a retrospective study of 127 patients of whom 94 percent were treated successfully for multiloculated empyema. Only 6 percent of the patients required a surgical approach.[108] This treatment should be carried out early in the course of parapneumonic effusion/empyema, before the adhesions

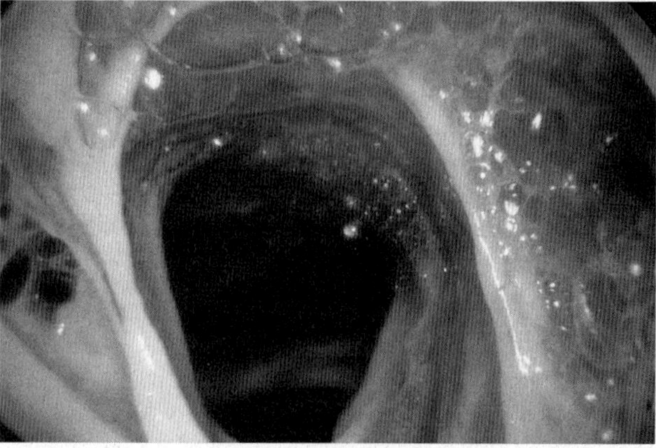

Figure 47.11 Thoracoscopic view of early empyema with fibrinopurulent membranes, which can be removed easily with the thoracoscopic biopsy forceps, thus restoring a single pleural space. (See also Color Plate 55.)

become too fibrous and adherent. Thus, if the indication for placement of a chest tube is present and if the facilities are available, medical thoracoscopy should be performed at the time of chest-tube insertion. For patients with complicated parapneumonic effusions, morbidity is lower in those who are treated with thoracoscopy or VATS than in those who received tube thoracostomy.[109] The consensus is to perform thoracoscopy earlier in patients with complicated parapneumonic effusions in whom tube thoracostomy and fibrinolytic therapy have failed.[110] Overall, medical thoracoscopy is a procedure similar to chest-tube placement, but enables the creation of one single pleural cavity, allowing much better local treatment.[48] However, prospective studies on the use of medical thoracoscopy in the treatment of early empyema have not yet been carried out.

SPONTANEOUS PNEUMOTHORAX

In spontaneous pneumothorax, medical thoracoscopy can be applied easily for diagnostic and therapeutic purposes, if the skills and facilities for this technique are available.[20,28,39,111,112] In particular, if a chest tube is introduced by the trocar technique, it is easy to use an optique for visual inspection of the lung and pleural cavity, before insertion of the chest tube through this cannula. On inspection during medical thoracoscopy, the underlying lesions can be directly assessed (Figure 47.12) according to the classification of Vanderschueren: stage I with an endoscopically normal lung; stage II with pleuropulmonary adhesions; stage III with small bullae and blebs (<2 cm in diameter); and stage IV with numerous large bullae (>2 cm in diameter).[113] In 1047 cases where medical thoracoscopy was used by three different teams,[114–116] pathological lesions were detected in approximately 70 percent of the cases with only slightly differing percentages for stages II to IV. Blebs and bullae were present in 45–62 percent. A false classification of stage I was shown at surgery in 8–28 percent of cases. Although the detection rates of blebs and bullae are higher (76–100 percent) in a series with VATS or thoracotomy,[111] it is unlikely that larger bullae and blebs or fistulae would not be detected during medical thoracoscopy. However, fluorescein-enhanced autofluorescence thoracoscopy detected more abnormalities compared with white light thoracoscopy.[117]

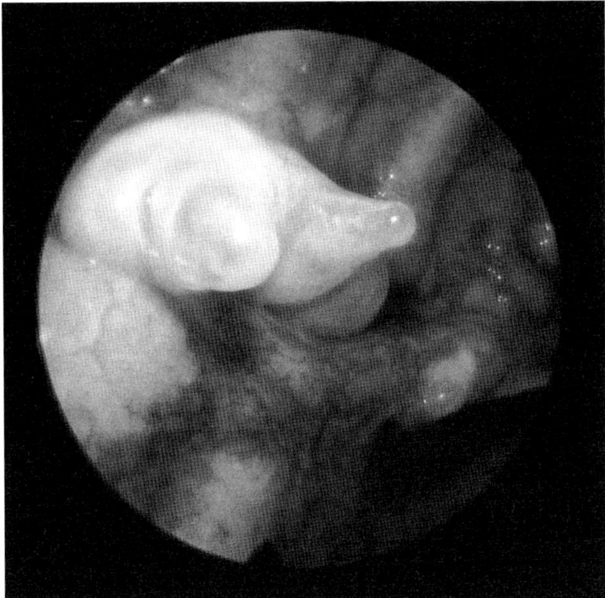

Figure 47.12 Thoracoscopic view of an emphysematous bulla in the apex of the right upper lobe (stage IV). (See also Color Plate 56.)

Medical thoracoscopy offers the possibility to combine chest drainage with coagulation of blebs and bullae as well as pleurodesis by talc poudrage.[39,109] Talc poudrage achieves the best conservative treatment results with recurrence rates below 10 percent.[39,118] Subsequent surgical intervention was necessary in 4–10 percent of the cases in the three above-mentioned series.[114–116] In stage IV with numerous large bullae, VATS or thoracotomy is usually indicated. These patients should be transferred directly to the surgical department after chest-tube insertion. Talc poudrage and/or coagulation of bullae are performed only in cases where surgery is contraindicated (e.g. because of respiratory insufficiency, secondary to severe bronchitis or other advanced pulmonary diseases).[119] Talc poudrage under thoracoscopy is safe, even in patients with advanced chronic obstructive pulmonary disease (COPD),[120] confirming previous studies.[112]

In our view, medical thoracoscopy is routinely justified in all patients with spontaneous pneumothorax where tube drainage is indicated, since several advantages are offered: precise assessment of underlying lesions under direct visual control, choice of best (conservative or surgical) treatment measures,[47] direct treatment by coagulation of blebs and bullae, and by severing of adhesions, if necessary, followed by talc poudrage, as well as selection of the best location for chest-tube placement.[28] In the case of recurrent or persistent pneumothorax, simple talc poudrage under medical thoracoscopy has been shown to be safe, cost-effective and no more painful than conservative treatment using a chest tube.[40]

For talc poudrage in pneumothorax patients, a mere 2–4 mL of talc are sufficient for effective pleurodesis.[39] No serious short-term complications have been seen if graded large-particle talc is used.[90,94,112] No long-term sequelae were observed 22–35 years after talc poudrage of pneumothorax: total lung capacity (TLC) averaged 89 percent predicted in 46 patients, whereas TLC was 97 percent predicted in 29 patients treated with tube thoracostomy alone.[121] None of the poudrage group developed mesothelioma over the 22- to 35-year follow-up. Although talc poudrage may result in minimally reduced TLC, as well as pleural thickening on chest radiography, these changes appear to be clinically unimportant. This is confirmed by a long-term follow-up study which showed that patients with successful talc pleurodesis had a median forced vital capacity of 102 percent and a median TLC of 99 percent at follow-up.[122] Since pleurodesis after talc poudrage is so effective, it may have some relative contraindications in patients who may become candidates for lung transplantation, although preceding talc pleurodesis is not considered an absolute contraindication to lung transplantation.[123]

OTHER INDICATIONS

The efficacy of forceps lung biopsy has been demonstrated in diffuse lung diseases,[20,21] whereas the results in localized lung diseases in chest wall lesions have been less positive.[5,20,124] Here, VATS is currently the preferred approach for these indications. However, medical thoracoscopy still maintains its efficacy for visceral pleura and peripheral lung biopsy, in particular in the presence of pleural effusion and lung disorders.[5,124]

A further therapeutic indication is thoracoscopic sympathectomy, which is minimally invasive and an accepted intervention for patients with a variety of autonomous nervous system disturbances. Essential hyperhidrosis patients and well-selected patients with other disorders can be helped with this procedure, which can also be performed by interventional pulmonologists.[124,125]

FUTURE DIRECTIONS

The most important role of medical thoracoscopy in the future will be mainly in diagnosing unexplained pleural effusions after non-diagnostic pleural fluid work-up. An exact early diagnosis for the pleural effusions will become even more important as more progress is made in the treatment of different entities (targeted cancer treatment, gene therapy, etc.).

Further indications for medical thoracoscopy as an important part of interventional pulmonology will be the application of talc poudrage for malignant or recurrent pleural effusion, and for the management of empyema in spontaneous pneumothorax.

Since thoracoscopy in many countries is performed by thoracic surgeons, usually as the much more invasive surgical procedure (VATS), training in medical thoracoscopy/pleuroscopy should become an intrinsic component of pulmonary training programmes. The development of semi-flexible pleuroscopes may facilitate the introduction of medical thoracoscopy into routine respiratory practice, at least in tertiary pulmonary centers.

KEY POINTS

- Medical thoracoscopy (pleuroscopy), compared with surgical thoracoscopy (VATS), has the advantage that it can be performed under local anesthesia or conscious sedation, in an endoscopy suite, using non-disposable rigid (or semi-rigid) instruments. Thus, it is considerably less expensive.
- The leading indications for medical thoracoscopy are pleural effusions, both for diagnosis, mainly in exudates of unknown etiology, or for staging in diffuse malignant mesothelioma or lung cancer, and for talc poudrage, which is the best conservative method today for pleurodesis.
- Spontaneous pneumothorax is an excellent indication for medical thoracoscopy, in particular if a chest tube is introduced by the trocar technique, which is very similar to the technique of medical thoracoscopy, the difference being that, before chest-tube insertion, an optique (the thoracoscope) is introduced through the cannula, which allows inspection of the pleural cavity including the lung surface, as well as therapeutic measures such as coagulation of blebs and bullae, and talc poudrage for efficient pleurodesis.
- In the same way, medical thoracoscopy can also be efficiently used in the management of early empyema.
- Medical thoracoscopy is a safe procedure which is even easier to learn than flexible bronchoscopy, provided that sufficient experience with chest-tube placement has been gained. However, as with all technical procedures, a learning curve is present before full competence is achieved.
- Medical thoracoscopy, as part of the new field of interventional pulmonology, should be included in the training program of chest physicians.
- In the above-mentioned indications, medical thoracoscopy can replace most of the surgical interventions, which are more invasive and more expensive.

REFERENCES

● = Key primary paper
◆ = Major review article
* = Paper that represents the first formal publication of a management guideline

●1. Jacobaeus HC. Über die Möglichkeit, die Zystoskopie bei Untersuchung seröser Höhlungen anzuwenden. *Münch med Wschr* 1910; **57**: 2090–2.
●2. Jacobaeus HC. The cauterization of adhesions in artificial pneumothorax therapy of tuberculosis. *Am Rev Tuberc* 1922; **6**: 871.

◆3. Mathur PN, Boutin C, Loddenkemper R. 'Medical' thoracoscopy: Technique and indications in pulmonary medicine. *J Bronchol* 1994; **1**: 228–39.

◆4. Loddenkemper R, McKenna RJ. Pleuroscopy, thoracoscopy and other invasive procedures. In: Mason, RJ, Broaddus, VC, Murray, JF, Nadel, JA. (eds). *Textbook of respiratory medicine*. Philadelphia: Elsevier Saunders, 2005: 651–70.

◆5. Loddenkemper R. Thoracoscopy – state of the art. *Eur Respir J* 1998; **11**: 213–21.

6. Dijkman JH, Martinez Gonzales del Rio J, Loddenkemper R, Prowse K, Siafakas N. Report of the working party of the 'UEMS monospecialty section on pneumology' on training requirements and facilities in Europe. *Eur Respir J* 1994: 1019–22.

7. Tape TG, Blank LL, Wigton RS. Procedural skills of practicing pulmonologists: a national survey of 1,000 members of the American College of Physicians. *Am J Respir Crit Care Med* 1995; **151**: 282–7.

8. Pastis NJ, Nietert PJ, Silvestri GA. Variation in training for interventional pulmonary procedures among US pulmonary/critical care fellowships – a survey of fellowship directors. *Chest* 2005; **127**: 1614–8.

9. Lee P, Lan RS, Colt HG. Survey of pulmonologists' perspectives on thoracoscopy. *J Bronchol* 2003; **10**: 99–106.

10. Burrows NJ, Ali NJ, Cox GM. The use and development of medical thoracoscopy in the United Kingdom over the past 5 years. *Respir Med* 2006; **7**: 1234–8.

◆11. Seijo LM, Sterman DH. Interventional pulmonology. *N Engl J Med* 2001; **344**: 740–9.

12. Piquet A, Giraud A. La pleuroscopie et la section des adhérences intrapleural au cours du pneumothorax thérapeutique. *La presse médicale* 1923; **23**.

13. Hoksch B, Birken-Bertsch H, Müller JM. Thoracoscopy before Jacobaeus. *Ann Thorac Surg* 2002; **74**: 1288–90.

◆14. Moisiuc FV, Colt HG. Thoracoscopy: origins revisited. *Respiration* 2007; **74**: 455–55.

◆15. Loddenkemper R. Medical thoracoscopy – historical perspective. In: Beamis JF, Mathur P, Mehta A (eds.). *Interventional pulmonary medicine*. New York: Marcel Dekker, Inc, 2004: 411–29.

◆16. Jacobaeus HC. Die Thorakoskopie und ihre praktische Bedeutung. *Ergebn ges Med* 1925; **7**: 112–66.

●17. Sattler A. Zur Behandlung des Spontanpneumothorax mit besonderer Berücksichtigung der Thorakoskopie. *Beitr Klin Tuberk* 1937; **89**: 395–408.

●18. Roche G, Delanoe Y, Moayer N. Talcage de la plèvre sous pleuroscopie. Résultats, indications, technique (A propos de 14 observations). *J Fr Med Chir Thorac* 1963; **21**: 177–95.

*19. Antony VB, Loddenkemper R, Astoul P, *et al.* Management of malignant pleural effusions (ERS/ATS Statement). *Am J Respir Crit Care Med* 2000; **162**: 1987–2001. *Eur Respir J* 2001; **18**: 402–19.

◆20. Brandt HJ, Loddenkemper R, Mai J. *Atlas of diagnostic thoracoscopy. Indications – Technique*. New York: Thieme Inc, 1985.

◆21. Boutin C, Viallat JR, Aelony Y. *Practical thoracoscopy*. Berlin: Springer, 1991.

◆22. Beamis JF, Mathur P, Mehta A. (eds.). *Interventional pulmonary medicine*. New York: Marcel Dekker, Inc, 2004.

◆23. Buchanan DR, Neville E. (eds.). *Thoracoscopy for physicians. A practical guide*. London: Arnold Hodder, 2004.

◆24. Lee P, Colt HG. *Flex-rigid pleuroscopy. Step-by-step*. Singapore: CMPMedica Asia Pte Ltd, 2005.

25. LoCicero J. Minimally invasive thoracic surgery, video-assisted thoracic surgery and thoracoscopy (Editorial). *Chest* 1992; **102**: 330–1.

26. Faber LP. Thoracoscopy: A surgeon's or a pulmonologist's domain. Pro surgeon. *J Bronchol* 1994; **1**: 155–9.

◆27. Harris RJ, Kavuru MS, Rice TW, Kirby TI. The diagnostic and therapeutic utility of thoracoscopy. A review. *Chest* 1995; **108**: 828–41.

◆28. Loddenkemper R, Boutin C. Thoracoscopy: present diagnostic and therapeutic indications. *Eur Respir J* 1993; **6**: 1544–55.

◆29. Maiwand MO. Video-assisted thoracoscopic surgery: Current applications, advantages, and limitations (review). *J Bronchol* 1997; **4**: 321–8.

30. Lewis JW Jr. Thoracoscopy: a surgeon's or a pulmonologist's domain; pro pulmonologist. *J Bronchol* 1994; **1**: 152–4.

31. Soffer A. Who should perform thoracoscopy? *Chest* 1992; **102**: 1553–5.

●32. Boutin C, Viallat JR, Cargnino C, Farisse P. Thoracoscopy in malignant pleural effusions. *Am Rev Respir Dis* 1981; **124**: 588–92.

●33. Janssen J, Boutin C. Extended thoracoscopy: a method to be used in case of pleural adhesions. *Eur Respir J* 1992; **5**: 763–6.

●34. Tassi G, Marchetti G. Minithoracoscopy. A less invasive approach to thoracoscopy. *Chest* 2003; **124**: 1975–7.

◆35. Mathur PN. How I do it. 'Medical' thoracoscopy. *J Bronchol* 1994; **2**: 144–51.

●36. Ernst A, Hersh CP, Herth F, *et al.* A novel instrument for the evaluation of the pleural space: an experience in 34 patients. *Chest* 2002; **122**: 1530–4.

37. Munavvar M, Khan MAI, Edwards J, Waqaruddin Z, Mills J. The autoclavable semirigid thoracoscope: the way forward in pleural disease? *Eur Respir J* 2007; **29**: 571–4.

38. Loddenkemper R. Thoracoscopy under local anesthesia. Is it safe? (Editorial) *J Bronchol* 2000; **7**: 207–9.

◆39. Boutin C, Astoul P, Rey F, Mathur PN. Thoracoscopy in the diagnosis and treatment of spontaneous pneumothorax. *Clin Chest Med* 1995; **16**: 497–503.

40. Tschopp J-M, Boutin C, Astoul P, *et al.* Talcage by medical thoracoscopy for primary spontaneous pneumothorax is more cost-effective than drainage: a randomised study. *Eur Respir J* 2002; **20**: 1003–9.

◆41. Colt HG. Thoracoscopy: a prospective study of safety and outcome. *Chest* 1995; **108**: 324–9.

42. Faurschou P, Madsen F, Viskum K. Thoracoscopy: influence of the procedure on some respiratory and cardiac values. *Thorax* 1983; **38**: 341–3.

43. Chhajed PN, Kaegi B, Rajasekaran R, Tamm MD. Detection of hypoventilation during thoracoscopy. Combined cutaneous carbon dioxide tension and oximetry monitoring with a new digital sensor. *Chest* 2005; **127**: 585–8.

◆44. Viskum K, Enk B. Complications of thoracoscopy. *Poumon Cœur* 1981; 37: 25–8.

●45. Boutin C, Rey F, Viallat JR. Prevention of malignant seeding after invasive diagnostic procedures in patients with pleural mesothelioma. A randomized trial of local radiotherapy. *Chest* 1995; **108**: 754–8.

46. Low EM, Khoury GG, Matthews AW, Neville E. Prevention of tumour seeding following thoracoscopy in mesothelioma by prophylactic radiotherapy. *Clin Oncol* 1995; **7**: 317–8.

47. Kaiser D. Indikationen zur chirurgischen Therapie beim Spontanpneumothorax. *Chir Praxis* 2000; **57**: 239–48.

48. Kaiser D. Indikationen zur Thorakoskopie beim Pleuraempyem. *Pneumologie* 1989; **43**: 76–9.

49. Collins TR, Sahn SA. Thoracentesis: Clinical value, complications, technical problems, and patient experience. *Chest* 1987; **91**: 817–22.

◆50. Light RW. Diagnostic principles in pleural disease. *Eur Respir J* 1997; **10**: 476–81.

◆51. Storey DD, Dines DE, Coles DT. Pleural effusion. A diagnostic dilemma. *J Am Med Assoc* 1976; **236**: 2183–6.

52. Menzies R. Charbonneau M. Thoracoscopy for the diagnosis of pleural disease. *Ann Intern Med* 1991; **114**: 271–6.

53. Enk B, Viskum K. Diagnostic thoracoscopy. *Eur J Respir Dis* 1981; **114**: 271–6.

54. Janssen JP, Ramlala S, Mravunac M. The long-term follow up of exudative pleural effusion after nondiagnostic thoracoscopy. *J Bronchol* 2004; **11**: 169–74.

55. Venekamp LN, Velkeniers B, Noppen M. Does 'idiopathic pleuritis' exist? Natural history of non-specific pleuritis diagnosed after thoracoscopy. *Respiration* 2005; **72**: 74–8.
●56. Chrysanthidis MG, Janssen JP. Autofluorescence videothoracoscopy in exudative pleural effusions: preliminary results. *Eur Respir J* 2005; **26**: 989–92.
●57. Ryan CJ, Rodgers RF, Uni UK, Hepper NG. The outcome of patients with pleural effusion of indeterminate cause at thoracotomy. *Mayo Clin Proc* 1981; **56**: 145–9.
●58. Lee P, Colt HG. Using diagnostic thoracoscopy to optimal effect. *J Respir Dis* 2003; **24**: 503–9.
●59. Rodriguez-Panadero F, Janssen JP, Astoul P. Thoracoscopy: general overview and place in the diagnosis and management of pleural effusion. *Eur Respir J* 2006; **28**: 409–21.
●60. Loddenkemper R, Grosser H, Gabler A, *et al.* Prospective evaluation of biopsy methods in the diagnosis of malignant pleural effusions. Intrapatient comparison between pleural fluid cytology, blind needle biopsy and thoracoscopy. *Am Rev Respir Dis* 1983; **127** (Suppl. 4): 114.
61. Oldenburg FA Jr, Newhouse MT. Thoracoscopy. A safe, accurate diagnostic procedure using the rigid thoracoscope and local anesthesia. *Chest* 1979; **75**: 45–50.
●62. Weissberg D, Kaufmann M, Schwecher I. Pleuroscopy in clinical evaluation and staging of lung cancer. *Poumon Coeur* 1981; **37**: 241–3.
63. Canto A, Ferrer G, Romagosa V, Moya J. Bernat R. Lung cancer and pleural effusion. Clinical significance and study of pleural metastatic locations. *Chest* 1985; **87**: 649–52.
●64. Boutin C, Rey F. Thoracoscopy in pleural malignant mesothelioma: a prospective study of 188 consecutive patients. Part 1: Diagnosis. *Cancer* 1993; **72**: 389–93.
●65. Boutin C, Rey F, Gouvernet J, *et al.* Thoracoscopy in pleural malignant mesothelioma. Part 2: Prognosis and staging. *Cancer* 1993; **72**: 394–404.
●66. Boutin C, Nussbaum E, Monnet I, *et al.* Intrapleural treatment with gamma-interferon in early stage malignant mesothelioma. *Cancer* 1994; **74**: 2460–7.
67. Goey SH, Eggemont AMM, Punt CJA, *et al.* Intrapleural administration of interleukin 2 in pleural mesothelioma: a phase I-II study. *Br J Cancer* 1995; **72**: 1283–8.
68. Boutin C, Schlesser M, Frenay C, Astoul PH. Malignant pleural mesothelioma. *Eur Respir J* 1998; **12**: 972–81.
●69. Boutin C, Dumortier P, Rey F, Viallat JR, DeVuyst P. Black spots concentrate oncogenic asbestosis fibers in the parietal pleura: thoracoscopic and mineralogic study. *Am J Respir Crit Care Med* 1996; **153**: 111–9.
●70. Levine MN, Young JE, Ryan ED, Newhouse MT. Pleural effusion in breast cancer: thoracoscopy for hormone receptor determination. *Cancer* 1986; **57**: 324–7.
71. Schwarz C, Lübbert HI, Rahn W, *et al.* Medical thoracoscopy: hormone receptor content in pleural metastases due to breast cancer. *Eur Respir J* 2004; **24**: 728–30.
●72. Celikoglu F, Teirstein AS, Krellenstein DJ, Strauchen JA. Pleural effusion in non-Hodgkins lymphoma. *Chest* 1992; **101**: 1357–60.
●73. Sanchez-Armengol A, Rodriguez-Panadero F. Survival and talc pleurodesis in metastatic pleural carcinoma, revisited. Report of 125 cases. *Chest* 1993; **104**: 1482–5.
●74. Antony VB, Nasreen N, Mohammed KA, *et al.* Talc pleurodesis. Basic fibroblast growth factor mediates pleural fibrosis. *Chest* 2004; **126**: 1522–8.
◆75. Rodriguez-Panadero F, Antony VB. Pleurodesis. State of the art. *Eur Respir J* 1997; **10**: 1648–54.
●76. Mares CC, Mathur PN. Thoracoscopic talc pleurodesis for lymphoma induced chylothorax, a case series of twenty two treated hemithoraces in eighteen patients. *Am J Respir Crit Care Med* 1997; **155**: A481.
●77. Janssen JP, Collier G, Astoul P, *et al.* Safety of talc pleurodesis with talc poudrage in malignant pleural effusion: a prospective cohort study. *Lancet* 2007; **369**: 1535–9.
78. Boutin C, Rey F, Viallat JR. Etude randomisée de l'efficacité du talcage thoracoscopique et de l'instillation de tétracycline dans le traitement des pleurésies cancéreuses récidivantes. *Rev Mal Resp* 1985; **2**: 374–8.
79. Fentiman IS, Rubens RD, Hayward JL. A comparison of intracavitary talc and tetracycline for the control of pleural effusions secondary to breast cancer. *Eur J Cancer Clin Oncol* 1986; **22**: 1079–81.
80. Hartmann DL, Gaither JM, Kesler KA, *et al.* Comparison of insufflated talc under thoracoscopic guidance with standard tetracycline and bleomycin pleurodesis for control of malignant pleural effusions. *J Thorac Cardiovasc Surg* 1993; **105**: 743–8.
81. Yin AC, Chan AT, Lee TW, Wan IY, Ho JK. Thoracoscopic talc insufflation *versus* talc slurry for symptomatic malignant pleural effusion. *Ann Thorac Surg* 1996; **62**: 1655–8.
82. Diacon AH, Wyser C, Bolliger CT, *et al.* Prospective randomized comparison of thoracoscopic talc poudrage under local anesthesia versus bleomycin instillation for pleurodesis in malignant pleural effusions. *Am J Respir Crit Care Med* 2000; **162**: 1445–9.
◆83. Tan C, Sedrakyan A, Browne J, Swift S, Treasure T. The evidence on the effectiveness of management for malignant pleural effusion: a systematic review. *Eur J Cardiothorac Surg* 2006; **29**: 829–38.
●84. Dresler CM, Olak J, Herndon JE, *et al.* Phase III intergroup study of talc poudrage vs talc slurry sclerosis for malignant pleural effusion. *Chest* 2005; **127**: 909–15.
85. Froudarakis ME, Klimathianaki M, Pougounias M. Systemic inflammatory reaction after thoracoscopic talc poudrage. *Chest* 2006; **129**: 356–61.
●86. Campos JR, Werebe EC, Vargas FS, Jatene FB, Light RW. Respiratory failure due to insufflated talc. *Lancet* 1997; **349**: 251–2.
87. Rehse DH, Aye RW, Florence MG. Respiratory failure following talc pleurodesis. *Am J Surg* 1999; **177**: 437–440.
●88. Ferrer J, Villarino MA, Tura JM, Traveria A, Light RW. Talc preparations used for pleurodesis vary markedly from one preparation to another. *Chest* 2001; **119**: 1901–5.
89. Ferrer J, Montes JF, Villarino MA, Light RW, Garcia-Valero J. Influence of particle size on extrapleural talc dissemination after talc slurry pleurodesis. *Chest* 2002; **122**: 1018–27.
●90. Maskell NA, Lee YC, Gleeson FV, *et al.* Randomized trials describing lung inflammation after pleurodesis with talc of varying particle size. *Am J Resp Crit Care Med* 2004; **170**: 377–82.
91. Weissberg D, BenZeev I. Talc pleurodesis: experience with 360 patients. *J Thorac Cardiovasc Surg* 1993; **106**: 689–95.
92. Viallat JR, Rey F. Astoul PI, Boutin C. Thoracoscopic talc poudrage pleurodesis for malignant effusions: a review of 360 cases. *Chest* 1996; **110**: 1387–93.
◆93. Cardillo G, Facciolo F, Carbone L, *et al.* Long term follow up of video assisted talc pleurodesis in malignant recurrent pleurals effusions. *Eur J Cardiothorac Surg* 2002; **21**: 302–6.
94. Noppen M. Who's (still) afraid of talc? *Eur Respir J* 2007; **29**: 619–21.
95. Nasreen N, Mohammed KA, Dowling PA, *et al.* Talc induces apoptosis in human malignant mesothelioma cells *in vitro*. *Am J Respir Crit Care Med* 2000; **161**: 595–600.
●96. Najmunnisa N, Mohammed KA, Brown S, *et al.* Talc mediates angiostasis in malignant pleural effusions via endostatin induction. *Eur Respir J* 2007; **29**: 761–9.
◆97. Loddenkemper R, Grosser H, Mai J, *et al.* Diagnostik des tuberkulösen Pleuraergusses: Prospektiver Vergleich laborchemischer, bakteriologischer, zytologischer und histologischer Untersuchungsergebnisse. *Prax Klin Pneumol* 1983; **37**: 1153–6.
98. Walzl G, Wyser D, Smedema J, Corbett C, van de Wal B. Comparing the diagnostic yield of Abrams needle pleural biopsy and thoracoscopy. *Am J Respir Crit Care Med* 1996; **153**: A460.

99. Wyser C, Walzl G. Smedema JP, *et al.* Corticosteroids in the treatment of tuberculous pleurisy. A double-blind, placebo-controlled, randomized study. *Chest* 1996; **110**: 333–8.

♦100. Diacon AH, Van de Wal BW, Wyser C, *et al.* Diagnostic tools in tuberculous pleurisy: a direct comparative study. *Eur Respir J* 2003; **22**: 589–91.

101. Aziz MA, Wright A, Laszlo A, *et al.* Epidemiology of antituberculosis drug resistance (the Global Project on Anti-tuberculosis Drug Resistance Surveillance): an updated analysis. *Lancet* 2006; **368**: 2142–54.

102. Sakuraba M, Masuda K, Hebisawa A, Sagara Y, Komatsu H. Thoracoscopic pleural biopsy for tuberculous pleurisy under local anesthesia. *Ann Thorac Cardiovasc Surg* 2006; **12**: 245–8.

*103. Maskell NA, Butland RJ, Pleural Diseases Group, Standards of Care Committee, British Thoracic Society. BTS guidelines for the investigation of a unilateral pleural effusion in adults. *Thorax* 2003; **58** (Suppl 2): ii8–17.

*104. Ernst A, Silvestri GA, Johnstone D, American College of Chest Physicians. Interventional pulmonary procedures. Guidelines from the American College of Chest Physicians. *Chest* 2003; **123**: 1693–1717.

●105. Sudduth C, Sahn SA. Pleurodesis for non-malignant pleural effusions. Recommendations. *Chest* 1992; **102**: 1855–60.

●106. Weissberg D. Pleuroscopy in empyema: is it ever necessary? *Poumon Coeur* 1981; **37**: 269–72.

♦107. Weissberg D. *Handbook of practical pleuroscopy.* Mount Kisko: Futura, 1991.

●108. Brutsche MH, Tassi GF, Györik S, *et al.* Treatment of sonographically stratified multiloculated thoracic empyema by medical thoracoscopy. *Chest* 2005; **128**: 3303–9.

109. Lee P, Colt HG. Thoracoscopy: an update on therapeutic applications. *J Respir Dis* 2003; **24**: 530–6.

*110. Colice GL, Curtis A, Deslauriers J, *et al.* Medical and surgical treatment of parapneumonic effusions. an evidence-based guideline. *Chest* 2000; **118**: 1158–71. (Erratum in: *Chest* 2001; **119**: 319.)

111. Schramel FMNH, Postmus PE, Vanderschueren RGJRA. Current aspects of spontaneous pneumothorax. *Eur Respir J* 1997; **10**: 1372–9.

♦112. Tschopp JM, Rami-Porta R, Noppen M, Astoul P. Management of spontaneous pneumothorax: state of the art. *Eur Respir J* 2006; **28**: 637–50.

●113. Vanderschueren RG. Le talcage pleural dans le pneumothorax spontané. *Poumon Cœur* 1981; **37**: 273–6.

114. vd Brekel JA, Duurkens VAM, Vanderschueren RGJRA. Pneumothorax: results of thoracoscopy and pleurodesis with talc poudrage and thoracotomy. *Chest* 1993; **103**: 345–7.

115. El Khawand C, Marchandise FX, Maynel A, *et al.* Pneumothorax spontané. Résultats du talcage pleural sous thoracoscopie. *Rev Med Resp* 1995; **12**: 275–81.

116. Hausmann M, Keller R. Thorakoskopische Pleurodese beim Spontanpneumothorax. *Schweiz Med Wochenschr* 1994; **124**: 97–104.

●117. Noppen M, Dekeukeleire T, Hanon S, *et al.* Fluorescein-enhanced autofluorescence thoracoscopy in patients with primary spontaneous pneumothorax and normal subjects. *Am J Respir Crit Care Med* 2006; **174**: 26–30.

118. Almind M, Lange P, Viskum K. Spontaneous pneumothorax: comparison of simple drainage, talc pleurodesis and tetracycline pleurodesis. *Thorax* 1989; **44**: 627–30.

119. Tschopp J-M, Brutsche M, Frey JG. Treatment of complicated spontaneous pneumothorax by simple talc pleurodesis under thoracoscopy and local anaesthesia. *Thorax* 1997; **52**: 329–32.

120. Lee P, Yap WS, Pek WY, *et al.* An audit of medical thoracoscopy and talc poudrage for pneumothorax prevention in advanced COPD. *Chest* 2004; **125**: 1315–20.

●121. Lange P, Mortensen J, Groth S. Lung function 22–25 years after treatment of idiopathic spontaneous pneumothorax with talc poudrage or simple drainage. *Thorax* 1988; **43**: 559–61.

122. Györik S, Erni S, Studler UI, *et al.* Long-term follow-up of thoracoscopic talc pleurodesis for primary spontaneous pneumothorax. *Eur Respir J* 2007; **29**: 757–60.

♦123. Judson MA, Sahn SA. The pleural space and organ transplantation. *Am J Respir Crit Care Med* 1996; **153**: 1153–65.

124. Tassi GF, Davies RJ, Noppen M. Advanced techniques in medical thoracoscopy. *Eur Respir J* 2006; **28**: 1051–9.

♦125. Noppen M. Medical thoracoscopy. Techniques for thoracic sympathectomy. In: Beamis JF, Mathur P, Mehta A (eds). *Interventional pulmonary medicine.* New York: Marcel Dekker, Inc: 2004: 483–502.

48

Surgery for pleural diseases

DAVID A WALLER, ANTONIO E MARTIN-UCAR

INTRODUCTION

Advances in surgery of the pleural cavity have been facilitated by the application of video-assisted thoracic surgery (VATS). This minimally invasive technique has not only prompted revision of standard selection criteria for surgery but has also extended the indications for surgery. VATS has also enabled pulmonologists to undertake simple invasive pleural procedures. Nevertheless, whilst basic diagnostic procedures are widely applicable, therapeutic VATS requires specialized training if basic surgical principles are to be adhered to. Thus, some VATS procedures are only performed by specialist surgeons and this specialization extends to some open pleural surgery which is carried out in only a limited number of centers. This chapter will address the whole spectrum of pleural surgery from procedures within the remit of general surgeons to those practiced in only a handful of centers worldwide.

SPONTANEOUS PNEUMOTHORAX

Indications for surgical intervention

PRIMARY SPONTANEOUS PNEUMOTHORAX

A recent consensus statement organized by the American College of Chest Physicians (ACCP) using the Delphi technique recommended surgical assement after the second episode of primary spontaneous pneumothorax (PSP) or a first episode with an air leak in excess of 4 days.[1] Delay in referral for surgery reduces the success of VATS due to the development of patchy pleural adhesions from pleural sepsis secondary to prolonged chest drainage.[2] Intervention in first-time PSP has not been validated but has been promoted in the presence of macroscopic blebs, larger than 5 mm on computed tomography (CT) scanning, which may predict recurrence.[3] However, it has been demostrated that even macroscopic blebs confirmed at routine thoracoscopy in first-time PSP were of no benefit in predicting recurrence.[4] In the ACCP consensus statement only 15 percent of panel members advocated surgical intervention to prevent recurrence after the first occurrence. Although there is some evidence that VATS is cost-effective when compared with intercostal drainage in first-time PSP,[5,6] intervention in this context is currently only recommended for special occupational or recreational needs, i.e. flying or deep sea diving.

SECONDARY SPONTANEOUS PNEUMOTHORAX

Secondary spontaneous pneumothorax (SSP) is an indication of an air leak from underlying pulmonary pathology (usually emphysema) which should be treated assuming the patient is fit for operation. In the previously mentioned ACCP consensus statement, 81 percent of the panel recommended an intervention to prevent recurrence after the first episode because of the potentially serious complications of a secondary pneumothorax.[1] Selection criteria for surgery in this group of typically elderly patients with emphysema include: absence of hypercapnia (partial pressure of CO_2 [PCO_2] < 7 KPa); maintained exercise tolerance (walk test >150 m) and absence of significant cardiovascular co-morbidity. Pulmonary function tests performed during the episode of SSP are likely to be inaccurate and do not contribute to patient selection for surgery. For patients with persistent air leaks, continued observation for no more than 5 days is recommended.

Surgical method

Prevention of persistent air leak or future recurrence requires initial identification of the source of the air leak, i.e. macroscopic blebs or bullae. Complete intrathoracic inspection requires division of all pleural adhesions since these often conceal the culprit lesion. The area of air leak is then controlled by any one of stapling, suturing or ligation. Obliteration of pleural space is then required to prevent recurrence in the likelihood of a new source of air leak or if a current air leak has not been identified. These procedures are either performed by VATS or by open thoracotomy. VATS is enabled by the insertion of a 5–10 mm video thoracoscope via a 2–3 cm incision in the lateral axillary line in the sixth intercostal space. Bleb excision and parietal pleurectomy or abrasion are then accomplished via two more similar incisions placed anteriorly and posteriorly in the fourth intercostal space. Instruments may be introduced via rigid or flexible tube cannulae or ports. Bleb excision or bullectomy is generally carried out with an endoscopic linear cutter which leaves up to three parallel rows of staples on the lung surface (Figure 48.1). When excising the emphysematous bulla the staple lines may be reinforced with material such as bovine pericardium to reduce post-operative air leak.

Parietal pleurectomy is performed by insertion of a long Roberts artery forceps into the extrapleural plane via the anterior incision under video control. The forceps are advanced towards the apex stripping off the pleural sheet with a sweeping motion. This process is then repeated from the posterior incision. Once the pleural sheet has been raised, its edge is grasped by the forceps and the sheet withdrawn from the chest using a twisting motion to wrap the sheet around the forceps whilst applying gentle traction (Figure 48.2). A single 24 or 28 F drain is left *in situ* via one port and usually connected to underwater seal drainage. Open surgery is usually performed via a form of muscle-sparing thoracotomy. A lateral or axillary thoracotomy via the fourth intercostal space preserving the fibres of latissimus dorsi and with minimal rib retraction has been used to good effect.[7] For any of these approaches the importance of double-lumen intubation and single-lung ventilation cannot be over emphasized. Spontaneous pneumothorax is a disease of the lung and not of the pleura, therefore optimal access to this organ is imperative to allow accurate identification of the source of pathology and therapeutic intervention.

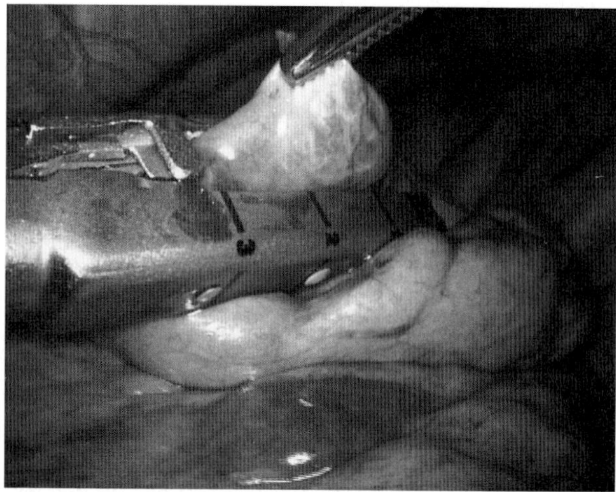

Figure 48.1 Stapled bleb excision by video-assisted thoracoscopic surgery in primary spontaneous pneumothorax.

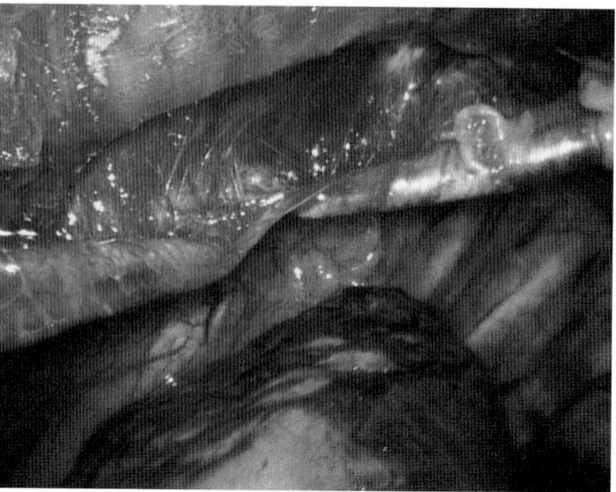

Figure 48.2 Video-assisted thoracoscopic surgery in parietal pleurectomy.

While VATS has potential benefits over thoracotomy in the elderly, it is more technically demanding in these patients than in PSP since there are more bullae and sites of potential air leak to be identified. We found in a randomized comparison with open surgery that the comparative initial results for VATS in SSP were therefore less successful than in PSP.[8] Operating time was longer and although less post-operative analgesia was required there were significantly more primary treatment failures requiring conversion to thoracotomy resulting in longer post-operative recovery. Nevertheless, VATS enables SSP to be treated surgically in patients who would not readily tolerate thoracotomy owing to poor respiratory function or age.[9] With increasing experience of the limitations of VATS, the proportion of operations for SSP has fallen.[10] A conservative alternative therapy may therefore be considered in the more high-risk candidates. The use of ambulatory in-dwelling chest drainage with a Heimlich valve system[11] has enabled early mobilization and hospital discharge in this group. Patients who do proceed to surgery can be considered for a form of lung volume reduction surgery (LVRS), i.e by removing more than just the culprit bulla. In light of the experience of the physiological benefits of reducing hyperinflation[12] by LVRS, we now evaluate patients presenting with stable SSP for this operation. Preoperative investigations may therefore include CT and radionuclide perfusion scintigraphy.

Is bleb resection necessary?

Failure to identify or ablate a macroscopic bleb at VATS has been found to be an independent predictor of recurrence.[13] Recurrence rates of 23 percent were reported compared with 1.8 percent when a bleb was ablated. Routine blind resection of the apex of the upper lobe together with a procedure to obtain pleural symphysis has therefore been advocated. An alternative method of dealing with a bleb is VATS ligation using a pre-tied Roeder slip knot introduced by an external applicator. Unfortunately, this technique was associated with a treatment failure rate of nearly 20 percent and is therefore not recommended.[14]

Which type of pleural procedure?

Whilst there has been a report of successful pneumothorax prevention by apical bullectomy without pleurodesis[15] it is accepted practice that a procedure to promote pleural adhesions is the norm.[1] Mechanical pleurodesis can be accomplished by parietal pleurectomy or pleural abrasion. In PSP when an apical source of air leak is the norm, an apical parietal pleurectomy is preferred. This theoretically allows the possibility of future thoracotomy for other indications. Pleural abrasion[16] is technically easier to perform then pleurectomy by VATS and preserves the extrapleural plane and is therefore favored by some surgeons. In a review of these two alternatives there was a slightly lower recurrence rate after pleurectomy than abrasion: 0.4 percent ($n = 752$) versus 2.3 percent ($n = 301$).[17]

In secondary SP, parietal pleurectomy may be avoided in favor of talc insufflation which may shorten the duration of anaesthesia, be less painful and for which there are less potential long-term problems in this age group.

Talc is the chemical sclerosant of choice with a lower recurrence rate than tetracycline in a comparative trial of 96 patients: 8 percent versus 13 percent.[4] In larger reviews the recurrence rate for talc pleurodesis alone was 10–15 percent and therefore mechanical methods should be preferred. The choice of pleural procedure in combination with bleb excision is less clear. Cardillo *et al.*[18] reported that the addition of talc poudrage rather than subtotal pleurectomy to stapled excision of the bleb by VATS carried a significantly lower recurrence rate. Their long-term experience of over 800 cases reported no adult repiratory distress and an overall recurrence rate of only 1.73 percent.[19]

Fibrin glue has also been used by insufflation to obtain pleurodesis but has been associated with high recurrence of up to 25 percent.[20]

Which surgical approach: VATS versus thoracotomy?

Video-assisted thoracoscopic surgery has been shown to be a less traumatic approach than thoracotomy as shown by the reduced release of inflammatory and vasoactive mediators after VATS. This may explain why VATS is better tolerated.[21]

In one of the few prospective randomized comparisons of the use of VATS versus open surgery (limited posterolateral thoracotomy) for spontaneous pneumothorax we found that stapled bullectomy and apical parietal pleurectomy could be performed equally reliably for PSP.[9] Operating time was no longer for VATS but the post-operative analgesic requirement and hospital stay were reduced. VATS resulted in less early post-operative respiratory dysfunction with a drop in FEV_1 (forced expiratory volume in 1 second) of 29 percent and in FVC (forced vital capacity) of 19 percent compared with falls of 43 and 39 percent, respectively, after lateral thoracotomy.

There has been no similar prospective randomized comparison of VATS and limited axillary thoracotomy (LAT). Whilst Dumont *et al.*[22] showed shorter stay, less pain and similar recurrence than LAT in a retrospective review of only 79 patients, Miller *et al.*[23] found no benefits from VATS. Similar findings have been described by other authors[24,25] who showed perioperative benefits from VATS but higher recurrence related to resection of fewer bullae than limited axillary thoracotomy. These findings may be explained by unfamiliarity with the newer technique of VATS. Indeed, the early comparisons of VATS with traditional methods may not have appreciated the technical difficulties in learning a new technique. It has been shown that VATS results improve with surgical experience with fewer complications[26] and a decrease in operating time and hospital stay;[10] in the largest reported series of VATS, the fact that the recurrence rates are slightly higher than the accepted rates for open surgery (Table 48.1) may be explained by this. In a systematic review of four trials of VATS versus thoracotomy in over 200 patients, Sedryakan *et al.*[27] found that VATS resulted in a reduced need for analgesia and length of stay.

Medical thoracoscopy

The use of video-assisted thoracoscopy in a spontaneously ventilating patient without double-lumen intubation has become to be known as 'medical thoracoscopy'. There are several proponents of this technique in the treatment of spontaneous pneumothorax with simple talc insufflation being the usual method employed. Indeed, there are proponents of its use in first-time PSP in preference to tube drainage alone.[28] Whilst early recurrence is reported to be low, recurrence is higher than open surgery when macroscopic bullae are present.[29] This results from a failure to treat the source of the air leak attributable to the absence of single-lung ventilation which precludes complete intrathoracic inspection. In the event of recurrence after initial medical thoracoscopic talc insufflations, subsequent VATS is precluded by patchy adhesions, thoracotomy is required and the benefits of VATS are lost. We do not

Table 48.1 Results of VATS for spontaneous pneumothorax

Author	Study	Number	Deaths	Conversion to thoractomy	Persistent air leak	Drain time (days)	Hospital stay (days)	Median follow-up	Recurrence
Liu *et al.*[102]	Multicenter	757	0	–	31 (4%)	–	4.5	30 months	16 (2.1%)
Cardillo *et al.*[18]	Retrospective	432	0	10 (2.3%)	6 (1.3%)	5.4	6.1	38 months	19 (4.4%)
Hurtgen *et al.*[103]	Multicenter	1365	2	–	39 (2.9%)	–	–	–	88 (6.5%)
Ohno *et al.*[104]	Retrospective	424	0	–	26 (6.1%)	–	–	31 months	40 (9.4%)
Yim[105]	Retrospective	224	0	–	10 (4.4%)	–	3	20 months	4 (1.8%)
Waller[10]	Prospective	180	2	0	–	–	4	24 months	12 (6.6%)
Bertrand *et al.*[106]	Retrospective	163	0	0	6 (3.6%)	4.4	4.4	24 months	3 (1.8%)
Freixinet *et al.*[107]	Multicenter	132	0	2	8 (6%)	–	5.6	1–3 years	8 (6%)
Naunheim *et al.*[13]	Multicenter	121	0	0	10 (8%)	–	4.3	13 months	5 (4.1%)
Chan *et al.*[108]	Retrospective	109	0	3	–	–	–	44 months	5 (5.7%)
Hatz *et al.*[109]	Retrospective	109	0	0	3 (3.1%)	–	4	53 months	5 (4.6%)

therefore believe that PSP is an indication for treatment by medical thoracoscopy.[30]

Special considerations

CYSTIC FIBROSIS

Although secondary spontaneous pneumothorax usually complicates emphysema, it may occur in other lung diseases. Cystic fibrosis may lead to pneumothorax late in the disease and is a marker of poor prognosis.[31] As lung transplantation is a future possibility in these cases, surgical treatment may need to be modified. Pleurectomy may prejudice selection for transplant due to potential technical difficulties in explanting the recipient lung.[32] Chemical pleurodesis, however, is acceptable as the extrapleural plane is preserved to allow future surgery.

CATAMENIAL PNEUMOTHORAX

This condition defines a cyclical pneumothorax which occurs in young females in relation to the menstrual cycle. Several causative theories have been forwarded including alveolar rupture secondary to the effects of raised prostaglandin F2 levels and ectopic foci of endometriosis in the lung.[33] The finding of diaphragmatic fenestrations supports a theory of the passage of free air from the peritoneal cavity due to absence of the normal cervical mucous plug during ovulation[34] and mandates surgical exploration. In a review of 154 operated cases in the published literature: endometriosis was found in 52 percent and diaphragmatic lesions in 39 percent.[35] Hormonal treatment (luteinizing hormone-releasing hormone analogue) alone, intended to treat pleural endometriosis as a cause, is not adequate since it will be appropriate in only 20 percent of cases where this condition coexists.[33] VATS should be used to exclude and treat an anatomical cause either by stapling of an apical bleb or a diaphragmatic fenestration (Figure 48.3) before hormonal treatment is commenced. An additional procedure to achieve pleurodesis at the level of the diaphragm is also advisable.[36]

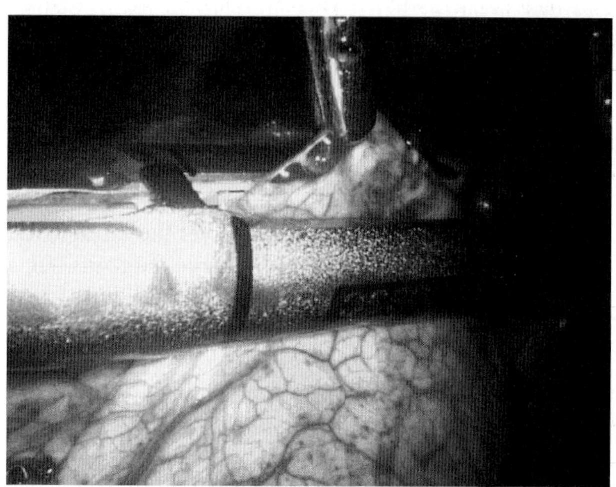

Figure 48.3 Stapled closure of a diaphragmatic pore in catamenial pneumothorax.

SPONTANEOUS HEMOPNEUMOTHORAX

This is defined as the accumulation of over 400 mL of blood in the pleural cavity associated with spontaneous pneumothorax. It occurs in up to 5 percent of cases[37] and is associated with hypovolemic shock in up to one in three cases. It is caused by the tearing of an arterial branch from the parietal pleural surface to the lung as the lung collapses following pneumothorax. Treatment may be successful by VATS and includes identification and either clipping or cautery of the feeding vessel.

PLEURAL EMPYEMA

Indications for surgical intervention

PARAPNEUMONIC EFFUSIONS

Recent guidelines for the management of parapneumonic effusions (PPE) have been produced by the ACCP[38] in which a risk categorization for poor outcome in PPE has been proposed based on pleural anatomy; pleural fluid bacteriology and chemistry. This approach differs from the traditional approach to categorizing PPE based on three phases: exudative, fibrinopurulent and organizing.

Four categories are identified: categories 3 and 4 require drainage and in these cases surgical referral should be considered since therapeutic thoracocentesis or tube thoracostomy alone are likely to be insufficient.

The clinical features defining category 3 PPE are: an effusion occupying more than half the hemithorax which may be loculated and in which the parietal pleura may be thickened; pleural fluid has a positive culture or Gram stain and pleural fluid pH < 7.2. Category 4 PPE is characterized by the additional finding of pus in the pleural cavity. The ACCP panel[38] concluded that there was evidence for the use of both surgery (by either VATS or thoracotomy) and percutaneous intrapleural fibrinolysis in category 3 and 4 PPE. (See also Chapter 26 on pleural infection.)

Surgical method

PRINCIPLES OF SURGERY

There are two main principles to surgical intervention in pleural empyema: debridement of the infected cavity and decortication of the underlying lung. The former contributes to the control of sepsis and the latter allows for re-expansion of the lung and obliteration of the empyema cavity.

SURGICAL APPROACH

There are three basic approaches to achieve the principles above: thoracotomy, thoracostomy or thoracoscopy. Thoracoscopy under direct vision has been used successfully in fibrinopurulent PPE[39] and more recently using VATS.

VATS treatment of pleural empyema

General anesthesia with double lumen intubation and single-lung ventilation provide the optimum operating conditions. However, we have successfully used VATS in a spontaneously ventilating patient. Intraoperative decortication of thickened visceral pleural cortex may be facilitated by the application of continuous positive airway pressure (CPAP) to the operative lung. The first 2-cm incision is usually placed just below the tip of the scapula with the patient placed in a lateral thoracotomy position. Insertion of the videothoracoscope may be preceeded by digital exploration of the incision to free local adhesions which would otherwise prevent scope insertion. Also, any free pleural fluid is suctioned via this port site prior to thoracoscopy. Two further port sites are usually required and their position is determined by the anatomy of the empyema cavity. They are sited under direct vision to prevent inadvertent parenchymal injury. Initial pleural debridement is performed by mechanical removal of fibrinous debris or by directed suction using a large-bore (>28 F) intercostal tube drain with an attached artery forceps (Figure 48.4). It is also possible to breakdown loculations by ultrasonic dissection by VATS.[40] Irrigation of the cavity with warm saline is also occasionally helpful. An assessment of lung expansion should then be made by reventilating the lung under direct vision. If the thickened visceral cortex prevents apposition of the two pleural surfaces, then decortication is required. It had been thought that removal of this peel could only be achieved via thoracotomy. However, we have successfully treated a series of patients with chronic post-pneumonic empyema by VATS. First, the cortex is incised across the circumference of the trapped lobe. Next, the two pleural sheets are elevated from the underlying visceral pleura by blunt dissection aided by simultaneous suction added to a mounted pledget (Figure 48.5). The elevated sheet is then excised and withdrawn via one of the port sites. We have used an aerosolized application of fibrin glue to the exposed visceral surface to reduce post-operative air leak.

Surgical results

VATS VERSUS FIBRINOLYSIS

Initial reports of the use of VATS in the management of the fibrinopurulent phase of empyema reported an imme-

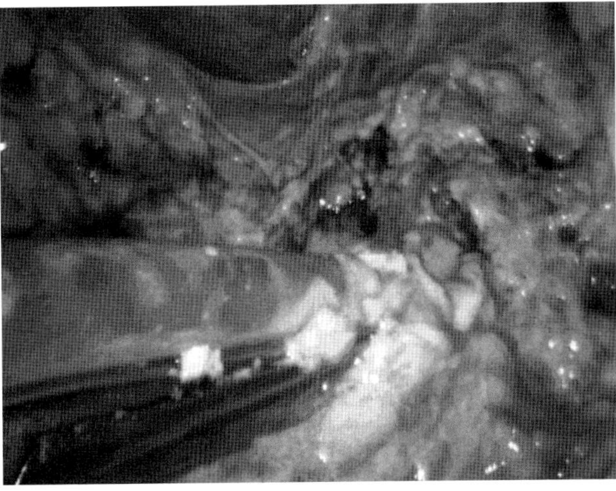

Figure 48.4 Video-assisted thoracoscopic suction debridement of fibrinopuruluent pleural empyema.

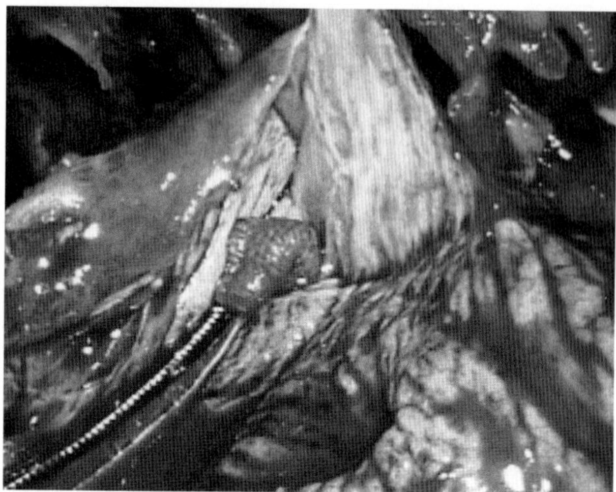

Figure 48.5 Video-assisted thoracoscopic decortication of a chronic parapneumonic empyema.

diate conversion rate of up to 28 percent due to the presence of an organized cortex.[41–43] There was also a late requirement for open surgery in 5–10 percent due to recurrent sepsis or failure to achieve full lung re-expansion.

Whether VATS mechanical debridement is preferable to intrapleural fibrinolysis and percutaneous catheter drainage is a topic of debate. A small but prospective, randomized trial found VATS to have a higher primary treatment success and shorter hospital stay with consequent cost savings in adults.[44] Certainly the use of fibrinolysis should be carefully monitored as delay in referral for surgical intervention reduces the likelihood of successful VATS due to the formation of fibrous pleural adhesions which prevent thoracoscopic access to the pleural cavity.[45,46] Empirical treatment with intrapleural fibrinolysis with early surgical drainage seems to offer a faster recovery than prolonged fibrinolysis and tube drainage.[47] However, the use of routine installation of fibrinolytics has been shown to be of no additional benefit when accurate and effective tube drainage has been established. The First Multicentre Intrapleural Sepsis Trial (MIST 1) showed no benefit in terms of mortality, need for surgery or hospital stay.[48]

In the treatment of paediatric pleural empyema, where tube drainage is often performed under general anaesthesia, VATS should be the primary therapy.[49]

VATS VERSUS THORACOTOMY

Pleural debridement by VATS has been shown to effectively treat fibrinopurulent empyema (Table 48.2). Some authors advocate VATS debridement as an initial, interim measure to limit the risk of toxic episodes and stabilize the patient prior to an elective thoracotomy and decortications.[42] When directly compared with thoracotomy in the management of fibrinopurulent PPE, VATS has been found to have comparable clinical effectiveness but advantages in terms of faster post-operative recovery.[41]

Percutaneous fibrinolysis is not effective once an empyema has become chronic and the inflammation organized and its use adds nothing to prevent the need for surgery despite apparently increasing the volume of drainage.[50] In the organizing phase of empyema (category 4), when the underlying lung has become entrapped, treatment is directed not only at pleural debridement but at removal of the thickened visceral pleural cortex by decortication. It has been thought that this procedure could only

Table 48.2 Results of video-assisted thoracoscopic surgery (VATS) for pleural empyema

Author	Early/ late[a]	Number	Conversion to thoracotomy	Reoperation	Drain time (days)	Hospital stay (days)	Mortality	Complications
Landreneau *et al.*[51]	Mixed	76	8 (17%)	5 (6%)	3.3	7.4	5 (6.6%)	2 (3%)
Solaini *et al.*[110]	Early	40	1 (2.5%)	–	4.8	–	–	–
Lackner *et al.*[111]	Early	17	4 (23%)	–	7	11	0%	–
Cassina *et al.*[112]	Mixed	45	8 (18%)	0	7	10.7	0%	5 (11%)
Waller *et al.*[53]	Mixed	36	15 (41%)	0	–	–	–	–
Lawrence *et al.*[42]	Early	31	3 (10%)	10 (32%)	4.3	6.8	1 (3%)	5 (16%)
Striffeler *et al.*[43]	Early	67	19 (28%)	3 (4%)	4.1	11.5	3 (4%)	–
Angelillo Mackinley *et al.*[41]	Early	31	3 (10%)	0	4.2	6.7	1 (3%)	5 (16%)
Cunniffe *et al.*[113]	Early	10	0	0	4.5	11	0%	
Ridley and Braimbridge[39]	Mixed	18	0	10 (55%)	10.7	–	2 (11%)	–
Wait *et al.*[44]	Early	11	0	0%	5.8	8.7	0%	–

[a]Late empyema defined as an empyema of more than three weeks delay to surgery.

be carried out by open thoracotomy. Landreneau *et al.*[51] found that 17 percent of his series required open decortication and in these patients 93 percent had an empyema for more than 3 weeks. Certainly, thoracotomy with decortication has an excellent success rate of around 95 percent in treating empyema at any stage with low associated morbidity and mortality.[52] Nevertheless, with technical refinement, VATS can successfully treat even the most chronic empyema. We have reported successful VATS decortication in patients with duration of symptoms of nearly 2 months.[53] With increasing experience in the use of VATS to treat all cases of chronic empyema primarily, we are currently successful in around 60 percent of cases.[54]

RIB RESECTION/THORACOSTOMY

Rib resection to drain the empyema cavity is indicated for patients at high-risk from more major surgery with thoracotomy or who could not tolerate single-lung ventilation. It may be performed with the patient spontaneously ventilating with the resection of a short segment of rib over the most dependent part of the empyema cavity to allow drainage of and limited breakdown of loculations in the infected space. A large bore tube is left *in situ*.[55] In patients in whom the empyema cavity is thought unlikely to close or to be sterilized, a permanent drainage site can be formed by resecting two to three ribs and by suturing the exposed parietal pleura to the skin of the raised cutaneous flaps. The cavity can then be easily irrigated and dressed as an outpatient. This procedure is described as the Eloesser flap drainage procedure.[56]

TUBERCULOUS EMPYEMA

The original description of thoracoscopy was for adhesiolysis for tuberculosis (TB).[57] VATS has been shown to be useful in the diagnosis of TB effusion and in the debridement of a TB empyema.[58] VATS decortication of the trapped lung in TB is also possible.

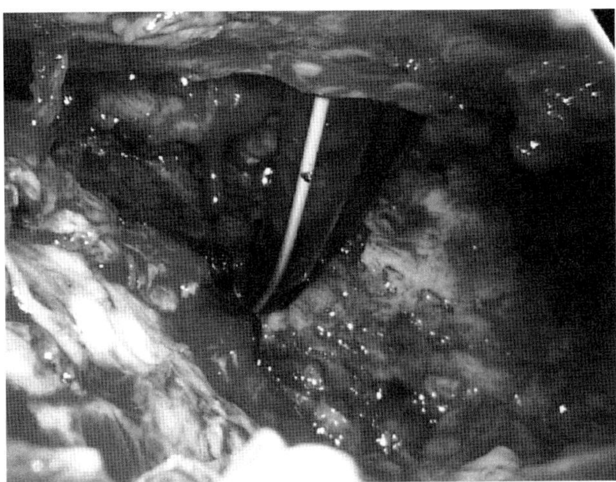

Figure 48.6 Video-assisted thoracoscopic debridement of a malignant pleural empyema.

MALIGNANT EMPYEMA

A malignant pleural effusion may become secondarily infected by percutaneous intervention or intrinsic pulmonary infection predisposed by collapse of the parenchyma (Figure 48.6). Repeated pleural aspirations render the patient particularly susceptible to secondary infection. Because of the frailty of these patients, fenestration may be all that is possible. However, the benefits of VATS are especially pertinent in this group of patients.

MALIGNANT PLEURAL EFFUSION

Indications for surgery

PLEURAL BIOPSY

Diagnostic pleural biopsy by VATS has a high sensitivity of over 90 percent[59] as it allows full inspection of the pleural surfaces under magnification and illumination. This procedure can be carried out in a spontaneously ventilating patient if the pleural disease is diffuse. If the patient is to be considered for more radical surgery, then the diagnostic pleural biopsy should be performed via as few incisions as possible (ideally in the line of a future thoracotomy incision) to minimize the risk of tumor implantation. Thoracoscopy is superior to closed pleural biopsy in the diagnosis of malignant pleural effusion.[60]

PLEURODESIS

Control of pleural fluid production can be achieved by inducing pleurodesis with talc insufflation administered by video-assisted or direct thoracoscopy and can be effectively administered in a spontaneously ventilating patient under local anesthesia.[61] Thoracoscopic talc poudrage is superior to talc slurry administered via tube thoracostomy.[62] In mesothelioma, cytoreductive parietal pleurectomy may have a longer lasting control of symptoms than chemical pleurodesis alone.[63] Cytoreductive pleurectomy may also have a survival benefit over pleural biopsy alone.[64] (Pleurodesis is also discussed in further detail in Chapter 46.)

TRAPPED LUNG

Once the visceral pleural surface has become involved by the malignant process, the underlying lung will not expand. Pleurodesis will not be successful if the pleural surfaces cannot be apposed. Repeated pleural aspiration may result in infection and empyema formation or tumor implantation. The goal of treatment is palliation by a single intervention which is reliable, causes little discomfort, avoids prolonged hospital stay and relieves symptoms during the terminal phase of the disease.

Surgical treatment is directed towards either evacuation of fluid from the thoracic cavity by the insertion of a pleuroperitoneal shunt or by attempting to re-expand the lung by visceral decortication. Whilst evacuation of the pleural space will improve dyspnoea, the patient will remain compromised by the collapsed lung.

Pleuroperitoneal shunts are usually inserted using VATS although mini-thoracotomy may be required if repeated prior aspiration has resulted in pleural adhesions. Operative complications are generally low but post-operative complications, such as infection, shunt blockage and tumor seeding at the port site, may occur in up to 15 percent of patients. However, effective palliation can be achieved in 95 percent of cases with no evidence of tumor seeding into peritoneum.[65]

We have found tumor decortication with visceral pleurectomy to be beneficial with symptomatic relief of dyspnea for over 3 months with acceptable operative mortality and morbidity.[66] Thoracotomy, however, should be reserved for those patients with epithelioid mesothelioma and before significant weight loss since post-operative recovery may significantly erode the remaining symptom-free survival. For this reason we have extended the role of VATS decortication to mesothelioma with survival benefit, especially in the elderly.[67]

Our current management protocol for malignant pleural effusion comprises early assessment by VATS and incorporates all the above treatment options (Figure 48.7).

RADICAL SURGERY

In selected cases, malignant pleural effusion secondary to malignant mesothelioma may be treated by extrapleural pneumonectomy. This operation is only advocated by a small number of surgical centers and is reserved for a selected number of patients. The indicators of favorable post-operative prognosis include epithelioid histology, clear surgical resection margins and the absence of extrapleural lymph node involvement.[68] Thus, careful preoperative staging is imperative. Malignant lymph node involvement cannot be accurately predicted from nodal uptake on positron-emission tomography (PET) scanning[69] or from nodal size,[70] therefore cervical mediastinoscopy is mandatory. Future preoperative selection may include biological markers of angiogenesis, i.e tumor microvessel counts or matrix metalloproteinase expression.[71]

The operation of extrapleural pneumonectomy (EPP) involves the *en-bloc* excision of the entire pleural surface with underlying lung and adjacent pericardium and hemidiaphragm. Mediastinal lymph node clearance is also advocated. The pericardium and diaphragm are replaced with prosthetic patches.The operation is usually performed via a lateral thoracotomy but we have found post-operative benefits from a median sternotomy approach.[72]

The initial reported operative mortality of 25 percent for extrapleural pneumonectomy[73] was initially thought to be preclusive but recent series reflecting improvements in perioperative care report operative mortality of as low as 3.8 percent.[68] Unfortunately, despite wider application, radical treatment has had little impact on overall survival from mesothelioma. The best 5-year survival figures are reported for those with the prognostic factors above and these represent a minority of those referred for surgery. With multi-modality treatment including radical surgery, radical hemithorax irradiation and chemotherapy median survival ranges from 33 to 51 months.[68,74] Despite these aggressive attempts at local disease control, including intracavitary chemotherapy,[75] survival from mesothelioma surgery is thwarted by distant disease progression,[76,77] commonly in the peritoneal cavity or the contralateral pleural cavity. Several authors therefore advocate radical pleurectomy/decortication, with preservation of the lung, in preference to EPP[78,79] as it is associated with lower operative mortality and potentially better functional status. We utilize this form of radical debulking in those with positive mediastinoscopy whose survival is limited.[80]

MISCELLANEOUS

Clotted hemothorax

A retained hemothorax may be expected in around 2 percent of patients with thoracic injuries.[81] CT is needed to predict the need for evacuation of the clotted blood as chest radiography alone is insensitive. VATS is effective in

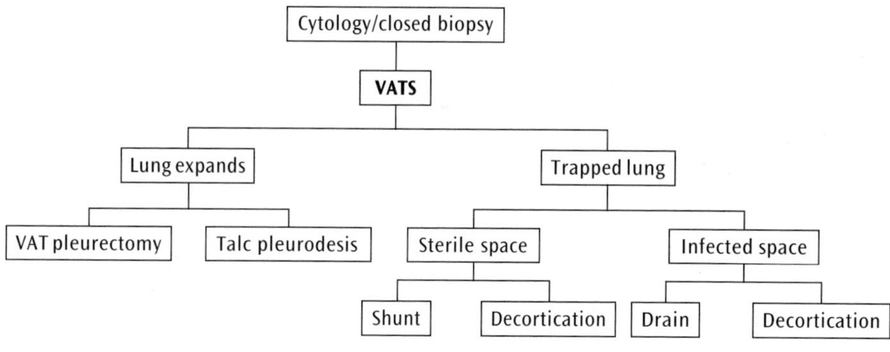

Figure 48.7 Surgical management protocol for malignant pleural effusion. VATS, video-assisted thoracoscopic surgery.

evacuating clotted hemothorax and preventing secondary infection and the development of an empyema.[51]

SURGICAL INDICATIONS

The optimum time for VATS evacuation is within the first week of the injury before the hematoma has become organized.[81]

SURGICAL RESULTS

Early VATS intervention has been shown to be a more efficient and economical strategy than intercostal tube drainage. A prospective randomized trial[82] found a reduction in hospital stay of around 3 days and a 40 percent saving in the cost of the hospital episode.

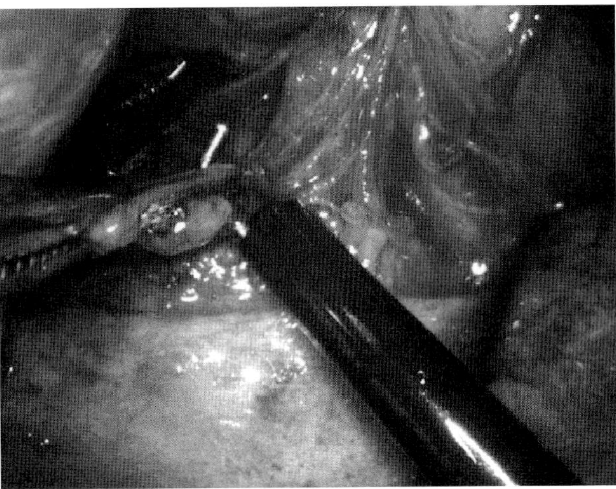

Figure 48.8 Video-assisted thoracoscopic control of thoracic duct in idiopathic spontaneous chylothorax.

Chylothorax

SURGICAL INDICATIONS

Approximately 50 percent of cases of chylothorax will not respond to conservative treatment of pleural drainage, intravenous feeding and fluid replacement.[83]

SURGICAL METHODS

Ligation of thoracic duct has been described in post-traumatic or post-surgical cases of chylous fistula. However, even ligation of a successfully identified duct may not fully control the leak due to the presence of lymphatic collaterals. In cases of intractable chylous fistula, identification of the fistula site or dissection of the thoracic duct may be avoided by supradiaphragmatic ligation of the lower end of the duct just above the cisterna chili.[84] To aid intraoperative identification of the site of chylous leak, the patient should ingest 50 mL of full-fat cream immediately prior to surgery. This will lead to the leakage of pure white chyle which is more easily seen. VATS has been successfully used to achieve ligation, suturing or clipping of the thoracic duct[85] (Figure 48.8). VATS talc pleurodesis may also be useful, particularly in cases where there is a diffuse chylous leak due to increased lymphatic pressure and may be superior to chemoradiation in lymphoma.[86]

Cirrhotic hydrothorax

The most likely mechanism for this condition, which develops in approximately 5 percent of patients with cirrhosis, is the passive collection of pleural fluid due to the movement of ascites along a pressure gradient through small diaphragmatic fenestrations.[87] Repeated thoracocentesis or tube drainage are contraindicated due to the resultant hypovolemia, protein loss and infection. Therapy should be directed toward reducing the formation of ascites by transjugular intrahepatic portosystemic shunting (TIPS). Attempts to shunt the ascites or pleural fluid into the venous circulation are prone to complications of shunt blockage or infection.[88] Chemical pleurodesis alone is prone to failure because the rapid reaccumulation of pleural fluid prevents adhesion. Control of diaphragmatic pores when present by suturing or stapling increases the efficacy of VATS talc pleurodesis to around 66 percent.[89] The best results are obtained by the primary control of portal hypertension and ascites production by TIPS.[90]

COMPLICATIONS OF SURGERY

Pleurectomy

Post-operative hemothorax occurs in less than 4 percent of patients after parietal pleurectomy.[91] Patients are at more risk from total rather than apical pleurectomy.[92] Chronic intercostal neuralgia has been reported after VATS;[93] in a small series of 60 patients (76 percent follow-up) 19 complained of chronic pain, in 12 of these mild pain only was reported related to trocar sites. Pain was greatest after pleurectomy. Horner's syndrome has been reported anecdotally after pleurectomy, possibly due to excessive traction on the apical pleural sheet.

Pleural biopsy

Malignant seeding of tumor cells in thoracoscopy port sites may occur in up to 40 percent of patients after biopsy of malignant pleural disease. A prospective randomized trial by Boutin and colleagues[94] demonstrated a preventive benefit from prophylactic external beam radiotherapy to these sites.

Talc pleurodesis

The fear of mesothelioma development as a long-term sequelae of talc poudrage is unfounded in the era of asbestos-free talc.[95] Long-term restrictive respiratory impairment is also not a major concern.[96] A potentially more serious risk from talc pleurodesis in the surgical setting is the development of acute respiratory distress after insufflations.[97] However, recent large series[19] have not seen this complication, particularly where large-particle talc is used.[98]

Decortication

Tumor decortication must ensure full lung re-expansion as these patients are particularly at risk from infection of any residual space with the formation of an empyema. In our own series we have found this complication in 4 percent of patients.[66] Other specific complications include an iatrogenic parenchymal lung injury with resultant persistent air leak, post-operative hemothorax and iatrogenic injuries to the azygos vein, thoracic duct or esophagus (the intraoperative placement of an esophageal bougie aids identification of the organ and reduces the risk of inadvertent injury).

Extrapleural pneumonectomy

Major morbidity is experienced by over 40 percent of patients undergoing this extensive operation,[99] most commonly supraventricular cardiac arrythmias. Specific technical complications include detachment of prosthetic patches, bronchopleural fistulae, esophageal rupture and post-operative hemorrhage. We have also observed rapid filling of the pneumonectomy space with serous fluid leading to mediastinal shift and hemodynamic compromise.[100] There is debate whether the use of induction chemotherapy increases the risk of post-operative complications.[100,101]

FUTURE SURGICAL DIRECTIONS

The following are areas of surgical practice which are under evaluation at present and which in the future may be incorporated into routine management protocols for pleural disease.

Spontaneous pneumothorax

- Surgical intervention by VATS after the first episode of primary spontaneous pneumothorax.
- Day case surgery by VATS with *in situ* Heimlich valve drainage system.
- Incorporating the principles of lung volume reduction surgery in patients presenting with secondary spontaneous pneumothorax.

Pleural empyema

- Earlier surgical intervention by VATS debridement rather than extended tube drainage or intrapleural fibrinolysis.
- Wider application of VATS to more chronic post-pneumonic and tuberculous cases.

Malignant pleural effusion

- Increased application of medical thoracoscopy with pleurodesis as the initial diagnostic procedure.
- Prospective randomized controlled trials of radical surgery in mesothelioma.
- Improved management of the trapped lung by VATS decortication.
- Prospective randomized controlled trials of VATS debulking surgery.

Hemothorax

The earlier use of VATS in the assessment of major thoracic trauma may prevent unnecessary thoracotomy from compounding the risks of the injury itself.

KEY POINTS

- Early surgical intervention by VATS is indicated in both spontaneous pneumothorax and pleural empyema to maximize the benefits of minimally invasive surgery.
- Percutaneous fibrinolytic treatment should not delay surgical intervention in pleural empyema.
- Multiple preoperative pleural interventions are unnecessary and may prejudice the outcome of surgery by inducing pleural sepsis and adhesions.
- VATS has many advantages over thoracotomy in the management of pleural disease but is subject to a learning curve.
- The role of VATS debulking in mesothelioma remains to be determined.
- The benefit of extrapleural pneumonectomy in mesothelioma remains to be proven.

REFERENCES

● = Key primary paper
◆ = Major review article

◆1. Baumann MH, Strange C, Heffner JE, *et al.* Management of spontaneous pneumothorax: an American College of Chest Physicians Delphi consensus statement. *Chest* 2001; **119**: 590–602.

2. Waller DA, McConnell SA, Rajesh PB. Delayed referral reduces the success of video-assisted thoracoscopic surgery for spontaneous pneumothorax. *Respir Med* 1998; **92**: 246–9.

3. Sihoe AD, Yim AP, Lee TW, *et al.* Can CT scanning be used to select patients with unilateral primary spontaneous pneumothorax for bilateral surgery? *Chest* 2000; **118**: 380–3.

4. Almind M, Lange P, Viskum K. Spontaneous pneumothorax: comparison of simple drainage,talc pleurodesis, tetracycline pleurodesis. *Thorax* 1989; **44**: 627–30.

5. Torresini G, Vaccarili M, Divisi D, Crisci R. Is video-assisted thoracic surgery justified at first spontaneous pneumothorax? *Eur J Cardiothorac Surg* 2001; **20**: 42–5.

6. Abdala OA, Levy RR, Bibiloni RH, *et al.* Advantages of video-assisted thoracic surgery in the treatment of spontaneous pneumothorax. *Medicina (B Aires)* 2001; **61**: 157–60.

7. Deslauriers J, Beaulieu M, Despres JP, *et al.* Transaxillary pleurectomy for treatment of spontaneous pneumothorax. *Ann Thorac Surg* 1980; **30**: 569–74.

●8. Waller DA, Forty J, Morritt GN. Video-assisted thoracoscopic surgery versus thoracotomy for spontaneous pneumothorax. *Ann Thorac Surg* 1994; **58**: 372–6.

9. Waller DA, Forty J, Soni AK, Conacher ID, Morritt GN. Videothoracoscopic operation for secondary spontaneous pneumothorax. *Ann Thorac Surg* 1994; **57**: 1612–15.

10. Waller DA. Video-assisted thoracoscopic surgery for spontaneous pneumothorax – a 7-year learning experience. *Ann R Coll Surg Engl* 1999; **81**: 387–92.

11. McManus KG, Spence GM, McGuigan JA. Outpatient chest tubes. *Ann Thorac Surg* 1998; **66**: 299–300.

12. Gelb AF, McKenna RJ Jr, Brenner M, Epstein JD, Zamel N. Lung function 5 years after lung volume reduction surgery for emphysema. *Am J Respir Crit Care Med* 2001; **163**: 1562–6.

◆13. Naunheim KS, Mack MJ, Hazelrigg SR, *et al.* Safety and efficacy of video-assisted thoracic surgical techniques for the treatment of spontaneous pneumothorax. *J Thorac Cardiovasc* Surg 1995; **109**: 1198–203.

14. Inderbitzi RG, Leiser A, Furrer M, Althaus U. Three years' experience in video-assisted thoracic surgery (VATS) for spontaneous pneumothorax. *J Thorac Cardiovasc Surg* 1994; **107**: 1410–15.

15. Ferguson LJ, Imrie CW, Hutchison J. Excision of bullae without pleurectomy in patients with spontaneous pneumothorax. *Br J Surg* 1981; **68**: 214–16.

16. Melvin WS, Krasna MJ, McLaughlin JS. Thoracoscopic management of spontaneous pneumothorax. *Chest* 1992; **102**: 1877–9.

17. Weeden D, Smith GH. Surgical experience in the management of spontaneous pneumothorax, 1972–82. *Thorax* 1983; **38**: 737–43.

18. Cardillo G, Facciolo F, Giunti R, *et al.* Videothoracoscopic treatment of primary spontaneous pneumothorax: a 6-year experience. *Ann Thorac Surg* 2000; **69**: 357–61.

19. Cardillo G, Carleo F, Giunti R, *et al.* Video thoracoscopic talc poudrage in primary spontaneous pneumothorax: a single-institution experience in 861 cases. *J Thorac Cardiovasc Surg* 2006; **131**: 322–8.

20. Guerin JC, van Derschueren RG. Treatment of recurrent pneumothorax applying fibrin adhesive under endoscopy. *Rev Mal Respir* 1989; **6**: 443–5.

21. Gebhard FT, Becker HP, Gerngross H, Bruckner UB. Reduced inflammatory response in minimal invasive surgery of pneumothorax. *Arch Surg* 1996; **131**: 1079–82.

22. Dumont P, Diemont F, Massard G, *et al.* Does a thoracoscopic approach for surgical treatment of spontaneous pneumothorax represent progress? *Eur J Cardiothorac Surg* 1997; **11**: 27–31.

23. Miller JD, Simone C, Kahnamoui K, *et al.* Comparison of videothoracoscopy and axillary thoracotomy for the treatment of spontaneous pneumothorax. *Am Surg* 2000; **66**: 1014–15.

24. Horio H, Nomori H, Fuyuno G, Kobayashi R, Suemasu K. Limited axillary thoracotomy vs video-assisted thoracoscopic surgery for spontaneous pneumothorax. *Surg Endosc* 1998; **12**: 1155–8.

25. Kim KH, Kim HK, Han JY, *et al.* Transaxillary minithoracotomy versus video-assisted thoracic surgery for spontaneous pneumothorax. *Ann Thorac Surg* 1996; **61**: 1510–12.

26. Jimenez-Merchan R, Garcia-Diaz F, Arenas-Linares C, *et al.* Comparative retrospective study of surgical treatment of spontaneous pneumothorax. Thoracotomy vs thoracoscopy. *Surg Endosc* 1997; **11**: 919–22.

◆27. Sedryakan A, van der Meulen J, Lewsey J, Treasure T. Video assisted thoracic surgery for treatment of pneumothorax and lung resections: systematic review of randomized clinical trials. *Br Med J* 2004; **329**: 1008–11.

28. Tschopp JM, Boutin C, Astoul P, *et al.* Talcage by medical thoracoscopy for primary spontaneous pneumothorax is more cost-effective than drainage: a randomized study. *Eur Respir J* 2002; **20**: 1003–9.

29. Tschopp JM, Brutsche M, Frey JG. Treatment of complicated spontaneous pneumothorax by simple talc pleurodesis under thoracoscopy and local anaesthesia. *Thorax* 1997; **52**: 329–32.

30. Waller DA. Video-assisted thoracoscopic surgery (VATS) in the management of spontaneous pneumothorax. *Thorax* 1997; **52**: 307–8.

31. Spector ML, Stern RC. Pneumothorax in cystic fibrosis: a 26 year experience. *Ann Thorac Surg* 1989; 47: 204–7.

32. Noyes BE, Orenstein DM. Treatment of pneumothorax in cystic fobrosis in the era of lung transplantation. *Chest* 1992; 101: 1187–8.

◆33. Joseph J, Sahn SA. Thoracic endometriosis syndrome: new observations from an analysis of 110 cases. *Am J Med* 1996; **100**: 164–70.

34. Fonseca P. Catamenial pneumothorax: a multifactorial etiology. *J Thorac Cardiovasc Surg* 1998; **116**: 872–3.

35. Korom S, Canyurt H, Missbach A, *et al.* Catamenial pneumothorax evisited. *J Thorac Cardiovasc Surg* 2004; **128**: 502–8.

36. Marshall MB, Ahmed Z, Kucharczuk JC, Kaiser LR, Shager JB. Catamenial pneumothorax: optimal hormonal and surgical management. *Eur J Cardiothorac Surg* 2005; **27**: 662–6.

37. Hsu NY, Shih CS, Hsu CP, Chen PR.Spontaneous hemopneumothorax revisited. *Ann Thorac Surg* 2005; **80**: 1859.

◆38. Colice GL, Curtis A, Deslauriers J, *et al.* Medical and surgical treatment of parapneumonic effusions: an evidence-based guideline. *Chest* 2000; **118**: 1158–71.

39. Ridley PD, Braimbridge MV. Thoracoscopic debridement and pleural irrigation in the management of empyema thoracis. *Ann Thorac Surg* 1991; **51**: 461–4.

40. Nakamura H, Taniguchi Y, Makihara K, Ohgi S. Ultrasonic pleural debridement of empyema. *Ann Thorac Cardiovasc Surg* 2001; **7**: 62–4.

41. Angelillo Mackinlay TA, Lyons GA, Chimondeguy DJ, *et al.* VATS debridement versus thoracotomy in the treatment of loculated postpneumonia empyema. *Ann Thorac Surg* 1996; **61**: 1626–30.

42. Lawrence DR, Ohri SK, Moxon RE, Townsend ER, Fountain SW. Thoracoscopic debridement of empyema thoracis. *Ann Thorac Surg* 1997; **64**: 1448–50.

43. Striffeler H, Gugger M, Im Hof V, *et al.* Video-assisted thoracoscopic surgery for fibrinopurulent pleural empyema in 67 patients. *Ann Thorac Surg* 1998; **65**: 319–23.

- ●44. Wait MA, Sharma S, Hohn J, Dal Nogare A. A randomized trial of empyema therapy. *Chest* 1997; **111**: 1548–51.
- 45. Waller DA, Rengarajan A, Nicholson FH, Rajesh PB. Delayed referral reduces the success of video-assisted thoracoscopic debridement for post-pneumonic empyema. *Respir Med* 2001; **95**: 836–40.
- 46. Lardinois D, Gock M, Pezzetta E, *et al.* Delayed referral and Gram negative organisms increase the conversion to thoracotomy rate in patients undergoing video-assisted thoracoscopic surgery for empyema. *Ann Thorac Surg* 2005; **79**: 1851–6.
- 47. Lim TK, Chin NK. Empirical treatment with fibrinolysis and early surgery reduces the duration of hospitalization in pleural sepsis. *Eur Respir J* 1999; **13**: 514–18.
- ●48. Maskell NA, Davies CWH, Nunn AJ, *et al.* UK controlled trial of intrapleural streptokinase for pleural infection. *N Engl J Med* 2005; **352**: 865–74.
- 49. Cohen G, Hjortal V, Ricci M. Primary thoracoscopic treatment of empyema in children. *J Thorac Cardiovasc Surg* 2003; **125**: 79–83.
- 50. Chin NK, Lim TK. Controlled trial of intrapleural streptokinase in the treatment of pleural empyema and complicated parapneumonic effusions. *Chest* 1997; **111**: 275–9.
- 51. Landreneau RJ, Keenan RJ, Hazelrigg SR, Mack MJ, Naunheim KS. Thoracoscopy for empyema and hemothorax. *Chest* 1996; **109**: 18–24.
- 52. Hoover EL, Hsu HK, Ross MJ, *et al.* Reappraisal of empyema thoracis. Surgical intervention when the duration of illness is unknown. *Chest* 1986; **90**: 511–15.
- 53. Waller DA, Rengarajan A. Thoracoscopic decortication: a role for video-assisted surgery in chronic postpneumonic pleural empyema. *Ann Thorac Surg* 2001; **71**: 1813–16.
- 54. Jutley RS, Coneybeare A, Rengarajan A,Waller DA. Video assisted thoracoscopic surgery for chronic post-pneumonic empyema: a missed opportunity? *Thorax* 2005; **60**: 31S
- 55. Samson PC. Empyema thoracis, essentials of present day management. *Ann Thorac Surg* 1971; **11**: 210.
- 56. Hurvitz RJ, Thucker BL. The Eloesser flap: past and present. *J Thorac Cardiovasc Surg* 1986; **42**: 958.
- 57. Jacobaeus H. The cauterization of adhesions in artificial pneumothrax treatment of tuberculosis under thoracoscopic control. *Proc R Soc Med* 1922–3; **16**: 45–60.
- 58. Yim AP, Izzat MB, Lee TW. Thoracoscopic surgery for pulmonary tuberculosis. *World J Surg* 1999; **23**: 1114–17.
- 59. Waller DA, Hasan A, Forty J, Morritt GN. Videothoracoscopy in the diagnosis of intrathoracic pathology: early experience. *Ann R Coll Surg Engl* 1994; **76**: 123–6.
- 60. Emad A, Rezaian GR. Diagnostic value of closed percutaneous pleural biopsy vs pleuroscopy in suspected malignant pleural effusion or tuberculous pleurisy in a region with a high incidence of tuberculosis: a comparative, age-dependent study. *Respir Med* 1998; **92**: 488–92.
- 61. Danby CA, Adebonojo SA, Moritz DM. Video-assisted talc pleurodesis for malignant pleural effusions utilizing local anesthesia and IV sedation. *Chest* 1998; **113**: 739–42.
- 62. Stefani A, Natali P, Casali C, Morandi U. Talc poudrage versus talc slurry in the treatment of malignant pleural effusion. A prospective comparative study. *Eur J Cardiothorac Surg* 2006; **30**: 827–32.
- 63. Waller DA, Morritt GN, Forty J. Video-assisted thoracoscopic pleurectomy in the management of malignant pleural effusion. *Chest* 1995; **107**: 1454–6.
- 64. Halstead JC, Lim E, Venkateswaran RM, *et al.* Improved survival with VATS pleurectomy-decortication in advanced malignant mesothelioma. *Eur J Surg Oncol* 2005; **31**: 314–20.
- ◆65. Genc O, Petrou M, Ladas G, Goldstraw P. The long-term morbidity of pleuroperitoneal shunts in the management of recurrent malignant effusions. *Eur J Cardiothorac Surg* 2000; **18**: 143–6.
- 66. Martin-Ucar AE, Edwards JG,Rengarajan A, Muller S, Waller DA. Palliative surgical debulking in malignant mesothelioma. Predictors of survival and symptom control. *Eur J Cardiothorac Surg* 2001; **20**: 1117–21.
- 67. Nakas A, Martin-Ucar AE, Barlow A, *et al.* The extent of surgery for malignant mesothelioma in patients over the age of 65: a therapeutic dilemma. *Thorax* 2006; **61**: 45S
- ●68. Sugarbaker DJ, Flores RM, Jaklitsch MT, *et al.* Resection margins, extrapleural nodal status, cell type determine postoperative long-term survival in trimodality therapy of malignant pleural mesothelioma: results in 183 patients. *J Thorac Cardiovasc Surg* 1999; **117**: 54–63.
- 69. Flores RM, Akhurst T, Gonen M, *et al.* Positron emission tomography predicts survival in malignant pleural mesothelioma. *J Thorac Cardiovasc Surg* 2006; **132**: 763–8.
- 70. Pilling JE, Stewart DJ, Martin-Ucar AE, *et al.* The case for routine cervical mediastinoscopy prior to radical surgery fro malignant pleural mesothelioma. *Eur J Cardiothorac Surg* 2004; **25**: 497–501.
- ◆71. O'Byrne KJ, Edwards JG, Waller DA. Clinico-pathological and biological prognostic factors in pleural malignant mesothelioma. *Lung Cancer* 2004; **45**: S45–8.
- 72. Edwards JG, Martin-Ucar AE, Stewart DJ, Waller DA. Right extrapleural pneumonectomy for malignant mesothelioma via median sternotomy or thoracotomy? Short and long-term results. *Eur J Cardiothorac Surg* 2007; **31**: 759–64.
- ●73. Butchart EG, Ashcroft T, Barnsley WC, Holden MP. Pleuropneumonectomy in the management of diffuse malignant mesothelioma of the pleura. Experience with 29 patients. *Thorax* 1976; **31**: 15–24.
- 74. Rusch VW, Rosenzweig K, Venkatraman E, *et al.*A phase II trial of surgical resection and adjuvant high-dose hemithoracic radiation for malignant pleural mesothelioma. *J Thorac Cardiovasc Surg* 2001; **122**: 788–95.
- 75. Richards WG, Zellos L, Bueno R, *et al.* Phase I to II study of pleurectomy/decortication and intraoperative intracavitary hyperthermic cisplatin lavage for mesothelioma. *J Clin Oncol* 2006; **24**: 1561–7.
- 76. Baldini EH, Recht A, Strauss GM, *et al.* Patterns of failure after trimodality therapy for malignant pleural mesothelioma. *Ann Thorac Surg* 1997; **63**: 334–8.
- 77. Stewart DJ, Martin-Ucar AE, Pilling JE, *et al.* The effect of extent of local resection on patterns of disease progression in malignant pleural mesothelioma. *Ann Thorac Surg* 2004; **78**: 245–52.
- 78. Rusch VW, Saltz L, Venkatraman E, *et al.* A phase II trial of pleurectomy/decortication followed by intrapleural and systemic chemotherapy for malignant pleural mesothelioma. *J Clin Oncol* 1994; **12**: 1156–63.
- 79. Pass HI, Kranda K, Temeck BK, Feuerstein I, Steinberg SM. Surgically debulked malignant pleural mesothelioma: results and prognostic factors. *Ann Surg Oncol* 1997; **4**: 215–22.
- 80. Martin-Ucar AE, Nakas A, Edwards JG, Waller DA. Case-control study between extrapleural pneumonectomy and radical pleurectomy/decortication for pathological N2 malignant pleural mesothelioma. *Eur J Cardiothorac Surg* 2007; **31**: 765–70.
- 81. Velmahos GC, Demetriades D. Early thoracoscopy for the evacuation of undrained haemothorax. *Eur J Surg* 1999; **165**: 924–9.
- ●82. Meyer DM, Jessen ME, Wait MA, Estrera AS. Early evacuation of traumatic retained hemothoraces using thoracoscopy: a prospective, randomized trial. *Ann Thorac Surg* 1997; **64**: 1396–400.
- 83. Milsom JW, Kron IL, Rheuban KS, Rodgers BM. Chylothorax: an assessment of current surgical management. *J Thorac Cardiovasc Surg* 1985; **89**: 221–7.
- 84. Patterson GA, Todd TR, Delarue NC, *et al.* Supradiaphragmatic ligation of the thoracic duct in intractable chylous fistula. *Ann Thorac Surg* 1981; **32**: 44–9.

85. Graham DD, McGahren ED, Tribble CG, Daniel TM, Rodgers BM. Use of video-assisted thoracic surgery in the treatment of chylothorax. *Ann Thorac Surg* 1994; **57**: 1507–11.
86. Mares DC, Mathur PN. Medical thoracoscopic talc pleurodesis for chylothorax due to lymphoma: a case series. *Chest* 1998; **114**: 731–5.
87. Strauss RM, Boyer TD. Hepatic hydrothorax. *Semin Liver Dis* 1997; **17**: 227–32.
88. Scholz DG, Nagorney DM, Lindor KD. Poor outcome from peritoneovenous shunts for refractory ascites. *Am J Gastroenterol* 1989; **84**: 540–3.
89. Milanez de Campos JR, Filho LO, de Campos Werebe E, Sette H Jr, Fernandez A, Filomeno LT, Jatene FB. Thoracoscopy and talc poudrage in the management of hepatic hydrothorax. *Chest* 2000; **118**: 13–17.
90. Lazaridis KN, Frank JW, Krowka MJ, Kamath PS. Hepatic hydrothorax: pathogenesis, diagnosis, management. *Am J Med* 1999; **107**: 262–7.
91. Thomas P, Le Mee F, Le Hors H, *et al.* Results of surgical treatment of persistent or recurrent pneumothorax. *Ann Chir* 1993; **47**: 136–40.
92. Weeden D, Smith GH. Surgical experience in the management of spontaneous pneumothorax, 1972–82. *Thorax* 1983; **38**: 737–43.
93. Passlick B, Born C, Sienel W, Thetter O. Incidence of chronic pain after minimal-invasive surgery for spontaneous pneumothorax. *Eur J Cardiothorac Surg* 2001; **19**: 355–8; discussion 8–9.
94. Boutin C, Rey F, Vaillat J-R. Prevention of malignant seeding after invasive diagnostic procedures in patients with pleural mesothelioma. *Chest* 1995; **108**: 754–8.
95. Chappel A, Johnson A, Charles J, *et al.* A survey of the long-term effects of talc and kaolin pleurodesis. Research Committee of the British Thoracic Association and the Medical Research Council Pneumoconiosis Unit. *Br J Dis Chest* 1979; **73**: 285–8.
96. Lange P, Mortensen J, Groth S. Lung function 22–35 years after treatment of idiopathic spontaneous pneumothorax with talc poudrage or simple drainage. *Thorax* 1988; **43**: 559–61.
97. Brant A, Eaton T. Serious complications with talc slurry pleurodesis. *Respirology* 2001; **6**: 181–5.
98. Janssen JP, Collier G, Astoul P, *et al.* Safety of pleurodesis with talc poudrage in malignant pleural effusion: a prospective cohort study. *Lancet* 2007; **369**: 1535–9.
●99. Sugarbaker DJ, Jaklitsch MT, Bueno R, *et al.* Prevention, early detection and management of complications after 328 consecutive extrapleural pneumonectomies. *J Thorac Cardiovasc Surg* 2004; **128**: 138–46.
100. Stewart DJ, Martin-Ucar AE, Edwards JG, West K, Waller DA. Extrapleural pneumonectomy for malignant pleural mesothelioma; the risks of induction chemotherapy, right-sided procedures and prolonged operations. *Eur J Cardiothorac Surg* 2005; **27**: 373–8.
101. Weder W, Kestenholz P, Taverna C, *et al.* Neoadjuvant chemotherapy followed by extrapleural pneumonectomy in malignant pleural mesothelioma. *J Clin Oncol* 2004; **22**: 3451–7.
102. Liu HP, Yim AP, Izzat MB, *et al.* Thoracoscopic surgery for spontaneous pneumothorax. *World J Surg* 1999; **23**: 1133–6.
103. Hürtgen M, Linder A, Friedel G, *et al.* Video-assisted thoracoscopic pleurodesis. A survey conducted by the German Society for Thoracic Surgery. *Thorac Cardiovasc Surg* 1996; **44**: 199–203.
104. Ohno K, Miyoshi S, Minami M, *et al.* Ipsilateral recurrence frequency after video-assisted thoracoscopic surgery for primary spontaneous pneumothorax. *Jpn J Thorac Cardiovasc Surg* 2000; **48**: 757–60.
105. Yim APC. Video-assisted thoracoscopic management of primary spontaneous pneumothorax. *Ann Acad Med Singapore* 1996; **25**: 668–72.
106. Bertrand PC, Regnard JF, Spaggiari L, *et al.* Immediate and long-term results after surgical treatment of primary spontaneous pneumothorax by VATS. *Ann Thorac Surg* 1996; **61**: 1641–5.
107. Freixinet J, Canalis E, Rivas JJ, *et al.* Surgical treatment of primary spontaneous pneumothorax with video-assisted thoracic surgery. *Eur Respir J* 1997; **10**: 409–11.
108. Chan P, Clarke P, Daniel FJ, *et al.* Efficacy study of video-assisted thoracoscopic surgery pleurodesis for spontaneous pneumothorax. *Ann Thorac Surg* 2000; **70**: 253–7.
109. Hatz RA, Kaps MF, Meimarakis G, *et al.* Long-term results after video-assisted thoracoscopic surgery for first-time and recurrent spontaneous pneumothorax. *Ann Thorac Surg* 2000; **70**: 253–7.
110. Solaini L, Prusciano F, Bagioni P. Video-assisted thoracic surgery in the treatment of pleural empyema. *Surg Endosc* 2007; **21**: 280–4.
111. Lackner RP, Hughes R, Anderson LA, *et al.* Video-assisted evacuation of empyema is the preferred procedure for management of pleural space infections. *Am J Surg* 2000; **179**: 27–30.
112. Cassina PC, Hauser M, Hillejan L, *et al.* Video-assisted thoracoscopy in the treatment of pleural empyema: stage-based management and outcome. *J Thorac Cardiovasc Surg* 1999; **117**: 234–8.
113. Cunniffe MG, Maguire D, McAnena OJ, *et al.* Video-assisted thoracoscopic surgery in the management of loculated empyema. *Surg Endosc* 2000; **14**: 175–8.

49

Gene therapy in pleural diseases

STEVEN M ALBELDA, DANIEL H STERMAN

INTRODUCTION

Gene therapy (the treatment of disease based upon the transfer of genetic material) involving the pleural space offers a number of potential unique advantages.[1] The pleural space has a large surface area lined by a thin layer of mesothelial cells, the ideal configuration for efficent gene transfer. Liquids or cell suspensions injected into the pleural space can disseminate rapidly and uniformly, potentially allowing a very large number of cells to be transduced. The patterns of fluid drainage from the pleural space through vascular and lymphatic channels ensure rapid systemic uptake. Access to the pleural space is relatively easy and safe through a needle-catheter system or a small indwelling tunneled catheter. Fusion of the pleural space is quite benign, and in some instances (i.e. where pleural effusions cause symptoms) may be desirable.

Gene transfer to the pleural space could be used in at least two possible scenarios. First, the cells of the pleural space could be used as factories to produce gene products that would be secreted and then transferred into the systemic circulation. Second, gene therapy could be used in the treatment of pleural diseases, in particular pleural malignancies, including primary tumors (malignant mesotheliomas) and secondary, metastatic tumors.

VECTORS USED IN PLEURAL GENE THERAPY

The first requirement for successful gene therapy is efficient gene delivery. A variety of viral and non-viral gene transfer vectors have been developed.[2] As summarized in Table 49.1, each of these vectors has certain advantages with regard to DNA carrying capacity, types of cells targeted, *in vivo* gene transfer efficiency, duration of expression and induction of inflammation.

The most widely used vector system in pleural gene therapy has been recombinant, replication-incompetent adenovirus. This vector system offers a high-efficiency transduction of target cells (including non-dividing cells) and high expression levels of the delivered transgene. However, gene expression is transient and accompanied by prominent local and systemic inflammatory responses. Mesothelial and mesothelioma cells in culture are quite easily transduced by adenoviral vectors. Adenoviral vectors have been injected into the pleural and peritoneal spaces in animal models where uniform and high-level gene transduction occurs.[3–6]

Adeno-associated virus (AAV) is a defective parvovirus with a single-strand DNA genome and a naked protein coat that persists in an episomal state that allows for stable, long-term gene expression, while potentially circumventing the safety concerns surrounding an integration event. Most of the initial studies of AAV were performed with serotype 2 (AAV2). However, many additional serotypes of AAV viruses have recently been identified.[7] These alternative serotypes use different entry mechanisms so that they have varying tissue tropisms.

PLEURAL GENE THERAPY FOR THE TREATMENT OF SYSTEMIC DISEASES

Pleural injection of plasmid/liposome or adenoviral vectors can produce biologically active proteins, but for only for brief periods of time (i.e. days).[8,9] In contrast, it has been recently demonstrated that intrapleural administration of AAV vectors can lead to high-level and persist-

Table 49.1 Characteristics of Gene therapy vectors and tumor-selective viruses

Vector	DNA-carrying capacity	Cell range	*In vivo* gene delivery efficiency	Duration of expression	Co-transfer viral gene elements	Inflammatory response
Retrovirus	<8 kb	Replicating cells only	Low	Stable integration	Yes	Low
Adenovirus	7–8 kb	Most cells	Moderate	Transient	Yes	High
Adeno-associated virus	<5 kb	Primarily muscle, liver, and brain – depends on serotype	Moderate	Long term	Minimal	Low
Lentivirus	<8 kb	Many non-dividing cells	Low	Stable integration	Yes	Low
Liposome	>10 kb	Most cells	Low	Transient	No	Moderate
Autologous transduced cell	unlimited	Fibroblast, myoblast, mesothelial	Moderate	Months	No	Low
Herpes virus	>10 kb	Most cells	Moderate	Transient	Yes	High
Vaccinia virus	>10 kb	Most cells	Moderate	Transient	Yes	High

ent systemic expression of transgenes.[1,10,11] De *et al.*[10] compared the efficiency of an AAV5-based vector expressing α1-antitrypsin (α1AT) with that of an AAV2 vector expressing the same transgene by intrapleural and intramuscular routes in mice and found that the AAV5 vector achieved lung (bronchoalveolar lavage) and serum levels that were 10-fold greater than the AA2 vector. At 40 weeks post-instillation, α1AT levels were a remarkable 900 μg/mL – 1.6-fold higher than the accepted therapeutic serum level of 570 μg/mL. In a follow-up study,[11] the same group performed a comprehensive screen of 25 AAV serotype vectors and showed the highest efficiencies were seen with AAV5, AAV8, AAV9 and AAV rhesus monkey-10 vectors. Application of this approach in non-human primate models is ongoing, but has not yet been published. Issues of importance would be how long the transfected mesothelial cells would remain alive and secretory, as well as development of potential immune responses against the transgene or AAV proteins. These studies raise the exciting possibility of using AAV gene delivery to the pleural space for genetic pulmonary diseases such as α1AT or other systemic diseases, such as hemophilia, lysosomal storage disorders or diabetes.[1]

GENE THERAPY FOR THE TREATMENT OF PLEURAL DISEASES

Non-malignant pleural diseases

It is currently difficult to envision a large number of clinical scenarios where pleural gene therapy would be both useful and cost-effective. The two large classes of non-malignant pleural diseases are those related to lung or pleural infection and those secondary to underlying systemic diseases (i.e. congestive heart failure), neither of which is particularly amenable to local therapy. However, one could image a situation, such as refractory air leaks, where it could be beneficial to introduce a gene (i.e. platelet-derived growth factor) that might accelerate healing of bronchopleural fistulae.

Malignant pleural diseases

In the near future, the most likely use for pleural gene therapy will be in the treatment of malignant diseases including malignant mesothelioma (MM) and metastatic pleural disease.[12] A number of clinical trials have already been performed (see below). Pleural tumors have several characteristics that make them attractive targets for gene therapy, including: (1) the absence of standard, effective therapy; (2) the accessibility of the pleural space for biopsy, vector delivery and analysis of treatment effects; and (3) the availability of therapeutic strategies that require only transient gene expression. MM is an especially attractive target since local extension of disease, rather than distant metastases, is responsible for much of its morbidity and mortality.

Preclinical studies

A large number of gene therapy strategies for pleural malignancy have been explored using cell culture and animal models (Table 49.2).

Table 49.2 Approaches for gene therapy of pleural malignancies

Principal	Examples
Suicide gene therapy	Herpes simplex thymidine kinase gene plus ganciclovir Cytosine deaminase gene plus 5-flurocytosine
Induction of apoptosis	p53, p16, p14^{ARF}, Bak, Anti-sense SV40-T antigen
Anti-angiogenesis	Soluble form of the VEGF receptor (Flt-1), anti-angiogenic pigment epithelium-derived factor
Immunogene therapy	
Cytokine therapy	Interleukin-2, interleukin-12, Type 1 and Type 2 interferons, GM-CSF
Non-specific induction of innate and acquired immunity ligand	Liposome/DNA complexes, mycobacterial heat shock protein gene (HSP-65), anti-CD40
Vaccination	SV40 T-antigen
Tumor-selective replicating virus	*Herpes virus*, *Vaccinia virus*, *Adenovirus*

GM-CSF, granulocyte macrophage colony-stimulating factor; SV40, *Simian virus 40*; VEGF, vascular endothelial growth factor.

INDUCTION OF APOPTOSIS

Delivery of the wild-type p53 gene has been the most frequent method of experimental gene therapy of solid tumors, since mutations in the p53 tumor suppressor gene account for the majority of genetic abnormalities in solid tumors. Even though most MMs contain wild-type p53, over-expression of p53 using an adenoviral vector has inhibited cell growth.[13] Other molecular approaches used in mesotheliomas have been re-expression of p16^{INK4a},[14] or the p14^{ARF} protein complex.[15] An alternate method of inhibiting MM cells is the introduction of 'downstream' promoters of apoptosis such as the pro-apoptotic Bcl-2 family member Bak.[16] The potential role for SV40 as a causative factor in MM oncogenesis and proliferation is the rationale for experiments by Schrump and colleagues showing that anti-sense oligonucleotides designed to abrogate *Simian virus 40* (SV40) Tag expression induce apoptosis and enhance sensitivity to chemotherapeutic agents in SV40-positive MM cells *in vitro*.[17]

Given that *in vivo* gene transfer is quite inefficient, a major limitation of all of these approaches is that inducing cell death in only the transduced cells (without bystander effects), will have only limited therapeutic efficacy.

ANTI-ANGIOGENESIS

Inhibiting tumor blood vessel growth as a treatment for cancer has been an area of active interest, resulting in a number of approved therapies, such as an anti-vascular endothelial cell growth factor (VEGF) antibody. Adenoviral vectors have been used to deliver a soluble form of the VEGF receptor (Flt-1) or the anti-angiogenic pigment epithelium-derived factor to the pleural space of mice with lung cancers or MMs with some success.[18,19] The short duration of expression of Ad (adenoviral) vectors will likely limit this strategy in the clinic, but development of AAV vectors expressing anti-angiogenic molecules (including antibodies) may be an effective primary treatment or chemotherapy adjuvant in the future.

SUICIDE GENE THERAPY

An attractive approach in cancer gene therapeutics is 'suicide' gene therapy where a neoplasm is transduced with a cDNA encoding for an enzyme rendering tumor cells sensitive to a benign agent by converting the 'prodrug' to a toxic metabolite. Enzymes used most commonly are the *herpes simplex virus*-1 thymidine kinase (HSV*tk*) gene which makes cells sensitive to the nucleoside analog ganciclovir (GCV) or the yeast enzyme cytosine deaminase which converts 5-fluorocytosine to the toxic 5-fluorouracil. Therapeutic efficacy in the former is enhanced by a 'bystander' effect that involves passage of toxic GCV metabolites from transduced to non-transduced cells via gap junctions or apoptotic vesicles and induction of anti-tumor immune responses capable of killing tumor cells not expressing the transgene.

The transfer of HSV*tk* DNA to target pleural or peritoneal tumor cells has been accomplished using a variety of delivery systems including carrier cells,[20,21] liposomes,[22,23] plasmid DNA–polyethylenimine complexes[22] and AAV2 vectors.[24] The most effective vector, however, has been adenovirus. Initial experiments demonstrated that replication-deficient adenoviral HSV*tk* vectors (Ad.HSV*tk*) efficiently transduced mesothelioma cells both in tissue culture and in animal models and facilitated HSV*tk*-mediated killing of human MM cells in the presence of low concentrations of GCV.[25] Subsequently, Ad.HSV*tk*/GCV gene therapy was used successfully to treat established intraperitoneal human MM tumors and lung cancers in immunodeficient mice[26] and in rat models of pleural MM.[5,27]

IMMUNO-GENE THERAPY

Innate and adaptive anti-tumor immune responses can be elicited by delivering non-specific immunostimulatory genes. Delivery of the immunogenic heat shock protein gene-65 via cationic liposomes showed efficacy in a syngeneic murine model of MM. This effect, however, appeared to be related to non-specific effects of lipid–pDNA complexes likely due to the unmethylated CpG motifs of the prokaryotic DNA in the vector plasmids that were sufficient to activate 'danger signals' and initiate innate and adaptive anti-tumor immune responses.[28,29]

Cytokines are known to have both direct anti-proliferative effects upon mesothelioma cells, as well as activating intrapleural and intratumoral immune effector cells *in vivo*. Several published Phase I and Phase II clinical trials have documented MM tumor responses to intrapleural infusion of interleukin-2 (IL-2), interferon beta (IFN-β), and interferon gamma (IFN-γ). The rationale for the use of gene therapy is that expression of cytokine genes by tumor cells generates high levels of intratumoral cytokines in a paracrine fashion, inducing powerful local cytokine effects without significant systemic toxicity.

Animal studies showing good anti-MM efficacy have been published using a variety of pro-inflammatory cytokines including IL-2,[30] IL-12,[31] granulocyte-monocyte-colony stimulating factor (GM-CSF),[32,33] IFN-γ[34,35], IL-24 (mda-7)[36] and CD40-ligand.[37]

Our group has explored the use of genes encoding type I (α, β) interferons. A single intraperitoneal (i.p.) injection of a recombinant adenovirus engineered to express the murine β-interferon gene (Ad.muIFN-β) eradicated syngeneic murine MM in >90 percent of animals tested.[38] Intraperitoneal Ad.muIFN-β gene therapy also resulted in a significant reduction of subcutaneous tumors at a distant site and was mediated by $CD8^+$ T lymphocytes.[39]

REPLICATING, TUMOR-SELECTIVE VECTORS

Although not technically 'gene therapy', an increasingly popular therapeutic strategy has been to adapt or engineer viruses so that they preferentially replicate within tumors, but not normal tissues. In addition, these replication-selective viruses can be 'armed' by inserting specific transgenes (i.e. a suicide gene or cytokine). This approach was pioneered using mutated adenoviruses and has led to a number of clinical trials in solid tumors, such as head and neck tumors and prostate cancers, although its use in MM has been limited to date to *in vitro* models.[40] Modified herpes viruses have been used to successfully treat mouse models of MM[41,42] and metastatic pleural cancer.[43] An IL-2-armed, replication-restricted vaccinia virus has been used in a clinical trial (see below).[44]

Clinical trials

A cell-transfer trial was conducted using an irradiated ovarian carcinoma cell line retrovirally transfected with HSV*tk* (PA1-STK cells). Cells were instilled via an indwelling pleural catheter followed by systemic administration of GCV.[21,45] Minimal side effects were seen; there were some post-treatment increases in the percentage of $CD8^+$ T lymphocytes in pleural fluid but no clinical responses were noted.

Sterman *et al.*[46–49] conducted a series of Phase 1 clinical trials of a replication-incompetent adenoviral vector encoding HSV*tk* (Ad.HSV*tk*) delivered intrapleurally (followed by ganciclovir) into more than 30 patients with pleural MM. Dose-limiting toxicity was not reached, side effects were minimal and gene transfer was confirmed in a dose-related fashion with clearly detectable gene transfer (indicated by immunostaining) at tumor surfaces and up to 30–50 cell layers deep (Figure 49.1). Anti-tumor antibodies and strong anti-adenoviral immune responses, including high titers of neutralizing antibody and proliferative T-cell responses, were generated, but with no obvious adverse clinical effects. Interestingly, a number of clinical responses were seen at the higher dose levels, including two patients that remain alive (one without disease) more than 8 years after vector instillation.[49]

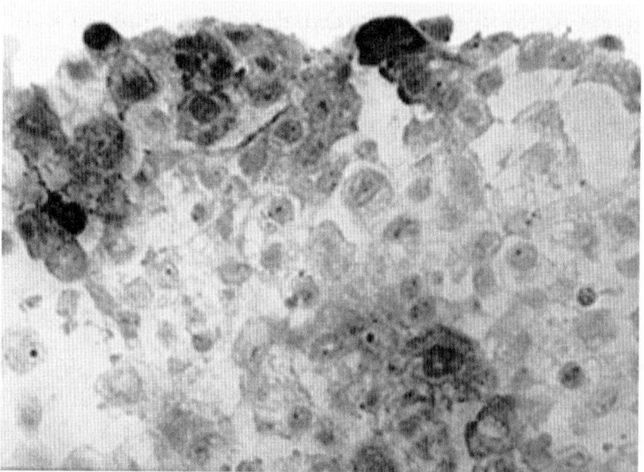

(a)

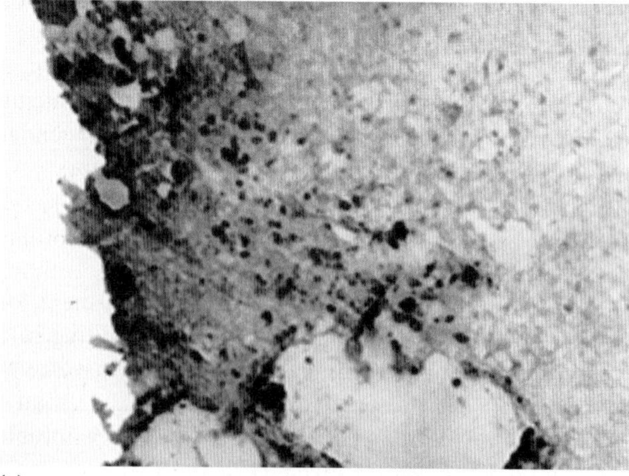

(b)

Figure 49.1 Gene transfer into mesothelioma. Forty-eight hours after intrapleural gene transfer, tumor biopsies were taken and stained for the transgene *Herpes simplex virus* (HSV)-thymidine kinase. Immunohistochemical staining (red color) showed clear expression in the surface layers of tumor cells in both nuclear (a) and cytoplasmic (b) locations. (See also Color Plates 57 and 58.)

Zarogoulidis *et al.*[50] treated six lung cancer patients with malignant pleural effusions intrapleurally with an adenovirus encoding the suicide gene cytosine deaminase followed by the prodrug flucytosine for 14 days. The treatment was well tolerated and inhibited pleural fluid reaccumulation in two patients, but no clear clinical responses were noted.

Vaccinia virus (VV) is a double-stranded DNA virus that relies primarily on its own proteins for DNA replication and mRNA synthesis, and so has minimal interactions with host proteins, facilitating production of daughter viral particles immediately after cell entry. Owing to its role in the eradication of smallpox, it has been used extensively in humans.[51] Mukherjee *et al.*[44] injected a replication-restricted recombinant VV expressing the human IL-2 gene intra-tumorally into patients with MM. Toxicities were minimal and there was no clinical or serological evidence of spread of virus to patient contacts. No significant tumor regression was seen in any of the patients and only modest intra-tumoral T-cell infiltration was detected. VV IL-2 mRNA was detected by reverse transcriptase-polymerase chain reaction (PCR) in serial tumor biopsies for up to 6 days after injection, but declined to low levels by day 8.

The use of a cellular vector to deliver the IL-2 gene in patients with pleural MM has been reported in abstract form.[52] Fourteen patients received intratumoral injections (four courses) of xenogenic fibroblasts (Vero cells) expressing IL-2. The treatment was well tolerated and circulating levels of IL-2 were detected in seven patients. One patient showed temporary tumor shrinkage and one had disease stabilization for 4 months, but this approach is not being pursued further.

Based on the preclinical data described above, our group at the University of Pennsylvania has recently completed a Phase 1 dose escalation study evaluating the safety and feasibility of single-dose intrapleural IFN-β gene transfer using an adenoviral vector (Ad.IFNβ) in seven patients with MM and three patients with metastatic pleural effusions (MPE).[53,54] Intrapleural Ad.INFβ was generally well tolerated. Gene transfer was documented in seven of the ten patients by demonstration of IFN-β message or protein in pleural fluid. Anti-tumor immune responses were elicited in seven of the ten patients, including humoral responses to known tumor antigens (SV40 virus large T-antigen and mesothelin) and unknown tumor antigens (seven patients). Four of ten patients showed meaningful clinical responses defined as disease stability and/or regression on fluorodeoxyglucose positron-emission tomograpy (FDG-PET) and computed tomography (CT) scans at day 60 post-vector infusion.[18]

Given these results, a second Phase 1 trial, using two doses of Ad.IFNβ separated by 2 weeks was conducted in 10 patients. Vector was generally well tolerated and induced similar anti-tumor humoral immune responses, along with two clinical responses. However, very high titers of neutralizing anti-Ad antibodies were induced after only 2 weeks, inhibiting transgene production after the second dose. Future plans are to administer two doses of Ad.IFNβ more closely together in time and in combination with chemotherapy for patients with MM and metastatic pleural effusions from non-small cell lung cancer (NSCLC). Based on other preclinical studies,[55] a neoadjuvant surgery trial is also being planned where vector would be given to patients with mesothelioma followed by a maximal debulking procedure and adjuvant chemo-radiotherapy.

CONCLUSIONS

Pleural gene therapy could potentially be used to treat systemic diseases by providing a large and easily accessible cellular target for gene transduction and protein secretion or for the treatment of a number of pleural diseases. Studies using novel AAV serotypes are especially promising in this regard. The other area where pleural gene therapy is likely to become useful is in the treatment of pleural diseases, especially pleural malignancies. A number of clinical trials in cancer patients have been completed that show the safety and feasibility of this approach.

Gene therapy has not yet been proven as a useful therapeutic tool for the treatment of pleural diseases. However, the field is less than 15 years old and great initial progress has been made. The authors have no doubt that gene therapy will be an important treatment strategy in the near future.

KEY POINTS

- Gene therapy (the treatment of disease based upon the transfer of genetic material) involving the pleural space offers a number of potential advantages and could be used to produce secreted gene products or in the treatment of pleural diseases.
- AAV vectors have been shown to lead to high-level and persistent expression of transgene and are being investigated for the treatment of α1-antitrypsin deficiency.
- The most likely use for pleural gene therapy will be in the treatment of malignant diseases including MM and metastatic pleural disease.
- A large number of gene therapy strategies for pleural malignancy have been explored using cell culture and animal models, including induction of apoptosis, anti-angiogenesis, suicide gene therapy, immuno-gene therapy and replicating, tumor-selective viruses.

- Clinical trials for pleural malignancy have been reported using cell transduced with the suicide gene Herpes simplex thymidine kinase (HSV*tk*), adenoviral vectors encoding HSV*tk*, a replication restricted vaccinia virus expressing interleukin-2, and an adenoviral vector expressing interferon-β. Anti-tumor immune responses and some clinical responses have been seen in the adenoviral trials.
- Gene therapy has not been proven yet as a useful therapeutic tool for the treatment of pleural diseases. However, excellent initial progress has been made and this modality will likely be an important treatment strategy in the near future.

REFERENCES

● = Key primary paper
◆ = Major review article

◆1. Heguy A, Crystal RG. Intrapleural 'outside-in' gene therapy: therapeutics for organs of the chest via gene transfer to the pleura. *Curr Opin Mol Ther* 2005; **7**: 440–53.
◆2. Young LS, Searle PF, Onion D, Mautner V. Viral gene therapy strategies: from basic science to clinical application. *J Pathol* 2006; **208**: 299–318.
●3. Smythe WR, Kaiser LR, Hwang HC, *et al.* Successful adenovirus-mediated gene transfer in an in vivo model of human malignant mesothelioma. *Ann Thorac Surg* 1994; **57**: 1395–401.
4. Brody SL, Jaffe HA, Han SK, Wersto RP, Crystal RG. Direct *in vivo* gene transfer and expression in malignant cells using adenovirus vectors. *Hum Gene Ther* 1994; **5**: 437–47.
5. Esandi MC, van Someren GD, Vincent AJ, *et al.* Gene therapy of experimental malignant mesothelioma using adenovirus vectors encoding the HSVtk gene. *Gene Ther* 1997; **4**: 280–7.
6. Smythe WR, Hwang HC, Amin KM, *et al.* Use of recombinant adenovirus to transfer the herpes simplex virus thymidine kinase (HSVtk) gene to thoracic neoplasms: an effective *in vitro* drug sensitization system. *Cancer Res* 1994; **54**: 2055–9.
◆7. Gao G, Vandenberghe LH, Wilson JM. New recombinant serotypes of AAV vectors. *Curr Gene Ther* 2005; **5**: 285–97.
8. Devin CJ, Lee YC, Light RW, Lane KB. Pleural space as a site of ectopic gene delivery: transfection of pleural mesothelial cells with systemic distribution of gene product. *Chest* 2003; **123**: 202–8.
9. Setoguchi Y, Jaffe HA, Chu CS, Crystal RG. Intraperitoneal *in vivo* gene therapy to deliver alpha 1-antitrypsin to the systemic circulation. *Am J Respir Cell Mol Biol* 1994; **10**: 369–77.
●10. De BP, Heguy A, Leopold PL, *et al.* Intrapleural administration of a serotype 5 adeno-associated virus coding for alpha1-antitrypsin mediates persistent, high lung and serum levels of alpha1-antitrypsin. *Mol Ther* 2004; **10**: 1003–10.
●11. De BP, Heguy A, Hackett NR, *et al.* High levels of persistent expression of alpha1-antitrypsin mediated by the nonhuman primate serotype rh.10 adeno-associated virus despite preexisting immunity to common human adeno-associated viruses. *Mol Ther* 2006; **13**: 67–76.
◆12. van der Most RG, Robinson BW, Nelson DJ. Gene therapy for malignant mesothelioma: beyond the infant years. *Cancer Gene Ther* 2006; **13**: 897–904.
13. Giuliano M, Catalano A, Strizzi L, *et al.* Adenovirus-mediated wild-type p53 overexpression reverts tumourigenicity of human mesothelioma cells. *Int J Mol Med* 2000; **5**: 591–6.
14. Frizelle SP, Rubins JB, Zhou JX, Curiel DT, Kratzke RA. Gene therapy of established mesothelioma xenografts with recombinant p16INK4a adenovirus. *Cancer Gene Ther* 2000; **7**: 1421–5.
15. Yang CT, You L, Uematsu K, *et al.* p14(ARF) modulates the cytolytic effect of ONYX-015 in mesothelioma cells with wild-type p53. *Cancer Res* 2001; **61**: 5959–63.
16. Pataer A, Smythe WR, Yu R, *et al.* Adenovirus-mediated Bak gene transfer induces apoptosis in mesothelioma cell lines. *J Thorac Cardiovasc Surg* 2001; **121**: 61–7.
17. Waheed I, Guo ZS, Chen GA, *et al.* Antisense to SV40 early gene region induces growth arrest and apoptosis in T-antigen-positive human pleural mesothelioma cells. *Cancer Res* 1999; **59**: 6068–73.
18. Mae M, Crystal RG. Gene transfer to the pleural mesothelium as a strategy to deliver proteins to the lung parenchyma. *Hum Gene Ther* 2002; **13**: 1471–82.
19. Merritt RE, Yamada RE, Wasif N, Crystal RG, Korst RJ. Effect of inhibition of multiple steps of angiogenesis in syngeneic murine pleural mesothelioma. *Ann Thorac Surg* 2004; **78**: 1042–51.
20. Schwarzenberger P, Harrison L, Weinacker A, *et al.* The treatment of malignant mesothelioma with a gene modified cancer cell line: a phase I study. *Hum Gene Ther* 1998; **9**: 2641–9.
21. Schwarzenberger P, Harrison L, Weinacker A, *et al.* Gene therapy for malignant mesothelioma: a novel approach for an incurable cancer with increased incidence in Louisiana. *J La State Med Soc* 1998; **150**: 168–74.
22. Aoki K, Yoshida T, Matsumoto N, *et al.* Gene therapy for peritoneal dissemination of pancreatic cancer by liposome-mediated transfer of herpes simplex virus thymidine kinase gene. *Hum Gene Ther* 1997; **8**: 1105–13.
23. Nagamachi Y, Tani M, Shimizu K, Yoshida T, Yokota J. Suicidal gene therapy for pleural metastasis of lung cancer by liposome-mediated transfer of herpes simplex virus thymidine kinase gene. *Cancer Gene Ther* 1999; **6**: 546–53.
24. Berlinghoff S, Veldwijk MR, Laufs S, *et al.* Susceptibility of mesothelioma cell lines to adeno-associated virus 2 vector-based suicide gene therapy. *Lung Cancer* 2004; **46**: 179–86.
●25. Smythe WR, Hwang HC, Elshami AA, *et al.* Treatment of experimental human mesothelioma using adenovirus transfer of the herpes simplex thymidine kinase gene. *Ann Surg* 1995; **222**: 78–86.
26. Hwang HC, Smythe WR, Elshami AA, *et al.* Gene therapy using adenovirus carrying the herpes simplex-thymidine kinase gene to treat *in vivo* models of human malignant mesothelioma and lung cancer. *Am J Respir Cell Mol Biol* 1995; **13**: 7–16.
27. Elshami AA, Kucharczuk JC, Zhang HB, *et al.* Treatment of pleural mesothelioma in an immunocompetent rat model utilizing adenoviral transfer of the herpes simplex virus thymidine kinase gene. *Hum Gene Ther* 1996; **7**: 141–8.
28. Lanuti M, Rudginsky S, Force SD, *et al.* Cationic lipid: bacterial DNA complexes elicit adaptive cellular immunity in murine intraperitoneal tumor models. *Cancer Res* 2000; **60**: 2955–63.
29. Rudginsky S, Siders W, Ingram L, *et al.* Antitumor activity of cationic lipid complexed with immunostimulatory DNA. *Mol Ther* 2001; **4**: 347–55.
30. Leong CC, Marley JV, Loh S, Robinson BW, Garlepp MJ. The induction of immune responses to murine malignant mesothelioma by IL-2 gene transfer. *Immunol Cell Biol* 1997; **75**: 356–9.
31. Caminschi I, Venetsanakos E, Leong CC, *et al.* Cytokine gene therapy of mesothelioma. Immune and antitumor effects of transfected interleukin-12. *Am J Respir Cell Mol Biol* 1999; **21**: 347–56.
32. Mukherjee S, Nelson D, Loh S, *et al.* The immune anti-tumor effects of GM-CSF and B7-1 gene transfection are enhanced

by surgical debulking of tumor. *Cancer Gene Ther* 2001; **8**: 580–8.
33. Triozzi PL, Aldrich W, Allen KO, *et al.* Antitumor activity of the intratumoral injection of fowlpox vectors expressing a triad of costimulatory molecules and granulocyte/macrophage colony stimulating factor in mesothelioma. *Int J Cancer* 2005; **113**: 406–14.
34. Gattacceca F, Pilatte Y, Billard C, *et al.* Ad-IFN gamma induces antiproliferative and antitumoral responses in malignant mesothelioma. *Clin Cancer Res* 2002; **8**: 3298–304.
35. Cordier Kellerman L, Valeyrie L, Fernandez N, *et al.* Regression of AK7 malignant mesothelioma established in immunocompetent mice following intratumoral gene transfer of interferon gamma. *Cancer Gene Ther* 2003; **10**: 481–90.
36. Cao XX, Mohuiddin I, Chada S, *et al.* Adenoviral transfer of mda-7 leads to BAX up-regulation and apoptosis in mesothelioma cells, and is abrogated by over-expression of BCL-XL. *Mol Med* 2002; **8**: 869–76.
37. Friedlander PL, Delaune CL, Abadie JM, *et al.* Efficacy of CD40 ligand gene therapy in malignant mesothelioma. *Am J Respir Cell Mol Biol* 2003; **29**: 321–30.
●38. Odaka M, Sterman DH, Wiewrodt R, *et al.* Eradication of intraperitoneal and distant tumor by adenovirus-mediated interferon-beta gene therapy is attributable to induction of systemic immunity. *Cancer Res* 2001; **61**: 6201–12.
39. Odaka M, Wiewrodt R, DeLong P, *et al.* Analysis of the immunologic response generated by Ad.IFN-beta during successful intraperitoneal tumor gene therapy. *Mol Ther* 2002; **6**: 210–8.
40. Zhu ZB, Makhija SK, Lu B, *et al.* Incorporating the survivin promoter in an infectivity enhanced CRAd-analysis of oncolysis and anti-tumor effects *in vitro* and *in vivo. Int J Oncol* 2005; **27**: 237–46.
●41. Kucharczuk JC, Randazzo B, Chang MY, *et al.* Use of a 'replication-restricted' herpes virus to treat experimental human malignant mesothelioma. *Cancer Res* 1997; **57**: 466–71.
42. Adusumilli PS, Stiles BM, Chan MK, *et al.* Imaging and therapy of malignant pleural mesothelioma using replication-competent herpes simplex viruses. *J Gene Med* 2006; **8**: 603–15.
43. Stiles BM, Adusumilli PS, Bhargava A, *et al.* Minimally invasive localization of oncolytic herpes simplex viral therapy of metastatic pleural cancer. *Cancer Gene Ther* 2006; **13**: 53–64.
●44. Mukherjee S, Haenel T, Himbeck R, *et al.* Replication-restricted vaccinia as a cytokine gene therapy vector in cancer: persistent transgene expression despite antibody generation. *Cancer Gene Ther* 2000; **7**: 663–70.
45. Harrison LH Jr, Schwarzenberger PO, Byrne PS, *et al.* Gene-modified PA1-STK cells home to tumor sites in patients with malignant pleural mesothelioma. *Ann Thorac Surg* 2000; **70**: 407–11.
●46. Sterman DH, Treat J, Litzky LA, *et al.* Adenovirus-mediated herpes simplex virus thymidine kinase/ganciclovir gene therapy in patients with localized malignancy: results of a phase I clinical trial in malignant mesothelioma. *Hum Gene Ther* 1998; **9**: 1083–92.
●47. Molnar-Kimber KL, Sterman DH, Chang M, *et al.* Impact of preexisting and induced humoral and cellular immune responses in an adenovirus-based gene therapy phase I clinical trial for localized mesothelioma. *Hum Gene Ther* 1998; **9**: 2121–33.
48. Sterman DH, Molnar-Kimber K, Iyengar T, *et al.* A pilot study of systemic corticosteroid administration in conjunction with intrapleural adenoviral vector administration in patients with malignant pleural mesothelioma. *Cancer Gene Ther* 2000; **7**: 1511–8.
●49. Sterman DH, Recio A, Vachani A, *et al.* Long-term follow-up of patients with malignant pleural mesothelioma receiving high-dose adenovirus herpes simplex thymidine kinase/ganciclovir suicide gene therapy. *Clin Cancer Res* 2005; **11**: 7444–53.
50. Zarogoulidis K, Kontakiotis T, Papagiannis A, Xafenias A, Kortsaris A. Management of resistant lung cancer malignant pleural effusion by intrapleural gene therapy. *J Clin Oncol* 2004; **22**: 3168.
◆51. Shen Y, Nemunaitis J. Fighting cancer with vaccinia virus: teaching new tricks to an old dog. *Mol Ther* 2005; **11**: 180–95.
52. Pitako J, Squiban P, Acres B, Digel W. A randomized phase II single center study of gene transfer-based non-specific immunotherapy of malignant mesothelioma (MM) by intratumoral injections of an interleukin-2 producing vero cells. *Proc Am Soc Clin Oncol* 2003; **22**(abstr 920).
●53. Sterman DH, Gillespie CT, Carroll RG, *et al.* Interferon beta adenoviral gene therapy in a patient with ovarian cancer. *Nat Clin Pract Oncol* 2006; **3**: 633–9.
54. Sterman DH, Recio A, Carroll RG, *et al.* A Phase I clinical trial of single-dose intrapleural interferon-beta gene transfer for malignant mesothelioma and metastatic pleural effusion: high rate of antitumor immune responses. *Clin Cancer Res* 2007; **13**(15 Pt1): 4456–66.
55. Kruklitis RJ, Singhal S, DeLong P, *et al.* Immunogene therapy with interferon-β before surgical debulking delays recurrence and improves survival in a murine model of malignant mesothelioma. *J Thorac Cardiovasc Surg* 2004; **127**: 123–30.

50

Future directions

YC GARY LEE, RICHARD W LIGHT

INTRODUCTION

Congratulations on arriving at the final chapter of this book!

The field of pleural disease includes a diverse range of clinical presentations that are both common and important. The significance and diversity of pleural diseases have been well covered in the clinical chapters of this text. In addition, it is an exciting field never short of new developments and controversies. For a long time pleural disease has failed to attract the same level of attention and interests as other medical fields of similar importance. The level of pleural research and the acquisition of new knowledge often lag behind other common clinical conditions. There is also a common misconception that pleural disease, when compared with other respiratory conditions, is less exciting or of less significance and as such many consider pleural disease research 'outside the mainstream'.[1]

This chapter discusses why pleural disease is relatively neglected and the possible measures that can promote pleural disease research and improve the clinical standard of management of pleural diseases. We highlight the recent advances in pleural disease management since the publication of the first edition of this text. We also provide our predictions on how pleural disease will evolve over the next couple of decades.

PLEURAL DISEASE IS COMMON AND IMPORTANT

Pleural disease is common in clinical practice. An estimated 3000 people per million population develop a pleural effusion each year. In the USA, up to one million patients develop parapneumonic effusions annually. Likewise, approximately 100 000 patients in the USA undergo pleurodesis for recurrent pleural effusions per year.

Pleural disease is important in clinical medicine. Tension pneumothorax is a medical emergency with potential fatal consequences. The correct diagnosis of a pleural effusion can change the outlook of the patient's prognosis and often alters management. For instance, the diagnosis of malignant involvement of the pleura affects the staging of patients with lung cancer and is an exclusion for surgical lung resection. It is important to establish the diagnosis of tuberculous pleuritis because untreated patients have a high risk of disseminated tuberculosis (TB) in subsequent years. Parapneumonic effusion, which occurs in up to 50 percent of hospitalized patients with pneumonia, must be managed appropriately to avoid the development of chronic pleural infection or a trapped lung requiring decortication.

Pleural diseases encompass a wide range of disorders as pleural involvement complicates most lung and systemic disorders. The diagnosis and management of pleural effusions and pneumothorax form the 'bread and butter' of pleural disease in clinical practice. Pleural malignancies, pleural fibrosis and pleuritic chest pain are also highly relevant. Pleural pathologies seldom exist in isolation, but often develop in association with pulmonary or extrapulmonary diseases: from the common maladies such as heart failure and lung cancer, to rare disorders such as yellow nail syndrome or body cavity lymphoma. The proper management of pleural diseases demands a broad range of clinical knowledge. As illustrated in this book, pleural involvement is not only common with internal medical conditions, but often crosses the boundaries of other specialities, such as obstetrics and gynecology, and frequently complicates surgical procedures. Thus, it is important that physicians of any specialty possess a good understanding of basic pleural anatomy, physiology and knowledge of common pleural pathologies. Unfortunately, clinicians often view pleural pathology as a 'side issue' of the principal diagnosis. Delays in the recognition and management of pleural involvement of various diseases are common occurrences in both primary and tertiary centers.

Pleural disease, as shown in the preceding chapters, is an exciting and dynamic field. New disease entities are continually being recognized. For example, pleural effusions are a recognized complication of organ transplantations and coronary artery bypass grafting (CABG), which are likely to be of greater significance as more of these operations are performed each year worldwide. The *Human immunodeficiency virus* (HIV) epidemic has seen a dramatic increase in effusions due to Karposi's sarcoma. The increasing application of *in vitro* fertilization has led to a new complication – the ovarian hyperstimulation syndrome – which often presents with large pleuro-peritoneal effusions.

The epidemiology of pleural diseases is dependent upon socioeconomical and geographic factors. The causative agents for pleural space infection and their sensitivities vary from region to region, and with time. In developing countries, TB pleuritis is significantly more common than in the developed countries. The incidence of asbestos-related pleural diseases, especially malignant mesothelioma, varies dramatically by geographic regions and reflects the level of asbestos mining or processing several decades before. It is for all these reasons that pleural disease remains a challenging field and for which a continuous update of knowledge is necessary.

RECENT ADVANCES AND CONTROVERSIES

Clinicians continue to strive for better management of pleural diseases with new strategies being developed constantly. Controversies continue to arise as new treatment options are developed. It is heartening to note that several large multi-center clinical trials have been completed since the previous edition of this book, all of which impact on clinical practice worldwide. The Multi-center Intrapleural Sepsis Trial (MIST)[2] randomized 454 patients with complicated parapneumonic effusions to intrapleural streptokinase or saline and showed no benefit from the streptokinase. This was corroborated by a smaller study from South Africa[3] which also showed no difference between the two groups at day 3 after treatment. Controversies exist, however, as there was a small benefit at day 7 in the latter trial favoring streptokinase. A large multicenter trial (MIST2) is presently under way in the UK which randomizes patients to tissue plasminogen activator (tPA), recombinant human deoxyribonuclease (rhDNase), both tPA and rhDNase, or placebo in the management of complicated parapneumonic effusions.

A randomized controlled study comparing talc slurry and talc insufflation for the treatment of malignant pleural effusions with more than 400 patients provided valuable data showing no differences between the two methods of talc delivery in the primary endpoints.[4] A randomized trial showed that small particle size talc induced pulmonary and systemic inflammation compared with talc preparations with larger median particle size.[5] The hypothesis that small talc particles are responsible for the inflammation is further supported by a large prospective observation study from 14 European and South African centers demonstrating no cases of acute respiratory distress syndrome (ARDS) following pleurodesis using calibrated talc preparations.[6] Another study is underway to compare the value of tunneled indwelling catheter (without pleurodesis) versus conventional talc pleurodesis as first-line treatment for malignant pleural effusions. This trial will use breathlessness score and quality of life measures as its key endpoints.

Malignant pleural mesothelioma continues to be an active area of research and controversies. Two large multicenter trials with 456 and 250 patients were the first randomized studies to demonstrate treatment (with pemetrexed[7] and raltitrexed,[8] respectively) can prolong survival in mesothelioma. The role of *Simian virus 40* (SV40) in mesothelioma development continues to be debated; new evidence casts further doubts on its role.[9] Prophylactic radiotherapy for pleural puncture sites in mesothelioma patients, once well accepted, is now being challenged after two randomized studies showed no significant benefits.[10,11]

The growth in clinical research in pleural disease is not paralleled by a significant increase in basic research of pleural pathologies. For example, little research has been undertaken in the pharmacokinetics of drug delivery to the pleural space. Likewise, despite the fact that genetic research is a flourishing area in modern medicine, there has been practically no research work performed on genetic aspects of pleural diseases, other than the genetics of mesothelioma development.

So why is pleural disease research being neglected? To start with, pleural disease is not commonly recognized as a sub-specialty of its own right. In most cases, pleural disease is managed by specialists who are involved with a narrow spectrum of the pleural involvement in their own specialty practice, who often see pleural disease as a 'side issue'. For example, oncologists are more likely to focus their research in management of the primary tumors than in malignant pleuritis; surgeons often regard post-operative pleural involvement as a nuisance rather than recognizing it as an important morbidity; infectious disease specialists caring for patients with pneumonia are more interested in selecting the proper antibiotics than draining the parapneumonic effusion.

Lack of commercial interest and drug company sponsorship is a significant disadvantage in pleural research, when compared with more 'marketable' conditions such as asthma or pneumonia. Many physicians also view pleural disease (especially malignant effusions) as a terminal event not worthy of efforts to improve its practice. The lack of funding and interest result in a lack of good research, making it difficult to attract funding and recruit talented young investigators. The net result is a vicious cycle in which pleural disease research continues to be ignored.

The pleural disease research community lacks a central organization to liase and put together investigators of similar interests. This partly explains the relative lack of large multi-center collaboration efforts. There exist no pleural disease interest groups within the major thoracic societies (e.g. the American Thoracic Society, European Respiratory Society or Thoracic Society of Australia and New Zealand), as there are for airways diseases, pulmonary vascular disease or lung fibrosis. There are no large patient support groups, such as those for asthma or lymphangioleiomyomatosis. No specialized forum exists for researchers in pleural disease to exchange ideas. Unlike for asthma or lung cancer, there are no scientific publications with a focus on pleural disease research. The *International Pleural Newsletter*, a free publication available at www.musc.edu/pleuralnews, is an attempt to provide useful knowledge on pleural diseases to the wider medical community, with the hope of promoting interests and research in pleural disease.

CURRENT STATE OF AFFAIRS

As a consequence of the relative lack of evidence-based medicine, clinical practices in pleural disease are commonly based on results of small trials, on 'traditional' practice or on anecdotal experience of individual physicians. Hence, there are major variations in practice among practitioners of different countries, or sometimes even different units within the same city.

Very often, adoption of advances in pleural disease management (e.g. thoracoscopy or using adenosine deaminase [ADA] to diagnose tuberculosis) is relatively slow by clinicians. The lack of interest and proper recognition of the importance of pleural disease are not without practical consequences. Around the world daily, there are patients whose pleural effusions are not investigated early. Delay in drainage or management of parapneumonic effusions happens regularly throughout the world, despite the repeated call that 'the sun should never set on a parapneumonic effusion'. Some clinicians are not comfortable in dealing with pleural diseases while others think it is a 'pure nuisance'. Hence, many clinicians tend to either ignore important clinical presentations or have a low threshold for referring patients to other specialists, including surgeons.

TO BRING FORWARD THE FIELD OF PLEURAL DISEASE

To improve the clinical practice of pleural disease, first and foremost we need to increase the awareness among physicians of the significance of pleural diseases, and the consequences of overlooking pleural abnormalities. This should take place in different levels simultaneously. Pulmonologists and thoracic surgeons should be encouraged to develop sub-specialty interests in the investigation and management of pleural diseases. Respiratory trainees should have mandatory experience and be competent in basic pleural procedures (e.g. thoracentesis, chest tube insertion and pleural biopsies). Junior staff, medical students and paramedical staff should be adequately educated to handle pleural emergencies, such as tension pneumothoraces, as well as to manage common pleural conditions such as the appropriate approach to a patient with a pleural effusion or the day-to-day management of chest tubes. Development of clinical guidelines for common pleural presentations may also help staff unfamiliar with these diseases.

In the long run, it is important that pleural disease be recognized as a specialty. Physicians should be encouraged to refer patients with difficult pleural problems to pulmonologists with a special interest in pleural diseases. In the bigger picture, developing a global league of interested physicians is the best way to raise the profile of pleural disease within the professional communities. Such an organization will facilitate the performance of multicenter trials often necessary to answer crucial clinical questions. Having regular and dedicated forums for discussion of current issues in pleural diseases, such as regular conferences and publications, is most worthwhile.

Improving funding and resources for pleural disease research is essential to improve its standards. Programs to raise public awareness will help attract research funding. Clinicians should work together with scientists, as the need to apply the latest technology in pleural research cannot be over-emphasized.

OUR PREDICTIONS FOR THE EVOLUTION OF PLEURAL DISEASE DURING THE FIRST PART OF THE TWENTY-FIRST CENTURY

Our first prediction is that at least 40 percent of what is written in this book will be proven wrong or at least outdated over the next 20 years. The difficult aspect is to predict which 40 percent is wrong. We readily admit that we are not clairvoyants and do not necessarily know any more than do other people who are interested in pleural disease. Nevertheless, we will offer the following predictions, albeit with some trepidation. Although authors of the clinical chapters have stated their own views about the future of their specific area of pleural disease, our predictions and their predictions differ on many occasions.

Indeed, the two editors do not necessarily agree in our predictions.

Overall predictions

The incidence of pleural diseases will continue to rise. This is because the general population will live longer and the elderly population is more likely to develop diseases associated with pleural effusions such as congestive heart failure, malignancy and pneumonia. As medical practice evolves, there are more interventions that lead to pleural disease (e.g. transthoracic needle aspiration and radiofrequency ablation causing pneumothorax; CABG surgery and fertility induction producing pleural effusions).

Historically, high-profile pleural researchers are predominantly based in the USA, from where a large proportion of high-impact clinical studies and cutting edge basic research on pleural diseases were published. With rising interests in pleural disease worldwide and globalization of technology, YCGL predicts that pleural research will be more evenly distributed around the world. European and Australian centers have already taken a lead in pleural infection and asbestos-related pleural diseases. It would be encouraging to see the number of centers with pleural interests continue to grow around the world.

Basic science predictions

1. There will be further increases in the recognition of the importance of resident pleural mesothelial cells in pleural diseases (e.g. inflammation, fibrosis, fluid accumulation). The differing roles of the mesothelial cells and pleural macrophages in the pleura will be defined. This contrasts with the focus of previous research, which tended to concentrate on cell types that are recruited into the pleural cavity (e.g. neutrophils and fibroblasts).
2. Cytokines and their manipulation will provide the most immediate areas of advances in understanding the pathophysiology of pleural disease in the next 10–20 years. This area will provide the basis for novel treatment options. Advances in the knowledge of intracellular signaling mechanisms will provide the focus for the next wave of basic science research in pleural disease, though clinical benefits from this knowledge remain to be seen.
3. Genetics in pleural diseases:
   i. Genetics is a broad new field of active research in all areas of medicine, yet few steps have been taken to apply the advances in genetics in pleural research. Why do some people develop pleural fibrosis and others do not following the same exposure to irradiation, asbestos or drugs? Why do certain patients develop effusions but others with the same condition do not? We predict that genetic predisposition will explain at least part of the differences in individual susceptibility to various pleural diseases. Pharmacogenetics may also help explain the differences in inter-individual responses to treatments of pleural diseases.
   ii. Powerful screening tools (e.g. microarray technology and proteomics) will be applied to hasten advances of our knowledge in the pathophysiology of pleural diseases. These tools may help diagnose the cause of pleural effusions, predict therapeutic responses and prognosis of patients with various conditions.
4. Gene therapy is only in its infantile stage and numerous hurdles lie ahead, but continual advances will be made towards large-scale clinical application. Gene therapy can potentially be applied: using the pleural space as a gene receptacle for systemic gene therapy; and using local gene therapy in the pleural space to treat pleural disorders such as mesothelioma or pleural metastases, or to produce pleurodesis.
5. The future direction for the management of pleural effusions should lie in targeting pleural fluid formation, rather than to manage the fluid after it is formed with procedures such as pleurodesis. We predict that significant advances will be gained in other disciplines (such as research in pulmonary edema) that target the fundamental control of fluid exudation.
6. There is an urgent need to elucidate the pharmacokinetics of the pleura. How best to deliver pharmacological agents to the pleura in adequate concentrations, and how to enhance removal of pleural substances are important yet unstudied questions. We are not entirely optimistic, however, that such questions would attract much interest (for the reasons outlined earlier in this chapter).
7. At present, basic research in mesothelioma accounts for a huge proportion of laboratory research in all pleural diseases. With the expected peak and the subsequent decline in the incidence of mesothelioma, the proportion of resources in pleural diseases that goes into mesothelioma research will eventually decrease.

Clinical practice predictions

Diagnosis of pleural disease:

1. The separation of pleural effusions into transudates and exudates will be forgotten. This division really is artificial. Instead, patients will be given a specific diagnosis, possibly by new diagnostic methods that allow the determination of the pleural fluid characteristics in a non-invasive fashion.[12] An example of this is using the NT-pro BNP levels to establish the diagnosis of congestive heart failure.
2. Non-radiologists, especially chest physicians, critical care physicians, emergency room physicians and thoracic surgeons will perform ultrasound more frequently

themselves for the diagnosis and management of pleural disease. This prediction has already been proven true since the last edition of this book.
3. Advances in laboratory diagnostic techniques (e.g. polymerase chain reaction, PCR) will allow identification of most infective organisms in parapneumonic effusions, pleural tuberculosis and pleural fungal diseases.
4. Many of the pleural effusions which are presently labeled as idiopathic will be proven to be due to viral infections by more sophisticated diagnostic technology.
5. Better imaging techniques will provide better delineation of the invasion of the underlying tissue in the pleura by malignancy. Such techniques will be used as part of the routine workup of possible pleural malignancies.
6. Identification of the cellular origin of metastatic pleural malignancies will become more important as more malignancies become amenable to chemotherapy.

Treatment of parapneumonic effusion:

1. RWL predicts that the combination of fibrinolytics and human recombinant DNAase, but not fibrinolytics by themselves, will be cost effective in the treatment of parapneumonic effusions.
2. RWL predicts that monoclonal antibodies or receptor agonists for the cytokines responsible for the fibrosis and pleural loculations will be used therapeutically to prevent pleural fluid loculation and fibrous covering of the visceral pleura. This treatment will follow the elucidation of the cytokines responsible for the pleural fluid loculations and pleural fibrosis that make treatment of this disease difficult. A leading candidate as an agent that is responsible for the loculations and fibrosis is transforming growth factor beta (TGF-β). YCGL is less optimistic along this vein and predicts that application of cytokine manipulation for therapeutic use would turn out to be very complicated due to the multifunctional nature of most of the cytokines.

Treatment of malignant pleural effusion:

1. RWL predicts that the increase in the use of outpatient therapy with indwelling cathers for malignant pleural effusion seen since the previous edition of this book will continue. This will be done with tunneled indwelling pleural catheters. When the amount of drainage with an indwelling catheter shows no strong tendency to decrease, attempts to create a pleurodesis will be made by injecting pleurodesing agents through the indwelling catheter. YCGL agrees with such an approach but predicts that general use of indwelling catheter treatment may prove difficult. Cost is likely to be a prohibitory factor in the near future. Such a catheter system requires either the patient or a dedicated caregiver to manage the drainage in an aseptic fashion, which is not always easy. Catheter blockage and bacterial colonization are concerns on the long-term use of indwelling catheters.
2. YCGL advocates that we should scrutinize our current concepts of management of malignant pleural effusions. The aim should be to improve quality of life, in part via preventing dyspnea from fluid accumulation. YCGL predicts that more clinical studies will adopt quality of life (instead of radiographic improvement) as principle endpoints. RWL believes that quality of life is very important but feels that studies on this are difficult because distinguishing symptom progression due to recurrence of the effusion or progression of the tumor is often difficult. Talc will gradually be replaced by other compounds. When talc is used, it will only be with large particle size talc. Talc is an inhomogeneous substance that is basically dirt and is associated with significant pulmonary problems. RWL maintains that in the third millennium we should be able to produce a pleurodesis with more sophisticated agents. YCGL believes that research efforts should focus on stopping fluid accumulation rather than secondary prevention such as pleurodesis.
3. RWL predicts that low doses of silver nitrate (20 mL 0.5 percent) or iodopovidone (Betadine) (100 mL 2.0 percent) will become the most common agents for pleurodesis in developing countries because they are effective, inexpensive, widely available and are associated with tolerable side effects. In developed countries, pleurodesis will be created by using more sophisticated agents (such as TGF-β) that can produce a pleurodesis without inducing pleural inflammation. YCGL would like to reserve judgment until more clinical data is available.
4. Therapies targeting the actual pathophysiology of pleural fluid formation, such as inhibitors of vascular endothelial growth factor, will be used to decrease pleural fluid production in malignant pleural effusions.

Management of pneumothorax:

1. RWL predicts that more patients with primary spontaneous pneumothorax will be initially managed with aspiration and not be hospitalized. YCGL notes that RWL is out of date and that this was already happening in many countries before the millennium. If this aspiration is successful, the patients will be sent home with a device which will measure the amount of air leak. Patients with primary spontaneous pneumothorax who are not initially managed successfully with aspiration or who have a recurrent pneumothorax will be subjected to early thoracotomy with stapling of blebs and pleural abrasion.
2. Iatrogenic pneumothoraces will be managed more frequently with observation or aspiration and less frequently with tube thoracostomy.
3. YCGL predicts that the underlying genetic or anatomical features that predispose to recurrence of pneumo-

thorax will be identified. Tests will therefore become available, either in the form of imaging or genetic/biochemical analysis, that identify the patient at high risk of recurrence who will actually need preventive therapy. RWL maintains that such a test is already available, i.e. does the patient smoke.

Thoracoscopy in the diagnosis and treatment of pleural disease:

1. YCGL predicts that thoracoscopy will be used more frequently in the diagnosis of pleural disease while RWL predicts that thoracoscopy will be used less frequently in the diagnosis of pleural disease as better non-invasive diagnostic tests will be developed.
2. Thoracoscopy will be used earlier in the treatment of parapneumonic effusions.
3. RWL predicts that more thoracic surgeons will become proficient with thoracoscopy and chest physicians will only perform the procedure where there are no thoracic surgeons trained for and interested in doing thoracoscopy. YCGL states that there are already increasing number of chest physicians performing thoracoscopy worldwide and predicts that increasingly surgeons will only be involved in complicated cases.
4. RWL believes that the demand for thoracoscopy will be relatively low (e.g. compared with bronchoscopy). As such, only a small percentage, but not the majority of chest physicians, will become proficient at thoracoscopy.

Diagnosis and management of other types of pleural effusion:

1. RWL notes that computed tomographic (CT) angiograms have replaced lung scans in the diagnosis of pulmonary embolism and believes the lung scan and the pulmonary arteriogram will be used less and less as better scanners are developed. YCGL notes the limitation of spiral CT in visualizing the smaller vessels makes it a good procedure if positive, but not good enough for exclusion of the diagnosis. It is still quite possible that the peripheral pulmonary emboli are the ones that cause effusions.
2. Controlled studies will be carried out evaluating various therapeutic modalities in the treatment of the post-CABG pleural effusions. YCGL notes that while such trials are useful, the level of interest from cardiothoracic sectors on post-CABG effusions is unlikely to be sufficient to lead to large proper clinical trials. This is partly because most post-CABG effusions are self-limiting with no long-term sequelae.
3. Unless new therapies for cirrhosis are found, hepatic hydrothorax will continue to be a very frustrating problem because patients with this problem have such severe underlying disease.

KEY POINTS

- Pleural diseases are common, but clinical interests and research in pleural diseases often fall below that of other respiratory illnesses
- The past few years have seen a significant increase in multi-center clinical studies that affect patient management. Large particle size talc preparations have been shown to be safer than small particle size ones. The effectiveness of talc, given as slurry or poudrage, does not differ significantly. Intrapleural streptokinase was not associated with significant clinical benefits in a large randomized trial. New anti-folate drugs can improve survival of mesothelioma patients.
- Pleural disease is never short of controversies: the best route of administration of talc (slurry versus poudrage), use of fibrinolytics in empyema, role of SV40 in development of mesothelioma and benefits of prophylactic radiotherapy in mesothelioma all remain controversial.
- Advances in pleural research and clinical disease management depend on raising the profile of pleural disease as a sub-specialty. Research collaborations among international centers and between clinical researchers and laboratory scientists are crucial.

REFERENCES

1. Lee YCG. Pleural disease: A forgotten frontier in respiratory research. *Respirology* 2006; **11**: 4–5.
2. Maskell NA, Davies CW, Nunn AJ, *et al.* UK Controlled trial of intrapleural streptokinase for pleural infection. *N Engl J Med* 2005; **352**: 865–74.
3. Diacon AH, Theron J, Schuurmans MM, Van de Wal BW, Bolliger CT. Intrapleural streptokinase for empyema and complicated parapneumonic effusions. *Am J Respir Crit Care Med* 2004; **170**: 49–53.
4. Dresler CM, Olak J, Herndon 2nd JE, *et al.* Phase III intergroup study of talc poudrage vs talc slurry sclerosis for malignant pleural effusion. *Chest* 2005; **127**: 909–15.
5. Maskell NA, Lee YCG, Gleeson FV, *et al.* Prospective randomized trials comparing the influence of talc of different particle sizes and tetracycline on lung and systemic inflammation after pleurodesis. *Am J Respir Crit Care Med* 2004; **170**: 377–82.
6. Janssen JP, Collier G, Astoul P, *et al.* Safety of pleurodesis with talc poudrage in malignant pleural effusion: a prospective cohort study. *Lancet* 2007; **369**: 1535–9.
7. Vogelzang NJ, Rusthoven J, Symanowski J, *et al.* Phase III study of pemetrexed in combination with cisplatin versus cisplatin alone in patients with malignant pleural mesothelioma. *J Clin Oncol* 2003; **21**: 2636–44.
8. van Meerbeeck JP, Gaafar R, Manegold C, *et al.* Randomized phase III study of cisplatin with or without raltitrexed in patients with malignant pleural mesothelioma: an intergroup study of the European Organisation for Research and Treatment of Cancer Lung Cancer Group and the National Cancer Institute of Canada. *J Clin Oncol* 2005; **23**: 6881–9.

9. Lopez-Rios F, Illei PB, Rusch V, Ladanyi M. Evidence against a role for SV40 infection in human mesotheliomas and high risk of false-positive PCR results owing to presence of SV40 sequences in common laboratory plasmids. *Lancet* 2004; **364**: 1157–66.
10. Bydder S, Phillips M, Joseph DJ, *et al.* A randomised trial of single-dose radiotherapy to prevent procedure tract metastasis by malignant mesothelioma. *Br J Cancer* 2004; **91**: 9–10.
11. O'Rourke N, Garcia JC, Paul J, *et al.* A randomised controlled trial of intervention site radiotherapy in malignant pleural mesothelioma. *Radiother Oncol* 2007; **84**: 18–22.
12. Lee YCG, Davies RJO, Light RW. Diagnosing pleural effusion: moving beyond transudate-exudate separation. *Chest* 2007; **131**: 942–3.

Index

Page numbers in **bold** denote figures, those in *italics* denote tables